PREVENTION'S
FOOD & NUTRITION

PREVENTION'S

FOOD & NUTRITION

The Most Complete Book Ever Written on Using Food and Vitamins to Feel Healthy and Cure Disease

By the Editors of ***PREVENTION*** Magazine Health Books
Edited by John Feltman

Rodale Press, Emmaus, Pennsylvania

Printed in the United States of America on acid-free ∞, recycled ♻ paper

If you have any questions or comments concerning this book, please write:
Rodale Press
Book Readers' Service
33 East Minor Street
Emmaus, PA 18098

Library of Congress Cataloging-in-Publication Data

Prevention's food and nutrition : the most complete book ever written on using food and vitamins to feel healthy and cure disease / by the editors of Prevention magazine health books, edited by John Feltman.
p. cm.
Includes index.
ISBN 0–87596–166–5 hardcover
1. Nutrition. I. Feltman, John. II. Prevention (Emmaus, Pa.)
III. Title: Food and nutrition.
RA784.P737 1993
613.2—dc20 92–39974
CIP

Distributed in the book trade by St. Martin's Press

2 4 6 8 10 9 7 5 3 1 hardcover

Notice

This book is intended as a reference volume only, not as a medical guide or manual for self-treatment. If you suspect that you have a medical problem, we urge you to seek competent medical help. Keep in mind that nutritional needs vary from person to person, depending on age, sex, health status and total diet. Information here is intended to help you make informed decisions about your diet, not to substitute for any treatment that may have been prescribed by your physician.

Contributors

Editor: **John Feltman**
Executive Editor: **Debora Tkac**
Contributing Writers: **Douglas Dollemore, Sara Henry, Matthew Hoffman, Marcia Holman, Brian Kauffman, Steven Lally, Gale Maleskey, Ellen Michaud, Joe Wargo, Pat Wittig**
Recipe Editor: **Jean Rogers**
Book and Cover Designer: **Lynn N. Gano**
Research Chief: **Ann Yermish**
Research/Fact-Checking Staff: **Susan Burdick, Christine Dreisbach, Melissa Gotthardt, Dawn Horvath, Paris Mihely-Muchanic, Debbie J. Pedron, Sally Reith, Anita Small, Bernadette Sukley**
Production Editor: **Jane Sherman**
Office Staff: **Roberta Mulliner, Julie Kehs, Mary Lou Stephen**

CONTENTS

PART 1: NUTRITION BASICS

CHAPTER 1 The Nutrition Revolution: An Introduction 3

CHAPTER 2 The Basic Three: Protein, Carbohydrate and Fat 10

CHAPTER 3 Vitamins and Minerals: The Essential Facts 23

CHAPTER 4 Meeting Your Nutrient Needs: The RDAs and Beyond 49

CHAPTER 5 Nutrient Robbers: You Can Guard against Them 60

CHAPTER 6 Special Nutrient Needs: Fine-Tuning Your Intake 71

PART 2: THE TOP DIETARY ISSUES

CHAPTER 7 Fiber: More for What Ails Us 85

CHAPTER 8 Low-Fat Eating: For All the Right Reasons 103

CHAPTER 9 Cholesterol: A Dietary Troublemaker 120

CHAPTER 10 Sodium: The Rewards of Moderation 133

CHAPTER 11 Calcium: For Healthy Bones and More 147

CHAPTER 12 Iron: Don't Get Caught Short 162

CHAPTER 13 Potassium: A Protector from Our Past 172

CHAPTER 14 Antioxidants: Dietary "Rustproofers" 184

CHAPTER 15 The 101 Healthiest Foods: Eat More of These 195

CHAPTER 16 Water: The Best Toast to Your Health 210

CHAPTER 17 Food Additives: A Mixed Blessing 217

CHAPTER 18 Ethnic Foods: Healthy Eating from Around the Globe 228

PART 3: ALL SYSTEMS ARE GO WITH GOOD NUTRITION

CHAPTER 19 The Brain: Food for Thought 244

CHAPTER 20 The Immune System: Defensive Dining 258

CHAPTER 21 The Heart and Arteries: Rolling Back the Risks 271

CHAPTER 22 Energy and Performance: Choosing the Right Fuel 289

CHAPTER 23 Staying Younger Longer: Anti-aging Nutrients 301

CHAPTER 24 Cancer Prevention: It Starts on Your Plate 309

CHAPTER 25 Sex and Reproduction: The Dietary Factor 322

CHAPTER 26 Nutritional Healing: An A-to-Z Guide 333

PART 4: USING FOODS WISELY

CHAPTER 27 Basic Strategies: Pick an Eating Plan You Can Live With 370

CHAPTER 28 Cooking Light: Techniques and Tips 383

CHAPTER 29 Restaurant Savvy: Dining Out without Damage 398

CHAPTER 30 Natural Food Stores: Naturally Better? 413

CHAPTER 31 Supplements: A Smart Buyer's Guide 424

PART 5: HEALING DIETS

CHAPTER 32 Weight Loss: What Really Works 437

CHAPTER 33 Vegetarianism: A Healthy Life without Meat 454

CHAPTER 34 Dietary Controversies: Going to Extremes 469

PART 6: IMPROVING YOUR EATING STYLE

CHAPTER 35 Quiz Time: Does Your Diet Measure Up? 485

CHAPTER 36 Eating Light, Eating Right: A Six-Week Program 505

INDEX 527

PART 1

NUTRITION BASICS

CHAPTER 1

THE NUTRITION REVOLUTION

AN INTRODUCTION

No doubt about it, it's an exciting time in nutrition. Okay, "exciting" and "nutrition" may not be two words you've ever linked together before—unless you count diving into Aunt Anne's Delectable Double Fudge Cake at the annual family reunion. But if there was ever a time to call nutrition exciting, it's now.

We all have at least a vague idea that good nutrition is important for good health. And we definitely know what happens when we eat *too* much: that uncomfortable stuffed feeling, which, if repeated too often, leads to the search through the recesses of our closets for roomier clothing.

So we've always recognized—to a certain extent—that there is a correlation between what we put in our mouths and how we look and feel (although we don't always let that *influence* what we put in our mouths). But never before has there been so much compelling evidence that what we eat has a direct relation to the occurrence of serious diseases ranging from cataracts to cardiovascular disease to cancer.

Food to prevent disease? Once most people would have hooted at the concept. "Just another crazy gimmick," they would have sniffed. But with the publication of numerous carefully controlled studies by respected researchers, the idea that nutrients can not only treat but prevent disease has moved steadfastly forward into the realm of acceptable science. And it's not just that good nutrition can let us live longer. It can also let us live *better.*

"As we go forward, we see more and more things that are nutritionally related that have to do with the quality of life, not just longevity," says Daniel B. Menzel, Ph.D., chairman of the Department of Community and Environmental Medicine at the University of California at Irvine.

NUTRIENTS TO THE RESCUE

They sound like something you should have studied in chemistry class, but they may turn out to be some of the best friends you'll ever make. "Antioxidants are probably one of the hottest areas in the coming decade," says Harinder S. Garewal, M.D., Ph.D., assistant director for cancer prevention and control at the University of Arizona Cancer Center in Tucson. "Excitement is high."

The antioxidants that have scientists and nutritionists so excited include beta-carotene—the stuff that makes carrots orange and that converts to vitamin A in the body—and vitamins C and E. In brief, antioxidants can scavenge and render harmless the free radicals in your body that are a result of normal bodily processes as well as exposure to x-rays, sunlight, ozone, smoke and other environmental pollutants. These free radicals may be part of what causes much of the deterioration we associate with aging—and our increased exposure to environmental pollutants such as nitrogen dioxide or ozone may *increase* our need for the antioxidants that can neutralize these free radicals, says Dr. Menzel.

Harvard Medical School researchers turned up astounding proof of the power of beta-carotene in a ten-year study of 22,000 male physicians: They found that men with a history of heart problems who received beta-carotene supplements every other day had *half as many* heart attacks, strokes and deaths as those who didn't take beta-carotene. (And *no* heart attacks occurred in a group who took both beta-carotene and aspirin.)

The antioxidants are also valiant anti-cancer crusaders. Some of Dr. Garewal's work showed that daily beta-carotene drastically reduced abnormal changes in the mouth that could lead to cancer. Another study of 189 women with cervical cancer and 227 cancer-free women showed that the risk of cervical cancer was only about half as great for those with high intakes of vitamin E, vitamin C and beta-carotene.

"The antioxidants really do work to reduce the incidence of cancer," says Dr. Menzel. "And people from all over the world in all different kinds of environmental circumstances showed these substances have very positive anti-cancer activities."

A LONG LIST OF PROTECTORS

Other nutrients have remarkable protective and healing powers as well. Folate, a B vitamin, can help fight cancer and has dramatically cut the rate of devastating birth defects.

Osteoporosis can be a crippling problem for the elderly, particularly women. But studies show that getting adequate amounts of dietary calcium can help women retain bone mass and possibly fend off this bone-weakening disease.

Vision-impairing cataracts are another plague associated with growing older, but just eating more fruits and vegetables may help prevent this problem. A U.S. Department of Agriculture (USDA) study found that people eating less than 1½ servings of fruit or less than 2 servings of vegetables daily were 3½ times more likely to develop cataracts than those who ate more.

"As you grow older, your risk for developing cataracts grows larger and larger," says Paul F. Jacques, D.Sc., an epidemiologist with the USDA's Human Nutrition Research Center on Aging at Tufts University in Boston.

A New Role for a New Vitamin D

Antioxidants, move over. Vitamin D is attracting new attention.

With the development of a new form of vitamin D that appears to circumvent a potentially serious side effect from large doses, the door may have opened to greatly expand this vitamin's use as a treatment.

"There are new roles for vitamin D that go way beyond its original activities in partnership with calcium," says Hector DeLuca, Ph.D., chairman of the Department of Biochemistry at the University of Wisconsin in Madison and a pioneer in vitamin D research. "Vitamin D isn't just for bones any more."

The classical role for vitamin D has been to help the body utilize calcium and build and maintain strong bones and teeth. Since 1985, scientists have suspected that vitamin D could also help fight cancer—but its use as a treatment was strictly limited because of side effects.

The problem is that high doses of vitamin D can raise blood calcium to excessive levels, which in severe cases can cause calcification of soft tissue, kidney failure and coma. "The window of safety between treatment and harm was very narrow," says Dr. DeLuca.

But this new form of D—technically referred to as an analog of dihydroxyvitamin D_3—*doesn't* mobilize calcium. This alleviates the risk of high blood calcium, dramatically increasing the feasibility of using vitamin D as a treatment.

The possibility of treating cancer is, of course, of primary interest, and research by Dr. DeLuca and others shows that D does help suppress the growth of cancer cells. But vitamin D has also been used to successfully treat psoriasis, a skin disorder, and it has a role in helping prevent osteoporosis. Other uses for this vitamin may be right around the corner.

"Eating a healthy diet may delay the usual aging of the lens of the eye, and so delay cataracts." Dr. Jacques thinks the secret may be the nutrient combination found in fruits and vegetables.

The list goes on. Zinc improves the immune system. There are some indications magnesium might help chronic fatigue syndrome. Vitamins E and C have slowed the progression of Parkinson's disease for some patients. Some physicians recommend eating more potassium-rich foods to control blood pressure and avoid stroke. Increased fiber in the diet may help lower cholesterol levels and cut risks of colon cancer and other gastrointestinal disorders.

"TAKE TWO ORANGES AND CALL ME IN THE MORNING"

Does all this mean that one day our doctors will be prescribing fruits, vegetables, whole-grain breads or nutrient supplements instead of drugs?

It's not a farfetched concept. In fact, the first line of attack for many problems is already diet-centered. Treatment for high blood pressure, high cho-

ALL THIS, AND CUT CANCER RISKS, TOO?

It was the ultimate controlled experiment—no late-night sneaking out to a 7-11 for a candy bar or Giant Gulp. While at sea for six months, crew members of the U.S. Navy's USS *Scott* were fed a diet that met the American Cancer Society's guidelines: low in fat, high in fiber, with lots of variety and plenty of fruits and vegetables. (No one expected to assess cancer risks during the six-month trial; the goal of the study was merely to test how well the guidelines could be adapted to everyday diets.)

The results:

- The crew averaged a weight loss of 12 pounds, while crew members of a sister ship served regular Navy fare *gained* 7 pounds.
- Average waist size decreased 2 inches, compared to an *increase* of 1½ inches on crew members of the sister ship.
- Seventy-four percent of those weighing 200 pounds or more lost weight, compared to 26 percent of the large-size group on the sister ship.
- Eighty-nine percent of crew members with above-acceptable body fat percentages showed a fat percentage decline.

You might not expect results this marked from a stay at a an expensive health spa! And as a side benefit, more than half the crew members liked their new diet, and many of them planned to continue similar eating habits on dry land.

lesterol and diabetes often depends heavily on dietary changes. And the American Cancer Society advocates a low-fat, high-fiber diet to help avoid cancer.

Some physicians actually prescribe specific nutrients for certain health problems. "Doctors use niacin to treat high triglycerides and high cholesterol," says Adrianne Bendich, Ph.D., senior clinical research coordinator in the Human Nutrition Research Division of Hoffmann-La Roche in Nutley, New Jersey. "They routinely use vitamin E to reduce the adverse effects of many cancer chemotherapies. Both calcium and vitamin D have a role to play against osteoporosis. There are strong indications that children hospitalized with measles should be given vitamin A to prevent complications. And I think the use of nutrients as preventive medicine is growing."

What It Means to You

Despite all the breakthroughs in nutritional research, deciding what and how to eat can still be enormously confusing. We're bombarded with information and misinformation about food and nutrition. One specialist says you can get all the nutrients you need in your daily diet; another one says you can't. Health food stores display a range of products that promise to replenish sexual vigor, vanquish migraines and a whole lot more. Meanwhile, supermarkets sell new food products for those concerned about heart disease and cancer. Cute tykes on television commercials lisp about the dangers of cholesterol, and "fat-free" has become the sell line of the decade. Many of us, confused by the barrage of information, abandon plans to renovate our diets.

And today is a hectic time. Just like 50 years ago, most of our meals are prepared by Mom—but today Mom is probably also juggling a 9-to-5 job, evening classes and workouts at the gym. Finding time to go to the supermarket can be a major task, let alone planning and preparing nutritious meals. More and more, we reach for prepared foods, or we dine out.

And the best of intentions, we all know, can fly out the window when you're faced with that all-you-can-eat breakfast buffet, the sumptuous potluck church supper or the fancy dinner at the boss's house.

But many of us are genuinely concerned about our health and the health of our families, and we want to eat better. If only we had more time . . . if only it were easier to keep track of nutrients . . . if only good nutrition didn't seem so complicated.

Eating Better Can Be Easy

We're not saying that nutrition is a simple issue, but eating healthy doesn't have to be complicated. Unless you're on a medically restricted diet, you don't have to carry a notepad and keep track of the nutrient content of everything you eat.

What's important, however, is understanding the basics of good nutrition

How We're Eating Now

Think about what you've eaten during the past week or two. Do you think you got your quota of vitamins and minerals, fruits and vegetables, protein and whole grains—and have you kept your fat intake down? Or do you *know* your diet is, well, less than perfect, but you just don't have the time or energy to do any better?

About a fourth of us are already very careful about what we eat, according to the Survey of American Dietary Habits, conducted by the American Dietetic Association. Another 38 percent of us know we should eat better, but either we don't want to give up our chips and ice cream or we think that a healthy diet takes too much time.

Another huge chunk of the population—presumably no one reading this book—just doesn't care what they eat. Thirty-six percent of American adults don't try to manage their diets. They eat out frequently and skip meals often.

The survey also showed that many of us are concerned about cholesterol, fat and vitamins and minerals—and while 52 percent knew that the recommended blood cholesterol is under 200, only 7 percent knew that the ceiling on fat intake recommended by the American Dietetic Association is 30 percent of calories.

So as a nation how are we doing, consumption-wise? A Nationwide Food Consumption Survey showed that most of us are consuming at least the Recommended Dietary Allowance of vitamins A, C, B_{12}, thiamine and riboflavin. We are a bit low on vitamin B_6 and vitamin E, but we're in no great danger of deficiency.

Our mineral status is more iffy, however. Females aged 12 to 50 take in only about two-thirds of the recommended iron levels; men and women both fall short on zinc and copper. Adult women consume less than the recommended amounts of calcium, and both men and women consume less magnesium than recommended.

When it comes to protein, we eat more than we need. Fat? It's no surprise that we overdo it in this category, considering our love affair with such fatty fare as ice cream and french fries. We average 35 to 37 percent of our daily calories from fat. Carbohydrate consumption is about one-fifth lower than recommended, and we don't get enough fiber.

In other words, while many of us are definitely *concerned* about nutrition, many of us also still need to improve our diets.

so you can make good choices throughout the day. That means altering your shopping, cooking and dining-out habits—but a little bit at a time.

In this book we explain today's hot issues: How nutrition really affects your heart, your brain, your blood pressure, your stamina and more. We examine all of the essential nutrients in foods, what they do and who needs more of what.

Ever enter the grocery store armed with a list of healthy foods and exit with things you really didn't intend to buy? We offer a guide for supermarket shopping and another for health food stores, plus tips on growing your own good foods. Wish you had an array of quick-and-easy healthy recipes? They're here. A week-by-week blueprint for improving your diet in all the critical areas? You've got it. A comparison of special diet programs offered by top clinics and spas? It's here.

It's all here, and more. You're holding in your hand a book that can guide you to enjoyable healthy eating—and a lifetime of good nutrition.

CHAPTER 2

THE BASIC THREE

PROTEIN, CARBOHYDRATE AND FAT

Oat bran won't do it, oranges won't do it, eggs won't do it. And neither will milk, cheese, steak, chicken, pretzels, potato chips, lima beans, peas, carrots or spaghetti. Even a sweet, soothing bowl of sherbet or a tempting tray of truffles won't do it. It's a basic fact of life: No single food can meet all of your nutritional needs.

"There is no one miracle food that has it all," says Elaine Kvitka, R.D., a nutrition consultant in Scottsdale, Arizona. "You need more than 40 different nutrients in your diet every day. In order to get those, you need to eat a wide variety of foods."

Even a breastfed baby isn't getting all of the necessary nutrients from Mom's milk. "Babies are born with built-up reserves of nutrients in their bodies that supplement breastfeeding," says Andrea Gardiner, R.D., a dietitian at the Hospital of the Good Samaritan in Los Angeles. "But after about four months, those reserves are depleted and the baby needs to begin eating food in order to survive."

There's no doubt that food is vital to our survival. That's because food does two important things. First, it provides us with essential nutrients, substances that the body can't produce for itself. Without those nutrients, we'd literally have no way of repairing cells or growing new ones. Without them, our bones would be brittle, our nerves and muscles wouldn't work well and thousands of other crucial jobs in our bodies, ranging from wound repair to heartbeat regulation, wouldn't get done.

Second, food serves as the fuel our bodies need to create heat and energy, says George Seperich, Ph.D., a food scientist and associate professor of agribusiness at Arizona State University in Tempe.

Without an adequate food supply, the body starts to burn anything, including muscle, to keep itself alive. If a person is undernourished for long enough, the body will even start breaking down muscle in the heart to feed itself.

"Your body actually starts to digest itself from the inside out," Dr. Seperich says. "Once it starts converting muscle cells to fuel, it gradually loses its ability to discriminate between heart muscle and less vital muscle. And of course, the minute you start weakening the heart muscle, you're in big trouble."

While famine and malnutrition are still facts of life in some parts of the world, most cultures long ago developed diets that have successfully fed millions. While these cuisines are diverse and often seem to have little in common, scientists now know that each contains the same basic components that every person needs to grow and stay healthy. If any one of these vital components is missing from a diet in sufficient quantities, it can lead to malnourishment and disease.

In some cases, scientists have determined that a lack of just one essential nutrient can cause disorders such as anemia or scurvy. In other instances, an excessive amount of one nutrient can actually cause malabsorption and deficiency of another nutrient. So eating well is a balancing act that requires not only that we consume all the necessary nutrients but also that all those nutrients work together as a team in our bodies so that we can live active and fulfilling lives.

In this chapter, we'll be looking at three of the most basic diet components: protein, carbohydrate and fat.

THE PROS AND CONS OF PROTEIN

In a sense, protein is the body's repairman and jack-of-all-trades. Found in every cell, protein builds and repairs everything from muscles and bones to blood vessels, hormones, hair and fingernails, says George L. Blackburn, M.D., Ph.D., associate professor of surgery at Harvard Medical School and chief of the Nutrition/Metabolism Laboratory at the Cancer Research Institute of New England Deaconess Hospital in Boston. Protein helps create enzymes that enable us to digest food and antibodies that fight off infections. In a pinch, it also can be used as a fuel by the body.

Chemically, protein is composed of varying combinations of 22 amino acids. Amino acids are compounds that contain carbon, hydrogen, oxygen and nitrogen, which happen to be the four elements necessary for life. To get a feeling for what a protein looks like, Dr. Seperich suggests that you imagine that you're making a bracelet and each amino acid is like a pop-it bead.

"Each bead has a little bulb that snaps into a hole in the bead next to it," he says. "When you snap all the beads together, you have a complete protein."

Most of these amino acids can be manufactured by the body, but nine essential ones can only be obtained from the foods that we eat. Lysine, one of these essential amino acids, is needed for the absorption of calcium, a mineral that strengthens bones and teeth. Others, such as phenylalanine, are needed for the production of important nerve hormones in the brain involved in learning and memory.

Animal proteins—meats, eggs and fish—were once considered superior protein sources because they have large amounts of proteins, and most contain all the amino acids. But scientists now believe that a mixture of animal and vegetable proteins is most useful to the body.

Eggs, for example, were once considered to be the perfect protein source. But scientists have found that if you replace a third of the egg protein with potato protein, the body actually uses the combination more efficiently than egg protein alone to build tissue or burn as fuel.

Although vegetable foods such as grains and beans also have some protein, they are considered lower-quality sources because they contain less of the nutrient than animal foods. In addition, most plant proteins contain just a few of the essential amino acids. The amino acids in plant proteins are still important, however. Rice and corn, for example, contain threonine, an amino acid needed for the formation of collagen, the substance that holds skin together. Beans and peanuts have significant amounts of methionine, an amino acid that promotes healthy skin and nails.

While any single plant food isn't likely to have all the essential amino acids, you can still get all the protein and essential amino acids you need from vegetables, fruits, beans and grains if you mix them right. Try to imagine making that bracelet of amino acids beads in the example given by Dr. Seperich. Only this time, you don't have enough beads to do the job.

"Each individual vegetable doesn't quite contain all of the beads you need to make a complete bracelet or protein. But if you use the amino acids from several plant foods, you can," he says.

If, for example, you take kidney beans, which are high in some amino acids and low in others, and combine them with rice, which is high in the amino acids that are lacking in kidney beans, then you'll end up eating a high-quality protein, says Elizabeth Somer, R.D., coauthor of *The Nutrition Desk Reference.* Rice and beans, in fact, is a dish served in the West Indies with the main meal.

But you don't necessarily have to eat those vegetable foods together, Dr. Seperich says. Thanks to the time it takes for your body to digest nutrients, the protein in the oatmeal you eat at breakfast can be combined with the corn you eat at lunch and the spaghetti you eat at dinner to create a high-quality protein containing all the essential amino acids.

How to Get the Right Amount

More than 700 million people are believed to suffer from protein deficiency worldwide, mostly in developing countries. Kwashiorkor and maras-

A User's Guide to Protein

Here's a sampling of protein amounts in common foods. A food is considered a good source of protein if it has at least 25 grams of the nutrient.

Food	Portion	Protein (g.)	Calories	Percent of Calories from Protein
Pork chop	3 oz.	30	231	52
Top round beef	3 oz.	30	178	67
Veal shoulder	3 oz.	29	169	69
Chuck roast	3 oz.	28	179	63
Chicken breast, roasted	3 oz.	27	142	76
Bluefin tuna	3 oz.	25	156	64
Tuna, canned in water	3 oz.	25	111	90
Turkey breast, roasted	3 oz.	25	133	76
Ground beef, lean	3 oz.	24	238	40
Ham	3 oz.	24	183	52
Porterhouse steak	3 oz.	24	185	52
Coho salmon	3 oz.	23	157	59
Shrimp	3 oz.	18	84	86
Low-fat (1%) cottage cheese	½ cup	14	82	68
Tofu, firm	3 oz.	13	117	43
Parmesan cheese	1 oz.	12	128	38
Skim milk	1 cup	10	100	40
Lentils, boiled	½ cup	9	115	31
Peanut butter	2 tbsp.	8	188	17
Spanish peanuts	1 oz.	8	162	20
Swiss cheese	1 oz.	8	105	30
Egg	1 large	6	75	32
Egg substitute, liquid	¼ cup	6	60	40
Yogurt, nonfat, plain	½ cup	6	63	38
Ice milk, vanilla	1 cup	5	184	11

mus, two common diseases caused by inadequate amounts of protein, can inhibit growth and impair mental capabilities. Symptoms include weight loss, irritability, swelling of the stomach and skin sores.

Both diseases are rare in the United States, Gardiner says. If anything, we're probably eating too much protein.

"I think that the myth that we have to have some protein at every meal is still around," says Melanie Polk, R.D., consulting nutritionist and author from North Potomac, Maryland. "Americans are probably eating twice as much protein as they really need."

The Recommended Dietary Allowance (RDA) of protein varies based on your age and weight. A 45-year-old woman weighing 139 pounds, for example, needs about 50 grams of protein daily. For a man of the same age weighing 174 pounds, the recommendation is for about 63 grams.

However, according to the National Research Council, adult women are consuming up to 70 grams of protein a day and some men are eating more than 90 grams. That's probably because it's easy to overload on protein on the typical American diet, Kvitka says. Just by eating an egg and a slice of sausage for breakfast, a quarter-pound hamburger for lunch and a three-ounce porterhouse steak for dinner, you've consumed 59 grams of protein that day.

Even if you eat more prudently, it's not hard to meet or exceed your RDA for protein. If you just eat ½ cup wheat cereal with 1 cup skim milk and two pieces of toast for breakfast, then have an apple, two ounces of cottage cheese, a three-ounce serving of salmon and ½ cup peas for lunch, you'll consume 60 grams of protein. That's nearly 120 percent of the RDA for a 25- to 50-year-old woman and easily meets the RDA for similarly aged man. And you haven't touched your dinner yet.

So what are the consequences of eating too much protein? High-protein foods, particularly meats, often are rich in calories and loaded with fat. If you meet your daily protein requirements, most of that protein will be used to build and repair muscle and some may be used as fuel by the body. But if you eat excessive amounts, any leftover protein that isn't burned for fuel will be stored as fat.

A diet high in animal protein may interfere with absorption of certain minerals such as calcium and may cause the excretion of more minerals in the urine.

Excessive protein also can overwork your kidneys. "If you give your kidneys more protein than they can handle—particularly animal protein, which is more difficult to process—it wears them down," Dr. Blackburn says. "Americans' obsession with getting enough protein may explain the fact the kidney disease is so common here." Here are a couple of tips to help you get the right amount of protein, but not too much.

Remember the 15 percent rule. Try to limit your protein consumption to less than 15 percent of your total calories, Dr. Blackburn suggests. To do that, women should eat no more than two three- to four-ounce servings of meat, poultry or fish a day. (A three-ounce serving roughly translates into one loin lamb chop, one-half chicken breast or four steamed jumbo shrimp.) Men need a bit more protein, but still should eat no more than two four- to six-ounce servings of meat, poultry or fish daily.

Take the spotlight off meat. Stop making meat the centerpiece of your meals, Somer says. In addition to all its protein, meat contains saturated fat and cholesterol, two things that contribute to heart disease. So instead of giving steak, pork chops and that teen idol—hamburger—a starring role in every meal, let meats play a bit part while dishes like spaghetti and beans make your taste buds swoon. "If we stopped planning our meals around meat and started planning them around grains and vegetables, we'd be much better off," Somer says.

FUEL UP ON CARBOHYDRATES

If you drove a high-performance racing car, would you fuel it with a substandard grade of gasoline? Of course not. Well, in a way your body is like that racing car, and the best fuel for it is carbohydrates.

"Your body works best when it's running on carbohydrates," Gardiner says. "Carbohydrates are like premium gasoline. They're the most efficient fuel your body can get."

Carbohydrates are sugars and starches that your body can easily break down into fuel. They also help break down fat and team up with proteins to form compounds that are essential for combating infections, lubricating joints and maintaining health of skin, bones and nails. Carbohydrates are found almost exclusively in plant foods such as beans, fruits and vegetables.

Unlike protein, which isn't broken down until it reaches the stomach, carbohydrate begins to be digested almost immediately after it enters the mouth. Saliva begins the process of breaking down the carbohydrate into glucose, the major form of sugar in the blood and your body's primary fuel. "Your nervous system and red blood cells will only use glucose. They won't use any other fuel. They need to have it," Gardiner says.

SIMPLE VERSUS COMPLEX

Basically, carbohydrates can be divided into two broad categories. Simple carbohydrates are tiny single or twin molecules of sugar found in such foods as table sugar, honey and molasses. The most common of these simple carbohydrates is glucose. Other types of simple carbohydrates include fructose, which is found in fruit, and lactose, which is found in milk. Simple sugars are a good energy source because they're already broken down into their component parts and are absorbed quite quickly into the bloodstream, Dr. Seperich says.

Natural sugars such as those found in fruit are the best form of simple carbohydrates because they have vitamins and minerals, which are not

THE WORLD'S BEST FOOD PROCESSOR

It slices. It dices. It even mashes, chops and churns. But your digestive system does something even the most expensive food processor can't do. It breaks food down into vital nutrients and absorbs them into your bloodstream.

This complex process is a bit like running an assembly line in reverse. "As we go along this disassembly line, there are different places where nutrients are broken down and absorbed," says Ronald L. Hoffman, M.D., medical director of the Hoffman Center for Holistic Medicine in New York and author of *Seven Weeks to a Settled Stomach*. Some carbohydrates, for example, can be easily disassembled by enzymes in the mouth, while most proteins need to be broken down by potent acids in the stomach. Fat, another major dietary component, isn't digested until after it is drenched with bile acid in the small intestine.

The first stop on this journey is the mouth, where your teeth chop the food into small bits and saliva mixes and softens the food into a digestible mush. After less than a minute, it enters the esophagus, a ten-inch-long muscular tube that connects the mouth to the stomach. In the esophagus, the food is mixed with more secretions that aid digestion. The trip though the esophagus can be quick—liquids often zip down it in less than ten seconds. Once in the stomach, the food is bathed in powerful secretions of hydrochloric acid, a substance so strong that it can burn holes in thick carpet. (Fortunately, your stomach has a self-protective mechanism that stops this acid from harming

found in sugars used in soft drinks, candies and other sweets, Somer says. Unfortunately, most of the sugar that we consume in this country is refined.

"The refined sugars are generally found in nutrient-poor foods. They typically are in foods that are high in fat and have a minimal amount of vitamins and minerals," Somer says. "The American diet is already marginal in terms of vitamins and minerals. So high-sugar foods just worsen that trend."

Complex carbohydrates, also known as starches, also supply your body with glucose. Commonly found in vegetables, fruits, beans and grains, complex carbohydrates are composed of groups of simple sugars stuck together in long molecular chains. To give you an idea of the size difference, think of a simple sugar as a tugboat. In comparison, a complex carbohydrate is like an aircraft carrier.

It takes your body longer to digest a complex carbohydrate because your

you). After six to eight hours of bombardment from these secretions, the food is transformed into a creamy, souplike substance called chyme. However, despite what you might think, the stomach doesn't absorb that many nutrients.

"Some absorption does occur in the mouth, and alcohol and some small chemical substances are absorbed to some extent in the stomach. But most of the absorption occurs in the small intestine," Dr. Hoffman says.

The small intestine is actually the major organ in the digestive tract. About 20 feet long, it is only called the small intestine because its diameter is less than that of the large intestine. After chyme leaves the stomach, it enters the small intestine, where most of the nutrients are extracted and absorbed into the bloodstream. That process can take more than nine hours.

Finally, the residue tumbles into the large intestine. About five feet long, the large intestine doesn't digest food, but it does absorb water and other fluids. It also is home to a variety of useful bacteria, yeasts and fungi that manufacture nutrients, such as vitamin K, that your body needs. As the waste travels through your large intestine, water is extracted and it becomes more and more solid until it is excreted from your body one to three days later.

The whole digestive process, depending on the meal and your metabolism, can take less than 18 hours or up to five days, Dr. Hoffman says.

digestive system must break it down into simple sugars. Because of that, complex carbohydrates also slow the absorption of glucose into the bloodstream. That's important for people with diabetes, who need to avoid extreme fluctuations in blood sugar levels.

In addition, complex carbohydrates are particularly important because they provide us with fiber, an indigestible substance in plant food that has a powerful punch. Researchers believe that fiber does a number of important things in the body, including help decrease constipation, lower cholesterol, and prevent colon and breast cancer.

Because it is indigestible, fiber goes through your digestive system like a big cotton ball absorbing water and sweeping stool, bile acids (which are made from cholesterol) and other fluids out of the body, Dr. Seperich says. Better yet, fiber may help you control your weight because it provides added bulk that fills your stomach and curbs your appetite.

MORE CARBS ARE NEEDED

Unfortunately, dietary experts say we eat fewer carbohydrates than we should.

At the beginning of the century, carbohydrate consumption in the United States and Europe hovered around 70 percent of our caloric intake. But since 1920, carbohydrate consumption in the United States has dropped by about 20 percent. Today, the average American diet consists of 46 percent calories from carbohydrates. And of those carbohydrates, half are the less desirable simple sugars. Not surprisingly, there also has been a sharp decrease in the proportion of energy provided by starches and a significant increase in the amount of fats and meats in our diet.

"One hundred years ago, we ate more carbohydrates than we do now. In particular, we ate fewer sweets and more starches. But social changes such as affluence have made it easier to get sweet things into our diet," says Maria Linder, Ph.D., a professor of biochemistry at California State University, Fullerton.

Some people have avoided carbohydrates because they have an undeserved bad reputation, Polk says.

"Many people still have a negative image of carbohydrates because they think if they eat lots of pasta, breads or potatoes, they're going to get fat," Polk says. "In reality, it's not those foods, but it's what you put on them that gets you in trouble."

A MUSCLE-BUILDING MEAL PLAN

If you believe the gym is the only place to start building muscle, think again. Replacing high-fat foods with lots of breads, grains, fruits and vegetables might help you create a solid, muscular body.

We know that a high-carbohydrate, low-fat diet can help us lose fat without the rigors of crash dieting. But research suggests a more unexpected benefit: It may boost lean body mass—muscle.

When researchers put 18 women on a high-fat diet for 4 weeks, and then on a low-fat, high-carbohydrate diet for 20 weeks, they found an 11 percent decrease in fat weight. But surprisingly, the women also had a 2 percent increase in lean body mass. Somehow the women had created new lean tissue without exercise.

"This is a very intriguing finding," says T. Elaine Prewitt, R.D., Ph.D., of the Department of Nutrition and Medical Dietetics at the University of Illinois at Chicago, who headed the study.

No, we're not suggesting that you drop your hand weights and pick up a fork instead. If anything, exercise adds even more to these benefits and helps maintain them over time.

"Carbohydrates are only fattening if you do things like load up your baked potato with butter and sour cream or if you smear cream cheese on your bagel," Kvitka says.

The consensus of the U.S. Department of Agriculture and the National Research Council is that at least 55 percent of your calories should come from carbohydrates. Here's how you can meet that goal.

It's simple—eat complex. The first thing you should eat at a meal should be a complex carbohydrate, Dr. Blackburn says. A small serving of pasta or soups that contain noodles or potatoes are good examples. Doing that might lessen your cravings for fatty foods, particularly if you eat slowly so that your meal lasts at least 20 minutes. That gives the carbohydrates time to activate enzymes in your intestinal tract, liver and brain, so you won't feel as much of a craving for fat.

Develop a passion for fruits, grains and vegetables. You should try to eat five or more ½-cup servings of vegetables and fruits daily and at least six servings of breads, cereals and beans.

"Six servings of grains sounds like a lot," Somer says. "But if you have a bowl of oatmeal and a couple pieces of toast for breakfast, you've already had three servings of grains. Then if you have a sandwich for lunch, that's two more servings. Finally if you have a baked potato or a ½-cup serving of rice with dinner, you have your six servings of grains for that day. It's really not as much as it sounds like."

FAT: FRIEND OR FOE?

There's no doubt that fat can be your enemy. But it may surprise you to know that fat, if eaten in moderate amounts, can be an important ally in your effort to stay healthy.

"It's absolutely essential that we have some fat in our bodies," Dr. Seperich says. "We spend a lot of time trying to get rid of it, but, in reality, your body needs a certain percentage of it to function properly."

Fats, also known as lipids, are hard to avoid because they're found in some form in virtually every food. In general, foods such as cheese or butter that are high in saturated fats are solid at room temperature, while unsaturated fats like vegetable oils are usually liquids.

Saturated fats—which have been linked to heart disease and high cholesterol—are primarily found in animal foods such as meat, poultry and dairy products.

The two types of unsaturated fat, polyunsaturated and monounsaturated, are usually found in plants and fish. Research suggests that these unsaturated fats, particularly omega-3 fatty acids found in fish, may help lower blood cholesterol levels and prevent heart attacks.

While there is no established RDA for fats, there are essential fatty acids that your body can't produce and that you must get from your diet. Of these, linoleic acid is the most important. Found in vegetable oils, nuts and

HOW FATS MEASURE UP

This table lists the percentage of saturated and unsaturated fat in commonly used cooking oils and fats. (The percentages may not add up to 100 percent since many of these fats have small amounts of other fatty substances.)

OIL/FAT	SATURATED FAT (%)	MONOUNSATURATED FAT (%)	POLYUNSATURATED FAT (%)
11 TERRIFIC COOKING OILS AND FATS . . .			
Canola oil	7	60	30
Safflower oil	9	13	76
Walnut oil	9	23	65
Sunflower oil	11	20	67
Corn oil	13	25	59
Olive oil	14	76	9
Soybean oil	15	24	59
Peanut oil	17	47	32
Rice oil	19	42	38
Wheat germ oil	19	15	63
Margarine	20	48	32
. . . PLUS 7 TO AVOID			
Coconut oil	89	6	2
Butter	64	29	4
Palm oil	50	36	9
Lard	39	45	11
Chicken fat	30	45	20
Cottonseed oil	26	18	53
Vegetable shortening	25	45	20

seeds, this polyunsaturated fat is important for growth and development as well as the production of hormonelike substances that regulate blood pressure. However, because we do eat so much fat, essential fatty acid deficiencies are extremely rare.

Of course, most of us have heard about the downside of fat. Eating excessive amounts of it has been linked to high cholesterol, heart disease, obesity and some types of cancer.

Yet fat still accounts for 43 percent of the total calories the average American is eating. That's about 80 to 100 grams of fat—equivalent to almost a whole stick of butter—every day.

"The number one thing that people can do to improve their waistlines, heart and overall health is cut the amount of fat in their diets," Somer says. "If that was the only thing they did, they would solve a wealth of problems."

But while dietitians stress that it's important to *cut* fat consumption to no more than 30 percent of your total calories, you shouldn't eliminate it from your diet entirely. That's because fat does some terrific things for you.

WHAT'S GOOD ABOUT FAT

Fat is a compact way for the body to store lots of energy until we need it, Dr. Seperich says. In fact, fats are capable of storing more than twice as much energy per gram as the same amount of carbohydrates.

"If we didn't have fat and stored all our energy as carbohydrates, we'd all have to be 12 feet tall and weigh 700 pounds to do it," Dr. Seperich says.

We also need fat for healthy skin and hair. And without it, we'd have a hard time regulating our body temperature. Fat deposited just below the skin acts like a thermal blanket to keep our body temperature constant, Dr. Seperich says.

Fat surrounds vital organs, such as the kidneys and the heart, protecting them from blows and trauma. Fat is also important to the nervous system because it acts like an insulator, coating nerves in a protective covering.

To squeeze the most benefits out of the fat you do eat, yet avoid the damage too much fat can cause, try these strategies.

Read between the grams. Probably the easiest way to ensure that you really are cutting the total fat in your diet to less than 30 percent of calories is to read labels on food packages, Kvitka says. In particular, be aware of the grams of fat in a food. "Percentage of fat is such a difficult concept for some people," she says. "But as you begin to read labels and become aware of fat grams, you'll learn that you can get to your goal by keeping your portions of meat down to two three-ounce servings a day, choosing low-fat or nonfat dairy products and getting five or six servings of fruits or vegetables a day."

Keep an immediate goal in sight. Take a long-term goal like reducing your fat consumption to 30 percent of calories and break it down into smaller goals, Somer says.

"Some people might want to start by eliminating butter from their toast in the morning. Others might prefer eating smaller portions of meat with every meal," Somer says. "There are a million ways to do it."

Cut back on all obvious fats in your diet. Bake, steam, broil or microwave your food, Kvitka says, and choose fried foods only occasionally. "High-fat foods like pizza and ice cream should only be eaten in moderate amounts," she says. "For example, have just one small scoop of ice cream, not an entire banana split. Better yet, try low-fat or nonfat frozen dairy desserts."

A Menu with the Right Mix

Here's a sample menu that illustrates how to fit the right proportions of carbohydrate, protein and fat into your day. For a total of 1,960 calories, this menu supplies 61 percent of calories from carbohydrate, 24 percent from fat and 15 percent from protein. This is in line with experts' recommendations that at least 55 percent of daily calories come from carbohydrates. You also should try to limit your protein consumption to 15 percent and reduce your fat intake to less than 30 percent of calories.

Food	**Portion**	**Calories**
Breakfast		
Cranberry juice	½ cup	65
Oatmeal	1 cup	145
Blueberries	½ cup	41
Yogurt, low-fat	1 cup	200
Lunch		
Sandwich made with:		
Wheat bread, light	2 slices	123
Tuna salad w/light mayonnaise	4 oz.	136
Alfalfa sprouts	¼ cup	3
Romaine lettuce	¼ cup	2
Tomato	½	13
Black bean soup	1 cup	218
Apple	1	81
Snack		
Air-popped popcorn, light	3 cups	75
Dinner		
Tossed salad	1 cup	32
Italian dressing	1 Tbsp.	32
Vegetable lasagna	11 oz.	400
Italian bread	2 slices	170
Margarine, diet	2 tsp.	33
Pear	1	98
Snack		
Raspberry frozen yogurt, nonfat	½ cup	93

CHAPTER 3

VITAMINS AND MINERALS

THE ESSENTIAL FACTS

So you pop your once-a-day every morning and never give the matter of vitamins and minerals another thought. Or maybe you just assume you get all the nutrients you need in the food you eat, and you don't think about vitamins and minerals at all.

But there's a lot more to vitamins and minerals than a little column of numbers running down the side panel of your cereal box.

The basic facts are easy: There are 13 essential vitamins. Recommended Dietary Allowances, or RDAs, have been established by the National Research Council for 11 of them: vitamin A, six of the B vitamins—B_6, B_{12}, folate, niacin, riboflavin (B_2) and thiamine (B_1)—vitamin C, vitamin D, vitamin E and vitamin K. There's less information for the two remaining vitamins, biotin and pantothenate, so instead of RDAs, there are "estimated safe and adequate" daily dietary intakes for these. In this chapter, values given for RDAs are those for women and men aged 25 to 50.

There's an established RDA for seven minerals—calcium, phosphorus, magnesium, iron, zinc, iodine and selenium—and suggested intakes for potassium, copper, manganese, fluoride, chromium and molybdenum. (Sodium is also essential, but as we generally consume too much of it, rather than not enough, deficiencies are rare.)

What's *not* so evident about vitamins and minerals is exactly what each nutrient does, who may need more, what happens if you don't get enough (or if you get too much) and what the best food sources are. In some cases it's also important to know a nutrient's protective intake range—usually a ballpark number that research suggests should put you in the right range for protective purposes. So here's your A-to-Z guide—from vitamin A to zinc.

VITAMINS

VITAMIN A AND BETA-CAROTENE

Chances are you've read a lot about beta-carotene in the news. Studies have shown that this substance can prevent oral cancer, delay cataracts and reduce the risk of heart attack and lung cancer. It's an antioxidant, a compound that may protect against disease by neutralizing unstable oxygen molecules, called free radicals, within the body.

Beta-carotene is a carotenoid (one of the group of compounds that makes up the red, orange and yellow pigments in plants) that's converted into vitamin A in the body. Unlike the preformed vitamin A from animal food sources, you essentially can't overdose on beta-carotene. It's converted to vitamin A on an as-needed basis, which is one reason it's the best way to get your vitamin A.

What does vitamin A do? It's involved in vision, growth, cell differentiation and reproduction. Night blindness and problems in bone growth can be caused by a vitamin A deficiency. It also shows dramatic effects in reducing the death rate from measles, and derivatives of vitamin A such as the

UNITS OF MEASUREMENT EXPLAINED

Vitamin and mineral amounts are usually expressed in *milligrams* (one-thousandth of a gram) or even smaller units called *micrograms* (one-thousandth of a milligram). These are commonly abbreviated *mg.* and *mcg.*, respectively. Another common measure is *international units* (I.U.). Vitamin D amounts, for example, are expressed in either mcg. or I.U. One microgram of vitamin D equals 40 I.U. Vitamin E is expressed in either I.U. or *alpha-tocopherol equivalents* (α-TE). One alpha-tocopherol equivalent equals 1 milligram of d-alpha-tocopherol (natural vitamin E). You may see vitamin A values expressed in a number of different ways. This nutrient was originally measured in I.U., but in 1974 the United States began using a measurement called *retinol equivalents* (REs). One RE equals either 3.3 I.U. of retinol (preformed vitamin A) or 6 micrograms of beta-carotene.

drugs Accutane and tretinoin can help clear up acne and psoriasis.

And even one daily serving of fruit or vegetables rich in beta-carotene may cut your risk for heart attack or stroke. "We've found a 22 percent reduction in the risk of heart attack and a 40 percent reduction in stroke for those women with high intakes of fruit and vegetables rich in beta-carotene compared with those with low intakes," says JoAnn E. Manson, M.D., project director for Brigham and Women's Hospital and Harvard Medical School.

Sources: For beta-carotene, fruit and vegetables (the deeper the color, the more vitamin A they provide); for preformed vitamin A, fish-liver oil, meat and milk.

RDA: 800 RE (4,000 I.U.) for women; 1,000 RE (5,000 I.U.) for men.

Protective range: As beta-carotene, 15 to 30 milligrams.

People with special needs: Those who are poorly nourished, have diabetes or are exposed to high levels of toxic chemicals and pollutants. Nursing mothers need an additional 400 to 500 RE daily.

Signs of deficiency: Night blindness, dry or rough skin, weak tooth enamel, diarrhea, loss of appetite.

Cautions: Very high doses of vitamin A (more than 50,000 I.U. in adults and 20,000 I.U. in children) can cause side effects such as headache, vomiting, blurred vision, hair loss, liver damage and aching bones. Vitamin A derivatives may cause birth defects if taken while pregnant.

VITAMIN A SOURCES

Superior food sources of vitamin A include:

FOOD	PORTION	VITAMIN A (RE)
Sweet potato, baked	1	2,488
Carrot, raw	1	2,025
Spinach, boiled	½ cup	737
Butternut squash, baked	½ cup	714
Fresh tuna, cooked, dry heat	3 oz.	643
Cantaloupe	1 cup cubes	515
Beet greens, boiled	½ cup	367

VITAMIN B_6

Of all the B vitamins, B_6, or pyridoxine, may be the most important for maintaining a strong immune system. A study of eight healthy elderly adults by the U.S. Department of Agriculture's (USDA) Human Nutrition Research Center on Aging at Tufts University in Boston found that deficiencies of B_6 adversely affected the immune system, but normal function returned when B_6 intake was increased.

B_6 is needed to help many enzymes function and for protein and nucleic acid synthesis. Severe deficiencies can cause anemia, nervous disorders and skin problems.

One study found that premenstrual symptoms were relieved in 21 of 25 women receiving 500 milligrams of B_6 daily—*and* that B_6 appeared to boost chances of conception. (Such a large dosage should only be taken under medical supervision.) Some women also find that B_6 alleviates morning sickness.

Some people have reported relief from carpal tunnel syndrome—a painful condition affecting the nerve that runs through the wrist—with B_6, but there's little medical evidence to confirm that.

Sources: Fortified cereals, whole grains, fish, chicken, soybeans, oats, peanuts, fruits and vegetables.

RDA: 1.6 milligrams for women; 2.0 milligrams for men.

Protective range: 2 to 10 milligrams.

People with special needs: Those taking oral contraceptives or those with carpal tunnel syndrome or diabetes. Women need an additional 0.6 milligrams if pregnant, 0.5 milligrams if nursing.

Signs of deficiency: Anemia, confusion, weakness, irritability, nervousness, poor coordination, insomnia, skin lesions, muscle twitching.

Cautions: Large amounts (2,000 milligrams a day) have resulted in nerve damage—consult a doctor before exceeding 50 milligrams daily. Reduces the therapeutic effect of levodopa, a drug for Parkinson's disease.

VITAMIN B_6 SOURCES

Superior food sources of vitamin B_6 include:

FOOD	PORTION	VITAMIN B_6 (mg.)
Banana	1	0.7
Potato, baked	1	0.7
Chick-peas, canned	½ cup	0.6
Chicken breast, roasted	½	0.5
Fresh tuna, cooked, dry heat	3 oz.	0.4

VITAMIN B_{12}

In the early 1900s, if you suffered from pernicious anemia, a blood disease that causes nerve tissue to degenerate, you were out of luck: The disease is fatal, and there was no cure. In 1926, however, researchers discovered an amazing cure—raw liver.

The curative powers of liver came from vitamin B_{12}, also called cobalamin. We need B_{12} to synthesize DNA (which carries the code of genetic information) and help make blood. Studies have also linked it to helping prevent heart disease, cancer and neurological problems.

If you're low in either B_{12} or folate (another B vitamin), your blood levels of an amino acid called homocysteine increase, notes Joel B. Mason, M.D., assistant professor in the divisions of clinical nutrition and gastroenterology at Tufts University School of Medicine—and high homocysteine is associated with an increased risk of cardiovascular disease. "Very modest increases in homocysteine can increase the risk of disease," says Dr. Mason.

What about cancer? A study of 73 men who smoked at least the equivalent of a pack of cigarettes per day for 20 years found that supplementing with vitamin B_{12} and folate decreased the number of precancerous bronchial cells.

Allergic to sulfites? One study showed that B_{12} can also help alleviate reactions to this common food additive.

Vitamin B_{12} deficiencies can cause some psychological problems and changes in mental function—and may be one of the reasons some older people seem confused, less alert and not well coordinated. Some people can't absorb vitamin B_{12} at a normal rate; doctors estimate that one in five people over age 60 just doesn't manufacture enough stomach acid to absorb B_{12}.

Vitamin B_{12} is found almost exclusively in animal food products. If you don't eat meat, fish, dairy products or eggs, you may need a B_{12} supplement. (There's some B_{12} in tempeh, a fermented soybean product, but amounts can vary and are small.) Vegetarian children are particularly at risk because they have no stores of B_{12}.

Sources: Fish, dairy products, eggs, beef and pork. While liver and other organ meats are rich in B_{12}, they are not recommended for frequent consumption because of their high cholesterol content.

RDA: 2 micrograms.

Protective range: 2 to 10 micrograms.

People with special needs: Strict vegetarians and alcohol or drug abusers. Women need an extra 0.2 micrograms daily if pregnant and 0.4 micrograms daily if nursing.

Signs of deficiency: Anemia, neurological problems, sore tongue, weakness.

VITAMIN B_{12} SOURCES

Superior food sources of vitamin B_{12} include:

FOOD	PORTION	VITAMIN B_{12} (mcg.)
Clams, steamed	20 small	89.0
Mackerel, cooked, dry heat	3 oz.	16.2
Oysters, steamed	6 med.	16.1
Atlantic herring, cooked, dry heat	3 oz.	11.2
Fresh tuna, cooked, dry heat	3 oz.	9.3

TWO KINDS OF VITAMINS

Nutrition scientists divide vitamins into two categories: fat-soluble and water-soluble. What's the difference?

Fat-soluble vitamins dissolve in fat, of course, and water-soluble ones dissolve in water. The significance of this is that the fat-soluble vitamins—vitamins A, D, E and K—are stored in your body, and because they accumulate, you can overdose on these vitamins if you take excessive amounts of supplements.

It's tougher to overdose on the water-soluble vitamins—vitamins C, B_6 and B_{12}, biotin, folate, niacin, pantothenate, riboflavin and thiamine—because excess intakes of these vitamins are excreted in your urine. This doesn't mean, however, that you *can't* overdose on a water-soluble vitamin: Nutritionists warn that doses more than ten times the RDA may cause problems.

BIOTIN

Biotin, a B vitamin, is produced in our intestines, so normally we have plenty of it. It's involved in the synthesis of fatty acids and glucose and the metabolism of several amino acids.

Deficiencies in biotin can cause skin problems and loss of hair, but there's no scientific evidence that biotin can help control normal hair loss.

Sources: Milk, vegetables, nuts, whole grains, organ meats, brewer's yeast and tuna.

Estimated safe and adequate daily intake: 30 to 100 micrograms.

People with special needs: Those who smoke, eat a lot of raw egg white, are on a poorly balanced diet or are taking oral antibiotics.

Signs of deficiency: Fatigue, depression, nausea, sleepiness, loss of appetite, muscle pain, hair loss, dermatitis.

VITAMIN C

C is for colds and cancer—fighting them, that is. Or so research scientist and Nobel laureate Linus Pauling has claimed for decades, and the latest evidence indicates that there's some truth to these claims.

Vitamin C's historical role, however, was alleviating scurvy, a serious disease marked by bleeding gums and swollen limbs that crippled navies and explorers. Also known as ascorbic acid, vitamin C helps form the dentin layer (just under the enamel) of our teeth and collagen in our connective tissue. It's also involved in amino acid metabolism and helps us use iron, calcium and folate.

There's strong evidence that vitamin C, an antioxidant that helps protect cells from damage by destructive oxygen molecules, helps prevent some forms of cancers. Vitamin C may act in conjunction with carotenoids and other substances in fruit and vegetables, according to Gladys Block, Ph.D., a professor of public health nutrition at the University of California in Berkeley. And colds: Studies at the University of Torino in Italy found that vitamin C protected against colds, hay fever and exposure to air pollution.

Meeting the RDA of 60 milligrams daily should be no problem. "If you meet the National Academy of Sciences guidelines and eat at least five servings of fruit and vegetables each day, you can't help but take in 120 milligrams of vitamin C," says Paul F. Jacques, D.Sc., an epidemiologist at Tufts University.

Vitamin C also may help prevent heart disease. Studies by Dr. Jacques found that women with higher levels of vitamin C in their blood were more likely to have higher levels of HDL (high-density lipoprotein) cholesterol, the "good" cholesterol—possibly because of C's work as an antioxidant.

Vitamin C helps protect against cataracts, a vision robber that affects nearly half of Americans aged 75 to 85. Eating 3½ servings of fruit and vegetables a day is enough to help lower the risk.

Sources: Citrus fruits, broccoli, spinach, strawberries and melons.

RDA: 60 milligrams.

Protective range: 100 to 500 milligrams.

People with special needs: Smokers and alcohol abusers. Women need an additional 10 milligrams daily if pregnant, 30 to 35 milligrams if nursing.

Signs of deficiency: Scurvy (weak muscles, swollen or bleeding gums, loss of teeth, fatigue, depression), shortness of breath, easy bruising, nosebleeds, anemia, frequent infections.

Cautions: Huge doses can cause side effects in some people; consult a doctor.

VITAMIN C SOURCES

Superior food sources of vitamin C include:

FOOD	PORTION	VITAMIN C (mg.)
Orange juice, fresh	1 cup	124
Broccoli, fresh, boiled	1 cup	116
Brussels sprouts, fresh, cooked	1 cup	97
Red bell peppers, raw	½ cup	95
Cranberry juice cocktail	1 cup	90
Cantaloupe	1 cup cubes	68

VITAMIN D

The great thing about vitamin D is that you can make it yourself: Your body forms vitamin D when your skin is exposed to the ultraviolet rays of the sun. You can also get D from foods such as fatty fish, liver, egg yolks and fortified milk.

The primary role of this vitamin is to help build and maintain strong bones and teeth (D is essential to help us absorb calcium, the bone-building mineral). The classic sign of deficiency is rickets, a disease that causes stunted, bowed limbs and unhealthy teeth in growing children. Deficiency has also been linked to osteomalacia, a bone formation defect.

Some studies have found that vitamin D helps in the treatment of psoriasis and may boost resistance to tuberculosis.

Vitamin D may have many other functions, however, which researchers are just starting to uncover. Some studies indicate that D may protect against colorectal and breast cancer and may help in treating other cancers.

"We can look for many new treatments and new functions of vitamin D in the future," says Hector DeLuca, Ph.D., chairman of the Department of Biochemistry at the University of Wisconsin in Madison. Research by Dr. DeLuca indicates that the hormonal form of vitamin D can suppress growth of cancer cells.

Who's likely to be deficient in D? The elderly tend to be at risk because they may have limited exposure to sunlight, eat few vitamin D–rich foods or take medications that interfere with vitamin D uptake or metabolism. Other high-risk categories are alcoholics, people who live in areas without much sun and people who don't eat dairy products. Studies have found cases of rickets in vegetarian children who did not eat eggs or drink milk.

You can get your vitamin D from food. Or you can give yourself a "dose" of sunshine three times a week: Spend five to ten minutes outdoors with your face, arms and hands exposed to the morning or late-afternoon sun, says Michael Holick, M.D., Ph.D., director of the Vitamin D and Bone Research Laboratory at the Boston University School of Medicine. Another option is a multivitamin supplement that supplies 200 to 400 I.U.

It *is* possible to get too much vitamin D, so read labels carefully if you use supplements. Too much D can cause hypercalcemia—high levels of calcium in the blood. If you have elevated blood calcium already, *don't* take supplemental D.

Sources: Fatty fish (mackerel, sardines, salmon), liver, egg yolks, fortified milk and sunlight.

RDA: 5 micrograms (200 I.U.).

People with special needs: Vegetarians, the elderly, alcoholics and those who avoid the sun or have kidney failure. Women need an additional 200 I.U. if pregnant or nursing.

Signs of deficiency: Rickets in children (bowed legs, malformed joints or bones, retarded growth, weak muscles, late development of teeth), osteomalacia in adults (pain in ribs, spine, pelvis, legs; muscle weakness; brittle bones).

Cautions: Overdoses may cause high blood levels of calcium (hypercalcemia). If you have elevated blood calcium, take supplemental D only under a doctor's direction.

VITAMIN D SOURCES

Superior food sources of vitamin D include:

FOOD	PORTION	VITAMIN D (I.U.)
Herring, pickled	3 oz.	578
Atlantic sardines, canned in oil	3 oz.	231
Salmon, chum, canned	3 oz.	190
Fortified milk	8 oz.	100
Edam cheese	3 oz.	72

VITAMIN E

Vitamin E, or tocopherol, is another of those magical antioxidants that protects your cells from damage by destructive oxygen molecules. Evidence is growing that it plays a role in preventing heart disease, cataracts and cervical cancer and improving the immune system. There's some suggestion that treatment with E can help people with Parkinson's disease and tardive dyskinesia, a movement disorder.

Most of us don't have to worry about actual deficits of vitamin E: The only people prone to deficiency are some premature babies and people who don't absorb fat normally.

But a Nurses Health Study involving more than 87,000 women found that about 100 I.U. of supplemental vitamin E daily was associated with a 36 percent drop in the risk of heart attacks. Low levels of E may also double the risk of angina, according to another study.

Another study showed that vitamin E can protect strenuously used muscles from damage. Vitamin E seemed to invigorate the substances that help repair the muscles. This protective process also occurs when your body fights an infection, says William J. Evans, Ph.D., chief of the Human Physiology Laboratory at Tufts University and coauthor of *Biomarkers: The 10 Determinants of Aging You Can Control.*

Sources: Vegetable oil, mayonnaise, corn-oil margarine, peanuts, whole grains, wheat germ and spinach.

RDA: 12 I.U. (8 milligrams α-TE) for women; 15 I.U. (10 milligrams α-TE) for men.

Protective range: 100 to 400 I.U. (67 to 268 milligrams α-TE).

People with special needs: Those over 55 and those who abuse alcohol or drugs or have hyperthyroidism. Women need an additional 2 milligrams α-TE daily if pregnant, 3 to 4 milligrams α-TE if nursing.

Signs of deficiency: Anemia, lethargy, apathy, inability to concentrate, muscle weakness, decreased sexual performance.

Cautions: High doses deplete vitamin A stores. Very high doses may impair sex functions, alter hormone metabolism and produce a bleeding tendency. Don't take vitamin E supplements if you are on anticoagulant drugs or have a vitamin K deficiency (which impairs blood clotting).

VITAMIN E SOURCES

Superior food sources of vitamin E include:

FOOD	PORTION	VITAMIN E (mg. α-TE)
Sunflower seeds, dried	¼ cup	18
Sweet potatoes, boiled	1 cup	15
Kale, fresh, boiled	1 cup	10
Yams, boiled or baked	1 cup	6
Spinach, boiled	1 cup	4

FOLATE

This B vitamin, also called folic acid, is involved in metabolism and all biological reactions in your body. A deficiency causes anemia similar to vitamin B_{12} anemia, with symptoms of weakness, fatigue and cramps, and possibly depression and schizophrenia.

In some patients with atherosclerosis, folate prevented the recurrence of heart attacks. And in several studies, folate supplementation improved the eyesight of elderly patients.

Low folate concentrations in the blood have also been linked with cervical cancer, points out C. E. Butterworth, Jr., M.D., with the Department of Nutrition Sciences at the University of Alabama in Birmingham. Research there also showed that oral doses of ten milligrams of folate plus 500 micrograms of B_{12} decreased the number of precancerous bronchial cells.

Sources: Fresh leafy green vegetables, wheat germ, mushrooms, oranges, beans, rice, brewer's yeast and liver.

RDA: 180 micrograms for women; 200 micrograms for men.

Protective range: 400 to 800 micrograms.

People with special needs: The elderly, those with sickle cell anemia or any condition involving high production of red blood cells, alcoholics, women taking oral contraceptives, people with intestinal malabsorption problems. Women need an additional 220 micrograms daily if pregnant, 80 to 100 micrograms if nursing.

Signs of deficiency: Anemia, irritability, weakness.

Cautions: People with B_{12} deficiency anemia should not take folate until the B_{12} deficiency is treated.

FOLATE SOURCES

Superior food sources of folate include:

FOOD	PORTION	FOLATE (mcg.)
Lentils, boiled	½ cup	179
Pinto beans, boiled	½ cup	146
Spinach, boiled	½ cup	131
Wheat germ, toasted	¼ cup	100
Orange juice, fresh	1 cup	75

VITAMIN K

K is for *koagulation*—the Danish word for coagulation. As you might suspect, vitamin K—which was discovered by a Danish scientist in 1934—plays a crucial role in blood clotting.

This vitamin can also help control bleeding in the brain of premature babies, whose immature blood vessels evidently can't handle the pressure surges that occur during birth. In one study of 92 pregnant women who were expected to deliver prematurely, half received vitamin K injections every five days until delivery. Of the babies born to mothers receiving vitamin K, only 16 percent suffered brain bleeding and none had severe bleeding. Thirty-six percent of the babies of mothers who didn't receive vitamin K had bleeding, however, and 11 percent had severe bleeding.

Vitamin K also plays a role in maintaining healthy bones and helping fractures to heal. "We think K may have a positive effect on bone transformation," says Cees Vermeer, Ph.D., of the Department of Biochemistry at the University of Limburg in the Netherlands. Many elderly people have an inadequate intake of vitamin K, he says. One Japanese study found that supplemental K reduced the loss of calcium—essential for healthy bones—by

18 to 50 percent in three postmenopausal women with osteoporosis. However, high doses of vitamin K can cause allergic skin reactions or liver problems, and supplementation above 100 micrograms daily is not encouraged.

Sources: Green leafy vegetables, fruits, root vegetables, seeds, eggs, dairy products, meat and alfalfa. Also synthesized by intestinal bacteria.

RDA: 65 micrograms for women; 80 micrograms for men.

People with special needs: Those with malabsorption problems, on very low calorie diets or being fed intravenously.

Signs of deficiency: Defective blood coagulation (can lead to nosebleeds, blood in urine and spontaneous black-and-blue marks).

Cautions: Doses over 500 micrograms may cause rashes, itching, flushing or possibly liver problems.

NIACIN

When scores of residents of small southern towns in the early 1900s fell prey to a disease marked by an uncomfortable combination of symptoms—dermatitis, diarrhea and dementia—at first no one suspected that the culprit was something missing from their diets.

The disease was pellagra, and the missing nutrient was niacin. This B vitamin is involved in the synthesis of protein and fat and the formation of DNA. It helps maintain your skin, nerves and digestive system. Niacin has other important uses: One study found that it reduces cholesterol and the recurrence of heart attacks by nearly 30 percent.

There are two forms of niacin: nicotinic acid and nicotinamide. Nicotinic acid, however, can cause "niacin flush"—a burning, itching feeling in the face, neck, arms or chest—when taken in large doses.

Sources: Brewer's yeast, meats, poultry, halibut, salmon, swordfish, tuna, peanut butter, sunflower seeds and legumes.

RDA: 15 milligrams for women; 19 milligrams for men.

People with special needs: Those over 55, alcoholics, those who participate in vigorous physical activity or have diabetes or hyperthyroidism. Women need an additional 2 milligrams daily if pregnant, 5 milligrams if nursing.

Signs of deficiency: Muscle weakness; fatigue; loss of appetite; red, swollen tongue; headaches; skin lesions; nausea and vomiting; diarrhea; irritability.

Cautions: Doses of nicotinic acid over 100 milligrams can cause burning; itching and tingling in face, neck, arms and upper chest; nausea; headache; cramps; diarrhea and altered heart rate. Extremely large doses may cause liver problems. People with diabetes, gout or gallbladder or liver disease should consult a doctor before taking niacin.

NIACIN SOURCES

Superior food sources of niacin include:

FOOD	PORTION	NIACIN (mg.)
Chicken breast, roasted	½	11.8
Light tuna, canned in water	3 oz.	10.5
Fresh tuna, cooked, dry heat	3 oz.	9.0
Halibut, cooked, dry heat	3 oz.	6.1
Turkey white meat, roasted	3 oz.	5.8

PANTOTHENATE

This B vitamin, also called pantothenic acid, is easy to find—all food groups contain some. It's involved in metabolizing carbohydrate, fat and protein. Deficiency may lower resistance to infection, and higher intakes may help you fight stress.

Sources: Organ meats, most fish, whole grains, blue cheese, brewer's yeast, corn, eggs, lentils, wheat germ, sunflower seeds, peanuts and peas.

Estimated safe and adequate daily intake: 4 to 7 milligrams.

People with special needs: Drug or alcohol abusers, athletes, pregnant or nursing women, those over 55, those on inadequate or low-calorie diets or smokers.

Signs of deficiency: May include fatigue, sleeping problems, loss of appetite, nausea, lowered resistance to infection.

Cautions: More than 10 grams daily could cause diarrhea and bloating. Don't take pantothenate if you are taking medication for Parkinson's disease.

RIBOFLAVIN

This B vitamin, also known as vitamin B_2, is essential for growth and tissue repair. Deficiencies have been linked to esophageal cancer.

Deficiency may be fairly common, particularly in youngsters who drink less than one cup of milk a day. Two cups of milk daily supply sufficient riboflavin, but you can also get it from fruit, vegetables and cereals.

If you do take a riboflavin supplement, take it with meals to dramatically increase the amount you'll absorb.

Sources: Milk, yogurt, cheese, wheat germ, whole grains, chicken, leafy green vegetables, almonds and fruit.

RDA: 1.3 milligrams for women; 1.7 milligrams for men.

People with special needs: Those who exercise regularly, eat only processed foods or are on low-calorie diets, have hypothyroidism or are alcoholics. Women need an additional 0.3 milligrams daily if pregnant, 0.4 to 0.5 milligrams if nursing.

Signs of deficiency: Cracks in corners of mouth, inflamed tongue and lips, sensitive eyes, itching and scaling of skin, trembling, dizziness, insomnia.

RIBOFLAVIN SOURCES

Superior food sources of riboflavin include:

FOOD	PORTION	RIBOFLAVIN (mg.)
Beef liver, braised	3 oz.	3.5
King mackerel, cooked	3 oz.	0.5
Nonfat yogurt	1 cup	0.5
Skim milk	1 cup	0.5
Swiss cheese	1 oz.	0.1

THIAMINE

This B vitamin, also called vitamin B_1, is involved in converting blood sugar into energy. It also helps form red blood cells and maintain skeletal muscle.

What it's most known for is preventing beriberi, a serious deficiency disease that causes confusion, weakened muscles, loss of appetite and quickened heartbeat. If not halted, the disease progresses either to "wet" beriberi, which causes swelling, accumulation of fluid in the heart muscle and eventual death, or "dry" beriberi, which causes serious nervous system problems and wasting away.

This was a common health problem in the mid-nineteenth century, particularly in countries where polished white rice was a staple of the diet. In the Philippines, where most of the thiamine present in rice is lost in milling, washing and cooking, beriberi is still the fourth leading cause of death.

Most of us in the United States get ample thiamine in our diets, but one group at risk for deficiency is alcoholics, because alcohol interferes with the absorption of thiamine *and* impairs the ability to store it. Many of the classic outward symptoms of alcoholism—confusion, vision problems and eye muscle paralysis—may be caused by thiamine deficiency.

But even marginal deficiencies can cause an array of unpleasant symptoms in older people. A study of 80 Irish women with moderate deficiency found that thiamine supplements improved their sleep patterns, decreased fatigue and restored appetite and sense of general well-being. The researchers suggest having your doctor check your thiamine levels with a blood test if you are over 65 and have these symptoms.

Sources: Pork, whole grains, wheat germ, brewer's yeast, legumes and seafood.

RDA: 1.1 milligrams for women; 1.5 milligrams for men.

People with special needs: Those on low-calorie diets, heavy coffee or tea drinkers, the elderly or alcoholics. Women need an additional 0.4 milligrams daily if pregnant, 0.5 milligrams if nursing.

Signs of deficiency: Loss of appetite, fatigue, nausea, vomiting, confusion, depression, gastrointestinal problems, fluid accumulation in arms and legs.

THIAMINE SOURCES

Superior food sources of thiamine include:

FOOD	PORTION	THIAMINE (mg.)
Pork center loin,roasted	3 oz.	0.8
Sunflower seeds, dried	1 oz.	0.7
Florida pompano, cooked, dry heat	3 oz.	0.6
Wheat germ, toasted	¼ cup	0.5
Spinach noodles, enriched, cooked	1 cup	0.4

MINERALS

CALCIUM

So you know all about calcium, you say. Try this quiz.

Calcium can help: (a) build and maintain strong bones and teeth, (b) lower blood pressure, (c) cut colon cancer risks, (d) ease menstrual discomfort, (e) reduce the number of premature births or (f) all of the above.

The correct answer is (f) all of the above.

People who miss out on enough calcium in their younger, bone-forming years may pay the piper years later. Around age 40, we begin to lose this mineral from our bones faster than it can be replaced. Women face especially large losses during menopause because of the lack of estrogen, which is necessary for their bones to absorb calcium. The result can be osteoporosis, with bones so weakened that they can break while just walking. Some studies have indicated that calcium can help even after the bone-forming years, however. According to several studies, calcium can help people with mild high blood pressure lower their levels to normal.

What role does calcium play in cancer prevention? For colon cancer, calcium may bind with possible cancer-causing bile acids that are produced in the colon.

A study of pregnant teenagers found that mothers who received supplemental calcium had markedly fewer premature births. And a 5½-month study by the USDA found that women who received higher calcium than a control group had fewer menstrual and premenstrual symptoms such as mood changes, cramps and backaches.

Sources: Dairy products, canned salmon and sardines (with bones), soybeans, tofu, kale, turnip greens and kelp.

RDA: 800 milligrams.

Protective range: 1,200 to 1,500 milligrams.

People with special needs: Those who avoid milk and other dairy products, are over 55 (especially women), are on low-calorie diets or are alcoholics. Women need an additional 400 milligrams daily if pregnant or nursing.

Signs of deficiency: Frequent fractures, hump in spine, seizures, muscle cramps, low backache.

Cautions: Avoid supplemental calcium if you have kidney stones or high blood calcium.

CALCIUM SOURCES

Superior food sources of calcium include:

FOOD	PORTION	CALCIUM (mg.)
Skim milk	1 cup	302
Sardines, canned	6	275
Mozzarella cheese	1 oz.	181
Salmon, canned (with bones)	3 oz.	181
Figs, dried	5	135

CHROMIUM

Yep, this is the stuff used to make the trim on your car glitter—but it's also an essential mineral linked to glucose tolerance, the ability to process blood sugar.

Glucose *intolerance* is a precursor of diabetes, and controlling it may prevent the development of that disease. In one study, glucose tolerance improved in 10 of 12 elderly people who were given chromium. Another study showed that supplementing with 200 micrograms daily improved glucose tolerance in people who were mildly glucose-intolerant.

What this means is that adequate chromium could keep many people who have mild glucose intolerance from becoming diabetic, says Richard A. Anderson, Ph.D., a biochemist with the USDA's Human Nutrition Research Center in Beltsville, Maryland. It's tough to get enough chromium in your foods, says Dr. Anderson. And he recommends a supplement. Another way to increase your chromium intake is to eat fewer foods that *deplete* chromium—such as cookies and pastries, with their simple carbohydrates. Complex carbohydrates such as pasta and potatoes, on the other hand, help *preserve* chromium.

You don't have to worry about overdosing on the chromium you get in foods. Toxicity can result, however, from overexposure to industrial processes involving chromium, such as electroplating, steel making and glassmaking.

Sources: Vegetables, whole grains, fruit, meat, cheese, oysters, fish, dairy products, beef, chicken and brewer's yeast.

Estimated safe and adequate daily intake: 50 to 200 micrograms.

Protective range: 100 to 200 micrograms.

People with special needs: Those who use alcohol or are on low-calorie diets, the elderly, pregnant women, athletes.

Signs of deficiency: Diabetes-like symptoms (overweight, fatigue, excessive thirst, frequent urination, urinary tract infections, yeast infections).

COPPER

Copper is necessary for the formation of red blood cells; it's also a catalyst for the storage and release of iron. It's involved in the production of collagen, the protein that makes bone, cartilage, skin and tendons all work. Copper also helps produce melanin, the pigment that gives color to our hair and skin. In animals, supplementary copper has been shown to protect against some cancers.

Some research indicates that copper deficiency is linked to heart disease. Leslie M. Klevay, M.D., research leader of the Clinical Nutrition Laboratory with the USDA Human Nutrition Research Center at the University of North Dakota in Grand Forks, notes that copper deficiency can raise cholesterol levels, lead to glucose intolerance, produce heart rhythm problems and increase blood pressure.

Many of us may not be getting enough copper: Two-thirds of Americans get less than the suggested minimum.

Sources: Nuts, fruit and legumes, oysters and other shellfish.

Estimated safe and adequate daily intake: 1.5 to 3.0 milligrams.

People with special needs: Premature babies and those taking high levels of zinc or vitamin C.

Signs of deficiency: Anemia, bone demineralization, low white blood cell count.

COPPER SOURCES

Superior food sources of copper include:

FOOD	PORTION	COPPER (mg.)
Oysters, cooked	12 med.	7.5
Alaskan king crab, steamed	3 oz.	1.0
Potatoes, baked, with skin	7 oz.	0.6
White beans, boiled	1 cup	0.5
Apricots, dried	½ cup	0.3

FLUORIDE

Scientists know that fluoride is incorporated into bones and tooth enamel, but they're not yet positive that it's nutritionally essential.

What they do know is that fluoride reduces dental cavities, particularly in children eight and younger, so many communities have fluoride added to the public water supply for that purpose. There's also some suggestion that fluoride may help protect bones in adults, apparently stimulating new bone growth and helping to make bone stronger.

Fluoridated water has one milligram of fluoride or less per liter; you can also get fluoride from foods, although the content varies.

Sources: Tea, canned salmon (with bones), mackerel and fluoridated water.

Estimated safe and adequate daily intake: 1.5 to 4.0 milligrams.

Cautions: High levels have caused mottling of children's teeth; huge doses may be toxic.

IODINE

You may have noticed that the salt you buy is fortified with iodine, but have you ever wondered why you need this mineral? Most of the iodine in your body is in your thyroid gland, and you need ample iodine to keep your thyroid hormones on track.

Deficiency can cause many disorders, including thyroid enlargement (known as goiter) and mental retardation. Iodine is present in both soil and water, but in some areas of the world levels are so low that iodine deficiency is common. The introduction of iodine into the salt supply in the United States in 1924 greatly decreased the occurrence of goiter, but it continues to be a major problem in Africa, Asia and South America.

Some studies suggest that iodine may help relieve fibrocystic breasts, painful or sore breasts common in premenopausal women.

Most North Americans get plenty of iodine in their diets, even without iodized salt. An exception may be people who eat lots of cruciferous vegetables such as rutabagas, cabbage, brussels sprouts and cauliflower. These foods are iodine antagonists—they block uptake of the mineral.

Sources: Seaweed, fish, shrimp, oysters and iodized salt.

RDA: 150 micrograms.

People with special needs: Those on low-calorie diets, who live in areas where soil is deficient in iodine and eat mostly locally grown produce, or those who eat lots of cruciferous vegetables. Women need an additional 25 micrograms daily if pregnant, 50 micrograms if nursing.

Signs of deficiency: Chronic fatigue, weight gain, intolerance to cold, goiter (enlarged thyroid gland).

Cautions: Too much iodine during pregnancy can result in thyroid enlargement, dwarfism or mental deficiency in the baby. Don't take supplements if you have elevated serum potassium or myotonia congenita (a hereditary disease that makes the muscles stiff). More than 50 milligrams daily can cause inflammation of the salivary glands.

IRON

Having trouble sleeping at night? You may not be consuming enough iron.

An insomnia study by the USDA found that people consuming one-third the recommended amount of iron woke more frequently during the night than people taking in adequate iron.

But contributing to a sound night's sleep is a minor role for iron. Iron produces the red blood cells that transport oxygen in our bodies. That's why a shortage of iron causes anemia. Low iron intake has been linked to learning problems in young children, and one study suggested that low iron levels adversely affected short-term memory and attention span in young women.

And iron deficiency is more common than you may think: Experts estimate that one-third to one-half of young American women are iron deficient. Even mild iron-deficiency anemia may cause you to feel depressed or lethargic. "If you're tired, listless and apathetic in a way you're not used to, you'd better check your iron levels," says Ernesto Pollitt, Ph.D., professor of human development at the University of California at Davis.

You should check with your doctor before taking iron supplements: One in 300 people may suffer from a genetic defect that causes iron overload, says James D. Cook, M.D., professor of medicine and director of the Division of Hematology at the University of Kansas Medical Center in Kansas City.

Sources: Red meat, clams, garbanzos, tomato juice and raisins.

RDA: 15 milligrams for women; 10 milligrams for men.

Protective range: 15 milligrams.

People with special needs: Menstruating women, those on restricted diets. Pregnant women need an additional 15 milligrams daily.

Signs of deficiency: Listlessness, heart palpitations on exertion, irritability, fatigue, pale skin, cracked lips and tongue.

Cautions: Don't take iron supplements if you have acute hepatitis, excess iron in your body, hemolytic anemia, or have had many blood transfusions. Iron supplements formulated for adults can be lethal for small children.

IRON SOURCES

Superior food sources of iron include:

FOOD	PORTION	IRON (mg.)
Clams, steamed	20 small	26.2
Cream of Wheat, cooked	¾ cup	7.7
Tofu	4 oz.	6.2
Soybeans, boiled	½ cup	4.4
Pumpkin seeds, hulled, dried	1 oz.	4.3

MAGNESIUM

Without magnesium, we wouldn't be here: This mineral is involved in every major biologic function in our bodies. It also may help prevent heart disease, kidney stones and gallstones, chronic fatigue syndrome and menstrual problems. Magnesium also acts as an antacid in small doses and as a laxative in large doses, and helps strengthen tooth enamel. Low magnesium can cause problems such as depression, irritability and confusion, says Daniel Kanofsky, M.D., assistant professor of psychiatry at the Albert Einstein College of Medicine of Yeshiva University in New York City.

Some researchers believe magnesium deficiency is a cause of cardiovascular disease. Death rates from heart disease are higher in areas with soft water—which, unlike hard water, doesn't contain appreciable amounts of magnesium. And magnesium given intravenously does help save the lives of heart attack victims.

Promising news for people who suffer from chronic fatigue syndrome (CFS) comes from a study in the United Kingdom. Of 15 CFS patients receiving a weekly intramuscular shot of magnesium sulfate for six weeks, 12 showed marked improvement—while only 3 of 17 patients who didn't receive magnesium said they felt better. "It may be worthwhile to check for magnesium deficiency in the blood—and if it's there, take the proper steps to fix it," says M. J. Campbell, Ph.D., senior lecturer at the University of Southampton General Hospital in the United Kingdom.

Sources: Wheat germ, sunflower seeds, leafy green vegetables, seafood, nuts, dairy products and meats.

RDA: 280 milligrams for women; 350 milligrams for men.

Protective range: 400 milligrams.

People with special needs: The elderly; those with diabetes, on low-calorie diets, taking diuretics or digitalis; alcohol drinkers; those who engage in regular strenuous exercise. Women need an additional 20 milligrams daily if pregnant, 60 to 75 milligrams if nursing.

Signs of deficiency: Nausea, muscle weakness, irritability, mental derangement.

Cautions: People with kidney problems, certain heart problems or ileostomy (a surgical opening in the small intestine) should not take magnesium supplements.

MAGNESIUM SOURCES

Superior food sources of magnesium include:

FOOD	PORTION	MAGNESIUM (mg.)
Pumpkin seeds, hulled, dried	1 oz.	152
Tofu	4 oz.	120
Sunflower seeds, dried	1 oz.	101
Wheat germ, toasted	¼ cup	91
Almonds	1 oz.	84

MANGANESE

There's still a lot of mystery about what manganese does for us, but scientists *do* know that it's essential. In animals, manganese is required for normal bone structure and glucose metabolism, and animals that are deficient in manganese sometimes have trouble reproducing.

Manganese helps enzymes break down carbohydrates and fats into fuel, and animal experiments suggest that it also works as an antioxidant, protecting cells from damage from destructive oxygen molecules. "Because manganese functions as an antioxidant, your intake may be important in terms of preventing a number of degenerative diseases like heart disease," says Sheri Zidenberg-Cherr, Ph.D., research nutritionist and lecturer at the University of California at Davis.

Most of us get adequate manganese in our diets, but if you're taking large doses of calcium or iron supplements, you could be significantly interfering with your manganese levels. There's some evidence that magnesium and phosphorus can partially block manganese absorption as well.

Overdosing on manganese in foods is unlikely, but people exposed to manganese dust—such as mine workers—can actually experience "manganese intoxication." Symptoms include delusions and hallucinations, followed by deep depression and an inability to stay awake.

Sources: Whole grains, nuts, shellfish, milk and organ meats.

Estimated safe and adequate daily intake: 2 to 5 milligrams.

People with special needs: Those on low-calorie diets or being fed intravenously or by tube. High intake of magnesium, calcium, iron or phosphate may decrease absorption of manganese.

Signs of deficiency: Slow growth and development in children.

Cautions: Consult a doctor before taking supplemental manganese if you have liver disease.

MOLYBDENUM

This mineral with the funny name is a part of the body's enzyme system. It also becomes a part of bones, liver and kidneys.

Molybdenum may play a vital role in protecting against esophageal cancer. A small region in China with soil very deficient in molybdenum has the highest rate of esophageal cancer in the world. Molybdenum is necessary for nitrates in the soil to change to the amines that are needed to nourish plants; without molybdenum, the nitrates change to cancer-causing forms instead. People in the region were also deficient in vitamin C, which helps detoxify those cancer-causing forms.

The happy ending to this story is that since molybdenum has been added to the soil and diets have been supplemented with vitamin C, the rate of esophageal cancer appears to be declining in China.

Molybdenum deficiency is quite rare, however. Studies show that most American diets supply between 75 and 250 micrograms, so chances are you're getting plenty.

Sources: Whole grains; legumes; dark green, leafy vegetables; milk; beans and organ meats.

Estimated safe and adequate daily intake: 75 to 250 micrograms.

People with special needs: Those on low-calorie diets or being fed intravenously or by tube.

Cautions: Don't take over 500 micrograms a day without a doctor's prescription. Consult a doctor before taking supplements containing molybdenum if you have high levels of uric acid or gout. Intake of 10 to 15 milligrams daily is associated with goutlike symptoms.

PHOSPHORUS

This mineral regulates the release of energy, helps transport nutrients involved in calcification of bones and teeth and helps regulate the acidity of body fluids.

It's an essential mineral, but because it's so plentiful in foods—daily intake in the American diet ranges from 800 to 1,500 milligrams—deficiency is rare. Phosphorus deficiency has resulted from taking antacids containing aluminum hydroxide, which binds with phosphorus and makes it unavailable for absorption.

Sources: Almost all foods.

RDA: 800 milligrams.

People with special needs: Alcoholics, those with gastrointestinal and kidney problems or diabetic ketoacidosis. Women need an additional 400 milligrams daily if pregnant or nursing.

Signs of deficiency: Bone loss, weakness, anorexia, pain.

POTASSIUM

We need potassium for many things—including maintaining a regular heartbeat and normal muscle contraction—but the exciting news is that, in some cases, this mineral can evidently lower blood pressure and help prevent heart disease and stroke.

"Strong evidence from a number of studies suggests that a diet low in potassium may lead to high blood pressure," says George Webb, Ph.D., associate professor of physiology and biophysics at the University of Vermont College of Medicine in Burlington.

In one study of 37 men and women with high blood pressure, one group took 2,340 milligrams of potassium daily, another group took the potassium plus magnesium, while a third group received a blank pill. After eight weeks, the blood pressure of both groups taking potassium dropped dramatically.

"A low potassium intake may substantially increase your risk of getting hypertension or, we now suspect, may make existing high blood pressure worse," says G. Gopal Krishna, M.D., associate professor of medicine at the University of Pennsylvania in Philadelphia.

Another study suggests that just one extra serving of fresh vegetables or fruit daily could reduce your risk of fatal stroke by 40 percent. That study, involving 859 southern Californian men and women ranging in age from 50 to 79, found that the 24 people who suffered stroke-related deaths had a markedly lower potassium intake than the others.

And if you're low in potassium, you actually retain more sodium—one of the enemies in the blood pressure battle—and *lose* more calcium, necessary to maintain strong bones.

Sources: Fresh vegetables and fruit, meat and milk.

Estimated minimum daily intake: 1,600 to 2,000 milligrams.

People with special needs: Those taking diuretics.

Signs of deficiency: Weakness, paralysis, low blood pressure, irregular or rapid heartbeat.

Cautions: People with impaired kidney function should avoid foods and supplements rich in potassium.

POTASSIUM SOURCES

Superior food sources of potassium include:

FOOD	PORTION	POTASSIUM (mg.)
Potato, baked	1	844
Apricots, dried	10 halves	482
Lima beans	½ cup	478
Banana	1	451
Skim milk	1 cup	447
Chicken breast, roasted	3 oz.	220

SELENIUM

We need this mineral only in very tiny quantities, but those minute amounts appear to help prevent some serious diseases—cancer and stroke.

Take a look at Rapid City, South Dakota, with the lowest rate of deaths from cancer in the United States. Rapid City *also* has the highest amount of selenium in its soil (and its crops). Now look at Ohio, with almost double the cancer rate as South Dakota and—you guessed it—the lowest soil selenium levels. Experiments show reduced rates of liver, skin, mammary and colon cancers in animals given selenium—and one study showed the cancer-fighting effect was more dramatic when rats received *both* selenium and garlic.

"From a practical standpoint, this means that people should eat foods that give them an adequate level of selenium," says Cornell University toxicologist Donald Lisk, Ph.D.

Areas of Georgia and North and South Carolina also have very low soil selenium—plus the highest rates of stroke and heart disease.

Like beta-carotene and vitamins C and E, selenium is an antioxidant. It latches onto harmful oxygen molecules, which may help explain its disease-fighting potential. Selenium may also increase immune responses, and it plays a role in sperm production and movement. Studies in China showed that supplementing with selenium can stop Keshan disease, which involves the degeneration of heart muscles.

Even moderately low levels of selenium can cause anxiety and tiredness. Researchers at the University College in Swansea, Wales, found that a supplement of 100 micrograms daily improved moods and anxiety levels.

Sources: Brewer's yeast, grains, fish, broccoli, cabbage, celery, cucumbers, onions, garlic, radishes and mushrooms.

RDA: 55 micrograms for women; 70 micrograms for men.

Protective range: 70 to 200 micrograms.

People with special needs: Women need an additional 10 micrograms daily if pregnant, 20 micrograms if nursing.

Signs of deficiency: Heart muscle disorders.

Cautions: Inorganic selenium (sodium selenite) may decrease absorption of vitamin C, so don't take them together. Toxicity has resulted from taking 1,000 micrograms of sodium selenite daily.

SELENIUM SOURCES

Superior food sources of selenium include:

FOOD	PORTION	SELENIUM (mcg.)
Tortilla chips	1 oz.	284
Corn chips	1 oz.	182
Tuna, canned	3 oz.	99
Cracked wheat bread	3 slices	67
Salmon, canned	3 oz.	64

ZINC

You can think of zinc as the bodyguard of your immune system, stalwartly fighting off invaders that threaten your health. But zinc moonlights at various other jobs, ranging from protecting your vision to reducing the duration of your colds.

Zinc is essential for normal growth and development; deficiencies can limit growth and delay sexual maturity. Zinc appears to slow down the advance of macular degeneration, a major cause of vision loss in the elderly. Low levels of the mineral have been linked with pregnancy complications and with low birth weight. Zinc may improve wound healing, particularly in people with a prior deficiency.

While serious zinc deficiency is rare, marginal deficiency may not be. Pregnant women are particularly at risk, and surveys show that zinc intakes of children are below minimal requirements. Many ingredients in our food—including fiber and other substances in plant foods, plus iron, calcium and copper—can reduce the availability of zinc. (On the other hand, protein and red wine can enhance zinc absorption.)

Because it can be difficult to consume enough zinc, Sheldon Saul Hendler, M.D., Ph.D., assistant clinical professor of medicine at the University of California at San Diego and author of *The Doctors' Vitamin and Mineral Encyclopedia,* recommends a daily supplement of 15 to 30 milligrams for adults and 10 milligrams for children. Because zinc can interfere with the absorption of copper and selenium, he suggests that along with zinc you take 1.5 to 3.0 milligrams of copper and 50 to 200 micrograms of selenium.

Sources: Wheat germ, wheat bran, whole grains, brewer's yeast, seafood, poultry and meat.

RDA: 12 milligrams for women; 15 milligrams for men.

People with special needs: Vegetarians, the elderly, athletes, dieters. Women need an additional 3 milligrams daily if pregnant, 4 to 7 milligrams if nursing.

Signs of deficiency: Moderate deficiencies can cause loss of smell and taste, slowed growth in children, rashes, loss of hair, vision impairment, irregular muscle movement, skin lesions, sterility, low sperm count, delayed wound healing. Serious deficiency can result in delayed bone maturity, enlarged liver or spleen, shrunken testicles, dwarfism.

Cautions: High doses (18 to 25 milligrams daily) of zinc may cause a copper deficiency; huge doses (300 milligrams daily) have adversely affected the immune system. Don't take supplemental zinc if you have stomach ulcers.

ZINC SOURCES

Superior food sources of zinc include:

FOOD	PORTION	ZINC (mg.)
Oysters, steamed	6 med.	76.4
Beef blade roast, braised	3 oz.	8.7
Alaskan king crab, steamed	3 oz.	6.5
Ribeye steak, broiled	3 oz.	5.9
Wheat germ, toasted	¼ cup	4.7

CHAPTER 4

Meeting Your Nutrient Needs

The RDAs and Beyond

It would be great if we all arrived on Earth with "care and feeding" tags like the ones that come with houseplants, listing exactly how much iron and vitamin A and selenium and so forth we need each day.

Unfortunately, we don't. Yes, much of our packaged food comes with little charts explaining nutrient content, and we can find larger charts telling us just how much of each nutrient we should be getting—but for most of us that still leaves plenty of unanswered questions.

What exactly do these figures mean? Are these *minimum* amounts or *maximum* amounts? And what about the exciting headlines on the newsstands about vitamins and minerals that might help prevent cancer, cataracts, high cholesterol, heart attacks and more?

Once we might have dismissed these headlines as farfetched and, well, *nuts*—but no one's laughing anymore.

"There was a lot of quackery in this field," says Harinder S. Garewal, M.D., Ph.D., assistant director for cancer prevention and control at the University of Arizona Cancer Center in Tucson. "But the work being done now is very sophisticated. It's now swinging back into acceptable science."

WHO DECIDES HOW MUCH?

The Recommended Dietary Allowances (RDAs) were established in 1941 to provide standards to serve as a goal for good nutrition.

These figures have been periodically revised by the Food and Nutrition Board of the National Research Council. A lot of different information is used to come up with these amounts, including studies that show how much of a nutrient is required to correct a deficiency and how much of a nutrient is normally consumed by people in good health. The figures also take into account that not all of each vitamin or mineral you ingest is actually usable by your body.

Because researchers are constantly getting new information from new studies, the RDAs evolve over time. The actual amounts may be raised or lowered, age groupings may be changed or nutrients may be added to the list. The 1989 RDAs, for example, included vitamin K and selenium for the first time, lowered folate and B_{12} requirements and increased calcium amounts for certain age groups. New tables are released every five to ten years.

WHEN MORE MIGHT BE BETTER

But what about going *beyond* the RDAs? These figures are judged to be adequate to meet the nutrient needs of most healthy people, but they often don't come close to the amounts that some scientists and nutritionists suggest could prevent or even help cure specific ailments. And it's possible that certain groups, such as the elderly—who often process nutrients less efficiently—have special needs.

"There is a growing number of studies that suggest that the RDAs are not really appropriate or sensitive to the changing nutritional needs of aging adults. Nor are they focused on the most important public health objective today—preventing chronic diseases like cancer and heart disease," says Jeffrey Blumberg, Ph.D., associate director of the U.S. Department of Agriculture's (USDA) Human Nutrition Research Center on Aging at Tufts University in Boston.

Some nutritionists believe that instead we should be given safe *ranges* of nutrients that we can consume in levels *beyond* the RDAs. "The American public should be advised about the reasonable doses of each of the vitamins—doses that have been associated with no adverse effects. I think the public is bright enough to use vitamin supplements safely," says Adrianne Bendich, Ph.D., senior clinical research coordinator in the Human Nutrition Research Division of Hoffmann-La Roche in Nutley, New Jersey.

"My own feeling is that there is a good likelihood that if all these studies continue to point in the same direction, then recommendations could be made for disease prevention in general," says Dr. Garewal.

THOSE AMAZING ANTIOXIDANTS

The unquestioned stars in the nutrient-as-treatment arena are the antioxidants—beta-carotene (which converts in the body to vitamin A), vitamin C and vitamin E. We all have within us something called free radicals, unstable molecules that can wreak havoc on cells and tissues. These harmful free radicals may be formed by natural processes in the body or by environmental influences such as cigarette smoke, sunlight or pollution. Antioxidants, however, neutralize these free radicals—and apparently help prevent (and in some cases treat) cancers, heart disease and respiratory problems.

Beta-carotene versus cancer. Some of Dr. Garewal's work has showed convincing results in the use of beta-carotene in fighting oral leukoplakia, premalignant lesions that may become cancerous. Seventeen of 24 people who took 30 milligrams of beta-carotene per day for six months showed major improvement. This is far more beta-carotene than the 4.8 milligrams (for women) and 6 milligrams (for men) needed to provide the RDA for vitamin A.

And there's an array of other convincing studies. Beta-carotene intake of over 6.2 milligrams per day in a Latin American study was associated with a 32 percent lower risk of cervical cancer than an intake of less than 2.3 milligrams per day. And in a Harvard Medical School study beta-carotene also dramatically cut risks of heart attack, stroke and death among men with prior heart problems.

"In my own mind, I like to get the very last trial nailed in before making definitive recommendations," says Dr. Garewal. "But there's a lot of convincing data about beta-carotene and other antioxidants that continues to accumulate. Hopefully, in the next few years evidence on which to base definitive recommendations will become available."

Vitamin C against colds and cancer. Vitamin C is another potential cancer blocker, according to Gladys Block, Ph.D., a professor of public health nutrition at the University of California at Berkeley. Thirty-three of 46 studies she reviewed found that C offered significant protection against cancers of the esophagus, larynx, pancreas, stomach, rectum, breast and cervix. "I do think the evidence is strong enough for me to say that for prevention of some cancers, vitamin C probably makes a difference," says Dr. Block.

And evidence suggests that vitamin C also helps protect against infections of the upper respiratory tract as well as bronchial problems caused by exposure to air pollutants. Researchers found that two grams (2,000 milligrams) of vitamin C daily helped protect people from the common cold, hay fever and effects of exposure to traffic fumes. (The RDA for men and women over age 25 is 60 milligrams.)

Research conducted in Torino, Italy, found that short-term exposure to air pollution decreases lung function and that treatment with C may coun-

RECOMMENDED DIETARY ALLOWANCES

Do you want to know specifically how much of each major nutrient you should be getting? Here are the amounts recommended by the Food and Nutrition Board of the National Research Council for various age groups, based on median heights and weights. These are average daily intakes—meaning that some days you could eat more and

					VITAMINS					
CATEGORY	AGE (yr.) OR CONDITION	WEIGHT (lb.)	HEIGHT (in.)	PROTEIN (g.)	VITAMIN A (mcg. RE)*	VITAMIN D (mcg.)	VITAMIN E (mg. α-TE)†	VITAMIN K (mcg.)	VITAMIN C (mg.)	THIAMINE (mg.)
Infants	0.0–0.5	13	24	13	375	7.5	3	5	30	0.3
	0.5–1.0	20	28	14	375	10	4	10	35	0.4
Children	1–3	29	35	16	400	10	6	15	40	0.7
	4–6	44	44	24	500	10	7	20	45	0.9
	7–10	62	52	28	700	10	7	30	45	1.0
Males	11–14	99	62	45	1,000	10	10	45	50	1.3
	15–18	145	69	59	1,000	10	10	65	60	1.5
	19–24	160	70	58	1,000	10	10	70	60	1.5
	25–50	174	70	63	1,000	5	10	80	60	1.5
	51+	170	68	63	1,000	5	10	80	60	1.2
Females	11–14	101	62	46	800	10	8	45	50	1.1
	15–18	120	64	44	800	10	8	55	60	1.1
	19–24	128	65	46	800	10	8	60	60	1.1
	25–50	138	64	50	800	5	8	65	60	1.1
	51+	143	63	50	800	5	8	65	60	1.0
Pregnant				60	800	10	10	65	70	1.5
Lactating	1st 6 months			65	1,300	10	12	65	95	1.6
	2nd 6 months			62	1,200	10	11	65	90	1.6

*RE = Retinol Equivalent
†α-TE = Alpha-Tocopherol Equivalent
‡NE = Niacin Equivalent

teract its effects. The research also indicates that vitamin C can help alleviate airway irritability, protect against the effects of air pollution and improve the prognosis for patients with chronic lung disease.

Vitamin E has many roles. Vitamin E has been nominated for a number of starring roles, including fighting cancer, helping heart attack victims and improving immune response. There are suggestions that it may slow

some days less—that are considered adequate to maintain good nutrition for healthy people under normal environmental stresses. The board recommends that you get these nutrients from a variety of foods to help supply other important nutrients for which RDAs have not been established.

					MINERALS						
RIBOFLAVIN (mg.)	NIACIN (mg. NE)‡	VITAMIN B_6 (mg.)	FOLATE (mcg.)	VITAMIN B_{12} (mcg.)	CALCIUM (mg.)	IODINE (mcg.)	IRON (mg.)	MAGNESIUM (mg.)	PHOSPHORUS (mg.)	SELENIUM (mcg.)	ZINC (mg.)
0.4	5	0.3	25	0.3	400	40	6	40	300	10	5
0.5	6	0.6	35	0.5	600	50	10	60	500	15	5
0.8	9	1.0	50	0.7	800	70	10	80	800	20	10
1.1	12	1.1	75	1.0	800	90	10	120	800	20	10
1.2	13	1.4	100	1.4	800	120	10	170	800	30	10
1.5	17	1.7	150	2.0	1,200	150	12	270	1,200	40	15
1.8	20	2.0	200	2.0	1,200	150	12	400	1,200	50	15
1.7	19	2.0	200	2.0	1,200	150	10	350	1,200	70	15
1.7	19	2.0	200	2.0	800	150	10	350	800	70	15
1.4	15	2.0	200	2.0	800	150	10	350	800	70	15
1.3	15	1.4	150	2.0	1,200	150	15	280	1,200	45	12
1.3	15	1.5	180	2.0	1,200	150	15	300	1,200	50	12
1.3	15	1.6	180	2.0	1,200	150	15	280	1,200	55	12
1.3	15	1.6	180	2.0	800	150	15	280	800	55	12
1.2	13	1.6	180	2.0	800	150	10	280	800	55	12
1.6	17	2.2	400	2.2	1,200	175	30	300	1,200	65	15
1.8	20	2.1	280	2.6	1,200	200	15	355	1,200	75	19
1.7	20	2.1	260	2.6	1,200	200	15	340	1,200	75	16

Parkinson's disease, help control epilepsy and reduce symptoms of premenstrual syndrome.

One study found that a group of nurses who took about 100 I.U. of vitamin E a day had 36 percent less risk of heart attack. And there's a possibility that E protects heart attack victims from further injury after the blood clots that triggered their attacks are dissolved. How? A major cause of heart attack and stroke is blood platelet blockage of arteries. But supplements of 400 I.U. a day of vitamin E greatly reduced the chance that platelets would stick to artery walls.

Vitamin E also apparently is involved in maintaining a healthy immune system. In one study of 32 healthy older adults, those who received 800 I.U. of E daily for 30 days—more than 50 times the RDA—showed markedly improved immune response. And other research showed that cervical cancer risk was about one-half lower for women who consumed high levels of vitamin E.

THOSE BUSY B VITAMINS

Not all the excitement in nutritional treatment is on the antioxidant front, however. The B-complex group of nutrients is also gaining a lot of attention.

Folate fights birth defects. One exciting role for this B vitamin is the prevention of neural tube defects. These can lead to spina bifida, a serious birth defect in which the covering of the spinal cord does not close com-

THE ALPHABET SOUP OF NUTRIENT REQUIREMENTS

So the label says the cereal you're eating is providing 100 percent of your RDA for seven important nutrients. Better make that U.S. RDA. Or maybe RDI. Are we confusing you?

The basic measure of daily nutrient intake is the RDA, or Recommended Dietary Allowance. If you take a closer look at that panel on the side of your cereal box, however, you'll see that nutrient amounts are listed as *percentage of U.S. Recommended Daily Allowances (U.S. RDAs)*. Actual RDAs vary according to how old you are, whether you're male or female and if you're pregnant or nursing. So how could one percentage be correct for everyone eating this cereal?

The answer is that it isn't. The U.S. RDAs were developed in 1968 by the Food and Drug Administration to give consumers some information about the nutritional content of the food they buy. But because it would be too awkward to list all the breakdowns by age and sex for each nutrient, the U.S. RDAs were pegged to the *highest* recommendation for any age and sex group (usually a male aged 15 to 18). So the percentage on your cereal box is most likely a percentage of the RDA for a teenaged male: Your own needs could very well be lower.

Following this so far? The RDAs are updated periodically to reflect new findings: Since 1974 they were changed twice, in 1980 and 1989. Logically, you'd think that the U.S. RDAs would have changed as well, to reflect the new values.

pletely, and anencephaly, where much of the brain is missing. When 81 Cuban women who had previously had children with neural tube defects (and hence were statistically more likely to have another child with the problem) were given five milligrams of folate daily from a month before conception to ten weeks after, *none* of them had babies with neural tube defects.

Large doses of folate may also help brighten the day for people with clinically diagnosed depression. Forty-one of 123 patients at an English hospital who were diagnosed with either major depression or schizophrenia were found to have some degree of folate deficiency. Twenty-two of the 41 were given a daily dose of 15 milligrams of a form of folate (the RDA for men is 200 *micrograms,* or 0.2 milligrams) and the other 19 were given blank pills. Over six months, the group supplemented with folate showed much greater improvement than the group without folate. (The patients were all receiving standard drug treatment as well.)

Some parts of the body may need more folate than others, according to Douglas C. Heimburger, M.D., of the Departments of Nutrition Sciences and Medicine at the University of Alabama at Birmingham. The result can

Wrong. The U.S. RDAs were never changed, presumably because of the amount of relabeling of products that would be required. So at least up until 1992, if your cereal box said that a serving supplied 10 percent of the U.S. RDA of protein, what it actually meant was that it supplied 10 percent of the amount of protein scientists thought a teenaged boy needed in 1968.

But in 1990, the Food and Drug Administration proposed replacing the U.S. RDAs with something called the Reference Daily Intake (RDI). Instead of being based on the highest possible need for any group, the RDIs would be based on an *average* of the needs of adults and children over the age of three. In most cases, the RDI would be lower than the previous U.S. RDAs. Many nutritionists didn't like the idea of the change, however, and wanted to stick with the old U.S. RDAs.

By the time you read this book, this issue may have been resolved one way or another: You'll either still be facing the U.S. RDA on the side panel of your cereal box, or you'll be looking at new RDI figures.

All this doesn't mean that the figures on your food labels are useless—only that they should only be used as a guideline, never an absolute. They provide a valuable tool for comparing one processed food to another. If you want to know *specifically* how much of each nutrient is recommended for your age group and sex, check the RDA table on page 52.

be a localized deficiency in that part of the body even though the folate level in the blood is normal. Such deficiencies can occur in smokers and may be a contributing factor in certain types of cancer, says Dr. Heimburger.

Move over, gelatin. Biotin is a B vitamin you may not have given a second thought to—unless you're troubled by splitting nails. Swiss research has showed that daily doses of biotin strengthen thin, fragile nails. In the study of 32 men and women, nail thickness increased by 25 percent in the group that received 2,500 micrograms of biotin daily for six to nine months. (Although no RDA has been set for biotin, it's estimated that a daily intake of 30 to 100 micrograms is normally adequate.)

"Biotin is absorbed into the bed of the nail, where it may encourage a better, thicker nail to grow," says Richard K. Scher, M.D., head of the Nail Section at Columbia Presbyterian Medical Center in New York City. But he recommends checking with your doctor before trying biotin supplements to cure your brittle nails.

The cholesterol fighter. Niacin has been used since the 1950s to lower cholesterol and triglycerides in the blood. Very huge doses were used at first, but results have been good with amounts ranging from 1,200 to 2,000 milligrams, still far higher than the RDA of 19 milligrams for men aged 25 to 50 (15 milligrams for women). Annoying side effects tended to limit its use, but researchers have found that enclosing the niacin in a wax honeycomb minimizes side effects. "Rapid absorption of the necessary high dose was what caused side effects," says Joseph M. Keenan, M.D., assistant professor and director of geriatric programs of the University of Minnesota in Minneapolis. "But waxed niacin greatly reduces those problems. Now it's the most effective slow-release form of the vitamin known."

A boost for your immune system. Supplements of B_6 can improve immunity in the elderly. In a study of eight healthy elderly adults at the U.S. Department of Agriculture's (USDA) Human Nutrition Research Center on Aging at Tufts University in Boston, the amounts of B_6 to correct immune impairments in most people were more than the RDA.

The RDA may be low for older Americans, particularly women, say USDA researchers. In another study they measured B_6 levels of 12 people aged 61 to 71 and found that women had to take in 1.9 milligrams a day to have enough B_6 in their bodies (the RDA is only 1.6 milligrams). For men, the RDA of 2.0 milligrams a day proved adequate—but might not be enough for people who are ill or who have increased needs.

TWO MORE VERSATILE VITAMINS

Researchers are also finding new uses for old standbys—in this case vitamins A and K.

A way to save lives. The death rate among hospitalized children suffering from measles drops substantially when they are supplemented with vitamin A. One study found that only about 2 percent of children with severe measles who received vitamin A died, compared with 10 percent of children receiving a blank pill. "Vitamin A status is one of the primary determinants affecting the virulence of measles," says Greg Hussey, senior specialist in the Department of Pediatrics and Child Health at the University of Cape Town in South Africa. "Our recommendation is that vitamin A be given as part of standard therapy to all children with measles in a hospital setting."

And a vitamin A–derived drug called tretinoin appears to help age cancer cells and hasten their demise. Nine of ten people with leukemia experienced complete remission when treated with tretinoin. When tretinoin was combined with chemotherapy, no patients relapsed. "This unique mechanism has broad implications for other types of cancer," says Raymond Warrell, Jr., M.D., at the Memorial Sloan-Kettering Cancer Center in New York City.

Extra help for bones. Vitamin K, which is involved in the formation and maintenance of bone, may also have a role in preventing and treating osteoporosis. Postmenopausal women who received vitamin K supplements showed much less loss of calcium in the urine, suggesting their bone mass was being depleted at a reduced rate. "This has implications for the RDA," says Cees Vermeer, Ph.D., of the Department of Biochemistry at the University of Limburg in the Netherlands. "We have to carefully re-examine this figure. We will probably find that the real need is much higher."

MORE BENEFITS FROM MINERALS

Minerals, too, are proving helpful in exciting new ways, often in amounts that challenge traditional thinking about RDAs.

Calcium to ease PMS. We've long known of calcium's role in building and maintaining strong bones and preventing osteoporosis, but this mineral appears to have significant other jobs as well. Strong evidence supporting calcium's role in curtailing symptoms of menstrual discomfort came from a 5½-month, live-in study by the USDA involving ten women who alternately received daily doses of either 1,300 or 600 milligrams of calcium. (The RDA for women aged 25 to 50 is 800 milligrams.) When women received the higher dosage, they reported fewer mood swings, cramps and back aches; when these same women received less calcium, they had more problems with work efficiency and concentration.

Hiking HDLs with chromium. Beta-blocking drugs are used to treat angina, hypertension and cardiac arrhythmias, but the beta-blockers can cause an undesirable drop in levels of high-density lipoprotein, or HDL, (good) cholesterol. Chromium, however, can *increase* HDL levels in people receiving beta-blockers, according to a North Carolina study of 63 men.

HIGH DOSES MAY BE HAZARDOUS

While in most cases it's difficult to overdose on vitamins and minerals in foods, you *can* overdose on supplements—with serious or even fatal consequences. Here are some areas of potential concern.

Vitamin A. Amounts even a few times greater than the RDA can be toxic, according to Jack Zeev Yetiv, M.D., Ph.D., author of *Popular Nutritional Practices: A Scientific Appraisal.* (And this is one nutrient you can overdose on from food, by eating large amounts of liver.) Effects can range from headache, vomiting, weakness and dry, rough skin to more serious problems such as liver damage, increased pressure in the brain, and bone and joint pain and damage. Toxicity is usually seen only with over 50,000 I.U. in adults and 20,000 I.U. in children, but how you react to high doses of vitamin A can depend on your health in general and particularly the health of your liver.

If you're taking A supplements, stop *immediately* if you have any symptoms such as nagging headaches, blurry vision, hair loss, nausea or aching bones, according to Sheldon Saul Hendler, M.D., Ph.D., assistant clinical professor of medicine at the University of California at San Diego and author of *The Doctors' Vitamin and Mineral Encyclo-*

One group received 600 micrograms of chromium daily—the estimated adequate daily intake is 50 to 200 micrograms—while the other group received look-alike pills with no chromium. The chromium-supplemented group showed significant increases in HDL levels.

Saving eyesight with zinc. A study of 151 patients with macular degeneration, a common eye problem that causes blindness, found that patients receiving 100 milligrams of zinc twice a day with their meals lost less of their vision than patients who received pills with no zinc. (The RDA is 12 milligrams for men and 15 milligrams for women.)

A WORD TO THE WISE

Enthused by all these studies, you may feel the urge to rush out and begin stocking up on vitamin and mineral supplements. Hold it right there. You should realize that all these studies were carefully controlled, and the people taking supplements were meticulously monitored. While some nutrients can generally be safely consumed in doses higher than the RDAs, there are others that are dangerous when taken in excess. On the other hand, certain conditions or drugs can affect your vitamin and mineral status and mean that you need *more* of certain nutrients. For these reasons, you

pedia. It's safer to consume beta-carotene instead, preferably in food, because studies have shown that it's not toxic, even in large amounts.

Vitamin D. This nutrient can be toxic in large doses, particularly for young children. It can cause high levels of calcium in the blood and excess calcium in the urine, deposits of calcium in soft tissues and kidney and cardiovascular damage. A dose as low as 45 micrograms (1,800 I.U.) per day has caused problems in children.

Niacin. Overdosing on niacin may cause flushing, headache and itching—or more serious problems such as heartbeat abnormalities, low blood pressure, liver damage and aggravation of peptic ulcers. Niacin also tends to increase blood sugar levels, which may cause problems for people with diabetes.

Vitamin B_6. Megadoses of 2,000 to 6,000 milligrams per day have caused nerve damage. You should stop taking supplemental B_6 if you have symptoms such as numb hands or feet or unsteadiness while walking.

Iron. This mineral can poison children who take adult supplements formulated for adults.

should always consult your doctor before considering supplementation at levels above the RDA.

And certainly don't think that practicing superb nutrition or taking preventive supplements will protect you against all ills or make up for other unhealthy lifestyle habits. "A nutrient is not a magic bullet," says Dr. Garewal. If you smoke cigarettes, for example, taking beta-carotene isn't the primary line of defense against disease, he says—stopping smoking is the more important change.

CHAPTER 5

NUTRIENT ROBBERS

YOU CAN GUARD AGAINST THEM

As you go unsuspectingly about your daily life, a stealthy band of thieving hoods is stalking you. And when they strike—deliberately or inadvertently—they'll inevitably deprive you of something valuable. We're talking about the nutrient robbers.

Sometimes they masquerade as a friend, such as aspirin, yet cat burgle with deliberate precision, snatching a single vital vitamin. Other times, such as when you're in the kitchen cooking, they loot and pillage indiscriminately, stealing varieties of nutrients. Often, as is the case with pollutants, they take from you the very key you need to lock your doors, latch your windows and protect yourself from their onslaught.

You're not defenseless against the nutrient robbers. You just have to know when they strike and what they're after.

SMOG ALERT

Coal, oil, shale, gasoline, diesel fuel—we depend on them for energy, transportation and light. "By far, cars are the dirtiest of the lot," says Daniel B. Menzel, Ph.D., chairman of the Department of Community and Environmental Medicine at the University of California at Irvine. As we tool down the road, nitrogen oxide and a little bit of unburned fuel dumps out of the tailpipe. Radiated by light, especially that from the ultraviolet spectrum, the mixture turns into nitrogen dioxide and ozone.

These potent poisons, Dr. Menzel says, are free radicals, meaning they have an extra electron attached to their molecular structure. Once free radicals get inside the body, they wreak havoc, initiating a chain reaction of damaged cells.

Nitrogen dioxide, the most common pollutant and the one found in the highest concentration, rapidly oxidizes vitamin C, Dr. Menzel says. Ozone seems to aim its destruction at fatty acids in cell membranes, where vitamin E is located. Both nutrients give themselves up to neutralize the free radicals so that body tissues either are saved or not injured as much.

So what should you do if you're regularly exposed to high levels of air pollution?

Replace what's been stolen. "Take some vitamin C, and take some vitamin E," says Dr. Menzel.

No one knows how much of the vitamins should be taken for best protection against pollution, he says. Studies he has conducted on animals suggest that adults should be taking between 150 and 200 international units (I.U.) of vitamin E every day. Compare that to the Recommended Dietary Allowance (RDA) of 15 I.U. for men and 12 I.U. for women.

As for vitamin C, while the government recommends ingesting 60 milligrams a day, Dr. Menzel personally feels that several hundred milligrams would be closer to reality, for better protection against pollution. You should check with your doctor, however, before taking any nutritional supplement at levels in excess of the RDA.

How Heat Can Deplete

If you really want to cook your goose nutritionally, turn the heat way up and let it bake for a long, long time.

That's the recipe for nutrient immolation. The higher the temperature and the longer the cooking time, the more you deprive yourself of the vitamins and minerals packed away in food. "Many are inactivated by heat," says Gertrude Armbruster, Ph.D., an associate professor in the Division of Nutritional Sciences at Cornell University in Ithaca, New York. "Heat changes the nature of nutrients so that they're not absorbed as well by the body." And nutrients may also leach out in cooking liquid.

Those emerald green broccoli florets, then, may not be quite the storehouses of vitamin C you believe them to be, depending on how you've cooked them. Anytime food is cooked—no matter what the method—nutrients are lost. Once in the kitchen, though, some cooking methods are more destructive than others. In general, "the less time food is cooked, the more nutritious it is," Dr. Armbruster says.

Of the dry-heat cooking methods, baking and grilling probably have the most negative impact on nutrients, Dr. Armbruster says. "They're long-time processes that expose food to high temperatures." All heat-sensitive nutrients—vitamin C, for example, some of the B vitamins, and possibly minerals—are vulnerable under those conditions. Broiling also subjects food to high heat, she says, "but it's a shorter cooking time, so it may not be as destructive."

Don't bake foods to a crisp. People often bake, broil and grill to brown food or make it crispy. While perhaps more appealing to the eyes and the palate, crispy brown food is less nutritious, according to Dr. Armbruster. "The browning process transforms protein in meat," she says. "It's effectively 'burned' and not absorbed as well as unburned protein."

Use wet heat wisely. Wet-heat cooking methods can be just as destructive to vitamins and minerals as baking and grilling. "In addition to the high heat, now you're adding water, which is another source of loss for all the water-soluble nutrients," Dr. Armbruster says.

Generally, pressure cooking preserves more nutrients in vegetables that otherwise would require a longer cooking time. Steaming, a wonderful no-fat alternative to frying, spares more vitamins and minerals than pressure cooking or boiling, but losses do occur.

When steamed, spinach, for example, loses almost 50 percent of its vitamin C, the most vulnerable of all vitamins. But boiling or pressure cooking destroys 60 percent. Broccoli loses about 55 percent of its vitamin C when boiled but only about 25 percent when steamed.

The B vitamin family is more thermally insulated. In most vegetables, niacin barely is affected by any cooking method. Thiamine, riboflavin, vitamin B_6 and folate are lost in smaller amounts when foods are steamed than when they are boiled.

Minerals in vegetables are especially susceptible. Even steaming can decrease availability of the potassium and calcium in spinach by half or more. Half of the iron and magnesium may be made unavailable, while the loss of zinc is about 30 percent. Boiling and draining remove even higher percentages of those minerals.

Perhaps the ultimate way to preserve nutrients is to eat vegetables raw in salads, Dr. Armbruster says. When that's not practical or desirable, steam them just until soft or boil them in as little water as possible. And make sure the water is boiling before you add the food.

Save that cooking liquid. When you steam carrots, do you pour the remaining orangish water down the sink? If you do, you're dumping cancer-combating carotenoids into the sewer system. After boiling potatoes, do you discard the broth? You're permitting valuable vitamin C to drip down the drain.

No matter how unappetizing it may initially look, use the nutrient-rich cooking water in other preparations. "There wouldn't really be significant

WAVE BYE-BYE TO COOKING LOSSES

Conventional stoves can drive off vitamins in droves. What's a health-conscious cook to do? Ride the microwave to the nutritional future.

"In some cases, you can get close to 100 percent nutrient retention with a microwave," according to Gertrude Armbruster, Ph.D., of Cornell University in Ithaca, New York. "It really minimizes nutrient losses."

Microwaves target water molecules in food, forcing them to vibrate and give off heat, which then cooks the food. "The energy gets to where it's supposed to go," Dr. Armbruster says. But when you cook on the stove, you're heating a lot more than you need to, and it takes a long time.

"Only 40 to 60 percent of the vitamins remain in vegetables cooked conventionally on the stove. Microwave cooking preserves significantly more, up to 50 to 100 percent. It makes a big difference."

losses if you keep that water," Dr. Armbruster says. "Although we recommend that, I'm told hardly anyone does it." The liquid can be used in soups, beverages, gravies and sauces.

STRESS: A NUTRITIONAL MESS

If you haven't stewed and steamed off your vitamins and minerals on the stovetop, you may once they enter your body. The frantic, frustrating exasperation of stress can rob you of nutrients at the same time it's increasing the need for them. "I wish we knew specifically how stress increases free-radical generation in the body, but there's evidence it does," says John Milner, Ph.D., head of the Department of Nutrition at Pennsylvania State University in University Park. The mental strain forces the body to secrete more hormones that speed up metabolism and the turnover of cells, he says. Fats also are altered and begin to turn rancid. Here's how to fight back.

Stick to a regular meal plan. Stress may send you to the refrigerator to soothe savaged nerves, so overeating could be a concern, Dr. Milner says. But under mental duress you also may skip meals or grab quick bites on the run. So in addition to worrying about whatever it is you're worrying about, you also must worry about maintaining your regular eating routine.

Fortify yourself with E, C and beta-carotene. To counteract any free radicals formed by stress, meals should provide adequate amounts of the antioxidant vitamins A, E and C, Dr. Milner says. "During stressful situations, the antioxidants serve as scavengers for free radicals generated in the body," he says.

Bounce back after trauma. Physiologic stress is an even greater danger to nutritional well-being. "The body's response to serious injury, complicated surgery or chronic inflammation such as rheumatoid arthritis creates a significant drain on energy and protein stores," says Joel B. Mason, M.D., an assistant professor in the divisions of clinical nutrition and gastroenterology at Tufts University School of Medicine in Boston. "It is not uncommon for a serious bodily injury to result in a loss of ten pounds of muscle and other critical organ tissues within a week; such a drain is not only harmful by itself but makes it considerably more difficult for the body to recover from the complications associated with the injury or disease.

"A common misconception, even among doctors, is that overweight patients have plenty of 'excess stores' to draw from and are therefore immune to the adverse nutritional effects associated with physiologic stress," says Dr. Mason. It is very important for anyone who has sustained a serious physiologic stress, regardless of whether or not they are overweight, to receive the additional calories and protein demanded by their condition.

Similarly, a person who has lost more than 10 percent of usual body weight due to disease and who is anticipating surgery will benefit from an aggressive attempt to correct some of the malnourishment before surgery. Adequate nutrient stores will improve the chances of a successful outcome. A well-trained dietitian can provide guidelines.

SOME HEALERS ARE STEALERS

What's worse—high blood pressure or impotence? Arthritis pain or anemia?

Many commonly used over-the-counter and prescription drugs can profoundly affect your nutrient needs. Some accelerate excretion of vitamins and minerals; others impede absorption. But if you understand how certain drugs interact with nutrients, you need not face damned-if-you-do-damned-if-you-don't alternatives.

ASPIRIN

Aspirin can ease pain and may even play a role in decreasing the chances of heart disease, Dr. Milner says. But if you're taking aspirin regularly, you may want to call your citrus supplier. That's because prolonged or excessive use forces the kidneys to excrete more vitamin C and potassium. In addition to depleting the body of those nutrients, you run the risk of developing iron-deficiency anemia, because aspirin can irritate the stomach lining and cause minor bleeding.

Aspirin also displaces folate in the body, and that could create a deficiency in those with poor diets, according to John Pinto, Ph.D., director of the

Nutrition Research Laboratory at Memorial Sloan-Kettering Cancer Center in New York City. "Arthritic individuals who take a lot of aspirin should be especially cautious," he says.

To counter depletion: Eat foods high in vitamin C, iron and folate.

LAXATIVES

Mineral oil, that old constipation cure, is a nutritional damnation in disguise. A lot of older people remain regular users of this regularity regulator, which also still is found in many commercial preparations, according to Arthur I. Jacknowitz, Pharm.D., chairman of the Department of Clinical Pharmacy in the School of Pharmacy at West Virginia University in Morgantown. Three other ingredients commonly found in laxatives—bisacodyl, phenolphthalein and senna—also can cause severe deficiencies in frequent users.

After ingesting laxatives containing any of these substances, among the

HIGH FIBER: AN EXTRA CHALLENGE

We know how fiber helps us. The natural laxative eases food through the body and reduces the possibility of colon and intestinal diseases. It also helps lower blood sugar levels in people with diabetes. But by rushing food through the system, fiber also cuts into the time the body needs to absorb nutrients.

"Especially at the extremes of life, for the very young and the old, fiber may create problems by interfering with absorption," says Benjamin Caballero, M.D., director of the Center for Human Nutrition at Johns Hopkins University in Baltimore.

The most significant interference is with calcium, needed in greater amounts by growing children and women to prevent later development of osteoporosis. "If you're just barely fulfilling the recommended calcium intake, a high-fiber diet will certainly affect calcium status," he says. "And it's not easy anyway to get all the calcium you need from foods. Women need at least 800 milligrams of calcium a day to prevent osteoporosis and probably should be taking supplements if they eat a lot of high-fiber foods."

Fiber also promotes excretion of vitamin B_6 and, at extremely high doses, causes out-and-out deficiencies of zinc, even if the diet contains adequate amounts of the mineral. But most healthy adults who eat well-balanced diets have little cause for concern, Dr. Caballero says. "The typical American diet has generous amounts of most nutrients and the fact that fiber decreases the efficiency of absorption probably has little relevance for healthy adults consuming a variety of foods."

things passing through your intestines more quickly will be all the fat-soluble vitamins—A, E, D and K—as well as phosphorus and calcium. Mineral oil traps fat-soluble vitamins and prevents their absorption, Dr. Jacknowitz says; the other drugs force the intestines to contract involuntarily, speeding food through too rapidly for proper absorption.

To counter depletion: Don't use mineral-oil laxatives frequently. Don't take a laxative containing any of the other three medications within two hours of any meal.

DIURETICS

What some laxatives do to fat-soluble vitamins, diuretics and other high blood pressure drugs do to their water-soluble counterparts—flush them from your system. "If you are well nourished, you shouldn't see appreciable vitamin deficiencies with diuretics," Dr. Pinto says, "but you could have a definite problem if you aren't or if your diet is at all marginal."

MAKING MEDICINE MORE EFFECTIVE

Some medications can cause significant disruptions in the body's vitamin and mineral balance. Conversely, some foods can interfere with the effectiveness of drugs. But the two aren't always antagonists. In fact, depending on what you eat and when you eat it, food sometimes can enhance the power of medications to make you feel better faster.

Generally, when a doctor instructs you to take your medicine with food, eat a meal high in carbohydrates, says John Pinto, Ph.D., of Memorial Sloan-Kettering Cancer Center in New York City. A high-carbohydrate meal will help the drug get into your system more quickly. A high-protein meal will reduce the effectiveness of the medication.

For example, in a study of children with asthma who were taking theophylline, Dr. Pinto says, bouts of wheezing were reduced when a high-carbohydrate (78 percent of calories from carbs), low-protein diet was eaten. The drug's power to control wheezing diminished when the kids began to eat high-protein, low-carbohydrate meals.

A low-protein diet also helps people with Parkinson's disease who are being treated with levodopa. The amino acids in protein compete with the drug for entry into the brain, Dr. Pinto says.

For treatment of urinary tract infections with the drug methenamine, therapy is much more effective if people increase the acidity of their urine by eating or drinking foods high in vitamin C—citrus juice, strawberries or broccoli, for example—two hours before taking the drug, Dr. Pinto says.

Potassium and magnesium are lost quickly through use of diuretics. Some medications, such as furosemide (sold under the brand name Lasix) and hydrochlorothiazide (sold as Esidrix) also speed the excretion of zinc, calcium and thiamine, Dr. Pinto says. Thiamine depletion alone caused by use of these drugs could cause cardiovascular problems. Regular use of diuretics also can elevate blood sugar levels by disrupting enzymes necessary for carbohydrate metabolism. Hydralazine, another high blood pressure medication, disrupts vitamin B_6 absorption, which could cause nerve and sensation problems in your arms and legs.

To counter depletion: Take the medication with meals and eat foods high in potassium (such as bananas and raisins) and thiamine (such as pork and whole-grain bread). Zinc, magnesium and vitamin B_6 supplements also may be required.

ANTIBIOTICS

Antibiotics and antibacterial drugs, used for everything from small cuts to major infections, impinge on the body's absorption of calcium, Dr. Pinto says. Excretion of riboflavin in urine increases as well with tetracycline. Magnesium, zinc and iron also are poorly utilized with this drug, and vitamin K and folate can be depleted. Neomycin blocks vitamin B_{12} absorption.

To counter depletion: Take antibiotics and antibacterial drugs on an empty stomach several hours before or after eating mineral-rich foods or dairy products.

ANTIDEPRESSANTS

Tricyclic compounds like chlorpromazine used to treat depression can devastate the body's stores of riboflavin, according to Dr. Pinto. In one study, urinary excretion of riboflavin rose markedly soon after treatment with chlorpromazine and continued for several days after drug use ceased. "A clinically significant riboflavin deficiency may result from the use of these agents," Dr. Pinto says, "despite a diet adequate in the vitamin."

To counter depletion: Eat foods rich in riboflavin, such as low-fat milk and yogurt, liver, broccoli and asparagus.

ANTACIDS

Plop, plop, fizz, fizz, oh, what a nutritional nuisance it is. If you can't believe you ate the whole thing, you won't believe the possible complications of your antacid cure for indigestion and heartburn. Over-the-counter antacids with ingredients such as aluminum hydroxide, sodium bicarbonate and magnesium trisilicate deprive the body of phosphorus. Mild phosphate depletion weakens muscles, and a more serious lack leads to a vitamin D deficiency. Extended use or high doses of antacids also destroys thiamine and skews absorption of the fat-soluble vitamins, particularly vitamin A. Iron absorption also is impeded.

To counter depletion: Don't eat the whole thing. Try to rely less on antacids, or take them only under your doctor's supervision.

WHEN NUTRIENTS COLLIDE

Vitamin E helps vitamin A, but too much E harms A. Too much zinc tarnishes iron; too much iron puts a chink in zinc. Too much protein muscles calcium out of the body, so you drink more milk to replenish your calcium stores. But milk is high in protein, which . . .

"What a bag of worms," sighs John Milner, Ph.D., of Pennsylvania State University in University Park when talking about how more of one nutrient can promote the body's use of another at the same time it creates a deficiency in still another.

Take vitamin C, for example. But not too much. Vitamin C aids the body in utilizing iron, especially as you age and stomach acidity decreases. But excessive levels of C inhibit absorption of copper. "And when you're talking copper, you're also talking about iron and zinc, because they're all interconnected," Dr. Milner says. "Excesses or deficiencies of one invariably lead to problems with the other two."

Here's a quick rundown of how some key nutrients may be affected by the status of another.

Vitamin A. Too little protein in the diet lessens absorption of vitamin A. Fat in the diet helps the body absorb beta-carotene, the vitamin A precursor. Except if it's polyunsaturated fat; that limits beta-carotene absorption. Vitamin E supplements raise blood levels of A in those with deficiencies of A, but too much E can decrease the amount of A in the blood.

Calcium. Some proteins may increase absorption but at the same time increase excretion of this bone-building mineral. Fat, so useful in

CHOLESTEROL-LOWERING DRUGS

Cholesterol-reducing medications, such as cholestyramine, don't sound like a lot of fun. They cause belching, bloating, flatulence and constipation, among other side effects. But because they work by interfering with fat absorption, they also interfere with the absorption of fat-soluble vitamins A, D, E and K. Deficiencies of folate also may result.

To counter depletion: Ask your doctor about water-soluble vitamin A and D supplements and about the need for supplementary vitamin K and folate.

WATCH OUT FOR THE ANTINUTRIENTS

They've been targeted as the bad guys, antinutrient chemicals in some otherwise exceedingly healthful plant foods that can rip you off nutritionally. But oxalate, phytin and tannins, while they deserve their nasty reputations, aren't as bad as once thought.

helping the body absorb beta-carotene, decreases calcium absorption. If calcium intake is low, zinc supplements slow calcium absorption, causing an even greater deficiency. But no effect is seen if calcium levels are normal. Salty diets also cause an increase in calcium excretion.

Vitamin B_6. Too much protein leads to more excretion of B_6 and lower levels of the vitamin in the blood.

Iron. Zinc supplements decrease iron absorption, and in a combined zinc/iron pill, the higher the ratio of zinc, the lower the utilization of iron.

Zinc. Virtually no zinc is absorbed from mineral supplements with high concentrations of iron. But heme iron, from animal foods, doesn't deter zinc absorption. However, nonheme iron, from plants, can interfere with zinc absorption. Calcium also inhibits zinc absorption. Animal protein helps the body use zinc, but unsupplemented soy protein causes a deficiency.

Confused? It's no wonder. But you really face no more of a disadvantage than the experts, who also have to sift through this nutritional morass. "I suppose what this shows is that you can't be overzealous with any of these nutrients, because what enhances one area may inhibit another," Dr. Milner says. "And it underlines the importance of a varied type of diet. By eating a wide variety of foods, you minimize the risk of imbalances and give yourself a greater chance of meeting *all* your nutrient needs."

OXALATE

The classic example always has been spinach, high in iron but in a form not absorbed easily by the body. The reason, researchers said, was the chemical oxalate in the plant. But newer studies suggest that all of the iron *naturally* occurring in spinach may, in fact, be available.

Because of how it's grown, spinach can show a misleadingly high iron content when analyzed, says William House, Ph.D., a research physiologist with the U.S. Department of Agriculture's (USDA) Plant, Soil and Nutrition Laboratory at Cornell University. Wind and rain splash spinach leaves with additional iron from the soil in which the plants are grown, Dr. House says. That dirt-derived mineral enters the leaves and drives up the measured iron content. But *that iron* cannot be absorbed by the body.

The assumption all these years was that oxalate in spinach inhibited iron absorption, Dr. House says. But when the USDA researchers grew spinach that didn't contain external iron from soil on its leaves in the laboratory, the plant turned out to be a fine source of iron for the body.

Oxalate, also found in rhubarb, "does appear to affect calcium utilization, though, by creating a calcium salt that's not soluble," says Dr. House.

PHYTIN

A substance that facilitates storage of minerals in seeds also interferes with the body's absorption of at least one of those nutrients, zinc. Phytin is found in almost all plant seeds, Dr. House says, and is especially high in legumes and cereal grains, such as wheat. "If you eat a lot of foods high in phytin, zinc availability will be depressed," he says, "but we don't think it's that important in most situations." People who suddenly switch from an omnivorous to vegetarian diet "may become a little zinc deficient temporarily, but studies do show that vegetarians still get enough zinc."

TANNINS

For people at risk of iron deficiency—menstruating women, young children and adolescents—tannins remain a concern, Dr. House says. These chemicals are found not only in coffee and tea but also in the hulls of some beans and in red wine. Rats fed bean hulls high in tannins show very little impairment of iron absorption, Dr. House says, but when the chemical is extracted and given to the rodents, "they show a small depression of iron absorption that is statistically significant."

Acquiring anemia from ingesting tannins probably isn't a major health concern, Dr. House says, but people should nevertheless try to get adequate iron in their diets.

CHAPTER 6

SPECIAL NUTRIENT NEEDS

FINE-TUNING YOUR INTAKE

So you think you're an average kind of person. Average height, average weight, average number of kids, average number of cars in the driveway. You have an average-looking dog in an average-looking yard, an average-looking cat napping on an averagely stuffed chair.

Well, your life may seem a lot like everyone else's, but there's a good chance your nutrient needs aren't. Your requirement for vitamins and minerals can change, depending on your personal habits, your activity level, even your age. Here's a closer look at some factors that may separate you or someone you know from the nutritional pack.

DIETING

Few dieters follow rational rules of repast as they attempt to lose weight. A significant cutback in calories or a fad diet with an unnatural reliance on one or two foods may hurl your body off its nutrient peak into the depths of deficiency.

"This business of periodically starving for calorie control or drastically reducing calories and not making appropriate adjustments in vitamin intake is risky," according to C. E. Butterworth, Jr., M.D., professor of nutrition sciences at the University of Alabama at Birmingham. But if you follow a few guidelines, losing weight doesn't have to be a nutritional bungee jump from a perilous precipice.

Don't void the vitamins. "Quality of the diet remains important," says Mindy Hermann, R.D., a spokesperson for the American Dietetic Association and a nutritional consultant in Mount Kisco, New York. "The main problem arises when a diet falls below 1,200 calories a day or if it's not well planned."

Most weight-loss programs do recommend taking some sort of supplement to meet the Recommended Dietary Allowances (RDAs) while curtailing caloric intake, she says.

The reason is that in cutting calories, "dieters cut the vitamins and minerals associated with those calories," according to Dr. Butterworth. "Unless they take supplements, they run the risk of getting transient vitamin deficiencies. They should be very careful."

Replenish the turnover. Of central concern are all the water-soluble vitamins, especially vitamin C and folate, that have a rapid turnover in the body. You're not getting enough of them because you've cut your meals, but your body continues to excrete them at a pretty good clip. Fat-soluble vitamins like vitamins A and E fade from the body more slowly, so no imminent deficiency danger exists, Dr. Butterworth says. But you still need to replace them over time.

Be nutritiously dense. In her classes at East Carolina University in Greenville, North Carolina, Kathryn Kolasa, Ph.D., head of the Nutrition Section in the Department of Family Medicine, likes to display a slide of a 450-pound woman. "The woman almost died of malnutrition," Dr. Kolasa says. "It always strikes people as odd to hear that, but it's true."

The slide-show subject was deficient in the whole array of vitamins and minerals as well as protein. What did she eat that caused malnutrition? Biscuits, snack crackers and other high-fat foods that are not nutrient-dense, Dr. Kolasa recalls. "She ate a lot of fatty meats and didn't eat vegetables."

The success of a weight-loss plan—to lose the flab forever and to remain healthy from a nutritional standpoint—depends on a diet teeming with nutrient-dense dishes—foods high in vitamins and minerals but relatively low in calories and fat. Examples include low-fat dairy products, whole-grain breads and cereals, beans, fruits and dark green vegetables.

Spice your life with variety. The days of single-food fad diets—eat nothing but grapefruit and lose pounds fast, for example—have fallen by the wayside. Which is good, because that's where they belong—in a ditch. An unnatural preponderance of a single food can easily create deficiencies of nutrients lacking in that food. "Whenever you do that," Dr. Butterworth says, "you're inevitably going to miss something you'd get in a mixed, varied diet of fruits and vegetables."

SMOKING

Smokers hit themselves with a nutritional double whammy, for compared to their cigarette-free peers, they typically ingest fewer of the very vitamins that nicotine destroys in their bodies.

Because of their habit and their diets, smokers may need more—but generally consume less—beta-carotene and vitamin C, the antioxidants that may provide some protection against smoke's cancerous effects, according to Linda C. Harlan, Ph.D., a National Cancer Institute researcher and coauthor of a study that examined the dietary habits of more than 11,000 smokers and nonsmokers.

Rise above the C-level. The most pronounced nutritional difference between smokers and nonsmokers is in vitamin C. Tobacco-users' bodies process C at a higher rate, either because smoke destroys it or because it is expended to counteract the carcinogens in smoke. While puffers seem to meet the RDA for C in their diets, "this level may not be high enough to counteract the increased vitamin C turnover resulting from their smoking habit," Dr. Harlan's study concluded.

And that's too bad, because not only does vitamin C help prevent carcinogens from forming and fight certain ones that do manifest themselves, it enhances the ability of vitamin E to combat cancer-causing agents—a two-pronged dose of protection.

In addition to the antioxidants, smokers also have a greater need for folate and vitamin B_{12}, according to Dr. Butterworth. Folate, essential for proper lung function, is damaged by smoke, he says.

Don't let meals go up in smoke. Blatantly bad eating habits compound smokers' nutritional nightmares. Compared to nonsmokers, they generally eat less, skip breakfast more, consume fewer nutritional supplements and drink more coffee and alcohol. They eat less poultry and fish, drink less skim milk and rely more heavily on luncheon meats.

As a result, they're shortchanging themselves even more on essential nutrients, such as beta-carotene, which has anti-cancer properties. "Our results," Dr. Harlan reports, "show that smokers, who may gain some protection from lung cancer by high carotenoid intake, are less likely than nonsmokers to be consuming carotenoid-dense food," such as yellow, orange and dark green leafy vegetables.

Get juiced up. Smokers' eating habits may change because tobacco can alter their predilections for certain foods. "It changes taste preferences," Dr. Harlan says. "Smokers don't, for example, like fruit and juices," all high in vitamin C. They generally don't like sweet things, and fruits tend to be sweet. If you find your sweet tooth souring a little, make it a special point to drink some juice at breakfast or as a thirst quencher at other times during the day.

Drinking

Alcohol does to drinkers what cigarettes do to smokers: It robs them of vitamins and minerals. And the poor dietary habits common in a booze-based lifestyle are likely to compound the damage.

"Drinking does destroy some nutrients," says Charles H. Halsted, M.D., professor of medicine and chief of the Division of Clinical Nutrition and Metabolism at the University of California, Davis, School of Medicine. It also interferes with the absorption of vitamins and minerals, he says.

Be careful with the B vitamins. Moderate and heavy drinkers typically suffer from deficiencies of three major nutrients—folate, which is important for blood formation and digestion; thiamine, which plays a significant role in brain and neurological function; and vitamin B_6, which also helps form healthy blood.

A thiamine deficiency is especially insidious because it could cause brain damage even before physical signs appear, some researchers assert. Diets fortified with thiamine and supplements can reverse the damage in its early stage, but once the harm advances, they don't have much effect.

Blood levels of riboflavin and C, as well as zinc, phosphate and magnesium, also may be depleted in moderate drinkers. Excessive consumers of

Keep the Beast in the Bottle with Good Nutrition

Recovering alcoholics are less likely to fall off the wagon if their carts are loaded with vitamin-rich vegetables and other complex carbohydrates, and unburdened of sugar and caffeine.

When the traditional Alcoholics Anonymous 12-step recovery program is supplemented with nutritional therapy that homes in on good eating practices, participants are more likely to resist the temptation to revert to the rye, according to researchers at Bowling Green State University in Ohio.

Two groups of new AA members were studied—one following the conventional 12-step program only, the other adding to that a comprehensive nutrition program that included menu planning, individualized nutrition counseling, weight management, shopping, label-reading and dining-out tips. They were put on a diet of high-complex-carbohydrate, low-sugar, no-caffeine meals. Vegetables, beans, grains and whole cereals all are high in complex carbohydrates.

"We just had them follow normal dietary guidelines," says Elsa A. McMullen, Ph.D., a professor in the Department of Applied Human Ecology at Bowling Green State University. "We made sure they were eating foods high in fiber and low in simple sugars. And we made sure

alcohol, who are at risk from liver disease, may also ail from a "substantial" lack of vitamin A, according to Dr. Halsted.

Eat—don't drink—your meals. Alcohol essentially is a high-calorie, high-carbohydrate substance—"liquid bread is what some people call it," Dr. Kolasa says. But this is a barren loaf, for alcohol is almost devoid of vitamins and minerals.

In addition to what they guzzle from the bottle, drinkers may or may not consume an adequate number of nutrient-dense calories from food to make up for the vitamins and minerals destroyed by alcohol. If they don't eat right, "tying one on" could refer to the nutritional noose they're slipping over their heads. Dr. Kolasa says, "If there are problems, it often is because of how drinkers have changed their diets, or rather how they've *let* their diets change."

Know your limit—and stop well short. Although not generally recommended, nonpregnant women probably can have up to three drinks a day and men up to six (a drink being defined as 12 ounces of beer or one shot of liquor) without risk of developing liver disease, provided their diets otherwise are nourishing, Dr. Halsted says. "Beyond that amount, risks for nutrient deficiencies and alcohol-related diseases increase, and they're set-

they ate those kinds of foods for snacks and desserts, too."

Four months into the programs, members of the nutrition therapy group reported no alcohol intake, less craving for a drink and less sugar consumption than those in the traditional group. Desire for alcohol seemed to relate directly to eating sugar: The cravings for alcohol decreased from 80 percent before treatment to only 17 percent among the newly nutritionally conscious, while cravings in the standard group actually increased, from 50 to 80 percent. The reduction in the ache for alcohol also seemed to be correlated to replenishing the body's supply of thiamine (vitamin B_1) and folate.

Diets lacking in nutrients but high in sugar and caffeine may stimulate a thirst for alcohol, the Bowling Green researchers theorize. And they point to other tests in which thiamine-deprived animals increased their drinking of alcohol. Diets lacking in the amino acid tryptophan, whose levels in the brain can be regulated by upping complex carbohydrate consumption, diminish the body's supply of serotonin, a brain neurotransmitter. Low levels of serotonin frequently are found within the brains of alcoholics.

ting themselves up for problems." Pregnant women should not drink at all, because we do not know the minimum level of alcohol consumption that is safe for the developing fetus.

EXERCISING

So you don't smoke. You don't drink. You don't chew tobacco, and you don't linger longer at the candy counter than you do in the produce section. In fact, you exercise. You walk, jog, bounce about in aerobics classes and lift weights. Supremely healthy and no chance of a dietary shortfall, right?

Actually, for a couple of reasons, physically active people have greater nutrient demands than their sedentary, couch-bound counterparts, according to John Milner, Ph.D., head of the Department of Nutrition at Pennsylvania State University in University Park. Whether it's walking or weight lifting, exercise stimulates the metabolism, burning calories and enhancing the turnover of nutrients. It also contributes to the generation inside your body of destructive, ravenous oxygen molecules.

Get enough food to burn. "If you don't consume enough food and you exercise, you'll end up in a malnourished state," Dr. Milner says. The body will burn not only food and fat but muscle, too. It'll begin to feed on itself to provide the energy you demand. Complex carbohydrates from breads, grains and vegetables can provide the fuel required to get you through your workouts.

But don't curb protein intake for those additional carbohydrates, Dr. Milner warns, for "there might really be a problem." You need more protein to maintain the lean muscle mass you have and to grow more muscle. "If you're physically active, protein is required in a little higher quantity than you typically take in for muscle maintenance and repair." And to properly metabolize the amino acids in protein, to break them down and make them available for use by the body, you need additional vitamin B_6, Dr. Milner says.

Calm free radicals with antioxidants. Every time you take a breath, a small portion of the oxygen generates highly unstable molecules, called free radicals. Free radicals can attack certain vital components in your body, damaging cells and turning fats rancid. The more you breathe, the more free radicals you generate. Huffing and puffing exercisers process much more oxygen and generate many more free radicals than your average couch potato. They also suck in more air pollutants with each breath, which gives birth to even more reactive molecules.

And if that isn't enough to make you rip up your gym membership card and stash your StairMaster in the attic, consider this: When you work out, blood is redirected to the working muscles at the expense of other organs. Free radicals are generated in these exercising muscles. Once the workout is over and oxygen-rich blood returns to the deprived organs, still more free radicals are generated.

Before ditching your dumbbells with the thought that you may be healthier if you don't exercise, try taking some antioxidant vitamins. Repeated studies show that beta-carotene, vitamin C and vitamin E protect the body against what's called the oxidative stress of working out.

Two weeks of vitamin E supplementation "significantly decreased" the oxidation of fats seen in people riding stationary bicycles. Another study using vitamin E, vitamin C and beta-carotene reduced oxidation during exercise and at rest.

AVOIDING MEAT

You shun fatty meats, eggs and dairy products. You also eat a lot of low-calorie, high-vitamin vegetables and fruits. And you consume a variety of high-fiber, complex carbohydrate foods. If you are a vegetarian, you may think you're following the perfect prescription for nutritional health. And you are—to a large extent. But especially if you are a vegan, a strictest-of-the-strict vegetarian who doesn't eat eggs or dairy foods, your diet may be lacking a few nutrients you cannot do without.

Don't forget the B_{12}. The most conspicuous concern for a true-blue vegan is vitamin B_{12}, which can be obtained only from animal foods, such as meat or dairy products. The bacteria from some fermented plant products—such as soybean-based tempeh—do produce a form of B_{12}, and it may even be labeled as such on the package. But debate exists over whether that B_{12}-like substance can be absorbed to meet the body's needs; B_{12} in supplement form is the best insurance.

Squeeze metal from a plant. Iron also may be deficient in an otherwise sound vegetarian diet. Meat, fish and poultry contain easily absorbable iron (the heme form), but plants possess a form not so readily utilized (called nonheme iron). In addition, plants contain fiber and chemicals called phytates that may interfere with absorption of the nutrient. Eating iron-fortified cereals might help balance the equation. Vegetarians also should eat more foods containing vitamin C, which facilitates the absorption of nonheme iron from plants.

Zone in on bone. Calcium is another nutrient that may be lacking. Oxalic acid and phytates in plants inhibit absorption of this bone-building mineral. Vegetarians should make a point of buying and eating foods fortified with calcium, such as certain brands of orange juice, Dr. Kolasa says.

PREGNANCY

When you're pregnant, you literally are eating for two—well, maybe one and a half. Requirements for many nutrients increase dramatically, and some more than double, to ensure proper fetal growth and the mother's needs.

Since you're in the expecting mode anyway, you should expect to gain between 25 and 30 pounds, and only a small portion of that, of course, will be your bouncing baby. The key to a healthy pregnancy, Hermann says, is ensuring that those extra calories come from nutrient-dense foods—vegetables, grains and legumes—not from ice cream and pickles or some other fanciful food cravings.

When you multiply, add vitamins. To supplement or not to supplement during pregnancy? "Theoretically, when you're pregnant you can get everything you need just from food," Hermann says. "In practice, it's much different," not just because of food aversions but because the nutrient demand is so great. Many doctors recommend taking multivitamins and multimineral supplements throughout the stages of pregnancy. If you want to take supplements during your pregnancy, however, you should do so only with the consent of your obstetrician.

High doses of one B vitamin, folate, Hermann says, have been shown to reduce incidence of neural tube defects, the most common of all birth defects, in which the baby's spinal cord closes improperly.

Lower risks of birth defects in general have been associated with regular multivitamin supplementation near the time of conception (at least three times a week before conception through at least the first trimester), according to Centers for Disease Control (CDC) researchers. In one study, they found that those women who reported using multivitamins from at least one month prior to conception through the first trimester were 60 percent less likely to give birth to a baby with brain or spinal defects.

In several cases, you have to double up. "The demand for vitamin D doubles," Hermann says, "and folate requirements more than double." Women also need much more vitamin E and C and all the B vitamins for their gestating sons or daughters. Among the minerals, extra calcium is critical. Iron demands double, and more zinc and magnesium are required, she says.

Keep sickness at bay. An aversion to certain foods is "one of the biggest problems during pregnancy," Hermann says. "I know there was not a lot I could eat when I was pregnant. Granted, I may have been in the minority, but nausea and indigestion from certain foods is a constant concern that could lead to deficiencies."

Severe nausea and vomiting during pregnancy apparently can be countered with supplemental doses of vitamin B_6, according to a group of researchers from the Obstetrics and Gynecology Department of the University of Iowa College of Medicine. A 25-milligram B_6 supplement taken every eight hours significantly improved symptoms of severe nausea in a study group of pregnant women but did little to alleviate mild or moderate nausea. B_6 at such high dosage levels should be taken only under a doctor's supervision.

INFANCY

Following birth, you're cradling a well-nourished baby. But the nutritional challenge isn't over yet. "A baby is like a growing puppy," Dr. Butterworth says. "Its nutritional needs are a lot greater and different from an adult's."

NUTRITION FOR NURSING

Even after the additional nutrient demands of pregnancy, a woman's vitamin requirements remain quite high after giving birth if she feeds her baby naturally.

"You still need more of many nutrients," says Kathryn Dewey, Ph.D., a professor in the Department of Nutrition at the University of California, Davis. A lactating woman should consume an extra 500 calories a day to get those nutrients and to compensate for the energy her body expends in producing breast milk.

Five nutrients—calcium, zinc, magnesium, vitamin B_6 and folate—are especially important, Dr. Dewey says, "not just because they're needed in higher amounts but because the diets of American women are particularly low in them." The needs for protein, vitamins A and D and fluids also are quite high during lactation. In fact, the level of vitamin D in breast milk is directly related to the amount of D in the mother's diet. If she eats a D-deficient diet or she is not often exposed to direct sunlight (which stimulates the body's own production of the vitamin), the American Dietetic Association recommends supplementation.

The requirements for vitamins A and D and fluids, however, can be fulfilled if the mother drinks two or three glasses of milk a day in addition to the two glasses a day that are normally recommended, according to Pat Harper, R.D., of the American Dietetic Association.

Make it mother's milk. Complete nutrition for those crying, cuddling, whining, wetting bundles of joy can best be provided by one food: mother's milk. While human and formula milk are comparable in many respects, healthy breast milk does have several nutritional advantages.

Early breast milk contains substances that bolster a baby's immune system to help fight off allergies and infections. Commercial formulas cannot reproduce these early protective effects but are very helpful after the first few weeks. Breast milk also is abundant in choline, a nutrient whose importance may not reveal itself until baby is old and gray. Some animal studies showed that rats exhibited less memory deterioration in later life if, when first born, their diets were high in choline. Infant formulas vary in choline content.

Infants should be fed breast milk or formula for the entire first year of their lives, with pureed solid foods offered only as a supplement, according to Pat Harper, R.D., a spokesperson for the American Dietetic Association and a dietitian in Pittsburgh. The exceptions are pre-term babies or those with low birth weights, whose nutritional needs may be significantly higher than what mother's milk can provide at that point. According to American

Dietetic Association recommendations, pre-term babies can be breastfed but may require special supplementation.

Don't cut out the fat—yet. Upon switching to commercial cow's milk, use whole, not skim or 2 percent, for the child's next year. "Babies need the extra calories, fat and cholesterol," Harper says. "It's the only time of their lives they need that." Their bodies are growing at an incredibly rapid rate, and the fat and cholesterol is vital for proper formation of cell walls and brain development.

THE TEEN YEARS

The teen scene is a time of revelry and rebellion, fast cars and fast food, growth spurts and the hormonal changes of puberty. The physiological growth spurt alone creates a greater nutrient demand, but the nutritional haphazardness of adolescence compounds the need. What's a teenager to do?

Bone up at a young age. While the requirement for almost all nutrients increases during the teenage years, calcium assumes a "critical importance," Harper says, especially for girls. Both young women and young men need at least the recommended 1,200 milligrams of the mineral. "In the teenage years and young adulthood, women build their maximum bone density and need extra calcium during that time. Strengthening their bones when young may help prevent osteoporosis later in life."

Turn on the iron. Both pubescent boys and girls need extra iron because their bodies are becoming bigger. For females that need continues: From age 11 through menopause, they require 50 percent more of the mineral (15 milligrams as opposed to 10 milligrams) than postpubescent males.

AGING

Eventually, time takes its toll on the body. It becomes harder to chew, harder to digest food, harder to absorb some of the nutrients—all of which means you have to work harder to ensure that your nutritional needs are met to keep you as healthy as possible.

Boost brain and body with B_{12}. At least one out of every five people older than 60 may need supplemental vitamin B_{12}. It's one of the more important nutrients affected by aging," says Robert M. Russell, M.D., a professor of medicine and nutrition at Tufts University in Boston. Extra B_{12} in the diets of senior citizens may help reverse senility-like lapses in memory and other neurological problems that disrupt muscle coordination and balance. Such symptoms often develop before the most apparent consequence of B_{12} deficiency, pernicious anemia.

Many older people won't need frequent visits to a doctor for B_{12} injections. B_{12} pills should do the job, Dr. Russell says.

As you age, your stomach may no longer secrete enough acid to separate B_{12} from protein. Or too much bacteria caused by the acid lack may interfere with absorption, a condition known as mild atrophic gastritis, says Dr. Russell, who also heads the gastrointestinal and micronutrient lab at the U.S. Department of Agriculture's Human Nutrition Research Center on Aging at Tufts.

"With mild atrophic gastritis, you can eat more foods containing B_{12} to get more B_{12} into your system," Dr. Russell says. Or you can take oral supplements which contain a crystalline (pure) form of the vitamin whose absorption is not impeded by a mild lack of stomach acids.

In severe cases of atrophic gastritis, though, no stomach acids at all are secreted, which means the body cannot produce another important absorptive aid called intrinsic factor. "No matter how much these people eat or take orally, it won't help them absorb vitamin B_{12}," Dr. Russell says. "These people would need injections of the vitamin."

Even though most older people with absorption problems can take B_{12} supplements, Dr. Russell advises that they take them only in consultation with a physician, who will be able to monitor blood levels of the nutrient and assess any deficiency damage.

Be selective about calcium supplements. Atrophic gastritis and other stomach difficulties can retard the absorption of the bone mineral calcium from its most common supplemental form, calcium carbonate. Older people should look for supplements made from calcium citrate, Dr. Russell advises, and they should take the pills with their meals.

Let B_6 help you get more out of a meal. A marginal deficiency of vitamin B_6 is commonly found in older people, compared to younger adults. This nutrient is needed for healthy blood and for proper functioning of the nervous system. It also seems to play a role in strengthening the immune system.

Vitamin B_6 also contributes significantly to metabolizing proteins. Based on studies analyzing vitamin B_6 and protein intakes, vitamin B_6 levels in the blood and excretion of vitamin B_6 matabolites in urine, a research team at Tufts University found that the minimum vitamin B_6 requirements of elderly men and women are about 1.96 and 1.90 milligrams per day, respectively. The current RDAs for elderly men and women are 2.0 and 1.6 milligrams per day, respectively. Since the RDAs are intended to "meet the nutrient needs of practically all healthy persons," the research team concluded that the current RDAs for B_6 are insufficient and should be reevaluated. Rich sources of B_6 include bananas, poultry and kidney beans.

Don't forget fluids. Many people worry about bladder control as they age, Dr. Kolasa says, and their thirst sensations diminish. For both these reasons, they may drink less fluids than they need. The result can be dehydration.

"Especially in the summer in the cities, elderly people die from dehydration," Dr. Russell says. "First they become confused; and if the dehydration persists, they slip into a coma."

Despite the extra danger, fluid requirements for older people don't differ drastically from those for younger adults. Everyone, Dr. Russell says, should be drinking between eight and ten glasses of fluid a day.

Ally yourself with the antioxidants. Because of evidence that the antioxidant vitamins help protect the body from age-related diseases and other health problems, Dr. Milner says, elderly people should make sure they're getting enough beta-carotene and vitamins E and C. In addition, they also need to boost their intake of iron, calcium, folate and the trace element selenium, he says.

Overcome reasons not to eat. For a number of reasons, elderly people are less likely to eat adequately, Harper says. They lose teeth and coordination. Their senses of taste and smell fade. They're generally weaker and may even find it uncomfortable to swallow. Many of them live alone and, thus, eat alone, either out of the house or at home with simple "meals" like tea and toast. "They're not concerned with the impact of decreasing nutrient intake, and if they are, they don't know what to do about it," Harper says.

"Simply because of the change in eating patterns," Dr. Milner emphasizes, "the demand for some nutrients is magnified." And if they or their loved ones don't ensure that they're getting enough of the right foods, the demand may not be met.

PART 2

THE TOP DIETARY ISSUES

CHAPTER 7

FIBER

MORE FOR WHAT AILS US

You can almost picture a snake-oil salesman selling this stuff from the back of a horse-drawn wagon, waving little brown bottles and shouting to the crowd: "Miracle substance! Cures just about any ailment! Easy to use!"

Instead of a traveling salesman, we have TV advertisers pitching the benefits of their fiber-containing products, plus magazines and newspapers that sometimes seem to have latched onto fiber as the cure-all of the decade. High cholesterol? Diabetes? Constipation? Overweight? Fiber has been touted as fixing them all.

But fiber *does* help with all these woes, and more. Studies indicate that fiber may also help with gastrointestinal problems, gallstones and ulcers. And it appears to help prevent colon and breast cancer. "We had never thought a food ingredient such as fiber could have the marked influence on diseases it does," says Sharon Fleming, Ph.D., associate professor in the Department of Nutrition Sciences at the University of California in Berkeley.

WHY ALL THE HULLABALOO?

What happened? Fifty years ago you didn't see people shaking bran flakes onto their cornflakes, or headlines popping off newspaper and magazine pages telling you about the amazing properties of oat bran.

FINDING FIBER IN FAST FOODS

So you try to work fiber into your diet—you really do—but somehow more and more often you find yourself at Wendy's or McDonald's or Taco Bell, gazing up at the neon-lit menu and trying to pick out something that's not *too* fattening or unhealthy.

Is there any fiber in fast food? Yes, but it's not always easy to find, says Marion J. Franz, of the International Diabetes Center in Minneapolis and author of *Fast Food Facts*. Most fast foods have so little fiber it's not even listed on those little nutritional sheets many restaurants provide. (You can forget about counting those few shreds of lettuce on your Jumbo Burger—lettuce is not a particularly good source of fiber.)

Where *can* you find fast-food fiber? In beans in chili, tacos or other Mexican foods, in vegetables at salad bars or atop pizzas, in whole-wheat rolls or buns and in baked potatoes (skin and all).

The salad bar is a sure bet, if you help yourself to a variety of vegetables and not just a pile of lettuce with a meager sprinkling of carrots and tomato. "In general, by the time people get through a salad bar, they've gotten two to three grams of fiber in all the raw vegetables," says Franz. A great way to add still more fiber to your salad is to

But 50 years ago people also weren't filling up on fiber-impoverished fast food and refined white-flour products, points out Dr. Fleming. They were much more likely to sit down to meals loaded with fiber: fresh or home-canned vegetables and fruit, whole-grain breads and a variety of grains and beans.

"As people became more affluent, a status factor came into play," says Dr. Fleming. People abandoned basic foods such as whole-meal bread and beans in favor of fluffy white bread, cakes, pastries, meat and highly processed foods. These days, hectic lifestyles have also taken their toll: "If you're eating TV dinners and fast foods rather than freshly prepared meals, you don't have much chance of getting enough fiber," says Dr. Fleming.

Today it's estimated that the fiber content of the typical U.S. diet ranges from 11.1 to 23.3 grams per day, down from around 40.0 grams a century ago. Fiber has no nutritive value, so at first no one thought taking it out of foods would hurt anything. But along with the drop in fiber intake came an increase in the incidence of chronic diseases.

The idea that there might be a *connection* between how much fiber we ate and these diseases came from British surgeon Denis Burkitt, M.D., and his landmark studies published in the 1970s. Dr. Burkitt pointed out that in places such as Africa, where the diet is heavy on cereals, legumes and root

add garbanzos, those little round, tan legumes also known as chick-peas.

Baked potatoes are another good choice at burger barns: A large potato, including the skin, offers about 4 grams of fiber. Beans in chili or Mexican fare usually will provide 3 to 4 grams, and corn on the cob, if you can find it, has between 2 and 3 grams. Choosing a wheat roll for your foot-long turkey sub at Subway will add 1½ grams of fiber to your meal, bringing it to nearly 6½ grams total. And two slices of a medium Pizza Hut pizza offer from 4 to 7 grams of fiber, depending on your toppings and the type of crust (the thin crust has less fiber). If you opt for an individual-size pizza heaped with vegetables, you get 8 to 9 grams of fiber.

So it's not *impossible* to get a reasonable amount of fiber from your fast-food meal. You can choose salad and chili, baked potato and a sandwich on a whole-wheat bun, a couple of bean burritos or two slices of pizza—all combinations that will give you seven to eight grams of fiber.

vegetables and includes 50 to 100 grams of fiber per day, there were fewer cases of colon and rectal cancer, intestinal diseases, hemorrhoids, gallstones and heart disease. In contrast, in Westernized countries with less fiber consumption, these diseases were increasing.

THE MIRACLE INGREDIENT

Despite the seemingly miraculous qualities of fiber, you can't just swig a fiber-containing drink or munch on a bran muffin and assume you're protected from disease. To reap the benefits fiber can offer, nutritionists recommend you get your fiber from a variety of foods and at several meals instead of one sitting.

Nor does fiber make up for eating *unhealthy* foods. "People tend to say to themselves, 'Gee, I've sprinkled bran on three things today, so I can eat these candy bars, these french fries and this deep-fried chicken,' " says Dr. Fleming.

What *is* great about fiber is that it requires no prescription and doesn't cost a lot—you can find it in many foods in your grocery store, many of them quite inexpensive.

Dietary fiber is the part of plants that resists digestion, so it passes through the system basically without being broken down. There are two

OAT BRAN: FACT OR FANTASY?

Oat bran: The wonder food, right? No, wait, that's the stuff that doesn't work, right?

It's no wonder that consumers are confused. First came a highly publicized study about 19 percent drops in cholesterol levels from eating oat bran. Then in 1990 came a study in the *New England Journal of Medicine* that concluded that oat bran had little effect on cholesterol.

So what's the word on oats? "The general feeling is that it's a good food, but it was put too high on the agenda in terms of expectations," says David Jenkins, M.D., Ph.D., of the University of Toronto in Ontario. "The trouble with the oat bran story is that it was pushed too many miles," he says.

"Oat bran is no better than other kinds of bran," says Barbara Harland, R.D., Ph.D., of Howard University in Washington, D.C. "It's ridiculous to limit your diet to one source of fiber."

In some cases you have to take closer looks at the studies. In the 19-percent-drop study, cholesterol was lowered by eating a bowl of oatmeal and five oat bran muffins daily *in combination with* a low-fat, low-cholesterol diet. And the study debunking fiber used inconsistent methods of comparing diets, and the subjects were all slender young women with normal cholesterol levels.

The bottom line, says Dr. Jenkins, is that oat bran is a fine food, with a definite effect on cholesterol—maybe not as large as first believed, but it's there, and it's valuable.

types of fiber, soluble and insoluble. Many foods contain both kinds of fiber, but some foods contain more of one type than the other.

Insoluble fibers—which include cellulose, lignin and some hemicelluloses—are linked to colon cancer protection and the prevention or alleviation of some digestive disorders. They also delay glucose absorption. You'll find insoluble fibers in wheat bran and whole grains and on the outside of legumes, fruits and seeds. Insoluble fiber is like a sponge, increasing the bulk of your stool and speeding it on its way through your intestinal tract.

Soluble fibers lower blood cholesterol and slow down how fast glucose gets into your bloodstream. Instead of hastening food's movement through you, soluble fibers decrease the pace. They're found in vegetables, fruits, brown rice, barley, oats and oat and rice bran, and include pectin, gums and some hemicelluloses.

A MULTITUDE OF BENEFITS

What exactly *does* this miracle substance accomplish? Although the jury is still out on some fronts, there is some consensus of opinion.

"The scientific community agrees that dietary fiber lowers cholesterol, relieves constipation, possibly reduces blood glucose response and may have a positive function in weight reduction," says David Jenkins, M.D., Ph.D., professor of medicine and nutritional sciences in the Department of Nutritional Sciences at the University of Toronto in Ontario. Dietary fiber can also help with gastrointestinal, gallbladder and gastric problems, according to the American Dietetic Association.

A diet high in fiber is often lower in fat and calories than one that is low in fiber, and some people argue that many of fiber's benefits can be attributed to the decrease in fat or calories. "The other factors may enhance the fiber effect," agrees Dr. Jenkins, "but that's not a bad thing."

Cutting Cholesterol

The link between cholesterol and fiber has gotten much media attention. Cholesterol is reduced primarily by soluble fiber, as in oat bran and psyllium, a seed used in laxative products such as Metamucil. According to some studies, fiber lowers harmful LDL (low-density lipoprotein) cholesterol without lowering good HDL (high-density lipoprotein) levels.

James W. Anderson, M.D., a pioneer in fiber research and professor of medicine and clinical nutrition at the University of Kentucky College of Medicine in Lexington, studied 105 men and women with elevated cholesterol levels. After taking psyllium for eight weeks, their LDL cholesterol had dropped nearly 9 percent more than while just eating a special cholesterol-lowering diet. In another study, a low-fat diet plus oat cereal lowered cholesterol 10 percent, while the same diet plus 13 grams of psyllium caused a *16 percent* drop.

Other studies confirm the cholesterol-lowering effect with other foods. In one study, a group of 41 men lowered their LDL cholesterol by eating 12 prunes daily (roughly six grams of fiber). In another study by Dr. Anderson, patients with high cholesterol experienced drops of more than 10 percent after three weeks of eating eight ounces of canned beans daily.

Curing Constipation

This is no laughing matter for the many people who suffer from it. The Western world's low fiber intake is the clear culprit here, say many doctors. Fortunately, fiber almost always provides relief. Fiber ranks high among *Prevention* magazine readers: 86 percent of respondents in a survey said bran and high-fiber cereal gave good results in relieving irregularity.

Insoluble fiber plus water forms a larger, softer stool that can pass easily and quickly. And when bacteria begin to break down the fiber, chemicals form that help things start moving.

If you're eating bran for a laxative effect, stick to coarse bran rather than finely ground bran, advises Jay Kenney, R.D., Ph.D., nutrition research specialist at the Pritikin Longevity Center in Santa Monica, California. "Finely ground bran has much less of an effect on constipation," he says. The laxative effect of wheat bran may also be reduced by cooking.

TO SUPPLEMENT OR NOT TO SUPPLEMENT

Adding fiber to your diet *does* require some time and planning, so you may be tempted to look for a quick-and-easy answer—such as fiber pills.

Most professionals urge caution when it comes to these pills. "Fiber pills are a disaster," says Sharon Fleming, Ph.D., of the University of California at Berkeley. "They're expensive, and, to a large degree, ineffective."

One problem is that fiber squeezed into a pill may not work the same as fiber in food. "The physical properties have been altered tremendously, and this can reduce the effectiveness of the fiber, gram for gram," explains Dr. Fleming. And you'd have to take a lot of pills to get substantial fiber: Five pills supply only about 2½ grams of fiber, about what you'd get in a small apple.

Even using bran as a supplement can be a mistake if you overdo it, says Dr. Fleming. "I would guard against sprinkling bran on everything," she says. Bran, whether in pills or the loose form, absorbs a lot of water, and without adequate liquid intake, Dr. Fleming points out, you're running the risk of impaction. If you like bran, don't eat it dry: Stir it into something wet, such as a bowl of oatmeal or a batter. Also use plenty of milk with high-fiber cereals, says Dr. Fleming.

Finally, if you're eating fiber only in concentrated forms, you're not getting the nutrients and minerals that generally accompany fiber when you eat it in foods. And because fiber *can* interfere with the absorption of minerals and vitamins, if you're increasing your fiber intake without increasing your nutrient intake—which is what happens when you pop bran pills or eat plain bran—you could put yourself at risk for deficiency.

Fiber can also help prevent hemorrhoids by eliminating constipation, which contributes to their formation. It can also make passing stools less painful when you do have hemorrhoids.

PREVENTING CANCER

Native Japanese, who eat less fat and more fiber than Westerners, have only about one-fifth our rate of breast cancer and colon cancer—but when Japanese immigrate to the Unites States and alter their diets, rates rise dramatically.

In colon cancer, fiber seems the most important factor. In Finland, where people eat as much fat as we do but also eat lots of whole grains and high-fiber foods, the rates of colon cancer are *one-third* of ours. And among the Hindu population in India, which eats a high-fiber diet, there's very little colon cancer. The Parsi community in Bombay, however, has a more Westernized diet—*and* colon cancer rates almost equal to those of Western countries. Closer to home, the Mormon population in Utah has a lower risk of colon cancer than the rest of the population: This group eats normally high American levels of fat but also eats cereal and breads made from stone-ground whole-grain flour.

How does fiber affect cancer risk? When we eat fat, some of the bile acids produced to process these fats develop into carcinogenic forms. Fiber can help by causing the stool to be bigger—which decreases carcinogen concentration in the stool—or it can bond with the carcinogens and carry them off. The oxygen produced in fiber fermentation may keep the bile acids from changing into their carcinogenic forms. Finally, fiber speeds the stool on its way, so if carcinogens *are* present, they'll spend less time in contact with the colon wall.

Insoluble fiber may lower estrogen levels in premenopausal women, which may help prevent breast cancer. In one study, 62 women ate wheat, oat or corn bran muffins, doubling their daily fiber intake to 30 grams. After two months, only the women eating wheat bran had significantly lower levels of circulating estrogen.

Effects have been seen in mammals of the four-legged variety. In a study of rats exposed to a carcinogen to induce mammary tumors, 90 percent of the animals eating a high-fat, low-fiber diet developed tumors, while only 66 percent of those eating a high-fat, high-fiber diet did.

Conclusion? "The most important thing the public can do is increase their overall dietary fiber intake from a variety of natural food sources," advises Bruce Trock, Ph.D., a cancer epidemiologist at Fox Chase Cancer Center in Philadelphia.

BATTLING THE BULGE

One reason fiber is successful in helping weight loss is simple: It fills you up. High-fiber foods make you feel full and tend to take longer to eat. They also tend to be low in fat.

Another benefit involves soluble fibers and insulin, the hormone that stimulates appetite and promotes fat storage. "The good news is that food fiber slows the body's insulin response," says Dr. Kenney.

DEALING WITH DIABETES

Diabetes, which is increasing annually by about 500,000 cases, according to Dr. Anderson, can be managed effectively by a high-carbohydrate, high-fiber diet. In some cases this regimen can alleviate the need for insulin: "Many diabetics don't need insulin. They need a diet program," says Dr. Anderson. Eating fiber also facilitates weight loss, which can help *avoid* diabetes.

Fiber can reduce glucose and insulin concentrations after meals, as seen in a study at the University of Virginia, where people with non-insulin-

FIBER CONTENT OF FOODS

Breads, fruits, vegetables and beans are generally your best fiber sources, but there are fairly large differences among individual foods, as this table shows.

FOOD	PORTION	FIBER (g.)
BREADS		
Whole-wheat bread	1 slice	2.1
Pumpernickel bread	1 slice	1.9
English muffin	1	1.6
Rye bread	1 slice	1.6
Bagel	1	1.2
Waffle	1	0.8
White bread	1 slice	0.5
FRUITS		
Strawberries, fresh	1 cup	3.9
Dates, dried	5 med.	3.5
Orange	1	3.1
Apple	1	3.0
Applesauce	½ cup	1.9
Pineapple, canned	1 cup	1.9
Banana	1	1.8
Prunes, dried	3 med.	1.8
Cantaloupe	1 cup cubes	1.3
Grapes	1 cup	1.1
Orange juice	½ cup	0.1

dependent diabetes received two 3.4-gram doses of psyllium fiber before breakfast and dinner. Their glucose levels were lower after those meals, and their serum insulin concentrations were reduced after breakfast and even after lunch.

Soluble fibers, such as those found in oat and rice bran, legumes and fruit and vegetables, seem to be the ticket. "The water-soluble fibers found in legumes, oats, barley and fruit, when eaten in a low-fat diet, have been shown to lower blood-fat levels," says Marion J. Franz, vice president of nutrition and publications at the International Diabetes Center in Minneapolis. Those fibers may also cause the sugar in your food to be absorbed more slowly, which gives your insulin a chance to keep your blood sugar on a more even keel.

FOOD	PORTION	FIBER (g.)
VEGETABLES		
Brussels sprouts, cooked	½ cup	3.4
Peas, frozen	½ cup	2.4
Carrot, raw 7½" long	1	2.3
Broccoli, cooked	½ cup	2.0
Green beans, frozen	½ cup	1.8
Mushrooms, boiled	½ cup	1.7
Tomato, fresh	1 med.	1.6
Beets, canned	½ cup	1.4
Iceberg lettuce, shredded	1 cup	1.4
Corn, canned	½ cup	1.2
Celery, raw, chopped	½ cup	1.0
BEANS		
Black-eyed peas, boiled	½ cup	8.3
Kidney beans, canned	½ cup	7.9
Chick-peas, canned	½ cup	7.0
Pork and beans, canned	½ can	6.9
Lentils, dried, cooked	½ cup	5.2
Pinto beans, boiled	½ cup	3.4

TREATING INTESTINAL ILLS

In diverticulosis, fairly common in adults 50 and older, small pouches form in the wall of the colon because of intestinal pressure. When the pouches trap feces, they can become inflamed. Some studies suggest that fiber may help *prevent* diverticulosis, and it may also help by reducing intestinal pressure and helping clear out existing pouches.

Fiber can be used to treat constipation problems in irritable bowel syndrome and has been used to treat some cases of duodenal ulcers. Crohn's disease involves inflammatory lesions in the intestines; after symptoms have subsided, small amounts of fiber can be added to the diet, according to the American Dietetic Association. Once the disease is under control, fiber can help keep it from recurring.

GALLING GALLSTONES

Fiber may help prevent gallstones by stimulating bile flow and preventing reabsorption of bile. It's also possible that gallstones *result* from low-fiber diets and that fiber can prevent their formation.

GUARDING THOSE GUMS

Chewing large volumes of fibrous foods helps massage gums and remove plaque, according to one study. All that chewing also stimulates the production of saliva, which helps clean teeth as well.

FITTING IN FIBER

Okay, you're committed. You *want* to increase the amount of fiber in your diet. Where do you start?

"First, a trip to the grocery store," says dietitian and nutritionist Barbara Harland, R.D., Ph.D., associate professor of nutrition in the Department of Nutritional Sciences at Howard University in Washington, D.C. Pause before you toss the Froot Loops or white Wonder bread into your shopping cart.

Go whole grain. You want to select whole-grain breads, crackers and muffins, advises Dr. Harland. This also means checking labels: Just because a loaf of bread is brown and labeled "wheat" doesn't mean it's whole grain. (Refined white flour is wheat, too.) Check the list of ingredients or choose items labeled "whole wheat."

Select your cereal. In the cereal aisle you'll find many cereals that will add to your fiber intake. Again, check the labels for the number of grams of fiber per serving.

Favor this food group. Stock up on fresh, frozen and canned fruits and vegetables.

Peruse the packaged goods. Instead of reaching for white rice, choose brown rice or another whole grain such as barley, bulgur or millet. Buy whole-grain pasta instead of the refined variety. You can also stock up on whole-wheat flour, which you can substitute for white flour in many recipes.

Bring on the beans. "A food high in fiber that people often neglect is legumes: dried beans, lentils, peas," says Dr. Jenkins, who supplements his diet with barley and beans. You can buy these canned or in soups, but dried is cheaper.

A PAINLESS PATH TO HIGH FIBER

The next step, of course, comes in the kitchen and at the dining room table. The first problem is lack of time. Say you come home from work tired and hungry. You're not likely to reach for raw vegetables and spend an hour preparing them before you can eat—you're going to reach for a fast and

THE LOWDOWN ON BREAKFAST CEREALS

Counting on your breakfast cereal to provide a chunk of your dietary fiber requirements? Here's the number of grams of fiber per serving.

CEREAL	PORTION*	FIBER (g.)
All-Bran	⅓ cup	9.0
All-Bran with Extra Fiber	½ cup	14.0
Bran Buds	⅓ cup	11.0
Cheerios	1¼ cups	2.5
Common Sense Oat Bran	¾ cup	3.0
Fiber One	½ cup	13.0
Fiberwise	⅔ cup	5.0
Frosted Bran	⅔ cup	3.0
Grape-Nuts	¼ cup	2.8
Nutri-Grain Wheat	⅔ cup	3.0
Product 19	1 cup	1.2
Puffed Rice	1 cup	1.2
Raisin Bran	¾ cup	5.0
Rice Krispies	1 cup	0.3
Spoon-Size Shredded Wheat	⅔ cup	3.0
Special K	1 cup	1.0
Total (wheat)	1 cup	2.0
Wheaties	1 cup	3.0

*Though serving sizes vary widely, all provide approximately 1 ounce.

easy food that quickly satisfies your hunger.

Have a plan. "Working fiber into your diet does take some effort," says Dr. Fleming. "It means planning ahead. It may mean cutting up your vegetables one night so you can have them the next night. It may mean eating at restaurants that offer salad bars with vegetables. It may mean making an effort—but it means taking care of ourselves."

Aim high. The American Dietetic Association recommends 20 to 35 grams of fiber daily (40 to 50 grams a day—or 25 grams per 1,000 calories—for people with diabetes). Don't, however, double your fiber intake overnight. Introduce fiber into your diet *gradually.* And if you have diabetes, always be sure to check with your doctor before making any dietary changes.

Pay attention to basics. These tips can help you increase your daily fiber intake.

MORE FIBER, LESS EFFORT

So you think fitting fiber into your diet means a complete revamping of how you eat? Changing your diet doesn't have to be tedious or difficult—sometimes small changes can make a big difference. Here's an example of how you can painlessly shift your menu to include more fiber in your diet. (The fiber values in the table are based on standard servings.)

FIBER IN YOUR OLD MENU . . .		AND IN THE NEW	
FOOD	**FIBER (g.)**	**FOOD**	**FIBER (g.)**
BREAKFAST		***BREAKFAST***	
Orange juice	0.1	Whole orange	3.1
Corn flakes	0.5	High-fiber cereal	9.0
Doughnut	negligible	Whole-wheat toast	2.1
LUNCH		***LUNCH***	
Hamburger on white bun	0.7	Chili	4.6
Fries	3.1	Baked sweet potato	3.4
Milk shake	negligible	Milk shake	negligible
DINNER		***DINNER***	
Lettuce salad	1.4	Lettuce salad with chick-peas, broccoli and mushrooms	6.1
Chicken	negligible	Chicken	negligible
White rice	0.2	Brown rice	1.7
SNACKS		***SNACKS***	
Apple	3.0	Pear	4.3
Potato chips	1.0	Popcorn (3 cups)	2.7
Daily Total:	**10.0**		**37.0**

- Eat whole fruit instead of drinking juice.
- Eat the skins of fruits and vegetables.
- Eat fruit with edible seeds such as kiwis, figs and blueberries.
- When preparing vegetables such as broccoli and asparagus, include more of the stem.
- Peel grapefruit and eat it like an orange instead of eating it with a spoon.
- Make your own bread crumbs or croutons from stale, whole-grain bread.
- Add beans, peas and lentils to soups, stews and salads.
- Scrub vegetables instead of peeling them.
- Add grated vegetables to meat loaf, casseroles and sauces.
- Use pureed vegetables instead of cream to thicken soups.

Resort to a super source. Still having trouble getting enough fiber? Try adding one of the following "supplements" per day—each offers four to five extra grams of fiber.

- Three dried figs
- One large pear
- Three medium plums
- Two medium peaches
- ½ cup cooked legumes (such as chick-peas, kidney beans or lentils)
- ⅓ to ½ cup bran cereal
- One tablespoon corn bran, three tablespoons wheat bran or four tablespoons rice bran, stirred into cereal, fruit or yogurt
- 1½ rounded teaspoons psyllium or 2 teaspoons soy fiber mixed with a beverage. (You should be aware that some people are allergic to psyllium: Stop using it if you experience rapid heartbeat or rapid breathing, swollen face or tight throat.)

Enough . . . or Too Much?

How concerned should you be about how much of your fiber is insoluble and how much is soluble? "What you should be concerned with is that you're eating the right foods," says Dr. Jenkins. If you eat a variety of fiber-containing foods, don't worry about how much of each type you're getting.

You may also wonder how to know if you're getting enough total fiber. Let's face it, few of us are going to keep track of how many grams of fiber we eat, day after day. A quick way to determine if you're getting enough fiber is by your stools, says Dr. Harland. "They shouldn't be very dark and hard to pass," she says. "A normal stool should be pale tan and soft."

If some fiber is good, a lot is better, you think as you heap bran on your oatmeal, pop fiber pills with lunch and snack on popcorn after dinner.

Hold it right there. Too much fiber, particularly in the form of bran or pills, can actually *clog you up*, says Dr. Fleming. Fiber absorbs a lot of liquid, and if you're eating fiber in a concentrated form and not taking in enough liquid, the fiber can literally form a plug inside you.

The second reason for not overdosing on fiber is that fiber binds some vitamins and minerals, decreasing their availability. For most of us, this isn't a problem. "If you're getting your fiber in foods, by increasing fiber, you're automatically increasing the nutrients," says Dr. Harland.

Who's in danger? People who take their fiber in forms such as fiber pills or fiber drinks, thereby adding fiber *without* adding nutrients; elderly people who exist on tea and toast; and some vegetarians, says Dr. Harland. Children who aren't eating a lot of calories may also be at risk, cautions the American Academy of Pediatrics.

Most of us, however, don't have to worry—as long as we're getting our fiber from a variety of foods. The "consumption of a complex, balanced diet

THE UNPLEASANT SIDE OF FIBER

Okay, we never said *everything* about fiber is great. In some people there are . . . well, certain unpleasant side effects. High-fiber foods can tend to be gas-producing, which at times can make you wonder if all that fiber is really worth the bother.

Don't despair! Even if previous forays into the world of high-fiber foods proved disastrous, there are ways to decrease your distress.

The first trick is to introduce fiber *gradually* into your diet, according to George L. Blackburn, M.D., Ph.D., associate professor of surgery at Harvard Medical School and chief of the Nutrition/Metabolism Laboratory at the Cancer Research Institute of New England Deaconess Hospital in Boston. Too much, too soon can result in gas and a bloated feeling. So if you're only eating 10 grams of fiber a day, don't rocket up to 25 grams a day all at once. Dr. Blackburn recommends adding fiber in 5-gram increments: Add 5 extra grams per day, and after five or six weeks, add another 5 grams, and so on.

Another simple trick is to soak beans before cooking, then pour off the water, and cook them in fresh water. This helps break down the sugars that cause the gas problem. Chewing thoroughly can also help.

And for those folks for whom all else fails, there's a secret weapon: a product called Beano. Much of the gas produced by high-fiber foods comes from hard-to-digest sugars, explains Luanne Hughes, R.D., manager of public relations for Beano. "When those sugars sit in your intestine undigested, bacteria feed on them." The results of this bacterial feast? Gas.

This is where Beano comes in: This bottled enzyme breaks down these sugars and substantially reduces the gas produced. Although it's named after the food that gives many of us trouble, the manufacturer claims it works on foods as diverse as flour, bran, brussels sprouts, squash, granola, peanut butter, tofu and more.

All you do is add drops of Beano to your first mouthful of gas-producing foods. Because not *all* the gas from fibrous foods comes from these sugars, Beano may not completely eliminate the problem, says Hughes, but it should substantially reduce it.

from a variety of food sources should not lead to overt vitamin/mineral deficiencies," states the American Dietetic Association.

Health professionals agree that it all comes down to a very simple formula: Eat a wide variety of fiber-containing foods.

HIGH-NUTRITION RECIPES

CHILI-TOPPED POTATOES

Beans are a treasure trove of fiber, so they deserve to make frequent appearances on your table. This simple entrée is equally good for lunch or dinner. You can vary it by substituting other beans and also by serving the chili over quick-cooking brown rice rather than potatoes.

4 large baking potatoes
2 teaspoons olive oil
1½ cups diced onions
1 cup diced sweet red peppers
1 cup diced carrots
1 clove garlic, minced
1 tablespoon chili powder
1 teaspoon ground cumin
⅛ teaspoon ground red pepper
1 can (28 ounces) whole tomatoes
1 cup defatted chicken stock
¾ cup mild or medium salsa
1 can (19 ounces) red kidney beans, rinsed well and drained
1 cup corn kernels

Pierce the potatoes all over with a fork. Place a paper towel directly on the floor of the microwave. Arrange the potatoes on it in a square pattern. Microwave on high for 5 minutes. Flip and rearrange the potatoes. Microwave on high for 5 to 7 minutes more, or until easily pierced with a fork. Cover with foil and let stand for at least 5 minutes.

Meanwhile, heat the oil in a 3-quart saucepan over medium-high heat. Add the onions, sweet red peppers, carrots and garlic. Sauté for 5 minutes, or until the vegetables are tender.

Stir in the chili powder, cumin and ground red pepper. Sauté for 1 minute, stirring constantly.

Drain the tomatoes, reserving ½ cup of the juice. Add the juice to the pan. Chop the tomatoes and add. Stir in the stock and salsa. Bring to a boil.

Reduce the heat to medium low and simmer for 10 minutes, stirring occasionally, until the mixture thickens slightly. Add the beans and corn. Simmer for 5 minutes.

Split the potatoes and lightly fluff the flesh with a fork. Serve topped with the chili.

Serves 4
Per serving: *352 calories, 5.8 g. fat (13% of calories), 12.3 g. dietary fiber, 0 mg. cholesterol, 578 mg. sodium*

ORANGE-RAISIN MUFFINS

Getting the recommended 20 to 35 grams of fiber a day into your diet can be a challenge. That's why you need to stoke up at every meal, including breakfast. Muffins are always a welcome addition to the morning meal. And they're portable, so those who don't have time for a sit-down meal can take them along to work or school. These muffins are especially good spread with apple butter, which contains both soluble and insoluble fiber.

2 cups shredded bran cereal, such as All-Bran or Fiber One
¾ cup boiling water
½ cup buttermilk
½ cup orange juice
¼ cup oil
¼ cup honey
¼ cup fat-free egg substitute
1 tablespoon grated orange rind
¾ cup golden raisins
¾ cup unbleached flour
½ cup whole-wheat flour
1½ teaspoons baking soda

In a large bowl, combine the cereal and water. Let stand for 5 minutes, or until the bran softens.

In a medium bowl, whisk together the buttermilk, orange juice, oil, honey, egg and orange rind. Stir into the bran mixture. Add the raisins and mix well.

In a small bowl, stir together the unbleached flour, whole-wheat flour and baking soda. Pour over the bran mixture. Stir just until the flour is moistened; do not overmix.

Coat 12 muffin cups with no-stick spray. Divide the batter among the cups. Bake at 400° for 18 minutes, or until lightly browned.

Makes 12

Tip: *These muffins are best served warm. To reheat them easily, slice in half, wrap in a damp paper towel and microwave one muffin at a time on high for 25 to 30 seconds. They'll be moist and soft, with just-baked flavor.*

Per muffin: *180 calories, 5.2 g. fat (23% of calories), 5.1 g. dietary fiber, <1 mg. cholesterol, 148 mg. sodium*

CHICKEN AND RICE CASSEROLE

One good way to increase your fiber intake is by using brown rice instead of white. Another is to up your consumption of high-fiber cereal. This delicious casserole combines both techniques to produce a nutty-tasting main dish. Serve with three-bean salad and whole-grain bread for even more fiber.

- **12 ounces boneless, skinless chicken breast, cut into 1" cubes**
- **1 cup diced onions**
- **¾ cup diced mushrooms**
- **2 teaspoons olive oil**
- **1¼ cups quick-cooking brown rice**
- **½ teaspoon dried thyme**
- **½ teaspoon ground black pepper**
- **2½ cups defatted chicken stock**
- **1 box (10 ounces) frozen peas, partially thawed**
- **1 cup shredded bran cereal, such as All-Bran or Fiber One**
- **¼ cup wheat germ or bread crumbs**
- **2 tablespoons grated Parmesan cheese**
- **1 cup nonfat yogurt or nonfat sour cream**
- **2 tablespoons minced fresh parsley**
- **⅛ teaspoon hot-pepper sauce**

Spread the chicken on a large, flat plate or in a 9" glass pie plate in as even a layer as possible. Cover with wax paper and microwave on high for 3 minutes. Stir, cover and microwave on high for 2 minutes, or until no longer pink. Set aside.

Meanwhile, in a large no-stick frying pan or Dutch oven over medium heat, sauté the onions and mushrooms in 1 teaspoon of the oil for 5 minutes, or until wilted. Stir in the rice, thyme and black pepper. Add 2 cups of the stock and bring to a boil. Cover and simmer over medium-low heat for 10 minutes. Stir in the peas, cereal, chicken and the remaining ½ cup stock.

Coat a 7" × 11" baking dish with no-stick spray. Spoon the chicken mixture into the dish. In a cup, combine the wheat germ or bread crumbs, Parmesan and the remaining 1 teaspoon oil. Sprinkle over the casserole. Bake at 350° for 15 minutes, or until the crumbs are lightly browned.

In a small bowl, stir together the yogurt or sour cream, parsley and hot-pepper sauce. Serve with the casserole.

Serves 4

Tip: *If you don't have a microwave, brown the chicken in a large no-stick frying pan that you've coated with no-stick spray. Also, if your frying pan or Dutch oven is ovenproof, you may simply sprinkle the crumbs over the chicken mixture and bake the casserole right in the pan—you'll have fewer dishes to clean up!*

Per serving: *400 calories, 6.7 g. fat (14% of calories), 13.2 g. dietary fiber, 53 mg. cholesterol, 531 mg. sodium*

SPICED FRUIT COMPOTE

Dried figs and prunes are especially high in dietary fiber. You can snack on them, or you can turn them into a delicious compote to serve over cooked cereal at breakfast or over nonfat frozen yogurt after dinner. Another idea is to mix fresh blueberries or raspberries into chilled compote, then top the mixture with nonfat vanilla yogurt and granola.

1 cup water
1 tea bag (preferably Earl Grey)
1½ cups cranberry juice cocktail
½ teaspoon vanilla
½ teaspoon ground cinnamon
¼ teaspoon grated nutmeg
12 dried figs, halved
12 bite-size pitted prunes
6 dried apricot halves, cut in half
¼ cup dried cranberries or currants

In a 2-quart saucepan over medium heat, bring the water to a boil. Remove from the heat, add the tea bag and let steep for 10 minutes. Remove the bag, pressing to extract the water.

Stir in the cocktail, vanilla, cinnamon and nutmeg. Bring to a boil. Add the figs, prunes, apricots and cranberries or currants. Cover and simmer over medium-low heat for 15 minutes, or until the fruit is plumped and soft. Serve warm or chilled.

Serves 6
Per serving: *221 calories, 0.6 g. fat (2% of calories), 5.6 g. dietary fiber, 0 mg. cholesterol, 10 mg. sodium*

CHAPTER 8

Low-Fat Eating

For All the Right Reasons

The last time was a charm for William J. Fanizzi. After surgeons inserted a balloon catheter into his chest to unclog his coronary arteries for a fourth time, Fanizzi finally vowed to get serious about cutting the fat out of his diet.

The 67-year-old former pediatrician was never what you'd call a high-fat fiend—his wife, Lucy, saw to that. But certain delicacies come with the territory when you're Italian: spicy sausages, pepperoni pizza, homemade meat and cheese lasagna and crispy garlic bread smothered with butter. Add to years of nutritional no-nos a family history of heart problems, and—Mama mia—you have the makings of a sick man.

Fanizzi's not alone. Many experts rate eating too much fat second only to smoking as the greatest threat to our health. More than 68 million Americans—over one in four—suffer some form of cardiovascular disease. As many as 34 million Americans are overweight—a condition linked to, among other conditions, arthritis, diabetes, gallstones, high blood pressure, high cholesterol and breathing ailments. Half a million Americans each year suffer a stroke. Roughly one in nine American women develops breast cancer. And *all* these diseases have been linked to fat.

But here's an offer you shouldn't refuse: Low-fat eating can dramatically improve your health—from lopping off excess pounds to actually lengthening your life. In fact, one study suggests that the number of Americans killed by heart disease could be cut by as much as 42,000 a year—if they reduced their fat intake a mere 7 percent. For most people, that's a goal that could be met (or even exceeded) by simply cutting out that daily doughnut.

"Most Americans who have health problems would not have them if they ate a low-fat diet," says William P. Castelli, M.D., director of the famed Framingham Heart Study.

THE TALE OF THE TARAHUMARA

For proof of the devastating—and rapid—effects of a high-fat diet, look no further than this unique study involving the superfit Tarahumara Indians of Mexico. World famous for their running ability, the Tarahumara—which literally means "fleet of foot"—are virtually untouched by fat-related diseases like heart disease. In fact, they're in such great shape, their favorite sport is a form of kickball that makes pro soccer look like a grade-school drill: The game covers no less than 100 to 150 miles. Their average meal is also a little different from ours: lots of complex carbohydrates like pinto beans and thick corn tortillas. If it's a holiday, they might also eat some meat.

A few years ago, researchers from Oregon Health Sciences University

FAT ON FILE

To plan your healthy eating strategy, you need to know what is low in fat and what is high. This chart can help you get started.

FOOD	PORTION	TOTAL FAT (g.)
Cornflakes	1 cup	0.0
Rice cakes	1	0.2
White rice	1 cup	0.4
Low-fat (1%) cottage cheese	¼ cup	0.6
Pretzel	1	0.7
Spaghetti, cooked	1 cup	0.9
Bagel (egg or water)	1	1.4
Half-and-half	1 Tbsp.	1.7
Pancake, from mix	1	2.0
Buttermilk	1 cup	2.2
Chocolate-chip cookie	1 small	2.2
Low-fat (1%) milk	1 cup	2.6
Turkey breast, roasted, without skin	3 oz.	2.7
Chicken breast, roasted, without skin	3 oz.	3.1
Low-fat yogurt	1 cup	3.5
Toaster pastry	1	5.7
Leg of lamb, trimmed, roasted	3 oz.	6.6

decided to see what would happen if the Tarahumaras ate some old-fashioned diner food. Of course, they don't have diners, so the food had to be specially provided: high-fat goodies like cheese, butter, lard and egg yolks. "In short, the same foods eaten by many Americans," says Martha P. McMurray, R.D., who spent two months with the Indians on the project.

In just five weeks, these formerly sleek, svelte Indians had gained an average of about 8.5 pounds. What's worse, their LDL (bad) cholesterol levels jumped an average of 31 percent—a danger sign for heart disease.

FAT FACTS

Why does life-threatening heart disease follow high cholesterol? Simply put, "a major determinant of one's cardiovascular health is diet," says Dean Ornish, M.D., author of *Dr. Dean Ornish's Program for Reversing Heart Disease* and director of the Preventive Medicine Research Institute in Sausalito, California.

Consider: Animal products like beef, milk and cheese, and tropical oils like coconut oil, contain saturated fat—the most dangerous kind, according to the American Heart Association (AHA).

FOOD	PORTION	TOTAL FAT (g.)
French toast, homemade	1 slice	6.7
Egg scrambled with milk and butter	1	7.3
Blue cheese dressing, regular	1 Tbsp.	8.0
Monterey Jack cheese	1 oz.	8.5
Instant chocolate-flavored breakfast drink	1 cup	8.8
Cream of mushroom soup, condensed, made with water	1 cup	9.0
Chocolate-covered peanuts	1 oz.	11.6
Beef frankfurter	1	12.8
Apple pie, homemade	4 oz.	13.1
Turkey sandwich on whole-wheat bread	1	13.1
Roast beef sandwich on rye bread	1	13.8
Ground beef, up to 30% fat	3 oz.	14.0
Almonds, dry-roasted	1 oz.	14.8
Chicken breast, batter-fried	1 piece	14.8
Pork sausage, smoked	1 link	21.6
Ham and cheese sandwich on rye bread	1	27.5
Chef salad with dressing	average	30.3

Corn oil and other vegetable oils like sunflower, safflower and soybean oil contain polyunsaturated fat. Canola and olive oils are high in monounsaturated fat. But, unlike saturated fat, both help reduce LDL cholesterol.

Your body does need some fat—it plays an important role in making up the membranes or coatings that protect your cells. But it doesn't need much. As a result, loading up on high-fat foods is the equivalent of a sludge spill in your cardiovascular system.

Fat and cholesterol from the meal is dumped into the bloodstream. The waxy mixture then circulates in the blood until an injury to the wall of an artery—caused by factors such as smoking or high blood pressure—causes some of it to collect.

As the cholesterol piles up over the years, the flow of blood is gradually reduced, narrowing and sometimes hardening the artery. This process is called atherosclerosis. The reduced blood flow forces the heart to work even harder, causing another common ailment: high blood pressure.

If the buildup severely slows or stops blood flow to the brain, a stroke occurs. If blood is cut off to the heart, the victim suffers a heart attack.

THE ORNISH APPROACH

At one time, it was thought that the devastating effects of heart disease, were, unlike love, forever: That is, unless surgery could undo the damage. But in fact, research by several doctors, including Dr. Ornish, shows that eating the right foods can not only stop heart disease in its greasy tracks but can actually reverse it.

To prove Dr. Ornish's theory, a group of patients with severely clogged arteries were divided into two groups. Those in the first group were directed to follow a commonly prescribed method of fighting heart disease—eat less red meat, more fish and chicken, margarine instead of butter and no more than three eggs a week; exercise moderately and quit smoking.

The rest were put on the ultimate low-fat diet, a strict vegetarian plan designed by Dr. Ornish that's 70 to 75 percent complex carbohydrates (rice, pasta, grains, beans, fruit and vegetables), 15 to 20 percent protein and no more than 10 percent of calories from fat. That meant no oils or animal foods, except egg whites and nonfat dairy products like skim milk. Even avocados, nuts and seeds were off-limits because of their high fat content. Caffeine and alcohol were also forbidden under the program.

The men who participated in the study were tested and then retested a year later. The results, confirmed by a special artery-viewing technique called angiography: In 82 percent of the men in the extreme low fat group, coronary artery blockages had diminished. No such reversal was evident in the other treatment group.

It's no surprise, then, that Dr. Ornish urges his patients not only to exercise, give up smoking and reduce stress but also to cut fat from their diets.

LOW FAT, LOW CANCER

Cutting fat may do more than just keep your heart healthy. An extraordinary study of 6,500 mainland Chinese suggests that it may also help keep you cancer-free.

In 1983, a group of researchers headed by T. Colin Campbell, Ph.D., of Cornell University in Ithaca, New York, in conjunction with the Chinese Academy of Preventative Medicine and Medical Sciences and the University of Oxford, began exploring the link between food, environment, social practices and diseases.

Although the study is expected to continue through the 1990s, early results, when contrasted by Dr. Campbell with disease data from the United States, shed new light on a likely fat/cancer connection.

While the Chinese actually average more calories daily (Them: 2,636, Us: 2,360), our diet is three times higher in calories from fat. Is it any coincidence that Americans have roughly five times the incidence of breast cancer? Not to Dr. Campbell. "Based on what we've found so far, a diet low in fat and animal foods is a diet that I would consider optimal for long-term health," he says.

An American study of 80,000 nurses failed to show a link between fat intake and breast cancer—at least between women consuming 38 percent of their calories from fat and those whose intake of fat was 29 percent of total calories. But that may be because the "low" fat levels weren't low enough. Many experts believe that protective benefits don't kick in until fat falls below 20 percent of total calories.

Another convincing piece of evidence on the fat/cancer connection comes from George L. Blackburn, M.D., Ph.D., associate professor of surgery at Harvard Medical School and chief of the Nutrition/Metabolism Laboratory at the Cancer Research Institute of New England Deaconess Hospital in Boston.

Dr. Blackburn says that the Japanese eat roughly half as much fat as we do, and their postmenopausal breast cancer rate is half ours.

His conclusion: "Studies that compare different cultures have found that people whose diets are the lowest in fat have the lowest breast cancer rates."

Researchers are also moving ever closer to linking fat with colon and rectal cancer. A Harvard study comparing the eating habits of 7,284 men found that those who ate low-fat, high-fiber diets were 3.7 times less likely to develop polyps in the colon and rectum polyps—tiny growths of tissue that can turn into cancer. However, men who regularly ate red meat instead of less-fatty chicken and fish had an 80 percent greater risk of developing polyps, the study shows.

Although more research needs to be done, cancer of the colon may just be another example of cell growth gone haywire from too much fat. Excess polyunsaturated fat (greater than 6 percent of daily calories) actually forces the colon cells to grow faster. Combine this with the lack of fiber commonly found in a high-fat diet, and the environment is right for the growth of potentially cancerous polyps, says Dr. Blackburn.

OBESITY: BIGGER, NOT BETTER

It's no secret that a high-fat diet will also make you a bigger (but not necessarily better) person.

What's less well known is that obesity itself is a killer. If you're 35 percent overweight, for example, your chances of premature death are 50 percent higher than normal. People who are 100 percent overweight are as much as 600 percent more likely to die prematurely.

THESE HEALTHIER FOODS PASS THE TASTE TEST

In the interest of science—and healthy eating, of course—the editors of *Prevention* magazine put their taste buds on the line to determine just how good those newly marketed nonfat versions of traditionally fatty foods really are.

The good news: You don't have to sacrifice satisfaction for security. Nonfat sour cream tastes great on a baked potato and has the same "mouthfeel" as the real thing. A fat-free, three-bean vegetarian chili with only 90 calories per serving proved zesty. A potato salad made with nonfat mayonnaise stumped half the staff when they were forced to choose between the nonfat version and one made with regular mayo. Nine out of ten preferred tuna salad made with water-packed tuna and nonfat mayo over the traditional version. Nonfat frozen yogurt, waffles and even pound cake all scored big on taste without the fat.

In checking out the "lite" fare at the local grocery, be aware that not all lite foods are low in fat. Lite potato chips may have less fat than regular brands but may still be high in fat. Lite bread can be the same old loaf—just sliced thinner.

To cut through the clutter, simply study the label. Many reduced-fat-and-calorie foods labels list nutrient information for both that product and their full-fat regular version. If not, you'll have to look for the full-fat version on the shelf and compare. In any case, calorie and fat amounts for the lite version should be reduced to about 25 percent of the original. Also important: Any food that delivers three grams of fat or less per 100 calories is a good choice, whether you see "lite" on the label or not.

What makes you pack on the pounds? Eating more calories than you burn. Here's the math: one gram of carbohydrate or protein is equal to four calories. One gram of dietary fat is equal to more than double that—over nine calories. Translation: A gram of fat takes twice as much effort to burn off as a gram of carbohydrate or protein.

Your body is also a tightwad as far as dietary fat is concerned; it would rather save (store) the fat than spend (burn) it. When it comes to storing fat, almost none of the fat you eat is burned in the conversion process from food to ready energy. By contrast, approximately 20 percent of complex carbohydrates disappear during the same transformation.

But your body *will* burn fat, provided you reduce the amount of fat you're eating, according to a Cornell University study. In fact, researchers found that women fed low-fat foods for 5½ months lost about ½ pound a week.

And no one was counting the calories of the food they were eating—feasts that included special low-fat versions of ice cream, cookies and pizza. But they were counting fat. All of the foods contained less than 25 percent fat as a percentage of total calories.

"The weight loss is relatively slow, but it's persistent and should result in a 10 percent loss of body weight per year," says David Levitsky, Ph.D., professor of nutrition and psychology at Cornell.

THE DIABETES CONNECTION

Life-threatening weight gain may seem bad enough, but unfortunately, obesity can also create another health hazard—diabetes. In fact, diabetes has been so closely linked to obesity that the American Diabetes Association coined the term "diabesity" to describe the connection, according to W. Stephen Pray, Ph.D., a professor of pharmaceutics at the School of Pharmacy at Southwestern Oklahoma State University, who's written extensively on the topic.

About 10 percent of diabetics are born with the disease, which can lead to blindness, kidney failure, even death. But most cases are caused by overeating, says Dr. Pray.

When you constantly eat too much—a common problem associated with a high-fat diet—your pancreas gets a workout. This large insulin-producing gland is treated like a factory that's added extra shifts to keep up. After years of overproduction, your pancreas may simply shut down, unable to produce the insulin your body needs to turn your food into energy, says Dr. Pray.

To get production in the insulin factory back in gear, says Dr. Pray, many people need only stop overeating. The pancreas may soon return to normal, eliminating the need for shots, pills, or other medication, he says. (If you have diabetes, always check with your doctor before making any changes in diet or medication.)

KNOWLEDGE IS POWER

By now you're probably convinced that eating a low-fat diet could be the best thing since shop-at-home television. But perhaps you're wondering if you can develop a low-fat eating plan and make it stick.

Don't worry. A landmark study for the National Cancer Institute shows that you can—if you're willing to apply your new-found nutritional knowledge.

Researchers divided 303 women into two groups. One received detailed nutritional information—like the kind found in this book. The other got no nutrition news.

Within six months, the amateur nutrition experts had slashed their dietary fat from 39 percent to 21 percent—an astonishing reduction! They were still sticking to their low-fat guns two years later. The no-nutritional-news crowd, however, showed virtually no improvement in their high-fat ways.

What follows is a collection of fat-busting techniques. Read them and select a particular diet or combine some of the tips to create your own personalized low-fat eating plan.

Whatever your approach, give yourself a chance to succeed: Changing lifelong habits takes time. Just ask William Fanizzi. "If I can stay away from Italian sausages, anyone can cut the amount of fat they're eating," he says.

ARE YOU READY TO TAKE THESE STEPS?

Although Step One and Step Two diets sound like a weight-loss program developed by Fred Astaire and Ginger Rogers, they're actually the AHA's approach to progressively reducing the amount of fat you're eating.

But be warned: Because it's less austere than other diets, some experts—like Dr. Dean Ornish—have criticized the AHA's approach. The AHA counters that many people are unable to make the dramatic dietary changes necessary to conform with harsh low-fat eating plans.

Before beginning either the Step One or Step Two diets, the AHA recommends that you have your cholesterol checked and then checked again, one to eight weeks after the first test.

Your cholesterol level is considered desirable if it's below 200. If it's between 200 and 239 milligrams, it's borderline high. If your cholesterol is above 240 milligrams, it's considered high.

STEP ONE

Under the Step One diet, total fat intake is set at less than 30 percent of calories. Saturated fat should be less than 10 percent of calories. Polyunsaturated fat should not exceed 10 percent of calories. Cholesterol intake should not exceed 300 milligrams a day. Carbohydrates should make up 50 percent or more of calories, with emphasis on complex carbohydrates. The rest of the calories should come from protein.

Within three months of starting the Step One diet, your cholesterol level should decline 10 to 15 percent.

A sample Step One diet supplying 1,600 calories a day includes:

Breakfast: Half a fresh grapefruit, 1 cup corn flakes, 1 nectarine, 1 cup 1 percent milk.

Lunch: 2 ounces broiled chicken thigh, one ear of corn on the cob with 1 teaspoon unsalted margarine, tossed salad (1 cup lettuce, 6 cucumber slices, Italian salad dressing), 5 slices melba toast, ½ cup strawberry frozen yogurt.

Dinner: 4 ounces round steak, ½ cup canned tomatoes, half a green pepper, 2 tablespoons diced onions, 3 steamed broccoli spears, carrot-raisin salad (made with ½ cup shredded carrots, 2 tablespoons raisins and 2 teaspoons mayonnaise), 1 whole-wheat dinner roll, 1 teaspoon unsalted margarine, 1 cup 1 percent milk, a small piece of angel food cake.

STEP TWO

If stronger dietary medicine is called for, the Step Two diet is designed to bring your saturated fat consumption to a new low, reducing it to less than 7 percent of total calories. Meanwhile, cholesterol is cut back to 200 milligrams a day. Depending on the specific foods chosen, total fat intake may also decline.

A sample Step Two, 1,600-calorie-a-day diet includes:

Breakfast: 1 cup cantaloupe cubes, 1 cup corn flakes, 1¼ cups strawberries, 1 cup skim milk, 1 slice whole-wheat toast, 1 teaspoon unsalted margarine.

Lunch: A turkey sandwich (made with 3 ounces turkey breast, 2 slices whole-wheat bread, 2 teaspoons mayonnaise, 1 lettuce leaf, 2 slices tomato), a tossed salad (made with 1 cup lettuce, 1 sliced tomato and 2 tablespoons French dressing), 1 apple.

Dinner: 3 ounces roast beef, ½ cup new potatoes, 1 teaspoon unsalted margarine, ½ cup steamed green beans, ½ cup steamed carrots, tossed salad (made with 1 cup romaine lettuce, 1 sliced tomato and vinegar), 1 cup skim milk, ⅔ cup orange sherbet.

THE PRITIKIN PLAN

To the late Nathan Pritikin—creator of the Pritikin Plan—fat and cholesterol were tantamount to arsenic. So it's no surprise that his program advocates one of the leanest diets around, allowing no more than 10 percent of calories from fat. Complex carbohydrates—like rice, pasta or beans—are supposed to take up a whopping 75 to 80 percent of the entire diet, while protein makes up 10 to 15 percent, according to Monroe Rosenthal, M.D., medical director of the Ocean View Medical Group at the Pritikin Longevity Center in Santa Monica, California.

The goal: to achieve a total cholesterol level of 100 plus your age, with 160 the maximum."There's no question that the data is out there to support

FIGURING YOUR FAT

Now that you've passed your own personal (your name here) Fat Reduction Act, you need to know how much fat you're putting in your mouth on a day-by-day basis.

There are two ways of keeping track. To figure the percentage of fat calories in any food, check the label for both grams of fat and calories per serving, then plug them into this formula: grams of fat × 9 ÷ total calories = percent of calories from fat.

For example: The label on a bag of potato chips indicates that each 160-calorie serving has ten grams of fat. Simply multiply those ten grams by nine (90), then divide by total calories (160), which gives you 0.56 or 56 percent fat.

If you're not a math whiz, you can keep track of the amount of fat in your diet by simply adding up the grams of fat you eat during the day. Most foods list the grams of fat per serving on the label.

To help you set your daily fat goals, we've done the calculations for you. They're based on 25 percent of your usual caloric intake. On average, nondieting women take in about 2,000 calories per day and men eat about 2,700.

If you find you're running over your fat budget at any time, simply cut back on the amount of fat you eat during the rest of the day in snacks and meals. Or if you've blown it for the day, cut back the following day.

CALORIE INTAKE	FAT (g.)
1,200	33
1,400	39
1,600	44
1,800	50
2,000	56
2,200	61
2,400	67
2,600	72
2,800	78

the dramatic benefits of a low-fat, low-cholesterol diet such as we advocate," says Dr. Rosenthal.

In the Pritikin Plan, foods are assigned to three categories: go, caution and stop, according to Dr. Rosenthal.

Go foods. These include fresh fruits, vegetables, whole grains, nonfat dairy products, legumes, fish and lean fowl or lean red meat, he says.

Caution foods. These foods, which should be eaten in moderation, include sweeteners like honey and molasses, decaffeinated coffee, tea, low-sodium soy sauce, low-fat dairy products, monounsaturated and polyunsaturated oils, unsalted nuts, avocados and olives.

Stop foods. These are forbidden because they significantly raise the risk of heart disease, he says. They include animal fats, butter, tropical oils, mayonnaise, fatty meats, whole dairy products, salt, coconuts and macadamia nuts, egg yolks and fried foods.

Daily allowances under the plan include two servings of nonfat yogurt or skim milk, six to eight servings of vegetables, three whole fruits, four to five servings of unrefined carbohydrates like whole-grain bread, pasta, rice, beans, peas or potatoes, and one 3½-ounce serving of lean meat, poultry or fish, Dr. Rosenthal says.

"The average participant gets a 23 percent reduction in total cholesterol in a period of three weeks. In the first week alone they usually get a 17 percent reduction. We frequently see people come in with high blood pressure and adult-onset diabetes who leave the center in a few weeks with normal blood pressure, normal blood sugar, no symptoms and no need for medication," he says.

FAT-FIGHTING TIPS

No matter what diet you choose, you can boost your chances of success by making low-fat choices at the supermarket or restaurant and in the kitchen by using these tips, suggested by the American Cancer Society, the American Heart Association and other experts.

SHOPPING

Make a map. Plan your trip to the supermarket by writing down the items you need on a list. Avoid impulse purchases.

Fill 'er up before you go. Never shop on an empty stomach.

Read the label, set a better table. Ingredients are listed in order of quantity—if you see fat or oil in the top four, be wary.

Get lean. When buying beef, choose either USDA Choice or Select for the leanest cuts. Because they have more marbling, USDA Prime meats contain more fat.

Avoid organ and lunch meats. Brains, heart, kidney, liver and sweetbreads are high in fat. Ditto for bologna, hot dogs and sausages.

DINING OUT

Drop a quarter. If a restaurant is unfamiliar to you, call and ask about their menu and cooking techniques.

Belly up to the bar. The salad bar, that is. Stay away from mayonnaise-based items and fatty dressings or condiments such as cheese, bacon bits and croutons.

Have it your way. Don't be afraid to special order entrées (broiled instead of fried) or substitute (salad instead of fries). Airlines also offer low-fat meals if you order ahead.

Bag it. Take home the remainder of a large portion of meat in a doggie bag and save it for another meal.

Say (no) cheese. Bag the cheese (and mayo) the next time you order a burger. Or get a chicken sandwich instead—just make sure it's not deep-fried.

Go topless. If an entrée is served with breading, topping or sauce, remove it before eating.

Be a crust-buster. If a fruit pie is served, avoid fat by eating the filling and leaving the crust.

REVISING RECIPES

Swap your sour cream. Puree low-fat or nonfat cottage cheese or light ricotta cheese. Mix in an equal amount of nonfat yogurt and a squeeze of lemon.

Substitute your white sauce. Puree low-fat or nonfat cottage cheese, thin with skim milk and mix with sautéed onions and garlic plus basil.

Banish eggs and oil. Buttermilk works just as well in Caesar salad dressing.

Quit putting cream in creamy soups. Cook your choice of vegetables with cubed potatoes or precooked white beans and defatted stock.

Discover herbs. Fresh cilantro, dill, garlic, parsley and chives are tasty replacements for those old, unhealthy standbys like oil and salt.

Stock up on chicken stock. Defatted chicken stock (scoop fat off the top after leaving in the refrigerator overnight) can be strained through cheesecloth and frozen in an ice cube tray for later use.

Whip up some (no-fat) whipped cream. Pour ⅓ cup skim milk into a small stainless steel or copper bowl. Set it in the freezer until ice crystals just begin to form (15 to 20 minutes). Thicken with a hand-held electric mixer by beating in ⅓ cup instant nonfat dry milk. Continue to beat on high until soft peaks form (about 2 minutes). If you like the cream sweetened, add 1 tablespoon honey and beat until stiff peaks form, about 2 minutes more. Use within 20 minutes.

COOKING MEAT

Start lean. After browning meat, make sure to pour off the fat. Ground meat is generally higher in fat than unground meat.

Make your burgers lose weight. To get really lean burgers, pick a piece of beef and then have your butcher trim the fat before grinding. Or put the piece of meat in the freezer briefly when you get home—even hidden fat turns white when chilled. Then trim it yourself and grind in a food processor.

Deal the right serving. Limit beef, pork and lamb servings to about 3½ ounces (a little larger than a deck of playing cards).

Marinate for your plate. Lean cuts don't have to be tough—marinate them in citrus juice and herbs, low-sodium soy sauce, vinegar or even yogurt. The acid in these marinades will help tenderize the meat and make it more tasty.

Rub it in. Basting meats with low-sodium broth, pineapple juice or low-sodium soy sauce will eliminate the need for added fat for cooking.

Do some stovetop grilling. Allow fat to drain during cooking by using a stovetop grill pan.

Broil (without oil). Position the pan so the meat is three to five inches from the heat, and use a broiling rack and drip pan.

Make the most of your roast. Larger, tougher cuts of meat undergo a change for more flavor in dry, 350° oven heat.

Don't brood—braise. Also good for tough, lean cuts. Braised meat is browned and then simmered in liquid for an hour or more.

Make clay. A clay cooker is a mini-oven in an oven, slowly roasting while sealing in moisture. The cooker and lid must be submerged in water before use. Don't preheat the oven—it could cause the cooker to crack. Allow the cooker to cool overnight before washing. Also, don't use soap during cleaning. The cooker may absorb the soap and then release it into food.

Wok this way. Stir-frying gives tough lean meat a second chance. Marinate before using.

Cut and fan. Slice meat thinly and then fan slices so it looks like you have an even larger serving.

Add crumbs. Adding one part fine bread crumbs for every two parts seasoned ground beef will cut down on the amount of fat you receive from each serving.

Cool it. After making stew or soup containing meat, refrigerate until the fat congeals and then scoop it off.

Favor chicken. Most poultry is lower in fat than red meat.

Add fish to your dish. Replace red meat with fish, which is lower in total fat. Among the best: cod, catfish, flounder, shark, haddock, perch and grouper.

Go meatless. Dry beans, peas, lentils and tofu are good alternate sources of protein if combined with low-fat dairy products.

CUTTING BACK ON OIL

Divide and conquer. Use half the amount of oil called for in a recipe. Most of the time it won't change the way the dish turns out.

Paint fat away. Instead of pouring cooking oil into a pan, apply it with a brush or paper towel. All you need to do is add a thin coating to prevent sticking.

Get serious about sautéing. Watch your technique when sautéing or stir-frying. If you keep the heat high and stir constantly, you will need little or no oil to keep food from sticking. Or simply use a nonstick skillet.

Hit the switch. Instead of using oil, sauté with broth, juice or water.

Bake the nonstick way. Coat muffin tins or cookie sheets with a no-stick spray instead of oil, or use no-stick baking pans.

Mix and match. In recipes that call for a very flavorful fat—like bacon fat—use one-quarter the required amount. Make up the rest of the measure by using one-quarter unsaturated vegetable oil like canola, and for the remaining half substitute water, vinegar or stock.

Pick a new flavor. Experiment with darker, less refined oils such as walnut, grapeseed or fruity olive oil in place of the blander, highly refined ones. You can use less of them because they have a definite flavor.

Get off the stick. Liquid margarine has less hydrogenated oil—a source of saturated fat—than stick margarine. And because you don't have to wait for it to melt on toast, you use less.

Don't get creamed. Cream substitutes like nondairy creamers, sour cream substitutes and whipped toppings are high in saturated fat, according to the AHA, because they often contain coconut, palm or palm-kernel oil. Avoid them.

Pop off. No oil is needed to cook popcorn when you use an air popper. Simply follow the manufacturer's directions.

HIGH-NUTRITION RECIPES

LIGHTLY BREADED HALIBUT

Fish should be a staple in the low-fat kitchen. If one of the ways you enjoy it is breaded and fried, you'll like this version, which gives the same crisp results with only a fraction of the fat. Serve the fish with corn on the cob, roasted or baked potatoes and coleslaw made using nonfat mayonnaise or nonfat yogurt.

1 pound haddock fillet
2 tablespoons unbleached flour
1 egg white
1 tablespoon water
½ cup dry bread crumbs
½ teaspoon dried oregano
¼ teaspoon paprika
¼ teaspoon ground black pepper

Rinse the fish and pat it dry. Cut it into 8 equal pieces. Dredge the pieces in the flour.

In a shallow bowl, whisk together the egg white and water until well mixed but not frothy.

On a sheet of wax paper, combine the bread crumbs, oregano, paprika and pepper.

Dip each piece of fish into the egg white, letting the excess drip off. Then dredge in the bread crumbs, coating the piece thoroughly.

Coat a no-stick baking sheet with no-stick spray. Add the fish, leaving space between the pieces. Lightly coat the top of the fish with no-stick spray. Bake at 375° for 10 to 12 minutes, or until the fish is crisp and flakes easily with a fork.

Serves 4
Per serving: *192 calories, 3.3 g. fat (16% of calories), 0.6 g. dietary fiber, 36 mg. cholesterol, 168 mg. sodium*

GRILLED PORK MEDALLIONS WITH BRAISED BEANS

You might think pork has no place in a low-fat diet, but many cuts are quite lean. The tenderloin, in particular, is very low in fat and makes an elegant dinner. This recipe was created by master chef Victor Gielisse for the American Cancer Society's educational program, the Great American Food Fight Against Cancer. The flageolets called for are tender French kidney beans that range in color from pale green to creamy white. They're available dried in many specialty stores. If you can't find them, substitute white beans, such as pea beans, haricots or canellinis.

- **1 pound dried flageolet beans, soaked overnight**
- **1 tablespoon canola oil**
- **1 leek, white part only, cleaned and chopped**
- **1 tablespoon sherry extract (optional)**
- **1 teaspoon dried tarragon**
- **1½ tablespoons chopped fresh parsley**
- **¼ teaspoon ground black pepper**
- **2¼ cups defatted chicken stock**
- **4 tomatoes, peeled, seeded and diced**
- **1 pork tenderloin (about 20 ounces), trimmed of all visible fat**
- **2 zucchini, julienned**
- **2 yellow summer squash, julienned**

Drain the beans and place in a 4-quart pot. Add cold water to cover. Bring to a boil, then simmer over medium-low heat for 1 hour, or until almost tender. Drain and set aside.

In a 2-quart saucepan over medium heat, warm the oil. Add the leeks and sauté for 1 minute. Add the sherry extract, if desired, and cook for 1 minute. Add the tarragon, parsley, pepper and 2 cups of the stock. Bring to a boil.

Add the beans. Reduce the heat to low and simmer for 20 minutes, stirring occasionally. Add the tomatoes and heat through; keep warm.

Meanwhile, cut the pork into 6 equal medallions. Grill or broil until just cooked through, about 4 minutes per side. Keep warm.

In a large no-stick frying pan over medium-high heat, warm the remaining ¼ cup stock. Add the zucchini and squash. Sauté for 3 to 5 minutes, or until crisp-tender.

To serve, arrange the zucchini mixture in a circle around the outer edges of dinner plates. Use a slotted spoon to ladle the bean mixture in the center. Top with the pork.

Serves 6

Per serving: *440 calories, 6.5 g. fat (13% of calories), 7.8 g. dietary fiber, 62 mg. cholesterol, 99 mg. sodium*

LEAN BEEF STROGANOFF

Beef stroganoff has a reputation for being high in fat, largely because of the rich sour cream it contains and the well-marbled cuts of beef used. This version uses ground top round, which is very lean, and a light sauce made with evaporated skim milk. If buying ready-ground meat, choose beef labeled 92% fat-free. This recipe was created by Houston chef Raymond Potter for the American Cancer Society.

- **12 ounces ground lean top round**
- **2 cups thinly sliced mushrooms**
- **1 cup diced sweet red peppers**
- **1 cup sliced scallions**
- **¼ cup diced onions**
- **1 tablespoon olive oil**
- **1 cup evaporated skim milk**
- **½ cup water**
- **¼ cup cornstarch**
- **½ teaspoon cracked black pepper**
- **12 ounces medium no-yolk egg noodles**
- **¼ cup minced fresh parsley**

In a large no-stick frying pan over medium-high heat, brown the meat, breaking up the pieces. Line a platter with a triple layer of paper towels. Spoon the beef onto the paper so any excess fat can be absorbed.

Wipe out the frying pan with a paper towel. Place the pan over medium-high heat, sauté the mushrooms, peppers, scallions and onions in the oil for 10 minutes, or until nicely browned. Add the drained meat to the pan. Pour in the milk and bring to a simmer over medium heat.

In a cup, combine the water and cornstarch until dissolved. Pour into the pan. Stir until the mixture thickens. Season with the pepper.

Meanwhile, cook the noodles in a large pot of boiling water until just tender. Drain and stir into the beef mixture. Sprinkle with the parsley.

Serves 4

Per serving: *490 calories, 9.6 g. fat (18% of calories), 4 g. dietary fiber, 67 mg. cholesterol, 164 mg. sodium*

CREAMY PASTA SHELLS

Most pasta sauces, such as Alfredo and béchamel, are loaded with fat from butter, cream and large amounts of cheese. This light sauce has a surprise ingredient: cauliflower, which has a mild taste and smooth texture when cooked and pureed.

12 ounces cauliflower florets
1 large onion, sliced into thin wedges
½ cup thinly sliced green peppers
1 teaspoon olive oil
12 sun-dried tomatoes, thinly sliced
1 cup sliced pimentos
½ teaspoon dried oregano
¼ teaspoon dried basil
¼ teaspoon ground black pepper
⅛ teaspoon grated nutmeg
1⅓ cups low-fat milk
1 tablespoon lemon juice
¼ cup grated Parmesan cheese
8 ounces medium pasta shells

Steam the cauliflower for 15 minutes, or until very tender.

Meanwhile, in a large no-stick frying pan over medium-high heat, sauté the onions and peppers in the oil for 5 minutes. Add the tomatoes and cook for 5 minutes. Stir in the pimentos, oregano, basil, pepper and nutmeg. Cover and keep warm over low heat.

Transfer the cauliflower to a blender. Add the milk and lemon juice. Blend until smooth. Transfer to a 2-quart saucepan and warm over medium heat. Stir in the Parmesan. Pour over the vegetables.

In a large pot of boiling water, cook the shells until just tender. Drain. Serve topped with the vegetable mixture.

Serves 4
Per serving: *361 calories, 5.9 g. fat (11% of calories), 5 g. dietary fiber, 11 mg. cholesterol, 192 mg. sodium*

CHAPTER 9

CHOLESTEROL
A DIETARY TROUBLEMAKER

The media howls about it. Your doctor warns you about it and your daughter tells you she watches for it as intently as if it were a mysterious stranger prowling the neighborhood.

In fact, it's pretty hard to find someone who *isn't* talking about their cholesterol. But what are we really doing about it? Apparently not as much as we should. While Americans are seemingly obsessed about this strange-sounding substance swimming around in their arteries, far too many of us are running around with cholesterol levels higher than 200—the number doctors agree is the safe limit for cholesterol in the blood.

And it's really not all that surprising, say some experts, considering the fact that cholesterol—while plenty talked about—is still one of the most misunderstood hot topics in health. After all, it's not easy to avoid something you can't even see. And then there's all that talk about good cholesterol and bad cholesterol. And about fat and cholesterol. Or wait, could it be that fat *is* cholesterol?

CHOLESTEROL DOES MAKE A DIFFERENCE

It's time to be in the dark no longer. We're about to set you on the strong and healthy path to cholesterol knowledge.

First, the hard truth. Eating too many foods rich in cholesterol, such as meat (especially organ meats), eggs and whole-milk dairy products, is a major contributor to heart disease, says Richard Shekelle, Ph.D., professor of epidemiology at the University of Texas Health Science Center in Houston.

And the evidence is spread far and wide.

In a classic 19-year follow-up study of 1,900 middle-aged men working at a Western Electric plant in Chicago, Dr. Shekelle and his colleagues linked dietary cholesterol to increased risk of fatal heart attacks. They found, for example, that if a man who was consuming 2,500 calories daily ate an additional 500 milligrams of cholesterol a day—the amount in two large egg yolks—he was 90 percent more likely to die of a heart attack than a man who didn't eat that extra cholesterol.

In addition, the researchers estimated that men who ate the lower amount of cholesterol had a life expectancy that was nearly 3½ years longer on average than that of men who regularly ate the higher amount of cholesterol.

"Our study and several other studies have found that dietary cholesterol does make a difference in the risk of developing a heart attack," Dr. Shekelle says.

In yet another major study, researchers followed the dietary habits of more than 8,000 Japanese-American men living in Honolulu. After ten years, the researchers concluded that, in addition to eating more protein, fat and saturated fat, the men who developed heart disease ate more cholesterol-rich foods than the men who didn't.

And, in a 20-year comparison study of men living in Ireland and Irish-Americans living in Boston, researchers found that those who died of heart disease were more likely to have consumed high amounts of saturated fat and cholesterol.

Overall, these studies indicate for every additional 200 milligrams of cholesterol you regularly consume per 1,000 calories, you increase your risk of heart disease by 30 percent, according to Jeremiah Stamler, M.D., a professor emeritus at the Northwestern University Medical School in Chicago.

The Good, the Bad and the Difference

Now you know you were right all along—you *should* be concerned about your cholesterol. But what exactly is it that makes it such a menace to the body? After all, you do remember learning in biology class that cholesterol is an essential component of life. And it's true. Your body needs cholesterol to make cell membranes, hormones and bile acids. But your body makes all the cholesterol it will ever need on its own. The rest—meaning the cholesterol in the food that you eat—is pure excess. Here's what happens.

Cholesterol gets around in your bloodstream wrapped in substances called lipoproteins—packages of protein molecules and triglycerides (a type of fat). Low-density lipoprotein, commonly called LDL cholesterol, is the bad kind of cholesterol you've been hearing about. Unfortunately, it typically makes up about 70 percent of the cholesterol in the body. It's the one responsible for forming the plaque that builds up on artery walls, creating dangerous blockages that may choke off the blood supply and cause a heart attack.

But, yes, there is a good cholesterol. It goes by the name high-density lipoprotein, or HDL cholesterol. As HDL circulates through your blood it heads for the liver. There it is converted into bile acids or excreted from the body. On its journey it picks up LDL cholesterol—but only as much as it can handle—and takes it along out of the body. That's what's so good about it. And that's why, researchers have found, that the more HDL you have, the

How Foods Measure Up

You can't see it, smell it or taste it. So how do you know when you're eating something that contains cholesterol? Well, here's a big clue: Cholesterol is found in any food of animal origin—including beef, chicken, fish, milk and eggs. The key is to limit the amount of those foods you eat and consume those that have the least amount of cholesterol and saturated fat. The following table ranks the cholesterol and saturated fat content of some common foods.

Food	Portion	Cholesterol (mg.)	Saturated Fat (g.)
Pork kidney	3 oz.	408	1.3
Beef liver	3 oz.	331	1.6
Beef kidney	3 oz.	329	0.9
Quiche Lorraine	1 slice	285	23.2
Egg	1	212	1.6
French vanilla ice cream, soft serve	1 cup	153	13.5
Veal cutlet	3 oz.	115	1.6
Waffle	1 (7")	102	4.0
Bearnaise sauce	½ cup	99	20.9
Hollandaise sauce	½ cup	94	20.9
Liverwurst	3 oz.	90	6.0
Chuck roast	3 oz.	86	2.7
Turkey bologna	3 slices	84	4.4
Corned beef	3 oz.	83	5.4
Lamb loin chop	3 oz.	81	2.9
Duck, without skin	3 oz.	76	3.6
Salmon	3 oz.	74	1.6
Chicken breast, roasted	3 oz.	73	0.9
Extra-lean ground beef	3 oz.	71	5.5
T-bone steak	3 oz.	68	3.5
Haddock	3 oz.	63	0.1

better off you will be. In fact, doctors now feel that the individual values of your HDL and LDL are a better indicator of heart health than total cholesterol. An HDL level of 70 or higher is considered protective against heart disease.

"Eating cholesterol raises cholesterol in your body. There's no question about that," says Daniel Eisenberg, M.D., a Los Angeles cardiologist and assistant clinical professor at the University of Southern California School of Medicine. And American cholesterol levels are typically too high because we eat too much cholesterol—an average of 400 to 500 milligrams per day in

FOOD	PORTION	CHOLESTEROL (mg.)	SATURATED FAT (g.)
Rainbow trout	3 oz.	62	0.7
Vanilla ice cream, regular	1 cup	59	8.9
Beef, eye of round, lean	3 oz.	59	1.5
Turkey breast	3 oz.	59	0.9
Whole-milk ricotta cheese	½ cup	58	9.4
Salami	3 oz.	55	7.7
Egg noodles	1 cup	53	0.5
Cod	3 oz.	47	0.1
Bran muffin, homemade	1	41	1.2
Snapper	3 oz.	40	0.3
Whole milk	1 cup	35	5.6
Halibut	3 oz.	35	0.4
Yellow layer cake w/icing	1 slice	33	2.8
Fig bars	4	27	0.9
Butter	2 tsp.	21	4.8
2% milk	1 cup	18	2.9
Cottage cheese, creamed	½ cup	17	3.2
Mozzarella cheese	1 oz.	16	2.8
Sherbet	1 cup	14	2.4
Low-fat yogurt, plain	1 cup	14	2.3
Buttermilk	1 cup	9	1.3
Cream pie	1 slice	8	15.0
Skim milk	1 cup	4	0.3
Pudding pops	1	1	2.5
Corn chips	1 oz.	0	1.5
Margarine, stick	2 tsp.	0	1.5
Popcorn, air-popped	1 cup	0	trace
Gelatin	½ cup	0	0

meats and animal products such as ice cream, cheese and butter. And the excess ends up exactly where we don't want it: on our artery walls. Experts estimate that for every 100 milligrams of dietary cholesterol consumed per 1,000 calories on a regular basis, blood cholesterol rises by about ten points.

The Fat Connection

Of course it's foolish to think that we can totally avoid cholesterol. But we can limit it. According to both the American Heart Association and the National Cholesterol Education Program, the safe limit for cholesterol consumption is less than 300 milligrams a day. And the easiest way to reach that goal is to restrict your intake of saturated fat. For saturated fat raises blood cholesterol even more than dietary cholesterol does. And both saturated fat and cholesterol are usually found in the same foods.

Studies show that adhering to a low-fat eating program has helped many people lower their cholesterol by 10 to 15 percent and reduce their estimated risk of coronary heart disease by 20 to 30 percent.

If you have any excess cholesterol in your body, it's safe to assume that two-thirds of it started out as saturated fat on your plate, says William P. Castelli, M.D., director of the Framingham Heart Study.

"My bias is that saturated fat is as bad or even worse for blood cholesterol levels than dietary cholesterol is," says Carl Lavie, M.D., a co-director of cardiac rehabilitation and prevention at the Ochsner Medical Institution in New Orleans.

"Fortunately, most foods that are high in saturated fat are also high in cholesterol. So if you avoid one type of food because of saturated fat, you're probably leaving cholesterol out of your diet, too," says Alan Chait, M.D., past chairman of the American Heart Association Nutrition Committee.

But there are some foods that have high amounts of cholesterol *without* saturated fat. Seafood and eggs are the best example. Eggs are very low in fat but, ounce for ounce, contain more cholesterol than any other food.

How to Avoid Shell Shock

The fact that eggs are laden with cholesterol is hardly news to anyone anymore. Egg consumption in the United States has dropped more than 20 percent since 1967. Americans have gone from eating 316 eggs annually per person to 249. That still averages out to more than 20 dozen eggs a year per person. Yes, you probably eat more eggs than you think. For even if you don't break eggs into a pan for your morning breakfast, you can still get more than your share in the baked goods and other prepared foods you eat every day.

And we're not just talking chickens here. Fish eggs such as roe or caviar also have large amounts of cholesterol.

Nature planned it that way. "Cholesterol is absolutely vital to creating

NIBBLE AWAY AT CHOLESTEROL

If you're serious about watching your cholesterol, then changing *how often* you eat may be as important as altering *what* you eat.

Small meals eaten frequently during the day may help keep your cholesterol under control and reduce your heart attack risk, according to researchers at the University of Toronto in Ontario.

In a preliminary study of seven men who each ate 17 meals totaling 2,500 to 3,000 calories a day, the researchers found that after two weeks total cholesterol levels dropped 9 percent and LDL cholesterol (the "bad" cholesterol) fell 14 percent.

The researchers believe that large meals cause the release of high levels of insulin. That, in turn, seems to stimulate cholesterol production by the liver. Eating frequent but smaller meals apparently short-circuits that process, says Thomas Wolever, M.D., Ph.D., a coauthor of the study and associate director of the Risk Factor Modification Center at St. Michael's Hospital in Toronto.

Of course, eating 17 meals a day isn't practical for most people—the men who did it ate prepackaged meals and carried alarm clocks to remind themselves when to eat. Moreover, Dr. Wolever thinks it would take discipline to avoid overeating. (In the study, a typical "meal" was either a couple of cookies, an apple or a half-sandwich.)

A later study of 2,000 people by researchers at the University of California at San Diego found drops in both total and LDL cholesterol in those eating four or more meals a day. "The key is taking whatever you're eating and spreading it out throughout the day. So eating five meals a day is probably better than eating less than three," Dr. Wolever says. "Many people tend to eat one big meal a day. I think that eating three evenly sized meals is fine. But if your three meals are a cup of coffee for breakfast, a muffin for lunch and a huge meal at dinner, that's the wrong way to go about it."

and maintaining cell walls," says George Seperich, Ph.D., a food scientist and associate professor of agribusiness at Arizona State University in Tempe. "So when you eat the egg of any species, you're consuming something that is going to have a high amount of cholesterol.

"Egg consumption is something you need to be aware of if you want to keep your cholesterol consumption in check," he says. Here's how.

Opt for a substitute. Some food manufacturers are marketing egg substitutes that are cholesterol-free and are lower in fat than whole eggs. They're all made with egg whites and have vitamins and minerals added to replace the nutrients of the yolk. Because these egg substitutes can be frozen, a package can be stored up to a year. They can be used in any dish requiring eggs, including casseroles, pancakes and desserts. Unfortunately, you have to be willing to pay: Egg substitutes can cost up to three times as much as regular eggs.

Try making your own. As an alternative, try making your own homemade substitutes, suggest William Connor, M.D., and his wife, Sonja Connor, R.D., authors of *The New American Diet System.* To do it, put six egg whites, ¼ cup powdered nonfat milk and one tablespoon oil in a mixing bowl and then blend until smooth. You can use the mixture for cooking and baking just as you would regular eggs. (About ¼ cup equals one whole egg.) You can store it in a jar in your refrigerator for up to one week, or freeze it.

Two halves are better than a whole. Another alternative when baking is to use two egg whites in place of each whole egg called for in the recipe. To replace some of the fat that would come from the yolk and may be needed for a successful outcome, add one teaspoon of vegetable oil for every yolk not used.

A healthier omelet. If you occasionally still want to use some whole eggs—to make scrambled eggs or omelets—then try using three egg whites with just one egg yolk.

KNOW THE HIDING PLACES

Once you get beyond eggs, knowing where to find the cholesterol in food tends to get a little difficult for most people, says Mary Felando, R.D., a cardiovascular nutrition specialist in Los Angeles. But it's really quite easy. Just think animal. Cholesterol is only found in foods derived from animal sources—such as beef, lamb, pork, poultry, fish, shellfish, milk, butter, ice cream. You name it.

"But some people aren't aware of that connection," says Felando. "Many people who come to see me think that chicken doesn't have any cholesterol. So they're eating half a chicken every day for dinner," she says. "But in reality, chicken is a very high cholesterol food." The fat/cholesterol connection in food isn't so strong that you can automatically assume that the less fat, the less dietary cholesterol. It's not that simple.

A three-ounce piece of broiled chicken, for example, has 73 milligrams of cholesterol. But the same size portion of broiled T-bone steak has about 68 milligrams of cholesterol, even though it has more saturated fat.

Organ meats hit the top of the list as the foods containing the most cholesterol. Pork kidneys, for example, have more than 400 milligrams per three-ounce serving.

Shellfish, particularly shrimp, have always taken a bad rap for being a bad-for-you food because of all their cholesterol. In fact, shrimp's pretty high on the list at 166 milligrams for a three-ounce serving. And other fish,

TAKE THE SURF OVER THE TURF

If you feel guilty about eating shellfish because it's high in cholesterol, here's good news.

"You're better off eating shrimp, lobster and crab than you are eating Cheddar cheese, beef, pork or lamb," says William P. Castelli, M.D., director of the famed Framingham Heart Study. "And the other shellfish—oysters, clams and scallops—are the best 'meats' you could possibly eat because they're the vegetarians of the sea and are very low in saturated fat and cholesterol."

In fact, researchers at the University of Washington who fed 18 men six types of shellfish for 21 days in place of cheese, meat and eggs found that some shellfish had a positive influence on blood cholesterol. Among the men who ate crabs, clams, mussels and oysters, levels of harmful LDL cholesterol, dropped. Levels of the good HDL cholesterol rose. Shrimp and squid didn't improve cholesterol levels, but they didn't harm them either. Overall, the researchers concluded that shellfish—especially when replacing fatty meats—are good for the heart.

And there's more good news for seafood lovers. Because of advances in testing methods, shellfish have been found to contain less cholesterol than was once believed.

Here's how the most popular varieties of shellfish stack up. For comparison, A three-ounce serving of lean ground beef has 74 milligrams of cholesterol and 6.2 grams of saturated fat.

SEAFOOD (3 oz.)	CHOLESTEROL (mg.)	SATURATED FAT (g.)
Shrimp	166	0.25
Oysters	93	1.07
Crab, blue	85	0.19
Lobster	61	0.09
Clams	57	0.16
Mussels	48	0.72
Scallops	28	0.07

such as salmon and pollock, have about as much cholesterol as chicken. But these fish and shellfish have an advantage that meat doesn't: They are all low in saturated fat. And remember, saturated fat is the primary cholesterol elevator in the bloodstream.

In fact, there is another reason to favor fish and shellfish over other cholesterol-laden foods. They also contain fish oil, also known as omega-3 fatty acids, which have actually been shown to have a cholesterol-lowering effect in the body.

Be Cholesterol Conscious

Unless you intend to become a strict vegetarian, it's almost impossible to avoid cholesterol entirely. But you can keep within healthy limits by becoming a savvy cholesterol watcher.

Cut back on meat. Of course, the most obvious way to beat dietary cholesterol is to eliminate meats from your diet entirely. Short of that, try eating less meat.

"If you want to include animal foods in your diet, you should limit them to three or four ounces a day. That's one serving about the size of a deck of cards," Felando says. "You should choose fish most often. I'd say eat it at least three times a week."

Concentrate on carbos. Eating lots of plant foods such as beans, oat bran, grains, fruits, vegetables and potatoes is a good dietary strategy because they contain no cholesterol unless they're prepared with dairy products such as milk, butter or cheese.

"If you're not eating a lot of starchy (carbohydrate) foods, you're not really following a low-fat, low-cholesterol diet. You should be having at least two to four servings of starches with every meal," Felando says. "I know it's hard for people to understand that because our mothers taught us to eat roast beef, but never to eat bread and mashed potatoes at the same meal. Even now, when my mother comes over and I serve corn and potatoes for dinner, she'll say, 'Isn't this two starches together?' But it's really okay because the people in nations that eat a lot of starches are the people who don't have problems with cholesterol."

And beans and oats add a special punch: Eating them has been shown to help bring cholesterol down.

Check out those label claims. When you're shopping, read food labels and be cautious about product claims, says Dr. Lavie. A product such as potato chips, for example, may be labeled cholesterol-free, but may contain significant amounts of saturated fat which you now know, raises the cholesterol level in your body.

"Only by being a skeptical and educated consumer can you cut through some of that. You need to be wary," says Karen Glanz, Ph.D., a professor of health education at Temple University in Philadelphia.

Be flexible. The secret is not to be too rigid about what you eat from day to day, suggests Karen Donato, R.D., coordinator of nutrition education and special initiatives for the National Heart, Lung, and Blood Institute in Bethesda, Maryland.

"It's not any one food, one meal or one day that's going to cause a high blood cholesterol problem," she says. "It's the cumulative effect that's the concern. In planning meals, you should try to average things out so that over a span of several days you're consuming less than 300 milligrams of

TAKE THE CHOLESTEROL PLUNGE

If making a few dietary changes can lower your cholesterol a bit, what kind of effort does it take to send your cholesterol diving?

"The key factor is diet," says Monroe Rosenthal, M.D., medical director of the Ocean View Medical Group at the Pritikin Longevity Center in Santa Monica, California. "When you push dietary cholesterol and saturated fat way down below a certain threshold, you'll see a dramatic linear response in the blood."

Exactly what that threshold is, no one knows for sure. But Dr. Rosenthal believes that it's less than 100 milligrams of cholesterol a day—a level that's consistent with the Pritikin Eating Plan, containing less than 10 percent of calories from fat. (The average American eats about 500 milligrams of cholesterol a day in a diet that contains about 40 percent fat).

"We do know that if someone switches from a high-fat diet to a somewhat modified diet, the effect on blood cholesterol is usually minimal," Dr. Rosenthal says. "But if that person then goes from a moderately reduced-fat diet to the Pritikin Eating Plan, in which cholesterol and saturated fat are drastically cut, blood cholesterol could take a steep drop."

On the Pritikin Eating Plan, participants are advised to consume no more than one 3½-ounce serving of lean meat, poultry, or fish and two cups nonfat dairy products per day. (Egg yolks and organ meats are not allowed.) Generally, the focus of the diet consists of fresh fruits and vegetables, whole grains, cereals, legumes and potatoes.

The results? The average cholesterol drop at the Pritikin Longevity Center in a 21-day period is a dramatic 23 percent. But many Pritikin participants do even better than that, Dr. Rosenthal says. In some cases, cholesterol levels have tumbled as much as 40 percent in three weeks.

dietary cholesterol daily. So if you have 600 milligrams one day, 200 the next, 250 the day after, and 150 the following day, it will still average out properly.

"That's the moral of the story here," she says. "We're not telling people that they can never eat eggs, cheese, meat or other foods that have saturated fat and cholesterol in them. We're not telling them that they have to totally revamp the way they eat. But there are some subtle dietary changes that they can make that will bring their cholesterol levels down."

HIGH-NUTRITION RECIPES

CHICKEN AND AVOCADO

Avocados have such a rich, creamy texture that you'd swear they were loaded with cholesterol—but, of course, only animal products contain the substance. This very easy recipe pairs them with chicken breasts, capers and quick-cooking brown rice. One thing you should know about avocados, though, is they contain a fair amount of fat, so you should save them for special occasions.

- **1¼ cups defatted chicken stock**
- **1 cup quick-cooking brown rice**
- **4 boneless, skinless chicken breast halves (4 ounces each)**
- **1 tablespoon unbleached flour**
- **1 tablespoon olive oil**
- **½ cup chopped pimentos**
- **2 tablespoons capers, rinsed**
- **½ cup lemon juice**
- **¼ cup minced fresh parsley**
- **½ avocado, thinly sliced**

In a 2-quart saucepan over medium heat, bring the stock to a boil. Add the rice. Cover and cook over medium-low heat for 10 minutes, until all the stock has been absorbed. Fluff with a fork and keep warm.

Meanwhile, dredge the chicken in the flour. In a large no-stick frying pan over medium-high heat, warm the oil. Add the chicken and brown for about 5 minutes per side, or until cooked through. Transfer to a plate and set aside.

Add the pimentos and capers to the pan. Sauté for 2 minutes. Add the lemon juice and cook over medium heat for 2 minutes, scraping up browned bits from the bottom of the pan with a wooden spoon. Stir in the parsley. Return the chicken to the pan and cook for 1 minute.

Serve with the rice and avocado slices.

Serves 4

Per serving: *347 calories, 10.1 g. fat (21% of calories), 3.1 g. dietary fiber, 66 mg. cholesterol, 203 mg. sodium*

LEAN CALIFORNIA BURGERS

Using ground turkey is an excellent way to cut back on fat when making burgers. This recipe uses the type of ground turkey readily available in supermarkets. For even leaner burgers, buy boneless turkey breast and grind it yourself in a food processor.

- **1 pound ground turkey**
- **½ cup dry bread crumbs**
- **2 tablespoons onion flakes**
- **2 tablespoons dried parsley flakes**
- **⅓ cup tomato sauce**
- **¼ cup fat-free egg substitute**
- **4 crusty hamburger buns**
- **4 thick tomato slices**
- **Lettuce**

In a large bowl, mix the turkey, bread crumbs, onion flakes and parsley flakes. Add the tomato sauce and egg. Mix well and form into 4 large patties.

Coat a broiler rack with no-stick spray. Place the patties on the rack and broil until browned on both sides and cooked through.

Serve on the buns topped with tomatoes and lettuce.

Serves 4
Per serving: *377 calories, 6.7 g. fat (16% of calories), 2.6 g. dietary fiber, 74 mg. cholesterol, 641 mg. sodium*

ORIENTAL SEAFOOD AND RICE SALAD

Even though seafood, such as shrimp and scallops, does contain cholesterol, levels are lower than previously thought. More important, these foods are very low in saturated fat, which doctors believe to be more of a dietary culprit when it comes to raising serum cholesterol. Combining a modest amount of seafood with rice and vegetables, as in this salad, produces a hearty main course that's quite low in cholesterol.

6 ounces bay scallops
4 ounces medium shrimp, peeled, deveined and halved lengthwise
1 cup frozen peas
2 cups cold cooked rice
1 cup diced carrots
1 cup diced sweet red peppers
½ cup thinly sliced scallions
1 tablespoon olive oil
1 teaspoon sesame oil
2 tablespoons cider vinegar
1 tablespoon low-sodium soy sauce
1 tablespoon grated fresh ginger
1 clove garlic, minced
Pinch of ground red pepper
2 tablespoons toasted sesame seeds

Bring about 1" of water to a boil in a large frying pan. Add the scallops and shrimp. Poach over medium heat for about 4 minutes, or until the shrimp is just beginning to turn pink; do not overcook. Stir in the peas, then drain immediately.

In a large bowl, toss together the rice, carrots, diced peppers and scallions. Add the seafood mixture and toss lightly.

In a small bowl, whisk together the olive oil, sesame oil, vinegar, soy sauce, ginger, garlic and ground pepper. Pour over the salad and toss well. Sprinkle with the sesame seeds. Serve immediately or chill.

Serves 4
Per serving: *318 calories, 8.2 g. fat (23% of calories), 3.3 g. dietary fiber, 57 mg. cholesterol, 315 mg. sodium*

BEEF AND MUSHROOM LASAGNA

Finely chopped mushrooms have a meaty texture and taste, so you can substitute them for part of the ground beef in many recipes. This lasagna uses skim milk and nonfat ricotta, both of which have less cholesterol than their full-fat counterparts, to further lower the cholesterol count.

- **9 lasagna noodles**
- **8 ounces extra-lean ground beef**
- **2 cups minced mushrooms**
- **1 cup finely chopped onions**
- **1 teaspoon dried basil**
- **¼ teaspoon ground black pepper**
- **2 cups skim milk**
- **2 tablespoons cornstarch**
- **1 cup nonfat ricotta cheese**
- **¼ cup fat-free egg substitute**
- **1¼ cups tomato sauce**
- **½ cup shredded part-skim mozzarella cheese**

Cook the lasagna in a large pot of boiling water for 12 minutes, or until just tender. Drain, rinse with cold water and set aside.

In a large no-stick frying pan over medium-high heat, brown the beef, breaking up the pieces. Add the mushrooms and onions. Cover the pan, reduce the heat to medium and cook for 3 minutes, or until the mushrooms have given up their liquid. Remove the lid and cook, stirring often, until the mixture is very dry. Stir in the basil and pepper; set aside.

In a 1-quart saucepan, whisk together the milk and cornstarch. Cook over medium heat, whisking frequently, until the mixture comes to a boil and thickens. Remove from the heat and whisk in the ricotta and egg. Stir into the beef mixture.

Coat a 9" × 13" baking dish with no-stick spray. Spread about ½ cup of the tomato sauce in the dish. Top with 3 of the noodles in a single layer and half of the beef mixture. Repeat with another layer of noodles and beef. Top with the remaining 3 noodles and ¾ cup tomato sauce. Sprinkle with the mozzarella.

Bake at 350° for 25 minutes. Let stand 10 minutes before cutting.

Serves 9

Tip: *The easiest way to mince the mushrooms is in the food processor. Halve or quarter about 8 ounces of mushrooms, then transfer to a food processor and chop with on/off turns. You'll end up with about 2 cups (don't worry if there's more; mushrooms have no fat and practically no calories, so you can use all you want in this casserole).*

Per serving: *244 calories, 6.9 g. fat (26% of calories), 1.3 g. dietary fiber, 20 mg. cholesterol, 269 mg. sodium*

CHAPTER 10

SODIUM
THE REWARDS OF MODERATION

Retired Pennsylvania steelworker Roy E. Rogers was the kind of person who thinks food without added salt is like champagne without the bubbles. Without salt, Roy believed, food would taste a little less tantalizing, a little too flat. But then he swapped his surplus sodium for something worthy of a champagne celebration: a new lease on life.

"As soon as the plate was set down, I'd pick up the saltshaker and go to town," Roy says. In the past, he wouldn't have dreamed of eating corn on the cob, a sirloin steak, a tomato salad or any other food on his plate without making it look like a snow-covered landscape.

But a super-high blood pressure reading and a strict warning from his doctor prompted Roy to mend his salty ways.

These days, Roy eats corn on the cob without a pinch of salt. He passes up mashed potatoes smothered in sauerkraut. Instead of salty sausage breakfasts at the fast-food restaurant, Roy has switched to whole-grain cereal. And when he feels the urge to toss a topping on his food, now it's more likely to be a sprinkling of herbs.

Roy's low-salt eating style has paid off. At his last checkup, his blood pressure had eased down an amazing 50 points, well within the normal, safe range. "I haven't had to take a single pill," he says.

A PRECAUTIONARY STEP

You don't have to wait until your blood pressure is sky-high to shake your salt habit and take a giant step toward better health.

There is mounting evidence to show that cutting back on dietary sodium may help keep your blood pressure in the safe zone and reduce your risk of heart attack and stroke.

That's the conclusion reached by three British researchers from the Medical College of St. Bartholomew's Hospital in London after analyzing published studies of blood pressure and sodium intake involving 47,000 people throughout the world.

After reviewing the data, the researchers made this stunning estimation: If all adults stopped eating highly salted processed food and adding salt at the table, the incidence of stroke could be reduced by 26 percent and heart disease by 15 percent.

"Few measures in preventive medicine are as simple and economical and yet can achieve so much," declared the researchers.

Does this mean we should confine ourselves to a menu of bland, boring food with as much flavor as a slice of cardboard? Are pretzels shimmering with white crystals never to cross our lips?

Let's not go overboard. "You should aim to limit *excessive* salt in your diet—not all salt," says Bonnie Liebman, a licensed nutritionist and director of nutrition for the Center for Science in the Public Interest in Washington, D.C.

Granted, there are some foods that aren't fit to eat without salt, she says. Cottage cheese containing no salt, for instance, is barely palatable. "The point is, once you've cut down on surplus salt by eating more foods with nonsalt seasonings, then there's room for some moderately salty foods."

A LITTLE SALT GOES A LONG WAY

Salt wasn't always regarded as the sinister white mineral in the black hat. In earlier days, salt was highly prized as a preservative for keeping meat and fish from spoiling and as a flavorful seasoning to cover up the taste of half-rotten food. So great was its value that sources were often depleted—wars were waged and lives were lost for salt.

Ironically, many people today are risking their lives over salt for the opposite reason: because it's so abundant in the foods we consume.

That's not to say we don't need any salt. Table salt, technically called sodium chloride, is the most common source of dietary sodium, a mineral our bodies need. Sodium's primary function is to regulate the proper balance of vital fluids and chemicals in our system.

But we can get all the sodium we need from the sodium naturally occurring in food without adding a pinch of salt. The estimated requirement is less than 500 milligrams a day—the equivalent of about ¼ teaspoon.

The problem is that the average American ingests anywhere from 3,000 to 6,000 milligrams of sodium—the equivalent of 1½ to 3 teaspoons of salt a day. That's more than ten times what we need.

Sound excessive? Actually, it can happen almost before you realize it. Consider, for example, that if you have nothing more than a pastry and two slices of Canadian bacon for breakfast (that's 1,800 milligrams of sodium), a serving of New England clam chowder for lunch (1,900 milligrams) and fast-food chicken with fries for dinner (1,100 milligrams), you've taken in almost 5,000 milligrams of sodium. Add a dill pickle and you gain nearly 1,000 milligrams more.

Many people seem to handle all that salt without any immediate detriment to their health. Their kidneys simply excrete the excess amount.

But for some people, the kidneys can't handle the overload. In these people, dubbed salt sensitive, the excess salt remains in the system. The blood-

DO YOU HAVE SALT WATER ON TAP?

You're careful about the foods you eat. Yet you may be getting more sodium than you'd find in a handful of corn chips each time you drink a glass of tap water.

Researchers have found that many U.S. communities exceed the 20 milligrams of sodium per liter limit for drinking water recommended by the American Heart Association for people on sodium-restricted diets. That could be a problem if you have high (or borderline high) blood pressure.

Scientists looking at drinking water in two communities showed that a higher level of sodium was related to higher blood pressure levels.

Keep in mind that sodium-rich drinking water doesn't always taste salty. To find out what your levels are, call your local health department. If your drinking water exceeds the recommended limit and you have high blood pressure, consult your physician. "The best advice for sodium-sensitive people may be to drink bottled water, which has no sodium," says Carolyn Hoffman, R.D., director of dietetics at Central Michigan University in Mount Pleasant.

You should also consider avoiding drinking water that has been softened by a home water softener. Water softeners replace calcium and magnesium (the minerals that make the water "hard") with sodium—a lot of sodium. Softening of water can increase the sodium content fivefold.

"If you use a water softener, you should run a separate pipe for your drinking water that bypasses the softening process," says Hoffman.

stream absorbs extra water to dilute the excess sodium, increasing the blood volume. Because the heart must pump harder to move this extra blood, pressure builds up in the arteries. Eventually, increased blood pressure (also called hypertension) can harden the arteries, making them susceptible to blockage. The result may be heart attack or stroke.

In this way, excess salt sets the stage for high blood pressure and possibly heart disease.

WHO IS SALT SENSITIVE?

Very specific medical tests are needed to accurately determine who is sodium sensitive and who isn't. But doctors say you could get a clue about salt's effects on your system from blood pressure measurements taken before and after going on a low-salt diet for six to eight weeks.

Your blood pressure measurement is a ratio of pressure that blood exerts against your arteries when the heart pumps (the systolic blood pressure) and when it's at rest (the diastolic blood pressure). Optimal blood pressure is 120/80 or less. High blood pressure is 140/90 or greater.

About half of the people with high blood pressure clearly are salt sensitive, according to G. Gopal Krishna, M.D., associate professor of medicine at the University of Pennsylvania in Philadelphia. Yet, there's emerging evidence showing that a lifetime of overdosing on salt could have unhealthy effects on most people's blood pressures.

To begin with, there's solid data showing that in salt-loving societies such as ours, blood pressure rises as we grow older. In a study called the Multiple Risk Factor Intervention Trial, for example, researchers measured blood pressure and then checked on the mortality rates of more than 350,000 men over a ten-year period. At the start, 80 percent of the men had above-optimal (greater than 120 systolic) blood pressure. And there were higher death rates for those who were above optimal—the higher the pressure, the higher the death rate.

In contrast, other studies reveal that in societies where very little salt is consumed, such as in remote parts of Brazil and parts of Africa, blood pressure does not rise significantly as people age. In fact, those populations rarely develop high blood pressure.

"Clearly, the evidence shows that an increase in blood pressure is not a natural phenomenon as we age," says Rose Stamler, professor of epidemiology and preventive medicine at Northwestern University Medical School in Chicago. "It's more likely that we're all genetically programmed—some more than others—to become 'salt sensitive' to today's high doses of salt."

This type of salt sensitivity, however, may not show up until our senior years, according to a lengthy study at the Indiana University School of Medicine's Hypertension Research Center in Indianapolis. In the study, people who had normal blood pressures did not show a sensitivity to salt until their sixth decade.

THE PRICE OF PLENTY

High blood pressure is the price many people pay for decades of ingesting 20 times more sodium than they need, says Stamler. For many, the kidneys and circulatory system just can't handle that kind of abuse.

In fact, says Stamler, "more than half of U.S. adults have high blood pressure by age 60." And while salt intake should certainly concern individuals with high blood pressure, she says, those with above-optimal (over 120/80) or borderline-high blood pressures also need to be careful. In one study, 20 percent of those people aged 30 to 44 who had high normal blood pressures and took no preventive measures moved up to definite hypertension in just five years.

The bottom line: "Most of us would benefit from reducing our salt intake, no matter what our current blood pressure," she says.

Other experts wholeheartedly agree. If your blood pressure is normal, cutting back on salt may keep it from rising, according to Norman Kaplan, M.D., professor of internal medicine at the University of Texas Southwestern Medical Center in Dallas. "Reducing sodium can't hurt; it may help and might even save your life," says Dr. Kaplan.

If your blood pressure is already high, most studies suggest that cutting your salt intake in half might lower your blood pressure several points, says Marvin Moser, M.D., clinical professor of medicine at Yale University School of Medicine.

If you're taking pills for high blood pressure, cutting back on salt might make it possible to go with less medication or none at all—though only your doctor can accurately advise you on this.

In the Hypertension Control Program study conducted jointly in Chicago and Minneapolis, patients with mild hypertension participated in nutritional therapy, including reduction of salt intake to not more than 4½ grams (1,800 milligrams of sodium) a day. After four years on this regimen, 39 percent of the patients were able to control their blood pressures without medication. As for those people who still required medication, salt reduction meant fewer pills and less side effects.

WHAT TO AIM FOR

The National Academy of Sciences says that we should consume no more than 2,400 milligrams of sodium a day. Ideally, we should aim for no more than 1,800 milligrams. That's the equivalent of just a smidgen less than a teaspoon of salt. (If you have high blood pressure, consult your doctor before making any dietary changes.)

To keep your salt intake at the one-teaspoon-a-day limit, you'll have to do more than swear off your saltshaker. Less than a quarter of our dietary sodium comes from salt sprinkled on food at the table and during cooking, studies show. More than three-fourths of our sodium intake comes from salt added by food manufacturers during processing.

Most convenience, or ready-to-eat, food is loaded with sodium, says Liebman. "Salt is a cheap way to add universally appealing flavor and sometimes increase shelf life," she says.

The more processing, the more sodium that's likely to be in the food. While 3½ ounces of raw potato contains just 7 milligrams of sodium, for example, the same amount of instant mashed potatoes dishes up 348 mil-

SODIUM LURKS WHERE YOU LEAST EXPECT IT

Which has more sodium: one homemade waffle or a pretzel? Incredibly, the waffle has over five times more sodium than the pretzel.

If you guessed wrong, it's no wonder. The presence of sodium isn't always easy to detect. Three-quarters of our dietary sodium is hidden in prepared foods. Surprisingly, waffles, bread, cereals and other grain products, not snack foods, are the leading source of sodium. Moreover, many salt-laced foods, such as pudding or diet soda, for instance, may not taste a bit salty. Yet one cup of pudding has more than 250 of milligrams of sodium. The soda contains about 35 milligrams.

Be on the lookout for these other sneaky sources of sodium.

FOOD	PORTION	SODIUM (mg.)
Chicken noodle soup	1 cup	1,106
Macaroni and cheese	1 cup	1,086
Low-fat (1%) cottage cheese	1 cup	918
Kidney beans, canned	1 cup	873
Tuna salad	1 cup	824
Roast beef sandwich	1	792
Turkey with gravy, frozen	5 oz.	787
Mushrooms, canned	1 cup	663
Tomato juice, canned	¾ cup	657
Potatoes au gratin, from mix	1 serving	601
Bologna	2 slices	578
Biscuits, from mix	1	350
Pizza with cheese	1 slice	336
Pancakes, from mix	2	322
Bacon	3 slices	303
Rice Krispies	1 cup	290
Beets, canned, cooked	½ cup slices	233
Nonfat yogurt	1 cup	174
Whole-wheat bread	1 slice	148
Shrimp, canned	3 oz.	144
Peanut butter	1 Tbsp.	76
Angel food cake	1 piece	58

ligrams. And the same weight of potato chips contains a whopping 469 milligrams. Likewise, a ½-cup serving of fresh peas contains only about 2 milligrams of sodium, while an equal amount of canned peas contains almost 100 times that much. Sodium even finds its way into our desserts: There are 147 milligrams in a piece of ready-to-eat apple pie compared to just a trace in a fresh apple.

The rule is: "Eat as close to fresh and 'from scratch' as possible," says Dr. Krishna.

Your menu should be laden with fresh fruits and vegetables, he adds, not just because salt is less abundant in these foods but also because they're rich in potassium.

"Potassium helps your body get rid of excess sodium," says Dr. Krishna. For optimum blood pressure control, he says, try to maintain a balance of potassium to sodium in your daily diet.

MAKE CUTBACKS GRADUALLY

Don't try to cut back on salt cold turkey. If you rush into low-salt eating, your taste buds will rebel and you'll be hunting for salty foods like a bear hunts down honey.

You can gently win your taste buds over to an appreciation of this new low-salt way of eating by mixing some low-sodium foods with higher-sodium ones. For example, you may not care for the bland taste of low-sodium cheese eaten alone. But the difference is not so noticeable if you blend low-sodium Cheddar and regular Swiss for melting on your homemade pizza. Here's another ploy: Try unsalted peanut butter atop a regular, salted cracker (or vice versa).

After three or four weeks of gradually decreasing salt, experts say you can expect your taste buds to be reformed and your salt cravings to wane. In a few months, you might even prefer less salty foods, one study suggests. Researchers compared the salt taste preferences of people on a low-sodium diet with those of people eating a normal diet. After five months, the low-salt group overwhelmingly chose less salty crackers while the other group had unchanged tastes.

AT HOME

The easiest way to begin trimming the salt from your diet is to cease sprinkling at the table or during cooking. Refuse to be a saltshaker robot—taste your food before salting it. Then if you still think it needs "a little something," read on.

Transform your saltshaker. Make it into a spice or herb shaker. Try filling it with dill, paprika and dried parsley—a great combo that can zip up everything from baked potatoes to meat loaf.

Use substitutes sparingly. Commercial salt substitutes contain potassi-

How to Season without Surrendering Flavor

If you're wondering how to appease your taste buds without salt, you need not worry. "There are hundreds of alternatives to salt," says Mary Winston, dietitian and author of the *American Heart Association Low-Salt Cookbook*. "Start by borrowing from some exotic cuisines: use items like curry, sesame seeds and ginger to create the taste of foods from India and China, for example. Or use table wines to impart a European flavor."

With a little imagination, you'll soon come to think of salty foods, as, well, salty. Here's how to add more spice to your life.

- **Experiment with herbal and spice blends.** For beef dishes, herbs such as marjoram, bay leaf and rosemary are naturals. For chicken, try curry powder, sage or savory. Allspice and turmeric are terrific on fish, while anise brings out the best in beets.
- **Mix and match tastes and textures.** Sweet foods matched with robust meats are particularly delicious, says Winston. Try roasting cinnamon-topped apple slices with pork chops. Or use mandarin orange wedges in a roast beef marinade.
- **Use fresh herbs whenever possible.** Prepare at the last moment and add them for "fresher, more 'alive' taste," says Winston.
- **Be prepared to pulverize.** Pound garlic, chilies and fresh herbs and spices with a mortar and pestle to release their flavors. And use a food processor to grate fresh horseradish, which packs more punch than the salted, bottled kind.
- **Treat yourself to dried toppings.** Mushrooms, tomatoes, cherries, cranberries and currants impart a more intense flavor when dried than when fresh, says Winston.
- **Discover citrus zest.** The zest of lemon, lime or orange is the part of the peel without the white pith. It actually holds the most intense flavor, says Winston. Grate it with a flat grater, to give just the right "bite" to foods.

um chloride. Adding a small amount of salt substitute to foods will make the food taste "salted," says dietitian Mary Winston of the American Heart Association in Dallas. But if you have high blood pressure and take medication, check with your doctor first. Potassium chloride can cause problems if you have kidney disease.

Be wary, too, of the so-called lite salts. The "lite" designation does not mean no sodium—just less of it.

Make friends with pepper. And pour on the garlic, onion and celery powders, too. (Just avoid the *salt* versions of these seasonings.)

Keep lemon juice handy. A drop or two from this perky fruit seems to have the same zesty effect on the taste buds as salt does, says Liebman. "Steamed broccoli dressed with lemon juice is delicious," she says.

Rinse canned goods. If you use canned foods, be sure to drain and rinse them. One study showed that rinsing canned green beans for one minute removed nearly half of their added sodium. Rinsing water-packed tuna for the same length of time reduces sodium by nearly 80 percent.

Switch to low-sodium baking ingredients. Cook and bake using unsalted margarine. Or use vegetable oil, which is salt-free. If a recipe calls for soup or bouillon, look for the low-salt variety. One regular instant bouillon cube contains 1,000 milligrams of sodium. That's almost half of the recommended quota for the day.

Experiment with homemade condiments. Most of those zippy commercial condiments can zap you with a heap of sodium. A single tablespoon of catsup or mustard has over 170 milligrams of sodium, for instance. A tablespoon of soy sauce has over 1,000 milligrams. One commercial chili seasoning for tacos has nearly 3,000 milligrams per one-ounce packet. A homemade version (made with paprika, crushed oregano, cumin, turmeric, garlic powder and ground red pepper) has virtually none.

When cooking from scratch, you can control the amount of sodium, says Winston. Here's how to give food zing without salt's sting.

- Mix mustard powder with water to make "a very sharp condiment that's just as powerful as the salty commercial kind," says Winston.
- Try a dash of aromatic bitters when making gravies, sauces or salad dressings.
- Sprinkle paprika on your popcorn.
- Drizzle flavored vinegars on garden greens. Rosemary-laced vinegar perks up radicchio and red-leaf lettuce, for example, with no oil needed. Flavored vinegars also provide great bases for making savory marinades for meats. Try tarragon vinegar mixed with a drop of hot-pepper sauce or unsalted liquid smoke. Pour it on chicken as it grills.

When Shopping

You've sworn off pickles, bacon and the other salty-tasting foods. That's the easy part. The fact is, most of our sodium is hidden in processed foods, commercial baked goods and fast foods. And often you can't rely on your tongue to steer you from these salt-laden foods; you must rely on your eyes.

Here's how to become a salt sleuth when you grocery shop.

Read labels with an eagle eye. Look for packaged products labeled "sodium-free" or "very low sodium." Under current Food and Drug Administration guidelines, products can only be called sodium-free if they contain less than 5 milligrams of sodium per serving; products labeled low sodium must not exceed 140 milligrams, and very low sodium cannot contain more than 35 milligrams of sodium per serving. On the other hand, a product labeled "one-third less" salt, such as Campbell's Healthy Request soup, for example, could still contain plenty of salt. In this case, one serving of chicken noodle has 420 milligrams less sodium than the regular version but still contains 460 milligrams.

Avoid products listing salt, or sodium chloride, or baking soda among the top five ingredients. In general, try to steer clear of items containing more than 150 milligrams of sodium per serving, suggests Stamler.

As far as avoiding foods containing other forms of sodium, such as monosodium glutamate, you don't have to be so careful, experts say. "Pre-

EXERCISE YOUR OPTIONS

With careful shopping, it's possible to choose many of your favorite foods in reduced-salt or no-salt varieties. Note the differences below.

FOOD	PORTION	SODIUM (mg.)
BUTTER		
Unsalted	1 Tbsp.	2
Salted	1 Tbsp.	117
CASHEWS		
Unsalted	1 cup	22
Salted	1 cup	877
CORN		
Fresh or frozen	1 cup	8
Canned	1 cup	646
CRACKERS		
Wheat	4	60
Saltines	4	125
GREEN BEANS		
Fresh	1 cup	4
Canned	1 cup	882
OATMEAL		
Cooked	1 cup	2
Instant	1 cup	285
PORK		
Pork chop	3 oz.	63
Canned ham	3 oz.	1,067
SWISS CHEESE		
Natural	1 oz.	74
Processed	1 oz.	390
TOMATO PASTE		
Unsalted	1 cup	170
Salted	1 cup	2,070

liminary studies seem to indicate that sodium chloride is the sole troublemaker in high blood pressure," says Dr. Krishna. "Other nonsalt sodiums don't seem to affect blood pressure."

Check out low-fat products carefully. Diet margarine, for example, has more sodium than regular margarine, according to Winston.

Look for low-salt versions of your favorite foods. Hundreds of low-sodium products from soups to nuts allow you to prepare your favorite meals without excess salt. If your traditional spaghetti recipe calls for a cup of marinara sauce, for example, substituting the reduced-salt type for the salted variety erases over 850 milligrams of sodium from your family's meal.

Sometimes these products are hard to find. Low-salt salsas, for example, might be relegated to the dietetic section of your supermarket. But the hunt is worth it. Here are some tips to set you in the right direction.

- Make a detour around the deli. Most deli items from prepared salads and dips to cold cuts are heavily salted. When possible, look for low-salt varieties. Request fresh cooked turkey or lean roast beef instead of precooked meats, for example.
- Steer clear of salt-laden dehydrated mixes for soups, sauces, salad dressings and puddings.
- Look for unsalted canned or frozen vegetables. Avoid those with sauces added.
- Ferret out the natural cheeses. Processed cheese and cheese spreads have up to 900 milligrams per two-ounce serving, while natural cheeses may have half that amount. Low-sodium cheeses, such as Colby and Monterey Jack, are available.
- Buy low-salt crackers. While many varieties of rice cakes contain no sodium, for example, four saltine crackers contain 125 milligrams.

DINING OUT

If you eat out frequently, you may have a tough time keeping a lid on your salt levels. Still, it's not impossible. All it takes is a little low-salt savvy.

Dine in restaurants where food is cooked to order. This way, you will have some control over salt, whereas in restaurants that have food prepared ahead of time, you don't, says Winston. A cooked-to-order broiled hamburger patty, for example, contains about 70 milligrams of sodium. The ready-to-eat fast-food version contains over twice that much.

Order sauces on the side. That goes for gravies and dressings, too. Be sure to ask for low-sodium dressings, or better yet, oil and vinegar—they're salt-free.

Hold the extras. A leading fast-food cheeseburger with "the works" has over 1,100 milligrams of sodium. You can cut the salt content in half if you tell the counter person to hold the cheese, mustard, catsup and relish.

Don't eat too many dinner rolls. Nearly 30 percent of our dietary sodium comes from bread and grain products. A single slice of enriched white bread or whole-wheat bread contains about 150 milligrams of sodium.

Remove fillings and breadings. If you order a fruit pie, remove the salty crust and eat only the filling. Ditto for breaded fish. Baked fish with breading gives you over 1,000 milligrams of sodium. With breading removed, it's 575 milligrams.

Steps like these may seem like deprivations at first. "But stick with it," Dr. Krishna says. "If you can follow your low-salt eating program for at least three to four months until you've had time to adjust, you should be all set."

HIGH-NUTRITION RECIPES

STUFFED CABBAGE

Tomato sauce can be a hidden source of sodium. Look for brands that are labeled either "low sodium" or "no added sodium." When cooking rice, as for these cabbage rolls, use either plain water or salt-free stock.

8 large cabbage leaves
1 cup finely chopped onions
2 teaspoons olive oil
8 ounces ground turkey
1 clove garlic, minced
½ teaspoon dried thyme
½ teaspoon dried oregano
1½ cups cold cooked rice
1 egg white
2 cups no-added-sodium tomato sauce

Blanch the cabbage leaves in boiling water for 1 minute. Drain and lay the leaves flat on a tray. Set aside.

In a large no-stick frying pan over medium heat, sauté the onions in the oil for 5 minutes, or until softened. Crumble the turkey into the pan and cook, breaking up the pieces, until browned. Stir in the garlic, thyme and oregano; cook for 1 minute.

Remove the pan from the heat. Stir in the rice, egg white and ½ cup of the tomato sauce. Let stand for a few minutes until cool enough to handle.

Divide the mixture among the cabbage leaves. Enclose the filling by tucking in the side edges and rolling up the leaves.

Coat a 9" × 13" glass baking dish with no-stick spray. Spread about ½ cup of the remaining tomato sauce in the bottom. Add the rolls, seam side down. Pour the remaining 1 cup tomato sauce over the top.

Cut a piece of wax paper to fit over the rolls. Then cover the pan tightly with foil. Bake at 350° for 30 minutes.

Serves 4

Per serving: *261 calories, 4.2 g. fat (15% of calories), 3.9 g. dietary fiber, 37 mg. cholesterol, 95 mg. sodium*

CHICKEN SAUSAGE LINKS

Besides being high in fat, regular sausage also contains lots of sodium. You can easily make lean, lower-sodium links or patties at home. These contain ground chicken and minced apples. You may also substitute ground turkey for a slightly different taste. (For the leanest patties, buy boneless, skinless chicken or turkey breast, cut it into cubes and finely chop in a food processor using on/off turns.) Serve with reduced-cholesterol scrambled eggs, homemade hash browns and low-sodium catsup for a special weekend brunch.

- **½ cup unsalted plain or seasoned dry bread crumbs**
- **¾ cup minced apples**
- **½ teaspoon dried sage**
- **¼ teaspoon ground black pepper**
- **Pinch of ground red pepper**
- **1 egg white, lightly beaten**
- **8 ounces ground chicken**

In a large bowl, combine the bread crumbs, apples, sage, black pepper and red pepper. Stir in the egg white. Add the chicken and mix well. Shape into 8 links measuring about 4½" × 1".

Coat a broiler pan with no-stick spray. Broil about 6" from the heat until lightly browned on the outside and cooked through, about 4 minutes per side. Drain on paper towels.

Serves 4
Per serving: *133 calories, 2.5 g. fat (17% of calories), 0.9 g. dietary fiber, 40 mg. cholesterol, 150 mg. sodium*

YAMS WITH HONEY TOPPING

This is a nice side dish that can double as a light lunch. Be sure to choose cottage cheese with no added sodium—regular types can easily contain over 450 milligrams per half cup. If you're in a real hurry, you may microwave the sweet potatoes—four take from 15 to 20 minutes.

- **4 medium sweet potatoes**
- **1½ cups unsalted dry-curd cottage cheese**
- **2 tablespoons honey**
- **⅛ teaspoon ground cinnamon**
- **⅛ teaspoon grated nutmeg**
- **1 tablespoon snipped chives**

Bake the sweet potatoes at 375° for 1 hour and 15 minutes, or until easily pierced with a fork.

In a food processor, blend the cottage cheese until smooth, about 3 minutes. Add the honey, cinnamon and nutmeg. Mix well.

Halve the potatoes and fluff the flesh with a fork. Top with dollops of the cottage-cheese mixture. Sprinkle with the chives.

Serves 4
Per serving: *215 calories, 0.6 g. fat (3% of calories), 4 g. dietary fiber, 4 mg. cholesterol, 25 mg. sodium*

CREAMY CARROT SOUP

Soups can be a challenge on a low-salt diet because most store-bought types are loaded with sodium. And making your own doesn't guarantee a low-sodium potage if you start with bouillon cubes or salty canned stock. Instead, either make your own stock or buy a brand that contains no added salt.

- **1 onion, diced**
- **2 teaspoons olive oil**
- **12 ounces carrots, thinly sliced**
- **4 ounces parsnips, thinly sliced**
- **½ teaspoon ground black pepper**
- **¼ teaspoon dried dill**
- **Pinch of grated nutmeg**
- **4 cups defatted low-sodium chicken stock**
- **2 cups cooked rice**
- **¼ cup nonfat sour cream**
- **Dill sprigs**

In a 3-quart saucepan over medium heat, sauté the onions in the oil for 5 minutes, or until lightly browned. Add the carrots and parsnips; cook for 5 minutes, stirring often.

Stir in the pepper, dill, nutmeg and 2 cups of the stock. Cover and simmer for 20 minutes, or until the vegetables are tender. Transfer to a blender and process until smooth. Return the mixture to the pan.

Stir in the rice and the remaining 2 cups stock. Heat through. Ladle into soup bowls and garnish each serving with a dollop of the sour cream and some dill.

Serves 6

Per serving: *182 calories, 2.8 g. fat (14% of calories), 3 g. dietary fiber, 0 mg. cholesterol, 84 mg. sodium*

CHAPTER 11

CALCIUM

FOR HEALTHY BONES AND MORE

When you were a kid you never thought twice about calcium—but chances are you were gulping three or four glasses of milk a day and guzzling ice cream whenever your mom would let you. You were getting plenty of calcium without even trying.

But times have changed. You have changed, and eating habits have changed. Many of us, ever aware of middle-age spread and how much fat we're eating, steer clear of calcium-rich foods such as cheese and ice cream. And instead of the milk we used to drink, many of us—young and old alike—swill soft drinks as if *they* contain some essential nutrient.

But the evidence is clear that we need calcium *throughout* our lives. Yes, it's crucial that children get ample calcium to build strong bones and teeth, but calcium can help keep your bones healthy long after childhood. And it has many other roles as well. It's involved with the functioning of your heart, blood, muscles and nerves, and in some cases it can help control blood pressure. Studies indicate that calcium also can alleviate many premenstrual problems, significantly reduce chances of premature births and lower chances of colon cancer and possibly breast cancer.

Fine, you say, but you eat a healthy diet and couldn't possibly be calcium deficient. Think again. The American Dietetic Association says you need a minimum of 800 milligrams of calcium a day, while children, teens, young adults and pregnant and breastfeeding women should take in at least 1,200

MILK: IT DOESN'T ALWAYS DO A BODY GOOD

Paul Wexler began experiencing puzzling symptoms soon after he was out of his teens: lethargy, bloating, diarrhea. He dragged himself from doctor to doctor while his symptoms worsened, and one doctor even suggested his problem was psychological. Finally a physician made a simple, quick, and accurate diagnosis: Wexler was lactose intolerant. He could not digest milk.

The story ended happily for Wexler, whose uncomfortable symptoms disappeared as soon as he cut out milk products. But for millions of Americans like him, milk spells distress with a capital *D*.

The culprit is lactose, the sugar in milk, which you normally break down with an enzyme called lactase. But if you don't produce enough lactase, you can't digest milk properly.

As babies, most of us produce plenty of lactase, but we produce less as we get older. And by the time we're adults, many of us—as many as 60 to 90 percent of Jews, Orientals, blacks, Mexican-Americans and native Americans—are lactose intolerant to some degree. The problem is less common among American whites, affecting only 5 to 20 percent.

So if milk turns your intestinal tract into a raging battle zone, how do you get enough calcium?

milligrams daily. Some professionals suggest that postmenopausal women need to consume even more. Many of us, however, don't come close.

When Paul Saltman, Ph.D., a biology professor at the University of California in San Diego, studied the food intake of 137 postmenopausal women—all well educated and with middle-class income—he found they weren't eating as well as they thought they were. "These were all women who said they were taking good care of themselves," says Dr. Saltman. "But the fact was, over two years, their calcium intake from food averaged only about 560 milligrams a day."

Nationwide, the average for all women aged 45 to 54 is only 474 milligrams daily. And more important, girls and young women seldom meet the daily requirements in their bone-forming years. Calcium intake is less of a problem for men and boys, who eat more and thus come closer to meeting minimum levels.

A MINERAL YOUR BODY DEMANDS

Calcium is an essential mineral that comes tidily packaged with other nutrients in a variety of foods—such as dairy products, leafy greens and canned sardines and salmon (with bones). The bulk of the calcium in our bodies, about 99 percent, is in our bones, and the rest is split evenly between our teeth and blood. And although it's a relatively small amount,

Settle for less. Being lactose intolerant doesn't necessarily mean you can't *ever* consume dairy products, says Liz Diemand, R.D., of Thornton, Colorado, spokesperson for the American Dietetic Association. Not everyone is as intolerant as Wexler.

"Try consuming dairy products in smaller portions," says Diemand. "Try just four ounces of milk, in combination with other foods."

Take a dairy detour. You can also try yogurt or aged cheeses, such as extra-sharp Cheddar, which are lower in lactose. "Many lactose-intolerant people can tolerate yogurt, because the bacteria help the digestion of lactose," explains Diemand. (But not all yogurts have live bacteria cultures—check the label.)

Try something special. You can also buy reduced-lactose milk, which contains 70 percent less lactose than regular milk, or lactase supplements that contain the lactase enzymes you're missing. These come in a liquid you can add directly to milk, or as chewable tablets.

Go with the green. You can load up on calcium-rich nondairy foods, such as broccoli, kale and mustard greens. "But if this is your only source of calcium, it's difficult to get enough in your diet," says Diemand. If you're consuming no milk products, she recommends that you ask your doctor about a calcium supplement.

the calcium in our blood is important: It's involved with many vital functions, including regulating muscle contractions, heartbeat, blood clotting and nerve transmission.

The calcium in your bones acts like deposits in a bank: Your body "borrows" calcium daily from your bones for your blood to use. But it also *re-deposits* calcium regularly from the foods you eat. This means that even during adulthood new bone is continually being formed—a process known as remodeling, which affects 10 to 15 percent of our bone surface at one time.

The system can go haywire, however, when you aren't supplying enough calcium in your diet to replace the calcium being withdrawn from your bones. Regardless of whether you're getting enough dietary calcium, your body will continue to "draw out" calcium from your bones. And if you are pregnant or breastfeeding and low on calcium, your body will also withdraw bone calcium to meet the baby's needs.

In general, we begin to lose bone around age 40 to 44. And to make matters worse, as we get older, we begin to lose some of our ability to absorb calcium—just as our intake of calcium is likely falling off, too.

It doesn't take a medical degree to figure out that if you keep sapping calcium from your bones without replacing it, you're going to run into trouble. (Just like when you make more withdrawals from your bank account than deposits.) Although it may take years for the effects of a serious defi-

CALCIUM AND ITS PALS

Calcium can't do its bone-building job without two companion nutrients—vitamin D and phosphorus.

Vitamin D. Generally the vitamin D you need comes from exposure to the sun, and most people make enough vitamin D in the sunny summer months to last through winter. But people who seldom or never get out of doors can be deficient in vitamin D—and this can be a problem for older people who may be housebound.

"It's increasingly my opinion that a major problem in the elderly—along with inadequate *calcium* intake—is insufficient vitamin D," says Lindsay Allen, R.D., Ph.D., professor of nutrition sciences at the University of Connecticut in Storrs. "Also, older people don't make vitamin D as well in their skin from sunlight as younger people." Studies support this: One study found that women who did not receive a vitamin D supplement lost more bone density than women who did get the supplement.

Two cups of milk fortified with vitamin D, however, will give you the recommended daily allowance of 200 international units. You can also increase your vitamin D level by going outdoors without sunscreen and exposing your face, arms and hands to the sun for five to ten minutes in the morning or late afternoon three times a week, says Michael Holick, M.D., Ph.D., director of the Vitamin D and Bone Research Laboratory at the Boston University School of Medicine.

If you can't handle either sun or milk, take a multivitamin supplement with 200 to 400 international units of vitamin D, says Dr. Holick. Or eat foods that supply vitamin D, such as sardines, salmon, tuna and cheese.

Phosphorus. Getting adequate phosphorus is seldom a problem, as this mineral abounds in cola-type soft drinks, processed foods, meats, dairy foods and poultry. Too much phosphorus in the diet, however, can interfere with calcium absorption, so if you're an inveterate soda-guzzler, you may want to cut back on your intake.

ciency to become apparent, eventually your calcium-starved bones become weak, porous, fragile and prone to break easily. This condition is known as osteoporosis, and it's common in postmenopausal women and some elderly men.

OSTEOPOROSIS: THE BONE WEAKENER

Remember when Grandma fell and broke her hip? Or more likely, broke her hip and fell? Chances are her bones had become thin and fragile because of osteoporosis, and her brittle hip shattered.

In people with osteoporosis, bones can break under their own weight. The complicating factor is that often the bone doesn't simply break—it shatters into pieces too small to be put back together. One-fourth of people over 55 who break their hips will not walk unaided again.

Osteoporosis affects primarily the hips, wrists and spine and results in about 1.3 million fractures a year. In many cases, vertebrae may compress and collapse. There are no early warning signs: The first indications may be a decrease in height or the formation of a "dowager's hump" as bone in the spine collapses.

Who gets osteoporosis? Many factors are involved, including how much bone mass you have to start with—which can be linked to race (black peo-

THE LINK WITH WHAT YOU DRINK

You could be taking in even *more* than your required levels of calcium—and still not have adequate calcium available. What gives?

How much calcium is available to you may be related to what you drink, whether it's coffee, alcohol or soft drinks.

Coffee. One study showed that the risk of hip fracture in middle-aged women who drank more than 6 cups of coffee a day was nearly three times higher than that of women who drank less than 1½ cups a day. Caffeine may harm bones directly, or indirectly by prompting calcium losses through frequent urination.

Alcohol. Alcoholic beverages can interfere with your ability to absorb and use calcium. And because women's ovaries are sensitive to the effects of alcohol, it may alter the hormonal balance necessary to maintain strong bones. And as if that's not enough, it's possible that alcohol's diuretic qualities promote calcium losses through the urine.

High levels of alcohol may counteract any beneficial effect calcium has on blood pressure. When researchers at the University of California Medical Center in San Diego studied data on 7,000 middle-aged men of Japanese descent living in Hawaii, they found that in light drinkers, higher calcium intake helped keep blood pressure levels down. In heavier drinkers, however, the calcium had no effect.

Soft drinks. Some studies suggest that soft drinks—because of their citric and phosphoric acid content—can decrease utilization of calcium or cause increased excretion. One survey found that athletic women who drank carbonated drinks had 2.3 times as many fractures as those who did not. Researchers are not all in accord, however. "It's debatable," says Elwood Speckmann, Ph.D., director of research programs at Shriners Hospitals for Crippled Children in Tampa, "but generally you should avoid extremes of nutrient intake. Inadequate calcium and excessive phosphorus is going to cause problems, just as too much calcium and not enough phosphorus would."

ple, for instance, have more bone mass than Caucasians) or to how much calcium you consumed and how physically active you were during your bone-forming years.

Risk factors you can't do much about include being light-skinned, having a delicate frame, undergoing early menopause or having relatives who have had osteoporosis. Factors you *can* control include being underweight or sedentary, eating a low-calcium diet, smoking and drinking more than two drinks per day.

Women are particularly vulnerable to osteoporosis partly because of calcium losses that can occur during pregnancy and menopause. If you don't consume enough calcium during pregnancy and nursing, it will be "robbed" from your bones. And drastic bone loss can occur during menopause when estrogen production falls off, because estrogen is necessary for bones to absorb calcium.

You can avoid this dramatic menopausal bone loss by hormone replacement therapy, which includes low doses of estrogen and progesterone. Women who have had breast cancer should not take estrogen, however.

WHO NEEDS CALCIUM SUPPLEMENTS?

So you need to take in more calcium. No problem, you decide, wheeling down the aisle and tossing a jumbo bottle of calcium supplements in your shopping cart.

What's wrong with this picture? A couple of things.

First, no one should *indiscriminately* take supplements, says Elwood Speckmann, Ph.D., director of research programs at Shriners Hospitals for Crippled Children in Tampa. Not everyone needs a supplement—you may be able to more effectively get your calcium from food—and people who do require supplements should pay careful attention to *how much* calcium is supplied and in what form.

Nutritionists believe the first approach to resolving a calcium deficiency should be to eat more foods containing calcium. "I don't like to see people rely on supplements and forget about what they're getting in their diets," says Liz Diemand, R.D., of Thornton, Colorado, a spokesperson for the American Dietetic Association. If at all possible, it's better to get your calcium along with other nutrients in a "package deal" in foods such as low-fat milk, yogurt, cheeses, broccoli and greens.

But in some cases you just can't take in enough calcium via food to meet your needs. Who's a candidate for supplements? People who can't digest milk or milk products; pregnant or nursing women, who have an increased need for calcium; and elderly people with limited appetites.

It's best to check with your doctor before adding a supplement,

And those with diabetes, asthma or heart disease may also be advised not to take hormones. Is osteoporosis and significant bone loss inevitable, particularly if you aren't starting out with a lot of bone mass? Not necessarily.

CALCIUM TO THE RESCUE

While you shouldn't think of calcium as a cure-all or sure-fire preventive for bone problems or osteoporosis—most professionals agree that additional measures are usually needed to halt bone loss—calcium *can* help. Researchers disagree on how much it helps and how much of its effect is due to other factors, but the bottom line is that some studies show that calcium may reduce the amount of bone you lose, help fend off osteoporosis and help prevent fractures.

"In preventing fractures, the evidence for calcium is strong," says Robert Heaney, M.D., chairman of the Congressional Office of Technology Assessment's scientific advisory panel on osteoporosis.

One study showed that men and women past 60 who took in more than

particularly if you have a family history of kidney stones. And always check the dosage of the supplement: Some people think if a little is good, a lot is better—but that's not always true. Calcium in excess of 2,500 milligrams a day can cause problems such as urinary stone formation and constipation and can interfere with absorption of iron, zinc and other minerals.

Another potential hazard of overdosing is hypercalcemia (excess calcium in the blood). Up to 2,500 milligrams of calcium a day won't cause a problem in healthy adults, but it *can* if you have a condition such as hyperparathyroidism or chronic kidney disease. And huge doses of calcium—four and more times the normal dose—can cause hypercalcemia in anyone.

Think you're getting your calcium from chewing antacids? You may be—but check those labels. Calcium-containing antacids such as Tums may have up to 500 milligrams of calcium, but antacids that contain aluminum and magnesium hydroxide can cause phosphate depletion and a *loss* of available calcium.

And don't assume that your calcium supplement is a fix-all for your bones. Calcium doesn't work alone: Vitamin D, lactose and protein all help calcium absorption, and regular weight-bearing exercise plays a crucial role in protecting bones.

Two final tips: If you're taking a calcium supplement, it's better to spread out the dosage throughout the day rather than taking it all at once, and to drink six to eight 8-ounce glasses of water a day.

765 milligrams of calcium a day had 60 percent fewer hip fractures than people getting less than 470 milligrams. Another study indicated that women with a lifetime calcium intake of 1,000 milligrams a day had 60 to 70 percent fewer hip fractures than women getting half that amount.

And a study at the University of Massachusetts Medical Center found that 30- to 40-year-old women who consumed 1,500 milligrams of the mineral a day from low-fat, calcium-rich foods had lost none of their bone mass over three years, while women consuming 800 milligrams a day had lost 3 percent.

Optimally, of course, you build strong bones in childhood and young adulthood and consume plenty of calcium *before* menopause. "Women who get enough calcium all their lives appear to have much less risk of losing significant amounts of bone after menopause," says Bess Dawson-Hughes, M.D., of the U.S. Department of Agriculture's (USDA) Nutrition Research Center on Aging at Tufts University in Boston. Studies suggest that calcium taken immediately after menopause is of no use in preventing bone loss.

This doesn't mean, however, that you should *neglect* your calcium intake during this period: Better late than never. "Even if you don't start taking

BEST AND WORST CALCIUM SOURCES

Some of the top sources of this important nutrient are listed here as well as a couple that just don't deliver.

FOOD	PORTION	CALCIUM (mg.)
A+ SOURCES		
Nonfat yogurt	1 cup	452
Skim milk	1 cup	302
Buttermilk	1 cup	285
Part-skim mozzarella cheese	1 oz.	181
Dairy products are by far the richest in calcium, and that calcium is also easily absorbed by the body. Depend on them to achieve recommended calcium intake.		
A SOURCES		
Sardines	6	275
Salmon, pink, canned (with bones)	3 oz.	181
Good supplementary calcium sources. They're high in calcium because of the tiny bones, but sardines can also be high in fat.		
B+ SOURCES		
Pinto beans, cooked	½ cup	118
Kale, chopped, cooked	½ cup	86
Bok choy, shredded, cooked	½ cup	79
Mustard greens, chopped, cooked	½ cup	52

extra calcium until early menopause, it will help prevent bone loss later, even if the results don't show up for five or six years," says Dr. Dawson-Hughes.

For two years, Dr. Dawson-Hughes studied 301 healthy postmenopausal women, some of whom received an additional 500-milligram supplement of calcium per day. The women who got less than 400 milligrams of total calcium per day lost 2 to 3 percent of their bone mass in the two years, while bone loss was greatly reduced in the women receiving supplements. The best results were found in women at least six years past menopause.

What about other therapies or additional strategies to avoid osteoporosis? Besides estrogen for menopausal women, vitamin D plays a vital role. And exercise is also crucial: All the calcium in the world won't stop or prevent bone loss if you don't exercise, says Dr. Heaney.

HELPING HIGH BLOOD PRESSURE

But calcium doesn't just affect bone health. Among other things, it may also help keep your blood pressure down.

A study by David McCarron, M.D., co-head of the Division of Nephrol-

FOOD	**PORTION**	**CALCIUM (mg.)**
Kidney beans, cooked	½ cup	43
Broccoli, chopped, cooked	½ cup	36

Greens and beans are moderately high in calcium, and that calcium is available to the body. Unfortunately, you'd have to eat mounds of them to meet the daily calcium levels that experts recommend. Depend on them as supplementary calcium sources.

Figs, dried	6	161
Almonds, toasted, unblanched	1 oz.	76
Hazelnuts	1 oz.	55
Brazil nuts	1 oz.	50
Prunes, dried	5	22

Like greens and beans, nuts and dried fruits are good as a supplementary source of calcium, but you'd have to cover your plate with them to meet daily requirements. Also, nuts are high in fat, and dried fruits are loaded with calories.

F SOURCES

Spinach, cooked	½ cup	122
Ground beef, lean, cooked	3 oz.	8

Spinach is high in oxalate, which makes its calcium unavailable to the body. Meats have insignificant calcium content.

ogy at the Oregon Health Sciences University in Portland, indicates that people with mild high blood pressure may be able to decrease their levels to normal by increasing their dietary calcium intake. Intake at or above 800 milligrams a day holds strong potential benefit for pregnant women and people who drink too much alcohol, according to Dr. McCarron.

And a 1991 study of 1,194 women in Argentina found that those in their twentieth week of pregnancy who took 2,000 milligrams of calcium a day had fewer problems with high blood pressure than did others who received a look-alike placebo with no calcium.

"Calcium is particularly good, it seems, in affecting normal age-related increases in blood pressure," says Jeffrey Blumberg, Ph.D., associate director of the USDA's Human Nutrition Research Center on Aging at Tufts University.

EASING MENSTRUAL PROBLEMS

For women who suffer from the monthly miseries of premenstrual syndrome or other menstrual problems, studies suggesting that calcium can ease much of their discomfort may be the best news they've heard in a long time.

Dramatic results were found in a 5½-month study by the USDA's Agricultural Research Service in Grand Forks, North Dakota. For 78 days, five of the ten women received 1,300 milligrams of calcium daily and the other five received 600 milligrams. For another 78 days of the study, the groups were switched.

"Women with higher calcium intakes showed a really dramatic decrease in a variety of symptoms," says research psychologist James G. Penland, Ph.D. On the higher levels of calcium, nine of the ten reported fewer mood changes such as irritability, tension, loneliness, and depression, and seven of the ten reported fewer cramps and backaches during the menstrual phase of the cycle. The women also reported retaining less water during the premenstrual phase of their cycle.

At the lower levels, says Dr. Penland, the women showed poorer work efficiency and overall efficiency. "They also slept more, avoided social activities and had an increase in concentration problems, insomnia, forgetfulness and accidents," he says.

And in another study at the Metropolitan Hospital in New York City, women suffering from PMS symptoms found they had fewer mood swings and less water retention and pain when they took 1,000 milligrams of calcium daily in addition to their regular diets.

CUTTING CANCER RISKS

Calcium against cancer? Possibly. Evidence is mounting that calcium at levels of 1,200 milligrams or more per day may lower the risk of colon cancer and possibly breast cancer.

"There are tentative findings that link higher levels of calcium intake with lower colorectal cancer risk in humans," says Martin Lipkin, M.D., head of the Irving Weinstein Laboratory for Gastrointestinal Cancer

Prevention at Memorial Sloan-Kettering Cancer Center in New York City.

The link between cancer and calcium was proposed in 1980 by brothers Cedric Garland, D.P.H., and Frank Garland, Ph.D., who found that colon and rectal cancer deaths were highest in areas with least sun, and later found a similar pattern with breast cancer. (Sunshine lets us make vitamin D, which in turn helps us absorb calcium.) They suggest that calcium intake levels of 1,800 milligrams per day for men and 1,500 milligrams per day for women are useful for reducing occurrences of colon cancer.

Although evidence linking calcium and breast cancer is far from conclusive, studies with rats suggest that low amounts of vitamin D and calcium and high levels of phosphate, increase the risk for mammary tumors when a high-fat diet is eaten.

How might calcium exert a protective effect? At least for colon cancer, a possible mechanism has been proposed: During the digestive process, bile acids that can be cancer-causing are produced in the colon. Calcium appears to bind with these acids and keep them from irritating the colon wall. One study found that calcium slows down the reproduction of immature cells taken from the colon wall, and helps make cancer cells "age" and die.

And Still More Benefits

A study at Johns Hopkins Adolescent Pregnancy Clinic found that calcium helped reduce the risk of premature births among pregnant teenagers. Only 7 percent of the teenaged mothers-to-be who received 2,000 milligrams of calcium daily from their fifth month on gave birth prematurely, while 21 percent of the group receiving a placebo had premature babies.

And of 2,000 respondents to a *Prevention* magazine survey, almost 74 percent reported that taking calcium helped reduce muscle cramps or spasms. "There may be a good physiologic basis for that," says Dr. Dawson-Hughes. "It is very well recognized that even slightly low potassium and low calcium levels cause muscle cramps." Seventy percent of readers also reported that calcium helped aching bones or joints, although there's no scientific evidence to back up this effect.

Looking Out for Your Needs

Where do you get your calcium?

Head for the dairy case. "The best sources are milk and dairy products," says Bettye J. Nowlin, R.D., Los Angeles dietitian and a spokesperson for the American Dietetic Association. Dairy products aren't all high in fat: You can choose low-fat or nonfat cheese, yogurt, and milk. "You can sprinkle cheese on a salad; use low-fat grated cheese in casseroles; add nonfat dry milk to meat loaf," advises Nowlin.

Eat a fair share of fish and broccoli. Other good sources are canned salmon and sardines (if you eat the soft bones as well), calcium-fortified orange or grapefruit juice, and broccoli. You can also find calcium in leafy greens such as kale, collard greens and turnip greens. Tortillas that are lime-

TEN QUICK TIPS TO BOOST YOUR CALCIUM INTAKE

1. Choose frozen yogurt, ice milk or puddings made with low-fat or skim milk for dessert.
2. Sprinkle Parmesan or Romano cheese on soups, salads, vegetables and popcorn.
3. Use low-fat or skim milk instead of water in canned soups and oatmeal and during baking.
4. Use plain yogurt in place of mayonnaise in salad dressing and other recipes.
5. Add a slice of cheese to sandwiches, or melt some on toast, English muffins or bagels.
6. Add one or two tablespoons of nonfat dry milk to hot cereals, stews, casseroles, meat loaf or mashed potatoes.
7. Use farmer's cheese, ricotta cheese or cottage cheese as a sandwich or toast spread.
8. Try tofu in place of beef or chicken in stir-fry recipes, or add it to soups and salads.
9. Choose broccoli, collards, kale, bok choy or turnip greens.
10. Have low-fat milk shakes instead of soft drinks.

processed (check the package) contain calcium, as does tofu.

Strive for three to four servings a day. Each serving of calcium-rich foods provides about 300 milligrams, says Nowlin. So if you aim for three or four servings per day, you'll be getting 900 to 1,200 milligrams. It's also best to spread out your calcium intake throughout the day, as your body can more efficiently absorb it in small doses.

YOUR DAILY QUOTA

Exactly how much is enough? There's no simple answer: The amount you need may vary according to your stage of life, and it can be different from person to person.

"Some women absorb only 15 percent of the calcium in their foods, while others absorb three times as much," says Dr. Heaney. People on high-fiber diets may absorb less, because fiber can bind calcium and make it less available. The rate also varies with age: As kids, we absorb about 75 percent of the calcium we take in. As adults, the amount typically drops to around 15 percent.

Calcium from a variety of foods is without a doubt your best bet. Generally, if you reach for three or four servings of calcium-rich foods a day—or five, if you're pregnant or nursing or in menopause—you'll be meeting your calcium needs.

AMOUNTS THAT PROTECT BEST

For best results in preventing osteoporosis, the National Osteoporosis Foundation suggests these daily intakes of calcium:

AGE/CONDITION	CALCIUM (mg.)
1–10	800
11–24	1,200
25–50	1,000
Pregnant women	1,200
Lactating women	1,200
Premenopausal women	1,000
Postmenopausal women	
If taking hormone replacement therapy	1,000
If not taking hormone replacement therapy	1,500
51+	1,000

HIGH-NUTRITION RECIPES

RASPBERRIES AND HONEY-YOGURT CREAM

Low-fat dairy products are a best bet when you're looking to increase your intake of calcium. This smooth yogurt sauce is easy to prepare and goes with most any fresh fruit.

1 cup nonfat yogurt
¾ cup nonfat sour cream
2 tablespoons honey
2 teaspoons grated orange rind
½ teaspoon vanilla
4 cups red or black raspberries

Spoon the yogurt into a yogurt-cheese funnel or a small sieve lined with cheesecloth. Place over a bowl, cover and let drain at room temperature for 1 hour. Transfer to a medium bowl. Whisk in the sour cream, honey, orange rind and vanilla.

Divide the berries among 4 dessert bowls. Top with the yogurt cream.

Serves 4
Per serving: *166 calories, 0.8 g. fat (4% of calories), 5.5 g. dietary fiber, 1 mg. cholesterol, 84 mg. sodium, 141 mg. calcium*

LOUISIANA SALMON CAKES

Most brands of canned salmon contain small edible bones, which are a good source of calcium. This recipe gets an extra helping of calcium from the nonfat ricotta cheese that's also incorporated into the patties. Serve the cakes with rice, noodles or baked potatoes and coleslaw.

- **¼ cup minced onions**
- **1 tablespoon water**
- **1 can (15½ ounces) salmon, drained well and flaked**
- **1 cup nonfat ricotta cheese**
- **¼ cup fat-free egg substitute**
- **2 tablespoons minced fresh parsley**
- **1 teaspoon Worcestershire sauce**
- **1 teaspoon Dijon mustard**
- **¼ teaspoon hot-pepper sauce**
- **1 cup seasoned dry bread crumbs**
- **1 teaspoon olive oil**

Combine the onions and water in a custard cup; cover with vented plastic wrap. Microwave on high for 1 minute, or until the onions are softened.

Transfer to a large bowl. Add the salmon, ricotta, egg, parsley, Worcestershire, mustard, hot-pepper sauce and ¾ cup of the bread crumbs. Mix well. Cover and refrigerate for at least 2 hours.

Form the mixture into 4 patties. Coat them with the remaining ¼ cup of the bread crumbs.

Heat the oil in a large no-stick frying pan over medium heat. Add the patties and brown on both sides.

Serves 4
Per serving: *261 calories, 7.5 g. fat (27% of calories), 1.2 g. dietary fiber, 46 mg. cholesterol, 747 mg. sodium, 214 mg. calcium*

KALE AND POTATO CASSEROLE

Many leafy greens, such as kale, contain good amounts of calcium. This easy kale and potato casserole gets extra calcium from buttermilk and low-fat cheese.

- **1½ pounds baking potatoes**
- **¾ cup buttermilk**
- **¼ cup fat-free egg substitute**
- **½ teaspoon ground black pepper**
- **¼ teaspoon dried dill**
- **1 large onion, thinly sliced**
- **1 teaspoon olive oil**
- **1 pound kale, coarse stems removed**
- **½ cup reduced-fat Cheddar cheese**
- **¼ cup seasoned dry bread crumbs**

Peel the potatoes and cut into 1" chunks. Place in a large saucepan with cold water to cover. Bring to a boil and cook for 15 minutes, or until the potatoes are tender. Drain and place in a large bowl. Mash with a potato masher.

Stir in the buttermilk, egg, pepper and dill. Set aside.

In a large frying pan over medium heat, sauté the onions in the oil for 5 minutes, or until softened.

Meanwhile, wash the kale in cold water and shake off the excess. Halve large leaves lengthwise. Cut the kale into crosswise shreds about ¼" wide. Add to the frying pan with the water clinging to the leaves. Cover and cook for 10 minutes, or until wilted.

Stir into the potato mixture. Fold in the cheese.

Coat a 2-quart casserole with no-stick spray. Add the potato mixture. Sprinkle with the bread crumbs. Bake at 400° for 15 minutes, or until the crumbs are lightly browned and the casserole is heated through.

Serves 4
Per serving: *297 calories, 5.4 g. fat (15% of calories), 2.4 g. dietary fiber, 9 mg. cholesterol, 211 mg. sodium, 245 mg. calcium*

TANGY TOFU SALAD

This luncheon or dinner salad contains three nice sources of dietary calcium: tofu, broccoli and kidney beans. For even more, you could toss in a bit of low-fat cheese or serve the salad atop shredded leafy greens, such as bok choy or kale. Although the percent of calories from fat in this recipe is a little high, it's largely due to healthy unsaturated fat—most of it coming from the tofu.

- **2 cups broccoli florets, lightly steamed**
- **1 can (15 ounces) kidney beans, rinsed and drained**
- **½ cup diced sweet red peppers**
- **½ cup thinly sliced scallions**
- **2 tablespoons minced fresh basil**
- **8 ounces firm tofu**
- **½ cup fat-free Italian dressing**

In a large bowl, toss together the broccoli, beans, peppers, scallions and basil.

Drain the tofu and gently squeeze out excess moisture using several thicknesses of paper towels. Cut the tofu into ½" or smaller cubes. Add to the bowl. Drizzle with the dressing and toss lightly.

Serves 4
Per serving: *172 calories, 5.5 g. fat (26% of calories), 5.8 g. dietary fiber, 0 mg. cholesterol, 282 mg. sodium, 169 mg. calcium*

CHAPTER 12

IRON

DON'T GET CAUGHT SHORT

"It's the fastest way to get iron in your diet," the sword swallower dryly jokes after sliding a two-foot-long saber out of his mouth. Having enough iron in the body is paramount to good health, but downing knives is hardly the way to get it. In fact, getting too much or too little iron is no joking matter.

Iron plays an absolutely vital role in every single cell of your body, says iron researcher Richard G. Stevens, Ph.D., an epidemiologist at Battelle Pacific Northwest Laboratories in Richland, Washington. It puts the red in red blood cells and makes it possible for those cells to deliver life-giving oxygen from the lungs to the rest of your body. Iron also helps the body release energy, grow and fight infections.

IRON AT WORK

Once iron enters the body, it tends to stay there for quite a while. When a bit of iron signs on with a red blood cell, it's guaranteed a job for the cell's entire working life, about four months. When the blood cell finally retires and breaks up, most of its liberated iron goes to the bone marrow. From there, most of it quickly becomes part of a new blood cell and goes back to work. The remaining iron goes either into storage or is used by other cell systems. If you're eating right, the amount of iron going into storage equals the amount of iron coming out. And, if you're eating right, you shouldn't come up short even if a little iron escapes, which it does. In fact, in women, a little iron is lost each month through menstrual bleeding.

"Usually, there's a balance between iron loss and absorption," says James D. Cook, M.D., professor of medicine and director of the Division of Hematology at the University of Kansas Medical Center in Kansas City. "When there's increased iron loss—through excess menstrual bleeding, for example—the body increases the rate of iron absorption."

Iron needs vary depending on a person's age and sex. In an average day, an average man needs to replace about 1 milligram of iron. Women in their childbearing years need to replace about 1½ milligrams per day.

IRON IN THE LIFE CYCLE

Young, old and in between, people need iron every day. But the amounts we need vary over the years. Here's a rundown of the changing daily Recommended Dietary Allowances for iron and the reasons that our iron needs change through the years.

AGE/CONDITION	RDA (mg./day)		MAJOR FACTORS
	WOMEN	MEN	
0–6 months	6	6	At 0–3 months the infant is still drawing on iron stored up while in the womb.
6 months–10 years	10	10	Growth requires greater iron usage.
11–18 years	15	12	Rapid growth in adolescence increases iron needs. Onset of menstruation in girls further increases need for iron.
19–50 years	15	10	Iron needs in women remain high until menopause. Men require less iron and maintain higher body iron stores than women.
Pregnancy	30		Increased blood volume and developing fetus demand high iron intake.
Lactation	15		Iron demands return to pre-pregnancy level.
51+ years	10	10	After menopause women need less iron.

The amount of iron that your body needs to replace every day is really small compared with Recommended Dietary Allowances (RDA). The RDA for women age 50 and under is a whopping 15 milligrams, for example. Why so much?

The answer lies in the difference between absorption and intake. When your body needs iron, it can absorb on average only about 10 percent of the iron you take in. Eat an iron-rich dinner that provides ten milligrams, and your body will absorb about one milligram, which is just about right—for many people.

DEFINING DEFICIENCY

It is fairly easy to get enough iron into your diet. But what happens if you don't? When a person doesn't eat enough iron-rich foods to replace iron losses, cells start double-dipping into stored iron, and deficiency begins.

Having "iron-poor, tired blood" (as TV ads used to call iron deficiency) means there's just not enough oxygen oomph in the blood to fuel the body and meet its energy needs. "People with low-level deficiencies are just not up to snuff," says Connie Weaver, Ph.D., professor of foods and nutrition at Purdue University in West Lafayette, Indiana. "They feel tired, and it's harder to fight off infections."

If deficiency deepens until iron stores are almost gone—as in anemia—red blood cells shrink, making it difficult for the body's cells to get enough oxygen. This means the heart and lungs have to work a lot harder. The resulting strain can cause a person to look pale and feel weak and fatigued, says Dr. Weaver.

There are, medical experts say, three general causes of iron deficiency: high blood loss, low iron intake and rapid body growth. As luck would have it, women are much more likely than men to have problems on all these counts.

Iron is lost during menstruation and needs to be replaced, explains Dr. Weaver. "Adequate iron intake is something menstruating women should be especially conscientious about," she says.

Adolescent girls and women on weight-loss diets need to be doubly concerned, she says.

Men are not immune to iron deficiency, but *nutritional* iron deficiency in men is rare, says Dr. Cook. "When iron deficiency does occur in men over age 18, it almost always means there's been blood loss of some kind," he says. Slow, internal bleeding that goes undetected—from long-term aspirin use, for example, or certain digestive diseases—can deplete iron stores.

MINING IRON (WITH A FORK)

For most healthy adults, nutritionists say, maintaining sufficient iron supplies is a snap. All it takes is eating the right kinds of foods.

Meat me at the dinner table. "By far, the most concentrated, most absorbable source of iron is red meat," says Janet P. Hunt, Ph.D., a research scientist at the USDA Human Nutrition Research Center in Grand Forks, North Dakota. "And red meat has even more highly available iron than white meats from poultry or fish," she says.

What's all this about "absorbable" and "available" iron?

Iron comes in two forms: heme and nonheme. Heme iron is the kind your body can most readily absorb and comes only from animal sources—red meat, poultry and fish, for example. Nonheme iron, which comes mostly from plant sources, is the hardest for the body to absorb. Meat contains both heme and nonheme iron.

Supply the ironworks. There's no need to go overboard at the butcher shop, however.

"Generally, eating a small (3½-ounce) serving of lean, red meat two or three times a week, plus poultry and fish two or three times, should be adequate for maintaining iron stores," says Andrew J. Silver, M.D., of the St. Louis University School of Medicine and Veterans Affairs Medical Center in Missouri. And lean meat actually has more iron than its fatty cousins.

Forget the liver. While liver used to be prescribed as the best antidote for iron deficiency, doctors no longer recommend it because it is so high in cholesterol. The trade-off just isn't worth it.

Please pass the vegetables. All this does not let you off the hook as far as eating your vegetables is concerned. Plant products, including beans and grains, are rich sources of nonheme iron.

ABSORB MORE

But getting iron from vegetables, legumes and grains is not as simple as popping them in your mouth. Your body must first change it into an absorbable form. Here's how.

Please pass the meat *and* vegetables. Stir-fry thinly sliced beef with broccoli and snow peas, or serve chicken with bean burritos, and you reap a double iron reward: "Meat increases the amount of iron your body can absorb from other foods eaten at the same time," says Dr. Hunt. "There is some as-yet-unknown factor in both red and white meats that can double or triple iron absorption from vegetable sources."

Think C. Add a few sections of orange or tangerine to your green salad. Citrus fruits provide vitamin C (ascorbic acid), which can help make nonheme iron more absorbable. "Make sure you have a source of ascorbic acid in your diet, especially if your iron is in nonheme form," Dr. Hunt advises. "It can easily double iron absorption."

To be effective iron enhancers, vitamin C–rich foods should be eaten at the same meal as iron-rich foods. A few other vitamin C sources that can help you mine the iron from meat and vegetable dishes are broccoli, peppers, tomatoes and potatoes.

Have a tomato juice cocktail. Drink vegetable juices to get iron and vitamin C in one big gulp. "Tomato juice is especially good because it contains high levels of both iron and vitamin C to help your body absorb it," says Dr. Weaver.

End on a high-C note. Top off a high-iron meal with a vitamin C–rich dessert. Citrus fruits, such as oranges and grapefruit, will do the trick, as will strawberries, raspberries and cantaloupe.

Adding to Your Supply

Your iron supplies are affected not only by what you eat but by how you prepare it as well. Here are a few kitchen tips to help you make sure that your iron supply doesn't run short.

Don't undress foods. Eat the jackets of baked potatoes and use whole, unpeeled fruits and vegetables to get the full iron punch they supply. Iron is often most concentrated in the skins.

Avoid overcooking. Eat raw vegetables when you can, or cook them for a short time in very little water. Recapture the iron that cooks out of vegetables by re-using cooking water in soups or sauces. (Note that heme iron from meat is less affected by cooking than nonheme iron.)

Cook in iron. Cook slow-simmering, acidic foods—like tomato sauce—in iron pots. Some foods absorb a small amount of iron from the pot. Researchers aren't sure how much iron your *body* will absorb from the food, says Dr. Cook, but there's apparently no harm in using iron cookware.

Iron Out the Wrinkles in Your Diet

There are also a few foods that can throw your iron absorption system out of sync if you eat them at the wrong time. These are perfectly fine foods, but they contain chemical components that can interfere with the body's ability to use iron. But you don't have to cross them off your menu. Here are some simple steps you can take to keep your iron-absorbing machinery working in tip-top fashion.

Choose brews with iron in mind. "Tea and coffee inhibit iron absorption," says Dr. Cook. Tea and coffee can rob you of half or more of the iron in foods. You don't have to forgo your coffee altogether. Just take your coffee break an hour before or after meals.

Go easy on the fiber. It's important to get fiber in your diet, but if upping iron absorption is your goal, you should be aware that fiber can push food through the digestive system so fast that iron doesn't have a chance to be absorbed. Also, many high-fiber foods contain phytic acid, a substance that traps and binds iron, making it unabsorbable. If you're eating a high-fiber diet, make sure you have lean red meat on the menu a couple times a week. And discuss your diet with your doctor.

Enriched and Fortified Food

So far, we've discussed making the most of naturally occurring iron in foods. Yet, almost any cereal, pasta, bread or baked good you buy contains flour that is enriched or fortified with iron. You might well wonder whether all that extra iron isn't more than enough?

The answer is a simple yes and no. Nutrition experts say that enriching commonly eaten, inexpensive foods has been a real boon, especially for people who can't afford or have trouble eating enough iron-rich meats and vegetables. Anemia in infants and children, for example, has declined drastically in the last two decades or so, thanks, in large part, to fortified foods.

But, while eating enriched foods may prevent severe iron shortages, it's not a cure-all for iron deficiency. Dr. Weaver explains why: "Not all the iron from fortified sources is well absorbed. Often, they use electrolytic iron, which is basically iron filings. Manufacturers use it because some of the

TAKING IT ALL IN: IRON-RICH FOODS

Planning menus that include high-iron foods will help you meet your daily iron needs, says Connie Weaver, Ph.D., of Purdue University in West Lafayette, Indiana. (Women 50 or younger need 15 milligrams of iron a day; older women and all men need 10 milligrams a day.) In general, iron from red meat, shellfish and fish is easiest for the body to use. But vegetables, dried beans, grains and iron-fortified cereals and breads are good sources of iron, too. The table below lists some of the best food sources to help you mine a bountiful supply of iron.

FOOD	PORTION	TOTAL IRON (mg.)
ANIMAL SOURCES		
Clams, cooked, moist heat	10 small	12.6
Oysters, cooked, moist heat	6 med.	5.6
Light tuna, canned in water	3 oz.	2.7
Top round beef, broiled	3 oz.	2.5
Pork tenderloin, roasted	3 oz.	1.3
Haddock, cooked, dry heat	3 oz.	1.2
Turkey, light meat, roasted, no skin	3 oz.	1.2
PLANT SOURCES		
Total cereal	1 oz.	18.0
Tofu, regular, raw	½ cup	6.2
Potato, baked	1	2.8
Kidney beans, cooked	½ cup	2.6
Blackstrap molasses	1 Tbsp.	1.3
Figs, dried	3	1.3
Oatmeal, cooked	1 cup	1.2
Raisins	¼ cup	0.8
Broccoli, cooked	½ cup	0.7

more absorbable forms of iron give food an off-flavor or odor, or cause the product to become rancid sooner."

So go ahead, enjoy your morning cereal. But don't assume that a cereal label that boasts 100 percent of the RDA for iron per serving guarantees complete protection. It's important to season your diet with the spice of life: variety. It gives you a better chance to get all the nutrients you need, including plenty of absorbable iron.

TESTING ONE, TWO, THREE

If your doctor suspects you're running low on iron because of a poor diet, he or she may order a blood test. "There's a wide range of symptoms related to iron that affect body tissues," says Dr. Cook, "but simple signs, like paleness or fatigue, are not reliable indicators of iron levels."

If diet and blood tests point toward iron deficiency, and if you are in a high-risk group, your doctor may prescribe iron supplements. Adolescent girls, pregnant women and growing children are the most likely candidates for supplements. "Their iron requirements are often higher than their diets

IRON OVERLOAD

Some bodies simply do not know when to say no to iron. Two or three people out of a thousand—mostly of northern European descent—inherit a disorder that allows their bodies to overload on iron.

Like mild iron deficiency, mild iron overload is virtually symptomless, says James D. Cook, M.D., of the University of Kansas Medical Center in Kansas City. This means that men with this condition would probably not know it before they're 40 years old. By then, they may have as much as 20 to 40 grams of iron in their bodies—ten times more than the average. Women who are prone to overloading usually don't know it until they are well past menopause.

But when symptoms of iron toxicity finally show up, they do so with a serious bang: "Liver disease, aching joints, darkening of the skin, early-onset diabetes, sexual dysfunction and heart problems are some of the signs of iron overload," says Dr. Cook.

The treatment? Surprisingly, it's not to consume less iron but actually to give blood. "After diagnosis, people give blood donations once or twice a week until the excess iron is removed. That can involve 50 to 200 donations in the first year or two of treatment. Thereafter, giving blood every two to three months is sufficient to take care of the amount of iron they absorb through diet," Dr. Cook says.

can meet, and their doctors may recommend supplements," says Dr. Cook.

But aren't iron pills or multivitamins with iron safe for everyone? The answer is a qualified no. While over-the-counter iron supplements are *probably* safe for most people, a decision to take them should certainly be discussed with your physician. "People—particularly men, as well as women beyond childbearing age—shouldn't take iron supplements for long periods of time without a physician's recommendation and supervision as well as a laboratory test to make sure that have a reason to take iron," says Dr. Cook.

Some studies have even raised the possibility that excess iron stores might increase the risk of cancer for some people.

"It is not wise to take supplements for years on end without a physician's approval," Dr. Silver agrees. "It's possible for iron supplements to mask a condition—such as slow, internal blood loss—that needs a different treatment. Taking iron unnecessarily in large amounts can also cause other problems, such as liver damage or iron toxicity."

If your doctor does recommend over-the-counter iron supplements, ask your pharmacist for a supplement of *ferrous* iron, such as ferrous sulfate, to assure maximum absorption, Dr. Hunt suggests. It's more easily absorbed than other types of supplements.

HIGH-NUTRITION RECIPES

APPLESAUCE CAKE

Blackstrap molasses contains lots of iron. One way to use it is in a moist spice cake, such as this one. If you really like blackstrap's flavor, you may use it exclusively instead of diluting it with light molasses.

1¼ cups unsweetened applesauce
½ cup blackstrap molasses
½ cup light molasses
¼ cup canola oil
¼ cup fat-free egg substitute
½ cup whole-wheat flour
½ cup unbleached flour
1 teaspoon baking soda
1 teaspoon ground cinnamon
½ teaspoon powdered ginger
½ teaspoon ground allspice
¼ teaspoon ground cloves

In a large bowl, whisk together the applesauce, molasses, oil and egg. Add the flours, baking soda, cinnamon, ginger, allspice and cloves. Mix well.

Coat a 9" × 9" baking dish with no-stick spray. Add the batter and smooth the top with a spatula. Bake at 325° for 45 minutes, or until the top center of the cake springs back when touched lightly. Cool before serving.

Serves 12
Per serving: *152 calories, 4.7 g. fat (27% of calories), 1.1 g. dietary fiber, 0 mg. cholesterol, 90 mg. sodium, 3.3 mg. iron*

HEARTY MEAT LOAF

Beef is an excellent source of dietary iron. But it can also contain lots of fat and cholesterol, so you don't want to eat too much. One way to strike a happy medium is to combine a modest amount of lean beef (such as ground top round) with plenty of vegetables and grains, as in this meat loaf.

1 cup finely chopped carrots
1 cup finely chopped onions
1 tablespoon water
1 pound ground lean top round
1 cup rolled oats
½ cup bran
¼ cup fat-free egg substitute
½ teaspoon dried basil
½ teaspoon dried marjoram
½ teaspoon ground black pepper
1 cup tomato juice

Combine the carrots, onions and water in a 1-quart glass measure. Cover with vented plastic wrap. Microwave on high for 4 minutes, or until the vegetables are just softened.

Transfer to a large bowl. Crumble the beef into the bowl. Add the oats and bran. Toss together lightly but thoroughly.

In a small bowl, whisk together the egg, basil, marjoram, pepper and ¾ cup of the juice. Pour over the meat and mix well.

Coat an 8" × 8" pan with no-stick spray. Add the meat and pat gently into a loaf shape. Pour the remaining ¼ cup juice over the meat.

Bake at 350° for 45 to 50 minutes, or until cooked through. If the top begins to brown too much, cover with a piece of foil.

Serves 6
Per serving: *198 calories, 4.2 g. fat (19% of calories), 4 g. dietary fiber, 43 mg. cholesterol, 214 mg. sodium, 3.2 mg. iron*

GINGERED BEEF AND VEGETABLE STIR-FRY

Here's another beef recipe, this one using the stir-fry technique. Marinating the lean meat before cooking it enhances its flavor and helps to tenderize it a bit.

1 pound boneless top round steak
2 tablespoons low-sodium soy sauce
1 tablespoon grated fresh ginger
1 tablespoon minced garlic
2 teaspoons sesame oil
1 cup julienned sweet red peppers
2 scallions, julienned
⅓ cup julienned celery
¼ cup plus 1 tablespoon water
1 cup snow peas
1 teaspoon arrowroot or cornstarch
3 cups hot cooked brown or basmati rice

Place the steak in the freezer until partially frozen, about 20 minutes. Trim off all visible fat. Slice the meat across the grain and on the diagonal to make thin (¼") strips. Place in a medium bowl. Add the soy sauce, ginger, garlic and 1 teaspoon of the oil. Mix well and let marinate while you cook the vegetables.

In a wok or large frying pan over high heat, heat the remaining 1 teaspoon oil. Add the peppers, scallions and celery. Stir briskly to coat the vegetables with the oil. Add ¼ cup water and cook for 2 minutes, stirring occasionally. Using a slotted spoon, transfer the vegetables to a plate.

Add the meat and its marinade to the wok. Cook, stirring frequently, for about 5 minutes, or until the meat browns slightly. Add the cooked vegetables and snow peas.

In a cup, combine the arrowroot or cornstarch and the remaining 1 tablespoon water. Add to the pan. Stir until the sauce thickens, about 1 minute. Serve over the rice.

Serves 4
Per serving: *372 calories, 8.6 g. fat (21% of calories), 4.1 g. dietary fiber, 65 mg. cholesterol, 379 mg. sodium, 4.2 mg. iron*

LINGUINE WITH CLAM SAUCE

Clams are a super source of iron. One classic way to enjoy them is over pasta. This recipe is an adaptation of one presented by heart researcher William P. Castelli, M.D., at a conference held by the American Diabetes Association. Each serving contains more than twice the Recommended Dietary Allowance for iron.

- **2 medium onions, diced**
- **2 cloves garlic, minced**
- **1 tablespoon olive oil**
- **2 cans (8 ounces each) minced clams**
- **½ cup apple cider or alcohol-free white wine**
- **3 tablespoons lemon juice**
- **½ teaspoon ground black pepper**
- **¼ cup chopped pimentos**
- **8 ounces linguine**
- **¼ cup chopped fresh parsley**
- **¼ cup chopped fresh basil**

In a large no-stick frying pan over medium heat, sauté the onions and garlic in the oil for 3 minutes, or until softened.

Drain the clams, saving the liquid. Set the clams aside. Add the liquid to the frying pan. Add the cider or wine. Bring to a boil and cook until the total volume is reduced by half, about 15 minutes. Stir in the lemon juice, pepper and reserved clams.

Cover the pan, reduce the heat to medium-low and simmer for 5 minutes. Stir in the pimentos.

Meanwhile, cook the linguine in a large pot of boiling water for about 8 minutes, or until just tender. Drain. Return the linguine to its pan. Add the clam mixture, parsley and basil. Toss to coat. Cover and cook over medium-low heat for 5 minutes.

Serves 4
Per serving: *453 calories, 6.7 g. fat (12% of calories), 0.5 g. dietary fiber, 76 mg. cholesterol, 138 mg. sodium, 35 mg. iron*

CHAPTER 13

POTASSIUM
A PROTECTOR FROM OUR PAST

Dateline: The Stone Age. Grok, a typical cave dweller, is preparing food for the day.

For breakfast, he eats a juicy cantaloupe smashed open against a jagged rock. He places a banana, some nuts and a squash in a goatskin sack for lunch. Then he's off to scrounge groceries—a few figs here, some potatoes there—to haul back to the cave, dodging wild beasts along the way.

Few of us would want to trade our condos or Cuisinarts for Grok's crude lifestyle. But if we *were* to return to our dietary roots and adopt his menu of potassium-rich plant foods, experts say we might at least be more likely to stave off modern-day diseases such as stroke, heart disease, diabetes and even cancer.

A QUESTION OF BALANCE

Louis Tobian, M.D., professor of medicine and head of the Hypertension Department at the University of Minnesota in Minneapolis, is the leading advocate for a return to an ancestral diet.

According to Dr. Tobian, the prehistoric cuisine, consisting mostly of vegetables, fruits, nuts, roots and occasionally wild game, contained very little sodium but lots of potassium. Both these minerals—in the proper ratio—are essential to health. When dissolved in body fluids, they carry on

THE PICKS OF POTASSIUM

Choosing a variety of potassium-rich foods can help you meet your daily goal of at least 3,000 milligrams easily and deliciously.

FOOD	PORTION	POTASSIUM (mg.)
Avocado	1	1,204
Raisins	1 cup	1,089
Acorn squash, baked	1 cup	891
Potato, baked	1	844
Spinach, cooked	1 cup	838
Cauliflower florets, raw	1 cup	795
Navy beans, cooked	1 cup	719
Apricots, fresh	1 cup	628
Plain nonfat yogurt	1 cup	579
Orange juice	1 cup	496
Cantaloupe	1 cup cubes	494
Skim milk	1 cup	447
Chicken breast, broiler/fryer	1	440
Sockeye salmon, fresh, cooked	3 oz.	319
Flounder, cooked	3 oz.	292
Ground beef, extra-lean	3 oz.	266
Turkey white meat	3 oz.	259
Turkey dark meat	3 oz.	247
Bran muffin	1	172
Pumpernickel bread	1 slice	145
Whole-wheat bread	1 slice	50

a sort of unceasing tug-of-war across the walls of cells, which ultimately determines the water balance inside the body.

Because humankind evolved for thousands of years on a potassium-rich diet similar to Grok's, our bodies have become very efficient at getting rid of any excess potassium. And because sodium was normally in short supply, our bodies have become programmed to store it up.

Where we've gotten ourselves in trouble, says Dr. Tobian, is by starting to eat the reverse of the prehistoric diet—one that's incompatible with the way we are biologically programmed. Today's typical diet skimps on fresh plant food. Instead it is laden with salty "factory food" that has had much of the potassium squeezed out during processing. And the closest some come to fruit is the prune filling inside a Danish. As for vegetables, we may eat lots of potassium-rich potatoes, but too often they're the salty, fried-in-fat kind.

We pay a high price for eating this lopsided, "unnatural" diet that is out of sync with our bodies, according to Dr. Tobian. "There's strong evidence suggesting that a lifetime of eating a typical modern diet can lead to heart disease and stroke," he says.

For example, researchers found that people in Scotland, who eat mostly low-potassium foods, have a greater incidence of heart disease than people in southern England, who eat higher amounts of potassium-rich food. In the United States, blacks in the southeast who typically eat potassium-poor diets have a higher stroke risk than any other group in the country.

KEEPING THE LID ON BLOOD PRESSURE

Laboratory studies show convincingly that a diet short on potassium boosts blood pressure—a leading cause of heart disease and stroke.

In a small but impressive study conducted at the Temple University School of Medicine and the University of Pennsylvania in Philadelphia, researchers placed ten men with normal blood pressures on two experimental diets, one providing normal amounts of potassium and the other low in potassium. Nine days on the normal potassium diet showed no significant change in blood pressure readings. But after going on the low-potassium diet, their blood pressures went up. The men also retained more sodium and fluid.

Similar results were found in people with high blood pressures. "Our research shows that when we feed people with either high or normal blood pressures a low-potassium diet, their blood pressures will increase in less than two weeks," says G. Gopal Krishna, M.D., associate professor of medicine at the University of Pennsylvania. One reason is that a low-potassium diet causes people to retain more sodium. Over time, this high sodium level attracts water, increasing blood volume and raising blood pressure.

But the good news, says Dr. Krishna, is that when these same people were put on a high-potassium diet, their blood pressures went down. "A high-potassium diet counteracts sodium's harmful effects on blood pressure," says Dr. Krishna.

Potassium even appears to be helpful for people with high blood pressures who take medication. Researchers at the University of Naples in Italy put a group of people on blood pressure medication on a potassium-rich daily diet of beans, fruits or vegetables for a year. The result: They slashed their drug intake by more than 50 percent.

The combined evidence makes one thing clear: "When it comes to controlling blood pressure, the amount of potassium in your diet may be more important than how little salt you eat," says Dr. Krishna.

HOLDING SODIUM IN CHECK

Potassium performs many jobs in the body. It is responsible for maintaining proper fluid balance within the cells, and it helps nerves transmit messages and assures proper muscle functioning. But the secret to its pro-

DON'T SWEAT OVER SPORTS DRINKS

It's mid-August, the second day of your hiking trip, and you're sweating like a racehorse near the finish line. Your hiking companions are swigging sports drinks like there's no tomorrow. Are you missing out on something?

Maybe so—if the drinks contain potassium.

When you perspire, you lose more than water. You also lose trace amounts of potassium and other electrolytes, important minerals that separate into electrically charged particles inside the body. Adequate potassium is needed to help muscles contract and relax. If your potassium level dips, your muscles may flex but not relax. The result: a cramp. What's more, a lack of potassium can impair your muscles' ability to use glycogen, the sugar that is their main source of energy.

In other words, a prolonged, sweaty workout could lead to weak, spasm-prone muscles. Worse, severe dehydration can lead to heatstroke.

Even so, many experts believe that, unless you are an endurance athlete competing in a hot environment, electrolyte sports beverages are probably unnecessary. That's because your body automatically rebalances its electrolyte levels through a regular diet of potassium-rich foods.

"For most exercisers, the important thing for preventing heatstroke and muscle cramps is getting fluid into your body," says Herman Johnson, Ph.D., of the United States Department of Agriculture's nutrition lab at the Presidio of San Francisco. "Plain water will do the trick."

But other experts argue that plain water is too "plain" for heavy exercise. "During a sweaty workout, more potassium may be depleted from the muscles than is measured by standard tests," says Robert Hackman, Ph.D., associate professor of nutrition at the University of Oregon in Eugene. When you're sweating heavily, he says, you need fluids containing potassium to prevent muscle cramps and fatigue.

These fluids need not be commercial sports drinks, however. "Sipping orange or grapefruit juice during and after a heavy workout is enough to make up for potential potassium losses," says Dr. Hackman. In between workouts, make sure you eat plenty of fruits and vegetables.

tective power against high blood pressure is its ability to police the amount of sodium in the body.

Both potassium and sodium are electrolytes, substances that separate into electrically charged particles called ions. A high-salt, low-potassium diet disrupts the proper electrolyte balance, throwing the fluid balance out of whack. The result: Blood flow in the arteries slows down.

As surplus salt attracts water, blood volume expands, boosting pressure in the arteries. This high volume begins to take its toll on your arteries. Over many years, high blood pressure damages these vessels in various areas, like the heart, brain or kidneys. Eventually, a heart attack or stroke can occur.

Enter potassium. It has the ability to regulate the amount of sodium trying to move into your bloodstream.

Exactly how potassium does its job is still a mystery. It is known, however, that potassium is necessary for proper cellular function and salt balance, says George Bakris, M.D., assistant professor of medicine and pharmacology at the University of Texas Health Science Center in San Antonio.

STROKE PROTECTION

Potassium also appears to be part of the armor against stroke-associated death. At least that's the conclusion of a long-term study conducted jointly by the University of California, San Diego, School of Medicine and the University of Cambridge School of Medicine in England.

After following the diets of 859 Californians for more than a decade, researchers found that those who consumed the least amount of potassium had the highest incidence of stroke-associated death. But not one stroke-associated death occurred among the people whose diets contained the highest levels of potassium.

Perhaps even more amazing is a study from India in which researchers found that potassium lowered both blood pressure and cholesterol (another stroke risk factor) in those with mild hypertension in just two months.

But such results are not surprising to Dr. Tobian. "I'm convinced that the best protection against aging arteries and modern diseases such as stroke and high blood pressure is to eat a primitive diet," he says. One with plenty of potassium.

A ROLE AGAINST CANCER?

A number of population studies, supported by preliminary studies in animals, indicate that there might even be a connection between potassium and cancer prevention.

"The potassium/sodium balance appears to play an important role in regulating cellular growth," says Birger Jansson, Ph.D., professor of biomathematics at the M. D. Anderson Cancer Center in Houston, where the research is taking place. When the balance tips toward a surplus of sodium, he explains, cells can grow abnormally and the likelihood of cancer increases. Ample potassium, however, appears to retard abnormal cell growth and lower the risk of cancer.

"We and scientists at other labs found that laboratory animals fed high-potassium, low-sodium diets had fewer tumors and a longer lifespan than rats fed the opposite diets," says Dr. Jansson. "While the study results are preliminary, I believe it's safe to assume that eating more fruits and vegetables and reducing the intake of salt helps reduce not only your risk of cardiovascular disease but also cancer."

How Much to Aim For

Of course, getting plenty of potassium doesn't mean you should be getting it by eating banana splits. "To protect against heart disease and stroke, you need to follow other good eating habits for maintaining healthy arteries," says Dr. Tobian. That means a low-fat diet and plenty of fruits and vegetables—Grok's main menu.

"A good diet and a regular program of aerobic exercise is as important as increasing potassium," says Dr. Tobian. "The more they become a part of you, the more potassium will benefit you."

Studies show that roughly 3,000 milligrams a day are needed to protect against stroke. "That's not hard to achieve when you consider that a typical balanced diet offers between 2,000 and 2,500 milligrams of potassium a day," says Dr. Tobian.

Indeed, in the California study, people who added only about 400 to 450 milligrams of extra potassium a day—the amount in one banana—to their normal diets were able to reduce their risk of stroke death by 40 percent.

But, if you're a fast-food fan or you generally don't eat plenty of fruits and vegetables, you'll have to work a little harder to get 3,000 milligrams a day.

And if you are at risk for high blood pressure or stroke, you may need twice that, says Dr. Tobian. But be sure to check with your doctor before taking any potassium supplements.

Potassium-Boosting Tips

Getting more potassium is a snap if you learn to follow a few rules and make some simple substitutions, according to Dr. Tobian.

Take a juice break. "Instead of a coffee break, I drink grapefruit juice three times a day. At 400 milligrams of potassium per cup, that's 1,200 milligrams right there," he says.

Take your mother's advice. "Vegetables are loaded with potassium," says Dr. Tobian. "They're really the key to eating a healthy primitive diet." Consider, for example, that a cup of cooked asparagus has 558 milligrams of potassium; a cup of baked butternut squash has 580 milligrams.

Go natural. As a general rule, go for more fresh food and less packaged, canned or fast food, says George Webb, Ph.D., associate professor of physiology and biophysics at the University of Vermont College of Medicine in Burlington. "The canning process usually involves boiling the food, which leaches out the potassium," says Dr. Webb. "The tasteless result is then flavored with table salt."

LESS PROCESSING—MORE POTASSIUM

The more a food has been processed, the more potassium it is likely to have lost. Compare the potassium content of the fresh or minimally processed foods below with their more processed versions.

FOOD (1 cup)	POTASSIUM (mg.)
BEETS	
Fresh	530
Canned	252
CAULIFLOWER	
Fresh	404
Canned	250
FLOUR	
Whole-wheat	444
White	109
MUSHROOMS	
Fresh	555
Canned	201
RICE	
Brown	137
White	57

Take peas, for instance. A half-cup of cooked fresh peas offers 217 milligrams of potassium and just 2 milligrams of sodium. But ½ cup canned peas delivers only 147 milligrams of potassium and 186 milligrams of sodium.

Go down to the farm. Although fruits and vegetables are the best sources of potassium, other sources are easy to find. Low-fat dairy products, fish, poultry and lean meat can also contribute to your daily intake.

Combine dishes to double your potassium. There are plenty of tasty ways you can bring potassium-rich foods together. Try a half cantaloupe with a scoop of ice milk, for example. Toss potassium-rich lentils in your spinach salad or bake fish with a layer of glazed apricots.

Season lightly with salt substitutes. Salt substitutes containing potassium chloride can help limit your salt intake while boosting your potassium intake. But you shouldn't rely solely on these products to meet your quota of extra potassium, warns Dr. Webb. "For one thing, we're not sure of chloride's role in blood pressure," he says. For another, potassium in food is absorbed more slowly and probably more effectively than man-made chemicals.

A note of caution: If you have kidney problems or take a potassium-sparing diuretic, you should avoid potassium chloride salt substitutes. Otherwise, you could be getting too much potassium. Check with your doctor.

You needn't go bananas. This sweet tropical fruit gets most of the attention as a prime potassium source. But it really isn't the highest source. While a banana has about 450 milligrams of potassium, a slice of watermelon has 602 milligrams and a cup of prune juice has over 700 milligrams.

Searching for something out of the ordinary? Try green plaintains. They look like unripe bananas but taste like potatoes and pack an awesome 716 milligrams per cup. Try baking them in their skins, or boiling and mashing them like potatoes.

Buy real juice. Some artificially flavored beverages are just chemical versions of juice. Others contain only about 10 percent real fruit juice. Look for juice labeled "100 percent fruit juice." Or squeeze your own freshly made juice complete with bits of healthy fiber.

Walk past the white bread. Choose whole-grain breads instead. A slice of white bread contains 26 milligrams of potassium; a slice of whole-wheat contains more than twice that amount. You can also buy whole-wheat flour for baking and whole-wheat bread crumbs for stuffing and mixing into meat loaf.

Stockpile potatoes. "People call milk the perfect food, but potatoes should really win that title," says Dr. Webb. For starters, they are great sources of potassium: one baked potato supplies more than 800 milligrams. They're also very low in calories, providing you avoid the fried kind and skip the butter topping.

For a treat, try potato pancakes. Simply shred one or two potatoes without peeling, add some minced onion, and brown in a nonstick pan. Serve with applesauce or a dollop of nonfat yogurt for even more potassium power.

Load up on legumes. Beans have a very high potassium content and make great additions to salads and stews. A cup of cooked pinto beans, for example, supplies 796 milligrams of potassium; the same amount of navy beans has 719 milligrams, and lima beans have 730 milligrams per cup.

Don't boil food. Boiling leaches out potassium. Researchers have found, for example, that boiled potatoes lose up to half of their potassium, while steamed potatoes lose only about 6 percent. Similar results were found with carrots, beans and peas. You're better off steaming, baking, microwaving or stir-frying.

Add a little blackstrap molasses. Two tablespoons of blackstrap molasses contain more than 435 milligrams of potassium. Try swirling it in hot cereal or using it instead of honey in recipes.

Toss in brewer's yeast. One tablespoon of this concentrated source of B

Easy Options for Extra Potassium

Here's some good news: High-potassium foods are great for your waistline. Here are some high-potassium substitutions for high-calorie fare.

- Instead of cream pie to satisfy your sweet tooth, have a pear for dessert. One juicy pear gives you 208 milligrams of potassium.
- Grill chicken or fish instead of frankfurters. A single chicken breast has less fat than a frank and gives you 220 milligrams of potassium compared to just 143 milligrams in the hot dog.
- Try fruit spreads in place of butter. Apple butter spread on your toast offers 38 milligrams of potassium per tablespoon and virtually no fat, versus 6 milligrams of potassium and 11 grams of fat per tablespoon of margarine.
- Instead of iced tea on a sweltering day, reach for frozen melon balls kept in the freezer. Substitute the frozen balls for ice cubes in fruit drinks. Or toss them in a blender for a refreshing slushy cooler. Honeydew melon, for example, contains 461 milligrams of potassium per cup; casaba has about 357 milligrams.

vitamins also gives you 152 milligrams of potassium. And you can add it to everything from soups and stews to blender drinks.

Mix in tofu. One cup of tofu contains 596 milligrams of potassium and 244 milligrams of calcium, another mineral that may do good things for blood pressure. Dice tofu and add to chili or substitute it for half the hamburger in lasagna.

Have a date or two. Ounce per ounce, dried fruits have even more potassium than fresh fruits do. That's because the water has been removed so the potassium is concentrated, says Dr. Webb. Three fresh apricots, for example, give you a respectable 314 milligrams of potassium. A cup of dried apricots, however, supplies a mighty 1,204 milligrams of the mineral. Try dried dates, prunes, raisins or figs on your morning cereal or as standalone snacks. They also make great substitutes for fatty sauces to flavor oven-baked poultry and pork.

Dried fruits, however, should be eaten sparingly—they're very high in calories.

Serve some soup. Homemade soup is an ideal way to bring lots of potassium-rich vegetables to your table—minus the high levels of added sodium found in many canned soups. In addition to old standbys like chicken or tomato soup, try pumpkin soup. A cup of canned pumpkin has 503 milligrams of potassium.

HIGH-NUTRITION RECIPES

CUBAN-STYLE PLANTAINS

Plantains are cooking bananas often featured in Caribbean cuisine. They're super sources of potassium, but unlike bananas, they cannot be eaten raw. Cooking softens their starchy texture and develops their flavor. Buy plantains that are fully yellow, firm and heavy. Use this recipe in place of potatoes when serving spicy chicken, fish or pork dishes.

4 plantains
¾ cup skim milk
¼ cup fat-free egg substitute
¼ cup minced scallions
3 tablespoons shredded low-fat Cheddar cheese
2 cups chunky salsa, heated

Peel the plantains using a sharp paring knife. Cut the flesh into ½" slices. Steam for 15 minutes, or until very tender. Place in a large bowl and mash with a potato masher. Stir in the milk, egg and scallions.

Coat a 9" pie plate with no-stick spray. Add the plantain mixture and smooth the top with a spatula. Sprinkle with the Cheddar.

Bake at 400° for 10 minutes, or until the mixture is heated through and the cheese is lightly browned.

Cut into wedges and serve topped with the salsa.

Serves 6
Per serving: *208 calories, 3.6 g. fat (13% of calories), 3 g. dietary fiber, 4 mg. cholesterol, 347 mg. sodium, 887 mg. potassium*

ORANGE SHAKE

Here's another high-potassium beverage—this one thick and creamy like a milk shake. (But it contains none of the fat found in regular shakes.) For variety, replace the dates with banana slices or strawberries.

About 1 cup orange juice
½ cup chopped dates
1½ cups frozen nonfat vanilla yogurt

In a blender, combine the orange juice and dates. Blend on high speed until the dates are very finely chopped. Add the yogurt and blend until just combined. If the mixture is too thick, thin with a little additional juice.

Serves 2
Per serving: *338 calories, 0.4 g. fat (1% of calories), 4.9 g. dietary fiber, 0 mg. cholesterol, 82 mg. sodium, 539 mg. potassium*

GERMAN POTATO SALAD

Potatoes are one of the best vegetable sources of potassium. But to help safeguard the nutrient, steam the potatoes rather than boiling them. Contrary to popular opinion, potatoes are not fattening. And neither is potato salad—as long as you stay away from fatty mayonnaise or oil-based dressing. This version has a tangy vinegar dressing and is served warm, in the German tradition.

- **2 pounds small potatoes**
- **2 ounces turkey bacon, cut into ½" pieces**
- **½ cup diced sweet red peppers**
- **½ cup diced red onions**
- **⅔ cup defatted beef stock**
- **⅓ cup apple-cider vinegar**
- **2 teaspoons honey**
- **½ teaspoon ground black pepper**
- **⅛ teaspoon celery seeds**
- **1 tablespoon cornstarch**
- **2 tablespoons water**
- **2 tablespoons minced fresh parsley**

Scrub the potatoes and cut into thin slices. Steam until tender but not mushy, about 10 minutes. Transfer to a large bowl.

Meanwhile, in a large no-stick frying pan over medium heat, cook the bacon, peppers and onions until the bacon is crisp, about 5 minutes. Add to the potatoes and toss lightly.

In a 1-quart saucepan, whisk together the stock, vinegar, honey, pepper and celery seeds. Bring to a boil over high heat. Reduce the heat to medium.

In a cup, dissolve the cornstarch in the water. Add to the pan and whisk constantly until the dressing thickens, about 2 minutes. Pour over the potatoes and toss gently. Sprinkle with the parsley. Serve warm.

Serves 6

Per serving: *174 calories, 3.5 g. fat (17% of calories), 3.2 g. dietary fiber, 9 mg. cholesterol, 231 mg. sodium, 870 mg. potassium*

GRAPEFRUIT COOLER

Fruit beverages are a tasty and easy way to get potassium into your diet. This citrus refresher combines potassium-rich grapefruit juice with orange or tangerine juice. You may serve the drink over regular ice cubes, but for an extra bonus of potassium, make cubes from additional grapefruit juice.

- **4 cups pink grapefruit juice**
- **½ cup orange or tangerine juice concentrate, thawed**
- **3 tablespoons lime juice**
- **2 cups sparkling mineral water**

In a large pitcher, mix the grapefruit juice, juice concentrate and lime juice. Stir in the mineral water. Serve over ice.

Serves 4
Per serving: *144 calories, 0.3 g. fat (2% of calories), 0.7 g. dietary fiber, 0 mg. cholesterol, 7 mg. sodium, 603 mg. potassium*

CHAPTER 14

ANTIOXIDANTS
DIETARY "RUSTPROOFERS"

Butter turns rancid. The iron gate rusts. Fire burns. Paint dries. Arteries harden. People grow old.

It's all the same, more and more scientists believe. The same chemical reaction—oxidation—that coats an unseasoned skillet with an orange film of rust is being implicated in such diseases as cancer, cataracts and atherosclerosis. Even aging may be caused by the same process.

If you slice an apple and leave it exposed to air, it will soon turn brown. But soak that sliced apple in a vitamin C solution first, and it will stay glistening white.

That's because vitamin C is one of a handful of nutrients with power to protect cells from the damage of oxidation. While the evidence still is inconclusive, it nonetheless strongly suggests that increasing dietary intake of nutrients known as antioxidants may help save the body from the ravages of certain diseases.

"It's only a hypothesis right now," says Balz B. Frei, Ph.D., an assistant professor of nutrition at the Harvard School of Public Health in Boston, "but there's a lot of good circumstantial evidence. While we still need to conduct more experiments, it's a good idea to have enough of the antioxidants around in your body."

AIRING THE ISSUE

Oxygen breathes life into our bodies; without it, every living thing would die. But the same process through which the body burns food with oxygen to generate energy also sparks a dangerous—albeit quite natural and common—side effect.

Eventually, the oxygen merges with hydrogen to form simple water molecules. But along the way, it also forms highly reactive molecularly unbalanced substances, called free radicals, that have the ability to attack and harm cells.

No, free radicals aren't some anachronistic throwback to the 1960s. A free radical is a wounded molecule that lacks an electron, and it lashes out violently at other molecules, stealing an electron to regain its balance. The victimized molecule itself becomes a free radical, initiating a chain reaction that can eventually destroy cells and organs.

"The problem is you have to get rid of that chain reaction," Dr. Frei says. "One or a few free radicals can oxidize a large amount of cells. The damage can spread very rapidly, especially in fats."

We can't totally escape from free radicals. They're everywhere—created in the body by ultraviolet light, radiation, pollution, car exhaust, cigarette smoke and alcohol—just to name the more common problems. The exposure is thought to be implicated in atherosclerosis, cancer, cataracts, degeneration of the retina in the eye and even aging.

"In each disease, the oxidation process is basically the same. It merely differs in what molecules are being attacked," says Denham Harman, M.D., Ph.D., professor emeritus of the University of Nebraska's College of Medicine in Omaha and executive director of the American Aging Association.

The body does have a defense system against the onslaught. Enzymes manufactured by cells, for example, interact and neutralize some free radicals, but we can do little to increase the amount of those enzymes in our bodies.

So attention has been focused on antioxidant nutrients, whose levels in the body *can* be increased by what we eat and by what supplements we ingest. The principal antioxidants—vitamin C, vitamin E and beta-carotene—do seem to offer protection. And scientists theorize that the higher their concentrations in body tissue and fluids, the better protected we may be against oxidative agents. If you put LDL—low-density lipoprotein, the "bad" cholesterol whose oxidation may initiate artery blockage—in a test tube and bubble air through it, "it won't oxidize appreciably until all the antioxidants are used up," says David Kritchevsky, Ph.D., a professor at the Wistar Institute in Philadelphia. If it works in a test tube, does that mean it works in humans? "We don't know," says Dr. Kritchevsky.

A POSSIBLE ROLE AGAINST CATARACTS

Seeing is believing, according to the cliché, and more people may be able to see more clearly without the obstruction of cataracts if they increase antioxidant nutrients in their diets.

Ophthalmologists are studying how vitamins may prevent or slow the age-related clouding of the eye's lens, a prime cause of blindness. Other research is attempting to determine if the same nutrients can prevent degeneration of the retina.

"The lens of the eye, unlike any other tissue in the body, is subject to the concerted insult of oxidation and light," says Allen Taylor, Ph.D., director of the Laboratory for Nutrition and Vision Research in the United States Department of Agriculture's Human Nutrition Research Center on Aging at Tufts University in Boston. "Because it is exposed almost constantly to the air and to light, it is a prime target for oxidation."

At the onset of cataract formation, the lens starts to harden, says Shambhu D. Varma, Ph.D., director of ophthalmology research at the University of Maryland School of Medicine in Baltimore. The lens cannot flatten or thicken to focus, and people become farsighted. People who are still relatively young can squint to adjust the eye's focal range and compensate for the rigidity of the lens. But as they age and the eye continues to be exposed to oxidative harm, small chalky spots begin forming on the lens. Light doesn't pass through it so easily, Dr. Varma says, and images sent to the retina are no longer clear and well

SACRIFICED FOR A GOOD CAUSE

In the test tube and in many animal studies, at least, the antioxidants work by sacrificing themselves to the oxidizing molecules. They're sort of suicide bombers for health, either sapping the oxidizing molecules of energy or offering them electrons before body cells can be attacked. In either case, the reactive oxygen is rendered harmless, but, unlike victimized body cells, antioxidants do not initiate or continue any destructive chain reaction. Nor do they become malignant.

Vitamins C and E are called scavengers because they react with free radicals before those troublemakers can reach body cells, Dr. Frei says. They are doubly effective because each vitamin molecule can donate two electrons, neutralizing two free radical molecules.

Water-soluble vitamin C circulates through the bloodstream and is found in all body fluids. Fat-soluble vitamin E collects in fat tissue and blood fats.

Beta-carotene's antioxidant power is different from that of vitamin E and vitamin C, according to Dr. Frei. "It's not clear why it has protective antioxi-

defined. Eventually, a white film coats the lens, and vision becomes cloudy.

Exposure of eyes and lenses to higher doses of antioxidant vitamins "seems to delay the onset or progress of cataracts," Dr. Taylor says. And Dr. Varma notes, "Slower development means prevention. We might be able to prevent cataracts or maybe delay their formation."

People with more beta-carotene and vitamin C in their blood often have lower incidences of cataracts, Dr. Taylor says. Vitamin E also seems to play a role.

The antioxidant trio also may be useful against macular degeneration, a disease that harms the membranes of the retina, where images fall and are sent to the brain. "When the central part of the retina begins to deteriorate, it can't transmit to the brain," Dr. Varma says. But preliminary research in animals suggests that vitamin C, beta-carotene and vitamin E may retard the degeneration.

Delivering antioxidants to where they're needed could run into a snag, though. "There's a general failure with eyedrops," Dr. Taylor says. "They are not a good way to get vitamins into the lens. The nutrients are not that stable in drop form, and the solutions that contain them could themselves be irritants."

The easiest and perhaps most effective way could be overall good nutrition, he says. "Increasing dietary consumption of the antioxidants can increase levels in the eye tissue."

dant properties," he says, because it does not scavenge free radicals and offer up electrons. It "quenches" reactive oxygen but does not chemically alter it. "It's an energy transfer," he says. "Beta-carotene takes up energy from the reactive oxygen molecules and dissipates it."

None of the antioxidant nutrients necessarily is a more potent protector than the others. In fact, in the case of vitamins C and E, they may even work in concert. "In different diseases or at different organ sites, one antioxidant may be more important than another, but they're all needed," says Gladys Block, Ph.D., a professor of public health nutrition at the University of California in Berkeley. While they probably act in unison, they usually are studied separately.

VITAMIN C: A KEY PROTECTOR

Heart disease. Vitamin C may be the body's most important guardian against atherosclerosis, according to Dr. Frei, who conducted laboratory tests on the subject. In the oxidative theory of hardening of the arteries, "if there's no oxidation, there's no atherosclerosis," he says. But if the arteries are left unprotected, oxidation eventually occurs. The "bad" LDL cholesterol in blood becomes trapped inside artery walls and slowly oxidizes. Once oxidized, it is taken up by cells in the artery walls at an extremely high rate and transforms into "foam cells," precursors of artery-narrowing plaque that Dr. Frei calls the hallmark of early atherosclerosis.

High-density lipoprotein (HDL) cholesterol, the "good" cholesterol, also is found in artery walls and may prevent LDL oxidation by removing it. But antioxidant vitamins seem to prevent oxidation even without removing the LDL, Dr. Frei says. In laboratory tests, vitamin C completely protected lipoproteins in human blood against a variety of oxidants, including smoke. Beta-carotene and vitamin E became activated only after all vitamin C in the plasma had been expended, and they only partially prevented oxidation.

Cancer. Scientists speculate that vitamin C's antioxidant properties may also play a role in cancer protection. Numerous studies show that people who have a low intake of vitamin C are almost twice as likely to develop cancer of the mouth, voice box or esophagus. In another study, people who consumed less than 90 milligrams of vitamin C a day were 1½ times more likely to develop lung cancer than those who ingested at least 140 milligrams of the nutrient.

And in a study of 55-year-old pack-a-day male smokers, those who consumed low amounts of vitamin C either through food or supplements had a 25 percent chance of dying from lung cancer. But those who ate a lot of foods high in vitamin C, particularly fruit, or who took supplements had only a 7 percent chance of dying from the disease.

High vitamin C intake also has been correlated with lower risks of stomach, pancreatic, cervical and rectal cancer. And postmenopausal women can reduce their risk of breast cancer by 16 percent, one study suggests, if they increase their consumption of the nutrient.

Low levels of vitamin C in men, according to researchers at the University of California at Berkeley, may offer a gateway to free radicals to damage sperm, possibly increasing the risk of birth defects.

Older people seem more likely to have low levels of vitamin C in their bodies. And, for reasons still not known, elderly men need to ingest more C than elderly women to maintain high levels of the vitamin in their bloodstream.

Where to find it. Good dietary sources of vitamin C include citrus fruit and juices, strawberries, red and green peppers, broccoli, cantaloupe, mangoes, tomatoes and tomato juice, watermelon, honeydew melon, brussels sprouts and cauliflower.

VITAMIN E: FREE RADICAL FIGHTER

Ischemia. During surgery, it often is necessary to cut off blood flow to an organ or a part of the body. This process, which is called ischemia, can also occur spontaneously because of disease, and when it happens in the heart, chest pain and even a heart attack could occur. In either case, when oxygen-rich blood flow is restored to the oxygen-starved tissue, free radicals are generated, and fats start to oxidize. That eventually could destroy vital organs. But, Dr. Kritchevsky says, "If vitamin E's around, this doesn't happen."

In people who received vitamin E supplementation 12 hours before heart bypass operations, hydrogen peroxide levels in their bodies—an indicator of oxidation—did not increase during surgery. Levels of the chemical did increase, though, in people who did not receive the supplement.

Other experiments have shown that vitamin E supplements diminish fat peroxides in blood and, in women, reduce the increase in blood clotting associated with long-term use of hormonal contraceptives.

Cancer. As with vitamin C, there is evidence that vitamin E may lessen

A Stop-Gap Measure for Smokers Who Can't Stop?

Smoke gets in your eyes, according to the song, but it also gets in your lungs and bloodstream, causing oxidative damage to cells.

The best approach to preventing lung cancer, emphysema and hardening of the arteries is, of course, to quit smoking. But if you're currently curled up with a Camel or musing with a Marlboro, you may take some comfort from what scientists are learning about antioxidant nutrients.

Vitamin E may be utilized by smokers to stave off the oxidation of fats in cells. A group of researchers from the University of Toronto Department of Medicine in Ontario suggests that "for smokers who cannot refrain from smoking, a possible means of reducing their total body lipid peroxidation is to administer additional antioxidants—vitamin E."

The authors of the study chose vitamin E because it appears to be the only fat-soluble antioxidant in blood and because it is generally safe even in large doses. Normal blood levels of the nutrient in smokers did not adequately prevent oxidation, but "substantial doses" of 800 milligrams a day did minimize the damage, according to the report.

Antioxidant treatment also holds out some hope for people who chew tobacco. Beta-carotene and vitamin A supplements given to a group of Indian fishermen over a six-month period resulted in remission of precancerous white patches in their mouths and prevented any new lesions from forming. Once supplementation ceased, the lesions reappeared, according to members of the British Columbia Cancer Research Centre in Vancouver. The good results are all the more startling, the researchers note, because the fishermen in the study continued to chew tobacco during the six months of the trial.

the risk of developing cancer, and not just because it scavenges free radicals. The nutrient may also bolster the body's immune system, enabling it to eliminate cells already damaged by oxidation. Vitamin E also seems to prevent the transformation of nitrite food additives into cancer-causing nitrosamines in the stomach.

Selenium, a nutrient that seems to work in conjunction with vitamin E, also possesses antioxidant properties. Experiments show that this mineral can reduce the size and growth of tumors in animals, perhaps by strengthening the immune system. But too much selenium in the body is toxic, and research shows that when vitamin E in the diet is adequate, selenium is of limited and perhaps no importance.

Where to find it. Good dietary doses of vitamin E include wheat germ, peanut butter, almonds, filbert nuts, sunflower seeds, shrimp, and vegetable oils. Green leafy vegetables also contain some vitamin E.

How Much Do We Need?

Way back in the early 1940s when the Recommended Dietary Allowances (RDAs) were first established for optimal nutrition, we needed guidelines for how much vitamin D was necessary to prevent rickets, how much vitamin C was required to ward off scurvy and how much vitamin B_1 would eliminate the chance of beriberi.

In the developed world today, we don't have to worry about pellagra, rickets and scurvy; we're plagued by cancer, atherosclerosis and diseases associated with aging.

"The RDAs have outlived their usefulness," says John H. Weisburger, M.D., Ph.D., of the American Health Foundation in Valhalla, New York. "There are no more deficiency diseases. We have enough nutrients to meet the RDAs. We need optimal amounts to prevent other diseases like heart disease, cancer and stroke."

What are those new, higher amounts? No one really knows for sure. But the levels, especially for the antioxidant vitamins, certainly are higher than the current RDAs. And partly because Americans don't eat anywhere near the recommended serving of fruits and vegetables, some experts say supplementation is a necessity.

"It's very clear that hardly anybody eats a well-balanced diet," says Gladys Block, Ph.D., of the University of California in Berkeley. According to one survey, about 17 percent of people eat no vegetables, only half eat a vegetable other than potatoes or a salad, and some 40 percent have no fruit or fruit juice. On any given day, only about a quarter of the American people eat fruits and vegetables rich in the antioxidant vitamins.

BETA-CAROTENE: THE A-PLUS NUTRIENT

Cancer. It once was thought that beta-carotene's principal benefit was that the body could convert it to vitamin A on an as-needed basis. (Overdoses of vitamin A can be toxic to the system.) No longer. As an antioxidant, beta-carotene seems to work its magic without its transformation into vitamin A. Moreover, while few studies point to an association between cancer protection and high levels of vitamin A in the body, research consistently demonstrates a significant link between high levels of beta-carotene and lower rates of certain cancers, especially in the lungs.

Of 11 studies of diet and lung cancer reviewed by one researcher, all found a decreased risk of disease with higher consumption of carotene-containing foods.

One of the most extensive long-term examinations of antioxidants and

"When we see what we're eating, we realize there are not a lot of the antioxidants in our diets," Dr. Block says. People should "dramatically increase their eating of fruits and vegetables because they have the E, the C, the beta-carotene. Those are very important agents in the body. Nature packaged them together, and we evolved on them."

The amounts of vitamins believed to be needed to counter oxidants in the body far exceeds the RDAs and may even go beyond what we're capable of ingesting through food. "The amounts in food are too small to get the values we're talking about," says Denham Harman, M.D., Ph.D., of the University of Nebraska College of Medicine and the American Aging Association. "You'd have to eat an awful lot of oranges, for example."

Dr. Harman suggests that people concerned about counteracting oxidants in their bodies take between 100 and 200 I.U. of vitamin E a day and 500 milligrams of vitamin C two to four times a day. (Supplementing at levels in excess of the RDAs should only be done in consultation with a physician.)

No optimal dietary amount has been established for beta-carotene, a lack that Dr. Weisburger calls "a gap in food and nutrition thought." He recommends between 10 and 20 milligrams of beta-carotene three times a week. "That gives you a certain blood level that is distributed to all tissues." Beta-carotene is not toxic and its dosage is "self-limiting," he says, because it isn't absorbed very well. Dr. Harman recommends 15 milligrams of beta-carotene every other day.

cancer, the Basel study of 2,974 men in Switzerland, determined that people with low blood levels of beta-carotene have "a significantly higher risk of death from [lung] cancer." Little correlation was found for vitamin A and lung cancer, and vitamin C was lower in most incidences of the disease. But beta-carotene levels were considerably lower in the men who had lung and stomach cancer. That led the researchers to "strongly encourage a higher intake of dietary carotenoids and carotene-containing supplements as a preventive measure against cancer."

Where to find it. Beta-carotene can be found in such foods as carrots, winter squash, pumpkin, sweet potatoes, apricots, cantaloupe, mangoes, peaches and dark green leafy vegetables such as spinach, kale and broccoli.

BRAKING THE AGING PROCESS

From wrinkling of the skin to degeneration of muscles and organs, growing old may be the cumulative bodily response to constant oxidation, experts like Dr. Harman propose. "The aging process may be simply the sum of the deleterious free-radical reactions going on continuously through the cells and tissues," he says. The reactions produce progressively more severe harm the longer they remain unchecked and the longer a person lives.

Doctors can't see free radicals; they can only infer their impact on aging by the clues they leave, such as age spots, the accumulation of oxidized blood fats and damage to organs. Theoretically, slowing oxidation of the

WHEN TO TAKE ANTIOXIDANTS

Most people take their vitamins—if they do, in fact, take their vitamins—at breakfast. They're swallowed with a few gulps of coffee or juice, perhaps accompanied by a piece of toast or a muffin. That's probably the worst meal of the day with which to take them, especially if you're looking for maximum protective benefits from the antioxidants.

The best time to take your vitamins is with the main meal of the day, says John H. Weisburger, M.D., Ph.D., of the American Health Foundation in Valhalla, New York, and it's better to swallow them at the end of the meal.

Beta-carotene and vitamin E are fat soluble, he says. "They won't be absorbed well in a nonfat meal." The typical breakfast of coffee or juice and perhaps cereal contains very little fat, he says, so the fat-soluble vitamins are whisked through the digestive system without being retained in tissue. Thus, there's no antioxidant benefit.

body—the onset of the process or the chain reaction it causes—should retard disease and extend life potential. And that might be achieved, Dr. Harman proposes, by increasing the amount of antioxidant chemicals in the body.

Maximum life span of the human species has not been extended so far, but aging could be slowed down and life extended by combating diseases that shorten life with antioxidants. That would permit humans to live closer to their maximum life potential, he predicts.

"Conquest of cancer and cardiovascular disease, the two main causes of death, would extend life expectancy by up to ten years," Dr. Harman says. "While most of the research suggesting that antioxidant nutrients could prevent those diseases involves animals, the human data we do have corroborate the animal studies."

HIGH-NUTRITION RECIPES

DIJON PASTA SALAD

This main-course salad is brimming with antioxidant nutrients: The peppers and broccoli have nice amounts of vitamin C; the carrots and kale are great sources of beta-carotene; and the shrimp, wheat germ and almonds contribute valuable vitamin E.

4 ounces tricolor rotelle
1 cup bite-size broccoli florets, lightly steamed
1 cup cooked baby shrimp
½ cup thinly sliced carrots
½ cup diced sweet red peppers
½ cup nonfat yogurt
½ cup nonfat mayonnaise
⅓ cup wheat germ
3 tablespoons white-wine vinegar
1 tablespoon Dijon mustard
½ teaspoon dried dill
½ teaspoon ground black pepper
Kale leaves
3 tablespoons sliced almonds

Cook the pasta in a large pot of boiling water until just tender. Drain and rinse with cold water. Place in a large bowl.

Add the broccoli, shrimp, carrots and red peppers. Toss well.

In a small bowl, whisk together the yogurt, mayonnaise, wheat germ, vinegar, mustard, dill and black pepper. Pour over the salad. Toss well.

Line individual plates with the kale. Divide the salad among the plates. Sprinkle with the almonds.

Serves 4
Per serving: *286 calories, 5.4 g. fat (17% of calories), 3.8 g. dietary fiber, 56 mg. cholesterol, 574 mg. sodium*

FRUIT SALAD SUPREME

What makes this salad supreme is its high complement of antioxidant nutrients: C, E and beta-carotene. The citrus fruits have plenty of vitamin C, the cantaloupe and mango kick in beta-carotene, and the nuts and seeds supply vitamin E.

1 pink grapefruit, peeled and sectioned
1 large navel orange, peeled and sectioned
1 mango, sliced
1 cup cantaloupe chunks
1 cup honeydew chunks
1 cup strawberry halves
½ cup raspberries
½ cup nonfat vanilla yogurt
2 tablespoons orange juice
1 tablespoon lime juice
1 teaspoon grated orange rind
¼ teaspoon poppy seeds
Lettuce
3 tablespoons sunflower seeds
3 tablespoons sliced almonds

In a large bowl, toss together the grapefruit, oranges, mango, cantaloupe, honeydew, strawberries and raspberries.

In a small bowl, whisk together the yogurt, orange juice, lime juice, orange rind and poppy seeds. Pour over the fruit and toss to combine.

Line individual plates with lettuce. Divide the fruit among the plates. Sprinkle with the sunflower seeds and nuts.

Serves 6
Per serving: *144 calories, 4.6 g. fat (26% of calories), 4.3 g. dietary fiber, <1 mg. cholesterol, 20 mg. sodium*

CHAPTER 15

THE 101 HEALTHIEST FOODS

EAT MORE OF THESE

Don't eat this. Don't eat that. Is this what most of today's nutrition advice sounds like to you—all negative?

Well, take heart. There are plenty of wonderful foods that are good for you and that also happen to taste divine. You would be doing yourself a favor if you ate them more often. That's why we came up with the 101 healthiest foods—our list of the foods that modern medical research smiles on for a whole lot of reasons.

What they have going for them (besides tastiness) are several nutritional factors that have been associated with lower risk of disease. Factors like dietary fiber, omega-3 fatty acids, beta-carotene, calcium and other health promoters that may help forestall the development of diseases such as cancer and heart disease. The evidence linking some of these factors to lower risk is strong; the evidence for others, though less conclusive, is promising.

In making our choices, we analyzed the nutritional content of more than 1,000 foods. In general, we tried to select foods that contain significant amounts of at least four essential nutrients that keep your body functioning at peak performance levels.

But we also chose some foods for what they *don't* have. To do that, we aimed for foods that have less than 200 calories and fewer than 100 milligrams of cholesterol and 200 milligrams of sodium per serving. In the meat category, our primary concern was selecting cuts that had less than 30 percent of calories from fat.

But of course, we're not suggesting that you should limit your diet to these 101 foods. "Variety and moderation are important factors in a well-rounded nutritional program," says George Seperich, Ph.D., a food scientist and associate professor of agribusiness at Arizona State University in Tempe. "It would be unwise to assume that these foods can provide absolute protection from health problems—no diet can do that. But eating meals based on this list may increase your odds of living a more energetic and healthy life."

FINFISH

You can't go wrong by including finfish in your diet. A terrific source of protein, fish is a good *lean* alternative to red meat. Flounder, for instance, has less than one-fourth the total fat of sirloin steak. Some species, like haddock, have hardly any fat at all. In any case, whatever fat the fish you select does have may actually be good for you.

Fish has something called omega-3 fatty acids, a type of polyunsaturated fat that may help prevent cardiovascular disease. In fact, some fatty fish might be dynamite secret weapons against high cholesterol and heart attack because they have extra large amounts of omega-3's. Population studies have linked high fish consumption with lower rates of heart disease and stroke among Greenland Eskimos and Japanese fishermen. But omega-3's are just one of many reasons why nutrition experts recommend that you eat at least two servings of fish a week.

Fish is a good source of iron, and that iron—which is in a form that is easier to absorb than iron from plants—helps fortify your blood and protect you against anemia. Most species also are high in magnesium and potassium, two minerals that help regulate blood pressure. Fish is also a good source of the B vitamins, particularly B_{12}, which is necessary for a healthy nervous system.

Flounder (1) with under 12 percent of calories from fat, and **haddock** (2) with under 8 percent, are among the trimmest fish in the ocean. But remember, fattier fish are not all bad, thanks to those heart-protecting omega-3 fatty acids. Although all fish have some omega-3's, among the smartest choices are **bluefish** (3), **mackerel** (4), **trout** (5) and **herring** (6). Two fish, **tuna** (7) and **salmon** (8), deserve special attention. The largest of the tunas, sometimes weighing in excess of 1,000 pounds, fresh bluefin tuna is an especially good heart protector and one of your best buys when available. Although they have somewhat less nutritional wallop, canned white and light tuna also are powerful dietary allies.

Another terrific source of omega-3's, canned salmon, if you eat it with the bones, provides ample amounts of bone-strengthening calcium and vitamin D.

HIGH-NUTRITION RECIPE

HERRING AND POTATO GRATIN

This fish dish would make a perfect brunch entrée. It features herring, which is a good source of healthy omega-3 fatty acids. Be aware that kippered herring contains a fair amount of salt, but you can remove some of it by rinsing and soaking the fish. You could also substitute poached or baked fresh herring.

2 cans (3¼ ounces each) kippered herring
2 large onions, thinly sliced
2 teaspoons olive oil
½ teaspoon ground black pepper
6 medium baking potatoes, thinly sliced
2 tablespoons unbleached flour
2 cups 1% low-fat milk
½ cup seasoned dry bread crumbs
3 tablespoons minced fresh dill

Drain the herring and place in a strainer. Rinse under cold water for 1 minute. Transfer to a medium bowl and cover with cold water. Set aside.

In a large no-stick frying pan over medium-low heat, sauté the onions in the oil for 15 minutes, or until limp and lightly browned. Stir in the pepper. Set aside.

Coat 6 (8-ounce) gratin dishes or ramekins with no-stick spray. Divide half of the potatoes among the dishes.

Drain the herring and flake with a fork. Divide among the dishes. Top with the onions, then with the remaining potatoes.

Place the flour in a medium bowl. Slowly whisk in the milk to make a smooth mixture. Pour into the dishes.

In a cup, mix the bread crumbs and dill. Sprinkle over the dishes.

Bake at 350° for 25 to 30 minutes, or until the potatoes are tender and have absorbed most of the milk.

Serves 6
Per serving: *300 calories, 9.4 g. fat (28% of calories), 3.9 g. dietary fiber, 6 mg. cholesterol, 274 mg. sodium*

SHELLFISH

Although shellfish contains lots of cholesterol, that is offset by the fact that it also is filled with the same type of omega-3 fatty acids found in finfish, which may actually help *lower* cholesterol levels in your body.

In addition, shellfish is extremely low in saturated fat. That's important because researchers now believe that eating saturated fat is a far greater risk factor for heart disease than consuming dietary cholesterol.

The importance of shellfish doesn't end there, though. Every time you crack into a crustacean or pry a mollusk apart, you're really opening a vault of hidden nutritional treasures. In fact, certain shellfish could vie for the title of "Nature's Mineral Depository" because of their abundance of calcium, zinc, magnesium and iron.

Clams (9), for example, are so high in iron, it's a wonder they don't rust. Twenty steamers provide over 160 percent of the women's RDA, 250 percent of the men's RDA. But more astounding, those 20 clams provide 45 times the daily recommendation for vitamin B_{12}.

Ounce for ounce, **oysters** (10) are among the best sources of zinc. Six medium oysters provide five times the RDA for men, more than six times the RDA for women. Oysters are iron-rich, too, but the Atlantic-bred variety is about 25 percent richer in iron than Pacific-grown types. **Mussels** (11) deserve recognition, in part because they are such an inexpensive source of good nutrition.

But as wonderful as shellfish is, "you should be cautious about eating it raw," says John Peters, a seafood processing specialist with the University of Washington Sea Grant Marine Advisory Service in Seattle. "Adequate cooking will kill any harmful bacteria that might be present." But whether you cook it or not, "be sure you buy only from a reputable source," he says.

POULTRY

Loaded with protein, poultry is lower in total fat and saturated fat than most red meat. That's important because saturated fat can raise blood cholesterol levels, and it plays a major role in the development of heart disease.

"If you remove the skin and trim the fat, poultry is great. It's probably one of the simplest and most versatile meats to prepare," Dr. Seperich says.

Poultry also is a good source of iron, zinc and niacin. In fact, some of the best sources of iron on earth can be found flying in the sky. Both **duck** (12) and **goose** (13) are high in the most absorbable type of iron.

For nearly as much absorbable iron, but much less fat, try **turkey** (14) and **chicken** (15). With turkey, dark meat's the most iron-rich part. But turkey breast is undeniably one of the leanest meat choices you can make. A three-ounce serving of skinless, roasted white turkey meat has 133 calories, 2.7 grams of total fat and less than a gram of saturated fat. Gobbling on turkey also provides nearly one-quarter of the daily recommendation for vitamin B_6. Chicken breast is a healthy choice, too. With only 19 percent of calories from fat, it also may help lower your risk of cancer. In a study of 88,751 women conducted over six years, researchers concluded that the women who consumed the most beef, pork and lamb had a higher risk of colon cancer than those who ate more skinless chicken and fish.

MEATS

Once considered America's all-star entrée, red meat is showing up on fewer plates these days because of concerns about saturated fat and cholesterol. It's true that many red meats are laden with those two heart disease-causing villains. In some cuts, more than 50 percent of the calories come from fat. But with proper selection and preparation, eating moderate three-ounce servings of lean red meat two to three times a week can be a good supplement to a low-fat, low-cholesterol diet.

It makes sense to include some red meat in your diet because it's one of the best sources of iron. Beef has 1½ times more iron than an equivalent serving of chicken or fish. Pork and lamb also contain more of this blood-strengthening nutrient than an equal amount of chicken. And, unlike the iron in vegetables, fruits or grains, the iron in red meat is readily absorbed by the body. Red meat also contains significant amounts of copper, manganese and zinc. These three minerals work together with calcium to build strong bones.

When buying meat, look for "select" grade—it has the least amount of fat. Before cooking be sure to trim all the visible fat off even the best cuts.

Preparation also is an important consideration. Broiling, for instance, is much better than frying because it allows fat to drip away from the meat. "If you bread and fry it, you're really undoing all the good that you did by

HIGH-NUTRITION RECIPE

SPICY VENISON STEW

Venison is a very lean meat that makes a tasty substitute for beef. This stew contains an interesting blend of spices that gives it a Middle Eastern flavor.

- **2 tablespoons unbleached flour**
- **1 pound boneless venison, cut into 1" cubes**
- **1 tablespoon olive oil**
- **2 cups diced onions**
- **1 teaspoon ground cumin**
- **1 teaspoon ground coriander**
- **½ teaspoon ground black pepper**
- **¼ teaspoon ground cinnamon**
- **¼ teaspoon red-pepper flakes**
- **1 clove garlic, minced**
- **3 cups defatted beef stock**
- **8 ounces medium no-yolk egg noodles**

Place the flour in a plastic or paper bag. Add the venison and shake the bag to coat the pieces.

In a 4-quart pot over medium heat, brown the meat in the oil. Stir in the onions, cumin, coriander, black pepper, cinnamon, red-pepper flakes and garlic. Mix well.

Add the stock. Bring to a boil. Cover and simmer for 1½ hours, or until the meat is tender.

Cook the noodles in a large pot of boiling water for 8 minutes, or until just tender. Drain. Serve topped with the stew.

Serves 4

Per serving: *464 calories, 8.4 g. fat (16% of calories), 3.7 g. dietary fiber, 96 mg. cholesterol, 102 mg. sodium*

buying that lean meat in the first place," says Margy Woodburn, Ph.D., professor and head of the Department of Nutrition and Food Management at Oregon State University in Corvallis.

While it's often difficult to find a cut of red meat that has less than 30 percent calories from fat, it's not impossible. **Pork tenderloin** (16), for example, gets only 26 percent of its calories from fat and provides 53 percent of the RDA for thiamine. With only 25 percent calories from fat, **top round steak** (17) is another tremendous nutritional bargain. A three-ounce serving of **eye round roast** (18) supplies nearly half the RDA for protein, yet only has 143 calories and 4.2 grams of fat. **Lamb foreshank** (19) is the leanest cut of lamb—29 percent calories from fat—and is a marvelous source of protein and zinc. On the wild side, **venison** (20) is low in both fat and cholesterol, and has less than 135 calories per serving.

BEANS

When Jack swapped his mother's cow for a handful of beans, he may have made the wisest trade in fairy tale lore. After all, beans (or legumes) are crammed with nutritious goodies, including fiber, which can promote regularity and help lower cholesterol. *Prevention* magazine adviser James W. Anderson, M.D., professor of medicine and clinical nutrition at the University of Kentucky College of Medicine in Lexington, advocates a diet high in legumes for cholesterol control. In small studies, Dr. Anderson has seen cholesterol levels drop 60 points in three weeks after adding beans to the diets of men with high cholesterol. In other studies, results indicate that beans help normalize blood sugar, which makes them a great dietary choice for those with diabetes.

Beans also are high in complex carbohydrates and low in artery-clogging fat, and they have no cholesterol. Compared to other plant foods, beans are loaded with protein and iron. Beans also are rich sources of B vitamins. Beans are a good choice for pregnant women because they are rich in folate, a B vitamin needed for healthy babies.

"Beans certainly deliver the goods," Dr. Seperich says. "The nice thing about them is there are so many varieties that you'll probably find at least one that appeals to your taste buds."

On the downside, beans—particularly dried ones—can produce a lot of flatulence. But using antigas products such as Beano can help relieve that problem.

Among the most popular dried beans are **pinto beans** (21), **kidney beans** (22), **lima beans** (23) and **lentils** (24)—not to mention **navy beans** (25), which have helped keep sailors going full speed ahead since the early nineteenth century. Like all other legumes, **peas** (26), **chick-peas (garbanzo beans)** (27) and tiny **adzuki beans** (28) are high in iron and other minerals. **Anasazi beans** (29) have a special attraction: all the nutrition of regular beans but less than 25 percent of the flatulence-causing sugars.

HIGH-NUTRITION RECIPE

WARM LENTIL SALAD

One way to enjoy fiber-rich lentils is mixed into an herb-scented salad, such as this.

8 ounces lentils, rinsed
3 cups water
¼ cup diced onions
1 clove garlic, minced
¼ teaspoon dried savory
Pinch of dried rosemary
1 bay leaf
1 cup diced yellow peppers
1 cup shredded carrots
2 tablespoons minced celery
2 tablespoons defatted chicken stock
2 tablespoons olive oil
2 tablespoons red-wine vinegar
½ teaspoon Dijon mustard
Shredded romaine lettuce

In a 2-quart saucepan, combine the lentils, water, onions, garlic, savory, rosemary and bay leaf. Bring to a boil. Partially cover the pan, reduce the heat to medium and simmer for 20 minutes, or until the lentils are tender but not mushy. Drain. Discard the bay leaf.

Transfer the lentils to a large bowl. Add the peppers, carrots and celery. Toss lightly.

In a small bowl, whisk together the stock, oil, vinegar and mustard. Pour over the salad and toss well. Serve warm over the lettuce.

Serves 4
Per serving: *281 calories, 7.6 g. fat (23% of calories), 8.4 g. dietary fiber, 0 mg. cholesterol, 46 mg. sodium*

DAIRY PRODUCTS

Rich in calcium and vitamin D, dairy foods are vital to growth and help us develop strong bones and teeth. In fact, there are no better natural sources of calcium than milk and other dairy products. Eating lots of dairy foods may prevent osteoporosis, the gradual loss of bone mass that can lead to fractures. In addition, studies indicate that low calcium consumption is a risk factor for high blood pressure. The problem with some dairy foods is that they tend to be loaded with fat and cholesterol as well as calcium. But there is a way around that problem—stick to low-fat varieties. After all, there are many to choose from.

Skim milk (30), with only about 6 percent of its calories from fat, is probably the best choice. "Like other dairy products, skim milk is packed with nutrients. Yet, unlike many other dairy products, it has virtually no fat and a minimum amount of calories, making it a super diet food," says George L. Blackburn, M.D., Ph.D., associate professor of surgery at Harvard Medical School and chief of the Nutrition/Metabolism Laboratory at the

Cancer Research Institute at New England Deaconess Hospital in Boston.

One percent low-fat milk (solids added) (31), with 20 percent of its calories from fat, **1 percent low-fat cottage cheese** (32), any other **low-fat cheese** (33) (such as sapsago or part-skim mozzarella) and **nonfat yogurt** (34) are other good high-calcium selections.

VEGETABLES

Eating plenty of vegetables every day won't make you invincible, but many of these plant foods certainly can be classified as dietary superheroes. Vegetables are the backbone of any good diet because they provide lots of complex carbohydrates and vitamins A and C. Yet veggies have virtually no fat and few calories, so they're great for weight-conscious eaters.

"If I had to choose just one vegetable to take with me on a long space flight, I wouldn't go because the nutritional value of vegetables is truly in their variety. By mixing them in your diet, you get a little bit of everything," Dr. Seperich says.

Vegetables contain fiber, which may help prevent a number of diseases including heart disease and colon and breast cancers. And some vegetables pack a mighty supply of calcium for rock-solid bones.

If you feel overly tired, particularly after exercise, adding more vegetables to your diet might help boost your energy. That's because most vegetables are high in magnesium and potassium, two minerals that combat weakness and fatigue. Better yet, eating veggies that have lots of potassium and magnesium may help prevent high blood pressure.

ORANGE-YELLOW VEGETABLES

This group of vegetables is an important source of beta-carotene, a substance that your body converts into vitamin A. Carotenes (including beta-carotene) may decrease the risk of lung, laryngeal, ovarian and other cancers. Researchers in California and Arizona also have found evidence that beta-carotene may prevent oral leukoplakias (precancerous sores inside the mouth). Carotenoids also might play a role in preventing cataracts by retarding oxidation of the lens in the eye.

Carrots (35), ounce for ounce, are one of the best sources of beta-carotene. **Winter squash** (36) (such as acorn, butternut and hubbard), **pumpkins** (37) and **sweet potatoes** (38) are delicious alternatives.

GREEN LEAFY VEGETABLES

Like squashes, carrots and other yellow-orange vegetables, greens are good sources of the carotenes your body uses to make vitamin A. In general, the greener the vegetable, the more carotenoids (including beta-carotene) it contains. Green leafy vegetables also have fair amounts of magnesium and potassium, which, along with calcium, may reduce the risk of high blood pressure. They also have moderate levels of vitamin C, a nutrient that may lower the risk of breast cancer.

Iron and calcium lurk in some greens, but our bodies can't use the minerals in these vegetables as efficiently as those from meats and dairy foods.

For a real nutritional boost, try **romaine lettuce** (39). A one-cup serving has more vitamin C than sweet cherries and twice as much folate as other types of lettuce. **Swiss chard** (40), a spinach look-alike, is actually a relative of the beet. For variety, try **endive** (41), **watercress** (42), **spinach** (43), **kale** (44), **arugula** (45) or **turnip greens** (46).

CRUCIFEROUS VEGETABLES

For a real anti-cancer diet, be sure to eat lots of cruciferous vegetables. These vegetables contain high levels of indole glucosinolates, compounds that are believed to have a variety of cancer-fighting effects. In particular, indoles may inactivate tumor-causing estrogen that targets the breast. Many of these vegetables are also high in insoluble fiber, vitamin C and folate.

When you think of cruciferous, think **broccoli** (47). This mighty veggie has loads of cancer-combating nutrients. Just ½ cup provides 100 percent of the RDA for vitamin C. One cup of raw broccoli has more vitamin C than an equivalent amount of cantaloupe.

Other major members of this family include **cabbage** (48), **bok choy (Chinese cabbage)** (49) and **cauliflower** (50). Thanks to modern horticultural wizardry, the best of cauliflower and broccoli are available in one plant: **broccoflower** (51). A serving of this hybrid crucifer has more vita-

HIGH-NUTRITION RECIPE

SESAME BROCCOFLOWER

Broccoflower combines all the nutritional benefits of broccoli and cauliflower in one handsome-looking package. Here it's sautéed with sesame seeds for a quick side dish—or even a main meal served over rice.

1 teaspoon canola oil
1 head broccoflower, cut into florets
¼ cup defatted chicken stock
1 tablespoon low-sodium soy sauce
1 teaspoon grated fresh ginger
1½ teaspoons toasted sesame seeds

In a wok or large frying pan over medium-high heat, warm the oil for 30 seconds. Add the broccoflower and stir-fry for 5 minutes. Add the stock, soy sauce and ginger. Cover and cook for 3 minutes, or until the broccoflower is crisp-tender. Serve sprinkled with the sesame seeds.

Serves 4
Per serving: *108 calories, 2.3 g. fat (26% of calories), 3.3 g. dietary fiber, 0 mg. cholesterol, 166 mg. sodium*

min C than broccoli and more beta-carotene than broccoli or cauliflower. Broccoflower has a sweet and mild flavor, without the cabbage taste that turns some people off to cauliflower.

Like broccoli, **brussels sprouts** (52) have a lot of calcium and iron for a plant source. The minerals aren't quite as easily absorbed as from animal sources, but some gets through nonetheless.

PEPPERS

Cruciferous plants are not the only vegetables that may have superb cancer-protecting qualities. Capsaicin, the substance that makes **chili peppers** (53) taste hot, may block the formation of cancer-causing compounds in cured meats. In addition, dieters may want to eat lots of foods seasoned with chili peppers, since capsaicin may help increase metabolism and hasten weight loss.

Brought to Spain from the New World by Christopher Columbus, **sweet or bell peppers** (54) are a phenomenal source of vitamin C. But if you really want a healthy dose of vitamins, then be sure to eat your peppers red. The ripened red pepper has about nine times as much vitamin A and twice as much vitamin C as the unripened green pepper.

ALLIUM VEGETABLES

Vegetables that are members of the allium family contain substances that seem to inhibit the formation of blood clots (a principal trigger for heart attacks). Some research suggests that eating a pound of allium vegetables each week may significantly reduce the risk of stomach and colon cancers.

Onions (55) and **garlic** (56) are probably the most familiar members of the allium family. Onions may help lower blood cholesterol. Garlic is a natural blood thinner and may help prevent clogged arteries. A favorite of the Roman emperor Nero, **leeks** (57) share the cancer-protective traits of other allium vegetables. Like onions, they also supply a fair amount of fiber.

HIGH-CARBOHYDRATE VEGETABLES

Potatoes (58) are a nutritionist's dream: good sources of vitamins C and B_6, copper, magnesium, phosphorus, potassium, iron and fiber. This low-calorie delight will also help keep your waistline trim, if you avoid the fatty toppings.

Corn (59) is no empty husk, either. The bran in corn may help lower blood cholesterol. And one ear of corn will give you nearly a fifth of the RDA of folate.

FRUIT

Fruit contains a healthy mixture of complex carbohydrates, natural sugars, fiber, vitamins and minerals. Like vegetables, fruit is a good source of beta-carotene and vitamin C, two nutrients that have been linked to reduced risk of breast and other cancers. Carotenoids such as beta-carotene also may reduce your risk of developing cataracts. Fruit is a good source of soluble fiber that helps control blood sugar levels and relieve constipation. Some soluble fiber may also help prevent colon cancer.

But fruit also is important because of what it doesn't contain. Most fruits have little or no fat. Excessive fat consumption has been linked to heart disease and breast and colon cancer. In addition, most fruit contains only a trace of sodium. That's important because salt may contribute to high blood pressure, a major cause of heart attack, stroke and kidney disease.

Remember that fruit as well as vegetables are less nutritious the longer they are stored or cooked. So your best bet is to eat fresh fruit raw.

CITRUS FRUITS

Citrus fruits are outstanding sources of vitamin C, carotenoids and other compounds that some researchers suspect may have natural cancer-fighting qualities. Most of us don't realize that citrus also is loaded with fiber, particularly in the stringy sections and inner peel. A day without an **orange** (60) is like a day without 116 percent of the RDA of vitamin C. Incidentally, oranges are the leading fruit crop in the United States. **Pink grapefruit** (61) gets its color from its stores of beta-carotene. Pink grapefruits have somewhat more vitamin C than white, but both are good sources of that important nutrient. Both orange and grapefruit juice, by the way, are especially good sources of vitamin C, magnesium and potassium.

Tangerines (62) have more beta-carotene than other citrus fruits. Civil War general Stonewall Jackson considered **lemons** (63) an indispensable part of his diet. He sucked on them incessantly—even as he rode toward battle. The Confederate hero could afford to indulge, since a ½-cup serving only has eight calories. Of course, few people these days suck on lemons, in part, because the acid in the raw fruit can erode tooth enamel. A better way to enjoy this tart fruit is diluted in lemonade or fresh-squeezed in sparkling mineral water. In the nineteenth century, British sailors were known as limeys because they ate **limes** (64) to prevent scurvy. Limes are an excellent way to add a tangy taste to fish and seafood.

HIGH-C FRUITS

The prime advantage of these fruits is their high vitamin C content. Most are also good sources of potassium. Once considered an exotic oddity from New Zealand, **kiwifruit** (65) is now grown in the United States and is popular worldwide. This fuzzy-skinned fruit with emerald green flesh is available year-round. One kiwi packs 124 percent of the RDA of vitamin C, which is 60 milligrams. **Acerola** (66), a West Indian fruit, is still a stranger to most Americans. It looks something like a cherry and tastes very tart, and just one contains 134 percent of the U.S. RDA. And don't forget other high-C contenders like **pineapples** (67), **honeydews** (68) and **pomegranates** (69).

BERRIES

Bursting with vitamin C, berries also are a great source of fiber. But remember that heat destroys vitamin C, so for the most nutritional benefits, try to eat uncooked berries whenever possible.

As sweet as a first kiss and as elegant as a Cole Porter tune, the **strawberry** (70) is one of nature's classic beauties. Strawberries also contain a substance called ellagic acid that seems able to fight off certain cancer-causing agents. But **blackberries** (71) and **blueberries** (72) can be equally delightful. Both are wondrous snacks, but blackberries have more vitamin E. Another great natural snack, **raspberries** (73) only have 60 calories per one-cup serving.

HIGH-FIBER FRUITS

Although most fruits are rich in fiber, some are naturally more hefty sources of this important dietary component that may relieve constipation, lower cholesterol and prevent colon and other types of digestive cancer. Most of the fiber in these fruits is pectin, which helps control appetite by creating a feeling of fullness in the stomach. In addition to their pectin, **apples** (74) have significant amounts of boron, a mineral that may help strengthen bones and keep you alert. **Pears** (75) and **bananas** (76) are two other top fiber sources. Bananas also have lots of vitamin B_6. Ten **cherries** (77) provide one gram of fiber, much of it soluble. Sour cherries have significantly more vitamin A and more vitamin C than sweet ones.

ORANGE-YELLOW FRUITS

These fruits, which include **cantaloupe** (78) and **apricots** (79), are good sources of beta-carotene, which may help prevent certain types of cancers. **Papaya** (80) has more vitamin C than oranges. **Mangoes** (81) are a great addition to yogurt, salads and vegetable dishes.

HIGH-NUTRITION RECIPE

ISLAND PARADISE SALAD

This delicious salad combines tropical fruit with lettuce, peppers and a citrus-based vinaigrette. Serve it as a light lunch on languid summer days. Here's a surprise: Papaya seeds are edible—they have a peppery flavor similar to radishes.

- **2 pink grapefruit**
- **1 papaya**
- **1 mango**
- **1 sweet red pepper, diced**
- **2 scallions, thinly sliced**
- **2 tablespoons minced fresh coriander or parsley**
- **3 tablespoons lime juice**
- **3 tablespoons nonfat yogurt**
- **2 tablespoons honey**
- **1 teaspoon olive oil**
- **¼ teaspoon ground black pepper**
- **Pinch of celery seeds**
- **Pinch of ground red pepper**
- **2 cups torn red-leaf lettuce**
- **1 bunch watercress**

Peel the grapefruit, removing the outer white pith. Working over a bowl to catch the juices, remove each segment from its surrounding membrane. Squeeze the membranes to extract extra juice. Measure out ¼ cup of juice and set aside.

Peel the papaya, halve and scoop out the seeds; reserve about 1 tablespoon of the seeds. Cut the flesh into cubes.

Peel the mango and carefully slice the flesh from the inner pit. Cut the flesh into cubes.

In a large bowl, toss together the grapefruit, papaya, mango, peppers, scallions and coriander or parsley.

In a small bowl, whisk together the reserved grapefruit juice, lime juice, yogurt, honey, oil, black pepper, celery seeds and red pepper. Pour over the salad and toss to combine.

Divide the lettuce and watercress among individual plates. Top with the salad. Sprinkle with the reserved papaya seeds.

Serves 4
Per serving: *148 calories, 1.7 g. fat (9% of calories), 4 g. dietary fiber, 0 mg. cholesterol, 18 mg. sodium*

DRIED FRUITS

Because the water has been taken out, dried fruits often have more calories than fresh fruits. But they also become concentrated storehouses for fiber and a variety of minerals, including copper, iron, magnesium, potassium and zinc. No sour grapes, please, when you speak of **raisins** (82). They have a combination of minerals that may help lower high blood pressure. Golden raisins have a bit more vitamin B_6 and riboflavin than darker varieties. Other outstanding dried fruits include **dried peaches** (83), **prunes** (84) and **figs** (85).

GRAINS

Any way you slice them, grind them or bake them, grains in some form should be an essential part of your diet. Whole grains are important sources of thiamine, iron, riboflavin, magnesium and vitamin B_6. Better yet, they're great low-fat, high-fiber foods loaded with complex carbohydrates. Even refined, processed grains such as the flour used in white bread are fairly nutritious when enriched with thiamine, riboflavin, iron and niacin.

Grains also can be one of a dieter's best friends. "Grains help satisfy your appetite. They make you feel like you've had a good meal. That's important because if you don't feel like you're full, you're more likely to snack on foods that have a lot of empty calories," Dr. Woodburn says.

Dietitians say we should be eating at least six servings of grains, cereals or breads daily. But remember that one serving is only a single slice of bread or ½ cup cooked cereal, rice or pasta. However, choosing the best grain foods could be a daunting task. Here's a sampling of some of our favorites.

Most grains aren't very high in calcium. But **amaranth** (86), a little-known, highly nutritious grain, is an exception. (It can be boiled and eaten like rice, popped like popcorn or ground into flour and used in hundreds of recipes.) Once an integral part of Aztec religion and culture, amaranth has more protein than most other grains. **High-fiber cereal** (87) and **whole-grain bread** (88) are usually fortified with calcium, iron and a variety of vitamins. The sprouting part of the wheat seed, **wheat germ** (89) really does deserve its reputation as a health food. Packed with vitamins and minerals, it can be added to many foods including breads, cookies, cereals and milk shakes. **Brown rice** (90) is more nutritious than white rice. Only the inedible outer husk has been removed. **Whole-wheat pasta** (91), **buckwheat** (92), and **barley** (93) are other superb grain foods. **Oatmeal** (94) and related foods have been shown to lower cholesterol. In South America, the Incas believed a steady diet of **quinoa** (95) ensured a long, fruitful life. It's one of the best plant sources of protein.

OILS

Cooking oils have one unfortunate thing in common—they're 100 percent fat. They also are incredibly calorie-rich (just one tablespoon of oil has at least 119 calories). But despite that, oils can remain a part of your diet if they're selected wisely and used sparingly. All oils are combinations of three types of fatty acids—saturated, monounsaturated and polyunsaturated. Saturated fats have been linked to higher cholesterol levels and increased risk of heart attack. Fortunately, liquid cooking oils are mostly polyunsaturated and monounsaturated fats.

Kudos for **olive oil** (96), which is high in monounsaturated fat and is excellent in salad dressings. It is also frequently used for cooking pastas and vegetables. And finally, three cheers for **canola oil** (97), also known as rapeseed oil. It is one of the few plant sources of heart-disease-fighting omega-3 fatty acids.

NUTS AND SEEDS

Yes, nuts and seeds are loaded with fat—up to 95 percent fat. But in most cases, much of that fat is either polyunsaturated or monounsaturated. But within their tiny shells, nuts and seeds have more than fat. A few nuts, such as **walnuts** (98) are also high in omega-3 fatty acids, the same heart-protecting substance found in fish. In addition, nuts and seeds are good sources of minerals, especially iron, potassium and magnesium. However, nuts should be eaten in moderation because of their high fat and calorie content. Barely a handful can contain more than 160 calories.

Chestnuts (99) are the exception to the high-fat, high-calorie tendency of nuts. With about 70 calories per serving, this lean nut derives less than 8 percent of its calories from fat. Fresh chestnuts usually are available from

September to February. You can roast them in the oven, but be sure to pierce the husk first to prevent the nut from exploding when it's heated. **Dried sunflower seeds** (100) get 78 percent of their calories from fat, but more than half of that fat is polyunsaturated. Sunflower seeds also are good sources of calcium, copper, iron, magnesium, potassium and zinc. **Dried pumpkin seeds** (101) are comparable to sunflower seeds but have slightly more zinc.

HIGH-NUTRITION RECIPE

SAVORY GLAZED CHESTNUTS

Chestnuts are one nut you can eat with abandon. That's because they contain only a trace of fat, unlike almonds, pecans and other common nuts. Although they're delicious as a snack when simply roasted, you can serve them as a vegetable.

12 ounces unshelled chestnuts
8 ounces pearl onions, peeled
1 cup defatted chicken stock
1 tablespoon maple syrup
1 tablespoon balsamic vinegar
1 teaspoon Dijon mustard
Pinch of dried marjoram

Cut an X in the flat side of each chestnut. Place in a 3-quart saucepan and cover with cold water. Bring to a boil. Cook for 1 minute. Remove from the heat.

Using a slotted spoon, remove 1 chestnut at a time. Remove the peel and inner skin. Set aside.

In a large no-stick frying pan, combine the onions, stock, syrup, vinegar, mustard and marjoram. Bring to a boil over medium-high heat. Cover, reduce the heat to medium-low and simmer for 5 minutes.

Add the chestnuts. Cover and simmer for 8 minutes, or until the chestnuts and onions are tender. Using a slotted spoon, transfer to a bowl.

Cook the remaining liquid over medium-high heat until it is reduced to about ¼ cup. Return the chestnuts and onions to the pan. Cook for another minute, until the liquid is reduced to a glaze and the chestnuts and onions are well coated.

Serves 4
Per serving: *183 calories, 2 g. fat (10% of calories), 3.4 g. dietary fiber, 0 mg. cholesterol, 57 mg. sodium*

CHAPTER 16

WATER

THE BEST TOAST TO YOUR HEALTH

The gray-haired honeymooners joked about their stamina as they raced each other through lush Hawaiian undergrowth. Finally, the waterfall appeared before them, plummeting hundreds of feet from the top of a green-shrouded cliff and crashing into a deep, shimmering pool. The pristine-looking, crystal-clear liquid invited the breathless couple to quench their thirst, but a small sign at the base of the fall stopped them. "Warning: Water not safe to drink."

The couple's desire to drink was thwarted, they later learned, by feral pigs running loose in the mountains. Like all living things, pigs need water. But by drinking from streams and excreting wastes in and near the water, the animals spread bacteria, like *Leptospira,* that can cause serious illnesses in humans. The lovers left, still thirsty but ready to swear off water for the rest of their trip.

It turned out to be a vow impossible to keep. No one on this "Water Planet" can live without that precious liquid for more than a few days. After all, we're made mostly of water. Sixty percent of most adult bodies are pure water. Infants are true "water babies," weighing in at 80 percent water. By retirement age, the ratio drops to around 50 percent. There is water in every cell of the body and in every type of body tissue, although, as you must suspect, teeth and bones harbor much less fluid than muscle, while blood is fully four-fifths water. Virtually every biological process going on inside us takes place in a watery medium as well.

WATER POWER

To help sort out its many functions, consider water's three major roles.

1. Transporter. Water in the body helps digest the salad you had for lunch and loads the blood with the dissolved nutrients, which it carries to each living cell. In the process, water helps carry toxins and waste products away from cells, to the lungs, skin or kidneys to be excreted. Water also helps solid wastes move through the intestines. Without water we would be poisoned by the by-products of life.

2. Temperature regulator. A healthy body's temperature hovers at 98.6°F—regardless of the weather outside or the great amount of heat generated inside us—thanks to self-adjusting blood vessel thermostats and the cooling effects of perspiration evaporating from the skin.

3. Lubricator. Without water to lubricate them, our joints would stop moving and we would stiffen up like statues. Our lungs would not be able to inflate or deflate.

TAKING IT ALL IN

Ironically, there is no "official" recommended daily allowance or requirement for water, yet all the other nutrients we require in a day could take a bath in the amount of water we need.

PERCHANCE TO DRINK, PER DAY, HOW MUCH?

"I see people carrying bottles of water everywhere today. It wasn't like that a few years ago," says Howard Flaks, M.D., a Beverly Hills weight-loss specialist and proponent of H_20. People are catching on to the wonders of water, but there is still some confusion about just how much they should drink.

To clarify things, specialists at the International Sportsmedicine Institute in Los Angeles worked out a "recipe" for refreshment and rehydration that anyone, from professional athlete to sedentary fan, can follow.

According to Leroy Perry, D.C., president of the Institute, a non-active, healthy adult, should be drinking ½ ounce water per day for each pound of body weight. A 160-pound person, therefore, should sip ten 8-ounce glasses of water throughout the day.

An active or athletic person will do well to drink ⅔ ounce for each pound of weight. In that case, a 160-pound person on the go should down 12 or 13 glasses of water throughout the day.

Experts say we need *at least* two quarts, or eight 8-ounce glasses, of water every day.

"Generally, a large percentage of the water we need comes from what we drink," says Howard Flaks, M.D., a Beverly Hills, California, weight-loss expert.

"Some of our fluid intake comes from solids in the diet," says Dr. Flaks. Yes, and he's not talking about ice cubes, either. It's no surprise that watermelon is 92 percent water, but lettuce swims in at 96 percent. Baked fish is still 76 percent H_2O. A potato? Seventy-five percent water. Surprisingly, that seems only a little drier than milk, at 88 percent.

"A small amount of fluids the body uses originate as products of metabolism released in the body," says Dr. Flaks. That is, when the body burns its carbohydrate, fat and protein fuels, energy and carbon dioxide are released, and water is produced. In a sense the water of metabolism is like ashes left after a fire, except the body uses this liquid by-product as a liquid asset.

So what's the best source of this liquid gold?

Make it pure and simple. Plain water may not be the best-tasting beverage around but it's the one experts recommend most. "I recommend drinking fluids in the form of pure water," says Dr. Flaks. "Eight glasses a day for a healthy person."

"Unfortunately, most of our fluid needs are met by flavored fluids with lots of calories without many nutrients," says George L. Blackburn, M.D., Ph.D., associate professor of surgery at Harvard Medical School and chief of the Nutrition/Metabolism Laboratory at the Cancer Research Institute of New England Deaconess Hospital in Boston. "We need to break that habit by consuming a cup of water before we drink the other," he suggests.

Fruit juices are not recommended because of their high sugar content. And forget coffee and cocktails as substitutes for filling your daily quota. Besides their obvious negatives (caffeine and alcohol), they also serve as diuretics, sometimes increasing your body's need for fluids.

Make it a habit. Most people do not tank up enough.Although the body *can* extract part of the water it needs from solid foods, many physicians prescribe eight to ten glasses of fluid *in addition to* the amount drawn from other sources. That may seem like a great deal, but the benefits from getting plenty of "hydro-power" can be great as well.

The full benefits may be best reaped, though, by spreading out your intake of water throughout the day. Drinking is not like showering. The inner body needs a steady supply of water, not a once- or twice-a-day dunking.

Letting It All Wash Out

What exactly does the body do with all the water it craves? "Just as we wash the outside of the body, we need to cleanse the inside of the body as well," explains Dr. Flaks. "We remove the stagnant, dirty water in the body by replacing it with fresh, clean water." It's like a circulating fountain. Water flows in, through and out. But instead of spouting from the tops of our heads, water leaves the body via four major routes: The kidneys and urinary tract, the intestinal tract, the skin and the lungs. Tear ducts and the nasal passages are a fifth, small-volume exit route.

Our average daily wastewater output is one to two quarts, and we eliminate most of it as urine. The water in urine spends much of its prior "internal" existence in the bloodstream, doling out nutrients to cells and collecting wastes in turn. Next, the blood races through the hard-working kidneys at a rate of about ½ cup per minute—that's up to 180 quarts per day—where waste products and extra water are filtered out. The kidneys pass the contaminated water to the bladder, where it collects until you urinate. If there is not enough water to handle the body's waste products, the kidneys may not be able to work efficiently, and wastes can contaminate the blood and tissues.

Although as much as eight to ten quarts of water pass in and out of the stomach and intestines every day, very little of it is excreted with the solid wastes it helps to form. In a healthy person only about 2 to 4 percent of the water output leaves the body through the intestinal tract.

Much more water than that exits through the skin in the form of perspiration. "Sweat is absolutely essential. It's a primary way your body regulates its internal temperature," says Norman Levine, M.D., professor and chief of dermatology at the University of Arizona Health Sciences Center in Tucson. When all systems are go, the body burns up nutrients and pumps out a lot of excess heat in the process. The body keeps itself cool by sending water through millions of sweat glands at the skin surface, where it evaporates, carrying heat away from the body.

Some of the body's water output also leaves through the lungs. Breathe in and the fluid between the outer and inner layers of the lung helps you collect air. Breathe out and away go carbon dioxide and water. You can see evaporated water leaving your body when you exhale in chilly air.

ABOVE AND BEYOND

Given the need to closely match water input with output, just how much should we really be drinking? As we've already noted, eight glasses a day is only a rule of thumb. There are actually almost as many exceptions to this rule as there are people.

Add such dehydrating factors as exercise, illness, hot or dry weather, stress, dieting and even air travel to the equation, and water needs change. You may need more water when you're menstruating or pregnant, if you're overweight or aged. Check with your doctor. In many cases, consuming extra water is absolutely vital to good health.

If you fit any of the following profiles, it is essential to keep a watch on your water consumption.

The aging. "Elderly people do not get enough water because they do not recognize thirst as well as they did when they were young," says Susan

Schiffman, Ph.D., a professor of psychology and psychiatry at Duke University located in Durham, North Carolina, who is an expert on the senses and how they change with age. And although increasing age brings a decreasing need for fluid, water and all its attendant functions are still prime concerns for the aged and people who care for them. Watch your loved ones for signs of water retention or dehydration, such as dry lips and skin, dwindling urination, confusion and high body temperature.

"I find that, for the elderly, offering flavored drinks is a better way to get them to drink water," says Dr. Schiffman, "because with their loss of the sense of smell—more so than the loss of their sense of taste—flavored drinks are more appealing. Water does not have a flavor, so there's less motivation to drink."

Exercisers. The old ticker starts humming, the limbs start swinging, and before long, the sweat starts flowing. A heavy-duty workout in hot weather could drain as much as six or seven quarts of water out of your body. A loss of—or failure to replace—just 3 or 4 percent of your vital fluid can definitely slow down all the action in your deprived cells.

There's no need to allow dehydration worries to dampen your fun. Just think—and drink—ahead. The experts typically recommend a hydrating routine like this: Before your workout, sip at least a cup of water. Every 15 to 20 minutes during your exercise, make it a point to chug ½ to ¾ cup, and soon after your routine is finished, enjoy another cupful.

The overweight. "Certainly, overweight people tend not to drink enough water," says Dr. Flaks. And that can actually make them look even heavier. "When people are not drinking enough, a lot of what appears to be fat is often retained water," he explains.

WATER WORRIES

It's easy enough to say we need to drink more water. But we're also aware that what looks cool, clear and inviting can also be downright dangerous—as the couple in Hawaii found out. In fact, pollution in drinking water is such a concern that the Environmental Protection Agency (EPA) has set safe-level standards for contaminants that may be health-threatening.

In fact, say the experts, some levels of contamination—though considered harmless—are hard to avoid. That's because there are so many water sources—surface waters such as rivers and reservoirs, ground water, municipal water companies and private wells and springs—and so many possible sources of contamination—industrial and mining by-products, agricultural chemicals, natural and man-made radiation, leaking underground fuel tanks, air pollutants washed down with rain, unlawfully dumped wastes, sewage and corroded plumbing.

"Any public water supply system that does not meet the requirements set by the EPA must inform the public and take remedial action," says Daniel Henry, information specialist with Geo/Resource Consultants working at the EPA Office of Ground Water and Drinking Water. If there is a problem, the water company will suggest temporary solutions to your drinking water supply problem until it is able to solve the problem. This may range from boiling the water to drinking bottled water at their expense.

Some forms of contamination, however, are much more likely to occur between the water plant and your spigot. The possibility of lead leaching from old water pipes is a prime example. Private wells or springs are also especially prone to contamination by bacteria. If it's been a while (a year or more) since you had your tap water tested or treated, now's a good time to call your state health office or department of environmental regulation for a list of EPA- or state-certified testing labs.

If your water proves to be tainted, or if it is safe but smells, tastes or

BETTER WATER FOUR WAYS

Choosing a water treatment system for your home can be mind-boggling. Here's how the four types of systems work to reduce undesirables in drinking water, according to Nancy Culotta, manager of the Drinking Water Treatment Program at NSF International, a nonprofit product testing foundation in Ann Arbor, Michigan.

Activated carbon. These filters work by passing water through a carbon bed that absorbs contaminants, including chlorine, volatile organic chemicals, and in some cases, lead, color, herbicides, hydrogen sulfide, pesticides and turbidity (fine, suspended particles). Carbon filters that attach directly to your faucet may cost around $100, while larger units range upward in price to $300.

Reverse osmosis. These systems force water through a membrane that rejects contaminants and stores the processed water in a tank. They help reduce arsenic, cadmium, chlorine, chromium, color, giardia cysts, iron, lead, nitrate, radium, sulfate and turbidity. Countertop and under-sink models range from about $200 to $500.

Distillation. By boiling off and then recondensing water, these systems remove contaminants such as arsenic, cadmium, chromium, giardia cysts, iron, lead, nitrate, sulfate and turbidity. Prices range from $400 for countertop models to around $2,500 for the largest models.

Water softeners. They replace the calcium and magnesium that make water hard with sodium to soften water. (If you are concerned about sodium intake, you may want to leave one cold-water tap unconnected to the system for drinking water.) They also may reduce the levels of cadmium, iron, and radium. Whole-house water-softening systems cost from $575 to $1,750.

NSF International, 3475 Plymouth Road, Ann Arbor, MI 48105, offers a free book listing certified treatment units to help you choose one that will suit your particular needs.

looks unacceptable to you, you may be a good candidate for an in-home water treatment system, especially if you have a private well. There are four basic types of units to choose from: activated carbon, reverse osmosis, distillation and water softeners. The type and brand of system you choose will depend on exactly which contaminants you want to get rid of.

IS BOTTLED WATER A GOOD BUY?

You may instead opt to get your water from the multibillion-dollar bottled-water industry. Whether you buy it in a supermarket or have it delivered to your home, you should know that bottled water is produced under rigorous quality control. Most bottled water sold in the United States is derived from natural springs and wells. About one-fourth of the bottled water sold comes from municipal water sources. In order to be sold as bottled water, however, water from these municipal sources must undergo additional treatment and quality control procedures.

Bottled spring, mineral and carbonated waters are all subject to the same EPA standards as any other publicly consumed water. Bottlers are not allowed to make health claims, and the products are sold primarily to people who like the way they taste . . . or *don't* taste, as the case may be.

If you purchase individual bottles of water at the market, you should take a few simple precautions to keep it wholesome.

"Bottled water is a food and should be handled as any other food product," says Lisa Prats, vice president of the International Bottled Water Association. Store bottled water in a cool, dry place, away from direct sunlight and household chemicals. After the bottle is opened, if all of the product is not consumed, be sure to recap the bottle and store it in a cool, dry location or in the refrigerator.

CHAPTER 17

Food Additives

A Mixed Blessing

Peter Gross, M.D., didn't believe in allergic reactions to food additives until he was doubled over with severe abdominal cramps.

Hospitalized four times in two years, the Hackensack, New Jersey, internist underwent nearly every conceivable test to determine the source of his agony. "All of them showed allergic reaction. The question was what was causing it," he says.

His wife, a health writer, suggested he keep a food and medicine diary. Sure enough, when Dr. Gross listed the ingredients of the items in the diary on a spreadsheet along with his symptom flare-ups, one common element stood out like a thug in a police lineup: Yellow Dye No. 6, an artificial coloring often used in drugs and processed foods.

Further testing confirmed the culprit. And since eliminating the foods and drugs containing the dye from his diet, Dr. Gross has been pain-free. "I just learned to read labels," he says.

Fortunately, most of us don't have to scrutinize lengthy ingredient listings *that* closely. If you're like most healthy Americans, those sometimes-ominous-sounding three-syllable food additives are harder to pronounce than to digest. Normally, research shows, our bodies have little trouble tolerating the smorgasbord of strange-sounding ingredients designed to keep

TV dinners oven-fresh, turn green citrus fruit sunshiny orange or tantalize our palates with ersatz flavors.

THEY'RE EVERYWHERE

In fact, chemical additives are so common in processed foods that more than 2,500 are approved for use by the Food and Drug Administration (FDA). And let's not forget that more familiar-sounding substances can be additives as well. Sugar, salt and corn syrup are the most common, found in everything from peanut butter to breakfast bars. And adding vitamins and minerals during processing sometimes takes nutrients where nutrients have never gone before.

Calorie-cutters like Simplesse, the revolutionary fat replacer, and Nutra-Sweet are the food additives of the future. Fat and sugar substitutes already top the list of some two dozen new additives heading for store shelves each year, says Manfred Kroger, Ph.D., professor of food science at Pennsylvania State University in University Park. "There's money to be made," says Dr. Kroger. "The public is buying diet products like wild."

Other additives—like MSG (monosodium glutamate), sulfites and certain colorings—are less popular, having been fingered for causing headaches, rashes and other reactions in an unfortunate, sensitive few.

In fact, the late Benjamin Feingold, M.D., an allergy specialist, made headlines during the 1970s by claiming there was a connection between hyperactivity in children and food additives. By following an additive-free diet, Dr. Feingold claimed, 50 percent of hyperactive and learning-disabled children would undergo a dramatic improvement in behavior.

Although Dr. Feingold's assertions have been questioned and disproven by his scientific brethren, for many people, concerns about the broader health risks of some food additives linger. Sodium nitrite, a common lunch meat preservative, for example, has long been suspected as a possible contributor to some cancers.

Of course, food manufacturers point out that any minute health threat created by additives pales in comparison to deadly diseases like botulism caused by spoiled (albeit preservative-free) food. Many health food purists, on the other hand, advocate avoiding additives at all costs, forcing you, perhaps, to forsake some of your favorite foods.

Perhaps the best approach, says Dr. Kroger, is "Know thyself." "If you have an individual sensitivity, once you know the effect a certain ingredient or food has on your health, you can try to steer clear of it. For example, if you're sensitive to alcohol, you should even check the label before buying a chocolate confection. The same with MSG, sulfites, caffeine, whatever." If you prefer to avoid as many additives as possible, stick to a healthy diet rich in fresh fruit, vegetables, whole grains, low-fat meats and dairy products. These are less likely to contain additives.

BETTER LIVING THROUGH FORTIFICATION

Among the most beneficial additives are vitamins and minerals blended into food. Not only do they enhance the nutritional value of many foods, in some cases added vitamins are also used to improve appearance and taste, according to the Institute of Food Technologists' Expert Panel on Food Safety and Nutrition.

Vitamin C, also called ascorbic acid, is perhaps the most versatile, improving bread, making wine and beer clear and enhancing the pink color of cured meat while inhibiting the formation of harmful substances. Because ascorbic acid is good at stopping oxygen's detrimental effects on foods, it's often added to sodas and fruit drinks. Vitamin E or tocopherols are antioxidants used in bacon, baked goods, butter, lard, margarine, rapeseed oil, safflower oil and sunflower seed oil.

Beta-carotene, a source of vitamin A, is used to add color to some margarines, shortening, butter, cheese, confections, baked goods, ice cream, egg nog, macaroni products, soups and juices.

The most common use of vitamins is to fortify, restore or enrich a food's nutritional value. In fact, the addition of vitamin D to milk and iodine to salt are credited with preventing major nutritional deficiencies like rickets and goiter in the United States.

The most frequently fortified foods: breakfast cereals. Even the most sugary breakfast concoctions are commonly fortified to provide at least 25 percent of the Recommended Dietary Allowance for ten vitamins and six minerals. Also on the list of fortified foods are bread, margarine, nonfat dry milk, evaporated milk, infant formulas, breakfast bars and liquid and solid meal replacements, according to the institute.

A surge of interest in fiber by consumers has led food manufacturers to add cellulose, pectin, starch, and other naturally derived fibers to foods. Although it may seem like a good idea, the FDA does not encourage indiscriminate food fortification. In fact, adding nutrients to fresh produce, meat, poultry or fish products, sugar, or snack foods is discouraged. However, fortifying is recognized as often necessary to restore nutrients lost in processing.

TAMING THE TINKERING

Additive use is a bit more sophisticated today, but there's nothing new about tinkering with food. The ancient Egyptians used sulfites to stop bacterial growth and fermentation in wine. They also used extracts from beetles for food coloring. Vegetable dyes from juniper fruits or beech-root juice were popular colorings in the Middle Ages, although wary kings began to

CHEMICALS WITH A MISSION

You've seen them in everything from cereal to salad dressings. But have you ever wondered just what those additives are doing in your food? Here's a short list with some of their job responsibilities.

Acetone peroxide. Used as a dough conditioner and bleaching and conditioning agent in many baked goods

BHA. Used alone or with BHT as an antioxidant to help stabilize fat in dehydrated potato shreds, dry beverage and dessert mixes, shortenings and potato flakes.

Calcium disodium EDTA. Used as a color or texture protector in canned soft drinks, canned white potatoes, dressings, beer, mayonnaise, processed dry pinto beans, cooked and canned crabmeat, clams and shrimp and lemon- or orange-flavored spreads.

Polydextrose. Used as a bulking agent, partial sugar replacer, formulation aid, humectant (helps maintain moisture) and texturizer in custards, pudding-filled pies, cakes, cookies, salad dressings and hard and soft candy.

Polysorbate 60. Used as an emulsifier (to ensure consistency) in whipped toppings, cake mixes, icings, dressings and milk and cream substitutes.

Sodium lauryl sulfate. Used as a whipping aid in marshmallows and angel food cake mix.

Sodium nitrate. Used as an antimicrobial agent and color fixative, with or without sodium nitrite, in smoked, cured meats, fish and poultry.

Sodium stearoyl lactylate. Used as a dough strengthener in pancakes and waffles, a formulation aid in dehydrated potatoes and an emulsifier in snack dips, cheese substitutes and gravies.

employ "garglers" to test their meals—perhaps for additives that did not originate in the kitchen. Saltpeter became the meat coloring and preservative of choice for aspiring chefs in Germany and Austria, according to seventeenth-century cookbooks.

But as time marched on, less scrupulous elements began their assault on the food supply. As early as 1887, muckraking journalists at *New York World* published a list of the additives that at the time appalled even the staid *Journal of the American Medical Association.* Observed *JAMA:* "On reading the list one is amazed at the ingenuity and dishonesty of civilized, Christian man." Among the ingredients found in milk by the *World:* "Water principally, flour or starch, boiled white carrots, milk of almonds, sheep's brains, gum tragacanth, carbonate of soda, chrome yellow for coloring."

On the heels of similar revelations, Congress passed the Pure Food and

Drug Act in 1906 and the Federal Food, Drug, and Cosmetic Act in 1938. While the laws were among the first attempts to regulate additives, they didn't pack much clout: In fact, it was up to the FDA, not the manufacturer, to prove an additive's "harmfulness."

The Food Additives Amendment of 1958 and Color Additive Amendments of 1960, however, solved this dilemma by requiring manufacturers to establish that their products were safe. The 1958 legislation led to the creation of a list of ingredients that were deemed free from the need for further investigation. These ingredients are called GRAS, or Generally Regarded As Safe. Another much-debated amendment, introduced by Representative Delaney in 1972 and passed by Congress, banned for human consumption any additive that caused cancer in lab animals.

But the cyclamate scare of 1969 raised questions about the coveted GRAS status. After research indicated that this artificial sweetener, already on the GRAS list, appeared to cause cancer in rats, cyclamates were taken off the GRAS list and disappeared from the U.S. marketplace. A White House Conference in 1969 led President Richard M. Nixon to order the FDA to review the entire GRAS list for potentially toxic substances.

Experts chosen by the Federation of American Societies for Experimental Biology reaffirmed the safety of 70 percent of the additives, while painting the rest varying shades of gray. Even though the last of their reports were issued in 1982, over 150 substances have yet to be reaffirmed as GRAS.

When animal tests showed that saccharin, an artificial sweetener, caused cancer, the FDA sought to remove it from the marketplace. But Congress chose, despite the Delaney Clause, to allow saccharin sales to continue, as long as the products included a warning label.

But for the most part, the only thing standing between you and these often helpful but sometimes harmful ingredients is still the FDA. The FDA alone is charged with the awesome task of policing our food supply.

So where does that leave the consumer? While the FDA attempts to police the industry, for your own peace of mind, it pays to have a bit of background on some of the most discussed additives.

ASPARTAME: A SWEET INNOVATION

Also known as NutraSweet brand sweetener, this additive appears in over 5,000 foods and beverages, from frozen desserts to diet soft drinks. There's little doubt about the reason for its popularity: Aspartame is 200 times as sweet as sugar with 95 percent fewer calories. And according to The NutraSweet Company, the additive—which is made from two naturally occurring amino acids, aspartic acid and phenylalanine—has been found safe in nearly 200 animal and human studies, making it "the most tested food ingredient ever approved by the FDA."

But the substance is not without some drawbacks. Products containing aspartame must carry a warning label "Phenylketonurics: Contains Phenylalanine" on the label. The notice is a red flag for about 1 in 15,000 Americans who has phenylketonuria, a disease that makes it nearly impossible for the individual to metabolize the amino acid phenylalanine. Diagnosed at birth, the disorder has been linked to mental retardation, epilepsy and other neurological problems.

The tip-off on the label is required by the FDA because many of the foods using aspartame would not normally contain phenylalanine. Other concerns have been raised about the safety of aspartame. Over 5,000 people have contacted the FDA in the 11 years since aspartame was approved for tabletop use, claiming that the product had caused a variety of symptoms. The FDA analyzed these complaints carefully and found no cause-and-effect relationship. In addition, clinical studies to investigate these complaints, conducted in U.S. and foreign medical schools, have confirmed the safety of aspartame.

MSG: The Invisible Additive

Sometimes even reading food labels isn't enough. Consider the case of the 32-year-old woman who suffered six moderate to severe migraines a month. The pain was so bad she missed at least one day of work a month for a year.

On the advice of her doctor, the woman avoided foods that had monosodium glutamate listed on the label, but her headaches continued. That is, until she learned that hydrolyzed vegetable protein and some natural flavors contain MSG naturally. Soon after switching to brands of mayonnaise and mustard without those mysterious ingredients and adopting other MSG-avoidance tactics, the woman's migraines decreased to one a month.

While some studies show that roughly 30 percent of people who eat Chinese food suffer from headache, tightness of the face, dizziness, diarrhea, nausea and abdominal cramps, this case shows that MSG reactions are no longer a problem strictly in Chinese restaurants. Purveyors of Oriental fare actually only account for a fraction of the 85 million pounds of MSG used in the United States each year—enough for five ounces per person.

Food manufacturers love the additive because it enhances flavor in processed products like frozen dinners, potato chips, soups, sauces, canned meats, lunch meats and broths.

And yet, ingredient labels that list pure MSG are rare. Manufacturers are aware that MSG occurs in hydrolyzed vegetable protein, hydrolyzed plant protein and some flavorings, so they are getting the flavor boost with these additives instead.

But a migraine is still a migraine. And researchers have demonstrated that three to five grams of MSG for those unable to tolerate the additive is enough to trigger severe headaches.

Nitrites: A Necessary Evil?

Scientists studying historical cookbooks and medical records discovered what may have been more than an interesting coincidence: The first detailed descriptions of large bowel cancer and multiple sclerosis in Germany and Austria did not appear until the early nineteenth century, a short time after the use of nitrates to color and preserve meat began.

There's little debate in the scientific community over the cancer-causing ability of nitrosamines, substances formed during the breakdown of nitrates and nitrites. Nitrites are the most commonly used preservative in meats. They are added to bacon, bologna, corned beef, frankfurters, sausages, ham and some fish and poultry products. The problem is that today there are no better alternatives. Nitrates are found naturally in vegetables like spinach, beets, celery and rhubarb.

The good news is that the way to prevent cancer-causing nitrosamines from forming from the nitrites in your morning bacon may be as close as your glass of orange juice. Further research is needed, but scientists have discovered that when nitrites are bathed in a solution containing vitamin C, the additive's ability to convert to nitrosamines is effectively blocked, says Leonard Cohen, Ph.D., head of the Section of Nutritional Endocrinology at the American Health Foundation in Valhalla, New York.

SIMPLESSE: THE FAT REPLACER

The introduction of Simplesse, the fat substitute developed by researchers at the NutraSweet Company, heralds a new era in food additives. Food manufacturers have replicated lots of flavors over the years—artificial flavors account for more than one-third of the taste in the marketplace today—but never that of fat.

"Nobody looking into their crystal ball can say whether this is good or this is bad. This is progress, and we ought to make the best of that," says Dr. Kroger.

Among the benefits: If used in the maximum number of applications, Simplesse could reduce the fat content in the U.S. diet by 14 percent, research shows. Among potential drawbacks: use of Simplesse could increase U.S. protein consumption, already higher than desired. Also, there have been no published long-term health investigations of human subjects who have eaten Simplesse.

Developed in 1982, Simplesse is the trade name for microparticulated protein, made by a patented process that shrinks the size of the protein in egg white or skim milk—without changing its chemistry, according to researchers. A similar but less advanced process is used to turn soybeans into simulated meat products.

If the transformation is less than spectacular, the results have drawn raves. In coffee ice cream taste tests, a product using Simplesse was rated nearly as high as fat-laden super premium ice cream. In fact, the participants rated the Simplesse product above super premium in aftertaste, color and "overall liking." Manufacturers credit the taste to Simplesse's "mouthfeel"—the closest thing to fat ever made in the lab.

And research shows that the fat content of foods with Simplesse drops

PESTICIDE RESIDUES LINGER ALONG WITH WORRIES

Pesticides aren't actually considered food additives. But judging from the results of the Food and Drug Administration's (FDA) own Market Basket Survey, they probably should be. According to the FDA, pesticide residue lurks beneath the bountiful exterior of roughly one-third of our produce.

The Environmental Protection Agency (EPA), however, contends that no more than 1 to 2 percent of all produce contains pesticide in amounts considered poisonous. Deaths from eating poisoned produce are almost nonexistent. But no one is sure about the long-term risks of cancer. While risks are generally considered very low, the cancer/pesticide connection is hard to establish.

But since the Alar apple scare of 1989 (sparked by claims by the Natural Resources Defense Council that the chemical, which was commonly used to make apples crisper, could cause cancer), consumers are more willing than ever to buy fruit and vegetables grown without the use of chemicals. In fact, 75 percent of consumers cited in a Rand Corporation study said they considered the use of pesticides, herbicides, additives and preservatives "a serious hazard." Those consumers who were most concerned indicated that they were willing to pay a "substantial premium to avoid these residues."

The EPA approves the use of pesticides and establishes residue tolerance levels for food. Residue tolerances are between 100 and 1,000 times lower than the level that caused "no effect" in test animals. The

dramatically. One tablespoon of traditional mayonnnaise-based salad dressing contains 12 grams of fat, while one tablespoon with Simplesse has less than 1 gram. A four-ounce serving of super premium ice cream that normally contains 15 grams of fat also has less than 1 gram of fat when made with Simplesse.

There are at least two groups of people who will never enjoy the benefits of this fat substitute: those allergic to eggs or milk. Studies show they'll also react to the Simplesse.

But that probably won't prevent the introduction of Simplesse into dozens of foods like cheeses, yogurts and salad dressings.

Already, several other companies are developing their own fat substitutes. Procter and Gamble, the consumer products giant, is attracting attention with Olestra, a nondigestible cooking oil additive. Hercules, a multinational chemical and aerospace company, has launched Slendid, a fat replacement made from citrus peels for use in baked goods, frozen desserts, soups, cheeses, sauces and yogurts, among other products.

EPA admits, however, that it's nearly impossible to determine how much residue might be harmful to humans.

Companies trying to get EPA approval for a pesticide's use must submit toxicology studies and pesticide residue reports that show how much pesticide is expected to remain in a crop.

To make sure that pesticide residue levels meet safety requirements, the FDA each year tests 15,000 to 18,000 shipments of food, including produce, seafood, milk and processed goods. Under another program, four times a year the agency buys more than 200 different supermarket food items from across the country that are representative of the diet of U.S. consumers. The foods are then prepared and analyzed for pesticide residues and other chemicals.

According to a 1991 FDA report, domestically grown items with the highest percentage of samples found containing residues include cranberries, grapefruit, lemons, oranges, peaches, nectarines, tangerines, pumpkins, strawberries, pears, fruit juices and barley.

The FDA says that the analytic methods used are capable of detecting only about half of the pesticides with established EPA tolerances, but the results are believed to be representative of residue levels.

Consumers can limit the amount of pesticide residues in foods by thoroughly washing fresh fruit and vegetables, removing the outer leaves of leafy vegetables and sometimes trimming the skin.

SULFITES: ASTHMATICS BEWARE

The reaction was sudden and alarming: Just two minutes after he was fed a mixture of sulfites and applesauce, the two-year-old asthmatic began to cough and wheeze. His pulse, blood pressure and respiratory rate all shot up. Because the boy was being closely monitored by a doctor, he was not in danger. But his reaction confirmed the diagnosis: sulfite sensitivity.

A common preservative primarily used to keep medicines potent and food looking fresh, sulfites are known by several names, including potassium or sodium sulfite, bisulfite, metabisulfite and sulfur dioxide.

Unfortunately, there was little government concern over the use of sulfites on fresh fruit and vegetables until after 17 unrelated deaths in 1985, most of which were connected to the use of sulfites at salad bars.

These deaths led the FDA to ban the preservative, which formerly had GRAS status, from nearly all raw or fresh fruits and vegetables in 1986.

"That's where most asthmatics were getting their exposure and having their reactions," says Ronald A. Simon, M.D., head of the Division of Allergy and Immunology at the Scripps Clinic and Research Foundation in La Jolla, California. "Then, because people became so aware of sulfites, the manufacturers began to pull them out of many other foods. Even in the foods they continue to be in, they are there in lower amounts."

But while sulfites do a remarkable job keeping food looking fresh, studies show that between two and five percent of asthmatics in the United States are extremely sensitive to sulfites.

Although it's unclear what actually triggers the reaction among asthmatics (one theory is individuals sometimes inhale the sulfur dioxide gas generated by the sulfites added to the food), there's no doubt about the consequences. Most reactions are characterized by severe bronchial spasms, which can occur within minutes after eating foods containing sulfites. During a reaction, sulfite-sensitive patients with asthma should immediately use their metered-dose inhalers and have epinephrine ready.

Although banned from nearly all fresh foods, the use of sulfites by food and beverage manufacturers continues. Foods that most commonly contain sulfites include shrimp, dried fruit, cider and vinegar. A single five-ounce glass of sweet white wine may contain up to 50 milligrams of sulfites. The only fresh vegetable that may still be sprayed with sulfites is potatoes.

To protect consumers, the FDA requires that packaged foods containing ten or more parts per million (ppm) of sulfites must say on the ingredient label that they contain sulfites. Foods with less than ten ppm should not be a problem even for the most sensitive patients.

Sulfites can be added during food manufacturing, processing or delivery

AVOIDING SULFITES? THEN START HERE

The following products often contain sulfites.

- Alcoholic beverages—beer, cocktail mix, red wine, white wine, wine coolers
- Condiments—olives, relishes, pickles, salad dressing mixes, wine vinegar, sauerkraut, pickled pearl onions
- Fresh fish and fish products—clams, crabs, lobsters, scallops, shrimp
- Processed fruit—dietetic fruit or juices, dried fruit, fruit juices and drinks, fruit pie fillings
- Processed foods—avocado mix; dried vegetables, including green vegetables and potatoes; pickled vegetables; vegetable juice; hominy; dry soup mixes
- Snack foods—apple bits, dried fruit, fruit-filled crackers, trail mix containing dried fruit bits

and are used as sanitizing agents for food containers and fermentation equipment.

However, most people do not have to be concerned about sulfites, says Dr. Simon. "There are these rare reported cases of hives or a more systemic allergic reaction we call anaphylaxis but they are so few and far between that I don't think the average person has to worry about it."

Anaphylaxis, the worst possible allergic reaction, often includes hives, throat swelling, low blood pressure, shock and perhaps even death. "In our opinion, those people who have that kind of anaphylactic reaction to sulfites probably are truly allergic to sulfites—not simply sensitive to sulfur dioxide gas," says Dr. Simon.

A simple skin test performed by any allergist can determine if you're sensitive to sulfites.

TARTRAZINE: COLOR IT POPULAR

Remember Dr. Gross, the internist from Hackensack? He's not the only one who's had trouble with food colorings.

Dr. Gross reacted to Yellow No. 6, the third most commonly used coloring. Red No. 40, commonly found in maraschino cherries, is the most popular coloring used by food manufacturers. Close behind, in second place, is tartrazine, or as it's known in the industry, Yellow No. 5.

By 1975, the number of reported cases of tartrazine reactions became large enough to make this dye "a major health concern," according to Joseph R. DiPalma, M.D., professor emeritus of pharmacology and medicine at the Hahnemann School of Medicine in Philadelphia. In 1980, the FDA, while still maintaining approval of tartrazine, issued new regulations that required listing of the dye on the labels of all drugs and food packages. The FDA estimates at least 50,000 Americans are sensitive to tartrazine.

The amount required to provoke tartrazine sensitivity varies from 25 milligrams down to as little as 0.00085 milligrams each day. Most people consume an average of 13 milligrams daily.

Products that may contain tartrazine include orange and lime drinks, ice cream and sherbets, gelatins and puddings, salad dressings, cheese dishes, cake mixes and icings, seasoned salts and confections.

Tartrazine has also caused its share of problems as a coloring in drugs. When a 50-year-old Milwaukee woman suffering from skin rash did not respond to treatment for six weeks, her physician recommended that she replace her estrogen tablets with others not colored with tartrazine. Soon after, the rash went away—until the woman was inadvertently served a relish containing tartrazine.

CHAPTER 18

Ethnic Foods

Healthy Eating from Around the Globe

In the days when Fords and Chevys ruled American roads and meat and potatoes ruled American menus, the closest many of us came to ethnic foods was chop suey from a can.

Today, Americans are as likely to drive a Honda as a Ford and as eager to feast on grilled Indonesian chicken saté or Spanish seafood paella as pot roast.

Yes, American food has gone global. And that's an international trade imbalance that can only result in a surplus—a surplus of health.

Unlike the Anglo-Germanic food that shaped the typical meat-and-milk American diet, this Asian-Mediterranean-Latin-influenced fare tends to be light and healthy. It's also infused with out-of-this-world flavor from tongue-tingling curries and chilies to sweetly sublime cinnamon and papaya.

You don't have to venture far to see evidence of the ethnic food boom. You can, for example, buy whole-grain Arabian pita bread at the local sandwich shop or dip into Lebanese hummus spread (pureed chick-peas) at the church buffet. Red-hot Mexican salsas outsell catsup in some parts of the country. In other areas, instant cup-of-Indian-style-lentils is giving chicken noodle soup a run for its money.

A stroll through almost any supermarket is a crash course in world gastronomy. Oriental bok choy, tofu and "tree ear" mushrooms are nestled next to the carrots and broccoli. Jade-tinged olive oil from Sicily and amber-colored sesame oil from China share shelf space with Crisco. Oodles of noodles stretch down the aisle with pastas ranging from whole wheat to buckwheat; there's skinny pasta for thick, Italian sauces and squiggly pasta for thin Japanese soups.

Open the newspaper and you'll see such tasty recipe alternatives to Tuesday's meat loaf as Moroccan orange pistachio couscous (cracked wheat) to Thai peanut-and-pepper grilled shrimp.

THE TIMING IS RIGHT

The explosion of ethnic food in America is a direct result of the influx of immigrants arriving from the Pacific Rim and Latin countries. And it couldn't be better timing, according to Aliza Minear, Ph.D., director of health and nutrition education at the Scripps Clinic in La Jolla, California. "People are seeking ways to cut back on calories, fat, salt and sugar and still have a satisfying, tasty meal. Eating ethnic foods fills the bill nicely."

Many ethnic diets are built around complex carohydrates—grains, greens and other plant foods, says Dr. Minear. They provide a lot less artery-clogging fat and a lot more cholesterol-busting fiber than you'd get from the traditional meat-and-dairy-based American diet. They also provide

SPICING IT UP: THE HEAT IS OPTIONAL

Spices can make low-fat, low-sodium dining a blast instead of a bore. A little salsa on a baked potato, for example, and you'll never miss the butter or salt.

Not all ethnic foods are fiery hot, though. For instance, while many Mexican dishes include palate-paralyzing chilies, others use subdued spices such as cinnamon and nutmeg along with a squeeze of tangy lime juice. A good cookbook with a spice chart can help you select flavor combinations to suit your palate.

On the other hand, if you can stand the heat, you may want to include a chili or two in your diet.

Capsaicin, the "hot stuff" in hot peppers, appears to lower cholesterol in lab animals in a way similar to some cholesterol-reducing drugs. After rats were fed capsaicin and other spices, it more than doubled the rate at which cholesterol was bound to bile acids, a process that helps whisk this troublemaker out of the body.

More hot food news for thought: It turns out that capsaicin not only burns your mouth but burns calories by increasing metabolism.

more disease-fighting nutrients. Among them: potassium to control blood pressure, nondairy calcium to stave off osteoporosis and beta-carotene to combat cancer.

Indeed, many nutrition experts believe that adopting ethnic food choices may be the ideal solution for combating obesity, heart disease, cancer and other chronic diseases linked to the usual American, high-fat, low-fiber diet.

Trying to "fix" our usual foods by engineering leaner hamburgers or fat-free cakes is not the best way to promote healthful eating, according to Marion Nestle, Ph.D., professor and chairperson of the Department of Nutrition, Food and Hotel Management at New York University in New York City. "People feel they are giving up something and may feel deprived."

But shifting to a plant-based cuisine that is highly flavorful makes eating light a whole new satisfying way of eating, not a sacrifice.

THE MEDITERRANEAN MODEL

You'd think that the country with the highest standard of living would produce the world's best diet. In fact, from a health standpoint, the standard American diet ranks among the world's worst.

Studies show that the healthy eating award goes to more "primitive" lands. As it turns out, countries in the Mediterranean Basin—the birthplace of civilization—have perfected one of the healthiest diets in the world.

Here, in the sun-drenched countries of Greece and Italy, for example, people still toil long hours in fields and dine on foods of their forefathers: fresh-picked green vegetables seasoned with garlic and olive oil, hearty minestrone soup laced with robust red beans, hunks of whole-grain bread, a plate of chewy pasta. It's also in this region that heart disease—America's number one killer—is as rare as marbled steaks and creamy milk shakes.

In a long-term landmark study begun some 40 years ago, Ancel Keys, Ph.D., of the University of Minnesota School of Public Health in Minneapolis, compared the mortality of men from Italy, Yugoslavia, Greece, Finland, the Netherlands, the United States and Japan. Dr. Keys found that the men living in countries with the highest fat intake—America and Finland—also had the highest death rate from heart disease. Among Greeks and Italians and other people in the Mediterranean Basin, however, the rate was only half that of Americans and Europeans.

And while the American/European meat-and-dairy diet is filled with saturated fat, the Mediterranean diet relies on olive oil, a monounsaturated fat that may actually lower cholesterol levels. Dr. Keys observed that these folks drizzled the "nectar of the olive" on tomatoes and pasta, sautéed zucchini in it and made marinara sauces with it.

Subsequent research has underscored olive oil's amazing health benefits. In one study involving 8,000 Italian men and women, for example, the regular olive oil users had significantly lower blood pressures as well as blood

A BUYER'S GUIDE TO OLIVE OIL

Heart-healthy olive oil may be used in place of other cooking oils. But *which* olive oil do you choose? Like fine wine, olive oil varies in bouquet, color and taste. Generally, the more full-bodied, the better the grade of olive oil. Mediterranean cooks prefer different grades to prepare different dishes. Here's a guide to the standard grades, set by international agreement.

Virgin olive oil. Oil that is pressed (never chemically extracted) from the fruit only, not the pit. In U.S.-produced oils, which account for less than 3 percent of the olive oil sold in this country, "virgin" means the oil is from the first pressing. Not to be used in high-temperature cooking (high heat breaks down flavor) but excellent for light sautéing and adding to cooked sauces and dressings.

Extra-virgin olive oil. Top quality, and most costly, oil from the first pressing. Acid levels are under 1 percent, and the oil has a greener color and richer flavor. Best used in cold pasta salads or drizzled over crisp greens, veggies or poached fish or chicken.

Pure olive oil. (Called refined oil in the United States.) Oil that's been refined and filtered to reduce acidity. Lighter in color and aroma, with less of an olive taste. Can be used in stir-frying.

Extra-light olive oil. An American invention, it's extra-refined and pale in color with a mild flavor, but it contains the same amount of fat (13 grams per tablespoon) and calories (120). Use it as you would any highly refined oil such as sunflower.

sugar levels, than those who used butter or polyunsaturated oil.

"Olive oil isn't a medicine," says Maurizio Trevisan, M.D., of the State University of New York at Buffalo School of Medicine and Biomedical Sciences who conducted the Italian study. You can't, for example, eat a greasy double cheeseburger and expect a salad drenched in olive oil to shield your heart.

Rather than adding olive oil to your usual diet, says Dr. Trevisan, you should use it sparingly as a *substitute* for saturated fat. "Your primary goal should be to reduce fat overall, eat a variety of vegetables and increase your intake of grains and fresh fruit," he says. Do this, and you'll truly be reaping the rewards of the Mediterranean diet.

THE LOW-FAT ASIAN WAY

Studies show that you'd also do well to take a few dietary tips from the Orient. Although Japan's high-tech industry has soared to heights matching

Mount Fuji's, many of her people eat the same simple, ultra-low fat diet consumed by the Japanese for centuries. This may be a big reason why Japan's people live longer than any other people on the planet and suffer fewer diet-related chronic diseases than people who regularly indulge in fatty foods.

In the Honolulu Heart Program study conducted by the National Heart, Lung and Blood Institute, researchers looked at 8,000 men of Japanese descent who lived in Japan or America. They found that the Japanese-American men had three to four times more heart disease than the men living in Japan.

The higher incidence of heart disease in Japanese-American men can be explained because they strayed from their low-fat diet of their ancestors, according to Grant N. Stemmermann, M.D., director of the Japan-Hawaii Cancer Study in Honolulu.

"In Japan, a person typically starts the day with rice and miso soup made from soybeans," says Dr. Stemmermann. "In contrast, a typical Japanese-American breakfast is ham and eggs." The saturated fat score? Japanese: one gram. Americans: six.

In similar studies from Stanford University School of Medicine comparing Chinese men in China with Chinese men in North America, the latter group had four to seven times more colorectal cancer than the former group. They also had more saturated fat in their diets.

MORE VEGETABLES, LESS MEAT

The most striking difference between the world's healthier diets and the standard American diets is this: Meat is not the centerpiece of meals.

Even meat-laden Italian dishes such as lasagna that Americans adore are reserved for celebratory feasts in the homeland. And in Third World locations, meat may be an even rarer treat. "Meat is expensive and hard to come by in many non-Westernized countries," says New York nutritionist Densie Webb, Ph.D., author of *The International Calorie Counter*.

An everyday Italian dish is more likely to be a plate of fiber-rich white beans and fresh-picked greens, for example. Or tomato and mushroom polenta (cornmeal mush). Unfortunately, many traditional dishes get "beefed up" once they cross U.S. borders.

A typical meal in China, for example, is a mound of steamed rice, lots of vegetables and a few bits of pork or beef. The Americanized version, however, serves the reverse: lots of meat, a little rice, with deep-fried egg rolls and enough soy sauce to send your sodium levels over the pagoda.

Likewise, a typical Americanized version of Mexican food is beef-stuffed burritos smothered in sour cream and Cheddar cheese. Authentic Mexican food is less artery-clogging. A common meal consists of cholesterol-fighting beans (like chick-peas or pinto beans), cabbage and corn or squash, for instance.

BEYOND BARBECUE SAUCE

Grilling using flavors from around the world is a mouthwatering way to prepare low-fat foods, according to Linda Burum, California ethnic food expert.

The soy sauces of the Orient, the balsamic vinegars of Italy, the limes of Latin American and yogurt dressings of the Middle East all naturally tenderize lean cuts of meat, chicken and fish. This means you don't need to add fat or rich sauces, says Burum.

Using these natural tenderizers as a base, you can add zip with almost any spice. To add a Latin-style flavor to shrimp, for example, soak in lime juice laced with cayenne pepper. Or grill chicken Thai-style, using rice vinegar, garlic and peanut-chili sauce. Flavorless, protein-rich tofu (soybean curd) takes on a delightful, meaty taste when marinated in Chinese hoisin sauce, (spicy brown paste from ground soybeans, garlic, sugar, vinegar and sesame sauce). Grill it, chop it and toss it in salads.

The bottom line: Most traditional ethnic cuisines could be classified as vegetarian or nearly so—and that may be their major health advantage, studies show.

Results from the Nurses Health Study from Harvard Medical School, involving 89,000 nurses, showed that the women who ate red meat infrequently had less than half the risk of colon cancer of their omnivorous colleagues.

Consuming certain vegetables may boost the health advantage even more. Take broccoli, for example. The people of Asia and Italy are fond of this bright emerald veggie and include it in countless stir-fried and pasta dishes. And they may be healthier for it.

The reason? Broccoli is higher in nutrients including vitamin C, iron and B vitamins than most other plant foods. What's more, broccoli, a member of the cabbage family, is a great source of beta-carotene. Studies show that regular consumption of beta-carotene-rich vegetables helps ward off heart attacks, strokes and cancers.

It's more than possible that Japan's lower incidence of lung cancer is because of their higher intake of beta-carotene-rich vegetables, from broccoli to seaweed, according to Dr. Stemmermann.

CALCIUM? PROTEIN? NO PROBLEM!

Except for some Indian dishes such as chicken masala that contain yogurt and butter, the world's healthiest cuisines are generally devoid of dairy products. You won't find the buttery sauces, creamy salad dressings, and mounds of cheese that typically blanket American food.

Yet, even with few milk-based foods, the people in many ethnic cultures manage to get enough calcium to keep their bones strong.

How? The answer, once again, is vegetables. Lots of them. In a study conducted at Creighton University in Omaha researchers found that the calcium in the Chinese vegetable bok choy, and also kale and spinach, is as readily absorbed as the calcium in milk. The bonus: There's very little fat. "Bok choy has the highest calcium-per-calorie ratio of any food," says the study's director, Robert Heaney, M.D., professor of medicine at Creighton. There's about 79 milligrams of calcium in a ½-cup serving, and only ten calories.

How do these cultures obtain protein without red meat? Often the answer lies in the deep blue sea. Fish favorites among the Japanese and Mediterranean peoples include mackerel and sardines, to name a few. Like all fish, these varieties are loaded with protein, but they also contain omega-3 fatty acids, a type of fat that has been found to keep cholesterol in check.

NOODLE KNOW-HOW

People from Italy to Asia have long known what Americans are now discovering: that pasta can be a nutritious, quickly fixed, low-calorie meal. (One cup is only 120 calories if you don't add creamy sauces.) Pasta is also the perfect companion for tossing with vegetables and bits of grilled seafood and for soaking up tomato-based marinaras or other savory sauces. There's a dizzying number of noodles on the market. Here's a bit of background to help you sort through them.

Italian pastas. Most are made with wheat flour, usually durum wheat, which is high in gluten, making the strands hard and firm. Semolina flour is durum wheat that is more coarsely ground than other what flours. It makes an even firmer, less elastic noodle, ideal for the curved "elbow" macaroni, for example. Semolina pasta also holds up to a thicker sauce. Pasta may also be made with flour from spinach, beets, corn, even Jerusalem artichokes. These flours add color but do not add much in the way of nutrition and may only impart a faint flavor.

Stir pasta while cooking to prevent sticking. It's done when it's *al dente* . . . chewy . . . not mushy. Rinsing is not necessary unless you're using the pasta in a cold salad.

FIBER HAS A STARRING ROLE

Unfortunately, most Americans get only half the protective amount of fiber they need. In contrast, high-fiber foods make up the bulk of the fare on most world menus.

Take Indian food, for example. You may associate this highly flavored food with the richly sauced lamb dishes typically served in Indian restaurants in this country. In India, however, rich meat dishes are reserved for royalty, according to Neela Paniz, owner of the Bombay Cafe in Los Angeles. A common everyday dish is dahl—a thick, split lentil stew served in dozens of ways and seasoned with a dazzling array of spices to suit every palate. Moong dahl, for example, is yellow split peas with fenugreek and cumin.

Lentils have virtually no fat and provide lots of protein and iron, and like other legumes they're super sources of soluble fiber. It's believed this type fiber may help flush out cholesterol before it builds up on artery walls. Studies conducted by James W. Anderson, M.D., professor of medicine and clinical nutrition at the University of Kentucky College of Medicine in

Asian pastas. Rice vermicelli, also known as rice sticks, are delicate in flavor and complement most Oriental meat, fish and vegetable dishes. Wheat noodles are made with or without eggs, and include ramen, somen and udon—each with a different shape for a different purpose. Ramen, for example is squiggly, and is often sold with packets of instant miso soup. Bean thread pasta, made from mung beans, is slippery, transparent noodles. They have little flavor but soak up tastes of everything they are cooked with, making them great in soups and stews. Buckwheat noodles, called soba, taste slightly nutty and can be eaten hot in broth or chilled and dipped in ginger-spiked soy-based sauces.

Try soba sprinkled with bits of broccoli, red pepper, carrots and other fresh vegetables. Just toss with light soy sauce, rice vinegar, sesame oil and ginger for a filling, low-fat meal.

"Don't overcook," says Linda Burum, California ethnic food expert and author of *Asian Pasta.* "Overcooking is the cardinal sin in noodle preparation." Place cooked noodles in a colander, drain, then refresh under running water, swirling in a colander. Place in a bowl and sprinkle with sesame oil.

Lexington found that adding 1½ cups of legumes a day to the diet lowered cholesterol 26 points in 30 days.

Grains are another potent fiber source in ethnic cuisines. Greeks eat chunks of crusty whole-grain bread at every meal. Mexicans eat cornmeal tortillas. In India, chapati, the flat whole-grain griddle-bread, is used in place of forks and knives to sop up every morsel of lentil stew. And in North Africa, couscous makes a complete high-fiber salad when combined with fresh oranges and dried figs.

Rice is the main ingredient in meals eaten by half the world's population. Rice types range from the chewy arborio in Italian risotti and the fluffy basmati in Middle Eastern pilafs to the sticky Asian rice, custom-made for chopsticks and dipping into fish sauces.

From Italy to Asia, there's literally pasta in every pot. Noodles come in all shapes and colors of the rainbow. In Japan, for example, noodles may be made from buckwheat or mung bean flour, and are served for breakfast, dinner and late-night snacks.

When mild-tasting grains and pastas are married with the melange of spices, spectacular dishes are born. Pesto, made with fresh-picked basil and pungent garlic, for example, can transform a simple plate of linguine into an unforgettable Italian feast.

Many of these seasonings have a health bonus of their own. Studies show that garlic, once believed to ward off evil spirits, may ward off heart attacks by reducing cholesterol and keeping blood clots from forming.

A Sweet Ending

Gooey Greek baklava aside, the healthiest cuisines generally feature Mother Nature's own dessert: raw fruit.

Melon and mangoes, popular meal-enders in Mexico and the Caribbean, for example, are chock-full of potassium. One study has found that adding about 400 milligrams of potassium to your daily diet—an amount easily supplied by a cup of cubed honeydew melon, for example—cuts your risk of fatal stroke almost in half.

Dessert or main course, we're not suggesting that all ethnic food is healthy, fat-free or low calorie. Thai mangoes and sticky rice made with coconut and cream, for example, packs a whopping 16 grams of fat. Miso and pickled vegetables, so popular in the Far East, can send your sodium levels into the ozone.

"The idea is to pick and choose the best foods from the world's banquet to create a healthy diet," says Dr. Minear.

Ten Ways to Eat Global Foods at Home

By adopting and adapting ethnic foods, you can trim fat, boost fiber and other nutrients and improve your health. Here are some tips.

1. Add new ingredients in small amounts. "Adapting your palate to new foods is like adapting to fine wine," says Sandy Kapoor, R.D., associate professor in the School of Hotel and Restaurant Management at the California Polytechnic Institute in Pomona. Introduce unfamiliar foods in small doses, says Dr. Kapoor. Instead of serving a lentil dahl dish as the main meal, try it as a side dish first. Toss some Asian noodles in your usual chicken noodle recipe. Throw in bok choy while steaming spinach.

SHOPPING FOR REAL ETHNIC FLAVOR

You're dying to try the recipe for Mexican spicy-chocolate chicken mole sauce, but where do you find ancho chilies in the middle of Maine? In your mailbox, of course.

Dozens of mail-order firms offer global ingredients that haven't yet made their way to your local supermarket, health food store or deli. We can't list them all here, but the sampling below will give you an idea of what's available.

Latin American. *G. B. Ratto and Company, 821 Washington Street, Oakland, CA 94607.* This one-stop "food hall" has been in the ethnic food business since 1897 and offers an impressive array of Mexican and Latin ingredients including quinoa, black beans, blue corn tortillas and Mexican chilies from mild to four-alarm hot.

Asian. *The Oriental Food Market, 2801 West Howard Street, Chicago, IL 60645.* If you can't find wasabi (Japanese horseradish), for example, or other ingredients for your Asian recipes, these folks will send it to you. Among their hundreds of mail-order offerings are more than two dozen types of teas, a multitude of noodles and canned, preserved and dried items from dried lotus root to boiled ginkgo nuts.

Italian. *Balducci's Mail Order Division, 11-02 Queen's Plaza South, Long Island City, NY 11101-1908,* is the Tiffany's of Italian food. They stock everything for your Mediterranean meal from polenta with sun-dried tomatoes to rare, aged balsamic vinegars.

Middle Eastern. *Sultan's Delight, P.O. Box 140253, 25 Croton Avenue, Staten Island, NY 10314.* Here you'll find everything from falafel, lentils, tabbouleh and tahini to ready-to-serve stuffed grape leaves and sweet-flower water. They can even send you belly dancing music and finger cymbals for dining entertainment (you provide the dancer).

Indian. *Cinnabar Specialty Foods, 214 Frontier Drive, Prescott, AZ 86303.* Their Barbados Honey Pepper Sauce can transform fish fillets or fresh vegetables into a meal to remember. Other homemade chutneys are made from mangoes, pears and peaches. And their Tandoori paste mixes with yogurt to infuse ordinary chicken with extraordinary flavor. A sampler pack offers you a choice of four products to try.

2. Substitute high-fiber, low-fat ingredients. Substitute whole-wheat tortillas for white flour varieties in Latin American dishes, for example. You can lighten up an Alfredo sauce by using Parmesan and nonfat yogurt instead of cream. Use polyunsaturated or olive oil instead of ghee (clarified butter) in Indian dishes and in place of lard when making Mexican refried beans.

3. Save meat for feasts. Three times a week, serve a hearty fish dish. A good one is Spanish paella, made with mussels and shrimp, crimson peppers and sunshine-yellow rice. Mussels provide about the same amount of protein as hamburger and are a better source of iron than sirloin. Their succulent flavor can satisfy without buttery sauces.

4. Go with the grain. Try tabbouleh salad made from bulgur, scallions, tomatoes, cucumbers, radishes, mint and a dash of lemon juice. One serving has less than 100 calories and less than a gram of fat, but it's packed with fiber as well as B vitamins, iron and calcium.

5. Invite a legume for lunch. Try a Greek salad made with white fava beans. Or puree chick-peas, to make a high-fiber dip for carrot sticks that's lighter and livelier than sour cream. Just blend with garlic and a squeeze of lemon.

6. Have butterless bread every day. To add a little zip, rub the surface with olive oil and lemongrass. Or try tahini, a peanut-butter-like spread made from ground sesame seeds. It's high in protein as well as vitamin E.

7. Phase in more fruit. Instead of coffee for breakfast, try a *licuado,* the Mexican nondairy version of a smoothie. Blend together potassium-rich cantaloupe with vitamin C–rich papaya, for example. (If the mixture is too thick for your liking, add a bit of juice.) Other great combos: strawberries and guava for double vitamin C punch. If you blend with a bit of watercress as they do in Mexico, it boosts the iron content.

8. Don't save the pumpkin for pie. This beta-carotene-rich vegetable is too good to reserve for just dessert. Try it in a dish like African pumpkin soup or Moroccan pumpkin-yogurt stuffing. For recipes, consult some ethnic cookbooks.

9. Go ahead, experiment. Ordinary vegetables come alive with a little creative cookery using exotic seasoning combinations. Transform steamed cauliflower into an Indian delight with cumin and cinnamon, for example.

10. Don't be afraid to mix and match. "Some of the best chefs now cross-pollinate cuisines," says California food expert and author Linda Burum, whose books include *Guide to Ethnic Restaurants in Los Angeles.* One popular restaurant combines Middle Eastern and Mexican food, for example. They grill Middle Eastern-style chicken with lemon, olive oil and rosemary, slice it and stuff it in a Mexican fajita (a thin, whole-grain tortilla). Topped with roasted chilies and a Middle Eastern yogurt-tahini sauce, it's fabulous!

HIGH-NUTRITION RECIPES

FETTUCCINE WITH PESTO SAUCE

Pesto is a much-loved Italian sauce made from fresh basil, garlic, olive oil, cheese and pine nuts. It's a wonderful change of pace from tomato sauce when on most any type of pasta. This recipe cuts back on the fat found in traditional recipes by substituting chicken stock for part of the oil.

1 cup tightly packed fresh basil
½ cup chopped fresh parsley
2 tablespoons grated Parmesan cheese
1 tablespoon pine nuts
2 cloves garlic, minced
1½ tablespoons olive oil
¼ cup defatted chicken stock
8 ounces fettuccine

Place the basil, parsley, Parmesan, pine nuts and garlic in the bowl of a food processor. Process with on/off turns until finely chopped. With the machine running, pour in the oil. Scrape down the sides of the container. With the machine running, slowly pour in the stock. Continue to process with on/off turns until a thick paste is formed.

Cook the fettuccine in a large pot of boiling water for 8 minutes, or until just tender. Drain and return to the pot. Off heat, add the pesto and toss to coat the pasta.

Serves 4
Per serving: *295 calories, 8.4 g. fat (25% of calories), 1.5 g. dietary fiber, 2 mg. cholesterol, 72 mg. sodium*

PORTUGUESE CHICK-PEAS

This hors d'oeuvre was enjoyed by one of our editors when she visited Lagos, Portugal. It also makes a great salad for two—serve it on a bed of mixed greens.

1 can (19 ounces) chick-peas, rinsed and drained
2 tablespoons diced onions
1–2 cloves garlic, thinly sliced
2 tablespoons red-wine vinegar
2 tablespoons minced fresh coriander
1 tablespoon olive oil
1 tablespoon water-packed tuna, mashed into a paste
4 thick slices crusty bread

In a large bowl, toss together the chick-peas, onions, garlic, vinegar, coriander, oil and tuna. Chill well. Serve accompanied by the bread.

Serves 4
Per serving: *151 calories, 5.4 g. fat (31% of calories), 4.2 g. dietary fiber, <1 mg. cholesterol, 395 mg. sodium*

PAELLA

This Spanish classic pairs modest amounts of poultry and seafood with rice and vegetables. Feel free to use other seafood, such as clams or small lobster tails.

- **2 teaspoons olive oil**
- **3 skinless chicken thighs, cut in half (see tip below)**
- **1 teaspoon fresh rosemary leaves**
- **2 cups medium-grain white rice**
- **4 cups defatted chicken stock**
- **1 can (28 ounces) plum tomatoes, drained**
- **½ teaspoon saffron threads**
- **12 large shrimp, peeled and deveined**
- **12 mussels, scrubbed**
- **1 cup peas**
- **2 canned pimentos, thinly sliced**
- **2 cloves garlic, minced**

In a very large ovenproof frying pan or paella pan, warm the oil over medium heat. Add the chicken and sauté for about 15 minutes, or until golden and almost entirely cooked through. Use tongs to transfer the pieces to a plate; sprinkle with the rosemary.

Add the rice to the frying pan and sauté over medium heat for 2 minutes. Add the stock, tomatoes and saffron. Stir with a wooden spoon to loosen browned bits from the bottom and also to break up the tomatoes. Bring to a boil.

Add the chicken (with any accumulated juices), shrimp, mussels, peas, pimentos and garlic. Bring to a boil and stir to mix the ingredients. Remove from the heat and cover the pan with a lid or foil.

Bake at 350° for 20 minutes. Remove from the oven and let stand, covered, for 20 minutes. Lift the chicken and shellfish to the surface of the dish to show them off.

Serves 6

Tip: *Cut the chicken thighs in half crosswise through the bone. Either use a sharp, heavy cleaver or ask the butcher at your supermarket to cut the thighs when you purchase them.*

Per serving: *390 calories, 5.2 g. fat (12% of calories), 2.5 g. dietary fiber, 58 mg. cholesterol, 166 mg. sodium*

COUSCOUS SALAD WITH ORANGES AND FIGS

Couscous is a staple of North African cuisine. This tiny pasta cooks up quickly and makes an ideal base for interesting salads. In the Moroccan tradition, we've combined the couscous with fresh oranges and dried figs. When fresh figs are in season, use them for a real taste treat.

1½ cups defatted chicken stock
¼ cup currants
1 teaspoon ground cumin
½ teaspoon turmeric
⅛ teaspoon ground red pepper
1 cup couscous
1 cup cooked peas
1 cup chopped orange sections
4 dried brown figs, quartered
2 tablespoons minced fresh parsley
1 tablespoon minced fresh mint
3 tablespoons lemon juice
2 tablespoons olive oil

In a 1-quart saucepan, combine 1¼ cups of the stock with the currants, cumin, turmeric and red pepper. Bring to a boil. Stir in the couscous. Remove from the heat, cover the pan and let stand for 10 minutes, or until all the liquid has been absorbed.

Fluff the couscous with a fork and transfer to a large bowl. Lightly toss with the peas, oranges, figs, parsley and mint.

In a cup, mix the lemon juice, oil and the remaining ¼ cup stock. Pour over the couscous mixture and toss to combine.

Serves 4
Per serving: *381 calories, 8.1 g. fat (19% of calories), 11.2 g. dietary fiber, 0 mg. cholesterol, 40 mg. sodium*

PART 3

ALL SYSTEMS ARE GO WITH GOOD NUTRITION

CHAPTER 19

THE BRAIN
FOOD FOR THOUGHT

When your boss breathes down your neck and steams up your collar, are you sometimes more capable of coping with the pressure and performing at your best? It could be because you first fed your head with breakfast. Do you feel mellow-minded or sleepy after eating spaghetti for lunch? It's probably because you've effectively injected your brain with a dose of a tranquilizing drug. Are your kids not performing as well as you'd like in school? It could be because they haven't taken their multivitamins.

You probably don't think about your brain the way you do about your heart or lungs or stomach or intestines. It is the essence of what you are. It defines your sense of self, what you think, what you believe, what you feel. But ultimately, it is an organ, just like any other in the body, and it needs to be adequately nourished to best do what it does.

What does it do? Technically, it coordinates the transmission of nerve impulses from one cell to another through the secretion of brain chemicals called neurotransmitters. The billions of nerve cells, called neurons, aren't wired together directly to interact; if they were, they'd be able to perform only one function. Instead, they're separated by imperceptibly thin gaps called synapses. Messages from one neuron to another travel across synapses through any of a number of neurotransmitters that are released from

LEAN BODY, FAT HEAD

You'd be smart to eat a low-fat diet, but you'd be stupid on a *no*-fat diet.

Fats and fatty acids are "absolutely essential" to the brain during development, according to Carol E. Greenwood, Ph.D., at the University of Toronto Faculty of Medicine in Ontario. And they're probably just as integral during the course of your lifetime.

The brain and nervous tissue have high concentrations of fatty acids, Dr. Greenwood says, but neuroscientists differ over how important fatty acids are once you're fully grown. Some say fat plays no role once the body is developed. But she argues that it does, citing the regeneration of all tissues (including the brain) over a person's life. "While the brain doesn't have any new cells developing once we have our full complement, these membranes still have to turn over and renew themselves," Dr. Greenwood says. "So we need fat for that. Damaged nerve cells also can repair themselves or sprout new terminals. All of these processes, while they won't require as much fat as we would developmentally, show that the brain will still have a degree of sensitivity to fat intake," she says.

All fats aren't born equal, of course, and new research suggests that nonanimal fats are better for the brain, Dr. Greenwood says. In tests she has conducted, she has found that rats fed soybean oil performed better at cognitive skills than those animals fed lard. She stops short of saying that lard-fed rats performed worse, though. The rats fed soy oil performed more like rats on the typical laboratory chow diet, whose fat content comes from nonanimal sources.

the nerve endings like a message in a bottle. How we feel, how we behave, and how well we do at our tasks depends on what neurotransmitters traverse the synaptic ocean to the neural shore on the other side, setting off a wave of reactions that triggers different responses in different parts of the brain.

To maintain the smooth firing of those neurotransmitters, the brain needs the whole array of vitamins and minerals. For energy, the brain requires glucose, sugar ingested from simple and complex carbohydrates. And for the production of some neurotransmitters as well as for repair and replacement of tissue, nerve cells and certain chemicals, the brain needs amino acids, which are obtained from protein.

From the digestive tract, glucose, protein, vitamins and minerals enter the blood, where they circulate to nourish the entire body. "But the brain gets them first," says John Fernstrom, Ph.D., professor of psychiatry and pharmacology at the University of Pittsburgh's School of Medicine. "The brain gets first choice of the nutrients available in the body."

Although it has the right of first use, the brain discriminates when it comes to what and how much of a certain element is allowed in. A buffering layer of cells, the blood/brain barrier, stands guard over the chemicals and nutrients in blood vessels like a bouncer at a nightclub, checking I.D.'s, rejecting riffraff that could cause problems and regulating the number so the room doesn't get too crowded.

The existence of that filtering system and the first-use concept traditionally led neuroscientists and psychologists to assert that the brain always is amply nourished and that individual meals and snacks never could influence mood or behavior by altering brain chemistry. But researchers are increasingly discovering that the quantity and quality of food can, in fact, tip the mental scale and—sometimes subtly, sometimes more obviously—affect behavior and mental performance.

Mind before Matter

There's no deficiency of irony in the fact that while Recommended Dietary Allowances (RDAs) for nutrients are based on avoiding physical impairment, the brain often shows signs of undernutrition long before the rest of the body. "What's enough to prevent physical symptoms of vitamin deficiencies may not be adequate to prevent impaired mental function," says Stephen Schoenthaler, Ph.D., who has studied the relationship between nutrition and behavior as a professor of sociology and criminal justice at California State University, Stanislaus in Turlock. "You can't assume subclinical malnutrition isn't there in the absence of physical problems."

The mental dysfunctions associated with vitamin malnutrition have been known, Dr. Schoenthaler says, since World War II, when the armed services experimented with conscientious objectors, systematically feeding them diets lacking in one specific nutrient to gauge the consequences. During the experiments, "impairment of mental function always occurred first," he says.

Today, under more stringent research standards, it's more difficult to quantify, analyze and verify the frequently subtle shifts in mood and behavior. Physical symptoms are easier to study, Dr. Schoenthaler says, which is one of the reasons why RDAs remain based on them.

Breakfast: For Champions

The connection between good nutrition and mental performance can be seen as early as the first meal of the day. Both children and adults perform better at school or at work if they've broken their night-long fast with a filling, nutritious meal. Generally, children who are reasonably well fed don't show any noticeable decline in school achievement if they miss an occasional breakfast, according to Bonnie Spring, Ph.D., a professor of psychology at the University of Health Sciences/Chicago Medical School, who's extensively studied the effects of food on behavior. "If the kids are basically well nourished," she says, "you see very minimal consequences. They can probably get away with skipping breakfast for the day, pull together and function okay. They have enough reserves."

But if the children are at all undernourished, missing breakfast "is not advisable," Dr. Spring says. If these kids miss the first meal of the day, by late in the morning, "they don't concentrate as well, and their problem-solving ability deteriorates." For them, "you do see improvements in school, which suggests there are long-term benefits of eating breakfast."

The mechanism behind the enhanced learning associated with breakfast is difficult to pinpoint, Dr. Spring says. "Who knows to what extent the benefit is due to nutrition or other factors that come along for the ride," such as better attendance because of less illness or better motivation because of a boost in mood and outlook. Whatever the reason, "there's enough evidence that something positive is happening when they eat breakfast."

A Smart Pill to Swallow

If your children can't always eat that breakfast, it may be wise for them—and you, too—at least to swallow a good multivitamin containing a full 100 percent of the RDAs for all essential nutrients. In a 12-week test of 615 children, Dr. Schoenthaler found that students who took a supplement offering a full day's supply of vitamins and minerals did significantly better on intelligence tests than those taking pills providing half that amount, twice that amount or nothing at all. The kids displayed improvement in "fluid" intelligence, the ability to reason and make analogies, but in pure rote learning or memory, the ability, say, to recall dates or facts.

The improvement—45 percent of the kids taking 100 percent of the RDAs gained at least 15 points on intelligence tests, as opposed to 20 percent of the children taking pills without nutrients—was seen even in pupils who otherwise would be considered well fed, Dr. Schoenthaler says.

The results raise intriguing questions, he says. Because the kids receiving 50 percent of the RDAs didn't perform as well as those receiving 100 percent, are the RDAs really adequate for optimal mental function? And if providing twice the RDA doesn't improve intelligence scores, is an excess of one vitamin interfering with the absorption of others, toppling the nutrient balance? "Getting more than is needed is not necessarily better," Dr. Schoenthaler says.

Students in another, much smaller study also scored gains in intelligence tests after taking additional vitamins and minerals. The authors of this British study theorize that pupils who increased their scores with supple-

(continued on page 250)

THE THINKING PERSON'S VITAMIN GUIDE

Every vitamin worth its alphabetic assignation is required by the brain for some mental function. Here are some of the most significant.

B_{12} before all. All of the B vitamins are especially important for optimal brain development and function, but B_{12} seems to be the most crucial. A dearth of the nutrient, also called cobalamin, has been linked to everything from paranoia, restlessness, irritability and manic depression to confusion, chronic fatigue syndrome, memory loss, phobias and insomnia. Mental problems often can develop long before the more physical sign—pernicious anemia—shows up in a blood test. The anemia itself can cause some of the same symptoms as well as listlessness, lower IQ, learning disorders and short attention span.

Why should a deficiency of B_{12} cause mental impairment? Researchers think it's because, along with dietary fat, B_{12} is vital to the growth and maintenance of the tissue that encases and protects the brain's nerve fibers, the myelin sheath. Without enough B_{12}, the myelin sheath degenerates, exposing the nerves and causing the mental disorders.

Few people, except some strict vegetarians, develop B_{12} deficiencies for dietary reasons; most people eat enough animal-derived foods, the only sources of the nutrient. Most deficiencies are caused by an inability of the body to absorb the vitamin, according to John Lindenbaum, M.D., a professor of medicine at Columbia University in New York City. People with atrophic gastritis, in which the stomach doesn't secrete a protein necessary for B_{12} absorption, and those who have had part of their colons removed are especially susceptible, Dr. Lindenbaum says.

Feeling better with folate. You're more likely to develop a deficiency of folate, or folic acid, than of B_{12}, although both these B vitamins interact in the body and a lack of either can bring on a case of the blues. Many psychiatric patients "show a high instance of folate deficiency," according to Simon Young, Ph.D., a professor in the Department of Psychiatry at McGill University in Montreal. Some association has been found between low folate in the body and depression-like symptoms. When people with such symptoms were treated with folate, Dr. Young says, their symptoms improved.

There also is a correlation with the neurotransmitter serotonin, whose presence in the brain seems to soothe and relax. Those with low serotonin levels in their brains have not only lower moods but lower amounts of folate in their bodies, according to Dr. Young. When supplemented with folate, these people lift both their serotonin counts and their spirits.

B_6 and the blahs. Many women who complain of premenstrual tension are deficient in vitamin B_6, says John Dommisse, M.D., a psychiatrist in private practice in nutritional and metabolic psychiatry in Portsmouth, Virginia. And the estrogen in some oral contraceptives and in the estrogen replacement therapy for postmenopausal difficulties and osteoporosis can cause a deficiency of this nutrient. Depression often is the result of a deficiency because, Dr. Dommisse explains, B_6 is needed to produce serotonin. Other mental signs of a B_6 deficiency include anemia-like symptoms, irritability and fatigue.

A need for niacin. This B vitamin also needed for a healthy myelin sheath, was used back in the 1950s and 1960s to treat schizophrenia, Dr. Dommisse says, but the connection today between niacin and the mental condition is regarded as unproven. Nonetheless, a chronic shortage causes the hallucinations, confusion and nervous disorders associated with the classic deficiency disease pellagra. Less severe niacin deficiencies can cause anxiety, fatigue, loss of short-term memory and depression.

Riboflavin for a better start. Riboflavin (vitamin B_2) deficiency can retard brain growth in children, leading to abnormalities in behavior as adults. Hypochondria, depression and lethargy could result from a marginal deficiency of riboflavin before other physical symptoms manifest themselves, according to some experts.

Thiamine versus the bottle. Heavy drinkers run the risk of developing a chronic deficiency of thiamine (vitamin B_1). People who frequently use aspirin or antacids also are especially susceptible to thiamine deficiency. That could be particularly dangerous because some researchers suggest that a thiamine deficiency causes brain damage even before overt signs of harm exist. Symptoms include fatigue, confusion, depression and loss of memory. Thiamine supplementation reverses the symptoms in very early stages, but once more advanced, the damage becomes irreversible.

Adrift without C. Scurvy, the classic vitamin C–deficiency disease, can result in depression, hypochondria and hysteria, Dr. Dommisse says, and less severe deficiencies have been shown to trigger edgy feelings of anxiety and overexcitement as well as depression and fatigue.

mentation may have had nutrient deficiencies because, while not malnourished, they may have been ingesting too many calories from junk foods.

ADULTS ARISE AND SHINE

While the impact of eating or missing breakfast has been examined extensively in children, comparatively few studies have assessed the intelligence and performance effects on adults. Nonetheless, there are several known consequences of not eating a morning meal. "As a general rule, when people eat breakfast, they are more alert by midday than they were when they first woke up in the morning," Dr. Spring says. "When they skip breakfast, they're about equal. In other words, they don't fully wake up." Alertness and reaction time suffers markedly on an empty stomach. "Breakfast skippers aren't sleepier than when they woke up," she says, "but they are no better than when they first rolled out of bed."

THE ELEMENTS OF BRAIN POWER

Minerals, too, are important for proper brain development and functioning. Research indicates that maternal mineral and trace element deficiencies before birth may cause irreversible brain damage in infants, while behavioral problems caused by malnutrition after birth can be reversed by supplementation.

Pump iron into the brain. Even without the low red blood cell counts found in anemia, a less-than-adequate amount of iron in the diet can cause mental problems, according to Harold H. Sandstead, M.D., of the Department of Preventive Medicine and Community Health at University of Texas Medical Branch in Galveston. Children have been examined more extensively in this regard than adults, he says, and most studies show that those who have problems in learning and comprehension are low in iron, which carries oxygen to the brain as well as to all other organs in the body.

"Iron is essential," Dr. Sandstead says. "Iron deficiency may be rather subtle—affecting attention, learning, concentration and other functions. But with iron repletion, things improve."

The possibility of iron deficiency should be considered if your children are hyperactive, have short attention spans and are irritable. Adults with an iron deficiency are often irritable and suffer from headaches.

Zinc to think. Researchers link zinc shortage to a variety of mood changes. A severe lack induces depression, lethargy and irritability, but supplementation reverses those problems, according to Dr. Sand-

Don't depend on coffee. The traditional wake-up call, coffee, may produce results similar to breakfast's effect, but with no nutritional benefit and actually at some nutritive cost. People profess to be more alert after drinking coffee, and it does help to keep you awake and to some extent sharpen reaction time. But controlled performance tests often don't confirm the stimulant effect. Chronic coffee and caffeine consumption can, of course, lead to coffee jitters, along with insomnia, anxiety and perhaps even paranoia or depression. There's evidence that heavy users may perform less well than light or moderate users or nonusers. And caffeine interferes with the body's absorption of iron, enough so that chronic intake could cause a potentially energy-robbing deficiency.

Although researchers don't know for certain, caffeine seems to work by blocking the brain chemical adenosine, a natural tranquilizer. It also stimulates production of the neurotransmitters epinephrine and norepinephrine, which stimulate the mind.

stead. Less drastic deficiencies impair memory, but "it's improved in certain areas with repletion."Low levels of zinc in the bloodstream also have been associated with more aggressive behavior, less curiosity, hyperactivity, mental retardation and dyslexia, says John Dommisse, M.D., a psychiatrist in private practice in nutritional and metabolic psychiatry in Portsmouth, Virginia.

More magnesium might be needed. Magnesium deficiency might be more common than most experts believe, Dr. Dommisse says, because processing removes much of this mineral from food. When the brain is low in magnesium, people could become depressed, agitated, confused and irritable. They also may experience tremors and twitches.

Low calcium and confusion. While calcium commonly is associated with strong bones, it also may bolster the brain, Dr. Sandstead suggests. Even short-term deficiencies of either calcium or magnesium can cause tremors in some people. When those two minerals are not in intravenous feeding solutions, he says, "hospital patients become confused."

Chromium puts a shine on stress. Because the brain gets its energy from glucose, this trace mineral plays an important role, for it is involved in the body's release of insulin for sugar metabolism. More related to behavior, though, chromium seems to help the body manage stress, Dr. Dommisse says.

Even though you may be sleepier without breakfast in your belly, comprehension and problem-solving skills late in the morning remain relatively unaffected—unless you're under emotional stress or the demands of deadline pressures. "When you're in a casual pace and not under any stress, you work fine" and there's no effect on intellect from not eating breakfast, according to Dr. Spring. "But if you add emotional stress or a deadline, you see an impairment in such things as math skills and reasoning skills." People also become more anxious and irritable, she says.

Aim for a balanced breakfast. The kind of breakfast you eat makes little difference, unless, again, you're under some form of duress or deadline demand. "There's some evidence that a balanced breakfast is better," Dr. Spring says. If working under stress, a meal comprised equally of carbohydrates and protein—for example, oatmeal or cereal for carbohydrates and a slice of lean ham or a large glass of skim milk for protein—offers a "significant advantage" in mental performance compared to the high-carbohydrate load of a bagel or two.

Serotonin: The Mood Maker

By the time the lunch hour rolls around, meal composition assumes a much greater importance to the brain, determining how you feel for the remainder of the day. While carbohydrates supply glucose necessary for the brain's energy, they also trigger the production of serotonin, a widely studied neurotransmitter associated with a variety of emotional states. It calms and relaxes, perhaps even inducing sleep under the right circumstances. It also tends to counteract feelings of stress and anxiety and enhances your ability to concentrate. Low brain serotonin, on the other hand, is associated with insomnia, depression, aggression, and hypersensitivity to sound, touch, heat and pain, according to Dr. Fernstrom.

No other neurotransmitter is as easily manipulated by food as serotonin, which the brain manufactures from the amino acid tryptophan. In a blatant bypass of the blood/brain barrier, the more tryptophan that reaches the brain, the more serotonin is produced. But you cannot raise brain tryptophan by eating high-protein food, because it has to vie against higher concentrations of all the other amino acids in the bloodstream rushing to the brain. Amid the competition, tryptophan is barely noticed and has little effect.

But it gets a virtual free ride up to the brain when you eat carbohydrates, which also contain small amounts of amino acids, including tryptophan. The reason is that sugars in carbohydrates stimulate the release of insulin, which draws most of the other amino acids into muscle cells. Tryptophan is unaffected by insulin's attraction, and so it freely cruises up to the brain, which then uses it to make more serotonin.

Until the Food and Drug Administration (FDA) took tryptophan supplements off the shelves of health food stores, there was a more direct way to

A Slave to the Crave?

Ever had a yen for orange juice or broccoli? Is it because you just like the taste, or is it because your brain is detecting a deficiency of vitamin C in your bloodstream? Is your mouth watering for a steak or seafood dinner? It may not be the atavistic carnivore in you at all. It simply may be the high-carbohydrate, low-protein lunch you had.

What you eat or don't eat not only sometimes determines your mood; it often determines what you'll ingest for your next meal. And the mood itself also plays a role in what you eat.

"You have to consider both," says Michael D. Chafetz, Ph.D., a clinical neuropsychologist and author of the book *Nutrition and Neurotransmitters*. "What you eat can determine your mood, and what your mood is directs what foods you eat. There's a change in eating pattern to feed the mood."

The precise mechanism is unknown, but the effect is seen all the time. When rats are given premeal snacks to judge later eating behavior, "we find that if it's a carbohydrate snack, the animals prefer a main meal of protein, and vice versa," says Carol E. Greenwood, Ph.D., at the University of Toronto Faculty of Medicine in Ontario.

"The signal," Dr. Greenwood says, "is serotonin," a neurotransmitter whose level in the brain is increased by eating carbohydrates and decreased by eating protein.

Anxious or depressed people often have lower brain levels of serotonin, and they seem to intuitively learn that eating high-carbohydrate foods as disparate as rice pilaf or chocolate cake improves their outlooks, eases the depression and soothes their nerves by increasing the production of the neurotransmitter. Similarly, people who receive medication to increase serotonin in their brains "tend to decrease carbohydrate intake," Dr. Chafetz says. They tend to want protein.

While serotonin plays a role, "it doesn't explain all of the phenomenon," Dr. Greenwood says. "We don't know yet what it is, but it's a whole-body issue dealing with the overall balance of the right foods for health."

That's obvious when you consider studies showing an innate desire for salt when the body is low in sodium, or for vitamin C when levels of that nutrient have dipped, Dr. Chafetz says. "We can't specify a mechanism like we can with carbohydrates, but it's suggestive." Perhaps, he theorizes, when your body is low or high in a nutrient, certain brain receptors aren't seeing enough of it in the blood or are gauging too much, and they send appetite-influencing signals accordingly.

deliver this amino acid to the brain. But a problem arose in the manufacturing of synthetic tryptophan by a certain company, according to Dr. Spring. "It's inaccurate to describe it as an impurity," she says, "but something unusual was done to it so that it caused a white blood cell disease in people

WHEN A RICE CAKE IS A SHOT IN THE ARM

If you're like most people, when you eat a high-carbohydrate, low-protein lunch or dinner, you calm down, relax a bit, get sleepy and sluggish.

But what if you don't? What if you find yourself invigorated after a heavy dish of spaghetti or a bowl of rice? Not to worry; you're just a carbo craver.

Some folks—often those suffering from premenstrual tension or seasonal affective disorder (wintertime depression), for example, "selectively overeat carbohydrates," says Bonnie Spring, Ph.D., at the University of Health Sciences/Chicago Medical School. "With unbalanced, high-carbohydrate meals, they get activated."

The reason, as with other triggers of food/mood reactions, is serotonin, a chemical in the brain that is responsible for feelings of serenity and placidness. The amount of serotonin in the brain can be increased by eating a high-carbohydrate meal.

People who crave carbohydrates "act as if they have a long-term deficiency in serotonin," Dr. Spring says. People who have a normal amount of serotonin get sleepy after eating a high-carbohydrate meal. "They trip the sleep mechanism because they're getting a rise in serotonin," she says. But those with a deficiency of the neurotransmitter feel better after a high-carbohydrate food because they're edging their serotonin level up to a normal level.

"They're giving themselves a high-carbohydrate load that is acting like a shot in the arm," Dr. Spring says. "It's correcting the deficiency in brain serotonin and improving their mood, almost as if they were self-medicating."

During midafternoon snacktime, if you find yourself habitually reaching for a carbohydrate food to make you feel better and get you through the rest of the workday, don't let your conscience bother you, Dr. Spring says. "You're probably one of those people who will get activated by carbohydrates." Your only concern should be to "keep the fat down. Eat ginger snaps or rice cakes or angel food cake," she says, "not potato chips."

who consumed it." The FDA pulled all brands of tryptophan from the market for its investigation merely as a precaution, but "there's little doubt it was the particular manufacturer." Increasing brain levels of the amino acid through eating should be no cause for concern because tryptophan is a common, natural substance in foods.

When most people eat a high-carbohydrate lunch, they become sleepy and sluggish by the middle of the afternoon. Eating some protein along with the carbohydrates, though, counteracts the serotonin slump, because the brain uses the amino acid tyrosine found in protein to produce norepinephrine and dopamine, two neurotransmitters associated with invigoration, motivation, mental acuity and quick thinking.

Early food/mood research suggested that a pure-protein meal would spike the neurotransmitter punch to give you vim and vigor for the rest of the day or evening, Dr. Spring says. Newer studies have found, though, that brain levels of tyrosine are not so readily affected, although enough reaches the brain to counteract tryptophan's production of serotonin.

What does this mental menu mean? Basically, you do have some options available to you.

Vary the protein/carbohydrate mix. If you want to fall asleep or feel lethargic after lunch or dinner, go for the high-carbohydrate, no-protein option. If not, "add meat sauce to the pasta or cream cheese to the bagel," Dr. Spring says. "You'll feel more invigorated and alert than if you ate a meal without protein."

Consider your timing. "On a day-to-day basis, with the kind of meal patterns most people have with protein and carbohydrates, it's unlikely we'd see a mood effect," notes Carol E. Greenwood, Ph.D., an associate professor in the Department of Nutritional Sciences at the University of Toronto Faculty of Medicine in Ontario. "But that doesn't mean we can't use the observations and play with them," altering performance by changing what we eat and when we eat it.

"Maybe that tells us that if we have dessert," she suggests, "it's better not to eat it with dinner but about half an hour before bed," when a carbohydrate punch will help us more easily greet the Sandman. "You're not changing the number of calories you eat in a day, but you're waiting for when you're most likely to get the positive benefit of carbohydrates."

Don't go overboard on calories. Just be aware of how much of everything you eat. High-calorie cramming will make you browse the drowse section of your mental folds regardless of your meal composition. "When you're eating a very high calorie lunch, all bets are off about protein or carbohydrates," Dr. Spring says. "We don't understand what the mechanism is, but you get about a 10 percent decline in performance after a high-calorie meal. No matter what you eat in that kind of meal, you're going to get sleepy."

Does Alzheimer's Start in the Womb?

If scientists ever find a nutritional way to avert Alzheimer's disease, the preventive path may start before birth.

Rats born to mothers fed extremely high doses of choline, a natural substance found in almost all foods, display better memory retention, and their brains seem to age much more slowly than rats not fed the nutrient.

"These are particularly exciting findings," says Christina Williams, Ph.D., an associate professor of psychiatry at Barnard College of Columbia University in New York City and part of a team of researchers studying, under a grant from the National Institute of Aging, how to prevent the brain deterioration of Alzheimer's. She says she hopes a variation of choline treatment one day could serve as an inoculation against memory loss in old age.

Choline's role in memory has long been examined because it is the precursor of the neurotransmitter acetylcholine, which courses through the cholinergic system, the memory and recall portion of the brain that appears to degenerate under Alzheimer's. Under certain circumstances, such as when the cholinergic neurons are being used actively to store memory, intake of exceedingly high doses of choline results in production of more brain acetylcholine.

Because of that, scientists initially thought that supplemental choline would help stave off or reduce the effects of the disease. A number of tests were conducted, many of them using lecithin, a choline-rich fatty substance found in soybeans and egg yolks, but "it's a relatively ineffective treatment," Dr. Williams says. "You can get a transient increase in memory, but you have to keep eating a huge amount of choline. And it doesn't work all the time in all people."

But because there are certain sensitive developmental periods during which memory-related parts of the brain form, it could be a question of *when* choline supplementation is started. And the answer to that may be found in mother's milk.

"In mother's milk, choline is remarkably high—more than in blood plasma," Dr. Williams says. And during the first week after birth, choline levels in mother's milk are exceptionally high. "Mothers are already supplementing choline to their kids," she says.

That at least says something about comparing labels on commercial infant formulas, which "differ quite dramatically in choline content," Dr. Williams says. (Soy-based formulas usually are highest in the nutrient.)

Instead of trying to treat aging adults already afflicted with a brain-degenerating disease or even trying to prevent it in adulthood, Dr. Williams and her colleagues decided to study choline supplements in unborn rats, giving them doses through the diets of their mothers, then testing their memories as they aged.

The rats fed choline prenatally performed 10 to 20 percent better on memory tests than their unsupplemented counterparts, Dr. Williams says. And as they aged, "they still behaved like a young adult," with memory retention between 20 and 30 percent better than their untreated peers.

"We're somehow strengthening the cholinergic system to withstand age-related changes," Dr. Williams says.

These experiments have been conducted exclusively on rats, and Dr. Williams foresees no human tests for quite some time. Dosages have been 10 to 20 times the amount of choline normally thought required by the body. "They're very high amounts, super amounts," she says, "but then choline is not lethal or toxic at all." But it's more than you can get from food alone.

Rather than rushing for the choline capsules just yet—the most common supplemental form is lecithin, which Dr. Williams says is "not good" because it primarily is fat—perhaps you should obtain more of the nutrient through diet. Almost all foods contain choline, according to Dr. Williams, but particularly good sources include spinach and other green vegetables, seaweed and eggs.

CHAPTER 20

THE IMMUNE SYSTEM

DEFENSIVE DINING

Imagine this urgent supply order from your body's front lines of defense: "Hey, what's the story? You forget we're here? We're just about out of zinc, our B_6 supply is going fast and we haven't had any vitamin E since you ate that avocado *last year!* Listen, we like pretzels and diet soda as well as you do, but we need some *real food!* Eat some bloody vegetables, will ya? And throw down a few oysters while you're at it."

Having a supply officer for your immune system's legions of infection-fighting white blood cells would certainly be a help. He would let you know in no uncertain terms just what you need to bounce back from a cold, the flu or other viral infections. You'd know what to pile on your plate to prevent infections after burns or surgery, perhaps even to avoid cell changes that can lead to cancer.

Just as real soldiers suffer serious morale problems when their C-rations are cut back, the cells of your immune system could go AWOL if they're not getting the high-quality nutrition they need to fight off infections and disease.

Researchers have known for many years that any nutritional deficit bad enough to produce classic deficiency diseases, such as kwashiorkor (caused by protein shortage) or scurvy (caused by lack of vitamin C), can also lead

A Formula for Peak Immunity

The limp lettuce and quivering gelatin on hospital dinner trays may not be what the immune system craves. But if you're sick enough to require a nasogastric feeding tube, you might be getting exactly the nourishment you need—or as close to it as researchers can now determine. This kind of nutritional support drips nutrients directly into your stomach through a tube inserted through your nose.

A few of the more than 300 feeding formulas now available contain "a veritable kitchen soup of everything that's known to enhance immune function," as one researcher puts it. Marketed as "immunostimulating" formulas, these liquids contain varying proportions of key ingredients.

Most contain fish oils and other omega-3 fatty acids that are thought to enhance immune response and dampen inflammatory response; arginine, an amino acid associated with enhanced immune function and preservation of body protein; nucleotides (bits of genetic material) whose restriction is thought to result in depressed immune function; and more than the Recommended Dietary Allowance of vitamins E, A, C, B_6 and other B-complex vitamins, zinc and copper, along with beta-carotene, selenium and a host of other essential nutrients.

How well do these formulas work? In a study at University Hospital in Philadelphia, surgical cancer patients receiving one such formula had less than a third as many infections and were released from the hospital five days sooner than patients receiving a standard liquid formula.

At Shriner's Burn Institute in Cincinnati, severely burned patients get feeding formulas made up just for them. "We give astonishing amounts of vitamin A, for example," says Michele A. Gottschlich, R.D., Ph.D., director of nutritional services. "A healthy person would develop a toxicity to such large doses, but we don't see toxicity in our patients because the need is so great. In fact, it boosts the immune system."

Because the nutritional needs of critically ill patients can vary, not everyone will do best on the same formula, Dr. Gottschlich says. "So ask your doctor about the formula he has chosen for you, and why."

to life-threatening drops in immune function.

And researchers are now finding that compromised immunity can also occur with borderline nutritional deficiencies and may even occur in people whose diets meet the current Recommended Dietary Allowances (RDAs).

"Some nutritionists get upset hearing this, but the fact is that the RDAs may not be the optimum amount to prevent certain diseases like cancer," says Ronald Watson, Ph.D., research professor at the University of Arizona College of Medicine in Tucson. Dr. Watson is studying the immunity-enhancing effects of beta-carotene, a compound in fruits and vegetables that is thought to help protect against cancer.

The list of nutritional deficiencies associated with poor immune function is long. It includes protein, vitamins A, E, C, B_6 and B_{12}, folate, beta-carotene, iron, and magnesium, plus the trace minerals selenium, copper, manganese and zinc.

Before detailing how some of these nutrients may enhance your immune system, though, we need to know how your body's defense works.

Members of a Mighty Army

Researchers—and writers—often find themselves using military terms to describe the immune system. They talk about invaders, attacks, counterattacks and defense systems. "In fact, the comparison is an accurate one," says Terry M. Phillips, D.Sc., Ph.D., director of the immunogenetics and immunochemistry lab at George Washington University's Medical Center and coauthor of *Winning the War Within*. "It seems the more we learn about the immune system, the more amazingly appropriate the army analogies become," Dr. Phillips says.

That system is a complex, total body system of cells that kill off bacteria, viruses, parasites and fungi and also detect and destroy virus-infested or damaged cells that may be or may become cancerous.

Cells of the immune system patrol the bloodstream, line our bronchial passages and lurk in our lymph nodes, just waiting for security to be breached. When it is, they spring into action. Some move into the area of infection, then call for reinforcements. Some multiply rapidly, producing several hundred thousand of their own kind in a single day. Some send out orders with a series of biochemicals (cytokines) that tell other cells what to do, where to go, even when to back off, Dr. Phillips says.

Digest and Conquer

Some cells are for general defense. They'll go after anything that isn't you, and they don't need to wait for orders from headquarters to do so.

General defense cells include all the "feeding" cells, called phagocytes. Two of the most common of these cells are neutrophils and macrophages.

"Neutrophils might be considered the foot soldiers of the immune system," Dr. Phillips says. They move quickly, swimming through your blood and oozing amoeba-like through the cells of your blood vessels to attack. A neutrophil flows around its prey, envelops it inside its body and then secretes digestive enzymes on it.

Macrophages are big eating cells, slow but tough. Each one can eat an

CAN YOU FIGHT THIS INFECTION WITH FOOD?

You're feeling miserable with a head-pounding cold, or is it really a touch of the flu you're battling? In any case, your nagging conscience is chiding: "No wonder you're sick. The way you eat."

So, since you're already laid up, does it matter what you eat *now?* You don't have much appetite anyway, so why not tickle your taste buds with that quart of Rocky Road in the freezer? Or would you feel better faster if you started drinking plenty of vitamin C–rich orange juice and scheduled some zinc-packed foods like oysters for supper?

"You *should* eat better, but realize that eating better over that short period of time is not going to cure your cold or flu," says Ananda Prasad, M.D., Ph.D., of Wayne State University in Detroit.

It's possible that eating well may provide some immediate immune system benefits, like maintaining fighting levels of vitamin C and zinc. (These nutrients tend to be used up fast during an infection.) But it's long-term good nutrition that improves immune function most, researchers say.

"If you have optimal nutrition status, you will be able to fight any infection better," Dr. Prasad says. "And optimal status takes at least several weeks to establish, and can take months, depending on your nutritional needs."

If a cold or the flu does rev up your resolve to eat better, make sure you continue to eat well even after you start to feel better, says Thomas Petro, Ph.D., associate professor of microbiology and immunology at the University of Nebraska Medical Center in Omaha. "That's because your body needs time to rebuild damaged tissue and restore a possibly battered army of immune cells, and unless it has the nourishment to do so, you're at risk for another infection soon down the road," Dr. Petro says.

infinite number of bacteria, as long as they don't eat them too fast. When a chemical signal brings an invasion to their attention, macrophages will ooze on over to see what the trouble is. Once they get into the fray, they liven up.

"Macrophages also do garbage detail. They devour the remains of invading microorganisms as well as the cellular casualties from your own immune system," Dr. Phillips explains.

After it digests a virus or bacteria, a macrophage burps out pieces of the offending substances (antigens) and puts them on its surface. It then presents the antigens to a different class of immune cells, known as lymphocytes, described below. When the lymphocytes get a look at the antigens, a whole different component of the immune system kicks in—one primed to go after specific targets, like that virus that's been percolating in your gut all day.

NATURAL KILLERS

The target-specific portion of the immune system includes two general types of lymphocytes: B-cells, formed in the bone marrow, and T-cells, formed in the thymus, a lymph gland behind the breastbone.

"B-cells are the admirals of your body's defense system," Dr. Phillips says. "They deploy antibodies into your bloodstream and other body fluids." (These Y-shaped protectors help to neutralize some invaders themselves, or work with a "chemical warfare" cohort, called complement, to subdue other foes.) B-cells also keep the war records of previous battles so that any repeat invasion by a former foe is immediately countered.

T-cells come in three types. Killer T-cells do the dirty work of killing any cells in your body that have been invaded by viruses. T-helper cells and suppressor T-cells regulate the magnitude of the immune response and help bring things back to normal when the infection in conquered.

Natural killer cells are closely related to killer T-cells but aren't as picky about what they'll go after. They can recognize cells infected by viruses, and some tumor cells, and kill them.

THE NUTRIENTS THAT MATTER MOST

All these specialized cells depend on what you eat to do their jobs: They need good nutrition to develop in the bone marrow or thymus, to multiply rapidly in response to an infection, to protect themselves during the heat of battle and to generate the biochemicals that orchestrate an effective immune response. Let's see why some of these nutrients are so important.

VITAMIN B_6: The Booster

Remember wheat germ, blackstrap molasses and brown rice? These perennial health food staples are chock-full of vitamin B_6. Your immune system may like them no better than you do, but eating them or other B_6-rich foods may do you both a lot of good.

Vitamin B_6 may help your immune system produce antibodies and your thymus to churn out the hormones that allow T-cells to mature into deadly, target-specific killers. B_6 and other B-complex vitamins are also needed for cells to replicate (make more of themselves). Low levels of some B vitamins means your body will be unable to produce the large numbers of immune cells it may need for a major attack, says Simin Meydani, Ph.D., of the U.S. Department of Agriculture's (USDA) Human Nutrition Research Center on Aging at Tufts University School of Nutrition in Boston.

Even though B_6 and other B-complex vitamins are found in whole-grain and fortified baked goods and cereals, some people don't get enough of these nutrients or may need more than the RDA for optimum immune function, Dr. Meydani says.

She and researcher Robert M. Russell, M.D., professor of medicine and nutrition at Tufts, discovered that when healthy elderly people had vitamin B_6 taken almost completely out of their diets, their immune response went down, as expected. What wasn't anticipated was the finding that the amount of vitamin B_6 needed to restore immune function was much higher than the current RDA of about two milligrams.

VITAMIN E: The Shield

Researchers know that vitamin E protects immune cells from what could be called stray bullets, harmful free radicals generated during immune system battles and the process of destroying bacteria and viruses. These battles involve chemical reactions that use oxygen—so they're called oxidative reactions. These oxidative reactions generate free radicals.

"As long as they have plenty of vitamin E incorporated into their outer membrane, immune cells are shielded from these reactions," explains Jeffrey Blumberg, Ph.D., chief of the Antioxidants Research Laboratory, also at the research center on aging at Tufts. "If immune cells lack sufficient antioxidant protection, however, their own reactions can injure or even kill them."

Vitamin E also affects the immune system by reducing the formation of a biochemical called prostaglandin E2 (PGE2), says Dr. Blumberg. PGE2 inhibits immune function. "So by giving vitamin E, we are turning one of the immune's system's 'off' switches back on," he explains. "We've also shown we get increases in interleukin-2, which is a T-cell growth factor, by giving vitamin E."

In one study, Dr. Blumberg found that older people given supplemental vitamin E had marked improvement in certain tests of immune response. One of the tests, a skin-patch test exposing the skin to certain toxins, measures the body's ability to fight antigens. (A poor response on this test is associated with increased death rates.) "However, after giving older people vitamin E supplements, their response to the skin-patch test was more like that of younger people," Dr. Blumberg says.

His subsequent research shows that vitamin E enhances immune response in older men after exercising. "That's important because this immune response helps repair tissue damaged during exercise; it may even be important in building new muscle," he explains.

VITAMIN C: The Protector

Do you naturally crave orange juice when you're feeling out of sorts? Maybe that supply officer's message *is* getting through. "Pour me a tall, cool one."

Like vitamin E, vitamin C is an antioxidant. So it helps to control the potentially damaging reactions that occur when immune cell meets bacteria, and the shooting starts. But because vitamin C is water soluble, not fat soluble, it provides protection not in the cell membrane, but in the watery fluid within cells, and surrounding cells.

"Vitamin C deficiency has been shown to weaken a number of immune system functions," says Adrianne Bendich, Ph.D., senior clinical research

SAVING LIVES WITH VITAMIN A

In some parts of the world, people die for lack of what we take for granted. That's because nutrition in some countries is so bad and the chances for all kinds of infections so good that a person's immune system never has a fighting chance.

Even in the face of across-the-board malnourishment, though, it appears that vitamin A can save lives.

In southern India, where vitamin A deficiency is rampant, the distribution to 15,000 preschool children of supplements that provided the Recommended Dietary Allowance of this nutrient reduced death rates by more than half in just one year. And in Nepal vitamin A cut children's deaths by a third.

"These children were dying mostly of pneumonia and fevers, or diarrhea and dysentery," says Keith West, Jr., Dr.P.H., director of the Vitamin A Project at Johns Hopkins Hospital in Baltimore. (The Vitamin A Project is aimed at solving health problems related to vitamin deficiencies in developing countries.) "We don't know all the details of how the vitamin A works, but we do know that it plays a role in a large number of activities within the body that involve defense against infection."

Vitamin A reduced death rates most dramatically in children who were the most poorly fed. "It seemed to work even in children whose growth was stunted, which would indicate chronic malnourishment," Dr. West says.

coordinator in the Human Nutrition Research Division of Hoffmann-La Roche in Nutley, New Jersey. "Cells just don't multiply, communicate or mature into target-specific fighters as well when vitamin C levels are low."

Studies show that when adequate vitamin C is present, the number of frontline infection fighters—T-cells and B-cells—increases. Studies with higher-than-normal intakes of vitamin C have had mixed results, Dr. Bendich says. "Some studies show improved immune response; others do not."

Research seems to show that vitamin C helps smokers and people with asthma retain immunity in the lungs, Dr. Bendich says. "Both cigarette smoke and the inflammatory response of asthma generate lots of free radicals that can damage lymphocytes in the lungs," she says. "Vitamin C seems to offer these cells some protection."

Studies show that certain immune cells, especially neutrophils, have concentrations of vitamin C up to 150 times the amount typically found in cells, and that vitamin C is quickly used up during infection fighting. So you may really need those extra glasses of orange juice when you're sick, researchers say.

BETA-CAROTENE: TUMOR DOOMER?

Do natural killer cells like a hearty lunch of carrots and sweet potatoes before resuming their day's work? Some research seems to indicate they do.

Those foods, along with other red, yellow, orange and dark green fruits and vegetables, are packed full of beta-carotene, a nutrient associated with reduced risk for several kinds of cancer. Some researchers believe beta-carotene may even reverse early cell changes that could lead to cancer.

In one study, Harinder S. Garewal M.D., Ph.D., assistant director for cancer prevention and control at the University of Arizona Cancer Center in Tucson, gave high doses of beta-carotene (30 milligrams a day) for six months to a group of 24 people with precancerous growths in their mouths. Seventeen responded to the treatment; their lesions decreased in size by at least 50 percent, and in several patients they disappeared altogether.

University of Arizona researcher Dr. Watson homed in on immune system changes in these same 24 people. "We found that 30 milligrams a day or more of beta-carotene caused significant increases in the number of natural killer cells and T-helper cells," he says. Both are important parts of the body's tumor surveillance and disposal system. "Levels of cells with interleukin-2 and transferrin receptors, both indicators of lymphocyte activation, also rose," he says.

"Theoretically, all those things should be good for cancer resistance," Dr. Watson says.

A typical American consumes about 5 milligrams of beta-carotene a day, about a carrot's worth.

Getting plenty of beta-carotene is also a safe, low-fat way to get enough vitamin A, a nutrient that has a profound impact on many immunological functions. Your body converts beta-carotene to vitamin A, but only as needed—thereby eliminating any potential for vitamin A overdose.

ZINC: THE VITAL LINK

Abraham Lincoln's army dined on Chesapeake Bay oysters and won the war. Your own internal army might thrive on an occasional serving of these tasty mollusks, too. Why? Because oysters are a great source of zinc, a mineral involved with many aspects of immune function.

"Our research shows that zinc is very important, especially for thymic-dependant lymphocyte functions," says Ananda Prasad, M.D., Ph.D., professor of medicine at Wayne State University in Detroit and a pioneer researcher in the role of zinc in immune function. "The thymus gland helps T-cells to mature and become target specific," Dr. Prasad says. These cells also hold the body's memory of an invader, which allows it to respond more quickly should an infection recur.

Zinc is also necessary for the frenzy of immune cell reproduction that takes place during infection, and for the production of cytokines, those biochemicals that whip immune cells into action, Dr. Prasad says.

Studies show that people deficient in zinc have a variety of immune system weaknesses and are much more prone to infection. "Adding adequate zinc to the diet has been valuable in improving immune response," Dr. Prasad says.

In the United States, some people get only 8 to 10 milligrams of zinc a day, well below the RDA of 12 to 15 milligrams, Dr. Prasad says. "Older people, dieters and people who eat little or no meat and lots of fiber are most likely to develop zinc deficiency–related immune problems," he says.

When Immunity Goes Astray

What do rheumatoid arthritis, multiple sclerosis and lupus have in common? All three are *autoimmune* diseases. Their symptoms are caused by misguided immune cells attacking the body's own tissue. In the case of arthritis, it's the joints that come under attack, for multiple sclerosis it's the central nervous system, for lupus it's the kidneys, skin, heart and joints.

"Little research has been done on nutrition and autoimmune diseases compared to nutrition and immunity in general, and most studies so far have been done in animals," says Carl Keen, Ph.D., professor of nutrition and internal medicine at the University of California at Davis. So researchers are extremely wary about making any kinds of dietary recommendations. Still, research suggests that in the future, dietary manipulation, along with other treatments, may help some of these diseases.

Among the findings so far: omega-3 fatty acids, found in fatty fish like mackerel and salmon, apparently help suppress the inflammatory reaction in autoimmune diseases and perhaps provide other, still-unknown benefits. "There are many different hypotheses about how these oils work in immune function, but the details have yet to be worked out," Dr. Keen says. "The few preliminary studies done so far in humans show some potential for benefit."

Antioxidants like vitamins A, E and C might also play a role in slowing organ damage from autoimmune disease, but research is needed to confirm that possible role, Dr. Keen says. "On the other hand, it's also possible that these nutrients could speed up damage in some cases by boosting immune function in a system out of control."

Animal studies also show that deliberately inducing deficiencies of nutrients needed for immune function, such as zinc or specific amino acids, sometimes prolong the lives of animals with autoimmune diseases. "But doing that sort of thing just wouldn't be at all advisable in people," says Dr. Keen, "since the nutritional deficiencies create all sorts of other problems."

AN EATING PLAN FOR IMMUNE POWER

How can you possibly eat everything you need for optimum immunity without overeating?

The goal is to choose a wide array of nutrition-packed foods that are low in fat and calories, says Susanna Cunningham-Rundles, Ph.D., associate professor of immunology at New York Hospital-Cornell University Medical Center in New York City. "That doesn't happen by chance. You need to plan meals, and know what to pick up at the grocery store or when dining out."

The single most important thing that most people can do to improve their nutrition? "Eat more fruits and vegetables," Dr. Cunningham-Rundles says. Aim for two servings of fruits and three servings of vegetables a day, she suggests. "You *can* expand your tastes by exposing yourself to foods you've never had before, in a cheerful way, not like it's medicine."

Once you've started to widen your dining horizons, here are some specific ways to zero in on what you need.

Snack on vitamin C–rich fruits and vegetables. These include grapefruit, oranges, strawberries, cantaloupe, honeydew melons, mangoes, watermelon, fortified fruit juices, red and green peppers, broccoli, potatoes (white or sweet), tomatoes, brussels sprouts and cauliflower.

Chow down on foods high in beta-carotene. Sweet potatoes top the list, along with carrots, spinach, winter squash, kale, cantaloupe, apricots, broccoli and other colorful fruits and vegetables.

Zero in on zinc. Add shellfish (oysters are your best source); beef; wheat germ; fortified, ready-to-eat breakfast cereals; chicken; turkey and pumpkin seeds.

Seek out vitamin E. Eat wheat germ, peanut butter, almonds, filbert nuts, sunflower seeds, shrimp and vegetable oils. Green leafy vegetables also supply some vitamin E.

Get your fair share of vitamin B_6. It's easy with chicken; fortified, ready-to-eat cereals; sweet green or red peppers; turkey; brown rice; soybeans; oats; whole-wheat products; peanuts; bananas; plantains and walnuts.

Add vitamin A. Eat the same foods that provide beta-carotene (in the body, beta-carotene is converted into vitamin A as needed) or with a low-fat source of preformed vitamin A such as fortified skim milk.

Fill up on folate. The list of foods that supply folate includes broccoli; green peas; fortified, ready-to-eat cereals; beans; baked potatoes and orange juice. Folate is needed to make all new cells, including the white blood cells of your immune system.

Add omega-3 fatty acids. Mackerel, salmon, bluefish, herring, trout and tuna are good sources. Fish oils rich in omega-3's help stop inflammation, and unlike some other fats, do not impair immune function. Indeed, they may enhance it.

Pump up iron intake. Lean red meats; fortified, ready-to-eat cereals; dark-meat chicken or turkey; fish; shellfish; beans; nuts and seeds are good sources. Iron plays a major role in the chemical reactions that allow immune cells to zap invaders.

Concentrate on copper. Shellfish, nuts, sesame seeds, mushrooms and whole-grain cereals are good sources. Copper, like zinc, plays an important role in making sure your T-cells and antibodies are working optimally.

For more help in formulating an immune-boosting diet and selecting appropriate supplements, if necessary, see a doctor knowledgeable in nutrition, or a registered dietitian. Especially if you're cutting calories or have frequent or chronic illness, professional help can be invaluable, experts say.

HIGH-NUTRITION RECIPES

SHRIMP CREOLE WITH BROWN RICE

This favorite Louisiana dish contains lots of immunity-bolstering nutrients, including vitamins C, B_6 and E, beta-carotene and copper.

3 cups defatted chicken stock
1 cup diced sweet red peppers
½ cup diced onions
½ cup diced celery
1 clove garlic, minced
1 tablespoon olive oil
1 tomato, seeded and diced
3 tablespoons unbleached flour
½ cup tomato sauce
½ teaspoon dried thyme
⅛ teaspoon ground red pepper
1 tablespoon sherry extract (optional)
1 pound small to medium shrimp, peeled and deveined
3 cups hot cooked brown rice

In a 1-quart saucepan over high heat, bring the stock to a boil. Keep warm over low heat.

In a 3-quart saucepan over medium heat, sauté the diced peppers, onions, celery and garlic in the oil for 5 minutes, or until the vegetables are wilted. Add the tomatoes and cook for 3 minutes.

Sprinkle with the flour and mix well. Stir in the stock, a little at a time, until it is well mixed with the flour, creating a smooth sauce. Stir in the tomato sauce, thyme, ground pepper and sherry extract, if desired. Cover and simmer over medium-low heat, stirring occasionally, for 25 minutes.

Add the shrimp. Cook for 5 minutes, or until the shrimp are pink and curled. Serve over the rice.

Serves 4

Per serving: *381 calories, 7.8 g. fat (19% of calories), 4.4 g. dietary fiber, 153 mg. cholesterol, 242 mg. sodium*

SWEET POTATO SALAD

Here's a nice change of pace from standard potato salads. The sweet potatoes add plenty of beta-carotene, which is not present in regular white spuds.

3 medium sweet potatoes (about 1 pound)
1 tart green apple, diced
½ cup chopped pineapple
¼ cup diced celery
2 tablespoons toasted slivered almonds
2 tablespoons minced scallions
½ cup nonfat mayonnaise
¼ cup nonfat yogurt
2 tablespoons lime juice

Scrub the potatoes and cook in boiling water to cover for 25 minutes, or until easily pierced with a knife but not mushy. Drain and set aside until cool enough to handle. Peel and cut into ¾" chunks. Place in a large bowl.

Add the apples, pineapple, celery, almonds and scallions. Toss lightly.

In a small bowl, whisk together the mayonnaise, yogurt and lime juice. Pour over the salad. Toss well. Chill before serving.

Serves 4
Per serving: *197 calories, 2.4 g. fat (11% of calories), 4.4 g. dietary fiber, <1 mg. cholesterol, 422 mg. sodium*

BREADED OYSTERS

Oysters are an awesome source of zinc, an indispensable mineral in the war against infections. Baking eliminates all the fat traditionally used in deep-frying.

24 large frying oysters
2 tablespoons unbleached flour
¼ cup fat-free egg substitute
1 tablespoon water
¼ teaspoon hot-pepper sauce
1 cup dry bread crumbs

Drain the oysters and pat them dry on paper towels. Dredge each oyster in the flour to lightly coat it.

In a shallow bowl, lightly combine the egg, water and hot-pepper sauce with a fork. Dip each oyster in the mixture to coat it lightly. Then dip it into the bread crumbs to coat it completely.

Coat a large baking sheet with no-stick spray. Place the oysters on the sheet with a little space between them. Mist lightly with no-stick spray.

Bake at 450° for 10 to 15 minutes, or until the coating becomes crisp.

Serves 4
Per serving: *175 calories, 3.4 g. fat (18% of calories), 1 g. dietary fiber, 46 mg. cholesterol, 299 mg. sodium*

PORK WITH APRICOTS

Vitamin B_6 is a major player on the immunity team. And lean pork—such as tenderloin—is a good source of the nutrient. Combining the meat with apricots adds other vital nutrients, such as beta-carotene and vitamin C. If fresh apricots are out of season, substitute drained canned halves.

- **1 pound pork tenderloin, trimmed of all visible fat and cut into 1" slices**
- **2 teaspoons olive oil**
- **½ cup defatted chicken stock**
- **2 tablespoons all-fruit apricot preserves**
- **1 tablespoon lemon juice**
- **½ teaspoon Dijon mustard**
- **8 apricots, halved and pitted**
- **8 ounces medium no-yolk egg noodles**

In a large no-stick frying pan over medium-high heat, brown the pork in the oil for about 2 minutes per side. Remove to a plate.

Reduce the heat to medium. To the pan, add the stock, preserves, lemon juice and mustard. Stir to mix thoroughly. Add the apricots. Cover and cook for 3 minutes, or until the apricots are soft but not mushy. Add the pork and keep warm over low heat.

Cook the noodles in a large pot of boiling water for 8 minutes, or until just tender. Drain. Serve the pork and apricots over the noodles.

Serves 4

Per serving: *401 calories, 6.6 g. fat (15% of calories), 3.7 g. dietary fiber, 74 mg. cholesterol, 116 mg. sodium*

CHAPTER 21

THE HEART AND ARTERIES

ROLLING BACK THE RISKS

Even though you know it probably isn't the healthiest lunch, you're in a hurry, so you decide to eat just one slice of gooey pizza covered with pepperoni and extra cheese. But it tastes so good that you appease your growling stomach with another piece.

You figure you're merely eating a quick meal packed with carbohydrates to keep yourself energetic throughout a busy afternoon. Of course, you know—or at least should know—that this pizza is loaded with cholesterol and saturated fat, two of your heart's worst enemies. But two slices of pizza aren't going to kill you. Or are they?

Well, it depends. "No, a slice or two of pizza now and then *isn't* going to hurt you," says Gregory Kay, M.D., a cardiothoracic and vascular surgeon at the Hospital of the Good Samaritan in Los Angeles. "But if it's part of a daily pattern of eggs, hamburgers and other fatty foods, then you're looking at trouble."

Heart disease isn't caused by one food, one meal or one day's menu. Heart disease often is the result of years of poor eating habits that include thousands of french fries, hundreds of eggs, hordes of hamburgers and yes, gobs of pizza.

Certainly there are other risk factors such as smoking, diabetes, lack of exercise and your family history that increase the risk of heart disease. But there's little doubt that over a lifetime what you eat does play a major role in determining your likelihood of suffering a fatal heart attack.

"In terms of the development of heart disease, 70 to 80 percent of your risk comes from what you eat," says Daniel Eisenberg, M.D., a Los Angeles cardiologist and assistant clinical professor at the University of Southern California School of Medicine.

CHOLESTEROL ISN'T COOL

Why? Well, let's take a look at what happened to that pizza you ate for lunch. As you ate those slices, you couldn't help but notice a few greasy spots on the napkin and pockets of oil floating on the pizza itself. All of that was fat—mostly saturated fat, the kind that your body uses to make cholesterol.

As this fat floated through your stomach, it was bombarded by acids in the stomach so strong they could burn a hole in your living room carpet. But as potent as they are, those acids aren't strong enough to break down that saturated fat. In fact, it wasn't until it entered your small intestine that the fat was battered into particles small enough to be absorbed by the bloodstream and transported to the liver. There, about 70 percent of it was made into low-density lipoproteins (LDL), the "bad" cholesterol that over time can clog and damage the arteries in your entire body, especially those to your heart. Fortunately, the liver transformed the remaining 30 percent of saturated fat into high-density lipoprotein (HDL), known as the "good" cholesterol because it helps transport the bad kind out of your system.

DOUBLE TROUBLE

As if that's not bad enough, in addition to the fat, that pizza also contains cholesterol from the milk and meat fat that goes *directly* into your bloodstream after you eat it. So when you ate the pizza, you were, in a way, getting a double dose of cholesterol: from the cholesterol in the pepperoni and cheese and from the fat these two foods contain.

Of course, saturated fat and cholesterol aren't just in pizza. Saturated fat is common in meats and animal by-products such as beef, chicken, lard, butter, sausage, whole milk and cheese. Cholesterol is found in most of those foods, too. In fact, it's hard to find a food high in saturated fat that doesn't have lots of cholesterol. The exceptions are solid and "hydrogenated" shortenings and tropical oils. These vegetable products contain saturated fat but no cholesterol.

Unlike fat, which you often can see, cholesterol is a microscopic, waxy substance that your body uses to make hormones and cell membranes. Sure, you need cholesterol, but your body manufactures all you'll ever need on its own. So what you eat is excess. And where does it go?

It circulates in your bloodstream and accumulates in the arteries and blocks blood flow to the heart. Fortunately, some of the good cholesterol latches onto some of the bad cholesterol and sweeps it out of the body. Unfortunately, there is usually much more bad cholesterol than the good can handle.

TRACKING DOWN THE CULPRIT

Certainly, a small amount of dietary cholesterol and fat probably won't harm you. But what happens to your arteries when you eat a steady diet of foods containing cholesterol and fats?

"Normally, as cholesterol circulates in the blood, it is constantly going in and out of cells in the artery walls," says Robert DiBianco, M.D., director of cardiology research at Washington Adventist Hospital and associate clinical professor of medicine at the Georgetown University School of Medicine in Washington, D.C. "But when you eat a steady diet of foods high in cholesterol and saturated fat, it can lead to a high concentration of "bad" LDL cholesterol in the blood. When that happens, there is more movement of cholesterol into than out of those cells and the excess cholesterol begins forming plaque deposits on the artery walls."

This is the beginning of a process known as atherosclerosis. As plaque builds up on the artery walls, it chokes off the blood supply. If this occurs in the arteries supplying the heart muscle, the result is angina, a tightness of the chest that indicates severe narrowing of the coronary arteries is taking place. Eventually, if enough plaque accumulates, it can block blood flow to the heart so completely that a heart attack occurs, Dr. DiBianco says. If the plaque buildup occurs in the arteries to the brain, it can result in a stroke.

Plaques are like having several cars double-parked on a street, making it difficult for traffic to pass. As traffic snarls up, the likelihood of an accident increases, explains George L. Blackburn, M.D., Ph.D., associate professor of surgery at Harvard Medical School and chief of the Nutrition/Metabolism Laboratory at the Cancer Research Institute at New England Deaconess Hospital in Boston.

So what do all those traffic jams in the arteries add up to? About 500,000 funerals a year, according to the National Cholesterol Education Program. Statistics show that 1.25 million Americans suffer heart attacks each year, and about one in three of those attacks are fatal. Another 6 million people in America are suffering loss of quality of life from symptoms including angina, cramps and pain in the lower legs, nausea and shortness of breath—particularly after modest physical exertion. All told, nearly 70 percent of adult Americans have some narrowing of their coronary arteries.

IT'S NOT TOO LATE

"Americans are throwing away huge amounts of their lives and spending a fortune on heart disease treatments that they wouldn't need if they took care of themselves," Dr. Blackburn says. "If people, working as a family unit, could be motivated to cut the fat out of their diets and to eat more of the foods that are good for their hearts, they'd be ahead of the game."

There is no question that the American diet needs some fine-tuning, says Dr. Blackburn. And he has plenty of reasons to believe that. Hundreds of studies conducted worldwide in the past 50 years have linked the consumption of fat- and cholesterol-laden foods—mainly highly processed foods and animal foods such as meat, cheese and eggs—to coronary diseases. What's more, many of those same studies are providing powerful evidence that changing what we eat can make an important difference.

In one classic study that began in 1965, researchers examined the dietary habits of more than 10,000 men of Japanese descent, many of whom had adopted an American diet. One group were native Japanese who had immigrated to Hawaii and begun eating the local diet, which is high in saturated fat and cholesterol. A second group were Japanese who had moved to California and adopted a diet that was even richer in saturated fat and cholesterol than that of the Hawaiian group. These two groups of immigrants were compared to a third group of people who lived in Japan and followed their country's traditional diet.

The men who moved to Hawaii and California weighed about ten pounds more, had higher blood cholesterol levels, ate 2½ times more total fat and about 4 times more saturated fat than Japanese men who remained in their native country and ate their native foods. And the researchers found that death from heart disease rose as the amount of saturated fat and cholesterol in the diet increased.

"The death rates from heart disease were lowest in Japan, intermediate in Hawaii and highest in the continental United States," says Millicent Higgins, M.D., associate director for epidemiology and biometry at the National Heart, Lung and Blood Institute in Bethesda, Maryland.

In one ongoing study that began in 1957, researchers have been following the eating and lifestyle habits of 12,763 middle-aged men in seven countries, including Greece, Italy, Japan, Finland and the United States. The men have been examined every five years and assessed for a number of coronary risk factors, including diet, smoking, blood pressure and weight. Among their many findings, the researchers have determined that the men who eat the least amount of saturated fat and cholesterol have a lower risk of developing heart disease compared to other men in the study, says Ancel Keys, Ph.D., of the University of Minnesota School of Public Health in Minneapolis, the lead author of the ongoing study and a pioneer in cholesterol research since 1947.

A study in India also shows the importance of limiting the amount of cholesterol and saturated fat in your diet. In this study, 228 people were asked to eat a low-cholesterol, low-saturated-fat diet that included fewer than 216 milligrams of cholesterol (just one medium-size egg has about 213 milligrams of cholesterol) and just 6 percent of calories from saturated fat daily—basically a vegetarian diet. (A porterhouse steak, by comparison, has 18 percent of calories from saturated fat and 45 percent from total fat).

The people in the first group were compared to 230 individuals who ate their usual diet, which contained an average of 318 milligrams of cholesterol and 11 percent saturated fat daily. In addition, the higher-fat group consumed twice as much animal protein, nearly 60 percent less fiber, a third less carbohydrates and fewer fruits and vegetables such as grapes, bananas, spinach, radishes and tomatoes.

After one year, the low-fat, low-cholesterol dieters had lower blood pressure and blood sugar levels and had fewer complications of heart disease including arrhythmia (irregular heartbeat), angina pain and heart attack than those who didn't eat a heart-protective diet. Overall, the low-cholesterol, low-fat dieters reduced their risk of heart disease by 32 percent.

In the United States, the famed Framingham Heart Study in Massachusetts also has shown that diet has a great influence on whether you will develop heart disease, says William P. Castelli, M.D., director of the ongoing study that has followed 5,127 men and women for more than 30 years.

"The average American family eats the same bloody stuff night after night, and it's just too rich in cholesterol and fat," Dr. Castelli says. "That's why about 80 percent of us end up with these deposits in our arteries, and about half of us die from that buildup."

SETTING THE TARGET

Based on the evidence, something has to change if heart disease is going to be knocked off the chart as the number one killer of Americans. According to Dr. Castelli, the average American male eats 80 to 100 grams of fat a day and almost 500 milligrams of cholesterol.

As a first step, the American Heart Association and the National Cholesterol Education Program recommend a diet that delivers less than 300 milligrams of cholesterol a day and limits total fat to 30 percent and saturated fat to less than 10 percent of your daily caloric intake.

If you have chronically high blood cholesterol (above 200), then your doctor may recommend that you restrict your consumption of saturated fat and cholesterol even more. Here's why.

The higher your blood cholesterol, the greater your risk of heart disease. And, although some people's bodies naturally produce more cholesterol than others, it's important to remember that the saturated fat and dietary cholesterol we eat also increases the amount of cholesterol in the bloodstream.

Most heart researchers agree that cholesterol becomes a risk when total blood levels are higher than 200, LDL levels go above 130, or HDL levels drop below 35. If your blood cholesterol level is higher than 240, your risk of developing heart disease is four times greater than if it were below 200, according to the National Cholesterol Education Program. Just dropping

THE DIET THAT *REVERSES* HEART DISEASE

It's strict and it includes comprehensive changes in diet and lifestyle, but the regimen prescribed by Dean Ornish, M.D., of the Preventive Medicine Research Institute in Sausalito, California, for his patients has become an important nonsurgical breakthrough in combating heart disease.

Research by Dr. Ornish indicates that diet and behavior changes can significantly reverse coronary blockages in just one year. The diet is far more restrictive than the diet recommended by the American Heart Association (AHA), which allows 30 percent of calories from fat and 300 milligrams of cholesterol daily. Instead, Dr. Ornish's diet is vegetarian and permits no caffeine, oils or animal products except for egg whites, nonfat milk and yogurt. It allows less than 10 percent of calories from fat and almost no cholesterol.

The participants are asked to practice an hour's worth of stress-management techniques, such as yoga, daily and to spend about three hours walking a week.

The dramatic result of Dr. Ornish's work was demonstrated in a study comparing 22 men who followed his diet for at least a year to 19 men who followed the guidelines of the AHA. About 82 percent of the people on Dr. Ornish's program had some reversal of their coronary blockages. The reductions were small—averaging about 5 percent—but even small changes can have significant impact on the amount of blood the heart receives, Dr. Ornish says.

your cholesterol level by 10 percent should lower your risk of coronary heart disease by 20 percent.

HEART-HEALTHY EATING TIPS

So how do you get started in your efforts to drive down your cholesterol levels and win the war against heart disease? Experts suggest these basic strategies.

Eat less cholesterol. Long before eggs became a staple and fast food became routine, our ancestors ate meals that were naturally low in dietary cholesterol. It's a lesson we need to relearn, Dr. Kay says.

"About 10,000 years ago, when humans were still evolving, they surely didn't eat a bunch of eggs. They ate fruits, nuts, vegetables and occasionally some meat," he says. "This phenomenon of eating two portions of beef every day, two eggs in the morning and a big scoop of ice cream every afternoon is fairly new. Unfortunately, many people think it's a lot easier and more fun to eat three eggs and three slices of bacon than it is to eat a well-balanced, heart-healthy meal."

Those who followed the AHA diet didn't experience the striking reversal of the Ornish diet group. Overall, the patients' disease appeared to worsen.

"Dr. Ornish's work is very significant because he has achieved with diet and relaxation the same kind of results other researchers have achieved with powerful cholesterol-lowering drugs," says William P. Castelli, M.D., of the Framingham Heart Study. "But the measures he uses are nontoxic, and you can do them forever."

However, some question if Americans are ready to embrace such a drastic lifestyle change.

"Personally, if I were a young man with coronary heart disease, I would be willing to try the Ornish approach," says Carl Lavie, M.D., of the Ochsner Medical Institution in New Orleans.

Dr. Ornish, author of *Dr. Dean Ornish's Program for Reversing Heart Disease,* thinks many Americans may be willing to choose lifestyle changes as an alternative to bypass surgery or a lifetime of cholesterol-lowering drugs.

"The reason for making changes in diet and lifestyle isn't necessarily to live longer but to live better," he says. "When people realize that the short-term benefits of changing can be so considerable—chest pain often decreases markedly, you feel better, you have more energy—and those benefits often occur within days or a few weeks after changing your lifestyle, then the choices become clearer."

Avoiding egg yolks and organ meats, such as liver, are two simple ways of slashing the amount of cholesterol in your diet. And since cholesterol is found only in animal foods, you also need to cut back on your consumption of meats and dairy foods.

Shed the fat. Slashing the amount of saturated fat you eat may be your best defense against high blood cholesterol, Dr. Eisenberg says.

"Saturated fat, milligram for milligram, has twice the cholesterol-raising effect as the same amount of dietary cholesterol," he says.

That's because the body easily converts saturated fat into cholesterol, Dr. Eisenberg says. No more than 1/10 of your total calories should be from saturated fat, common in meats—such as beef and chicken—and dairy products—such as whole milk and cheese.

But the most prudent way to reduce your saturated fat intake is to lower your consumption of *all* fats, Dr. Castelli says. "If you reduce all dietary fat, you automatically knock down saturated fat intake, because about half of the fat we eat is saturated fat."

To get going in the right direction, consider using low-fat alternatives

STARTING OVER

If you want to reduce the cholesterol and fat in your diet, but aren't sure how to begin, this table may give you some ideas.

IF YOU USUALLY EAT . . .	A BETTER CHOICE IS . . .
Butter	Tub or soft margarine
Cakes	Angel food cake
Chocolate	Cocoa
Creamed salad dressing	Oil and vinegar
Fried foods	Broiled, baked or steamed foods
Goose or duck	Chicken or turkey without the skin
Hamburger	Salad or pasta
Ice cream	Sherbet
Mayonnaise	Nonfat mayonnaise or low-fat yogurt
Potato chips	Pretzels or rice cakes
Scalloped potatoes	Rice
Shortening	Unhydrogenated vegetable oil or olive oil
Sour cream	Low-fat yogurt or cottage cheese
Steak	Fish
Toast with butter	Toast with jelly only
Vegetables with butter	Vegetables with herbs, citrus juice
Whole-egg omelet	Three egg whites and one egg yolk
Whole milk or cream	Skim or low-fat milk

when preparing food. Start substituting 1 percent milk for whole milk, for example. Use low-fat yogurt, buttermilk or evaporated skim milk instead of sour cream, cream or cream cheese.

"There are a lot of imitation and low-fat products that are on the market now," says Andrea Gardiner, R.D., a dietitian specializing in cardiac rehabilitation at the Hospital of the Good Samaritan in Los Angeles. "With careful label reading, you can find products that are fat-free, too. Also you can easily make your own versions at home. For a sour cream substitute, for example, you could mix nonfat yogurt with nonfat cottage cheese in a blender. You should always consider using creative solutions like this."

Whenever possible, use nonfat mayonnaise or mix nonfat yogurt with low-fat mayonnaise when making tuna or chicken salad, she says.

Make the switch. Switching from saturated fats such as butter to monounsaturates such as olive oil or polyunsaturates like corn oil also might help lower your total cholesterol and raise your HDLs.

In a study of 4,903 Italian men and women, researchers concluded that increased consumption of butter was associated with significantly elevated blood pressure and serum cholesterol in men and higher blood sugar levels on both men and women. All three are risk factors for coronary heart disease. But eating more foods made with olive oil and vegetable oil *lowered* those risks in both sexes.

"It looks like olive and other vegetable oils have very similar effects. Olive oil seems to be stronger with regard to blood glucose and blood pressure, while polyunsaturates seem slightly stronger than olive oil with regard to serum cholesterol," says Maurizio Trevisan, M.D., author of the study and an associate professor at the State University of New York at Buffalo School of Medicine and Biomedical Sciences.

"When you're cooking at home, you're always much better off using a liquid oil rather than melting butter, margarine or shortening because those are solid fats and are more saturated," Gardiner says.

It's important to realize, however, that even though monounsaturates are healthier, they still need to be used sparingly. After all, they're still fats and can easily increase your total fat intake. A rule of thumb: Use no more than one teaspoon in any dish.

Count on the grams. Counting grams is the easiest way to monitor your fat consumption because that's how most food manufacturers label their products.

Most doctors suggest that you should reduce saturated fat in your diet to no more than 10 percent of your total calories. To translate that percentage into grams of fat, take the total number of calories you eat each day and multiply that by 30 percent. That will give you the total number of calories of fat you can eat each day. Then divide by 9 (that's the number of calories in a gram of fat). That will give you the total grams of fat you want in your diet. Finally, divide by 3. That will give the maximum number of grams of saturated fat you can eat each day.

So if you eat 2,000 calories a day, for example, that means you should be eating a maximum of 600 calories or 67 grams of total fat each day. Divide that by 3, and you'll find that you should eat no more than 22 grams of saturated fat daily (that's one-third of your total fat calories).

Knowing the grams of saturated fat allowed in your diet will help plan meals more wisely, Dr. Castelli says. So if you do eat 2,000 calories a day and gobble up 3½ ounces (100 grams) of the fattiest hamburger for lunch, you've just consumed about 20 grams of saturated fat. In other words, you've basically just used up your daily allowance of saturated fat in one meal, Dr. Castelli says. However, if you eat 3½ ounces of select grade hamburger, you'll be getting only 4 grams of saturated fat. "Theoretically, you could have a select grade hamburger for breakfast, lunch and dinner and still have 10 grams of saturated fat to spend that day," Dr. Castelli says.

Lean toward lean meats. Buy the leanest cuts of meat you can, Dr. Castelli advises. Almost half the fat in some cuts of beef, for example, is saturated. So choosing the leanest grades of beef is crucial to maintaining cardiovascular health. Of the three grades of beef, select is your best choice, Dr. Castelli says. Only 10 percent fat by weight, it only has about 4 grams

THIS HERB MIGHT BE YOUR ARTERIES' ALLY

So you think eating garlic isn't going to make your heartthrob want to get romantic. But breathtaking findings that this bulb can help ward off coronary disease may give you compelling reasons to persuade your favorite person that snuggling with a garlic lover isn't so bad.

In a study of 40 people with elevated cholesterol levels, readings dropped an average of 21 percent in 20 people taking 900 milligrams of powdered garlic daily for 16 weeks. The cholesterol levels of the 20 people who didn't get garlic only fell 3 percent.

In a larger study, 221 people with high cholesterol were given either 800 milligrams of garlic powder or a look-alike placebo. After four months, those who took garlic pills daily had overall reductions in their cholesterol averaging 12 percent. The placebo group's cholesterol only dropped an average of 3 percent.

In five other studies, garlic also reduced artery-clogging cholesterol, kept blood platelets from clumping (a process that can lead to dangerous clots) and lowered heart attack risk.

But it remains unclear how much garlic is needed to produce a protective effect on the cardiovascular system. In some studies, the equivalent of 7 to 28 cloves of garlic a day were needed to get results.

Another problem is that cooking, drying or steaming may destroy some of the active ingredients—allicin and ajoene—that fend off heart disease.

of saturated fat per 3½-ounce serving. (About 28 grams equal an ounce). In comparison, choice beef, the next grade, ranges from 15 to 35 percent fat, and a 3½-ounce serving can have 10 to 15 grams of saturated fat. Prime beef, the fattest grade, is 35 to 40 percent fat by weight and has about 20 grams of saturated fat per 3½ ounces.

One is the healthiest number. To really keep your heart disease risk low, it's probably wise to have no more than one serving of lean meat, fish or poultry a day. "If you eat only one 3½-ounce serving of meat, fish or poultry each day, that means you are eliminating at least two fatty meat meals from your diet," Dr. Kay says. "It's that simple. It's just another easy way of minimizing your fat consumption."

Don't count on alcohol. Is an after-dinner drink a great way to protect your cardiovascular system? "Some studies suggest that people who drink one to two glasses of alcohol a day do slightly better from a cardiovascular standpoint than people who don't drink at all," says Carl Lavie, M.D., co-director of cardiac rehabilitation and prevention at the Ochsner Medical Institution in New Orleans. "But once you get beyond three drinks a day, the risk of heart disease goes way up."

While it's still too soon to declare garlic a proven therapy, the herb may deserve more prominence in your diet, says Yu-Yan Yeh, Ph.D., associate professor of nutrition at Pennsylvania State University in University Park, who has done preliminary research that shows that garlic can lower cholesterol levels in laboratory rats.

"In general, I think that it is safe to say that if you consume garlic regularly, even just one to two cloves a day, you could be getting some beneficial effects," Dr. Yeh says.

To do that, try mincing garlic and sprinkling it on salads and vegetables, or add it at the very end of preparing pasta sauces.

Garlic also can be served as a side dish. Cut off the tops of the garlic heads to expose all the cloves. Fit the heads snugly in a baking dish. Dot each clove with margarine, then pour about ¼ teaspoon olive oil over each head. Sprinkle with thyme and pepper to taste. Cover and bake at 300° for 30 minutes. Uncover and bake for another hour until the garlic is tender. The husk should be golden brown and the cloves soft enough to squeeze out.

Of course, if you want to take the bite out of heart disease without pungent breath, odorless garlic capsules are available in many drug and health food stores. In general, one to two capsules of dried, odorless garlic powder equal one clove, Dr. Yeh says.

But for many reasons, including the potential risk of alcoholism, doctors are reluctant to advise patients to drink, he says. "There are so many problems associated with alcohol in this country that you really can't recommend that," Dr. Lavie says. "But it is reasonable to tell people who are drinking more than two drinks a day to cut back. It is also reasonable to tell people who are drinking one to two drinks that there is no reason, from a cardiovascular standpoint, to stop doing that."

He suggests that alcohol drinkers limit their consumption to no more than 2 ounces of whiskey, 8 ounces of wine or 24 ounces of beer a day.

ADDING TO SUBTRACT FROM THE RISK

But don't fall into the trap of thinking that eliminating foods from your diet is the only way that you can make a difference. *Adding* some of foods to your menu can to ensure your heart's health, too.

It does seem like people are always being told to eat less of this or less of that, says Warren Thompson, M.D., an associate professor of internal medicine at the University of Tennessee Graduate School of Medicine at Knoxville."My feeling is that people shouldn't feel like they're punishing themselves. So I always try to emphasize that people should eat more of certain foods like fruits and vegetables that taste good, are enjoyable to eat and will protect their hearts."

To improve your chances of keeping your arteries clear and your heart pumping for many years to come, try adding a few of these foods to your diet.

If it swims, eat it. Substituting fish for red meat is probably one of your best choices. A serving of cooked Atlantic salmon (one of the fattiest fish) has less than one-third the total fat of the same size serving of broiled rib-eye steak. In addition, fish such as mackerel, salmon, tuna and cod all contain high amounts of omega-3 fatty acids, a type of fat that may lower total cholesterol levels, raise HDLs and decrease the risk of heart disease.

Eating fish also helps keep arteries pliable, say researchers at Monash University in Melbourne, Australia. The researchers tested the blood vessels of 53 people and found that folks who ate one or more fish meals a week had more flexible arteries, a signal that their cardiovascular systems were healthier than those of people who ate no fish.

In another small study of 28 South Africans, fatty fish significantly lowered blood cholesterol levels when substituted for red meat.

If eating fish regularly doesn't appeal to you, then you might try taking a fish-oil supplement containing 300 milligrams of omega-3 every day, says William S. Harris, Ph.D., an assistant professor studying dietary fats at the University of Kansas in Kansas City.

"It's better to try to get your omega-3's through your diet than supplements, but you have to live with reality," Dr. Harris says. "And in reality, many people don't like to eat oily fish."

Health is a thing with feathers. "Poultry is an excellent alternative to red meat," says John Paraskos, M.D., an associate director of cardiovascular medicine and professor of medicine at the University of Massachusetts in Worcester. That's because chicken, turkey and other fowl usually contain fewer calories and less saturated fat than red meat.

To avoid adding unwanted fat to the meal, broil or bake fowl instead of frying it in cooking oils, he says. You can leave the skin on while cooking to help the meat retain moisture, but since the skin is high in fat, it should be removed before eating.

You also should eat dark meat sparingly because it more fat than white meat, Dr. Paraskos says.

Make room for fiber. Soluble fiber found in certain grains, fruits and vegetables such as oat bran, green peppers, citrus fruits, beans and psyllium seeds may lower blood cholesterol by 10 to 20 percent.

"Soluble fiber is important. It has many beneficial effects," Dr. Lavie says. "Increasing soluble fiber consumption lowers your risk of coronary disease. It probably also decreases cancer risk, particularly for colon cancer."

Soluble fiber dissolves in water, but resists digestion in the gastrointestinal tract. It's still unclear how the process works, but some scientists theorize that as soluble fiber moves through your system, it bonds to bile acid (a digestive fluid that is made with cholesterol) and excretes it from the body. In order to replace those lost bile acids, the liver removes cholesterol from the bloodstream to make more bile.

"Besides that effect, people are probably benefiting in other ways," Dr. Lavie says. "Because soluble fiber is a filler, it satisfies the appetite. It makes people less hungry so they avoid eating foods that are high in saturated fat and cholesterol."

Get a load of oat bran. Of all the fibrous foods, oat bran has clearly been the star. Numerous studies have shown that oat bran significantly lowers serum cholesterol.

In one study of 140 men, researchers found that those who ate two to three ounces of oat bran a day reduced their LDL cholesterol levels 11 to 15 percent in six weeks. In a smaller study, 20 men who ate about four ounces of oat bran daily decreased their total and LDL cholesterol levels by 12 percent in just three weeks.

But while most researchers are convinced that oat bran is an effective way to reduce blood cholesterol, there has been some controversy because of the broad range of results from some studies. A few studies have found that the bran has virtually no effect, while others have shown reductions in blood cholesterol up to 26 percent.

To settle this issue, researchers at the University of Minnesota analyzed 12 previous studies of oat products, including oat bran, conducted since 1985. The researchers concluded that eating a daily dose of three grams of soluble fiber from oat products did cause a modest 2 to 3 percent reduction in blood cholesterol. That's still significant, because every 1 percent drop in blood cholesterol lowers your risk of dying from heart disease by 2 percent. Overall, the Minnesota study backs up the good things that other researchers have been saying about oat bran for a long time.

"If you go off bacon and eggs and substitute any whole-grain cereal with skim milk, you'll lower your cholesterol 6 to 8 percent. That's mainly due to what you took out of your diet," Dr. Castelli says. "But if you eat an oat bran-enriched cereal, you'll drop your cholesterol another 3 to 5 percent. We know that soluble fiber like oat bran does that.

"You'd be hard-pressed to find something else for breakfast that would be such a good first step in a total dietary program of controlling blood fats," he says.

Eat a hill of beans. Not only are beans low in artery-clogging fat, they are a good source of soluble fiber, which may help lower blood cholesterol, says James W. Anderson, M.D., professor of medicine and clinical nutrition at the University of Kentucky College of Medicine in Lexington. To get the heart-saving qualities out of legumes, try eating ½ to 1 cup beans, such as kidney beans, lentils, lima beans or pinto beans, a day. For variety, you can mix beans with rice, pasta or small amounts of chicken, meat or fish.

Pump up on pectin. Pectin, a type of soluble fiber found in apples, oranges and other fruits and vegetables, has lowered serum cholesterol about 8 percent in human studies at the University of Florida College of Medicine in Gainesville.

"It not only helps lower cholesterol levels, it also reduces the risk of coronary heart disease by reducing the amount of atherosclerosis in the arteries," says Frank Robbins, a biological scientist studying the effects of grapefruit pectin in conjunction with James J. Cerda, M.D., a professor of medicine in gastroenterology at the university.

As little as 15 grams of pectin a day—the equivalent of eating two to three grapefruit—might be enough to lower your heart disease risk, Robbins says.

KEEP YOUR ARTERIES "RUST-FREE"

Some researchers suspect that antioxidants such as vitamins C and E and beta-carotene may be an overlooked solution to heart disease.

These vitamins may combat oxidation, the same chemical process that rusts metals and turns butter rancid, which also alters cholesterol in harmful ways inside the body. Once LDL cholesterol is oxidized, cells in the immune system called macrophages ingest it. The macrophages become overloaded with fat globules and are transformed into foam cells. These foam cells collect in artery walls and begin the development of atherosclerosis. Some researchers suspect that this is the point where antioxidant nutrients exert their protective effect.

In the Nurses Health Study of 87,245 women, aged 34 to 59, researchers at Harvard University compared the vitamin intake levels of healthy nurses and those who had suffered heart attacks. The nurses who ate the most beta-carotene (a plant pigment that our bodies convert to vitamin A) had a 22 percent lower risk of heart attack risk than the nurses who ate the least. Fresh fruits and vegetables such as apricots, carrots, spinach, squash and sweet potatoes provided the beta-carotene. In fact, just one carrot, containing 15 to 20 milligrams of beta-carotene, can make a difference.

In addition, high amounts of vitamin E caused a 34 percent reduction in heart disease risk. Consuming slightly more than 100 I.U. of vitamin E daily could lower heart disease risk, according to the study. Vitamin E is found in nuts and green leafy vegetables. Here are a few simple ways to get more of these antioxidants into your diet.

Swallow the C. Men who consume lots of vitamin C have half the death rate from heart disease of men who don't get as much of the vitamin, says James Enstrom, Ph.D., an epidemiologist at the University of California, Los Angeles, who studied the vitamin consumption of 11,348 men and women. Women who take high doses of vitamin C seem to get less benefit from it than men do, but still have a 25 percent lower death rate from heart disease than women who don't take any. The protective effects of vitamin C appear to kick in at about 50 milligrams. That's equivalent to drinking about four ounces of orange juice a day. The maximum benefit occurred in those people who took about 300 milligrams.

Heavy smokers and people with diabetes probably need to consume about 120 milligrams—about ten ounces of orange juice—each day, says Ishwarlal Jialal, M.D., a researcher studying antioxidants at the University of Texas Southwestern Medical Center in Dallas. That's because these groups tend to have low blood levels of vitamin C and are at higher risk for heart disease.

Get a daily supplement. Denham Harman, M.D., Ph.D., professor emeritus at the University of Nebraska College of Medicine in Omaha and executive director of the American Aging Association, believes that vitamin supplementation is a good way to get the necessary amounts of antioxidants into your diet. "What it comes down to is how much you should take, and I don't think anybody really knows that answer right now," Dr. Harman says. "But what I tell people is to take 500 milligrams of vitamin C two to three times a day and 100 to 200 milligrams of vitamin E daily. I don't know if that will be sufficient. But in all probability, it will be beneficial to the heart and won't be harmful."

TAKING THE EXTRA STEP

For most people, making the dietary changes we've just suggested will be enough to dramatically lower their heart disease risk. But if a person's cholesterol level remains elevated despite making these dietary changes, or there is evidence of heart disease or extensive artery blockage, then a stricter approach may be necessary.

In fact, ongoing work by Dean Ornish, M.D., director of the Preventive Medicine Research Institute in Sausalito, California, indicates that some people with symptoms of atherosclerosis who make dramatic behavioral changes, including adopting a vegetarian diet that limits total dietary fat to less than 10 percent of calories, can reverse dangerous blockages in their coronary arteries.

"Some people still question the connection, but I think if you go on a very vigorous diet that lowers fat consumption to 10 percent of calories and cholesterol intake to less than 50 milligrams a day, you really can reverse atherosclerosis," says Dr. Lavie.

Finally, keep in mind that diet is just one part of a comprehensive plan that includes exercise, stress reduction and smoking cessation to keep your heart healthy. Just walking for 15 minutes at four miles per hour, three times a week, can make a difference.

"It's a matter of how you want to live your life," Dr. Kay says. "If you think it's important to eat junk food, smoke and lounge around, then you can sit back and say, 'Oh well, I'm going to die anyway.' But if you want to lead an active life for many years, you need to exercise, eat healthy foods and stop smoking."

WHAT'S THE SCOOP ON COFFEE?

Does drinking coffee really increase your chances of heart disease, as some scientists once suggested? Probably not, according to research.

Much of the hoopla that swirled around coffee a few years ago was generated by studies conducted in Scandinavia, where coffee is boiled rather than paper-filtered as it is in the United States. In those studies, researchers found that boiled coffee does significantly raise blood cholesterol and increases the likelihood of death from heart disease. "The coffee story is becoming a little clearer. We now know that it's the method of preparation used in Scandinavia that extracts compounds from coffee that are bad for cholesterol levels. Regular coffee, as it's prepared in America, probably does nothing like that," says Alan Chait, M.D., past chairman of the American Heart Association Nutrition Committee.

So a cup or two of coffee a day isn't the heart-stopping hazard some once imagined. "Although large amounts of caffeine can cause arrhythmia [irregular beats] in the upper chambers of your heart, moderate consumption won't give you too much grief," says Thomas Kottke, M.D., a cardiologist at the Mayo Clinic in Rochester, Minnesota.

HIGH-NUTRITION RECIPES

SPICED CARROTS

Carrots have more going for them than you may suspect—especially in regard to heart health. They're high in soluble fiber, which has been shown to help lower cholesterol. And they're a wonderful source of beta-carotene, which doctors believe may also offer some protection against heart disease. This recipe gives cooked carrots a new, Middle Eastern twist. And it contains both olive oil and garlic, two more foods that may help ward off heart problems. Serve this dish with roast chicken or lemon-broiled fish.

1 pound carrots, thinly cut on the diagonal
3 cloves garlic
2 tablespoons lemon juice
2 teaspoons olive oil
½ teaspoon ground cumin
Pinch of ground red pepper
2 tablespoons minced fresh parsley

Steam the carrots and garlic for 5 minutes, or until the carrots are just tender. Remove the garlic and set aside. Transfer the carrots to a large no-stick frying pan.

Mash the garlic and place in a cup. Whisk in the lemon juice, oil, cumin and pepper. Pour over the carrots. Toss over medium heat for 2 minutes. Sprinkle with the parsley.

Serves 4
Per serving: *75 calories, 2.6 g. fat (31% of calories), 3.7 g. dietary fiber, 0 mg. cholesterol, 42 mg. sodium*

SEA SALAD

Sardines are among those fish that are high in heart-healthy omega-3 fatty acids. If you're looking for a new way to incorporate them into your diet, this very easy salad should fill the bill. Serve it with crusty, whole-grain rolls. You'll notice that the percent of calories from fat in this salad is high, but that's because practically all the calories come from the beneficial omega-3's and monounsaturated olive oil—the vegetables are very low in calories. Keep in mind that it's the overall level of fat in your diet that's crucial for heart health, not the amount in any single dish.

1 sweet red or yellow pepper, thinly sliced
1 large tomato, seeded and chopped
1 cup thinly sliced carrots
½ cup thinly sliced scallions
2 tablespoons white-wine vinegar
1 tablespoon olive oil
1 teaspoon Dijon mustard
½ teaspoon dried basil
Red and green leaf lettuce, torn into bite-size pieces
2 cups alfalfa sprouts
1 can (3¾ ounces) water-packed sardines, drained and cut into bite-size pieces

In a large bowl, toss together the peppers, tomatoes, carrots and scallions.

In a cup, combine the vinegar, oil, mustard and basil. Pour over the vegetables and toss to coat.

Line individual dinner plates with the lettuce. Top with the sprouts, then the vegetables. Arrange the sardines on top.

Serves 4
Per serving: *129 calories, 8.6 g. fat (60% of calories), 2.6 g. dietary fiber, 40 mg. cholesterol, 144 mg. sodium*

GINGER-SCENTED MACKEREL

Mackerel is another champ in the omega-3 department. (And don't forget that it's the heart-healthy fats that make this such a super fish, so don't be alarmed by the amount of fat in this dish.) This oriental way of preparing mackerel is so simple you'll want to have it often. Serve it with steamed green beans.

- **1 pound mackerel fillet, divided into 4 equal pieces**
- **½ cup thinly sliced scallions**
- **¼ cup minced fresh coriander**
- **Juice of 1 lemon or lime**
- **1 tablespoon low-sodium soy sauce**
- **1 tablespoon grated fresh ginger**
- **½ teaspoon ground black pepper**
- **4 cups hot cooked brown rice**

Coat an 8" × 8" baking dish with no-stick spray. Place the mackerel in a single layer in the dish.

In a small bowl, combine the scallions, coriander, lemon or lime juice, soy sauce, ginger and pepper. Spoon over the fish.

Cover the dish tightly with foil. Bake at 450° for 20 minutes, or until the fish flakes easily with a fork. Serve with the rice.

Serves 4

Per serving: *481 calories, 17.7 g. fat (33% of calories), 4.8 g. dietary fiber, 80 mg. cholesterol, 265 mg. sodium*

CREAMY MASHED POTATOES

Here's a way to get lots of garlic into your diet. But don't fret that the generous amount will overwhelm the rest of your meal. Parboiling tames garlic's flavor, so it blends in nicely with the mashed potatoes.

- **2 heads garlic (about 30 cloves), unpeeled**
- **2 pounds baking potatoes, peeled and cut into 1" cubes**
- **1 cup buttermilk**
- **2 tablespoons minced fresh parsley**
- **2 tablespoons butter-flavored sprinkles**
- **½ teaspoon ground black pepper**

Separate the cloves and drop into boiling water. Boil for 2 minutes. Drain and slip off the peels.

Place potatoes in a 3-quart saucepan and cover with cold water. Add the garlic. Bring to a boil and cook for 15 minutes, or until the potatoes are tender. Drain, then return the vegetables to the pan and stir over medium heat for 2 minutes to evaporate excess moisture.

Using a food mill or potato masher, mash the potatoes and garlic. Beat in the buttermilk, parsley, butter-flavored sprinkles and pepper.

Serves 4

Per serving: *214 calories, 0.9 g. fat (4% of calories), 2 g. dietary fiber, 2 mg. cholesterol, 181 mg. sodium*

CHAPTER 22

ENERGY AND PERFORMANCE

CHOOSING THE RIGHT FUEL

There he was, fitness and nutrition director for SportsMind, a Seattle-based company charged with boosting the performance of employees at Fortune 500 firms—and some of Larry Burback's charges were falling asleep in class. The rigors of lectures, obstacle courses and assorted team-building exercises were just too physically demanding for those who had tried to re-energize at lunch with a burger, fries and a coffee chaser.

But then SportsMind stopped merely talking about the importance of nutrition during its training sessions and began serving chicken fajitas, pita sandwiches stuffed with turkey, vegetarian lasagna and other low-fat meals and snacks.

They're not nodding off now. In fact, says SportsMind founder Chris Majer, the executives often report *increased* energy—even before completing the course. "It's a fairly common experience for them to tell us that their energy has been enhanced."

You may not be a captain of industry, but if you're like most of us, your ship of state could probably use a little extra steam. In fact, having enough get-up-and-go just to get through the day—without feeling like you've run a grueling marathon—would probably make you happier than winning a gold medal.

Fortunately, experts say that if you're willing to feed your body the right fuel at the right time while including a moderate amount of exercise in your daily routine, you're on your way to the winner's circle.

For more proof, look no further than the role of nutrition in competitive athletics. "If you look at an athlete competing against another athlete of the same age, equal ability and equal training, at that point, diet can make a 100 percent difference in who claims the victory," says Ann Grandjean, Ed.D., chief nutrition consultant for the U.S. Olympic Committee.

Remember, your quest for more energy doesn't have to be a heroic struggle. The right nutritional choices can help boost stamina and make you a better performer at home, at the office or in the gym.

Energy Essentials

A crowd packed elbow-to-elbow at a buffet table is evidence enough that many people live to eat. But actually, we're supposed to eat to live. Although your body can produce some of the chemicals needed to keep you healthy, it's your mouth's sometimes-delicious job to supply what are called essential nutrients. Among them: carbohydrates, protein, vitamins, minerals—even some fat.

You've probably seen essential nutrients listed on cereal boxes and can labels under such assumed names as the U.S. Recommended Daily Allowance. But there's no secret about their task. Essential nutrients help promote growth and repair of skin and internal organs, regulate critical body processes, and—equally important—boost your energy.

When you're energetic enough to vacuum the rug, wash the windows, do the laundry and cook dinner as a warm-up for an evening of transmission repair, you've supplied your body with just the right mixture of these nutrients: Roughly 60 percent carbohydrates, 25 percent fat and 15 percent protein, experts say.

But when you can't even get yourself into first gear, you may be suffering the consequences of any number of energy-sapping eating sins, according to Liz Applegate, Ph.D., sports nutrition columnist for *Runner's World* magazine and author of *Power Foods.* Perhaps the worst: Missing a meal and then trying to compensate with a sugary snack.

"Any time you deprive your body of the fuel you need, you're setting yourself up for a fall," Dr. Applegate says. "And if you love sugary things, you're better off eating them after a meal. That way, your body gets the important nutrients instead of only empty calories from sugar." Or better yet, Dr. Applegate says, turn your sweet tooth into a craving for the energizer of the sports world—complex carbohydrates.

Stamina from Starch

The days of starch-bashing are definitely over. Elite athletes and weekend warriors have known the energy-boosting benefits of complex carbohydrates for years.

WHERE ARE THE CARBOHYDRATES?

If you're a moderately active male who weighs 150 pounds, you need to consume about 350 grams of carbohydrates each day. A variety of foods and their carbohydrate values are listed below.

FOOD	PORTION	CARBOHYDRATES (g.)
Raisins	1 cup	114.8
Dates	10	61.0
Potato, baked	1	51.0
Peanut butter and jelly sandwich	1	44.6
Spaghetti	1 cup	39.7
Bagel	1	31.0
English muffin	1	30.0
Apple juice	1 cup	29.0
Apple	1	21.1
Roll	1	19.6
Whole-wheat bread	1 slice	13.8
Low-fat milk	1 cup	11.7
Graham cracker	1	10.4
Saltine crackers	5	10.2
Carrot	1 med.	7.3
Spinach	½ cup	3.4
Coffee	¾ cup	0.7
Egg	1	0.6
American cheese	1 oz.	0.5
Diet cola	1½ cups	0.4

But the merits of carbs actually came to light in the 1930s, says William Fink, assistant to the director of the Human Performance Laboratory at Ball State University in Muncie, Indiana.

While breakthroughs were occurring in chemistry, physics and biology, two Swedish researchers studying amateur athletes like cyclists and skiers pushed exercise physiology to the edge of a new frontier by simply adding a little starch.

During their experiment, some athletes were fed potatoes and bread, foods loaded with carbohydrates; others were fed low-carbohydrate fare. Later, both groups were required to ride a bicycle to exhaustion. The results, repeated hundreds of times since that first test, were astonishing: The athletes who ate the high-carbohydrate foods rode significantly longer than their counterparts, Fink says.

But it wasn't until later that scientists learned *why* carbohydrates boosted athletic endurance. And why complex carbohydrates like pasta, potatoes and bagels provide a more even-burning fuel than simple carbohydrates like jelly beans and sugary soft drinks.

Just as your fuel choices at the pump determine whether your car will be burning regular or premium gas, your food choices at the table determine whether you'll be getting the important nutrients your body needs for better performance, such as fiber, minerals, vitamins and complex carbohydrates, Dr. Applegate says.

Complex-carbohydrate foods, such as whole-wheat bread, pasta, grains, rice, vegetables and beans, are packed with nutrients and fiber.

Simple carbohydrate foods, such as candy, cookies, honey, presweetened cereals and soft drinks, are generally low in fiber and nutritional value.

The body burns both kinds of carbohydrates for energy. Simple carbohydrates are metabolized rapidly. Most complex carbohydrates contain fiber

PASTA: THE PRE-RACE FAVORITE

Here's a fact to keep in mind next time you feel pressured preparing a spaghetti dinner for your family: The athletes at the U.S. Olympic Training Center in Colorado Springs eat more than ½ *million* pounds of pasta a year, according to Terri Moreman, food service manager for the U.S. Olympic team.

The reason, in part: carbo-loading. Research shows that by stuffing themselves with starchy, high-carbohydrate foods like pasta each day for two to three days before an endurance event, athletes can essentially supercharge their bodies with energy to levels roughly twice those of a normal person. First developed in the late 1960s and early 1970s, carbo-loading is popular today with marathon and distance runners, cross-country skiers, cyclists and triathletes.

Before the technique was perfected, researchers thought it was necessary for athletes to consume a low-carbohydrate diet for three days before carbo-loading. The idea behind first dropping the carbs: Depleting the body of glycogen would make it hungry for even more. The unintended result: Athletes with low blood glucose levels were irritable and unable to train.

However, research by William Sherman, Ph.D., of the Exercise Physiology Laboratory at Ohio State University in Columbus, showed that three days of eating a moderate amount of carbohydrates prior to loading worked just as well as depletion—and without the side effects.

Today, endurance athletes are encouraged to rest two to three days before the event while consuming eight to ten grams of carbohydrates daily for each kilogram (2.2 pounds) of body weight. And that's the equivalent of a lot of pasta—roughly a 2-pound plateful.

and pulp and take longer to break down into glucose, providing even, longer-lasting energy.

Some of the digested carbohydrates are recombined to form glycogen, which is stored in your liver and muscles as a reserve energy source that can be called upon for additional glucose as needed during a workout. Your brain is powered almost exclusively by glucose.

If you're engaged in moderate or intense athletic activity—running or bicycling, for example—your muscles' glycogen stores will be depleted in about an hour or two. Through such techniques as carbo-loading, however, an athlete can significantly increase the body's ability to store glycogen and, as a result, improve endurance.

You don't have to be a triathlete to benefit from complex carbohydrates. One of the most promising findings linking food and energy levels in regular folks came from a study at the University of California at Los Angeles. After nearly a month of eating a high-carbohydrate, low-fat diet—lots of bran, rice and vegetables and a little fish or fowl—and walking twice a day, the participants—all in their seventies—significantly improved their performance on a treadmill, according to James Barnard, Ph.D., vice chairman of the Department of Physiological Science at UCLA. His conclusion: "People can significantly improve their work and health by switching to a high-complex-carbohydrate, low-fat diet and undertaking a walking program."

There's only one side effect associated with eating lots of carbohydrates. Research has shown that they may have a calming or relaxing effect in some people.

Don't Forget the Protein

A small amount of protein eaten with your carbohydrates could be just what the doctor ordered to prevent any carbohydrate calming tendencies that might occur and help keep mental performance at its peak, according to brain researcher Judith Wurtman, Ph.D., at the Massachusetts Institute of Technology.

The production of three important chemical neurotransmitters in the brain—serotonin, dopamine and norepinephrine—is influenced by the foods we eat, says Dr. Wurtman, in her book, *Managing Your Mind and Mood through Food.* Dopamine and norepinephrine help keep our mental performance up to speed. Serotonin, a calming chemical, makes us relax.

Eating protein prompts the creation of dopamine and norepinephrine, which keeps you more alert, Dr. Wurtman's research shows. Eating carbohydrates, though, sparks creation of serotonin—making you more relaxed.

The ideal interaction between the physical performance benefits of carbohydrates and mental performance benefits of protein is activated by this simple technique: Include three to four ounces of protein at lunch or dinner. The trick, Dr. Wurtman says, is to have several bites of protein with the carbohydrates.

Some good sources of protein, according to Dr. Wurtman, are shellfish, fish, chicken, veal, very lean beef, low-fat cottage cheese, skim or low-fat milk, low-fat yogurt, dried peas and beans, lentils and tofu.

FAT'S ROLE IN FATIGUE

For an essential nutrient, fat has a terrible reputation. The problem is, we eat way too much fat for our own good. On the average, Americans get 37 percent of their calories from fat. Think of it: Fat accounts for over a third of what we put in our mouths—while we only need roughly 2 percent to survive.

While the health problems associated with fat are well known, researchers are only beginning to understand what effect fat has on our energy levels.

There's strong evidence to suggest that high-fat meals slow digestion. As a result, you may feel sluggish, says Judith Hallfrisch, Ph.D., research leader for the Carbohydrate Nutrition Laboratory at the U.S. Department of Agriculture's (USDA) Human Nutrition Research Center in Beltsville, Maryland.

Once digested, some of the fat makes its way into the blood, actually making it thicker. According to Dr. Barnard, thicker blood slows circulation, reducing the amount of oxygen delivered by the blood to the rest of the body. Think of it as a raging river reduced to a slow-moving stream. Does less oxygen mean less energy? Could be, says Dr. Barnard. "That may be one of the reasons people are so lethargic in this country," he says.

But a study conducted by the Pennington Biomedical Research Center, a division of Louisiana State University in Baton Rouge, perhaps sheds the most light on the fat/energy debate. Researchers studying the effects of dietary fat on the energy levels of 44 women discovered that those who were getting fatter actually became less active after putting on the weight. "It appears to be a chain reaction," says Don Williamson, Ph.D., director of the Psychological Service Center at Louisiana State University.

In any case, the U.S. Army isn't taking any chances. Army officials have enlisted the aid of experts at Pennington to slash fat, cholesterol and sodium from the menus of soldiers stationed at forts and garrisons across the country, according to Catherine Champagne, Ph.D., Pennington's assistant professor of research. "I think they feel that if the soldiers are in better shape, they'll get more out of them," Dr. Champagne says. "A healthier person is a more productive person."

FIVE-MEAL-A-DAY PLAN

Before you get your own marching orders, make sure you've made plans to provide the food you need to fuel your day. And make sure you get that food at regular intervals. Skipping meals is a lot like writing your mind and

EATING FOR ENERGY MADE EASY

To ensure fuel for your busy day, sports nutrition columnist and author Liz Applegate offers these top ten eating tips.

1. Begin with breakfast. Skipping breakfast can undercut reading skills, memory and the ability to concentrate. Children who miss breakfast, research shows, have poorer school performance.

2. Carb-up. Complex carbohydrates such as beans, whole grains and vegetables, start to enter your system almost immediately, but because they break down slowly, they provide a steady stream of energy.

3. Cut the caffeine. Not only can caffeine let you down after a initial surge of activity during the day, but if you consume too much, you might even have trouble falling asleep at night.

4. Lunch lightly. Mental performance test scores were lower for subjects fed over 1,000 calories at lunchtime. Remember to eat slowly; it takes 20 minutes for your brain to get the message that your stomach is full.

5. Schedule mini-meals. Eat at least a little something every three to four hours to keep energy flowing. Snacking throughout the day will give you the fuel you need to keep going, but only if you choose healthy items such as sport bars, rice cakes, plain popcorn, unsalted pretzels and muffins and bagels without butter.

6. Pull your sweet tooth. Or at least wait until the end of your meal to indulge. That way, normally fast-burning simple carbohydrates will mix with what's already in your stomach and be digested more slowly.

7. Pump up your protein. Carbohydrates are a great energy source but you also need some protein to increase alertness. Chicken, fish, and low-fat cottage cheese are good sources.

8. Replace a missed meal. If you do have to skip a meal, don't hold off until the next one to make up for the lost calories. Try a high-carb snack containing 200 to 300 calories, such as a sport bar, a bagel with fruit, or nonfat yogurt with pretzels.

9. Set your watch. Consistency pays. Eating frequently, every three hours or so, can keep energy levels up and prevent you from overeating.

10. In case of hunger, break glass. Always keep some emergency high-carb snacks on hand.

body a bad check. And, boy, do they bounce! Your body is forced to rely on insufficient reserves of glycogen in the liver and muscles to fuel your activity, leaving you hungry, tired, and sapped of brain power, Dr. Applegate says. If you skip breakfast, for example, you're likely to concentrate less effectively in the late morning, work or study less efficiently, and then binge at lunch, she says. The experts who were interviewed all favored the idea of eating at least five times a day—even if some of those "meals" are quite small.

Breakfast. You want to use this opportunity to get your day off to a power start. Executives participating in SportsMind's early-morning training sessions fuel up on oatmeal, pancakes, fruit and fruit juices, and potatoes. Noticeably absent: runny eggs and high-fat bacon or sausage. "They're not going to get any of that stuff here," says SportsMind's Burback. If you're in a hurry, Dr. Applegate recommends a small stick of low-fat string cheese, a whole-wheat bagel and a can of orange-pineapple juice. "Whether you eat it in the car or while you're getting dressed, it doesn't matter," she says. "Just make sure you eat something good for you."

Midmorning snack. Eating something light at this point can help keep your performance at a peak until lunchtime. An apple is a common midmorning snack for Dr. Barnard. "I keep the apple machines here at UCLA in business," he says. Dr. Grandjean prefers cantaloupe.

Lunch. The idea here is to keep it lean and include some protein to heighten mental performance. Dr. Applegate suggests a chicken sandwich, along with whole-grain crackers and fruit. Chicken fajitas, pita-bread turkey sandwiches and soup are common lunch entrées at SportsMind, says Bruback.

Midafternoon snack. A modest repast here helps ensure against any post-3:00 P.M. droop. Midafternoon snacks range from Dr. Grandjean's yogurt to Dr. Applegate's sport bars. Also popular with our crew of experts:

DECISIONS, DECISIONS

Next time you have a choice between a diet soda and a chocolate bar, choose candy if you have an afternoon of pencil pushing planned. But yogurt would be even better.

That's the finding of a study at Tufts University in Boston that measured the mental performance ability of college men fed an afternoon snack of either diet soda, chocolate or fruit-flavored yogurt.

"The basic conclusion is that a calorie snack in the late afternoon had a beneficial effect on memory tasks and on the ability to pay attention," according to Robin Kanarek, Ph.D., professor of psychology and author of the study.

The men solved significantly more math problems in less time an hour after eating yogurt than they did after eating candy or drinking diet soda. Their visual reaction time was also better after eating either the yogurt or the candy, Dr. Kanarek says.

Rice cakes, bagels, muffins, hard pretzels, even sports drinks.

Dinner. Depending on what you've eaten earlier in the day, supper may be your main meal—or something less. In any case, the goal is the same: power for your evening activities. Dr. Barnard indulges in lean chicken or beef, while SportsMind serves vegetarian lasagna. Dr. Grandjean often restricts this meal to cereal with 1 percent milk.

ENERGY ROBBERS

When a dawn-to-dusk schedule puts your dining in doubt, don't put your energy at further risk with the wrong kind of quick pick-me-up. Some energy boosters can actually backfire, becoming energy robbers that steal your spunk in the long run. In other cases, shortfalls of key nutrients can put the brakes on your go-power even more insidiously.

Caffeine. A proven short-term eye-opener, caffeine has even been found to enhance endurance in some athletes, Dr. Applegate says.

But the more coffee you drink over time, the more you'll need to just keep you going, let alone give you a boost, according to Dr. Applegate. Two cups a day isn't bad, she says. Once you're making hourly pilgrimages to the percolator, though, you know its time to cut back.

"Caffeine for a lot of people really is an energy robber because they become dependent on it," she says. "They make their day around various cups of coffee."

Just stopping what you're doing to fetch a cup cuts productivity. And many heavy coffee drinkers complain of such problems as anxiety, irregular heartbeat, insomnia, shaking and nervousness.

Sugar. It does have a reputation as a short-term energy booster. But turning to sugary snacks like cookies, cake and candy bars when your go-power sags isn't a wise move, says Dr. Applegate.

"The concern is that these high-sugar foods, which are devoid of important nutrients, like B vitamins and fiber, will displace more nutritious foods from your diet. So in that sense they rob you of what you could have had," says Dr. Applegate.

By choosing a snack with less sugar and more complex carbohydrates—carrot sticks, for instance—you'll gain the benefit of extra nutrients. If the urge to splurge on something sweet is still too great, compromise, says Dr. Applegate.

"When eating a high-sugar food like candy or cookies, its best to moderate the amount and throw in something additional that will enhance performance like a muffin or a bagel," she says.

Nutritional deficiencies. Fatigue can also be the result of things that we fail to do, like not getting enough vitamins and minerals. For example, thiamine—a B vitamin found in breads, cereals and beans—is essential for energy. Without enough, you may feel lethargic and lose your appetite, experts say.

On the mineral front, iron deficiency can lead to anemia and corre-

POWERING UP WITH SPORTS DRINKS

Drinking and athletics rarely go together—unless you're talking about sports drinks. Once limited to Gatorade, no fewer than a half-dozen sports drinks are now common in America's locker rooms.

Amateur athletes and researchers have apparently made the same discovery: A sports drink made with the right proportion of carbohydrate (about 6 percent) moves into the bloodstream as quickly as plain water—and does a better job of enhancing energy.

And it may even be better than carbo-loading at giving a pre-race boost. Researchers from Ohio State University, Virginia Military Institute and the University of Wisconsin working together discovered that pre-race loading with a sports drink containing maltodextrin, also known as glucose polymer, helped endurance runners perform as well as those who feasted on precompetition meals of pasta—with less stomach discomfort.

sponding fatigue, weakness, irritability and shortness of breath.

"At least 10 percent of the female population is iron deficient, and 60 to 80 percent have reduced iron stores. That's pretty scary. That tells you that there are lots of people walking around with marginal iron status," Dr. Applegate says.

Among the chief nutritional causes of iron deficiency: cutting back on meat (a superior iron source). In addition, runners, menstruating women and pregnant women are all susceptible to iron deficiency. Runners may lose extra iron when they sweat in large amounts. Menstruating women lose iron along with blood. And during pregnancy, a woman's body is programmed to put her baby's iron needs ahead of her own. Most women need 15 milligrams of iron a day (30 milligrams during pregnancy), men require just 10.

To pump up your iron, eat lean beef and other low-fat cuts of meat as well as enriched or whole-grain cereals. The caffeine in coffee and tea interferes with iron absorption, so it's best to avoid them. Instead, have a glass of orange juice. The vitamin C in citrus fruits helps iron absorption. Cooking in a cast-iron skillet can also boost your iron intake.

Whatever approach you develop to maximize your energy level, avoid what some executives have done. "They seem to have a fairly high level of nutritional knowledge," SportsMind's Majer says, "but they are relatively poor at acting on what they know."

HIGH-NUTRITION RECIPES

POACHED SALMON WITH POTATO PANCAKES

When you need a steady boost of energy, combine some protein and complex carbohydrates. In this recipe, the salmon supplies the protein, and the pancakes kick in carbohydrates from the potatoes and apples they contain. This is a good way to use up leftover baked potatoes. You'll notice that the percent of calories from fat is a little high, but that's because salmon is a very good source of heart-healthy monounsaturated fat. When you combine the fish and pancakes with low-fat side dishes, the total percent for the meal will be reduced.

2 tablespoons lemon juice
½ teaspoon ground black pepper
4 salmon steaks (about 5 ounces each)
2 large cold baked potatoes, peeled
1 tart green apple, peeled and cored
¼ cup fat-free egg substitute
1 small onion, minced or shredded
2 tablespoons grated Parmesan cheese
½ teaspoon dried tarragon
Pinch of grated nutmeg or crushed caraway seeds
1 teaspoon olive oil
1 cup mild or medium chunky salsa

In a 8" × 8" glass baking dish, mix the lemon juice and pepper. Add the salmon and turn to coat both sides. Set aside.

Coarsely shred the potatoes into a large bowl. Then shred the apple into the bowl. Stir in the egg, onions, Parmesan, tarragon and nutmeg or caraway. Form the mixture into 8 flat pancakes about ½" thick.

Coat a broiler rack with no-stick spray. Add the salmon steaks. Broil about 4" from the heat for 5 minutes. Flip and broil for 5 to 7 minutes more, or until cooked through.

While the salmon is cooking, heat ½ teaspoon of the oil in a large no-stick frying pan over medium heat. Add 4 of the pancakes and sauté until browned on both sides. Repeat with the remaining oil and pancakes. Serve with the salmon and salsa.

Serves 4

Tip: *Baked potatoes are easier to shred if they're cold. If you don't have any leftovers, bake potatoes in the microwave then chill for at least 30 minutes.*

Per serving: *332 calories, 12.3 g. fat (33% of calories), 2.8 g. dietary fiber, 34 mg. cholesterol, 366 mg. sodium*

TURKEY PITA SANDWICHES

A turkey sandwich pairs high-quality protein with complex carbohydrate–rich bread. If you use pita bread, the sandwich will be nicely portable—take a half sandwich along to work for a midmorning energy boost.

2 cups diced or shredded cooked turkey breast
½ cup diced sweet red peppers
½ cup diced carrots
¼ teaspoon dried thyme
¼ teaspoon ground black pepper
½ cup fat-free mayonnaise
¼ cup nonfat yogurt
4 whole-wheat pitas, halved
1½ cups alfalfa sprouts

In a large bowl, combine the turkey, peppers, carrots, thyme and black pepper. Stir in the mayonnaise and yogurt.

Spoon into the pita pockets. Top each half sandwich with sprouts.

Serves 4
Per serving: *260 calories, 3 g. fat (11% of calories), 1.5 g. dietary fiber, 49 mg. cholesterol, 656 mg. sodium*

CHAPTER 23

Staying Younger Longer

Anti-Aging Nutrients

Imagine old age without arthritis, cataracts, osteoporosis and memory loss. Imagine being able to stave off cancer and heart disease indefinitely. You may not need to have a rich imagination to picture a healthy old age. You may be able to live it.

Welcome to nutrition's "brave new world." Ongoing research, much of it done at the U.S. Department of Agriculture's (USDA) Human Nutrition Research Center on Aging at Tufts University in Boston, may yet make it possible to grow old gracefully, without growing chronically ill and infirm. The Human Nutrition Research Center is the only research center in the country whose sole purpose is to study the relationship between nutrition and the aging process.

Through proper diet—with the right amounts and kinds of nutrients—we may be able to remain healthy throughout the life that medical research and technology is prolonging.

No Magic Bullet

With everyone looking for an easy answer, how close are we to an anti-aging supplement? "I wish I could say, 'We're almost there,' but I don't think we'll ever find a single magic bullet. Life is more complicated," says Jeffrey Blumberg, Ph.D., associate director of the research center and a leading authority on aging and nutrition.

"However, I must say vitamins E and B_6 are showing a lot of promise in our anti-aging research. We have done some exciting studies with these two nutrients; it appears that they affect the health of the immune system. Generally, immunity declines somewhat as we get older, making us more

YOUTH-FULL NUTRIENTS

Research on the aging process—like that coming out of the U.S. Department of Agriculture's Human Nutrition Research Center on Aging at Tufts University in Boston—suggests that maximizing the nutritional quality of your diet may slow down or prevent age-related problems that many people think are inevitable. The following are top food sources of key nutrients that have shown promise in anti-aging research. (Since a number of these nutrients are destroyed by light and air, store foods in airtight containers and avoid light exposure. Also cook foods for as short a time and in as little water as possible.)

Vitamin E. (RDA: 10 milligrams for men; 8 milligrams for women) Good sources: wheat germ, peanut butter, almonds, filbert nuts, sunflower seeds, shrimp and vegetable oils. Green leafy vegetables also supply vitamin E.

Vitamin C. (RDA: 60 milligrams for men and women) Good sources: citrus fruits and juices, strawberries, red and green peppers, broccoli, cantaloupe and fortified juices. Also, potatoes (white and sweet), mangoes, tomatoes and tomato juice, watermelon, honeydew, brussels sprouts, snow peas and cauliflower.

Beta-carotene. (RDA: none) Good sources: carrots, winter squash, pumpkin, sweet potatoes, dark green vegetables (like spinach, kale and broccoli), apricots, cantaloupe, mangoes and peaches.

Vitamin B_6. (RDA: 2 milligrams for men; 1.6 milligrams for women) Good sources: chicken, fish, lean pork and eggs. Also, whole-grain rice, soybeans, oats, whole-wheat products, peanuts, bananas, plantains and walnuts.

Vitamin B_{12}. (RDA: 2 micrograms for men and women) Good sources: lean meats and fish. Also, milk products and eggs.

Folate. (RDA: 200 micrograms for men; 180 micrograms for women) Good sources: legumes, such as lentils, kidney beans and black-eyed peas; citrus fruit; whole-grain products and vegetables, particularly spinach.

Calcium. (RDA: 800 milligrams for men and women) Good sources: dairy products, broccoli, kale, collards and sardines.

Note: Fortified cereals may provide fair amounts of some or all of these nutrients. Check the labels, since products vary.

susceptible to bacterial and viral infections as well as certain diseases most common among the elderly, like cancer, arthritis and heart disease.

"Several studies have shown that certain nutrients may slow or prevent the decline in immunity," says Dr. Blumberg. "Our most striking work in this area was with vitamin E supplements in older people. We found that high doses markedly improved certain tests of immune function." For example, when they did a skin-patch test exposing the skin to certain toxins, the person normally would have reacted with a red swelling (caused when the immune system increases its output of white blood cells that surround and destroy the toxin). The reaction is an indication that the immune system is responding and fighting the antigen. "In older people, we found this response didn't occur because their immune systems are less vigorous," he says. "However, after giving older people vitamin E supplements, their response to the skin patch test was like that of younger people."

Researchers found that vitamin B_6 might play a role in the proper functioning of the immune system, too. Robert M. Russell, M.D., professor of medicine at Tufts Medical School, and Simin Meydani, Ph.D., of Tufts School of Nutrition, discovered that when healthy elderly people had vitamin B_6 almost completely taken out of their diets, their immune response went down, as expected. What wasn't anticipated was the finding that the amount of vitamin B_6 needed to restore immune function was much higher than the Recommended Dietary Allowance (RDA) of about two milligrams. And when the study participants were given higher than the RDA levels, their immune function was even better than it was before the study started! A word of caution, however: Vitamin B_6 can be toxic at high doses.

OLDER PEOPLE ARE SPECIAL

The Tufts findings suggest that the RDA for certain vitamins might not be high enough to put the brakes on the illnesses that accompany aging. "I believe that, for some nutrients, the RDAs should probably be increased as we age," Dr. Blumberg says. "In other cases, however, the RDAs may need to be lowered for older adults since the need for certain nutrients seems to decrease as we age."

Remember that the RDAs are nutritional guidelines designed to help prevent deficiency symptoms in the average healthy person. But there is a growing number of studies that suggest that the RDAs are not really appropriate or sensitive to the changing nutritional needs of aging adults. Nor are they focused on our most important public health objectives—preventing chronic diseases like cancer and heart disease.

"In most cases, the RDAs are extrapolations based on studies of younger people," Dr. Blumberg says. "If you look at the current RDAs, you'll see that although there are special amounts for children and young adults, there really aren't special amounts for people over age 51. But we're finding that the needs of younger adults are not the same as those of people in their sixties, seventies and eighties.

"Take the vitamin B_6 study as an example. While it was only a preliminary study, it does suggest the need for vitamin B_6 may increase with age and even higher amounts of vitamin B_6 might prevent or delay age-related changes in the immune system. More research needs to be done, however, before we can make any specific recommendations."

THE WEAR-AND-TEAR FIGHTERS

Certain nutrients, called antioxidants, have been shown to slow down the deterioration that accompanies aging. These nutrients, which include vitamins E and C and beta-carotene, may slow down or prevent damage from chemicals called free radicals. Free radicals occur naturally, for instance, when the fat and proteins you eat interact with the oxygen in your body to form toxic compounds. When there are too many free radicals, they can attack parts of your body's cells, like cell membranes, causing them to break down.

"There is a theory that aging is the result of accumulated damage from free-radical reactions, Dr. Blumberg says. "Fortunately, Mother Nature has provided a natural way to cope with free radicals, in the form of these antioxidants. Antioxidants help inactivate free radicals and prevent them from attacking cells. Each one seems to work in a different way to counteract free-radical damage, so they're all important."

Even if free-radical reactions don't cause aging per se, a growing body of evidence suggests they are involved in immune-function decline as well as in causing common age-related diseases, including heart disease and cancer. Based on experimental studies, some researchers believe antioxidants may help prevent these ailments.

As a case in point, a Harvard Medical School study revealed that 333 men with heart disease who were given beta-carotene supplements for an average of six years had fewer heart attacks and heart-related deaths than did men not given the supplements.

Researchers speculate that there may be a way to get a jump on stalling the aging process by increasing our intake of certain nutrients while in middle age. "My feeling is that if we can retard or reverse a phenomenon like the decline in immunity with nutritional intervention in older adults, then it's reasonable to speculate that we can slow age-related changes by having a relatively high intake of these nutrients in the middle years," Dr. Blumberg says. "Since research in this area is still in early stages, however, it will be years before we know whether certain vitamins—and what amounts—slow aging. We do know changes in the immune system—and in nutrient needs—are gradual. So I think it makes sense to pay special attention to your diet, increasing intake of nutritional foods, before you reach old age."

HOW TO GET MORE FROM LESS

With weight control a growing concern for many of us as we grow older, the question is: How do we eat more foods without consuming more calories?

Make the most of every mouthful. The most obvious way is to focus on foods that contain the greatest concentration of nutrients with the least amount of calories and fat. Most fresh fruits and vegetables, whole grains, lean meats and fish and low-fat or nonfat dairy products do that. Don't waste your calories on sugary soft drinks, sweet confections or alcohol—the so-called empty-calorie foods.

Burn more to eat more. Exercise can also help. By virtue of the fact that you're burning off more calories, you can eat more food than someone who doesn't exercise. When you eat more food, you have a better chance of getting more vitamins and minerals. Exercise can also optimize the way the body handles certain nutrients. "Calcium, for instance, seems to be incorporated into bone more efficiently if you exercise regularly," Dr. Blumberg says.

Consider extra vitamin E. Getting adequate amounts of vitamin E and other fat-soluble vitamins, which are found in polyunsaturated fats, can be difficult on a low-fat diet. "This is a major problem," Dr. Blumberg says. "Not only are many health-conscious people cutting back on fats of all types, but the polyunsaturated fats that are on the market tend to have less vitamin E than they used to because of processing methods. In fact, a study published in the *Journal of the Canadian Dietetic Association* indicated that people who went from a diet containing more than 30 percent fat calories to one providing less fat experienced a drop in vitamin E intake that placed them well below RDA levels. Even RDA amounts may not be enough to optimize immune function as we grow older. This may be one case when supplementation may be in order. Many vitamin E researchers suggest supplements of 100 to 400 I.U. per day; however, there aren't enough studies yet to be more specific than that."

CAN YOU BE TOO THIN?

Some newspaper reports have suggested that being underweight may actually prolong life. But Dr. Blumberg isn't convinced. "As far as longevity is concerned, I don't think that there's much sound evidence that being underweight prolongs human life. Yes, numerous studies in rats and mice show that animals fed diets that are deficient in calories but adequate in protein, vitamins and minerals tend to live longer than animals fed normal diets. The problem is that these studies have only been done in animals that have very short life spans, and the findings may or may not apply to humans. We'll have a better answer years from now when ongoing studies in monkeys (which have much longer life spans and are biologically more like people) are completed by the National Institute on Aging (NIA)."

FIVE STEPS TO AN ANTI-AGING DIET

1. Decrease fat to less than 30 percent of your overall calorie intake.
2. Increase fiber to between 20 and 35 grams a day.
3. Eat foods rich in the antioxidants—vitamins E and C and beta-carotene.
4. Consume low-fat foods high in calcium.
5. Take a multivitamin/mineral supplement to ensure you're getting at least the Recommended Dietary Allowances.

In the meantime, Dr. Blumberg doesn't recommend cutting back on calories if you're trying to stay younger longer. "I don't recommend caloric restriction because it's very experimental," he says. "Animals in caloric restriction studies are 'undernourished, but not malnourished.' They're on carefully planned diets that assure the animals are getting the right nutrients. People who try this on their own could easily become malnourished. I've already pointed out how important it is to have a nutrient-rich diet if you want to slow aging. That becomes much tougher if you cut way back on calories."

That doesn't mean, though, that it's okay to get fat as you grow older. "We're not talking about becoming obese," Dr. Blumberg explains. "This just suggests that maybe it's good to have a little fat reserve when you're older so that if you do develop some sort of disease, you have something to draw upon. Being a little heavier may also act as a hedge against the natural decline in appetite that tends to occur as we age. I'd say that if you were not overweight when you were younger, then you certainly shouldn't panic if you weigh up to 5 percent more than your youthful weight during middle age."

No matter what you weigh, your goal should be to keep up your muscle tissue by exercising. Since muscle tissue burns fat but fat tissue doesn't, that should help boost your calorie requirement. Thus, if you're exercising, you can afford more calories.

William J. Evans, Ph.D., chief of the Human Physiology Laboratory at Tufts, and his coworkers have done a series of studies to examine the impact of fairly intensive exercise training—involving a combination of activities like bicycling, walking and weight lifting—on people of various ages. "Not surprising, they found that people who exercised more were the most physically fit—whether they were young or as old as 90. What came as a surprise was the finding that the extent to which exercise helped a person maintain muscle mass seemed to depend on how "nutritionally fit" he or she was.

The researchers put people on an exercise program and gave them a liquid supplement containing a variety of vitamins and minerals as well as protein. They found that this regimen seemed to increase both muscle mass and strength in older people, but made no difference in young adults. "Since the supplement contained many different nutrients, we don't know which one or ones might have been responsible for the improvement," Dr. Blumberg comments. "But the fact that the participants were all eating pretty well balanced diets indicates that getting extra amounts of one or more nutrients might optimize the effect of exercise in middle-aged and older adults."

Keeping the Mind Sharp

There's also evidence that good nutrition might be able to keep our brains as healthy as our aging bodies. That's encouraging because many people fear the loss of mental acuity more than they fear some of the killer diseases.

"There's some exciting research going on aimed at keeping the brain young," Dr. Blumberg says. "For a long time we've known that people who are seriously deficient in B vitamins start to develop mental or cognitive troubles as well as other problems, such as anemia. But we now have sophisticated new tests that tell us when people are just borderline-deficient—when they show no outward or obvious signs of deficiency—in vitamins B_6, B_{12} and folate."

When someone is borderline-deficient in any of these nutrients, levels of an amino acid called homocysteine become elevated. "There's evidence that a small but significant number of elderly people have elevated homocysteine levels that return to normal when the mild deficiencies are corrected with B-vitamin supplements," says Dr. Blumberg. "Not only that, but preliminary studies suggest some people show improvement in memory and learning ability after B supplementation."

So what does this mean for younger people who want to stay sharp into a ripe old age? "Based on the limited evidence we have, I'd say that changes in cognitive function are gradual," Dr. Blumberg explains. "So you want to make sure that your diet is rich in these three nutrients—vitamins B_6, B_{12} and folate—because they seem to be particularly vulnerable to the aging process. I don't mean to imply, however, that taking B vitamins will prevent or reverse all cognitive changes related to aging."

Conserving Your Vision—And More

Speaking of keeping sharp, what about the eyes? Is there any dietary way to preserve your vision as you grow older?

Most people don't realize that cataracts afflict virtually everyone who lives long enough. The process, which results in loss of transparency of the lens of the eye and eventual loss of vision, usually starts around age 60. Cataracts can be easily corrected with surgery, but who wants to go through the trouble and expense if you can avoid it?

"Since we now know that cataracts develop because of free radical damage to the lens—for example, as a result of exposure to ultraviolet light from the sun—it makes sense that antioxidants would play a protective role," says Dr. Blumberg. Indeed, studies of older people by Paul F. Jacques, D.Sc., an epidemiologist at Tufts, showed that those with higher blood and dietary levels of vitamins E, C and beta-carotene had the lowest incidence of cataracts. But Dr. Blumberg points out there are no guarantees: I want to stress that this refers to a reduction in risk—some people who had high antioxidant levels also had cataracts. It may be that these people had more exposure to UV light when they were younger.

So what's the bottom line for people who want to do everything in their power to put the brakes on aging through nutrition? "In essence, eating a super high quality diet is crucial if you want to do all you can to stay young longer," Dr. Blumberg says. "It's especially important to key in on good food sources of vitamins E, C and beta-carotene. It's interesting that it keeps coming back to these antioxidants—whether we're talking about immune function, cardiovascular disease or cataracts. I'd work on eating good sources of B vitamins and folate as well. In addition, I'd go so far as to advise people who want to take steps to slow down the aging process to take a daily multivitamin/mineral supplement."

Research so far suggests that if you're an older adult, you should take a multivitamin/mineral supplement formulated at one to two times the RDA levels, plus eat a diverse diet low in fat and high in fiber. The idea behind this is that then you can die 'young'—as late as possible.

CHAPTER 24

Cancer Prevention

It Starts on Your Plate

"I give up! Everything causes cancer!" Each time we read about a new cancer-causing substance in our diets we may react that way—feeling like it's hopeless. We might as well go ahead and eat, drink and be merry, we tell ourselves, because we all know what's next, and it's no fun at all.

But the truth is, not everything we eat or drink causes cancer. As researchers find out more about the things that cause cancer, they are also discovering foods and substances in foods that help to *prevent* cancer. In fact, some foods may be so good at discouraging cancer that the suspected beneficial components in these foods are being studied as potential anticancer *drugs*.

"In many cases, the foods that cut our risk for developing cancer are the same ones that protect us from other big killers—heart disease, diabetes and stroke," says Daniel Nixon, M.D., the American Cancer Society's vice president for detection and treatment. These foods, part of an all-around healthy diet, include fruits and vegetables, whole grains, beans, low-fat dairy products, fish and lean meats.

Looking for Clues

So far, much of what we know about food and cancer comes from population studies. These studies evaluate the health and eating habits of large

HOLD THE HAM

Baked ham with honey mustard. Beef jerky. Franks at the ballgame. Your idea of a treat? Better make it an occasional one.

Both the National Cancer Institute and the American Cancer Society suggest you limit your intake of salt-cured, smoked and nitrite-preserved foods such as ham, hot dogs, bacon and some varieties of sausage, cold cuts and fish. These foods contain a number of compounds chemically similar to the carcinogenic tars present in tobacco smoke. In population studies, people whose diet is top-heavy with such foods are more likely than normal to develop stomach or throat cancer.

What's considered a safe amount of these foods to be eating? "No one knows for sure, but if you consume a serving of something from this group once a week or less you're probably within a safe range," says Daniel Nixon, M.D., of the American Cancer Society.

groups of people. Some follow groups over many years to see who develops cancer; others look at people who already have cancer and work backward, asking questions about dietary habits in the past or analyzing nutrient levels in blood samples taken earlier. Both look for associations between what people eat, or don't eat, and the kinds of cancer they develop.

"It's these types of studies that have suggested that certain types of fruits and vegetables may help protect against mouth and throat cancer, for instance, or that point an accusing finger at high-fat diets when it comes to colon cancer," Dr. Nixon says.

Such studies lead researchers to estimate that about 35 percent of all cancer deaths are related to diet, and another 5 percent to alcohol consumption. That's an impressive percentage. It means that what we put in our stomachs may account for more cancer deaths than pollution, tobacco and occupational exposure to chemicals *combined.* And some types of cancer may have an even stronger dinner-plate connection. Some researchers believe that most cases of colon cancer and breast cancer may be food-linked.

THE KEY DIETARY FACTORS

Exactly what foods are cancer researchers most interested in, and why?

Fats. A high-fat diet seems to work in a number of ways to increase the risk of colon, pancreatic, breast, prostate and most likely other cancers. "A high-fat diet in general, and polyunsaturated fats specifically, are implicated," says Leonard Cohen, Ph.D., head of the Section of Nutritional Endocrinology at the American Health Foundation in Valhalla, New York. Monounsaturated fats (found in olive, peanut and canola oil) seem to be neutral, Dr. Cohen says. They neither promote nor protect. And fish oils seem to have a protective effect, But researchers don't know just why this is so.

Fiber. A low-fiber diet seems to promote colon and rectal cancer and may also contribute to the development of breast cancer, Dr. Cohen says. Populations eating high-fiber diets show reduced breast and colon cancer rates, and in animals, high-fiber diets are associated with decreased tumor development.

Fruits and vegetables. Diets low in fruits and vegetables have been associated with increased risk for colon, breast, prostate and other types of cancer. "Fruits and vegetables contain a multitude of possible cancer-preventing vitamins, minerals, fibers and other compounds," Dr. Nixon says.

Dairy products. A calcium-rich diet has been tentatively linked with reduced risk of colon cancer. Vitamins A and D in milk and other foods also seem to promote normal cell growth, experts say.

With those general points in mind, let's take a more detailed look at several specific cancer sites.

Colon Cancer

We'll start with colon cancer, which most researchers agree has the best evidence backing up its nutritional connection.Your colon is directly exposed to the consequences of a poor diet. Too much fat, especially saturated fat from animal foods, and not enough fiber from foods like whole grains, beans, fruits and vegetables, have made colon and rectal cancer all too common these days. Most population and animal studies show that diets high in fat and low in fiber increase the risk for colon cancer.

One study, by researchers at Harvard University, found that people who normally ate beef, pork or lamb every day could halve their risk of colon cancer by eating red meat just once a week and substituting fish or chicken on other days. Fat itself isn't carcinogenic, scientists say. But it sets off a chain reaction in the digestive system that can produce cancer-causing substances.

The typical American diet dishes out almost 40 percent of its calories from fat, or about 67 to 89 grams of fat a day. The current National Cancer Institute recommendation is to reduce fat intake to no more than 30 percent of calories. "An increasing number of researchers, though, believe an optimum cancer-protecting level is closer to 20 to 25 percent of calories," Dr. Cohen says. That translates to just 33 to 56 grams of fat a day, based on a daily intake of 1,500 to 2,000 calories.

A Bulking Effect

Fiber helps prevent colon cancer in several ways. It bulks up the stool, increases acidity in the colon and creates an environment that reduces the concentration of potential carcinogens. "And it may have other whole-body effects, such as reducing blood levels of hormones like estrogen, which could mean it can also fight breast cancer," Dr. Cohen says.

Some studies suggest that wheat bran and rye bran are most effective at reducing cancer risks. "Most cancer experts say that simply eating more fiber-rich foods—grains, legumes, fruits and vegetables—is the most important thing to do," says Moshe Shike, M.D., director of clinical nutrition at Memorial Sloan-Kettering Cancer Center in New York City. Dr. Shike is also director of the hospital's Diet Colon Polyp Prevention Program.

The average American consumes just 11 to 12 grams of dietary fiber a day. But you'll be well on your way toward the 20 to 30 grams recommended by the National Cancer Institute if you eat a bowl of high-fiber cereal, three slices of whole-grain bread, four servings of fresh vegetables and two pieces of fruit a day, says Abby Bloch, R.D., coordinator of clinical nutrition research at Memorial Sloan-Kettering. (Check the label on the cereal; it must provide at least 9 grams of fiber per serving to be considered high-fiber, Bloch advises.)

A Role for Calcium?

Some evidence also shows that certain vitamins and minerals may help protect against colon cancer. Calcium seems to be the most promising of these. A few studies link higher levels of calcium intake with a lower rate of colon cancer.

Like fiber, calcium seems to bind bile acids, which prevents them from irritating the colon wall. And it may help normalize growth and development of the cells lining the colon wall. Research indicates that a daily calcium intake of 1,200 milligrams or more is linked to decreased colon cancer risk.

"For right now, though, I'd say it's important to simply get the Recommended Dietary Allowance (RDA) of calcium—800 milligrams," says Dr. Shike. About one-third of all men and more than half of all women in the United States get less than 70 percent of the RDA for calcium, studies show.

The Cabbage Connection

Diets rich in fruits and vegetables may halve your risk for colon cancer, according to several studies. "It's true that fruits and vegetables are markers for a low-fat, high-fiber diet, but it's probably more than that, because we know that fruits and vegetables also very good sources of the dietary antioxidants," says Jeffrey Blumberg, Ph.D., who in addition to being the associate director of the U.S. Department of Agriculture's (USDA) Human Nutrition Research Center on Aging at Tufts University in Boston, also heads the Antioxidants Research Laboratory there. Antioxidants are substances that help block the formation of harmful oxygen breakdown products in the body.

In both animal and population studies there seems to be an independent protective effect for the antioxidants, Dr. Blumberg says. "Across the normal range of intake of fats and fibers—high or low—increasing intakes of the antioxidants provides additional cancer protection."

Vitamins E and C are two antioxidants that may play a direct role in neutralizing cancer-promoting nitrosamines in the stomach, Dr. Blumberg says. Nitrosamines are produced during the digestion of nitrates and nitrites, compounds found in especially high concentration in preserved meats.

How many servings of fruits and vegetables do *you* eat in a day? (Catsup doesn't count.) Try keeping track for a few days. If you are like a lot of people, you are lucky if you come anywhere near the five daily fruit or vegetable servings that would move you into the recommended consumption range. One survey of nearly 12,000 consumers found that only 9 percent met the USDA guidelines recommending five servings of vegetables and fruit a day.

COULD A CLOVE A DAY KEEP CANCER AT BAY?

For folk healers around the world, garlic is a revered remedy for everything from intestinal parasites to heart disease.

And evidence that this odiferous globe may also fight cancer has been mounting steadily. Two studies found reduced rates of stomach cancer, and another showed reduced rates of colorectal cancer in people who indulged liberally in garlic-laden foods. Another found that rats that ate the equivalent of about 20 cloves of garlic a day had a marked decrease in mammary cancer.

The sulfur-containing substances that give garlic its pungent, elevator-clearing aroma are also what probably give it its anticarcinogenic activity, says Daniel Nixon, M.D., of the American Cancer Society. These compounds may inhibit the body's production of harmful biochemicals; they may also enhance immune system function so that carcinogens can be intercepted before they can damage cells, Dr. Nixon explains. "And some components of garlic may also have the potential to stimulate the liver to clear toxins out of the body," he says.

Both raw and cooked garlic may have beneficial effects, although the raw may be somewhat more potent. No one knows how much you'd need to eat to see a protective effect. And little cancer-related research has been done with deodorized garlic extracts available at health food stores, Dr. Nixon says.

If you like garlic, indulge in good health. (And invite your friends to join you. If they're eating it, too, they'll never notice *your* breath.) One serving suggestion: Roast whole cloves, then squeeze the insides onto toasted Italian bread lightly brushed with olive oil and fresh rosemary. Enjoy!

BREAST CANCER

High-fat diets have also been implicated in the case of breast cancer, and in animal studies, the connection is particularly strong, Dr. Cohen says. (Some population studies find little linkage between breast cancer rates and levels of dietary fat, apparently because *all* the people in the study—even those eating the least fat—have a relatively high-fat diet—30 percent fat or more, Dr. Cohen says.)

Researchers are making the same tentative recommendations regarding breast cancer as they are for colon cancer: reduce your fat intake down to 20 to 25 percent of calories.

"We believe that cut would result in a significant decrease in the breast cancer rate," Dr. Cohen says. "We've seen in animals that there doesn't seem to be a continuum of gradually decreasing risk between fat intake and breast cancer. Instead, there seems to be a point somewhere—we don't know exactly where—between 25 and 30 percent of calories or lower, where the promoting effect of fat switches on."

TAMING ESTROGEN

Fiber—wheat bran in particular—seems to play a special protective role in breast cancer. How? High-fat diets appear to raise blood levels of estrogen, a female hormone that stimulates breast cell growth and may contribute to the development of breast cancer. Fiber reduces blood levels of estrogen, even in the face of a high-fat diet, researchers at the American Health Foundation have found.

"And in animals, when you combine a low-fat diet with a diet high in wheat bran, you reduce the rate of mammary cancer even further than you do with a low-fat diet alone," Dr. Cohen says. Here again, the suggestion is to double your fiber intake, to about 30 grams a day.

Diets high in fruits and vegetables also seem protective against breast cancer. Such diets are naturally low in fat and high in fiber. And there are also potentially protective constituents in these foods, says Dr. Blumberg.

Vitamins C, E and A and beta-carotene (a vitamin-A precursor found in many fruits and vegetables) and selenium (a trace mineral found in grains and seafoods) may all play a role. "Low intake of any one of these nutrients has been associated with higher rates of breast cancer," Dr. Blumberg says. "The link so far is strongest for beta-carotene and vitamin C and weakest for vitamin E, even though pharmacological doses of vitamin E have been used to treat fibrocystic breast disease, and there has been some success along those lines."

In one study, breast cancer risk was almost twice as high in women eating the fewest carotene-rich foods, compared with women eating lots of those foods. (The low beta-carotene group ate less of the following: tomato juice, vegetable juice cocktail, tomatoes, corn, asparagus, strawberries, apples, grapefruit, lemons and limes.) The risk appeared to drop off signifi-

EASY DOES IT WITH ALCOHOL

Do alcoholic beverages cause cancer? Scientists can't say for sure. Studies do consistently show that people considered "heavy drinkers" (more than one or two drinks daily) have higher than normal rates of cancer of the mouth and throat. Heavy drinking has been less strongly linked with cancer of the esophagus, stomach, pancreas and liver. (Some studies show an association; others don't.) "Since heavy drinkers have notoriously poor eating habits and often smoke cigarettes, it's hard to say exactly what's causing what," says Clark Heath, M.D., the American Cancer Society's vice president for epidemiology and statistics.

If alcohol does promote cancer, it may do so by compromising the liver's ability to detoxify potential cancer-causing substances, by irritating the mouth and throat in a way that makes them more susceptible to cancer or by carrying cancer-causing substances produced during distillation. (Darker liquors, such as rum, bourbon and scotch are more likely culprits here.)

"When it comes to moderate or light drinking, the picture is even murkier," Dr. Heath says. One well-publicized study by Harvard researchers showed an increase in breast cancer in women who had even a few drinks a week. But while most researchers agree that the more a woman drinks, the greater her risk for breast cancer, many say that for the average woman drinking alcohol in moderate amounts (one drink or less a day), that risk is so small there's no need to stop drinking. "And risks for other cancers with light to moderate drinking seem small, too," Dr. Heath says.

What's a safe ceiling? According to the American Institute for Cancer Research, under no circumstances should you drink more than 1.5 ounces of pure alcohol a day. You'd get that amount in two 12-ounce beers, 8 ounces of table wine or two shots of straight spirits.

cantly once women reached a beta-carotene intake of more than 5,824 I.U. per day, the researchers note.

LUNG CANCER

In population studies, one category of nutrient stands out as being consistently associated with reduced rates of lung cancer: It's the carotenoids (including beta-carotene)—the pigments found in green leafy vegetables such as kale and yellow and orange fruits and vegetables such as carrots and cantaloupe.

Other nutrients—vitamins A, E and C and selenium—may also cut your risk for lung cancer, but in population studies, these nutrients are less consistently associated with reduced rates of lung cancer than are carotenoids, says Jerry McLarty, Ph.D., of the Department of Epidemiology and Biomathematics at the University of Texas Health Science Center at Tyler.

Dr. McLarty is directing in a clinical trial using beta-carotene and vitamin A (retinol) in a group of people at up to 100 times the normal risk for lung cancer—smokers who have been exposed to asbestos. The study will see whether large amounts of these nutrients (equivalent to several pounds of carrots a day) reduce these men's risk. Several other studies using varying doses of these nutrients are being conducted around the country.

"We realistically should expect that some of these trials won't come up with positive results, but that doesn't mean the idea isn't a good one," Dr. McLarty says. "One of the problems all of us have had to face is that we don't know how much of these nutrients to give and how long to give them. We know that years of the right kind of diet has been shown to protect people, but can you overcome a lifetime of asbestos exposure and cigarette

A Reason to Drink Green Tea?

Could an Eastern passion for green tea be one reason Japanese men can smoke more than American men but still have lower rates of lung cancer? Researchers studying the tea think it may.

In one study, consumption of green tea cut the lung cancer rate by 45 percent in mice exposed to one of the most potent cancer-causing components in cigarette smoke. Other studies in animals suggest that drinking green tea could cut the rates of stomach and liver cancer as well.

"Many constituents in green tea are capable of blocking cell mutations which could set the stage for cancer," says Chi-Tang Ho, Ph.D., professor of food sciences at Rutgers University in New Brunswick, New Jersey. "The tea contains a wide variety of antioxidant compounds that have demonstrated significant cancer-preventive activity in animals."

Green tea is made from the same plant as the black tea commonly used in western countries. But the leaves undergo less processing. (Black tea is known to contain much lower amounts of certain protective antioxidants than green tea.)

Many Japanese researchers are encouraging people to drink up and live long. American researchers say one or two cups of green tea a day won't hurt you, but that more research is needed to confirm any health benefits—or risks.

smoking with just a short period of supplementation, even at fairly high levels? We don't know."

Until results are in, "we can only recommend what we know—diets that are high in fruits and vegetables." And no dietary changes reduce your risk for lung cancer as much as not smoking, Dr. McLarty emphasizes. "Smoking increases your risk tenfold. With these nutrients, at best, we may be able to cut that risk in half."

CANCER-PROOFING YOUR DIET

So, to sum up, what overall strategies can you take to minimize your risk of developing cancer?

Carve away fat. Cut a quarter, a third or even half of the fat calories in your diet. "Cutting down on total fat should be your main concern, and you may also want to cut back on polyunsaturated fats," says Bloch.

Try substituting broiled fish, skinned chicken breasts, ground turkey burgers or a vegetarian main dish for red meat. And when you do eat red meat, reduce your serving size to about three ounces (about the size of a deck of cards.) Switch to 1 percent fat or nonfat milk. Sauté foods in fruit juice or vegetable stock instead of oil or butter. Use reduced fat or nonfat versions of cheeses, salad dressings, mayonnaise, ice cream, yogurt and sour cream. Use nonfat butter-flavored sprinkles such as Butter Buds instead of the real thing.

Fill up on fiber. Many cancer prevention specialists believe we would do well to double our average fiber intake to 30 grams or more a day. To do that, you need to eat high-fiber foods throughout the day: Eating three or four servings of whole grains and beans and five servings of fruits and vegetables a day will provide plenty of fiber. "If you've been on a low-fiber diet, avoid intestinal problems by increasing fiber intake gradually," Bloch says. "Your system needs time to get used to handling and processing fiber."

Bran cereals (nine or more grams per serving) and beans (with up to seven grams) are significantly higher in fiber than other food sources. A slice of whole-wheat bread has about two grams of fiber, and so does a serving of broccoli. Most fruits and vegetables have two to four grams of fiber per serving.

Fruits highest in fiber are dried figs, peaches and apricots; prunes; raisins; kiwi; pears (with skin); raspberries; oranges; blackberries and apples (with skin). Vegetables highest in fiber are artichokes, brussels sprouts, potatoes (with skin), corn, peas, carrots and sweet potatoes. Real rye bread, usually found in delicatessens, is also high in fiber. So are most rye biscuits or wafers.

Go for the orange, green and red. Dark leafy greens and orange, red or yellow fruits and vegetables are generally rich sources of carotenoids, including beta-carotene, Bloch says. Top choices: sweet peppers, carrots, winter squash, pumpkin, sweet potatoes, spinach, kale, broccoli, apricots, cantaloupe, mangoes and peaches. Hold the iceberg lettuce; it's mostly water and doesn't have much beta-carotene or fiber. Other good leafy greens are romaine, buttercup or red sail lettuce; radicchio; endive and collard or mustard greens.

Crunch on the cruciferous crowd. Broccoli, cauliflower, cabbage, bok choy, brussels sprouts, rutabaga, watercress and some of the new hybrids like broccoflower and orange cauliflower are all in this group. These vegetables contain high levels of indole gluosinolates (indoles for short), compounds that appear to have a variety of cancer-fighting talents. They seem to block carcinogenic changes in the colon and other organs.

For maximum indoles, eat them raw. Or make low-fat coleslaw, borscht, ground-turkey-and-rice-stuffed cabbage rolls or an apple-cabbage side dish.

Bone up on calcium. Eat a cup of low-fat or nonfat yogurt, with 452 milligrams of calcium. Drink a glass of skim milk, with 302 milligrams of calcium per cup. Stock up on sardines. One can of Atlantic sardines offers 351 milligrams of calcium, plus 1.4 grams of omega-3 fatty acids, which may have their own anti-cancer talents.

Add antioxidants. Vitamins E and C, beta-carotene and the trace mineral selenium, are antioxidant nutrients. They help to protect cells from membrane and chromosome damage that can lead to cancer, Dr. Blumberg explains. They may also neutralize some carcinogens you may eat, inhale or produce in your body.

Vitamin E is found in almonds, sunflower seeds, wheat germ, peanut butter, filbert nuts, shrimp and vegetable oils. "These foods are all high in fat, though, so don't go overboard eating them," Bloch points out. Citrus fruits and juices, strawberries, red and green peppers, broccoli, cantaloupe and fortified juices are all great sources of vitamin C. Orange and yellow vegetables and fruits are good sources of beta-carotene. Sources of selenium include fish and shellfish (tuna, salmon, oysters, shrimp) and Brazil nuts. Whole grains can be a good source if they're grown in selenium-rich soil. Grains grown in the United States are generally good sources of selenium, Bloch says.

Go easy on smoked foods. Salt-cured, smoked and nitrite-preserved foods like hams, hot dogs and bacon contain compounds similar to the carcinogenic tars in tobacco smoke. In population studies, these foods are associated with a rise in throat and stomach cancers. "Eat these foods only on special occasions," Bloch suggests.

Put a ceiling on the hard stuff. Never drink alcohol when you're thirsty. Start with water or juice to satisfy your thirst. "Dietize" any alcohol you do consume by ordering diluted drinks such as wine spritzers (wine mixed with sparkling water and ice.) At parties, eat before you drink and while you're drinking to help limit the amount you drink. Don't allow your drinks to be continually "freshened up" with alcohol. It's an easy way to drink more than you planned.

HIGH-NUTRITION RECIPES

OVEN-ROASTED TOMATO SOUP

When the American Cancer Society geared up for its third annual Great American Food Fight against Cancer, it enlisted the help of top chefs—professionals who could create truly delicious recipes that people would enjoy. One of the chefs was Victor Gielisse, owner of the acclaimed Actuelle restaurant in Dallas. Among his culinary creations were the following recipes. This unusual tomato soup could be a wonderful first course or a light lunch.

- **20 Italian plum tomatoes**
- **1 teaspoon canola oil**
- **1 tablespoon minced fresh parsley**
- **1 teaspoon dried basil**
- **1 teaspoon dried tarragon**
- **4 cups defatted chicken stock**
- **1 teaspoon ground cumin**
- **1 teaspoon ground coriander**
- **½ teaspoon ground black pepper**
- **1 teaspoon chopped fresh coriander**

With a small sharp knife, lightly score the peel on each tomato. Halve lengthwise and scoop out the seeds. Place the tomatoes, cut side down, on a baking sheet. Rub with the oil and sprinkle with the parsley, basil and tarragon. Bake at 250° for 1½ to 2 hours, or until softened.

Puree the tomatoes in a blender or food processor. Transfer to a 3-quart saucepan. Add the stock and bring to a boil over high heat. Stir in the cumin, ground coriander and pepper.

Ladle the soup into bowls and garnish each serving with fresh coriander.

Serves 6

Per serving: *57 calories, 2.2 g. fat (34% of calories), 1.4 g. dietary fiber, 0 mg. cholesterol, 64 mg. sodium*

PAN-SEARED LAMB

Although this individual recipe gets a fairly high percent of its calories from fat, the actual grams of fat are reasonable for a red-meat dish. And serving it with Tuscan Beans (page 321) brings the figure down to 30 percent.

- **1 pound lamb loin, trimmed of all visible fat**
- **2 tablespoons canola oil**
- **1 teaspoon minced garlic**
- **1 teaspoon minced shallots or onions**
- **1 teaspoon mustard seeds**
- **½ teaspoon red-pepper flakes**
- **½ teaspoon ground black pepper**
- **¼ teaspoon dried thyme**
- **¼ teaspoon dried basil**

With a sharp knife, cut the lamb crosswise into 6 medallions.

In a 9" × 13" baking dish, combine the oil, garlic, shallots or onions, mustard seeds, red-pepper flakes, black pepper, thyme and basil. Add the lamb and turn to coat both sides. Cover, refrigerate and allow to marinate for 2 hours.

Preheat the oven to 375°. Heat a large no-stick frying pan over medium-high heat until hot. Add the lamb and sear on both sides until golden brown. Transfer to a baking dish and bake for 6 to 10 minutes, or until just cooked through.

Transfer to a platter. Cover and chill. To serve, cut into very thin slices.

Serves 6
Per serving: *149 calories, 9.2 g. fat (56% of calories), 0.1 g. dietary fiber, 53 mg. cholesterol, 59 mg. sodium*

RIGATONI IN MUSHROOM BROTH

You may serve this as a soup or as a "brothy" main dish. Chef Gielisse likes a mixture of mushrooms, including porcinis, shiitakes and morels, but you may use whatever kind you prefer. For variety, you may add some protein such as cooked chicken, turkey or seafood.

- **1 pound rigatoni or other tubular pasta**
- **1 red onion, thinly sliced**
- **1 tablespoon minced shallots**
- **1 teaspoon minced garlic**
- **2 tablespoons canola oil**
- **¾ cup finely diced mushrooms**
- **4 cups defatted chicken stock**
- **1 tomato, seeded and finely diced**
- **2 tablespoons sherry extract (optional)**
- **3 tablespoons chopped fresh basil**
- **¼ teaspoon ground black pepper**
- **3 tablespoons grated Parmesan cheese**

Cook the pasta in a large pot of boiling water until just tender. Drain and set aside.

In a 3-quart saucepan over medium-high heat, sauté the onions, shallots and garlic in the oil for 2 minutes. Add the mushrooms and sauté for 5 minutes.

Stir in the stock, tomatoes and sherry extract, if desired; bring to a boil, stirring often. Reduce the heat to low and simmer for 5 minutes. Add the basil and pepper. Stir in the pasta and heat through.

To serve, ladle into soup plates. Sprinkle with the Parmesan.

Serves 6
Per serving: *378 calories, 7.8 g. fat (19% of calories), 1.9 g. dietary fiber, 2 mg. cholesterol, 121 mg. sodium*

TUSCAN BEANS

Fiber has been shown to help prevent various types of cancer, especially those of the digestive tract. Beans are loaded with fiber, so including them in your diet makes plenty of sense. This salad can be made ahead and marinated overnight. If you neglected to presoak the beans, you may take this shortcut: Place them in a 2½-quart glass casserole and cover generously with cold water. Microwave on high for 15 minutes. Stir, cover and let stand until the beans have swelled up, about 15 minutes. Drain and proceed with your recipe.

18 ounces small white dried beans, soaked overnight
1 large carrot, diced
1 celery stalk, diced
1 red onion, diced
¼ cup diced green, sweet red or yellow peppers
2 tablespoons snipped chives
2 tablespoons minced fresh parsley
½ cup rice-wine vinegar
3 tablespoons olive oil
¼ teaspoon ground black pepper

Drain the beans. Cook in fresh water until tender, about 1 hour. Drain and rinse with cold water. Cover and refrigerate until well chilled.

In a large bowl, combine the beans, carrots, celery, onions, peppers, chives and parsley.

In a small bowl, whisk together the vinegar, oil and pepper. Pour over the bean mixture and toss to combine. Let marinate at room temperature for 2 hours before serving.

Serves 6
Per serving: *364 calories, 7.9 g. fat (20% of calories), 8.8 g. dietary fiber, 0 mg. cholesterol, 22 mg. sodium*

CHAPTER 25

SEX AND REPRODUCTION
THE DIETARY FACTOR

Who'd ever think that the orange juice you toss down at breakfast or the grilled chicken breast you sink your teeth into at lunch has anything to do with your sex life?

That's right. Your *sex life.*

It only makes sense that what you eat has an impact on your sexual self. Your reproductive system depends on good nutrition to function optimally, just as the rest of your body does.

Hormone-producing glands like the ovaries and testes slow down or shut down if the proper building materials—protein, fat, certain vitamins and minerals—aren't available in needed amounts. Some areas with high cell turnover, such as the cervix and testes, show signs of abnormal or slowed cell growth when they're low on nutrients like folate or zinc.

In fact, several aspects of reproduction—from sex drive to fertility to delivering a healthy baby—may depend on adequate nutritional status.

BOY MEETS GIRL

For all the time and trouble we go through to prevent it, you'd think pregnancy would happen naturally if we just let it. For most couples, that's the case.

But about one of every six couples has trouble conceiving. They have

CAN FAT KILL ROMANCE?

A steady diet of cheeseburgers, french fries, cheesecake and other fatty foods may leave some men uninterested in sex. That, at least, is what researchers are theorizing after their study suggested that fatty meals may actually curb the production of testosterone, a hormone that can influence sex drive.

Four hours after serving fatty shakes to a group of eight men, the researcher saw the men's blood levels of testosterone decrease by 30 percent. When the men drank a low-fat drink of carbohydrates and protein or a nonnutritive drink instead, this sex hormone was unaffected.

"We looked only at the immediate result of one high-fat meal, though it may be hypothesized that after some time a high-fat diet could lower testosterone and weaken a man's sex drive," says A. Wayne Meikle, M.D., professor in the Division of Endocrinology and Metabolism at the University of Utah in Salt Lake City.

Testosterone levels can also affect a woman's sex drive, but this study only looked at men.

tried, without success, for a year or more, to produce a baby. Often the problem can be diagnosed and corrected. But sometimes the problem is not so obvious and seems to be related to hormonal or metabolic imbalances. That's where it might pay to see if your eating habits and lifestyle are thwarting your chances for parenthood, experts say.

Stress, alcohol and cigarettes are well-known monkey wrenches when it comes to making babies, for both men and women. Improper nutrition has long been recognized as a factor in infertility, too, but when it comes to understanding the details, "We know more about cows than we do humans," says Earl Dawson, Ph.D., associate professor of obstetrics and gynecology at the University of Texas Medical School at Galveston.

In men, infertility sometimes means that sperm are too few, too slow or downright defective, Dr. Dawson explains.

Several different nutrients have been recommended over the years to improve a man's "batting average." Two of the more commonly recommended—zinc and vitamin C—are both highly concentrated in semen and play an important role in male sexual functioning.

Ask your doctor to check your zinc status. "We proved long ago that zinc deficiency prevents or delays sexual maturation in men," says Ananda Prasad, M.D., Ph.D., professor of medicine at Wayne State University in Detroit and a leading researcher on the health effects of zinc. "It's also known that, in adult men, zinc deficiency leads to reduced levels of testosterone, the main male hormone." Low testosterone levels lead to impaired fertility.

In one study, Dr. Prasad and colleagues found that men on diets deliberately made low in zinc had significant drops in testosterone levels and in sperm count. When the men's zinc intake was restored to levels on a par with the Recommended Dietary Allowance (RDA), both the testosterone levels and sperm count slowly came back to normal in 6 to 12 months.

Since low sperm counts can be caused by many things, Dr. Prasad doesn't routinely recommend zinc supplements as a quick fix for male infertility. "But if a man is zinc deficient and has low testosterone levels, he may benefit from additional zinc," Dr. Prasad says.

The RDA for zinc, 15 milligrams, is thought to be more than adequate to keep up zinc stores in healthy young men. In one study, though, people

TURN-ON FOODS?

How about a nice steaming bowl of sea slug soup? Some ginseng tea? A plate of raw oysters?

For centuries, people around the world have turned to these and other foods, herbs and concoctions in an attempt to fuel sexual desire and perk up performance. But do they really work?

Overblown claims and lack of proof led the Food and Drug Administration in 1990 to prohibit interstate sales of any over-the-counter product that claims to act as an aphrodisiac or to restore sexual vigor. In this government agency's eyes, there's no such thing.

But some think a few of these foods may actually have something going for them.

Oysters and other shellfish, which have long been considered to have aphrodisiac properties in many cultures, are a rich source of zinc, which plays a major role in male testosterone production. For a man lacking this mineral, oysters might indeed be fuel for love.

Ginseng, a plant whose gnarled root is dried, ground and powdered, has a 5,000-year-old reputation as a cure-all. Some studies report ginseng steps up mating behavior in rats, but its effects on humans have not been proven.

Yohimbine, which is really a chemical, not a food, is derived from the bark of the African yohimbe tree. It has a long history as a "love potion" and is now used as a prescription drug to treat male impotence. Just how it works isn't understood. Some investigators think it acts directly on the central nervous system, others through complex hormonal pathways. In studies, it has consistently improved symptoms in about one-third of men with physical or psychological impotence.

who got only 10 milligrams a day showed blood zinc levels dropping by 1 to 2 milligrams a day. Most people get 10 to 15 milligrams of zinc a day, studies show. Try oysters, wheat germ, pumpkin seeds, beef, lamb and shiitake mushrooms for good amounts of zinc.

Keep sperm moving with vitamin C. Vitamin C plays a much different role in male fertility. It maintains sperm function.

A lack of vitamin C makes sperm clump together, a problem called agglutinization that is readily apparent when sperm are examined under a microscope. "You can see them all stuck together, head to head, tail to tail, head to tail," Dr. Dawson says. The stickiness keeps the sperm from wriggling their way to an egg.

Adding enough vitamin C to a man's diet can correct the problem, Dr. Dawson has found.

Many reputed aphrodisiacs, however, probably operate only by power of suggestion, if at all. "If you believe a particular food or herb is going to work, it may just work for you," says University of Florida anthropologist George Armelagos. And the rarer and more expensive the food, the more powerful its suggestive force. Whole species of animals (like rhinos and sea turtles) have been hunted to near-extinction just for their horns, penises or sex glands, says Armelagos, coauthor of *Consuming Passions*.

Some health food stores carry both male and female "formulas" that imply that they can improve sexual performance. These products have a variety of ingredients, including vitamins, minerals and herbs. The male potency versions may include yohimbine, ginkgo (added for its alleged ability to increase peripheral vascular circulation) and saw palmetto (a palm used in European herbal remedies for prostate problems).

"In small amounts, these products are unlikely to hurt you," says William J. Keller, Ph.D., head of the Division of Medicinal Chemistry and Pharmaceutics at Northeast Louisiana University's School of Pharmacy in Monroe.

But as with any other product, it's important to read the label and understand what's in the product, Dr. Keller says. "One potential danger is that, by relying on an over-the-counter remedy to treat your symptoms, you may be neglecting a problem that needs medical treatment," he says. "Impotence can be an early sign of diabetes or peripheral vascular disease. And lack of sexual desire can be caused by depression. Both symptoms are frequent side effects of certain prescription medicines."

In one study, a group of 30 men, all with sperm agglutinization problems and all unsuccessfully trying to get their wives pregnant, were divided into three groups. Two groups got vitamin C, either 200 or 1,000 milligrams a day. The third group got a placebo (blank pill.) At the end of 60 days, every one of the men taking vitamin C had impregnated their wives; none of the placebo group reported a pregnancy.

In another study, researchers found that men who cut back on vitamin C from 250 to 10 or 20 milligrams a day had 2½ times the amount of genetic damage to sperm. When the men increased their intake of vitamin C to 60 to 250 milligrams a day, the genetic damage dropped.

"We know now that if your dietary intake of vitamin C gets below about 60 milligrams a day, you get into trouble," says researcher Bruce Ames, Ph.D., of the Division of Biochemistry and Molecular Biology at the University of California, Berkeley. "And smokers, who have lots of damage-causing oxidants in their bodies, may have genetic damage even at higher intakes." In fact, smokers may need two to three times as much vitamin C, up to about 180 milligrams a day, "just to keep even with nonsmokers," Dr. Ames says.

To be safe, Dr. Ames recommends eating two fruits and three vegetables a day. "That gives you not just the vitamin C you need, but also folate and lots of other protective nutrients," Dr. Ames says. "It will benefit you and your children yet to be born."

Find your most fertile weight. Doctors who specialize in infertility have known for ages that women who are too thin or too thick have more trouble than usual getting pregnant.

"That's because body fat plays an important role in estrogen levels in the body," says reproductive endocrinologist G. William Bates, M.D., professor of obstetrics and gynecology at the Medical University of South Carolina College of Medicine in Charleston.

Body fat stores estrogen and can convert other hormones into estrogen, Dr. Bates says. Thin women may have too little estrogen, and overweight women too much, for a successful pregnancy, he says.

Dr. Bates has found that women who reach their normal body weight, either by dieting or gaining weight, increase their changes of becoming pregnant.

"We've seen women who were trying to conceive for years, and they gain some weight, and they conceive," he says. "We expect pregnancy within six months of attaining normal body weight."

Thin women need to gain an average of 8½ pounds to become fertile; overweight women don't need to become svelte, but they do need to lose enough weight to allow their periods to normalize. "The target weight for most obese women is 140 to 160 pounds," Dr. Bates says.

Women gaining weight are encouraged to temporarily load up on high-fat, high-calorie goodies like cheesecake, pastries and ice cream. This regimen puts pounds on fast; once the weight is gained, the women go back to healthy foods. Those losing weight are steered toward a moderate weight-loss and exercise program that allows them to shed a pound a week.

"I'm amazed how often body fat causes infertility problems," Dr, Bates says. "As many as 15 percent of couples may have an overweight or underweight problem. And I am amazed at how often it is overlooked."

MOTHER-TO-BE

Eating for two? A successful pregnancy can also benefit from good nutrition, from the moment of conception to the day of delivery—and even beyond if you are breastfeeding. A balanced diet helps prevent certain complications of pregnancy. And it may also guard against low birth weight and infant mortality.

A healthy diet provides the raw materials your body needs to produce a baby, which weighs an average of seven pounds. It also supplies the building blocks for the extras that go along with pregnancy. Increased blood and fluid volume, the placenta, amniotic fluid and bigger breasts, not to mention those "fat stores" the body stashes away during pregnancy for future breastfeeding, add up to 25 to 35 pounds of new tissue, all manufactured during pregnancy.

That comes to an average of about 300 extra calories a day, or a total of about 81,000 calories over the course of a pregnancy, says Elyse Sosin, R.D., supervisor of clinical nutrition at Mount Sinai Medical Center in New York City.

Those calories need to be chosen carefully. Pregnant women need extras of just about everything, including vitamin A, thiamine, riboflavin, folate, vitamin B_{12}, calcium, phosphorus, magnesium and iron.

But dietary surveys indicate that pregnant women tend to come up short, consistently getting well below the RDA for eight nutrients—vitamins B_6, D and E, folate, iron, zinc, calcium and magnesium. "If it's severe enough, any one of these deficiencies can pose dangers for both mother and fetus," says John Repke, M.D., associate professor of obstetrics, gynecology and reproductive biology at Harvard Medical School.

Many obstetricians *do* recommend prenatal supplements. If your doctor hasn't, you may want to bring the topic up at your next visit.

PREVENTING BIRTH DEFECTS

Good nutrition is important right from the start . . . even *before* the start! Why? Because certain serious defects that have been linked with poor diet are present by the fourth week of pregnancy. That's about the time most women first realize they're pregnant, Sosin says.

Neural tube defects, for instance, have been strongly linked with a deficiency of folate, a B-complex vitamin. Neural tube defects can be deadly—they result in spina bifida (failure of the spinal column to close) or anencephaly (failure of the brain to develop.)

In a large study, researchers found that adding four milligrams of folate to pregnant women's diets cut by 72 percent their risk of having a baby with neural tube defects. These women were considered at high risk, because they'd already had one baby with this defect.

Ask your doctor about folate—before you become pregnant. The Centers for Disease Control recommend that women who've had one baby with neural tube defects start taking four milligrams of folate daily starting *at least six weeks prior to attempting to become pregnant.* All other women of childbearing age are advised to take 0.4 milligrams (400 micrograms) of folate daily.

AVOIDING ANEMIA

It's hard enough hauling around that extra baggage. If you're anemic as well, your pregnancy can be a time of bone-weary, tail-dragging fatigue.

Iron requirements double during pregnancy, from 15 to 30 milligrams daily. The National Academy of Science recommends a daily 30 milligram iron supplement, beginning in the fourth month, because it's so hard for a pregnant woman to get all the iron she needs through diet. Most pre-

CRAVINGS: FOODS PREGNANT WOMEN CAN'T RESIST

For one expectant mom, it was chicken liver pâté; for another, M&Ms—plain, not peanut; a third couldn't get enough ice cream—but it had to be strawberry, and only one brand would do.

Food cravings are common during pregnancy. Studies show that as many as 75 percent of women find certain foods irresistible. The cravings often begin in the first few months of pregnancy, when levels of appetite-stimulating hormones are highest, and for many, continue until childbirth.

What foods do women desire most? That varies from study to study, but milk, ice cream, salty foods and snacks, sweets, chocolate and fruit seem to top most lists, says researcher Judith Brown, Ph.D., at the University of Minnesota's School of Public Health.

Apparently these hankerings can be fairly intense. In one study, women indicated they'd be willing to steal the food items they craved.

Pregnant women also tend to develop aversions to some foods: colas, coffee, alcohol, fried foods and meat seem most likely to cause turned-up noses.

One theory proposes that women are gravitating naturally toward foods that contain nutrients they need: pregnant women who crave salty foods, for instance, really may need more salt. That theory is shaky, though, since women don't always pick the food richest in a

natal vitamins contain at least some iron.

Ask your doctor about iron supplements. Some obstetricians recommend iron supplements from the start of a pregnancy, based on a woman's iron status. Others, though, wait until iron stores begin to dip. "During the 16th through 24th week, a woman's hemoglobin is at the lowest point ever during her pregnancy, and that's often why iron supplementation is started at this point or a little before," Sosin says.

KEEPING A LID ON BLOOD PRESSURE

Pregnancy-induced high blood pressure, with its accompanying bloating and protein breakdown, can be risky to both mother and baby. Some doctors believe this condition is caused by poor nutrition. Many, though, claim the cause is unknown. Some studies do suggest that pregnancy-induced hypertension is linked with an imbalance of minerals—too little calcium, magnesium or potassium and too much salt. The link currently is strongest for calcium.

Bone-building calcium demands shoot up to 1,200 milligrams a day for a pregnant woman, the amount found in about a quart of milk. Most studies

particular nutrient. "If a woman craves chocolate because she needs more magnesium, why doesn't she crave a better source of it, like green vegetables?" Dr. Brown asks.

As for aversions, some researchers think the distaste (often to the point of nausea) some women develop for some foods may be their bodies' reaction to substances that are potentially harmful to their babies. A distaste for alcohol and coffee, for example, often occurs early in pregnancy. Alcohol's harmful effects on an unborn baby are well known. In moderation, though, caffeine seems to do no harm. So the aversion theory, too, remains to be proven.

What should a pregnant woman do about cravings? "If it's for a healthy food, like milk or fruit, indulge and don't think yourself strange," Dr. Brown says. "If it's for a food that's giving you mostly empty calories, like chocolate or ice cream, try to limit portions." If you are having a hard time avoiding unhealthy foods or find yourself craving nonfood items, such as ice, clay or laundry starch (strange as it seems), it may pay to have a nutritional analysis done, she says. And make sure you discuss it with your health-care provider. Some researchers believe these nonfood cravings are the result of nutritional deficiencies, especially iron deficiency, which is common in pregnant women who are not taking iron supplements.

show women coming up short on calcium. "We found poor pregnant women got about 65 percent of their RDA," Dr. Repke says.

In one study by Dr. Repke and others at Johns Hopkins Hospital in Baltimore, women who were given two grams of calcium a day had lower blood pressure and a lower incidence of pregnancy-induced high blood pressure, than women not receiving calcium supplements. They also were less likely to have premature or low-birthweight babies. "We felt calcium supplementation provided some protection from this disorder," Dr. Repke says.

Ask your doctor about calcium supplements. Most pregnant women need to add calcium-rich foods to their diet or take calcium supplements, Dr. Repke says. The average prenatal vitamin contains only about 20 percent of the RDA. The National Academy of Science recommends calcium supplements for pregnant women who consume only one serving of calcium-rich food a day.

Make sure you're getting enough of other minerals. Several preliminary studies suggest that pregnancy-induced hypertension may also be influenced by levels of magnesium and zinc. "Right now, though, most doctors believe evidence supporting those links is weak," Dr. Repke says. Intravenous magnesium sulfate is given to stop pregnancy-induced hypertension (also called preeclampsia) from progressing to eclampsia, a full-scale medical emergency that may include seizures.

Avoid salt-laden foods. Pregnant women do need extra salt, so a severely salt-restricted diet is less likely to be used these days to control pregnancy-induced hypertension. Still, doctors do nix very salty foods like pickles, potato chips and pepperoni.

Food Tamers for PMS

Could what you eat ease or exacerbate the irritability, bloating, breast tenderness and fatigue some women have in the week or so prior to menstruation? Could certain nutrients, such as vitamin B_6, influence a woman's production of hormones promoting premenstrual syndrome (PMS)? No one knows for sure, but there's some evidence to indicate that good nutrition may ease this rough spot in a woman's monthly cycle.

Along with countless theories about the causes of PMS have come many remedies, from hormones to psychotherapy. Special diets, and sometimes nutritional supplements, have been popular treatments for PMS for years, even though studies that would conclusively support such measures are few and far between.

Vitamin B_6, vitamin E, evening primrose oil and a certain "PMS formula" multivitamin/mineral supplement all seem to show some benefits, according to studies and clinical experience. Eliminating caffeine and alcohol and cutting back on sugar have also been shown to help in some studies, says Susan M. Lark, M.D., author of *The Premenstrual Syndrome Self-Help Book*

GOOD NUTRITION FOR BREASTFEEDING MOMS

You don't necessarily have to eat right to have health-giving breast milk, but you *do* need a balanced diet if you don't want to rob your body of nutrients while you're breastfeeding.

"A woman's body will see to it that most of the nutrients needed in the milk get in the milk, even if it means robbing minerals, fat or protein from other parts of the body to do so," says Judith B. Roepke, R,D., Ph.D., associate provost, dean of continuing education and professor of home economics at Ball State University in Muncie, Indiana, and a member of the La Leche League International professional advisory council.

If you're not getting enough calcium (1,200 milligrams a day) to meet your breastfeeding needs, your body will borrow it from your bones. The price you pay may be osteoporosis later in life. You don't necessarily have to drink milk to make milk, Dr. Roepke says, "but it is true that milk is an easily absorbed source of calcium."

Breast milk uses up to 0.5 to 1 milligram of iron a day, Dr. Roepke adds. Over a month that adds up to less than the amount lost during menstruation. However, many doctors recommend that breastfeeding mothers continue to take an iron supplement to build up their iron stores after pregnancy.

Breastfeeding is also an energy-intensive activity. You'll need 500 extra calories a day, 200 more than you did while you were pregnant, to keep up with the calorie needs of breastfeeding. This will slowly use up the eight or so pounds of fat your body stored during pregnancy just for this use. "Women who breastfeed generally lose a pound or two a month, so that by the time the baby is four to six months old, they are back to their prepregnancy weight," Dr. Roepke says.

Breastfeeding also requires extra fluid. "But the only rule of thumb is: Drink to satisfy your thirst," says Betty L. Crase, La Leche League International's director of scientific information. "Women who force themselves to drink large amounts of milk or water can overload their bodies, which can be just as detrimental to milk production as dehydration."

According to the American Academy of Pediatrics, a good breastfeeding daily menu includes 5 servings of milk or milk products and 4 two- to three-ounce servings of protein foods such as meat, chicken or fish. The U.S. Department of Agriculture also recommends at least 3 to 5 servings of fruits and vegetables and 6 to 11 servings of breads, cereals, rice and pasta.

and director of the PMS and Menopause Self-Help Center, in Los Altos, California.

Based on research studies and her own experiences, Dr. Lark has designed a PMS diet that she says many women find offers across-the-board symptom relief.

"It emphasizes the same kind of healthy eating habits recommended to most people these days," she says.

The PMS diet cuts out what several studies have suggested are PMS-aggravating foods: coffee, refined sugar, chocolate, alcohol, salty and fatty fried foods and anything that qualifies as "junk food" (few nutrients, lots of calories and/or fat). It emphasizes whole-grain complex carbohydrates, including whole-grain cereals, breads, crackers, pancakes, waffles and pasta; legumes, such as lentils and kidney beans; lean meat, especially chicken and fish; raw seeds and nuts; vegetables, especially root vegetables and leafy greens; fresh fruits; and cold-pressed oils such as sesame, olive, corn and safflower oil.

"By reducing simple sugars and caffeine and increasing fiber and complex carbohydrates, this diet helps to stabilize blood sugar, which may play a role in PMS," Dr. Lark says. "It also provides nutrients thought to be important in the management of PMS—B-complex, vitamin E, various minerals and certain types of vegetable oils."

SAILING THROUGH MENOPAUSE

Today, many symptoms of menopause, especially hot flashes and vaginal dryness and thinning, are treated with hormone replacement therapy. But some doctors recommend dietary changes and vitamin/mineral supplements, both for their patients taking hormone replacement therapy and for those who can't or won't take hormones.

What's a menopause diet like? "It's a basic, healthy diet," says Dr. Lark, in her book *The Menopause Self-Help Book.*

The menu is packed with whole grains, vegetables and fruits, leaves plenty of room for fish, allows small portions of meats and poultry, emphasizes vegetable oils over saturated fats, and edges out sugar, high-fat foods, caffeine and alcohol.

Dr. Lark also recommends a range of vitamin and mineral supplements, including calcium and magnesium, which help prevent osteoporosis and may help relieve fatigue, nervousness and irritability; vitamin E, which in some older studies seemed to help reduce the frequency and severity of hot flashes; and bioflavonoids (found in the membranes of citrus fruits), which older studies show also help to reduce hot flashes.

"For women with fibroid tumors, endometriosis or some other condition that prevents them from taking estrogen when they reach menopause, I find that vitamin E and other nutrients are the answer to their problem," Dr. Lark says.

CHAPTER 26

NUTRITIONAL HEALING

AN A-TO-Z GUIDE

"Take two zucchini and call me in the morning." Imagine your doctor scribbling out such a prescription. You might think he's blown a fuse from filling out endless medical insurance forms.

But studies show that dietary changes can sometimes be as effective as drugs in the treatment of certain illnesses—without potentially harmful side effects.

High blood pressure, gout, indigestion and headaches are just a few examples of the health problems that may be completely controlled in some cases with a few judicious dietary adjustments. Even when a health problem requires medical care, proper nourishment often adds a healing advantage. And when it comes to preventing diseases such as cancer and heart disease, studies clearly show that dietary factors—plenty of fruits and vegetables, for instance, and fewer fatty foods—can help provide protection.

In this chapter you'll read about a number of disorders that respond to dietary changes, along with key research findings that detail exactly how to eat for maximum benefits.

In some cases, as we've indicated, good nutrition is considered secondary to proper medical care. In other cases, such as cancer, dietary changes play a purely preventive role; they are not considered part of treatment.

ACNE

Just about anyone who's made it through adolescence is familiar with the bumps and embarrassment of acne. These blemishes occur when skin pores clog up and become infected, usually just before a big event. Hormones, stress and genetics are involved.

White medications—benzoyl peroxide products, topical or oral antibiotics and vitamin A–derived drugs (Retin-A, Accutane)—are the cornerstone of medical treatment, poor diet has long been thought to play a part. And although its role more recently has been downplayed, it hasn't been totally dismissed.

Several studies done during the 1970s and 1980s showed that people eating what's considered a typical Western diet (high in fat and salt and low in fiber) were more likely to have acne than people eating the traditional diets of their region. One study showed that Eskimos who changed to a Western diet developed a number of new diseases, including acne. Another found less acne among blacks in Kenya eating a traditional low-fat, high-fiber diet than among blacks in the United States.

If diet does aggravate acne, no one knows for sure what components are to blame. The usual list of suspects includes chocolate, shellfish, iodized salt, cheese, fatty foods and colas. But studies have failed to show that restricting these foods clears up acne, and most dermatologists now simply advise their patients to eat a well-balanced diet and eliminate only those foods that consistently cause flare-ups. Those foods vary from person to person.

Other nutritional recommendations for acne include:

Get more zinc. Two studies showed that people with acne had lower zinc levels than people without acne. In four studies, supplemental zinc led to fewer breakouts.

Get enough vitamins A, E and B_6, folate, selenium and chromium. All have been found to reduce acne breakouts in some studies.

ALCOHOLISM

Problem drinkers (people who have three or more alcoholic drinks a day) also tend to eat poorly. So their bodies have to endure a double insult—from overindulgence and malnourishment. The combination can be deadly.

The usual treatment for alcoholics trying to stop drinking is to substitute tranquilizers for alcohol, then slowly reduce the dose over time. These drugs ease symptoms of withdrawal. In some cases, nutritional therapy may be included to counteract alcohol's toxic effects and to restore severely depleted nutrients. Some addiction experts believe good nutrition can reduce craving for alcohol, making it easier to stay on the wagon. Their recommendations:

Take a good multivitamin/mineral supplement. Thiamine, folate, magnesium, potassium and calcium are just some of the nutrients alcoholics often lack. Most doctors give supplements until a person is stable and eating well.

Add extras of some vitamins to reduce alcohol's harmful effects. Vitamins C and E, zinc and selenium may help protect the liver; thiamine may help prevent nerve damage; and vitamin E may protect the heart. Discuss dosages with your doctor.

Upgrade your diet. Make sure you're getting enough protein, fruits and vegetables and whole grains. Research is limited, but several animal studies suggest alcohol craving is stronger when it's compounded by poor diet. And one study shows that alcoholics getting nutritional support (individual nutritional counseling and a menu designed by a dietitian) are more likely to abstain than those getting traditional therapy.

ALLERGIES

Does your immune system get all worked up over nothing? Allergies are an overreaction by the immune system to substances normally considered harmless. People with allergies are usually advised to avoid whatever is causing their symptoms, to take drugs that suppress symptoms or to get desensitizing shots.

Diet usually isn't addressed in allergy treatment unless a person reacts to a particular food or food additive, such as sulfites. But some doctors believe certain nutrients may aid the sneeze-prone by tempering allergic response. Their suggestions:

Add vitamin C. Studies show that people with low vitamin C levels have higher-than-normal blood levels of histamine, a biochemical that produces allergic symptoms. In one study, adding extra vitamin C to allergy sufferers' diets resulted in reduced histamine levels.

And vitamin E. In another study, this nutrient dampened histamine-related allergic response.

Try flavonoids. These compounds, found in the membranes of citrus fruits, and in other fruits, vegetables, nuts and seeds, also seem to inhibit some allergic responses. "Data indicate that a number of flavonoids inhibit *in vitro* [test tube] allergic reactions, and may have an influence on many immunologic actions," says Elliott Middleton, Ph.D., of the State University of New York at Buffalo School of Medicine and Biomedical Sciences. Flavonoids are not considered to be vitamins. One widely marketed flavonoid is Quercetin.

ANGINA

Nobody likes getting shortchanged, and when it's your heart running low on oxygen, the result is downright painful.

Angina pectoris is chest pain that occurs when blood flow to the heart is impaired, so heart muscles don't get enough oxygen. Angina usually occurs during physical activity, which increases oxygen needs. Rest or nitroglycerin (which opens arteries, improving blood flow) both relieve angina. Dietary changes can help keep blood vessels clear of fatty deposits and make them less likely to go into spasms. Recommendations include:

Eat low fat. The same lean menu that prevents heart disease can help ease symptoms of angina by preventing further buildup of artery-choking fat deposits. (And a very low fat diet may *shrink* deposits.) A low-fat diet also makes blood cells less likely to clump together or to adhere to blood vessel walls.

Take vitamin E. In one study, low levels of vitamin E were associated with more than double the risk of angina. Although no clinical trials have been done to show vitamin E helps prevent angina, there's good reason to think it might. It has been proven to reduce symptoms of intermittent claudication, a kind of "angina of the leg."

Add magnesium. In several studies, magnesium given intravenously was effective in stopping *variant angina,* spasms in the coronary arteries that are not related to a permanent blockage. It's not the drug of choice in hospitals but magnesium seems to work by relieving the spasms that occur with this type of angina. However, at normal dosage levels it does not seem to help people with *stable effort angina,* which is caused by a permanent blockage. Ongoing research shows that getting adequate magnesium in the diet can be helpful in preventing complications from heart disease.

ANOREXIA NERVOSA

If you think you can't be too thin or too rich, you're only half right. People with anorexia nervosa are obsessed with the fear of becoming overweight. They may eat so little they need to be hospitalized.

Most people who develop anorexia nervosa are women between the ages of 12 and 18. The condition is classified as a psychiatric disorder. It is treated with psychotherapy and a structured eating program. Nutritional recommendations include:

Eat right with a professionally designed diet. Nutrition therapy includes a carefully balanced diet that offers enough calories to first regain weight, and then maintain normal body weight. Monitoring the minerals that control heart rate and blood pressure—potassium, calcium, magnesium and sodium—is particularly important. Imbalances can cause serious problems.

Get adequate zinc in your diet. Some researchers believe correcting a zinc deficiency can help break the cycle of chronic anorexia.

Studies show that women with anorexia nervosa are more likely than normal to be low in zinc. That's important because a zinc deficiency can produce symptoms similar to anorexia nervosa—lack of appetite, depression, changes in taste and smell, cessation of menstrual periods.

"A woman who goes on a weight-loss diet low in zinc may slowly become zinc deficient," explains Laurie Humphries, M.D., associate professor of psychiatry at the University of Kentucky Medical Center in Lexington. "That may lead her into a vicious cycle. She eats less, becomes even more zinc deficient and finally loses her appetite altogether."

Studies also show that women with anorexia nervosa tend to become *more* zinc deficient during refeeding if they are getting only the RDA of zinc. (That's because extra zinc is needed to metabolize the extra calories.)

"Even if an anorexic woman is not clearly zinc deficient when she begins treatment, she can become zinc deficient within 30 days of refeeding unless she gets adequate supplemental zinc," Dr. Humphries says. "Even if they regain weight, women who remain zinc deficient may go back to their old eating habits."

ANXIETY

Anxiety is considered a psychological state—a mix of fear and anger—but it has a definite physical dimension. Along with clammy hands comes rapid heartbeat and fast, shallow breathing, the result of adrenaline pouring into your system.

Traditional treatment includes psychological counseling and anti-anxiety drugs such as tranquilizers. Nutritional recommendations involve avoiding foods that may heighten the physical aspects of anxiety. They include:

Sidestep symptom producers. Anxiety-provoking food components may vary from person to person, but they often include caffeine, alcohol and sugar. Caffeine is a known stimulant. Alcohol is often considered a mild tranquilizer, but when it's abused, withdrawal symptoms can include anxiety. And sugar and other refined carbohydrates can lead to a quick rise, then a big drop in blood sugar. It's the drop that generates anxiety in some people.

Rule out nutritional deficiencies. Some studies suggest that B-vitamin deficiencies can cause anxiety-related symptoms. And some researchers contend that calcium and magnesium deficiencies can cause jumpiness and frayed nerves. But experts in this area say that more research is needed.

ASTHMA

Air may be one of the best things in life that's free, but perhaps you're having trouble getting your fair share. Coughing, wheezing and shortness of breath are the trademarks of asthma.

Anti-inflammatory and other inhalant spray drugs that relax bronchial passages, allergy shots and avoidance of environmental triggers are the usual medical treatments for asthma.

Nutritional therapy is based on eliminating the foods and food additives (such as sulfites) that may cause attacks, and adding nutrients some doctors believe make the lungs less reactive. Recommendations include:

Add vitamins C and E. Some doctors recommend these nutrients as a way to protect the lungs from damaging air pollution and to help tame "twitchy" bronchial muscles.

Havva cuppa java. (Better make that two.) A study suggests drinking coffee regularly may reduce the number of attacks you have. Although not a substitute for medication, a couple of cups of strong coffee might have a short-acting beneficial effect on asthma, adds one allergist. Caffeine and the popular asthma drug theophylline are almost identical, although the latter is much more powerful.

BLADDER INFECTIONS

Burning pain when urinating and the unpleasant sensation of having to go, go, go, even when you've just gone are familiar signs to some people. They could mean a bladder infection is brewing.

Most bladder infections happen when *E. coli* bacteria normally found in the colon make their way into the bladder and multiply, infecting the lining and causing pain and, sometimes, bleeding.

Most bladder infections are easily treated with antibiotics. To help prevent chronic bladder infections, some doctors suggest dietary changes in addition to drug treatment.

Drink plenty of fluids. Urinating frequently helps flush bacteria out of the bladder and stops them from multiplying. Drink enough water and other fluids to make your urine clear; if it's a deep yellow color, you aren't drinking enough, experts say.

Try a cranberry chaser. Although it's controversial and not scientifically proven, many stand by the claim that cranberry juice can help get rid of a bladder infection. The theory: It contains substantial vitamin C, which acidifies the urine and inhibits bacterial growth.

Toss down some vitamin C. Doses of 1,000 milligrams a day are sometimes recommended to deter chronic infections.

CANCER, BREAST

Breast cancer shares top billing with lung cancer as the leading cause of cancer deaths among women. Despite that, premenopausal breast cancer is considered to respond well to medical treatment, especially when the tumor is detected early. Breast cancer appears to have some links with diet, and many experts believe women can cut their risk with changes in eating habits. Their recommendations:

Eat a low-fat diet. Some researchers suggest you try to keep fat intake at 20 to 25 percent of total calories. High-fat diets have been implicated as a cause of breast cancer; in animal studies, the connection is particularly strong.

Fill up on fiber. Preliminary studies suggest that fiber (cereal fiber in particular) reduces blood levels of estrogen, even in the face of a high-fat diet. Too-high blood levels of this hormone seem to promote the development of breast cancer. Aim for 30 grams of fiber a day.

Include vitamins C, E and A, beta-carotene and selenium. In animal studies low intakes of each of these nutrients has been associated with an increased risk of breast cancer.

CANCER, CERVICAL

Thanks to the Pap smear that detects cell changes *before* they become cancerous, the death rate for cervical cancer is at its lowest ever. And healthy eating may pare your risk of developing cervical cancer. Studies indicate cervical cancer is less common in women who get adequate amounts of certain nutrients. Recommendations include:

Fill up on folate. Researchers have found that the risk of cervical cancer climbs sharply in women whose diets are low in this B-complex vitamin found in green leafy vegetables. They speculate that sufficient amounts of folate protect genetic material in cervical cells from virus-induced damage.

Color away risk. In some studies, women who filled up on carotenoid-rich red, yellow and green fruits and vegetables had a reduced risk of cervical cancer.

Add vitamins C and E. Deficiencies of either vitamin have been associated with a higher risk of invasive cervical cancer. Citrus fruits are your best dietary source of vitamin C; for E, it's nuts and vegetable oils.

CANCER, COLON

Of all the types of cancer thought to have dietary links, colon cancer stands out as one of the most obvious. Researchers speculate that most cases of colon cancer cases are linked with diet. Their findings point to these dietary changes.

Eat low fat and high fiber. Fat itself isn't carcinogenic. But it sets off a chain reaction that enhances the development of tumors. Some researchers suggest cutting fat back to 20 to 25 percent of calories. Fiber may help prevent colon cancer a number of ways—decreasing bowel transit time, diluting toxins and carcinogens, lowering blood levels of hormones and binding with cancer-promoting secondary bile acids. Experts suggest increasing fiber intake to about 30 grams a day (double what most people get.)

Drink your milk. A calcium-rich diet has been tentatively linked with reduced risk of colon cancer.

Add vitamins A and D. Both promote the normal development of cells in the colon.

Disarm toxins with vitamins E and C. Both help protect the colon by neutralizing cancer-promoting nitrosamines (chemicals produced during the digestion of nitrates, which are found in preserved meats and some other foods).

Cancer, Lung

Cancer occurs when a cell mutates and starts mutiplying out of control, eventually crowding out or taking over vital organs, causing them to fail. In lung cancer, delicate lung tissue turns into a fibrous tangle that can no longer absorb oxygen. By the time signs of cancer (bloody sputum, persistent cough, shortness of breath) are present, the disease is usually advanced. Treatment involves surgery and chemotherapy. Prevention includes avoiding cigarette smoke and asbestos, both well-known lung cancer promoters. Prevention may also be linked to diet.

Treat your lungs to a salad. Researchers don't know for sure yet if certain nutrients can protect people at high risk for lung cancer. They're studying that right now. But they *do* know that lung cancer rates are lower in people who eat several servings a day of foods high in carotenoids, including beta-carotene, found in green leafy vegetables such as kale and spinach, and in yellow, orange and red fruits and vegetables such as carrots and cantaloupe.

Add vitamins A, E and C and selenium. These nutrients may also cut your risk for lung cancer, although they don't seem to offer as much protection as carotenoids.

Canker Sores

One good thing about canker sores: They're *inside* your mouth, not on your lips where everyone can see them. These small, painful ulcers are common, but doctors can't seem to figure out what triggers them. Injury to the mouth, stress and certain foods may play a role in triggering these lesions, but an altered immune response appears to be the most plausible explanation. Topical antibiotics can rid the sore of the accumulated bacteria that can prolong healing. Astringents, antiseptics or a baking soda rinse may also help in reducing pain.

Nutritional recommendations include:

Check for dietary shortcomings. Iron, vitamin B_{12} and folate deficiencies have been linked to canker sores in some people, according to a study from Scotland. Supplementation for six months improved symptoms in most of the people studied. However, these findings could not be duplicated in several other studies.

Ferret out food sensitivities. They may be associated with canker sores. In one study, about 18 percent of people with canker sores traced their occurrence to eating specific foods. Citrus, chocolate and nuts are the most common offenders.

Cardiac Arrhythmia

In a love song a wild heartbeat may signal romance, but in real life it signals trouble. Cardiac arrhythmia means your heart is beating out of sync, making this vital pump much less efficient at moving blood throughout your body.

Arrhythmia can be caused by many things, including damage to heart muscles caused by heart attack, reactions to heart drugs and an imbalance of heartbeat-regulating minerals known as electrolytes (sodium, calcium, magnesium and potassium).

Cardiac arrhythmias are usually treated by correcting an electrolyte imbalance or by using drugs that help stabilize heart rhythm. Sometimes doctors remove tissue in the heart that is causing the erratic electrical impulses, or implant a pacemaker or other device capable of delivering an electrical impulse to the heart. Nutritional measures include:

Make sure a doctor checks your electrolyte balance. A potassium deficiency is the most commonly diagnosed electrolyte problem. Intravenous or oral potassium supplements (available only by prescription) may correct the problem. Intravenous magnesium sulfate can sometimes correct serious arrhythmias when potassium alone will not work. That's one reason some researchers believe a magnesium deficiency can contribute to heart arrhythmia. A calcium deficiency, or too much calcium can also cause arrhythmia.

Cut back on coffee. Too much caffeine seems to set some hearts aflutter, especially if abnormalities already exist.

Be on the lookout for food instigators. Foods or food additives are a rare cause of heart irregularities in some people.

CARPAL TUNNEL SYNDROME

The carpal tunnel is a sheath of bones and tendons in your wrist that normally protects a major nerve to your hand, the median nerve. If this tunnel collapses and begins to squeeze the nerve, you have carpal tunnel syndrome.

Numbness, pain, weakness and a pins-and-needles sensation in the thumb, index finger and middle finger are your first clues. If untreated, the pain can radiate to the elbow, upper arm and even the shoulder. Eventually, the nerve can be permanently damaged.

Carpal tunnel syndrome seems to go hand in hand with jobs that require repetitious manual motions. Meat cutters, data processors, cashiers and assembly-line workers are especially vulnerable.

Splints that keep the wrist straight, physical therapy, cortisone injections and surgery that cuts ligaments to free the nerve from any underlying adhesions are all standard medical treatments. A few doctors have only one nutritional recommendation.

Take vitamin B_6, with medical supervision. The vitamin is thought to help preserve the integrity of synovian, the thick, slippery sheath that surrounds the bones and tendons in the wrist.

Fairly large doses of B are used (100 to 300 milligrams daily.) Since large doses may *cause* sensory nerve problems, it's important to have your treatment monitored by a doctor. Improvement from B_6 supplementation is said to start within a few weeks, with a complete cure in 8 to 12 weeks for 85 percent of patients.

CATARACTS

Cataracts occur when proteins in the lens of the eye lose their crystal-clear properties, becoming opaque and hard to see through.

Smoking, years of exposure to sunlight, damage to the eyes or an accumulation of sugar in the lens (usually associated with diabetes) can all contribute to cataract development.

Several dietary strategies seem to help shield eyes from the damage that causes cataracts. Recommendations include:

Become a fruit and vegetable fan. In one study, people who ate more than 3½ servings per day of fruits and vegetables had only one-sixth the risk of developing cataracts as people who ate fewer than 3½ servings a day.

Take C and see. Another study found that people taking supplements of vitamin C had a 70 percent reduction in their risk of developing cataracts, compared to the general population.

Make "E" stand for eyes. Research in animals has demonstrated that vitamin E is able to prevent cataract formation to some degree. In one study, people taking 400 I.U. of vitamin E a day reduced their risk for cataracts by more than 50 percent.

CELIAC DISEASE

Bread may be the staff of life for most of us, but for people with celiac disease, it means trouble.

People with this disorder are sensitive to gluten, a sticky protein found in wheat, rye, barley and oats. When they eat gluten, the lining of their intestine is damaged. They develop bloating, cramping and diarrhea and can become malnourished because they have trouble absorbing nutrients. Celiac disease often becomes apparent as soon as cereal is introduced into an infant's diet. Sometimes, though, the first signs of the disorder appear in adulthood.

Steer clear of gluten. A diet that completely eliminates gluten is standard treatment for celiac disease. That means no food that contains wheat, rye, barley or oats. Symptoms usually improve within days or weeks.

Do a temporary bypass around dairy foods. Some people with celiac disease develop lactose (milk sugar) intolerance as well, so these foods may be restricted initially, and slowly added back as the bowel recovers. (Some people will continue to have problems digesting dairy products, and may need to permanently limit their intake.)

Replace missing nutrients. Celiac disease often causes malabsorption, which can create vitamin and mineral deficiencies even in people who are eating well. (The only way to minimize malabsorption is to keep the disease under control with a gluten-free diet.) Using blood tests, your doctor can determine if you are developing nutritional deficiencies. Anemia, especially, may be a tip-off that you need to get more iron, B_{12} or folate.

COMMON COLD

The symptoms—head congestion, sneezing, coughing, runny nose and eyes—begin a few days after your nose is invaded by a virus. You probably know the signs of a common cold all too well, even if you go years between bouts.

Antibiotics are considered inappropriate treatment for a cold. Most doctors suggest you simply let it run its course, or use over-the-counter drugs to ease symptoms. Nutritional suggestions range from symptom-soothing soups to virus-fighting vitamins. They include:

Opt for oranges. Some doctors dispute its effectiveness, but there's no doubt vitamin C remains a popular remedy for colds, perhaps with good reason. One study found that men taking large doses of vitamin C (2,000 milligrams a day) had half the symptoms of men taking look-alike sugar pills. Vitamin C is known to boost immune system response.

Suck on zinc. In one study, cold-infected volunteers who sucked on zinc gluconate lozenges every two hours had less nasal secretion than those using sugar pills. Like vitamin C, zinc is important for boosting immunity.

Go Italian. Dine on garlic, a tasty bulb with proven virus-taming talents.

Turn up the heat. Season foods with chili peppers, curry or cumin, spices with head-clearing, mucus-thinning effects.

Load up on liquids. Plenty of fluids, especially hot soups and herbal teas, may help clear your head by thinning mucus and opening airways.

CONSTIPATION

In medical-ese, constipation is "the infrequent and difficult passage of stool." What's considered infrequent? Less than three times a week. What's considered difficult? Well, if you keep a copy of *War and Peace* by the toilet, and are finding time to read it, you may have a problem.

Drugs, iron supplements, dehydration, poor diet and laxative abuse can all block you up. Knowing what's causing your constipation is important: You may need medical treatment.

If poor diet is contributing to your problem, however, it's time to revamp your habits.

Eat more fiber. Slowly increase your intake of whole-grain breads and cereals, prunes, figs, raisins, corn and other sources of insoluble fiber, giving yourself time to adapt, until you're regular. Also eat foods high in soluble fibers—beans, oat bran, barley, peas, carrots, apples and citrus fruits. Insoluble fibers add lots of *bulk*, moving things along faster. *Soluble* fibers dissolve in water to form a gel that helps keep stools soft.

Drink lots of liquids. Experts suggest one to two quarts a day. That's especially important because fiber needs to absorb fluid before it can have its bulking effect on the stool.

Once you start such dietary measures, always answer nature's call without delay. Even with a high-fiber diet, stools kept "on hold" in the colon become dry and hard.

CROHN'S DISEASE

Crohn's disease is a chronic inflammation that can occur anywhere in the intestine. Most often, it attacks the lower bowel. Diarrhea, cramping, fatigue, loss of appetite and weight loss may all be symptoms. Typically, Crohn's disease starts at around age 25, with attacks every few months. If the disease continues without treatment, the bowel gradually deteriorates.

Most people do get better if they eat no solid food at all, so that treatment is sometimes suggested. They go on an elemental diet, fed through a naso-gastric tube, that puts all the nutrients they need, already broken down, into the intestine. Anti-inflammatory drugs are another treatment option. Dietary recommendations include:

Throw out the junk. Some studies suggest diets low in sugar and refined carbohydrates help people with Crohn's disease. One study, by researchers in Sweden, found that people who ate fast foods at least twice a week were 3½ times more likely to develop Crohn's disease than people who ate these foods less frequently. It also found that people who ate more than 55 grams of sugar per day (the equivalent of about 13 teaspoons) were 2½ times more likely to develop Crohn's disease.

But most U.S. doctors don't think a low-sugar diet would help much. "Unlike celiac disease, Crohn's is not a classic allergy condition. There's no standard diet that's proven to work," says Theodore Bayless, M.D., director of the Meyerhoff Digestive Disease Center at Johns Hopkins Medical Institutions in Baltimore. Dr. Bayless works with patients individually to eliminate symptom-aggravating foods such as milk, and makes sure they eat nutritious meals with adequate protein and calories.

DEPRESSION

It's normal to be sad sometimes. It's part of being human. What's called clinical depression, though, goes beyond sad. Its symptoms include troubled sleep, fatigue, tearfulness, weight loss or gain, and the lost capacity to experience pleasure. Clinical depression is *not* something you can talk yourself out of, or shake off with a smile.

These days, depression is usually treated with drugs that treat brain chemistry imbalances as well as by psychotherapy.

Many nutritional deficiencies have depression as a symptom, but doctors treating depression do not usually test for nutritional deficiencies because normally there's no reason to. Some doctors, however, *do* consider nutritional deficiencies as a possible factor in depression. Their recommendations include:

Ask your doctor if it's appropriate to test for nutritional deficiencies. Especially if you also have fatigue, muscle weakness or irritability. Depression has been associated with deficiencies in folate, vitamin B_{12}, vitamin C, iron, magnesium and potassium.

Cut out caffeine, sugar and refined carbohydrates. Studies suggest avoiding these foods can improve mood in some depressed people.

DIABETES

Diabetes occurs when the body produces too little insulin (called insulin-dependent diabetes) or when it becomes resistant to insulin (called non-insulin-dependent diabetes).

Insulin is needed to break down glucose for energy. When insulin isn't available, this sugar builds up in the bloodstream and organs, causing damage to blood vessels, eyes and kidneys.

Nutritional recommendations for diabetes are designed to maintain normal blood sugar level and to reduce the risk of cardiovascular disease, which is higher-than-normal in those with diabetes. They include:

Reduce to the lean side of normal. Since 85 percent of diabetics are overweight at the time of diagnosis, weight loss is an important part of treatment. They can often keep their blood sugar levels in line with a weight-reducing diet.

Say "no thanks" to dessert. Although restrictions on carbohydrates have been eased, keeping sugar intake to a minimum is still recommended for most people with diabetes. That means you may even need to limit fruit intake.

Put some balance in your diet. Balanced meals with a mix of protein, high-fiber complex carbohydrates and fat are recommended.

Ward off damage with vitamins. There's evidence that vitamin C can help prevent blood vessel damage in those with diabetes. And some studies suggest that B-complex vitamins can help prevent diabetic nerve damage.

Monitor your minerals. Chromium deficiency may be at fault in the development of non-insulin-dependent diabetes. Chromium must be present for the body to move glucose out of the blood and into cells; chromium is also needed for cells to metabolize glucose. In one study, supplementation with 200 micrograms chromium daily brought both high and low blood sugar back toward normal.

Potassium deficiency (associated with the use of some diuretics) is a well-known cause of insulin resistance. In many cases, insulin resistance occurs even though the body is producing plenty of insulin, but it's not being properly utilized by the body's cells.

DIVERTICULOSIS

Diverticulosis occurs when pouches form in the walls of the colon, likely as a result of constipation. Trying to pass hard, dry stools creates so much pressure on the colon walls that they develop permanent pockets. These pockets or pouches can become inflamed or infected. That condition is called diverticulitis.

Large, soft stools help prevent diverticulosis, and tame inflammation in people who already have the disorder. Dietary recommendations include:

Bulk up on fiber. Include both soluble fiber sources (like oat bran, barley, apples, citrus fruits and prunes) and insoluble fiber sources (such as wheat bran, corn bran and vegetables).

Avoid fiber, though, during an acute attack of diverticulitis. In fact, your doctor may want you to avoid solid foods altogether for a few days.

Wash it all down with lots of fluids. Fiber absorbs fluid, so to keep things moving smoothly, it's important to drink plenty of water. Try for eight big glasses a day.

Steer clear of seeds, such as poppy or sesame, and popcorn. Some doctors suspect that small, hard particles such as these can become lodged in the pouches, causing inflammation.

EPILEPSY

If you have been diagnosed with epilepsy, consider yourself lucky to have been born during this day and age. Exorcism will not be considered one of your treatment options.

In epileptics an electrical misfiring of cells in the brain can cause a variety of seizures—from convulsions to vacant staring. More than 50 percent of all cases are considered idiopathic—that is, doctors don't know the cause. Antiseizure drugs are standard treatment for most forms of this disorder.

Most cases of epilepsy are *not* treated with dietary changes. But some are, quite successfully. Dietary recommendations include:

Ask your doctor to check for nutritional deficiencies. Low levels of calcium, magnesium and vitamin B_6 may make some people more seizure-prone. And certain epilepsy medications make nutritional deficiencies more likely.

Make sure you get enough folate. Antiseizure drugs can deplete the body of this important B vitamin. Check with your doctor if you are taking drugs. Folate deficiencies have been associated with serious birth defects.

Check out vitamin E. In a study by researchers at the University of Toronto in Ontario, children with epilepsy whose seizures could not be controlled by medication were given 400 I.U. of vitamin E daily over a period of three months, along with their regular medication. The frequency of seizures was reduced by more than 60 percent in 10 of the 12 children. Six of them had a 90 to 100 percent reduction in seizures.

Vitamin E may protect brain cell membranes from the damaging effects of oxygen or toxic chemicals, making the cells less prone to seizures, researchers say. And it may work in adults as well. (Adults weren't included in this study since they are much less likely than children to have severe epilepsy.)

FATIGUE

Feel like your get-up-and-go got up and went? Join the crowd. Twenty-five percent of all the people in the United States say their tails are dragging. Because there are so many possible causes, the real reason for your fatigue may be hard to pinpoint.

Many nutritional deficiencies have tiredness as a symptom. In some people, multiple deficiencies work together to cause fatigue, so a complete dietary overhaul is in order. Aging, dieting, pregnancy, heavy menstrual periods, absorption problems and, of course, poor eating habits can all set the stage for weariness.

Have your doctor check your iron status. Especially if you are a menstruating woman, iron deficiency is a common and easy-to-diagnose problem.

Beef up your vitamin B intake. Deficiencies of folate, B_6, pantothenate and B_{12} are all associated with fatigue and sometimes also with depression and nerve problems.

Make sure you're getting enough magnesium. This mineral is essential for biochemical reactions that allow the body to burn carbohydrates. In one study, people with chronic fatigue syndrome had low quantities of magnesium in their red blood cells. Receiving magnesium injections to boost their intake improved symptoms in 12 of 15; those with the least energy improved most.

FIBROCYSTIC BREASTS

Breast lumps that ebb and swell with the menstrual cycle are not unusual. They can be the size of peas, grapes or even golf balls. And they can hurt! This condition used to be called fibrocystic breast disease. But since it's so common, the "disease" label has been dropped.

Studies that looked at diet's role in triggering fibrocystic breasts have had mixed results. Still, some doctors suggest their patients try making dietary changes. Among their suggestions:

Avoid coffee, tea, chocolate and cola. These foods contain compounds called methylxanthines. In several studies, women who completely eliminated these foods from their diets had a significant reduction in symptoms.

Eat a low-fat, high-fiber diet with a calorie count that maintains your ideal weight. This kind of diet helps to reduce body levels of estrogen, a known breast-tissue stimulant that is stored in body fat. It may reduce your risk of breast cancer. And some doctors say it can help relieve breast pain. (Some women say avoiding fat-rich dairy products is especially helpful.)

Take vitamin E. Several studies have shown that vitamin E seems to ease monthly breast pain and swelling perhaps by reducing levels of certain biochemicals implicated in the disease. In one study, improvement was found in 15 of 17 women with fibrocystic breast condition who took 600 I.U. of vitamin E daily for two months.

Gallstones

One good thing about gallstones: They develop in an organ you can afford to lose.

The gallbladder is a pear-shaped sac tucked beneath the liver. It holds bile, an important digestive fluid formed by the liver. When food reaches the small intestine, the gallbladder squirts bile through a duct into the intestine. The bile breaks food down into particles small enough to be absorbed.

Bile carries large amounts of cholesterol, which helps digest fats and other foods. Gallstones form when the excess cholesterol in bile "precipitates." Instead of remaining fluid, the cholesterol forms tiny, waxy spheres that slowly become larger and larger, until they are the size of stones. Gallstones may happen because of obesity, diet or a genetic tendency. Not eating for long periods of time also tends to concentrate cholesterol in bile.

Gallstones may be symptomless; if they lodge in a duct, however, the pain will be memorable. These days, stones can be dissolved with drugs or removed by surgery. More frequently, the entire gallbladder is removed.

Dietary measures to sidestep gallstones include:

Stay lean and trim. The more overweight you are, the greater your chances of getting gallstones. Researchers at Harvard University found that women who were slightly overweight had a 70 percent greater risk than ideal-weight women of developing gallstones. And those who were very obese had a 600 percent greater risk.

If you're losing weight, do so gradually. Overweight people who lose weight rapidly on a very restricted diet may be at special risk of forming gallstones, according to a study from Cedars-Mt. Sinai Hospital in Los Angeles.

Up your fiber intake. Fiber, especially water-soluble fiber, escorts cholesterol-laden bile from the body and may also lower your risk for gallstones.

Be a grazer. Small, frequent meals may pare your risk for gallstones by regularly emptying the gallbladder of bile, researchers have found. In one study people who regularly went about 14 hours without eating were more likely to develop gallstones.

Gout

You're in good company if you have gout—Michelangelo, Leonardo da Vinci and Henry VIII all had this disease.

A form of arthritis, a gout attack starts when crystals of uric acid form in the fluid surrounding joints. (Gravity puts the big toe first in line for an attack, but other joints may follow.) The sharp crystals cause painful swelling.

Dietary therapy is designed to reduce body levels of uric acid. That can best be achieved by losing weight. It's also advisable to avoid foods containing purine, an amino acid that breaks down in the body to form uric acid.

Steer clear of purine-containing foods. Anchovies, asparagus, consommé, gravies, organ meats (kidney, liver, heart, sweetbreads), herring, mincemeat, mushrooms, mussels and sardines are all high in purines. Beans, cauliflower, fish (other than those mentioned above), nonorgan meats and poultry are moderately high sources.

Go easy on alcohol. Beer, especially, is high in purines. Moderate beer drinking causes increases in uric acid levels, which may contribute to gout, British researchers have found.

Try cherries. This popular home remedy for gout has been around for a while, and some people claim it does work. Unfortunately, no research has been done on cherries or any of this tasty fruit's components to prove this one way or another. One study indicated that vitamin C improved uric acid clearance from the kidneys, but there are better sources of vitamin C than cherries.

HEADACHE

A headache is a *symptom,* not a disease in itself. Most can be traced to stress-related muscle tension or migraine problems. Some headaches, though, may be linked with food sensitivities, dehydration or caffeine withdrawal.

Toss out your trouble foods. Red wine, caffeine, chocolate, aged cheeses, eggs and milk are all known headache causers for some people. So are foods containing additives like monosodium glutamate (MSG, a flavor enhancer that may be found in many processed foods), nitrates and nitrites (found in preserved meats like hot dogs, salami and bacon), tartrazine (yellow dye #5) and yeast (found in wine and raised baked goods).

Bathe your brain. If the throbbing in your head comes after too much fun and sun or too much alcohol, it is probably due, in part, to dehydration. After a night on the town or a day on the beach, a big glass of water before bed may help avert "morning after" symptoms.

Beware of withdrawal symptoms. Not getting your normal fix of caffeine may cause a headache. If you're trying to cut back or stop drinking coffee, cola or tea, do so gradually to avoid head-pounding symptoms.

HEARTBURN

Considering the strange assortment of foods we toss down, it's no wonder our stomachs sometimes rebel. A bout of heartburn occurs when hydrochloric acid escapes from the stomach into the esophagus, the tube between the stomach and mouth. That produces smoldering pain behind the breastbone and an acrid taste in the mouth. If the condition becomes chronic, the acid can actually erode the esophagus. Changing how you eat is an important part of treatment.

Know when to stop. Stuffing yourself silly is the main cause of occasional heartburn. Your stomach becomes so distended that its contents are pushed back up the esophagus. So eat smaller, more frequent meals. When you're eating out, ask for a doggie bag.

Avoid flame-fanning foods. South-of-the-border dishes are the prime trigger of heartburn, a poll reports, followed by Italian cuisine. In addition to spicy foods, some people have problems with acidic foods like tomatoes, orange or grapefruit juice and red peppers. Others find that grease-laden burgers and French fries, chocolate, alcoholic beverages or peppermint fan their flames. These foods relax the ring of muscles around the lower esophagus that normally keep stomach acid in its place.

HIGH BLOOD PRESSURE

High blood pressure is a serious problem that requires a doctor's attention. Often pressure-lowering drugs are prescribed. But dietary changes are a proven way to prevent or reduce high blood pressure in many people. Among the most important:

Shake the salt habit. This is often recommended as the first line of defense for high blood pressure, with good reason. The sodium in salt makes the body retain water, and too much fluid retention causes blood pressure to rise. Studies show that Americans get up to 20 times as much salt as they need—the equivalent of 2 teaspoons a day, when ⅛ teaspoon would suffice.

Make sure you're getting enough potassium, calcium and magnesium. These minerals, along with sodium, help to regulate the amount of fluid retained in your body. A well-balanced diet generally provides proper amounts of all four minerals and is necessary for normal blood pressure. But studies show that, all too often, potassium, calcium and magnesium come up short. Adding these minerals back by a change in diet away from high-salt foods to more fresh vegetables, grains and fruits often leads to a drop in blood pressure.

Shed pounds. Obese people are three times as likely to have high blood pressure as people of normal weight. In some cases, even losing just half that excess weight normalizes blood pressure.

Add fiber. Some studies show that adding fiber to the diet helps reduce blood pressure.

Eat low fat. Steering away from fatty foods may lower blood pressure directly, and it helps prevent heart disease, a cause of high blood pressure.

Do it all. Studies show a combined approach works best—a low-salt, low-fat, high-fiber, high-potassium, high-calcium, high-magnesium diet. That translates into lots of fruits and vegetables, whole grains, lean meats and low-fat dairy foods.

HYPERACTIVITY

Most of us wouldn't mind having a bit more pep, but people (usually children) who are hyperactive have more energy than they can handle.

Hyperactivity (also called attention deficient hyperactivity disorder) includes many symptoms: fidgeting, excitability, impulsiveness, poor sleep habits, short attention span, compulsive aggression, and memory, reasoning and reading problems.

No one knows for sure what causes hyperactive behavior. Some people believe that, in those vulnerable to hyperactivity, certain compounds found naturally in foods or added to foods play an important activating role.

The Feingold diet, developed by the late Benjamin Feingold, M.D., is a dietary program that eliminates foods containing these compounds. Many pediatricians and food industry spokesmen contend there's little evidence to support the Feingold diet's recommendations. But a National Institutes of Health Consensus Panel Report stated that there were enough individual instances of improvement to warrant a trial of the Feingold diet for one to two months, "after thorough and appropriate evaluation of the child and family—including consideration of other possible therapies." Here's what's involved:

Avoid certain food additives. Avoid *all* food colorings, *all* artificial flavors and three preservatives (BHA, BHT and TBHQ). And avoid medicines containing artificial colors or flavors.

Forgo foods containing salicylates. These naturally occurring substances are found in almonds, apples (also cider and cider vinegar), apricots, all berries, cherries, cloves, coffee, cucumbers and pickles, currants, grapes and raisins (also wine and wine vinegar), nectarines, oranges, peaches, peppers (bell and chili), plums and prunes, tangerines, tea, tomatoes and oil of wintergreen. Aspirin also contains salicylates.

INFERTILITY

About one of every six couples has trouble conceiving. They have tried, without success, for a year or more, to produce a baby. There are lots of reasons for infertility. But when it's not associated with something obvious, infertility may sometimes be traced to poor nutrition.

Check your vitamin C intake. If you're a man, make sure you're getting at least the RDA of 60 milligrams of vitamin C daily. (Smokers should aim for more than 100 milligrams.) Vitamin C helps prevent sperm from sticking together, which keeps them from wriggling toward an egg. It also protects them from genetic damage that can cause birth defects.

Get enough zinc. In adult men, zinc deficiencies lead to reduced levels of testosterone, the main male hormone. And low testosterone levels reduce sperm production. Improving zinc status can normalize testosterone levels, but it may take months.

If you're a woman, maintain your normal weight. Being too thin, or seriously overweight, upsets female hormones and may cause infertility, researchers have found. Gaining or losing weight may be all it takes to become pregnant.

INFLUENZA

It's almost impossible to avoid meeting up with at least a few of the viruses that cause the flu. But whether or not you get laid low is determined in part by your immune system's ability to fight back. And that depends on good nutrition.

Bone up on the Bs. B_6 and other B-complex vitamins play a vital role in immune function. They help produce the cells and chemicals that allow your body to gear up for an attack.

Zero in on zinc. This mineral is important for the proper functioning of the thymus, a gland that produces immune cells. People deficient in zinc have a number of immune system weaknesses that makes them much more prone to infection.

Add vitamin E. This antioxidant shields immune cells from the oxidative reactions that are part of the battle against viral infections.

Stock up on vitamin C. Like vitamin E, vitamin C protects frontline infection fighters. Some immune cells have up to 150 times the amount of vitamin C found in other cells. Vitamin C is used up quickly during infections and is not stored in the body, so it's important to get a fresh supply every day.

Toss down some carrots. Beta-carotene, a pigment found in carrots, sweet potatoes, cantaloupe and other orange-yellow vegetables and fruits, seems to have potent immune-stimulating powers. One study found that about 30 milligrams a day of beta-carotene (about four carrots' worth) produced significant increases in natural killer cells and T-helper cells—two types of immune cells.

IRRITABLE BOWEL SYNDROME

Some people are fussy; they want things to be *just so,* and when they're not, they grumble and have trouble adjusting. Well, some innards react like that, too. A day full of rude people or the wrong foods produces pain, cramps, gas and diarrhea.

This condition, known as irritable bowel syndrome, does not stem from a *physical* problem. There's no inflammation or ulceration of the intestines, for instance. But there is a *functional* problem. Instead of moving food along with coordinated waves of muscle contraction, the bowels go into spasms.

Dietary changes are usually the first course of treatment for irritable bowel. Often, careful eating is all that's needed to relieve symptoms.

Find out if you're lactose intolerant. Lots of people with irritable bowel syndrome are really lactose intolerant. They have a hard time digesting lactose, the sugar found in dairy products. A breath hydrogen test is the surest way to determine if you have this problem.

Fence off the worst offenders. Besides dairy foods, these other foods top the list of culprits: alcoholic beverages, fatty foods, beans, cabbage, onions, spicy or acidic foods, coffee and other caffeinated beverages and foods containing sorbitol or fructose (mostly fruits). Try avoiding these items for a week or so to see if your symptoms ease up.

Take the high-fiber route. A high-fiber diet can soothe spastic intestines. Just make sure you chase the fiber with a big glass of water. (Note: You may need to avoid some high-fiber foods, such as beans, which contain a hard-to-digest starch that can cause gas.)

Opt for acidophilus. Some people with irritable bowel find yogurt or acidophilus tablets helpful. Both contain bacteria that tend to normalize bowel function.

KIDNEY STONES

The majority of kidney stones form as a result of excess calcium in the urine. The calcium combines with other substances, oxalates or phosphates, to form crystals. The resulting stones cause pain in the middle back that radiates around the abdomen toward the genitals.

Some people simply inherit the tendency to form kidney stones, but eating habits also play a role. Dietary measures cannot remove already-formed stones. But they may cut your chances for a recurrence.

Float 'em. Kidney stones can start to form during a single incident of dehydration. So don't let yourself get too dry; drink at least eight glasses of fluid a day.

Factor in fiber. Fiber helps to reduce the amount of calcium in your urine, a major risk factor for calcium oxalate stones, the most common kind.

Save a steer. Vegetarians have a 50 to 60 percent decreased risk of kidney stones compared to meat eaters. Animal protein increases calcium excretion.

Avoid oxalates. Limit these oxalate-containing foods: beans, cocoa, instant coffee, parsley, rhubarb, spinach and tea.

Make sure that you are getting enough magnesium and vitamin B_6. Deficiencies have been associated with an increased tendency for stone formation.

Shake the salt habit. Salt increases calcium excretion in urine.

Don't be too sweet. Sugar also increases urinary calcium concentration.

Cut back on caffeine. Caffeine increases urinary excretion of several minerals, including calcium.

Lupus

Most of the time a raring-to-go immune system is just fine. It keeps your body from becoming "home sweet home" to an array of opportunistic microbes.

With lupus, though, as with other autoimmune diseases, the immune system becomes overzealous. It begins to attack the organs and joints of the body, causing inflammation and tissue damage. One form of the disease, systemic lupus erythematosus, can be fatal. Another form, discoid lupus erythematosus, can cause disfiguring skin problems. Both types flare up, then go into remission. The drugs used to treat lupus often have their own serious effects.

In animal studies, low-fat, low-calorie diets help stop flare-ups. "But these are basically starvation diets that no doctor would recommend to a patient," says Daniel Wallace, M.D., an inflammatory disease expert at the University of California, Los Angeles, UCLA School of Medicine.

Put fish on the menu. Lupus is an inflammatory disease, and several studies indicate that the omega-3 fatty acids found in fatty fish such as salmon, mackerel and sardines can help reduce inflammation. Only a few studies so far have looked at fish oil and lupus. But all showed a beneficial effect. Dr. Wallace suggests his patients eat at least two fatty fish meals a week.

Avoid alfalfa. You can thank the monkeys at the Washington Zoo for this tip. Turns out that they all came down with lupuslike symptoms after eating a diet consisting mostly of alfalfa sprouts. These sprouts contain an immune-system stimulating chemical—enough, apparently, to trigger symptoms in lupus-prone individuals.

Macular Degeneration

Age spots on your skin are easy to see. But age spots of a different sort can appear on the retina at the back of your eye. They're called *drusen,* and they're only visible to a doctor examining your eye. These yellow spots indicate that the cells in the middle of the retina—the macula—are dying, making your central vision fuzzy.

Simply getting old is the biggest risk factor for macular degeneration. The risk increases, though, if you're light-eyed and fair-skinned. And exposure to sunlight may also play a role.

Dietary suggestions for macular degeneration are meant to keep retinal cells healthy and ward off sunlight-related damage.

Make sure you're getting enough zinc. In one study, a group of healthy older people taking zinc supplements had significantly less loss of vision due to macular degeneration than a group taking blank pills. Zinc supplements should only be taken with medical supervision. Large doses interfere with other minerals such as copper.

Protect your retinas with vitamins C and E, beta-carotene and selenium.

Results from studies using these nutrients show a significant retardation of vision loss in people with macular degeneration. Damage seems to be cut by about one-third.

MITRAL VALVE PROLAPSE

Normally, the valves that regulate the flow of blood through the heart close neatly, snapping shut with the sounds—*lub-dub*—that we recognize as a heartbeat.

With mitral valve prolapse, though, an additional click is added to the heartbeat, as the valve strains against the pressure of blood, almost like a parachute being snapped in the wind. If the valve lets some blood leak backward into the chamber of the heart from which it's just come, you have a heart murmur.

Mitral valve prolapse usually produces no symptoms. In some people, though, it's associated with chest pain, fatigue, heart palpitations, muscle cramps, episodes of low blood pressure and anxiety. Most doctors treat their patients with beta-blockers, drugs that help regulate heart rate. Some, however, prescribe magnesium, a mineral vitally important for proper functioning of the heart muscle.

Ask your doctor to check your red blood cell magnesium levels. Several studies have found that a high percentage of people with mitral valve prolapse have lower than normal magnesium levels.

In one study by researchers at the University of Alabama School of Medicine, people with mitral valve prolapse and low magnesium levels showed a marked improvement in symptoms after taking supplemental magnesium. Muscle cramps decreased by 90 percent, and chest pain was cut by 47 percent. Palpitations were also markedly diminished.

MOTION SICKNESS

There's no doubt that stomachs prefer terra firma. Send them spinning, bouncing or bobbing for too long and they're likely to get plenty upset.

Even though the symptoms settle in the stomach, motion sickness doesn't start there. It starts in your head, when your brain gets confused between motion your inner ears sense and motion your eyes see. The result is an unpleasant mix of dizziness, sweating, nausea and anxiety.

Some people are more sensitive than others, but a bumpy ride in the back of a pickup truck, a spin on the twirly-whirl or boating in choppy surf can eventually turn most stomachs sour. Drugs to prevent motion sickness are available in pill and patch forms, but there are also self-care cures.

Go gingerly. Pleasant, spicy ginger has proven antinausea effects. Some experts suggest taking two capsules (450 milligrams each) of powdered gingerroot at least ten minutes before movement begins, and more as needed. (The effects do not last very long.)

Travel on half a tank. Stomachs stay calmer if they have a bit of food in them, experts say. An empty stomach creates worse motion sickness symptoms. Try munching on soda crackers, a piece of bread or a hard pretzel.

Stick with quease-free foods. Foods that make you mildly queasy when you're standing still can bring on a case of the roaring heaves when they're combined with motion sickness, experts say. So save those foods for the times when your stomach has nothing else to contend with.

Save the martinis for port. Too much alcohol can disrupt the balance mechanism in your inner ear, setting your head spinning. That's enough in itself to make you sick, and it's likely to turn the tide against you when you're battling motion sickness. Sip ginger ale or a cola instead. Both have stomach-settling potential.

MUSCLE CRAMPS

They can grab you just about anywhere, but muscle cramps are most likely to go for your calves or feet, two body parts that do much of the work when you walk, and so are more likely to suffer abuse. These painful, prolonged contractions can be caused by various things: overuse, dehydration, muscle injuries or tightness, mineral inbalances and poor circulation.

To prevent muscle cramps, warm up with light exercise, such as easy walking, followed by stretching, before beginning a vigorous workout. Soothe cramped muscles with stretching and massage.

Nutritional recommendations to prevent muscle cramps are designed to maintain normal body levels of fluid and minerals, two factors vital to properly functioning muscles. They include:

Drink up. Drink a cup or more of water before you begin an exercise routine, and ½ cup every half-hour or so, whether you're thirsty or not. Drink more if it's hot and you're sweating a lot. Dehydration is a common cause of exercise-related cramps. Diuretics (drugs often used to control high blood pressure) can cause dehydration.

Make sure you're getting enough calcium, magnesium and potassium. These minerals are involved in muscle contraction and relaxation; too little, or too much, of any one can make muscles weak, trembly or quick to cramp. Calcium supplements have been shown to relieve leg cramps during pregnancy. Sodium is important, too. If you're on a low-sodium diet and have persistent muscle cramps, talk with your doctor.

Try vitamin E. A few studies suggest that supplemental vitamin E improves symptoms of intermittent claudication, a leg-cramping condition caused by poor blood flow. It seems to enhance the body's oxygen delivery system. Oxygen is important to hard-working muscles.

NAIL PROBLEMS

If you're using your fingernails as screwdrivers or staple removers, or nibbling on them for an afternoon snack, you already know why they're so beat up. If you have brittle or disfigured nails for no apparent reason, though, it's possible you may need a nutritional boost. Like skin and hair, fingernails can be a indicator of general nutritional status.

Ask your doctor about biotin. Veterinarians give this B vitamin to horses with problem hooves, and it works wonders. So Swiss researchers decided to try it out on people with brittle and splitting fingernails. After three to four months of daily treatment, their nail flexibility was boosted significantly. Good sources of this nutrient include cauliflower, lentils, milk and peanut butter.

Check for other nutritional deficiencies. Horizontal furrows across a nail or spoon-shaped nails may indicate low iron status.

OBESITY

Those of us whose battle of the bulge has turned into the longest standoff in history know at least one basic rule: To lose weight, we need to consume fewer calories than we burn up as energy. Sounds simple, but when it comes down to rationing out the Melba toast, most of us are soon ready to shout "Surrender!" We're *hungry.*

So what's the trick to successful weight loss? Here's what experts suggest.

Take aim at fat, not calories. Limit your intake of fats such as butter, mayonnaise, marbled meats, oils and most baked goods so that you aren't getting more than about 25 to 30 percent of calories from fat. Fats are the most concentrated source of calories; it's also easier for our bodies to make fat from fat, than from protein or carbohydrates.

Satisfy your hunger with fiber. High-fiber foods like oatmeal, carrots and beans fill you up, not out. Some doctors recommend raw vegetables with a meal or as a snack.

Don't go too low. Diets that offer fewer than 1,200 calories a day for women, or 1,400 for men, can backfire because they provide too few calories. Metabolism (calorie burning) slows down. It's much better to eat a few more calories and make exercise a regular part of your day. That way you build muscle mass and shed fat.

OSTEOARTHRITIS

Do your knees snap, crackle and pop when you kneel? It could be that your joints are developing some painful rough spots. Smooth, rubbery cartilage is wearing away; what's regrowing may be rough and hard. Doctors call the problem osteoarthritis, and it's considered an inevitable consequence of aging. By age 70, almost everyone has it.

Nutritional recommendations for osteoarthrits are meant to help repair cartilage and keep underlying bone strong.

Drop a load. Being overweight is a well-established risk factor for osteoarthritis of the knees. One theory is that obesity puts the squeeze on weight-bearing joints. Some patients who lose weight have less pain.

Eat an orange; better yet, eat two. Vitamin C is important for the formation of collagen, a fibrous material that's used to make both bone and cartilage. In animal studies, adequate vitamin C slowed the development of osteoarthritis. Some doctors advise their older patients with arthritis to take about 1,000 milligrams of vitamin C a day.

Check your calcium. Calcium helps maintain the underlying structure of the joint—the bones. Many people with osteoarthritis also have osteoporosis, and say that extra calcium helps ease their bone pain.

OSTEOPOROSIS

Imagine bones as weak and fragile as a termite-infested log. That's what can happen with osteoporosis. Instead of being strong and dense, the bones become porous, light and frail. The least blow, sometimes even the weight of your own body, can cause them to snap.

Postmenopausal women are at highest risk for osteoporosis. Nutritional recommendations are meant to enhance the bone-preserving effects of estrogen replacement therapy, which slows bone loss.

Bone up on calcium. Get at least the RDA of calcium during the premenopausal years. That's 800 milligrams daily for women aged 19 to 50. Studies indicate most women fall far short. After menopause, some doctors recommend 1,000 to 1,500 milligrams daily.

Make sure you're getting adequate vitamin D. This nutrient is essential for calcium absorption and utilization. Two cups of milk provide the RDA of 200 I.U. of vitamin D. Sunlight also allows the body to produce vitamin D.

Add other minerals. Manganese, magnesium, zinc, copper, boron and other nutrients also play a role in the formation of bone. The best way to get these nutrients? Eat a varied diet of wholesome foods, including nuts and seeds; leafy greens; sea vegetables such as nori, laver and kombu; fruits; whole grains; beans; shellfish and lean red meat.

Limit coffee to two cups a day. Studies show that caffeine increases urinary and fecal calcium loss.

PARKINSON'S DISEASE

Imagine being trapped in a body that balks at the simplest tasks. That's what can happen with Parkinson's disease. Brain cells that produce an important chemical messenger slowly die; the result is slowness and reduced movement, rigid muscles, trembling and balance problems.

Parkinson's disease may be caused by a combination of factors: exposure to toxins or viruses, genetic vulnerability, even aging. Only recently has nutrition been thought to play a possible role. Researchers suspect some nutrients may help delay or prevent the brain cell death that causes symptoms.

Add antioxidants. A preliminary study suggests that large amounts of antioxidant nutrients—vitamins E and C—slow the progression of Parkinson's disease, delaying by 2½ to 3 years the time when a symptom-reducing drug, L-dopa, is required.

If you're taking L-dopa, watch daytime protein. High-protein meals may interfere with your body's ability to use L-dopa. One dietary program saves high-protein foods (meats, fish, eggs, legumes, dairy products) for your evening meal, eaten shortly before bedtime. That way, amino acid levels peak while you're asleep, blocking L-dopa when it matters least.

PERIODONTAL DISEASE

Periodontal means "around a tooth" and it refers to any disorder of the gums or other supporting structures of the teeth. In periodontal disease, sticky deposits of bacteria, mucus and food particles, called plaque, accumulate on teeth. Plaque causes the gums to become infected and swollen, forming pockets between teeth that trap even more plaque. The infection can eventually cause teeth to loosen as it eats away the bone in the jaw. Gum disease is usually treated with professional cleaning, antibiotics to treat infection, and sometimes, surgery to remove infected gum tissue and and reshape the bone.

Nutritional treatment to control gum disease includes avoiding foods that promote plaque formation, and adding foods that help fight infection and rebuild gum and bone tissue.

Avoid dental enemy number one. That's sugar. When you eat it, you set the stage for plaque-forming bacteria to take over your mouth. If you do eat sugary foods, eat them as part of a meal, not as snacks. And brush afterward.

Eat an orange. Even a borderline deficiency of vitamin C increases your chances of developing bleeding, infected gums. And if you're vitamin C deficient, studies show that increasing your intake may help reduce gum inflammation.

Say Mo-o-o-o-o-o-o. . . . Teeth need calcium to stay anchored in the jawbone. Calcium deficiency is associated with bone loss around the tooth. In addition to making teeth wobble, that makes room around the gumline for bacteria to move right in.

Balance your act with other nutrients. Folate, vitamins A and E, zinc and magnesium are also important for healthy teeth, gums and jawbone.

PREMENSTRUAL SYNDROME

Premenstrual syndrome (PMS) includes an array of physical and psychological changes, including bloating, breast tenderness, headache, fatigue, anxiety, depression and food cravings. These symptoms are associated with hormonal shifts in a woman's body, but just why one woman suffers so much while another breezes through this time of month is a mystery.

Studies show mixed results when it comes to any particular dietary regimen, but many women say they feel better following a special nutritional program. Most emphasize well-balanced, low-fat, high-fiber meals, along with nutritional supplements.

Dietary recommendations include:

Axe PMS-aggravating foods. Certain foods seem to aggravate PMS symptoms. Coffee, sugar, chocolate, alcohol and salty and fatty fried foods stand out as the main culprits in some studies; you may need to do some experimenting to determine which, if any, affect you.

Eat all-around healthy foods. One very popular PMS eating program, designed by Susan M. Lark, M.D., author of *The Premenstrual Syndrome Self-Help Book,* fulfills all the requirements of a healthy diet. It offers whole-grain cereals, breads, crackers, pancakes and waffles and pasta; legumes, such as lentils and kidney beans; lean meat, especially chicken and fish; raw seeds and nuts; vegetables, especially root vegetables and leafy greens; fresh fruits and oils such as sesame, olive, corn and safflower. A diet featuring these foods, followed conscientiously—not just before your period—may help alleviate some of the symptoms of PMS.

Ask your doctor about supplemental nutrients. Vitamins B_6 and E, calcium and a certain PMS formula multivitamin/mineral supplements all seem to show some benefits, according to studies and clinical experience.

PROSTATE ENLARGEMENT

Enlargement of this walnut-size gland, located just below the bladder, is the most common prostate problem. The growth, called benign prostatic hyperplasia, occurs in more than 80 percent of men older than age 60. If you have an enlarged prostate, you may need to get up to urinate at night or have trouble completely emptying your bladder. You may develop bladder infections, or, with prolonged urinary obstruction, kidney problems. The enlargement is thought to be due to hormonal changes that occur as a man ages.

Any prostate problem deserves a doctor's diagnosis and monitoring. That's because prostate cancer is one of the most common cancers among men and the second leading cause of cancer deaths.

Most doctors treat benign prostate enlargement with drugs that shrink the gland or surgery that removes excess tissue blocking the urinary passageway. However, a few doctors may suggest a trial of nutritional therapy first.

Ask your doctor about zinc. Some doctors suggest their patients with benign prostatic hyperplasia take zinc sulfate. (Zinc gluconate, the more common form of zinc supplements, apparently does not reach the same level of absorption in the prostate.) There's some clinical evidence (but no studies with a control group of men not taking zinc) that indicates zinc may be helpful for benign enlargement. But zinc apparently does not help the firm, nodular variety of prostate enlargement. (A urologist can easily feel the difference between the two types.)

One urologist who prescribes zinc sulfate for his patients with benign prostatic hyperplasia recommends a preparation that also contains vitamin

C, magnesium and B vitamins. He says these nutrients seem to help the body absorb and use the zinc more efficiently.

PSORIASIS

The dry, silvery scales that sometimes characterize psoriasis most commonly appear in spots on the scalp, elbows and knees, back or buttocks. In more severe cases, the scales may cover the entire body.

One out of three cases of psoriasis is thought to be inherited. Scaling occurs because the cells that produce skin, called epidermal cells, have cranked up production. Instead of taking 28 to 30 days to produce a new layer of skin, they take only 6 to 8 days. The result: a birthday suit with plenty of quantity but little quality.

Tar ointments, cortisone creams and ultraviolet therapy are the usual treatments.

Psoriasis generally is *not* considered to be caused by poor nutrition. Nevertheless, nutritional intervention has offered relief in some cases.

Ask your doctor about fish oil . . . In some studies, omega-3 fatty acids found in fish oil improved symptoms of people with psoriasis. (In one study, it also improved symptoms of psoriatic arthritis, a related condition.) The fish oil worked best when used in addition to other treatments; by itself, improvement was only modest.

. . . And about new synthetic vitamin treatments. In several studies, either topical or oral forms of vitamins A and D have reduced scaling in people with psoriasis. Since these experimental drugs can have serious side effects, their use requires medical supervision. Over-the-counter versions of vitamins A and D are not considered to help psoriasis and can be harmful in large amounts.

RAYNAUD'S SYNDROME

It's normal for blood vessels in your hands and feet to constrict somewhat when they are exposed to cold, or when you're under stress. Most of us don't even notice it. With Raynaud's syndrome, though, the response is exaggerated. Blood flow is severely restricted and sometimes stops completely. The condition can cause discomfort, numbness, even pain.

In severe cases, hands change color—from white, as blood leaves, to blue, as venous blood pools, to deep red, at the end of the attack as freshly oxygenated blood rushes in. The whole process can last from less than one minute to as long as several hours.

Most cases of Raynaud's are mild and have no known cause. They are usually treated simply by taking care to keep hands warm. More serious cases may be caused by a connective tissue disorder or repeated physical stress, especially vibration. These cases may be treated with drugs that help maintain normal blood flow.

Mild cases, with no known cause, may respond to a dietary addition: fish oil.

Take a mackerel to lunch. The omega-3 fatty acids concentrated in fatty fish seem to help keep blood vessels open in some people with Raynaud's syndrome.

In one study, symptoms stopped altogether in 5 of 11 people taking fish-oil capsules daily for 12 weeks. The other 6 extended the time they could keep their hands submerged in cold water from 31 to 46 minutes (an increase of 50 percent) before blood flow to their fingers shut down. In a comparison group of 9 other people with Raynaud's taking olive oil, only 1 showed any improvement.

Restless Legs Syndrome

You're not camping out under the stars, but you feel like a whole forest of creepy crawlers is attacking your legs. Unfortunately, even the strongest insect repellents won't help. The strange, crawling sensation is a neurological condition called restless legs, so named because the odd feelings (people describe them as "like writhing worms" or "crawling with ants") make the urge to move your legs irresistible.

People with restless legs syndrome notice these sensations most often when they're at rest—often in bed. Walking seems to ease symptoms.

Although restless legs is considered a malfunction of the nerves in the legs, doctors find no apparent neurological abnormalities or other evidence of disease. The disorder is most likely to develop in people with higher-than-normal blood levels of uric acid, including people on kidney dialysis and those with diabetes. Pregnant women sometimes develop restless legs; the condition usually disappears after delivery.

Some cases of restless legs respond to a variety of muscle-relaxing or antiseizure drugs; others, to nutritional therapy.

Make sure you're getting enough iron. Restless legs syndrome has long been associated with iron-deficiency anemia. Menstruating women and older people who are taking drugs for rheumatoid arthritis may have low iron status.

Check your folate intake. Restless legs sometimes includes symptoms of pain or numbness. Studies suggest that folate may help these symptoms.

Junk the java. Doctors report that some patients who stop drinking caffeinated beverages get relief.

Rheumatoid Arthritis

For decades, some people with rheumatoid arthritis have contended that eating certain foods made their joint pain and swelling worse, and that avoiding those foods eased their symptoms. Some doctors listened, but most pooh-poohed the idea. More recently, there has been enough hard evidence to help sort fact from fiction and provide some nutritional guidance when it comes to arthritis relief. Even the Arthritis Foundation, a longtime holdout against the notion of a diet-arthritis link, now says, "There are some scientific reasons to think that diet might affect certain kinds of arthritis in some patients."

Dietary changes seem to work best used along with such standard treatments as exercise, heat or cold and medications.

Dietary strategies seem to help rheumatoid arthritis in some patients by reducing joint tenderness. Avoiding bad flare-ups is important; it may spare your joints from additional damage.

Talk to your doctor about fish oil. Several studies have shown that the omega-3 fatty acids found in highest concentrations in fatty fish like salmon, mackerel and sardines help reduce tenderness, possibly by reducing inflammation. Some doctors suggest eating fatty fish a few times a week.

Rule out food flare-ups. Some people with arthritis have increased joint pain soon after they eat particular foods. (That's one reason short-term fasting or vegetarian diets seem to help some people.) Since just about any food—or component of food—can be implicated, it's important to work with a doctor who can help you pinpoint your symptom-producing foods, if any.

Make sure you're eating extra well. Nutritional deficiencies might exacerbate rheumatoid arthritis in some people: Studies from researchers around the world suggest that copper, selenium, zinc, vitamins C and E and pantothenate may all play a role in this disorder.

STROKE

The results of a stroke can be devastating. Because it's your brain that's injured, you may lose the ability to move parts of your body. You may also lose the capacity to see, feel or speak. Imagine not being able to converse with people you've known all your life, or being unable to say the words "I love you."

A stroke is usually caused by a blood clot that disrupts blood flow to parts of the brain, allowing brain cells to die, or by a hemorrhage that destroys brain tissue. Some people have a mini-stroke, which does little damage but is a serious warning that a full-blown stroke may be coming. It is possible to reduce your risks of a major stroke by reducing blood pressure, not smoking, lowering high cholesterol, losing weight, if necessary, and improving your eating habits.

Cut the fat. Eighty-four percent of strokes are caused by a blockage of the blood supply to the brain, either from a blood clot or fatty plaque that obstructs the cerebral arteries. This obstruction causes a kind of a "heart attack of the head." Reducing blood cholesterol by cutting back on dietary fat can reduce your risk of this kind of stroke.

Toss your salt shaker. High blood pressure can dramatically increase your risk of stroke, especially hemmorhagic strokes. For many people, a high-salt diet sends blood pressure creeping upward.

Eat an extra serving of fruit or vegetables each day. In one study, one additional serving of fresh fruit or vegetables a day was associated with a 40 percent reduction in the risk of a fatal stroke. It is believed that the high levels of potassium in fruits and vegetables are responsible. This mineral plays a vital role in the regulation of blood pressure.

Lay off the hard stuff. Several studies have shown that drinkers, and especially heavy drinkers and binge drinkers, are more likely to have the kind of stroke caused by hemmorhaging within the brain.

TASTE IMPAIRMENT

Some people might think it would be just dandy if they couldn't taste foods. Then they wouldn't be lured into overindulgence by their mouth-watering response to flame-broiled burgers or fresh-baked brownies.

The fact is, though, that people who can't taste—or who have a distorted sense of taste—often lose their appetite altogether and become malnourished. Plus, they make terrible cooks!

Nasal viruses and exposure to toxic chemicals are common causes of taste (and smell) disorders. They may cause a temporary problem, but sometimes the effects are permanent.

One nutrient—zinc—has been associated with taste and smell disorders.

Ask your doctor to test for zinc deficiency. Zinc deficiency is a possible cause of taste and smell impairment. Zinc-depleting drugs, poor eating habits, alcoholism, kidney disease or the stress of surgery or severe burns can all set the stage for zinc deficiency. Even if your blood zinc level is normal, your doctor might detect a deficiency with a 24-hour urinary zinc excretion test.

If they're going to work at all, zinc supplements should improve symptoms within weeks. In studies, 440 milligrams of zinc sulfate (equivalent to 176 milligrams of elemental zinc) or 15 to 25 milligrams of zinc acetate or gluconate were effective. Some doctors recommend their patients continue to take supplements for a few weeks after their symptoms improve, then cut back to RDA levels—15 milligrams for men, 12 milligrams for women.

TINNITUS

Experts estimate that 40 to 50 million Americans experience the internal jangle of hums, roars, buzzes, clicks or, of course, ringing, that characterizes tinnitus.

For most, the sounds are barely noticeable annoyances that last from a few minutes to a few days. For others, though, the noise becomes increasingly loud and persistent, to the point where it disrupts their lives and sends them on the search for treatment. Ringing ears can be caused by loud noises, drugs, allergies or health problems. In some cases, symptoms can be relieved with a small electronic device, known as a masker, which is usually combined with a hearing aid. The masker produces a competitive but pleasant sound that for some people masks the tinnitus.

Most dietary recommendations for tinnitus are designed to address some of the whole-body ailments that can contribute to the problem: high blood pressure, high cholesterol or diabetes. A few recommendations, however, address tinnitus directly.

Avoid caffeine and alcohol. In people who already have tinnitus, overindulging in these foods can make symptoms worse. Red wine, in particular, can turn up the volume for some people. (Nicotine, although not a food, does the same thing. So do aspirin-containing drugs.)

Hold the MSG. In some people, this common food additive causes ears to buzz.

ULCERATIVE COLITIS

This serious inflammatory bowel disease strikes the colon, causing the intestinal wall to break down. Bloody diarrhea, mucus, pain and fever signal a flare-up. Treated promptly with anti-inflammatory drugs, symptoms usually subside.

Dietary treatment for ulcerative colitis involves avoiding foods that aggravate symptoms, and filling up on those that help.

Go fish. In one study by researchers at the University of California at Davis, daily doses of inflammation-fighting fish oil soothed the symptoms of ulcerative colitis. Eleven men who took 4.2 grams of fish oil a day for three months had a 56 percent decline in the severity of the disease, while another group taking a placebo (harmless blank pill) had only a 4 percent decline. Eight of the men taking fish oil were able to reduce or eliminate their medication. There were no side effects from the fish oil.

Pinpoint trouble foods. Foods aren't thought to cause ulcerative colitis, but once you have developed the disorder, certain foods seem to make symptoms worse. One study found that people with ulcerative colitis had developed a sensitivity to cow's milk. In another, 10 of 13 ulcerative colitis patients on a dairy-free diet remained symptom-free, compared to 5 of 13 people on a control diet that contained dairy products. Fatty foods also seem to cause problems for lots of people. Raw fruits and vegetables, along with other high-fiber foods such as popcorn and bran, are often restricted, too.

Ask your doctor about pectin. Doctors often restrict solid food during a flare-up. In one study, people with ulcerative colitis fed a liquid diet containing pectin (a soluble fiber found in fruits and used to thicken jellies) fared better that those fed the usual liquid diet.

ULCERS

Doctors used to think gastric ulcers were caused by too much stomach acid or a combination of acid and stress. Treatments were designed to decrease or neutralize stomach acid, one way or another. Bland diets were often recommended.

Now, though, it's thought that the development of gastric ulcers is more complex. Researchers believe bacteria (*Helicobacter pylori*) that lodge in the stomach and upper intestine are probably involved in the development of some, if not most, cases of ulcers. The bacteria, thought to secrete chemicals that attack the lining of the stomach or intestine and make it vulnerable to acid erosion, can be found in more than 50 percent of people age 60 or older. Although most people who have the bacteria *do not* develop ulcers, those who do are much less likely to have a recurrence if the bacteria is eradicated with a combination of drugs.

Dietary recommendations are designed to help minimize symptoms while an ulcer is healing and to provide the materials a body needs to heal properly. They include:

Aim for optimal nourishment. Vitamins A and C, zinc and other nutrients are essential for wound-healing. In one study, large amounts of vitamin A helped ulcers heal faster. In another, extra vitamin A reduced formation of ulcers in people with severe burns, injuries or postoperative complications. And in another, zinc supplements resulted in faster healing and reduced pain. In an animal study, vitamin E reduced the occurrence of stress ulcers. Several studies suggest vitamin C helps ulcers heal faster.

Eat full-size meals at regular intervals. "Snacking stimulates stomach acid production but doesn't provide enough food to buffer the additional acid," explains William Ruderman, M.D., chairman of the Department of Gastroenterology at the Cleveland Clinic in Fort Lauderdale, Florida. "I tell my snackers to become meal eaters."

Eat whatever you want, but avoid foods that have given you an upset stomach in the past. Coffee and strong tea stimulate gastric acid secretion, irritating an already fussy stomach. Spicy hot foods have pretty much gotten a bum rap—they don't *cause* ulcers. But if they upset your stomach, stick with tamer fare.

Don't count on milk to soothe your stomach. Initially, it may neutralize acid and you may feel better. But milk actually stimulates acid release: Thirty minutes or more after drinking milk, your acid level goes up. Rely on antacids instead.

VAGINAL YEAST INFECTIONS

The main sign of a vaginal yeast infection is an itch that won't quit in a place that's never scratched in polite company.

Yeast is normally found in the vagina, but with a yeast infection, it grows out of control. Antibiotics, birth control pills, even semen can upset the vagina's slightly acidic balance and allow yeast to flourish. The yeast can be killed with over-the-counter creams designed just for this purpose. The creams are very effective, with few side effects.

Nutritional therapy is not meant to cure an existing infection. But it can help reduce the number of infections a woman gets. It's aimed at edging the yeast out with beneficial bacteria and restoring the vagina's normal acid balance, which helps keep the yeast population in check.

Eat a cup of live-culture yogurt every day. Yogurt is a popular home remedy for vaginal infections—women eat it or apply it topically. A study confirms that eating yogurt really does work, and even helps women with chronic, drug-resistant vaginal yeast infections. In the study, women who ate one cup a day of yogurt containing live *Lactobacillus acidophilus* (a beneficial type of bacteria that colonizes the vagina and colon) had a clear-cut reduction in symptoms of itching, burning and discharge. During a six-month yogurt-eating period, the average number of infections in the group fell from 2.5 per woman to less than 1.

PART 4

USING FOODS WISELY

CHAPTER 27

BASIC STRATEGIES

PICK AN EATING PLAN YOU CAN LIVE WITH

In *The Wizard of Oz,* Dorothy asks Toto the way to the Emerald City. The Scarecrow, hanging nearby, points in *both* directions.

Americans, when it comes to their diets, are a lot like Scarecrow. We want to be healthy *and* feast on pizza, lose weight *and* grab some ice cream. In other words, we not only worry about our cake, we eat it, too.

A Gallup poll perfectly illustrates our yes/no relationship with nutrition. According to the poll:

- Nearly three in four Americans worry about nutrition.
- More than half of all adults say they have significantly changed their eating habits in recent years.
- More than half of grocery shoppers say they read the labels on new foods most or all of the time.

Are we on the road to nutritional health? Not quite. When the people polled were asked to plan a "perfect" meal, nutrition wasn't necessarily the first thing on their minds. Like their parents before them, they craved steak and potatoes, followed by cheesecake or ice cream for dessert.

There's quite a difference between what we think we should eat and what we actually eat, says Marion Nestle, Ph.D., professor and chairperson of the Department of Nutrition, Food and Hotel Management at New York University in New York City.

"The general attitudes toward dietary change in this country reflect a one-third, one-third, one-third trend," adds C. Wayne Callaway, M.D., associate clinical professor at the George Washington University Medical Center in Washington, D.C. According to Dr. Callaway, one-third of people learn about nutrition and make changes in their diet. Another third know they should change their habits, but don't. The last group, unconvinced of the merits of dietary reform, are best described as the still-alive club: "I ate hamburgers and fries yesterday and I'm still alive."

Making Nutrition Work for You

Whichever group you belong to, launching a healthy-eating lifestyle can be a confusing process. "There are so many guidelines out there, it's easy for people to throw up their hands and shout, 'I give up,' " says Jeannette Miller, R.D., a nutrition consultant and newspaper columnist in Carbondale, Illinois. "But if they pick just one sensible set of guidelines that they can follow and live with, they'll have a much easier time of it."

In a bit, we'll discuss some of the specific guidelines that can help you plan a nutritious, eminently enjoyable diet. But first let's look at some general rules that can help make your path (whichever one you finally choose) as easy as possible.

Be creative. "There are many ways to eat an adequate diet," says Paul R. Thomas, R.D., Ed.D., project director of the Food and Nutrition Board of the National Academy of Sciences in Washington, D.C. "Make sure you eat a wide variety of grain products, fruits and vegetables. Flexibility is the key." If you usually eat spaghetti, for example, try some spinach fetuccine, instead. Instead of a three-bean salad, make it with four or five types of beans.

Expand your horizons. There's no reason for a nutritionally sound meal to be a culinary snooze. Let your imagination fly. Have you ever tasted low-fat cheese with a tart green apple? Try topping your grapefruit half with thinly sliced kiwi. Or sprinkle warm spinach leaves with lemon and hard-boiled egg whites for a unusually tasty breakfast treat.

Take one step at a time. "Never expect your family to make a lot of big changes all at once," Miller advises. "For example, don't give skim milk to someone who is used to drinking whole milk. Give them 2 percent milk for a few weeks, then 1 percent milk and eventually, skim. If you walk away from something gradually, you won't miss it."

Banish temptation. Even staunchly sensible eaters occasionally are tempted by cookies, ice cream and the many other "diet traps" that will sabotage the best of intentions. Protect yourself by stocking the pantry with foods you know you should eat—not those you can't resist. "If good food is in the house, that's what you'll eat," Miller says.

Watch the big picture. The best-laid schemes, said poet Robert Burns, often go awry. That's especially true for dietary improvement plans. Nearly

(continued on page 374)

SETTING YOUR PRIORITIES

Of all the hundreds of dietary habits you can possibly adopt, which ones are the most powerful for preventing disease and promoting optimum health? Should you put a lot of energy into reducing the amount of cholesterol in your diet? Or is it more important to avoid alcoholic beverages? Where exactly is the biggest health payoff?

The question was posed to more than 300 top nutrition experts in a poll conducted by Medical Consensus Surveys, a research arm of *Prevention* magazine. These black belts in nutrition were asked to rate 44 nutritional actions (all purported to benefit health) as follows: extremely important, very important, important, not important but may help or probably worthless.

The nutritionists' responses were then compiled and statistically weighted to create a list of dietary "top priorities" for preserving and boosting your health.

PRIORITY/RANKING	ACTION
VERY HIGH PRIORITY	
79	Control calorie intake to control your weight
76	Reduce all dietary fats
75	Control fat intake to control your weight
HIGH PRIORITY	
71	Increase physical activity to enable greater nutrient intake
71	Enjoy your food
70	Balance your diet among the four food groups
69	Ensure adequate intake of vitamins and minerals to meet the RDAs
65	Replace saturated fats with monos and polys
65	If not pregnant or trying to conceive, limit your alcohol intake to one or two drinks per day
63	Replace whole-milk products with low-fat and nonfat dairy products
63	Avoid raw eggs, raw meat and raw seafood
62	Increase total fiber to at least 20 grams per day
62	Eat more complex carbohydrates, such as grains, rice, beans, potatoes, bread and pasta
61	Eat more fish in place of meat
59	Ensure adequate intake of soluble fiber
57	Avoid very low calorie diets
56	Cut meat portions to three to four ounces
55	Reduce dietary cholesterol
54	Ensure adequate intake of insoluble fiber

54	Eat at least five fruit and vegetables per day
54	Eat breakfast
51	Reduce sodium intake
MODERATE PRIORITY	
49	Increase intake of cruciferous vegetables, such as broccoli, cauliflower, kale and others
49	Avoid eating large meals and snacking excessively in the evening when activity levels tend to be low
48	Switch from butter to margarine
48	Restrict intake of tropical oils
47	Drink six to eight 8-ounce glasses of water (or decaffeinated, low-calorie and low-fat fluids) every day
47	Avoid nitrates and nitrites (smoked and cured foods)
44	Reduce trans-fatty acids (e.g., stick margarine, hydrogenated vegetable shortening)
43	Reduce sugar intake
41	Eat three square meals a day with a minimum of snacking in between
41	Eat only when you're hungry (regardless of whether it's mealtime or not) and only to satiety
40	Limit your daily caffeine consumption to the amount in four cups of coffee
38	Peel or wash fruit before eating to avoid pesticides
37	Increase beta-carotene intake
37	Switch from stick margarine to soft (tub) and liquid margarine
35	Have a regular nutritional assessment
30	Eliminate alcohol from your diet
29	Restrict your intake of phosphorus
LOW PRIORITY	
24	Increase intake of vitamin E beyond the RDA without exceeding safe limits
23	Increase intake of vitamin C beyond the RDA without exceeding safe limits
16	Make breakfast the biggest meal of the day
14	Avoid irradiated foods
13	Avoid overgrilled (i.e., charred) or blackened foods

NOTE: The numbers in the left column represent the relative importance of each positive action, based on a scale of 0 (not important) to 100 (extremely important).

everyone occasionally indulges in a sugary snack or "forgets" and has two helpings of steak. "People should think about their food intake over time and not just focus on single food items," says Dr. Callaway. "You need to look at your food intake the way you look at your checkbook—it's something you have to balance over weeks, months, years and a lifetime."

Now that you understand the basics, it's time to take a look at some of the different plans nutritionists recommend for healthy eating. Each approach has its own strengths and weaknesses. Which you ultimately pick is entirely up to you. Let's begin this discussion by looking at the grand-daddy of nutritional guidelines, the Basic Four.

FOUR GROUPS, THOUSANDS OF CHOICES

In 1956 the U.S. Department of Agriculture divided the wide world of foods into four groups: grains, meats, dairy products and fruits and vegetables. For Americans to have a balanced diet, experts said, they need only eat several daily servings from each of the groups. They called this plan the Basic Four Food Groups.

Imagine a cube or circle divided into four equal sections. The dairy group typically is represented by a wedge of cheese or a milk bottle. In the meat compartment goes a pork chop or a chicken and an egg. A carrot and peach may represent the fruit and vegetable group, while a loaf of bread typifies the grain group.

The Basic Four is to nutrition what the three Rs—reading, writing and 'rithmetic—are to education: A strong foundation to support a lifetime of good habits. "There was an understanding early on that what one ate had a strong influence on one's health," says Dr. Thomas.

PUTTING THE PLAN TO WORK

Now that you understand the Basic Four, you can begin "building" nutritious meals from each of the four groups. Keep in mind the minimum recommended number of servings: two dairy products; two servings of meat, fish, poultry or eggs; four helpings of fruits and vegetables; and four servings of bread, flour or whole-grain cereals.

To get your daily allotment of grains, for example, you could eat a bowl of cereal, two slices of whole-wheat toast, a serving of rice and a zesty bowl of tabbouleh during the course of your day. The fruit and vegetable category offers even more variety: apples, oranges, melons, berries, peas, beans and spinach are among the foods that you can choose from. There's just as much variety in the meat and dairy groups. You could eat different foods seven days a week and always have a square meal!

Indeed, eating different foods can be a nutritional boon, Dr. Thomas says. "The greater the variety of foods you eat, the better you'll do." By contrast, the more limited the variety, "the greater the risk of not getting enough nutrients."

SERIOUS OMISSIONS

Although the Basic Four provides an easy-to-follow framework for healthy eating, some nutritionists worry it's a bit too simple. Yes, by following the guidelines you're unlikely to become malnourished. But what about eating too much? When it comes to dietary *excess,* Dr. Nestle says, the Basic Four is basically silent.

Foods that are high in calories, fat, salt or sugar and low in nutrients may appear in any of the four groups, and no distinction is made between them and more healthful options. For example, cheesecake might be found in the dairy category, although few people would suggest it's the nutritional equal of yogurt. Similarly, a slice of sponge cake might appear in the grain category, although it's scarcely a rival for seven-grain bread.

The same problem occurs with "related" foods that have vastly different nutritional values. For example, both broccoli and iceberg lettuce occupy the vegetable niche, yet broccoli contains a great deal more fiber, vitamins A and C and other nutrients, says Dr. Nestle. In short, it's a superior food, athough you wouldn't know this if your only information came from the Basic Four.

Despite these "crimes of omission," doctors agree the Basic Four is a use-

SQUARE MEALS OR WISHFUL THINKING?

Mmmmm. I'll have the 16-ounce steak, onion rings and chocolate cake with vanilla ice cream, please. Meat? Check. Vegetable? Yep. Grain? Check. Dairy? Check. Okay—now I have all four of the Basic Four Food Groups. Must be a good, square meal, right?

Hardly. But with wishful thinking, "virtually any food can be made to fit into one of the food groups," says Paul R. Thomas, R.D., Ed.D., project director of the Food and Nutrition Board of the National Academy of Sciences in Washington, D.C.

Take the meal above. Technically it meets the requirements for the Basic Four plan. But the meal is so heavy on protein and fat, and so light on healthful grains and vegetables, it's probably worse than following no plan at all.

When you begin "building" meals based on the Basic Four, try to be realistic, Dr. Thomas advises. The idea isn't to fool yourself but to lay down a healthy foundation of grains, vegetables and fruits with smaller amounts of dairy products and meat or meat alternatives such as legumes. Once you have a firm base, then you can treat yourself to the occasional potato chip or strawberry sundae. What's the category? Just call them the *fun* food group!

ful guide on the road to good nutrition. For more detailed guidelines, look at the plan below.

The National Dietary Guidelines

In many parts of the world, people are more likely to get too little food than too much. In this country, the opposite is true. Dietary excesses are a leading cause of obesity, diabetes, heart disease, high blood pressure and many other serious diseases.

To check our tendency to overindulge, experts have formulated the *Dietary Guidelines for Americans.* The guidelines aren't meant to replace the Basic Four. What they do is encourage people to concentrate on healthy foods, says Dr. Callaway.

"Rather than come at it from a restrictive point of view and tell people what they shouldn't eat, the Dietary Guidelines emphasize the positive: the delicious foods people can add to their diets," he says.

Seven Steps to Health

The guidelines are simple: Eat more fruits, vegetables and grains, and limit your consumption of sugar, fats, alcohol and salt. Specifically, experts say:

1. **Enjoy nature's bounty.** There are more than 40 nutrients that are essential to good health. The best way to get enough of these nutrients is to regularly eat many foods, says Dr. Nestle. So experiment. Try new foods in new combinations. Instead of eggs for breakfast, have a grapefruit. Follow your noon sandwich with an apple or pear. Have turkey breast instead of pot roast. Add several vegetables to the dinner menu, and follow up with fruit for dessert. The more healthful foods you try, she says, the less likely you are to come up short—or overweight.

2. **Be a lean machine.** Study after study has shown that diets high in fat contribute to everything from diabetes and cancer to high blood pressure and heart disease. If you do eat meat, stick to lean cuts such as flank steak or chicken breast (without the skin). A low-fat diet is the best short-cut to keeping your cholesterol low, your arteries clear and your weight down.

3. **Plan to eat more plant foods.** On the nutritional road to good health, the plant kingdom should be your first stop. Most fruits, vegetables and cereal grains are low in fat, high in fiber and positively packed with important vitamins and minerals.

The guidelines call for three servings of vegetables, two servings of fruit and six servings of grains every day. This may sound like a mountain of food, but it's all in a normal day's dining. For example, a single slice of whole-grain bread takes care of one of your grain servings. A bowl of oatmeal and a small biscuit take care of two more. Add to this a grapefruit, an apple and several servings of salad or cooked vegetables, and you've fulfilled one part of the guidelines. The others are just as easy.

4. Sack the sugar. It's unfortunate, but many of the foods we love the best—cookies, candy bars and ice cream, to name just a few—don't love us back. The arithmetic is simple: Processed sugar, whether packed into peanut butter fudge or stirred into coffee, adds up to empty calories. To satisfy your sweet tooth *and* protect your waistline, get your sugars the natural way—from grapes, watermelon and other fruits.

5. Go lightly on salt. In small amounts, sodium and chloride—the main ingredients in table salt—are essential nutrients for good health. Taken in excess, however, they can cause high blood pressure and a host of other problems.

Salt is tough to avoid. Even if you shun the shaker on your table, it's found in everything from canned soups to store-bought bread. That's why you *must* read the labels, experts say. Whenever possible, buy foods that have little or no added salt. In the kitchen, don't add salt while you're cooking. In time you'll lose your "salt tooth," and your health will be the winner.

6. Maintain a healthy weight. Doctors agree that obesity is one of the leading causes of disease and early death. If you've tried to lose weight and can't, see your doctor. When you succeed, the benefits will last a lifetime.

7. Drink only in moderation. There simply are no great benefits to be had from drinking alcohol, and there are plenty of risks. If you do drink, doctors say, do so in moderation—no more than one to two drinks a day. And remember: The calories in alcohol are "empty." As the drinks go down, your weight may go up.

THE FOOD GUIDE PYRAMID

Here's still another approach to healthy eating. Designed by the U.S. Department of Agriculture, the Food Guide Pyramid displays the types of foods you should eat each day: grains, vegetables, fruits, meats and dairy products. (Fats, oils and sweets are included but are optional.) The Pyramid also lists the recommended number of servings for each group.

Did you just hear an echo from the Basic Four Food Groups? The plans are similar. However, the Food Guide Pyramid doesn't treat the food groups equally. (You'll remember this was a complaint leveled against the Basic Four.) Instead, it recommends eating more of some types of foods and less of others. Let's take a look.

Like the Egyptian landmark, the Food Guide Pyramid is a triangle planted wide-end down. The inside is divided into four tiers, with the broadest at the bottom and the smallest at the top. The size of each tier corresponds to the amounts of food you should eat. For example:

Begin with grains. Rice, pastas, breads and cereals occupy the Pyramid's largest tier, and with good reason: They represent the *foundation* for your diet. These foods give you a firm base of complex carbohydrates, B vitamins, protein and fiber. The plan calls for 6 to 11 servings a day.

Then add fruits and vegetables. These form the second tier of the Pyra-

PYRAMID POWER

Let's compare your diet to the Food Guide Pyramid. First count the servings you eat every day from each of the different groups. Then compare them to the daily servings recommended below. This will help you decide which foods you need more of, which you may cut back on and which are just right.

FOOD GROUP	SERVINGS PER DAY	SERVING SIZE EXAMPLES
Bread, cereals, pasta, other grain products	6–11 (include several whole-grain products every day)	1 slice of bread ½ hamburger bun or English muffin 1 small roll, biscuit or muffin 4 small or 2 large crackers ½ cup cooked cereal, pasta, rice or other whole grain, such as barley or buckwheat 1 ounce ready-to-eat cereal
Fruits	2–4	1 med. apple, orange or banana ½ grapefruit 1 melon wedge 6 ounces fruit juice ½ cup berries ½ cup cooked or canned fruit

mid. Fruits (two to four servings daily) and vegetables (three to five servings) will help you meet your daily requirements for fiber, vitamins C and A and many other important nutrients.

Add some protein. The third tier of the Pyramid includes red meat, poultry, fish, dry beans, eggs, cheese, milk and yogurt. Nutritionists say you should eat two to three daily servings of the meat, bean and egg group, and the same number of servings of dairy products. Together, these groups will give you an abundance of protein, B vitamins, calcium and other minerals.

Watch out for fats. Unlike the Basic Four, the Pyramid doesn't ignore fats, oils and sweets. Instead, they're perched on the Pyramid's pinnacle—along with a warning to use them sparingly.

TOO MANY CHOICES?

As with the Basic Four and the Dietary Guidelines, the Food Guide Pyramid offers a complete, easy-to-understand guide for a lifetime of healthy eating. So long as you properly apportion your diet among the four tiers, you can eat pretty much everything you want—within your caloric limits,

FOOD GROUP	SERVINGS PER DAY	SERVING SIZE EXAMPLES
		¼ cup dried fruit, such as raisins, apricots or prunes
Vegetables (dark green or yellow vegetables, potatoes, dry beans and peas or other legumes)	3–5	½ cup cooked vegetables ½ cup chopped, raw vegetables 1 cup raw, leafy vegetables, such as spinach or lettuce
Meat, poultry, fish and alternates (eggs, dry beans and peas, nuts and seeds)	2–3	Servings should total 5 to 7 ounces of cooked lean meat, poultry or fish per day 1 egg, ½ cup cooked beans or 2 tablespoons peanut butter count as 1 ounce of meat
Milk, cheese or yogurt	2 (3 for pregnant women)	1 cup milk or yogurt 1½ ounces natural cheese 2 ounces processed cheese
Fats, oils, sweets and alcohol	—	Avoid too many fats and sweets. If you drink alcoholic beverages, do so in moderation.

of course! "The actual foods you choose are a matter of personal preference," says Dr. Thomas. In other words, the Pyramid emphasizes groups—you pick the foods.

For beginners, however, the Food Guide Pyramid can seem daunting. They may wonder, "Must we stuff ourselves with up to *11* servings of breads, cereals and grains? Is there enough time in the day to eat as many as *9* helpings of fruits and vegetables? Won't we burst?"

The servings quickly add up, Dr. Thomas says. "Just a sandwich can give you a third of the minimum six servings of grain products," he explains. In fact, if you drink juice in the morning, add dried fruit to your cereal, snack on fruits and vegetables and add carrots and potatoes to your casserole, you're well on your way.

THE NEW FOUR FOOD GROUPS

Doctors have known for a long time that people who base their diets on high-fiber, low-fat foods tend to be healthier than those who fill up on pizza, hamburgers and shakes. Large studies such as the Framingham Heart

WEED OUT TEMPTATION

So you're ready to begin cutting fat, adding fiber and otherwise improving your diet. Where to begin?

For starters, nutritionists say, take a look at the foods in your larder. Are white bread and salted crackers really the best choices for one of your food groups? Do you have to buy hamburger, or would lean flank steak do as well? The next time you go shopping, nutritionists say, begin replacing inferior foods with their more nutritious counterparts. For example:

LOW FIBER	HIGH FIBER
White bread	7-grain bread
White rice	Brown rice
Spaghetti	Whole-wheat pasta
Instant pilaf mix	Lentils and chick-peas
Corn flakes	Corn bran cereal
Fruit juice	Oranges and apples
Watermelon	Fresh berries
HIGH SODIUM	**LOW SODIUM**
Canned beans	Dry beans
Canned vegetables	Frozen or fresh veggies
Mix-n-eat oatmeal	Regular oatmeal
Cold cuts	Fresh cuts of meat and poultry
American cheese	Low-salt Swiss cheese
Soy sauce	Lemon juice
HIGH FAT	**LOW FAT**
Ice cream	Low-fat frozen yogurt
Whole milk	Skim or 1 percent milk
Cheddar cheese	Skim-milk cheese
Corned beef	Lean roast beef
Spareribs	Skinless chicken breast
Sardines	Tuna packed in water

These are just a few examples to help you begin your nutritional make-over. Before long, stocking your pantry with low-fat, low-sodium and high-fiber foods will be second nature.

Study, the China Health Study and work by Dean Ornish, M.D., all have shown that diets based on plant foods can help cut the risk of cancer, diabetes, heart disease and high blood pressure. That's why experts nearly are unanimous in recommending that people eat fewer meats and more grains, fruits and vegetables.

The New Four Food Groups plan takes this approach a step further. Designed by the Physicians Committee for Responsible Medicine, it recommends that people build their diets from whole grains, legumes, vegetables and fruits. No meat. No sweets. No dairy products.

"The New Four Food Groups do not mean you should *never* eat meat or dairy products," explains Neal Barnard, M.D., president of the physicians committee. "What we are saying is that they should be considered options, not essentials."

People should have five servings a day of breads, pastas, rice, corn or other grains, Dr. Barnard says. Three servings a day each of beans, vegetables and fruits completes the requirements.

Because the plan represents quite a departure from the traditional American diet (hot dogs and hamburgers come to mind), it may be a challenge for people who aren't seriously motivated, Dr. Thomas says. And if they don't plan carefully, they may put themselves at nutritional risk. Those who succeed in making plant foods the center of their dietary circles, however, may be well rewarded—with lower cholesterol, healthier arteries and perhaps slimmer waistlines, too.

FIVE A DAY FOR HEALTH

The Five-a-Day Plan, which is being promoted by the National Cancer Institute, focuses on the disease-fighting power of fruits and vegetables, says Elizabeth Pivonka, R.D., Ph.D., director of nutrition and sciences for the

WE HAVE A LONG WAY TO GO

Though Americans have become increasingly savvy about nutrition, we still have room for improvement, says Marion Nestle, Ph.D., of New York University in New York City. Polls have shown:

- About 36 to 38 percent of Americans' calories come from fat. That's down slightly from the 1960s, although it is well above the recommended 30 percent or less.
- We still eat a lot of steak, hamburger and pot roast, despite warnings about the health risks of eating too much red meat.
- Only 33 percent of Americans ate the recommended minimum of five servings of fruits and vegetables on the day they were surveyed. In fact, 7 percent said they ate *no* fruits or vegetables.

It doesn't have to be this way. According to Paul R. Thomas, R.D., Ed.D., of the National Academy of Sciences in Washington, D.C., people can make healthful changes in their diets without going crazy. "Making relatively minor changes in the diet—for example, decreasing the size of the meat portion and including a fruit or vegetable in each of your meals—can lead to substantial changes toward healthier diets," he says.

Produce for Better Health Foundation in Newark, Delaware. "It's a completely positive message—we're not telling anyone what *not* to eat," she says.

The idea is simply to eat a minimum of five servings of vegetables and fruits daily as part of a low-fat, high-fiber diet.

"The Five-a-Day program is something that everybody should feel really comfortable about supporting," says Dr. Nestle. "Eating five fruits and vegetables every day would make a big difference in the American diet." Adds Dr. Pivonka, "The plan is easy to remember, easy to follow, and it's tasty." It's also an easy way to pump healthy amounts of fiber and vitamins A and C into your daily diet.

Don't be lulled into a false sense of security, though, by adding a few extra vegetables and fruits to your diet and doing little else. You can't *really* keep the doctor away with an apple a day—not if every day you eat three eggs for breakfast, fast food for lunch and greasy pizza for supper.

Still, some people aren't prepared to change their entire diet, Dr. Pivonka says. For them, adding a few oranges, green salads, broccoli and other fruits and vegetables might make a big difference.

CHAPTER 28

COOKING LIGHT

TECHNIQUES AND TIPS

Your shelves may bow under packages of dry beans and pasta, but the benefits they bestow can be overwhelmed in dishes that ooze butter or cheese.

Your refrigerator bins overflow with fresh vegetables, which, in turn, overflow with vitamins, but their nutrients can be nullified by boiling them away.

Your freezer is packed with poultry and fish, but their low-fat goodness will be lost if you coat them with batter and deep-fry them.

Cooking methods that obliterate foods' nutritious goodness are sheer folly when your priority is to give your diet a healthful lift. The not-so-healthful techniques that scarcely deserve a good-bye wave as you usher them out of your kitchen include boiling vegetables into green-gray mush, deep-frying and extra oily sautéing, butter-based baking, marinating and basting with fat and salty sauces, and adding fat- and salt-drenched gravies and toppings to otherwise healthful dishes. Good riddance.

Clear your culinary thinking of those poor preparation choices and you're left with a rich array of cooking methods that lend such flavor and variety you'll never miss your old ways. The good news is that you can begin today to take control of your healthful eating strategy by adopting cooking methods like these.

STEAMING

It's hard to resist the fresh flavor of steamed vegetables cooked to perfection, splashed with lemon juice, sprinkled with basil, dill or any fresh herb and presented without a hint of added fat. Although vitamin-robbing boiling water is the cooking agent in this method, foods never actually touch it, so more of the vitamins in fresh and frozen vegetables are yours to keep, as long as steaming time is short, says Susan Witz, R.D., Director of Nutrition at Heartland Health and Fitness Retreat and Spa in Gilman, Illinois.

Put a lid on it. For the best steaming results, bring about an inch of

HOW LONG SHOULD YOU STEAM?

Steaming vegetables is an imprecise art, because of the great ranges of sizes and densities. You can use this table, though, to gauge the time at which you should begin checking the food for doneness.

TIME (min.)	VEGETABLE
3	Asparagus
	Broccoli rabe, whole leaves
	Greens, beet, kale, etc.
	Peas, shelled
	Snow pea pods
5	Beans, green or wax
	Beans, lima
	Corn, off the cob
	Snap pea pods
7	Broccoli, medium stalks
	Corn on the cob
	Potato chunks
	Summer squash chunks
8	Cabbage, quarter heads
10	Brussels sprouts
	Carrot chunks
	Fennel, quarter heads
	Parsnip chunks
12	Cauliflower florets
	Turnips, quartered
15	Eggplant slices, peeled
18	Potatoes, whole, medium
20	Winter squash chunks
30	Artichokes, whole

water to a boil in a pot with a tight-fitting lid. Place vegetables in a steaming basket that fits into the pot without getting dunked, and cover. To conserve color and vitamins, steam vegetables until they are tender, but no longer. Steaming is an excellent, no-fat-added, quick way to cook broccoli, summer squash, asparagus, carrots and spinach. It is also a better choice than boiling for longer-cooking vegetables such as potatoes, turnips and parsnips.

"Some people might think steamed vegetables are going to be tasteless; they want a sauce on everything," says Nancy Leicht, former sous chef at Heartland. "But steaming lets us get down to the essence of eating fresh foods. It's a matter of learning that we don't need all those rich calories to enjoy them."

POACHING

"A lot of people feel they don't have time to cook," Leicht points out. Yet you can quickly prepare healthful and elegant foods by starting with fresh, high-quality ingredients that don't need a lot of time-hungry cooking methods or embellishments, she says. Poaching is a quick, gentle, no-fat-added method that rivals the results of much more elaborate techniques.

Depend on these liquid assets. Poach foods by briefly simmering them in a shallow pool of whatever liquid you choose: water, broth, fruit or vegetable juice. No-fuss poaching works especially well for delicate fillets of fish, such as sole, that cook in minutes, and for fragile fruits, such as ripe, skinned pears. The water, broth or juice in which the food is cooked can then be seasoned and reduced—boiled down to a fraction of its original volume—to intensify its flavor, then poured over the food for a light, refreshing sauce.

STIR-FRYING

Stir-frying vegetables, meats and fish with little or no added fat is one of the fastest ways to put a remarkably healthful meal on the table. "The basic idea behind stir-fry cooking is to cook at high heat for a short amount of time, which retains vitamins and keeps food intact so it doesn't become limp or lose its appeal," says Leicht.

Bring on the vegetables . . . any vegetables. You can cook colorful, delicious and nourishing vegetable masterpieces in minutes by stir-frying. Almost any combination of vegetables—oriental cabbages, carrots, onions, peppers, snow peas, squash, broccoli, asparagus, you name it—can be whipped up in a hot wok or large sauté pan.

"The key to easy stir-frying is cutting the foods up into similar sizes beforehand so that it all cooks evenly and is ready at the same time," says Leicht. Vegetables are done when they take on an intense color but have not lost their crispness. "Carrots or other hard vegetables should be cooked for a few minutes before most of the other foods go in, and you can throw pea pods in at the last moment to prevent them from being overcooked," she suggests.

A dab of cooking oil guarantees a stick-free dish, but for the ultimate low-fat vegetable stir-fry, try tossing your vegetables with a few tablespoons of water, wine, broth or fruit juice, says Joanne D'Agostino, R.N., author and low-fat-cooking consultant based in Easton, Pennsylvania. Stir-frying without oil is a no-stick snap as long as your wok or sauté pan is large enough to keep the food sizzling hot and moving rapidly. "I really find

Getting into Hot Water

Despite the reputation that boiling has as a vitamin robber, there are a few types of foods on your healthy-eating menu that just have to be cooked in hot water: Pasta, grains and dry beans.

Pasta. To take full advantage of the low-fat, high-carbohydrate, low-sodium nature of pasta, unlearn the urge to cook it in salted water with a layer of anti-stick oil floating in it. Cook dry or fresh pasta in rapidly boiling, plain water. Use enough water for the pasta to swim freely when you gently stir it once or twice during cooking to avoid sticking.

"Any pasta dish can also be made with the colorful pastas that are available, although there is so little spinach, tomato or other vegetable added to them for color that they're not significantly more nutritious than plain, white pasta," says Susan Witz, R.D., of Heartland Health and Fitness Retreat and Spa in Gilman, Illinois. "Whole-wheat pasta does have a little more fiber and protein, though, and there are various types of high-gluten, high-protein pastas that do provide more of that nutrient."

Grains. If boiling a batch of white rice is your idea of grain cooking, be prepared to widen your horizons. "Two of the most popular healthy grains are bulgur and millet, and they're both very easy to prepare," says vegetarian cookbook author Mollie Katzen, of Berkeley, California. Bulgur is chopped, or cracked, pre-steamed, whole-wheat grains. "To cook bulgur, put some in a bowl, pour in up to twice as much boiling water, cover and wait 15 or 20 minutes for the grains to absorb the moisture," says Katzen. The result is a pleasantly chewy, nourishing grain dish that can be used instead of rice as a bed for stir-fried vegetables. Or serve it cold, mixed with parsley, tomato, garlic, olive oil, mint and lemon juice, as tabbouleh, a healthful Middle Eastern salad.

that vegetables taste better without the oil, and they stay crisper," says D'Agostino. Go easy on salt in your vegetable stir-fry by splashing on a reduced-sodium soy sauce, if you like. Or, skip the salt altogether by adding a dash of ginger juice. Finally, your amazingly healthful and colorful creation is ready for a bed of rice, barley or pasta. Or add a side dish of cooked, dried beans instead of meat for a vegetarian stir-fry feast.

Add lean meat, poultry or fish and wok away from fat. "In traditional Chinese and Asian cuisine, meat is used as a flavoring ingredient or as a supplement or condiment rather than a main ingredient," says Martin Yan,

Millet is another quick-cooking, nutritious whole grain that is ideal for pan toasting, a low-fat method that gives grains a nutty flavor and keeps them from turning mushy when simmered as a base for fluffy pilaf. Toast the pale yellow spheres of millet over low to moderate heat in a large, heavy pan, stirring frequently until the grains turn tawny. Add boiling water or fat-free stock to the grains, and whatever seasonings and vegetables you like, such as diced onions, peppers and carrots. Cover the pan tightly and simmer until all the water is absorbed. Fluff it with a fork and your perfect pilaf is served. "You can do this with just about any grain or combination of grains to add flavor and interest to them," says Katzen, "but the amounts of water and cooking times will vary."

Most other whole grains—long- or short-grain brown rice, whole-oat groats, wild rice, barley and cracked corn grits also turn out very well when you simply measure the grain, add it to the correct amount of boiling water or broth in a heavy saucepan, cover it tightly and simmer it very gently for the called-for amount of time. No peeking or stirring while it cooks or the grain may turn out underdone or sticky. To add flavor to the grains without adding salt, fat or calories, try adding lemon pepper, Italian seasonings or curry powder to the water. To cut most grains' cooking times in half, simmer them in a pressure cooker, instead.

Beans. Because they, too, must be reconstituted, many of the cooking methods for dry beans and lentils are similar to those for grains. They can also be simmered in slow cookers or crock pots or speed cooked (relatively speaking) after overnight soaking. Follow the directions on dry bean packages for the best results. Cooking with canned or precooked, dehydrated beans are instant ways to add these high-fiber, low-fat little wonders to your healthy diet.

chef, food consultant and public television cooking show host. A little bit of marinated meat, poultry or firm-fleshed fish can go a long way when it is stir-fried with lots of crisp vegetables. "You don't need a lot of oil, whatever you stir-fry," says Yan.

For stir-fried combination dishes, cook the meat or fish first until it is almost done, before adding vegetables, which need only a quick toss in a hot wok. "You don't want to worry about thinly sliced peppers being overcooked while the chicken or shrimp is still raw in the center, for example," says Leicht. "Another way to hasten the cooking of chicken, shrimp and scallops in a stir-fry is to marinate them in an acid, such as lemon or lime juice, with some herbs. The marinade adds flavor and also actually firms up the flesh so that when you put it in the wok it will cook faster because it's already on its way."

For an exciting change of pace, add diced apples, orange segments or pineapple chunks to your next stir-fry.

GRILLING AND BROILING

Almost any food would do well to jump *out* of the frying pan and into the fire—or at least *close* to the fire—from a grill or broiler. Grilling and broiling have similar advantages: Foods cook over or under direct, high heat, and neither method calls for adding fats. Any fats that do cook out of foods fall into the grill or are drained away into a pan beneath the broiling rack. The idea is to keep fat levels down as much as possible, so barbecued ribs and other fat-laden items are out. To keep grilled or broiled foods moist and flavorful, marinate or baste them with citrus fruit juice, defatted broth or fat-free sauces.

Keep it simple. Poultry, lean cuts of meat and firm-fleshed fish are naturals on a grill or under a broiler. "Grilling, by its nature, is a healthy style of cooking because it produces a lot of flavor on its own, and it doesn't call for a lot of accompaniments," says Chris Schlesinger, chef and co-owner of the East Coast Grill in Cambridge, Massachusetts. "For example, you can grill a piece of plain fish or beef and that's all you need; no herb butter, no cream sauce," he explains.

Or, perhaps you like to show off your flair for dressing up foods. There are plenty of ways to do so without reaching for fatty or salty barbecue sauces. "Top grilled meat or fish with fruit relishes, salsas or chutneys instead," Schlesinger suggests. "And you can add lime juice, ginger, garlic and other spices to fish, rather than loading it down with rich sauces."

Take special care with fish. Firm fish, such as swordfish and tuna can stand up to just about any cooking style, but more tender types of fish need a bit more care in their handling, says Leicht. "When you grill or broil fish such as salmon or trout, the heat of the grill and the amount of cooking time are the most important factors to consider. The coals should be medium hot. That means they're not flaming anymore and are powdery on the surface," she says. "When you put a small piece of fish on a grill that is so hot, it won't take very long at all to cook, so watch it closely.

"The appearance and feel of the fish are important indicators of doneness. When a dense fish, like salmon, is approaching the overdone point, a white residue appears on the surface and tells you it is definitely time to get the fish away from the fire. More delicate fish, like sole, turn from a translucent state to a pure white state and take on a firmness when they are done," she explains.

If you have been shy about grilling fish because of its delicate nature, try cooking fish steaks, rather than fillets. They're a bit easier to handle. Also, fish does have a tendency to stick to grills, and could be hard to turn or remove, says Leicht. "To prevent that, brush or spray a little bit of canola oil on the grill or on the fish itself and there won't be any problem," she suggests.

Try meatless kabobs. You need not put your grill away if you rarely eat meat. Most vegetables can easily and quickly be broiled or grilled. Leave small veggies—such as cherry tomatoes, mushrooms, small onions and pea pods—whole and grill them in a mesh rack, or skewer them on shish-kabob spears. Large vegetables, such as summer squash and potatoes, can be sliced diagonally to give them a large surface area for resting on the grill. Marinate or baste vegetables with lime or orange juice or with low-fat salad dressing to keep them moist while they cook.

For a special, fruity treat, try grilled or broiled sliced apples, bananas, pineapple, oranges, peaches, or pears. Season them with ginger, cinnamon or lemon or lime juice. Wrap fruit in foil for grilling or broil it directly. Or thread chunks of fruit onto skewers and enjoy grilled or broiled fruit kabobs.

BAKING AND ROASTING

Baking and roasting might conjure images of belt-busting holiday feasts, but your oven is also a great place to prepare lots of everyday foods in a healthful way.

Curtail fat without fuss. Most meats and poultry can go directly from the refrigerator into the oven, without much fuss, after a quick rinse and dry-off with paper towels, and certainly without adding fats, oils or salt. Place meats and poultry on a rack in an ovenproof pan to melt away and drain off much of the fat you cannot trim off. Once the food is put in the oven at the recommended temperature, it is basically on "automatic pilot," thriving on minimum attention until your oven timer goes off.

Make it moist with marinade. For added flavor interest, and to help meat and fish stay moist, baste them with broth, fruit juice or a low-fat marinade. Marinating can be a flavor and moisture boon to low-fat foods that could otherwise become dry or tough when you bake or roast them. "Marinating can be especially healthful if you limit the oil. Use just a scant amount of olive oil in marinades or eliminate it altogether. Concentrate more on herb-lemon or herb-vinegar blends for marinating. There are virtually no calories in these, but there is a lot of flavor," says Leicht.

Be quick with fish. "Slow roasting is one method that does not usually lend itself well to fish. It's better to bake fish quickly, at relatively high heat, so that it doesn't become tough," says Leicht. "The more delicate a fish is in flavor and texture, the more you must guard against taking away from that delicacy. You can bake delicate fillets of sole or flounder, if you do it carefully. Denser fish, like salmon or tuna, can be baked, too, but they also stand up to cooking by just about any method," she explains.

"Overcooking by just a few minutes can make fish dry, and you can't reverse overdoneness," Leicht says. To prevent that, check the fish frequently when it is approaching the time limit called for in recipes.

Don't stop with just potatoes. "Roasting and baking are slow-cooking methods that can be used for dense vegetables, such as potatoes and sweet potatoes, winter squash, onions and garlic," says Leicht. Baking vegetables can be as simple as washing them, pricking the skins to prevent steam buildup, which can cause vegetables to explode, and placing them on a baking sheet in a hot oven. Vegetables are done when they can easily be pierced to the center with a fork.

Moisture-lending vegetables, such as zucchini and pumpkin, are quite at home in flavorful, baked quick breads and muffins, too, says D'Agostino. They give baked products a moist texture that can make people forget egg-enriched or butter-burdened cakes.

Bake some sweet treats. Various fruits, such as apples, bananas and pears, can be baked whole for simple, warm desserts. Add a sprinkle of cinnamon or nutmeg for a spicy flavor boost without added calories.

Baked goods that include fruit for flavor, sweetness and moisture can be the crowning glory of low-fat cooking. Apples, bananas, pears, peaches and other sweet, moist fruits can be used in breads, quick breads, cookies and muffins to replace eggs and fats and to add fiber and nutrients. Fresh or frozen berries as well as raisins, chopped figs or other dried fruits are sweet, fiber-rich delights when you add them to fruit tarts, cobblers, pies and crisps. The concentrated sweetness of very ripe berries and dried fruits can replace some of the sugar in many dessert recipes.

Fiber-up with flour power. Baking breads, quick breads, cakes, muffins, waffles and cookies using whole-grain flours is a good way to add fiber to your diet. You can do it in an extra healthful way by cutting in half (or better) the amount of butter, margarine or oil called for in recipes that contain fruit, vegetables or other moistening ingredients, such as nonfat yogurt, says D'Agostino.

You can also give your baked goods a fiber lift by adding wheat germ or bran to your recipes, replacing an equal amount of flour. The secret to working with bran, says Linny Largent-Mayer, executive chef at the Los

A Little of This, Instead of That

When you begin cooking in more healthful ways, usually you need not deprive yourself by giving up your favorite dishes. In many cases, you can substitute healthful ingredients for less healthful ones and come up with a dish that satisfies both your hunger for the foods you like and your desire to eat in the most healthy way possible.

"The first thing you can do to any recipe is find the source of fat in it, and reduce it. Cut it in half, or just eliminate it, in most cases," says Joanne D'Agostino, R.N., a low-fat-cooking consultant in Easton, Pennsylvania. "When a recipe calls for butter or shortening, use a whipped, diet, polyunsaturated margarine and use a third to a half less," she suggests. "Or, if a recipe calls for oil, as many muffin recipes do, substitute half as much corn syrup or honey in place of the oil and decrease the amount of sugar."

"In most cases, you can substitute turkey for red meat in recipes without making any other changes," says D'Agostino. Use ground, skinless turkey in meat loaf, chili or spaghetti sauce. And, turkey breast cutlets can be marinated and poached or used in low-fat, stir-fried dishes, for example.

The representatives of Project LEAN (Low-fat Eating for America Now), based in Chicago, and other cooking experts, suggest these additional fat-busting, salt-reducing substitutions.

If the Recipe Calls for . . .	**Substitute**
Milk	Skim or 1% milk
Light cream	Equal portions 1% milk and evaporated skim milk
Baking chocolate (1 oz.)	3 tablespoons cocoa plus 1 tablespoon vegetable oil
Sour cream	Blend 1 cup low-fat (1%) cottage cheese with 1 tablespoon skim milk and 2 tablespoons lemon juice
Eggs	Two egg whites for one whole egg
Salt	Lemon or lime juice
	Fresh herbs
	Spicy salt substitutes
	Low-sodium hot sauce
High-fat sauces	Fat-free mayonnaise mixed with nonfat yogurt
	Fruit or vegetable salsas
	Chutney
	Reduced stocks or fruit juice

Olivos Grand Hotel near Santa Barbara, California, is to soak it in hot water for at least 10 minutes to soften it. This will make your fiber-rich baked goods much lighter and moister.

BRAISING

Braising, like baking, takes place in an oven. It is a slow, moist cooking method in which foods simmer in a covered pan in a moderately hot oven. Braising is a good way to tenderize dense vegetables, such as whole potatoes, quartered rutabagas, whole onions and large carrots as well as some of the leanest cuts of meat, such as fat-trimmed flank cuts, which can be tough.

Sear first, simmer later. Braising is especially healthful as long as meats are well trimmed and no fats are added to the pan. Prepare meat for braising by first searing it in a hot, heavy pan on top of the stove. Cook off as much fat as possible and drain it off. Searing browns and seals the surface so the meat stays moist. Then, place the meat, along with whatever vegetables and seasonings are called for in your recipe in a covered, oven-safe dish or roasting pan. Add enough liquid to cover about a third of the food, and cook it according to your recipe's instructions. The result is a medley of flavors that meld and blend like the voices in a barbershop quartet.

MICROWAVING

Microwaving is probably the next best thing to eating foods raw. Vitamins are conserved especially in vegetables, because cooking times are short and little or no water is needed. Also, added fat is not necessary.

Let your veggies ride the waves. "Vegetables in the microwave are marvelously healthful because they cook in one-fourth the time needed for other methods and require only two tablespoons of added water per quart of fresh vegetables," says Joan Toole, certified home economist, cookware designer, author and microwave-cooking instructor in Wilmington, Delaware.

Toole offers a few more rules of thumb for making microwaved vegetables as healthful and appealing as possible: Cut vegetables into uniform slices, always cover and vent them and cook on high power for six to seven minutes per pound, depending on the liquid content of the food. Low-moisture veggies like carrots take longer. To cook vegetables with different densities or sizes, such as peas and carrots, start the carrots a few minutes before adding the peas.

Because microwave energy heats liquid first, drain the liquid from canned vegetables before heating them in the microwave. For the same reason soups and very saucy dishes with chunks of vegetables or meats will not cook evenly unless you carefully follow the directions in a good microwave cookbook.

DAILY DAIRY DELIVERY—WITHOUT THE FAT

Low-fat milk, yogurt and cheeses have found their way into your fridge. Now here are many ways to help them find their way into your daily diet in place of the fattier products called for in many recipes. "In most recipes that call for milk or cheese, you can substitute low-fat or nonfat milk products with no changes to the recipe," says Melanie Polk, R.D., consulting nutritionist and author from North Potomac, Maryland.

"In some cases you won't get the same result, however," she warns. "Sometimes people need to use a little experimentation and creativity. For example, I've had lots of luck making lasagna with nonfat cheeses, but pizzas did not work out too well. My recommendation is to use the lowest-fat product that will give the results you find acceptable. Some products will work well in some dishes, but not in others."

Cheeses. "When you use a nonfat cheese, in many cases, you should use a lower cooking temperature or the cheese will get tough," says Polk. "Regular cheese is made of protein and fat, but if you take away the fat, all that's left is protein, which toughens when it's subjected to high heat." If possible, when you use nonfat cheese in a recipe, wait until near the end to add it.

Yogurt. "When you use yogurt—low-fat or otherwise—instead of sour cream in soups, dips or casseroles, add the yogurt at the end and stir it into hot foods gradually, or the yogurt will curdle," Polk warns.

Milk. "When using low-fat or skim milk in packaged puddings or custards, the finished product will be very similar to the versions made with whole milk. There's no reason to change your cooking method in that case," says Polk. What could be easier?

Stuffed, baked potatoes in ten minutes? It's possible in a microwave, says Toole. "First, pierce a potato all the way through, bake it on high power for about five minutes, then wrap it in a paper towel and let it finish cooking on the counter while you prepare low-fat cheese sauce (see page 394) and broccoli: Roll chopped broccoli in a damp, white, paper towel and put it on a paper plate. Into the oven it goes for two minutes. Split and fluff the potato with a fork, stuff it with broccoli and pour the cheese sauce over it," Toole says. "It's fun, delicious and fast."

Don't strain over grains. The time-cutting wonder of microwave cooking will not hasten grain cooking. "Rice and other grains have to be reconstituted, which takes almost as much time in a microwave oven as on the stove," says Toole. "They do come out beautifully, though, because they are not likely to stick to the cooking vessel," she explains, "and you *can* shave down the cooking time a little by starting them in very hot water."

Oatmeal and other whole-grain cereals, such as rolled barley, Wheatena and buckwheat kasha or mixed-grain Kashi, on the other hand, can be microwave-cooked right in a bowl, at 70 percent power, in about a third of the time it takes to cook them on a stove. It's quick, and there is no pot to scorch or scrub, which might encourage people to eat a hot breakfast when they might otherwise be inclined to skip it, says Toole.

Satisfy your sweet tooth. "Low-fat cakes, quick breads and muffins also can be quickly cooked in a microwave oven with good results, provided the recipe calls for fruit or low-fat yogurt. You don't really need lots of oil or egg yolks to get good results," says Toole.

"Fruits are just fabulous in the microwave, too" says Toole. Four or five baked apples, cored and stuffed with raisins and cinnamon, take just eight minutes to cook on high power, in a covered, vented dish. To make quick, no-sugar-added apple, pear or peach sauce, just chop the fruit, add a little water and some cinnamon, if you like, and cook on high power, stirring every three or four minutes, Toole recommends. Fruit sauce can be added to baked goods as a no-fat ingredient for a tasty topping.

Make the most of meat, fish and fowl. "To microwave meat, fish and poultry, it's very important to begin with food that is the same temperature throughout," says Toole. "To cook fish in the microwave oven, place it in a microwave-safe dish and tuck under any thin tails of flesh on fillets so that the fish has a uniform thickness. As for meat, face the heavier pieces toward the outer edges of the oven, where the microwave energy is most powerful."

Say cheese. "Foods with cheese in them should be cooked in a microwave set at only 70 percent power. If you cook low-fat cheese at high power for too long, it will come out like rubber," says Toole. In most cases, however, grated, low-fat cheeses can be sprinkled on microwaved foods—such as a vegetable medley of red onions; green, red and yellow peppers; squash and broccoli—after cooking, during the standing time, and it will melt just fine.

Joan Toole's low-fat, microwaved cheese sauce: "Stir together ½ cup low-fat, imitation mayonnaise, ½ cup skim milk and ⅓ cup grated, low-fat cheese in a glass measuring cup covered loosely with plastic wrap, cook it at 70 percent power for 2½ minutes, stirring it every 60 seconds, and that's it. Pour some of it over your baked potato stuffed with broccoli (see page 393), stick the rest in the refrigerator, grab a beverage, and you can sit down to eat in about 10 minutes," Toole exclaims.

HIGH-NUTRITION RECIPES

MICROWAVE LASAGNA

This recipe takes a lot of the fuss out of preparing lasagna. You can brown the ground turkey (or lean beef, if you prefer) in the microwave. Then you assemble the dish without cooking the noodles first. This recipe was created by Anita Hirsch, a nutritionist at the Rodale Food Center.

- **8 ounces lean ground turkey**
- **4 cups tomato sauce**
- **½ cup water**
- **1½ cups nonfat ricotta cheese**
- **¼ cup fat-free egg substitute**
- **2 tablespoons minced fresh basil**
- **2 tablespoons minced fresh parsley**
- **½ teaspoon ground black pepper**
- **9 lasagna noodles**
- **8 ounces nonfat mozzarella cheese, shredded**
- **¼ cup grated Parmesan cheese**

Crumble the turkey into a large glass bowl. Microwave on high for 2 minutes. Break up the pieces and stir well. Microwave on high for 1 minute, or until the turkey is cooked through. Drain well. Stir in the tomato sauce and water.

In a medium bowl, mix the ricotta, egg, basil, parsley and pepper.

Spoon about 1 cup of the tomato mixture into the bottom of an 8" × 12" glass baking dish.

Top with 3 of the noodles. Spread with about ½ cup of the ricotta mixture. Sprinkle with some mozzarella and Parmesan. Top with about 1 cup of the tomato mixture. Repeat the layering procedure twice to use all the ingredients.

Cover with wax paper. Microwave on high for 4 minutes. Give the dish a quarter turn. (If your microwave isn't deep enough to hold the dish sideways, give it a half-turn.) Microwave on high for 4 more minutes.

Turn the dish again. Microwave on medium-low (30% power) for a total of 30 minutes; stop every 10 minutes to turn the dish.

Let stand 15 minutes before serving.

Serves 9

Per serving: *191 calories, 1.5 g. fat (7% of calories), 1.8 g. dietary fiber, 22 mg. cholesterol, 371 mg. sodium*

Mahi Mahi with Jamaican Tartar Sauce

Poaching is a very easy, low-fat way to cook fish. This recipe was developed by Tom Ney, director of the Rodale Food Center. You may substitute other types of firm fish, such as salmon, cod, snapper or sablefish.

⅓ cup finely chopped papaya
⅓ cup nonfat mayonnaise
¼ cup thinly sliced scallions
2 tablespoons finely chopped lime flesh
1 tablespoon minced fresh coriander
½ teaspoon hot-pepper sauce
2 quarts water
3 tablespoons white-wine vinegar
3 lemon slices
4 bay leaves
1 tablespoon pickling spices
¼ teaspoon celery seeds
1 pound mahi mahi fillet

In a small bowl, mix the papaya, mayonnaise, scallions, lime, coriander and hot-pepper sauce. Cover and refrigerate for at least 1 hour.

In a large frying pan, combine the water, vinegar, lemon slices, bay leaves, pickling spices and celery seeds. Bring to a boil, then reduce the heat to medium-low and simmer for 10 minutes.

Add the mahi mahi to the pan. If necessary, add more water to the pan to cover the fish. Simmer for 15 minutes, or until the fish is just cooked through.

Use 2 metal spatulas to remove the fish from the liquid without breaking it. If desired, remove some of the spices from the fish (but they're edible, except for the bay leaves). Serve with the papaya sauce.

Serves 4
Per serving: *120 calories, 0.8 g. fat (6% of calories), 0.2 g. dietary fiber, 83 mg. cholesterol, 355 mg. sodium*

Savory Roasted Onions

Roasting gives onions a sweet, mellow flavor, making them a delicious side-dish vegetable for fish, poultry or meat.

4 large onions
¼ teaspoon olive oil
¼ teaspoon dried savory
2 teaspoons balsamic vinegar

Peel the onions and cut in half lengthwise. Coat with the oil and sprinkle with the savory. Place, cut side down, in a shallow baking dish. Bake at 350° for 50 minutes, or until tender. Sprinkle with the vinegar before serving.

Serves 4
Per serving: *66 calories, 0.5 g. fat (7% of calories), 2.6 g. dietary fiber, 0 mg. cholesterol, 5 mg. sodium*

SCALLOP STIR-FRY

Stir-frying is a quick cooking method that retains the fresh flavors of foods. And it's very adaptable to whatever is in your pantry. In this recipe, you may replace the scallops with shrimp or strips of chicken breast. And you may use other vegetables, such as broccoli florets, mushrooms, onions, snow peas or peppers.

- **1 pound medium sea scallops**
- **1 tablespoon cornstarch**
- **¾ cup orange juice**
- **2 tablespoons low-sodium soy sauce**
- **1 tablespoon honey**
- **1 tablespoon minced fresh ginger**
- **¼ teaspoon red-pepper flakes**
- **2 large carrots, thinly sliced on the diagonal**
- **1 celery stalk, thinly sliced on the diagonal**
- **½ cup sliced water chestnuts**
- **2 teaspoons peanut or canola oil**
- **3 cups hot cooked rice**

Cut the scallops crosswise into rounds about ⅓" thick. Pat dry on paper towels and set aside.

In a small bowl, dissolve the cornstarch in the orange juice. Stir in the soy sauce, honey, ginger and red-pepper flakes. Set aside.

In a wok or large frying pan over medium-high heat, stir-fry the carrots, celery and chestnuts in 1 teaspoon of the oil for 5 minutes, or until crisp-tender. Remove with a slotted spoon and set aside.

Add the remaining 1 teaspoon oil to the pan. Add the scallops and stir-fry for 2 minutes, or until just cooked through. Return the vegetables to the pan. Pour in the orange sauce. Stir until thickened, about 2 minutes.

Serve over the rice.

Serves 4
Per serving: *359 calories, 4.6 g. fat (12% of calories), 4.3 g. dietary fiber, 37 mg. cholesterol, 515 mg. sodium*

CHAPTER 29

RESTAURANT SAVVY

DINING OUT WITHOUT DAMAGE

If calories consumed were dollars spent, a not-so-unusual restaurant meal for two of chicken wings, New England clam chowder, tossed salad with blue cheese dressing, prime rib with sour cream and horseradish sauce, twice-baked potato stuffed with Cheddar cheese, buttered corn-on-the-cob, garlic bread, deep-dish apple pie à la mode and Irish coffee would cost almost enough to buy the restaurant owner a gold Rolex.

Lucky thing that's not the case. But a meal like this *can* cost you plenty in terms of your calorie, salt, fat and cholesterol budget. Dining out—whether breakfast with the boss, a fast-food jaunt with the kids, lunch in the company cafeteria or a romantic dinner can be a nourishing adventure, though, when you take your healthy eating habits with you.

Before you leave the house and head for the neon signs that virtually cry out, "Eat here, eat here," there are two general guidelines to keep in mind about dining out without damage. They apply to all types of establishments, including diners, pizza parlors, sandwich shops, cafeterias, convenience stores, full-service restaurants, bar-and-grills, fast-food places and even other people's homes.

First, be on the lookout for meals that fulfill both your flavor *and* nutrition needs. They can be found almost anywhere, but it's easier to select a healthy and tasty balance of foods in eateries that offer a wide variety of dishes.

Next, strive for moderation in your eating habits, even though many restaurants make it all too easy to overindulge. You can hold the line on calories, salt, fat and sugar even when you're not doing the cooking. It's just a matter of making smart choices and sticking to them.

CHEFS WHO CARE ABOUT HEALTH

The healthy bandwagon is traveling at a dizzying pace as more and more people like you jump on. Restaurant owners and chefs are not only among the wagon-hopping crowd—they're often leading the band. "It's become the responsibility of restaurateurs to educate and show customers that there's a healthy way to eat without giving up the excitement of the restaurant experience," says Michael Franks, proprietor of several West Coast restaurants, including Chez Melange in Redondo Beach, California.

Franks is national chairman of the chefs' committee of Project LEAN, a group whose objective is to creatively reduce fat in the American diet. Innovative chefs around the country are finding substitutes for and cutting back on offending ingredients; devising menus that depend less on fatty meats and more on vegetables, grains and other heart-smart items; and borrowing pearls of healthful wisdom from the cuisines of other cultures. A peek into a few inspired chefs' kitchens will show you how they do it.

At Chez Melange, the game, in many cases, is substitution, Franks explains. "We try to replace high-fat items with low-fat items. Nonfat yogurt replaces sour cream. We also cook with reduced stocks in place of butter. Instead of rich sauces we use fresh, nonfat salsas. We often replace fatty meat, like hamburger, with a low-fat protein like ground turkey. We try to replace things while still giving customers what they're used to. And we do it by using products that are fresh and natural."

Are you afraid that by going to a health-oriented restaurant you might be faced with boring, tasteless dietetic foods? One taste of a typical Chez Melange lunch—peppered fresh tuna with Japanese salsa over oriental greens, with basmati rice and steamed vegetables—may quell your fears. This dish weighs in at just 240 calories, 25 milligrams of cholesterol and 4 grams of fat.

TEACHING THE RIGHT TECHNIQUES

Some chefs emphasize moderation, rather than eliminating certain ingredients altogether, explains Robert Briggs, a chef instructor at the Culinary Institute of America in Hyde Park, New York, where students attend classes in nutritional cooking as well as gourmet cooking. "We're teaching students who are going to be chefs to use ingredients they're already comfortable with, but to use less of them when they can. For example, we show them how they can do a lot with a lot less butter than usual. One way to drasti-

A CAFÉ THAT'S REALLY SPECIAL

Nutrition education for chefs is a trend for the 90s and beyond. The Culinary Institute of America, in Hyde Park, New York, teaches low-fat cooking and nutrition to its future chefs during a three-week course conducted at St. Andrew's Cafe, one of the school's four public restaurants. The healthy philosophy there calls for moderating calories, fats, sodium and cholesterol, while bolstering complex carbohydrates. "Meals at the café provide about 800 to 1,000 calories each, compared with a typical restaurant meal's calorie load of 2,000 to 2,200 calories," explains Catherine Powers, R.D., a nutritionist at the institute.

The menu reveals a roster of treats that sound anything but depriving. How about an appetizer of warm smoked duck with pasta, radicchio and shallot vinaigrette, followed by Michigan white bean soup scented with rosemary and sage, an entrée of roast chicken stuffed with fresh herbs, served with garlic-potato ravioli, glazed root vegetables and a salad of baby mixed greens with champagne herb vinaigrette?

Leave room for dessert. There's saffron-poached pears with rice pudding and kiln-dried cherry sauce. Or perhaps you prefer the fresh-baked Hudson Valley pear strudel with amaretto glacé. If you haven't drooled all over this page, you may want to show it to your favorite chef as an example of the lavish, yet healthful heights to which restaurant fare can soar.

cally reduce the amount of melted butter we use is to put it in a spray bottle," Briggs explains. In many cases, just a spritz can boost flavor without significantly increasing calories from fat.

At the institute, student chefs are taught techniques for cutting fat in everything from salad dressings to desserts: "Normal salad dressing, for example, is about 75 to 95 percent fat," Briggs says. "But we can cut that by about two-thirds by using a small amount of very high quality fat—like avocado puree—that has a lot of flavor. Then we replace the fat we've taken out with juice, stock or water and thicken it lightly with cornstarch or arrowroot, so it's the same consistency as oily dressing. By adding vinegar or citrus juice and whatever seasoning we want to that basic recipe, we can make an infinite number of different dressings, and no one knows they're lower in fat."

The four basic sauces in traditional cooking—velouté, bechámel, brown and hollandaise—make up another fat-laden area that lends itself well to the institute's method. "The basic sauces can all be made low-fat by using evaporated skim milk instead of cream and by thickening them with a plain starch instead of roux or egg yolk. By adding flavorings like mustard, defatted chicken stock or fish stock, the possibilities are limitless," says Briggs.

Chefs at the institute who teach the health-wise classes have even developed a low-fat version of crème anglaise—the creamy basis for many rich desserts—from a mixture of ricotta cheese, nonfat yogurt and sugar, corn syrup or honey. By adding gelatin and meringue to the base, rather than real cream, it is transformed into low-fat Bavarian cream. In another metamorphosis it becomes a rich-tasting frozen delight.

Another way some chefs cater to their guests' health concerns is to offer low-fat options in addition to a "regular" menu. "We have a separate menu insert that lists all our reduced-fat items together with the amount of total fat, calories and percentage of calories from fat in each dish," says Richard Wright, senior chef at Hawk Prairie Inn in Olympia, Washington. For example, guests can order a 'typical' prime rib roast beef dinner or another beef dish featuring meat that was raised and processed to contain less fat.

A World of Low-Fat Cuisines

Another way chefs are helping Americans change the way they eat is by borrowing ingredients and cooking techniques from the global community. "International cuisines are frequently built around rice or other grains, and they use more naturally low-fat foods, such as fish, lentils and beans," says Franks.

"In traditional Chinese and Asian cuisine, meat is not served on a daily or even monthly basis," explains Martin Yan, chef, food consultant, and host of the PBS-TV series "Yan Can Cook." "Meat, when it is available, is mainly used as a flavoring ingredient or as a supplement to a variety of vegetable dishes. It's more of a condiment than a main ingredient. A lot of dishes are made by combining several vegetables that are in season."

We're not talking about piles of flavorless, boiled string beans with canned pearl onions, either. Innovative American chefs are combining colorful, crisp veggies from here and abroad with Mediterranean whole grains, pastas and fruits. Beans and seeds dance to a Latin beat, or they're dressed in lemongrass from Thailand, curries from India, ginger from China and sauces from Indonesia and Vietnam. Marco Polo himself would have been thrilled to sample the flavors that are flying in from around the world and landing in American restaurants.

"International foods are usually only healthy if they're prepared and eaten the way they are in their country of origin, though," says Franks. "The trouble comes when foods become too Americanized." To bypass that snag, many restaurants with a healthy bent borrow cooking techniques and philosophies as well as ingredients from international kitchens.

"The healthiest techniques in Chinese and Asian cuisine, for example, are steaming and stir-frying, with occasional braising and stewing," says Yan. "Deep-frying is rarely used. Stir-frying uses a minimum amount of oil, and the wok is heated before the oil and food are added. When meat is stir-fried, the heat sears and seals in its juices. By steaming, the food cooks in its own juice and moisture and never touches water or oil, so the food retains its original flavor and character."

THE BEST AND WORST AT ETHNIC EATERIES

Living in a melting pot like the United States means you can have a taste of different cultures without traveling very far. Some of the world's healthiest fare comes from afar, too. The listings below, arranged according to restaurant type, will help you choose wisely when you explore the world with your fork.

CHINESE

Dig into: Steamed rice; boiled, steamed or stir-fried veggies with little oil; skinless poultry; fish and shellfish (in moderation); tofu (not fried).

Steer clear of: Fried rice, salty soups, too much soy sauce, MSG, fried noodles, crispy duck, egg dishes and soups, sweet-and-sour dishes (they're deep-fried first), pickled foods.

MEDITERRANEAN AND MIDDLE EASTERN

Dig into: Pita bread; legumes like lentils, chick-peas and broad beans; hummus; roast eggplant (babaghanouj) and olive oil in moderate amounts; wheat or cracked-wheat foods like couscous and bulgur; yogurt or pima; grape leaves.

Steer clear of: Too many olives and anchovies and too much feta cheese (use just a little of these as flavorings), baklava and other phyllo-dough dishes (except tiny servings), fatty lamb dishes, fried eggplant.

JAPANESE

Dig into: Rice (except fried), fish, raw vegetables, tofu, miso soup, yakimono (broiled foods), sukiyaki (stir-fried meat dish).

Steer clear of: Too much soy sauce or peanut sauce, deep-fried tempura, teriyaki, too many pickled foods.

INDIAN

Dig into: Yogurt-based curry sauce, salads, chutneys, raita (yogurt with shredded vegetables), tandoori chicken and fish (request no butter-basting), seekh kabab with lean lamb only, dal (lentils),

READY TO TRY SOMETHING NEW?

Finally, there are chefs who believe the best way to change the way you eat is to change the way you think about food. "Instead of taking a dish that's meant to be very rich and trying to turn it into a healthy dish, I say just forget that dish altogether and go have something completely different," suggests Chris Schlesinger, chef and co-owner of the East Coast Grill in Cambridge, Massachusetts.

rice, breads like pulkas and nan.

Steer clear of: Ghee (clarified butter), deep-fried meats.

ITALIAN

Dig into: Pasta with vegetables or marinara sauce, garlic, salads and antipasto without oily dressing or too many meats, crusty bread without butter or oil, steamed leafy vegetables like kale and broccoli raab, zucchini, fresh tomatoes and fresh (unsalted) mozzarella, broiled or grilled meat or fish dishes, Italian ices.

Steer clear of: Cream-, butter-, or oil-and-wine-based sauces; meatballs and sausage; veal scaloppine; Parmesan-style or cheese-stuffed dishes; fried eggplant; spumone or tortoni ice creams; cappuccino.

MEXICAN

Dig into: Whole beans and rice, salsas, grilled chicken or fish, corn or flour tortillas in moderation (most are made with oil), seviche (marinade-cooked fish), colorful soups and stews, salads, onions and peppers, sliced avocado garnishes, fruit and fruit ices.

Steer clear of: Ground beef and pork dishes, heavy cheese, sour cream and guacamole fillings and toppings, chimichangas, refried beans cooked with lard, deep-fried churros (doughnuts) and other sweet breads.

FRENCH

Dig into: Salads with dressings on the side, steamed mussels, crusty baguettes without butter, fresh fruit, steamed vegetables, some "nouvelle" dishes, bordelaise and other light wine sauces in moderation, crêpes with fruit or lightly sautéed seafood.

Steer clear of: Pâtés; duck or goose with skin; au gratin dishes; hollandaise, béchamel, béarnaise, and other cream, egg, butter and high-salt sauces; buttery omelettes, croissants and pastries.

"Look to fundamental change, not to substitutes," Schlesinger continues. "Eat something different, like grilled shrimp in tomatilla pineapple salsa with rice and beans. Or try grilled squid with lo mein noodles and ginger, garlic and lime juice. Don't just stop eating certain things. Instead, introduce a wider variety of foods into your diet."

Wide variety is truly the spice of life in cities like New Orleans, a place famed for spice and excitement. Just ask Emeril Lagasse, formerly executive chef at Commander's Palace, now owner of Emeril's. He strives to bring Creole dishes into the health-conscious 90s. "To do this, we start with the best ingredients and work from scratch. That way, we can really control the quality of the food we serve our customers," says Lagasse, a chef who really keeps pace with what his customers want.

"There's a growing interest in vegetables and vegetarian dishes," Lagasse observes. American poll-takers, ever alert to changes in the nation's pulse, concur. About one-third of all adults surveyed in one study said they are likely to order vegetarian meals if available. At Emeril's, their search would not be in vain.

"We do a lot of things with vegetables. For example, we offer a creative vegetable dish that consists of about 14 to 16 seasonal vegetables that are grilled, roasted, baked or pureed. In fall, for example, there may be two or three different types of baby beets, roasted sweet corn, roasted garlic, puree of two or three root vegetables or squashes and more-typical vegetables like zucchini, yellow squash, onions and stewed tomatoes with garlic. The foundation of the plate is a vegetable pasta tossed with herbs," Lagasse says.

Your Table Is Waiting

Makes you want to hop a plane just to sample the healthy fare in one of these restaurants, doesn't it? Well, you may not have to. An enlightened chef or restaurateur—or one who's willing to learn—may be right around the corner. Here's what you need to do.

Call ahead. To find such a restaurateur, call ahead, not just to make reservations or ask about prices, but to learn how well the establishment can serve your health needs. Ask for a few examples from the regular menu. If nothing stands out, find out if the chef is willing to make simple changes—such as serving sauces on the side, poaching or broiling fish or meat, preparing meatless dishes or omitting salt or butter. In response, the manager or chef may suggest a particular time when custom-made orders will be easiest to fulfill. Sudden demands for unusual fare at seven o'clock on a hectic Saturday night may find a less than flexible chef and staff. If they know your needs in advance, though, you will most likely be well accommodated, so don't be an anonymous caller. And if you enjoy your customized meal, a little praise for the staff and recommending the restaurant to others afterward, will go a long way toward making you a welcome and honored guest.

Take responsibility. Finding a restaurant that offers a variety of foods from which you may order a healthy meal is at least half the battle. But few restaurants—outside of health spas—offer nothing but low-fat, low-sodium, high-fiber foods. No matter how varied the offerings, there is only one person who can control the real impact this dining experience will have on your body. You guessed it. That person is you. And the decisions you make about how much and what types of foods you will order begin before you even look at the menu.

Eat something in advance. Don't risk a gut-splitting pigout by starving yourself before you get to the restaurant. Stifle an urge to overindulge by eating normally earlier in the day. Otherwise, you may not be as resistant to high-fat appetizers and hors d'oeuvres, salty munchies or gigantic portions. A snack of bread or fruit may be helpful if dinner or lunch will be served very late.

ARE YOU READY TO ORDER?

Here are a few guidelines for making your way through a typical restaurant meal. We'll begin at the top, with a health-smart cocktail and the free tongue ticklers that often get to the table before you do.

Drinks. An elegant meal need not begin with a high-calorie, alcohol-based drink. To quench your thirst or give your hands something to do before your meal arrives, you may wish to order fresh-squeezed orange juice, a glass of ice and a bottle of sparkling water to mix your own fruit spritzer. Or try sparkling water with a dash of bitters. Many mixed drinks can also be prepared "virgin-style" (without alcohol) as well.

Finger foods. Delve right into the relish tray, if one is offered. It may contain crisp, raw snow peas, red peppers, cauliflower, baby corn, carrots, celery, radishes or other colorful tidbits. Be wary of most other free hors d'oeuvres, however. Popcorn, crackers with pâtés or spreads, and hot hors d'oeuvres are usually loaded with fat and salt. They will entice you to drink. In this case, restaurants are not concerned so much about your health as they are about their own bottom lines.

Appetizers. "Stay away from anything deep-fried," advises Dotty Griffith, cookbook author, food editor of the *Dallas Morning News* and participant in Project LEAN. That includes fried vegetables, cheese or fish appetizers. "And anytime you find a dish that's had a lot done to it—if it's breaded, fried, sautéed in butter, pureed or has a sauce or other ingredient on it—chances are, the stuff they add is made of fat, because fat carries flavor," says Griffith. Better selections are simple appetizers, like smoked fish, roasted fresh vegetables or fruit.

Soups. "Cream soups are another thing to watch out for," says Griffith. Where there's a choice, go with clear soups that are hearty with vegetables, grains or pasta.

Salads. "Salads are not really healthy selections if they're globbed up with a lot of cheese or high-fat dressing," Griffith warns. Instead, look for salads that are topped with fresh herbs or crunchy treats, such as baby corn, water chestnuts or snow peas. A salad like that doesn't need to be overdressed. "A dash of herb vinegar or lemon or lime juice goes a long way," says Griffith.

Entrées. When you are ready to order your main course, you may wish to glance back at the menu's earlier course offerings. Some restaurants offer separate pasta courses in appetizer sizes, which you could order as an entrée, instead. Regardless of the portion size, you will probably have your

MENU WARNING SIGNALS

To help you sort through the appetizer, soup, entrée and dessert offerings on a typical restaurant menu, here are two lists. These contain some common buzzwords that may tip you off to foods that could tilt your fat and sodium scales in the wrong direction.

HIGH-FAT WARNING WORDS

- Rich
- Creamy
- Au gratin
- Cheesy
- Fried, including "pan-fried"
- Fritter
- Gravy
- Saucy
- Breaded
- Crunchy
- Crispy
- Scalloped or escalloped
- Buttery
- Flaky
- Pastry

HIGH-SODIUM WARNING WORDS

- Smoked
- Pickled
- Barbecued
- Broth
- Bouillon
- Cocktail sauce
- Soy sauce
- Teriyaki
- Cured
- Marinated

Remember, these are just clues. If there is any doubt about how a food is actually prepared, ask your server.

choice of sauces: There's always marinara sauce, which is healthiest because there's very little fat in it, says Joanne D'Agostino, R.N., cookbook author and Pennsylvania-based restaurant consultant. Alfredo sauce, made mostly from cream and cheese is probably out of the question. Meat sauces may not look fatty, but often the meat and all the fat that cooks out of it go directly into the sauce without draining, D'Agostino explains. "Seafood sauces are healthier because the amount of fat that leaves the fish and cooks into the sauce is minimal and, chances are, there won't be a tremendous amount of oil added."

As for more traditional entrées, if you have a choice between deep-fried and poached seafood, or between a fatty steak and a grilled chicken breast, the healthy selections are obvious. But if the choices are not so clearly spelled out, you may need to use a more savvy approach.

"If the restaurant does not mark the menu in some way to indicate which items are low-fat and which are not, it becomes incumbent on customers to know what kinds of ingredients they need to avoid," says Wright. "Then they need to decide which items on the menu are going to be good for them and which aren't, and start asking if certain ingredients can be withheld." For example, many sautéed or broiled meat or seafood dishes incorporate a lot of fat in the cooking process, or receive a shower of butter just before leaving the kitchen. The customer must learn to ask if there is a lot of butter, oil or salt in a dish and, if so, whether the chef can hold those ingredients, Wright explains.

"You can take this advice into any restaurant," advises Yan. "If you go into an Italian restaurant and there's too much olive oil in your pasta dish, next time ask them to use less. But ask with courtesy," he cautions. "You want to develop a working relationship with the chef and the staff in the restaurant. Most restaurateurs will gladly accommodate your request. Besides, they want your business, especially if you are a longtime customer. If they are unwilling to cooperate, it is time to switch to another restaurant and develop a working relationship there. After all, it is your health that matters most."

HEARTS ON MY MENU

They're popping up on menus all over the country: Little red heart-shaped symbols that signal heart-healthy items. Who decides which foods will have a heart? Many restaurants are joining forces with hospital-sponsored or independent dietitians to help customers find foods that promote good health.

"We sponsor area restaurants that use recipes that are lower in fat, cholesterol and sodium," explains Vickie L. Spillane, R.D., who reviews menus to determine how well they fit with the HEARTCHECK Program of Our Lady of Lourdes Medical Center in Camden, New Jersey. Some of the parameters for eligibility in this program and others like it include:

- Preparing foods with two teaspoons or less of a polyunsaturated or monounsaturated oil or margarine per serving.
- Using low-fat cooking methods, such as baking, broiling, roasting, grilling, poaching and steaming instead of frying.
- Preparing foods without adding salt or MSG.
- Preparing broth-based soups.
- Serving polyunsaturated margarine as an alternative to butter.
- Trimming all visible fat from meat and limiting portion size to six ounces.
- Providing skim or 1 percent milk as an alternative to whole milk.

Dining in restaurants sponsored by hospital-based programs like HEARTCHECK takes the guesswork out of healthy dining. What could be easier?

Whatever entrée you decide upon, the next challenge is controlling the amount you eat. For meat or fish entrées, one way to gauge the generally recommended three- to four-ounce serving is to use the "palm method," says Sheri Shansby Boyden, R.D., a dietitian at the Mayo Medical Center in Rochester, Minnesota, who advises diabetic patients about healthy eating. "The average woman's palm, without fingers, is about the size of a correct portion," she explains. "So, when the food arrives, a woman can discreetly compare the portion of meat, fish or poultry to her palm and decide how much she should actually eat." Men may wish to envision a deck of cards as their size guide, instead, experts say.

Others advise simply deciding beforehand not to overeat and relying on willpower to avoid getting carried away. One technique to avoid overeating that works for many people is to chew more. "Relax, eat slowly, chew your food thoroughly and let dinner last a long time," D'Agostino advises. "Chewing and really tasting food brings a lot of satisfaction. And extending the amount of time it takes to eat helps to overcome the tendency to stuff ourselves because it gives the stomach a chance to tell the brain that it's had enough."

Side dishes. Now that you are adept at entrée selection, you're ready for this side-dish quiz: Which of the following side dishes are good selections for a vitamin/mineral/fiber boost without excess fat?

- Fresh-cut French-fried potatoes
- Herbed new potatoes
- Cheese-stuffed baked potato
- Sliced tomatoes with basil
- Creamy coleslaw
- Broccoli florets marinated in dill vinegar
- Asparagus spears with hollandaise sauce
- Garden-fresh peas with pearl onions

Answer: Every other one, beginning with the second selection, is a healthy choice. Enjoy.

Bonus question: Which of the less-healthy dishes above can be modified most easily and how should you relay your request to the cook?

Answer: It's the asparagus, and one good way to phrase your special request is: "I'd like the asparagus, please. But will you ask the chef to put the hollandaise on the side so that I can use just a taste of it? Thank you."

Congratulations! You've won a chance to read about dessert.

Desserts. "When you have a choice, lean toward fruit desserts," advises Briggs. "They will generally be healthier. And it doesn't just have to be a poached pear or baked apple. Today, there are many frozen fruit yogurts and sorbets. Beware, though, that some can be loaded with sugar, even though they may be lower in fat than ice cream. A phyllo dough basket filled with fruit and served with fruit sauce is another possibility," he suggests.

"Fruit cup from the appetizer menu, and low-fat frozen yogurt or sherbet can be combined to make a low-fat sundae," D'Agostino suggests. "Angel food cake with fresh fruit is another good choice. And, if I really can't find anything else on the menu, I'd order fruit pie, but skip the crust and just eat the filling."

Even chocolate cake is okay to order once in a while, especially if you ask for just one piece to share among several people. This kind of mini-indulgence has become the norm, rather than the exception, in many restaurants.

The healthy dining methods above cover a lot of territory, and many are useful whether the meal is breakfast, lunch or dinner. The two earlier meals of the day have some interesting challenges all their own, however.

RISE AND SHINE

Breakfast. It's often called the most important meal of the day, yet it's the meal most often skipped. It's also the meal least frequently eaten out, although more and more people are eating breakfast away from home these days.

Many traditional diner-style breakfast foods have no-no reputations: triple-egg omelettes oozing cheese; pancakes, french toast and waffles slathered with butter and syrup; bacon, sausage, ham, pork roll and scrapple; plus home fries, corned beef hash and hash brown potatoes sizzling in the grease left on the grill. A long, slippery list, but it's easily countered by yes-yes breakfast dishes with a host of saving graces.

Fresh berries over crispy, buckwheat waffles, steaming oatmeal with raisins and cinnamon; a lightly toasted bagel with strawberry jam; oven-browned garlic-and-parsley potatoes; sweet slices of cantaloupe and honeydew melon; even yolkless omelettes stuffed with sweet red peppers, mushrooms, onions and broccoli are great eye-openers. And with someone else doing the cooking, a healthy breakfast away from home can really light up your morning, says Tracy Ritter, a chef and owner of Vitality Cuisine, a food consulting firm in San Diego.

Breakfast and brunch buffets are especially easy places to eat too much. Here's where Clean Plate Club members may face their biggest challenge. Heaps of greasy sausage and eggs, mountains of deep-fried French toast, tray upon tray of home fries and buckets of steaming grits with tubs of butter and thick gravy beckon with oversized serving spoons and beg to be eaten or . . . gulp . . . go to waste. It may take gargantuan willpower, but reject the challenge to use up a whole stack of fresh plates by yourself. Remember, there are lots of people in line behind you who will help empty the tureens of cheese sauce. You don't have to do it alone.

Breakfast and brunch buffets offer a wide selection of foods, and if your main objective is to "get your money's worth," you can certainly do it without sending your cholesterol count through the ceiling. Take a good look down the line at the array of offerings before you fill your plate with the items closest to you. It's okay to shuffle along with an empty plate until you reach the cereals, fruits, juices and breads. With so many delicious and healthy ways to start the day, making it through to lunch should be a snap.

The Lunch Whistle

If you are one of the lucky few who have a company dining room or cafeteria that has leaped onto the healthy bandwagon, you know the joys of

In the Fast Lane

For occasions that find you in fast-food places, here's a short guide to items with some of the lowest proportions of fat.

Food	Calories	Fat (g.)	Percentage of Calories from Fat
Breakfast Foods			
Hardee's Three Pancakes (with syrup and margarine)	292	8	25
McDonald's Hotcakes (with margarine and syrup)	440	12	25
Roy Rogers Pancake Platter (with ham)	506	17	30
McDonald's Egg McMuffin	280	11	35
Burgers			
McDonald's McLean Deluxe	320	10	28
Wendy's Jr. Hamburger	270	9	30
Hardee's Hamburger	260	10	35
Roast Beef			
Roy Rogers Roast Beef Sandwich	317	10	28
Hardee's Regular Roast Beef	280	11	35
Chicken			
Chick-fil-A Chargrilled Chicken Deluxe Sandwich	266	5	17
Carl's Jr. Charbroiler BBQ Chicken Sandwich	310	6	17
Hardee's Grilled Chicken Sandwich	310	9	26
Long John Silver's Batter-Dipped Chicken Sandwich	410	16	35

bean, vegetable or pasta salads and low-fat hot entrées that look good, taste great and keep you going strong all afternoon. If not, take some tips from Terri Seewald Klein, R.D., a Havertown, Pennsylvania nutrition consultant specializing in helping businesses improve their employee food and fitness services.

"First of all, do some advance planning," Klein says. "Look over the week's menu before you even walk into the cafeteria, and have some decisions made before you're confronted with items that may tempt you.

FOOD	CALORIES	FAT (g.)	PERCENTAGE OF CALORIES FROM FAT
FISH			
Long John Silver's Light Portion Fish (2 pieces, with lemon crumb, rice and small salad)	270	5	17
Long John Silver's Baked Fish (3 pieces, with lemon crumb, rice, green beans, coleslaw and roll)	570	12	19
POTATOES			
Roy Rogers' Plain Baked Potato	211	0.2	0.9
Wendy's Plain Baked Potato	300	<1	<3
Carl's Jr. Lite Potato	290	1	3
Arby's Plain Baked Potato	240	2	8
MEXICAN			
El Pollo Loco Pinto Beans	110	1	8
Taco Bell Bean Burrito with red sauce)	458	14	28
El Pollo Loco Chicken (with corn tortillas and salsa)	530	20	34

"Look for hot entrées that are steamed, broiled or grilled. Anything in a cream sauce or deep-fried will be higher in fat. If the vegetables are steamed and you have the option of ordering them without butter or with sauce on the side, that's preferable," says Klein.

Eating your vegetables this way is a good way to increase your fiber intake. The sandwich and salad bar is another good place to bulk up on high-fiber items. "Salad bars have really been a great addition to company cafeterias," says Klein. They are also important parts of many restaurants and supermarkets as well. Wherever you graze, the general guidelines are the same: Select items like beans, tomatoes, peppers, sprouts, cauliflower, broccoli and spinach. Spinach is a better choice than iceberg lettuce as a base for your salad because of the additional vitamins and minerals it contains. Things to watch out for are potato salad, coleslaw, egg salad: Anything prepared with lots of added fats. That includes croutons. Many croutons are prepared with additional fat. "Another word of caution about salad bars concerns dressings," Klein adds. "They can really add a lot of fat to the diet. Good alternatives are reduced-calorie or fat-free salad dressing, lemon juice or vinegar with a little bit of oil."

Next stop is the sandwich line. "When you have a choice in the sandwich line, select whole-grain breads, " Klein advises. "And steer clear of high-fat cold cuts, like salami and bologna. More heart-healthy choices are lean meats like turkey or lean ham. But, anyone on a salt- or sodium-restricted diet has to watch out for many deli items, which are processed with salt," she warns. What is the health rating of other standard sandwich fillings? "Anything that's prepared with mayonnaise will add a lot of fat to the diet. Some cafeterias or sandwich shops give you the option of reduced-calorie mayonnaise as a spread. Or opt for mustard, catsup or vinegar with just a splash of oil."

If fast food is more your speed, check out a burger joint that also serves up baked potatoes (hold the sour cream, cheese and bacon, though). Or, seek out a place with salads or a salad bar and follow the guidelines above. Hold the fries and think twice about having fried chicken or fish unless you *at least* remove the skin and crust.

Nearly anywhere and anytime you choose to eat out, you have at least some healthy options, and they're increasing as rapidly as new restaurants are opening. With a bit of communication and cooperation between restaurant owners, chefs and customers, it is becoming ever easier for *every* meal to be healthy as well as satisfying.

CHAPTER 30

Natural Food Stores

Naturally Better?

You wouldn't know it from the cramped shelves and less-than-posh decor, but chances are, your neighborhood natural food store contains the foods of the future.

Many of the nutritionally superior foods gracing supermarket shelves today got their start in health food and natural food stores. Among them are granola, herbal teas, ice cream substitutes, pita bread, rice cakes, salsa, sports drinks, soy meat and dairy substitutes, wheat bran and yogurt. "Really just about any innovative product you can think of," says Jeffrey Bland, Ph.D., a clinical nutritionist in Gig Harbor, Washington, and a senior investigator for the American Association of Clinical Scientists.

And then there are the natural food store items that perpetuate the convenience-store-to-the-counterculture mystique: mysterious potions, wacky literature (One actual headline: "Your Astrology Diet") and dubious supplements that promise to boost energy, renew your sex drive and build muscle—simultaneously.

"You have to be careful," says Kim Galeaz-Gioe, R.D., a spokesperson for the American Dietetic Association. "Just because something is sold in a health food store doesn't automatically mean it's healthy."

In fact, the average natural food store carries several hundred items—from herbs to organic peanut butter—each with its own purported health merits.

But once past the questionable products, your taste buds and body are in for an adventure: A smorgasbord of healthy foods await that you can't find in most supermarkets . . . *yet*.

NOT JUST FOR HEALTH NUTS ANYMORE

Here, overprocessed foods loaded with additives and refined sugar are out and products made with whole, natural and often organically grown ingredients are in.

And who's buying? Diabetics avoiding added sugar. Wheat- and yeast-sensitive people trying to find bread that doesn't make them feel bad. People with lactose intolerance turning to soy milk. Moms who want to give their kids nutritious snacks. Aspiring body-builders searching for a competitive edge. Not just folks with ailments, but folks who want to eat healthier.

"It just makes sense. The closer you can get to consuming food in its natural state, the better," says Mark Messina, Ph.D., a nutritionist with the National Cancer Institute's Diet and Cancer Branch in Bethesda, Maryland.

Health foods stores are definitely a hit: Americans now spend over $4 billion a year at natural food stores, according to the National Nutritional Foods Association, the industry's leading trade group.

Growth in popularity of natural foods has also meant growth in the sizes of stores. Over the past decade, nearly 200 supermarket-size health food stores have sprouted across the country, including chains like Mrs. Gooch's Natural Market in California, Kathy's Ranch Market in Las Vegas and Salt Lake City, and Massachusetts-based Bread and Circus. The nation's largest: Unicorn Village Marketplace, a 28,000-square-foot behemoth that includes a restaurant and a gift store, located in the posh Aventura section of North Miami Beach.

In addition to offering an even wider selection than mom-and-pop-size health food markets, these superstores often stock private-label products, organically grown produce (fruit and vegetables grown without the use of synthetic fertilizers or pesticides) and beef and poultry from grain-fed animals that have not been treated with growth hormones.

HEALTHY HUNT: FINDING A STORE YOU LIKE

But big or little, there are certain basic requirements for *any* good natural food store, says Sandy Gooch, owner of Mrs. Gooch's, one of the country's leading natural foods retailers. "If the establishment doesn't have a wide selection of supplements, whole grains, cereals, legumes, spring water, fresh juices, natural yogurts, tofu, soy milk, healthy snacks, organically grown produce, and in some cases, fresh-prepared foods, you're in the wrong place," she says.

What if you feel daunted by that dizzying array of new or unusual products? Just browse and read the fine print, says Janet Savage, an Oakland,

California, nutritionist who leads groups—from seniors to school kids—on educational tours of natural food stores. "We have to take time to find out what's going into our bodies," Savage says.

And if you're on a tight budget, you may also have to take the time to check the prices. In most cases, you'll pay at least 10 percent more for an item than for its nearest counterpart in a traditional grocery store. Reasons vary: Fewer preservatives usually mean a shorter product shelf life; most of the products are made by small companies with higher costs; small retailers can't always buy in larger quantities to get price breaks. The obvious exception: Bulk bins that sometimes offer deep discounts on dried fruits, beans, nuts and other items, while allowing you to select just the right quantity. But health food advocates suggest any short-term added expense is worth it in the long run. "It comes down to how much you are willing to pay for an improved quality of life," says Martie Whittekin, president of the National Nutritional Foods Association.

But before you reach for your wallet, join us for an exploratory trip down the aisles.

BEANS: THE HIGH-FIBER CULTURAL EXPERIENCE

One of the biggest advantages of shopping at natural food stores is exposure to a wide variety of healthful ethnic foods. In addition to offering the usual dry beans like lentils, chick-peas, red kidney beans and black beans, many stores also stock a few types that may make you feel like a globetrotter.

But beans offer more than just an inexpensive cultural dining experience. Says Dr. Messina: "Beans as a whole are high in fiber and low in fat. If you have a chance to try some different ones, it's going to add some healthful variety to your diet."

Among the most unusual:

Adzuki beans. Small, red, kidney-shaped beans that do not need soaking before preparation, adzukis are popular in Japan and often used in confections.

Anasazi beans. These small palomino-colored, kidney-shaped beans, popular in Mexico and the American Southwest, are sweeter and meatier than most and contain generous amounts of protein and iron.

Mung beans. Tender and slightly sweet, mung beans are popular in China and India. They're most often green but may be yellow or black. Primarily used for sprouting, mung beans do not have to be soaked before cooking.

Soybeans. Perhaps the world's most versatile bean—used for making oil, tofu, soy sauce, soy milk and other products—the small round soybean is also great cooked for dinner. High in protein, soybeans contain fiber, calcium, iron, zinc, magnesium, thiamine, riboflavin and niacin, plus high concentrations of compounds that demonstrate anti-cancer properties, according to researchers.

Breads: Man Does Not Live by White Alone

Official natural food store bread tip number one: Don't look for a bread rack. Because most of the breads here don't contain preservatives, they're kept on ice in the freezer. An exception: Space-age packaging and a half-dollar-size "oxygen absorber" allow at least one brand of brown rice bread to reside in the store refrigerator.

But locating these whole-grain feasts isn't nearly as much fun as sampling them. Most natural food stores stock a flavorful selection of whole-grain, rye, sourdough and sprouted breads that are so heavy and dense you'll need a steak knife to carve off a slab. And nobody has to feel left out: most stores stock wheat- and yeast-free loaves for those with allergies.

Whole-grain breads also retain more vitamins and fiber than those using refined ingredients—a healthful plus of which cancer experts approve. Some breads combine as many as 12 grains; others, like macrobiotic brown rice bread, are made from organically grown grain.

Sprouted breads are made from grains like rye or wheat that have been sprouted just before baking. "You know the grains are wholesome if they're able to sprout a plant," says Whittekin.

Sea Vegetables: Produce from the Deep

Harvesting vegetables from the ocean may seem like a relatively new concept, but the Japanese have been doing it for centuries. Don't be concerned, however, if you don't take to sea vegetables like Jacques Cousteau: With their salty, fishy flavor, they're definitely not for everyone.

But if you enjoy the taste, natural food stores often stock a variety of dried sea vegetables. Here are some examples of what you might find.

Arame. A vegetable side dish that need only be rinsed and soaked for five minutes before cooking.

Dulse. A popular ingredient in stir-fries, sandwiches and soups.

Hijiki. A black, erect sea grass that can be added to soups and salads.

Kelp. Rich in iodine, it can be used in salads and as wrapping for other dishes.

Kombu. Can add flavor to beans or vegetables and simultaneously prevent the rice from sticking to the bottom of the pan during cooking.

Nori. Used to wrap sushi, comes in toasted strips which are a zesty complement to rice or vegetables..

Most breads available in natural food stores contain baking powder free of aluminum for those concerned about a possible link between high amounts of that metal and Alzheimer's disease. And sourdough preparations allow many people with yeast allergies to enjoy bread worry-free, Whittekin says.

Flat, round, whole-wheat chapatis—often sold by the dozen—look like tortillas, but they're actually unleavened breads; they do not contain any yeast.

And if you can't find a bread you like, why not bake your own? A wide variety of flour is generally available, including organic barley, buckwheat, millet, oat, rice, rye and teff.

Used to make injera, an Ethiopian flat bread, teff is the smallest grain in the world. Yet it has more bran ounce per ounce than any other grain.

Multigrain flour combines the goodness of wheat, barley, pinto beans, green lentils, millet, rye and other ingredients. And what about bake mixes that make oat bran, blue corn and seven-grain pancakes? There's even high-lysine corn flour that has a nutty flavor, crunchy texture and a naturally sweet taste along with its enhanced protein content.

CEREALS: SOMETHING NEW FOR YOUR BOWL

They may come in boxes similar to those on supermarket shelves, but these cereals usually contain fewer additives, not to mention less sugar and salt. "Some cereals on the market today have more salt than a bag of potato chips," says Whittekin.

Varieties range from oatmeal and millet to crispy brown rice and muesli. You'll find corn, wheat and other flakes, too. The sweeteners of choice: fruit juice concentrate and honey.

Once the darling of the natural foods industry, granola has also enjoyed mainstream success in supermarkets. To fight back, health food stores are now stocking fat-free granolas that claim to be the best you can buy.

Amaranth cereal, often with whole wheat and barley added as well, is a tasty, high-protein breakfast alternative made from this newly rediscovered grain.

First introduced in Europe, muesli is the cereal with a strong following in natural food stores. It's easy to see why: Muesli is a rich, tasty collection of unsweetened, whole grains like oats, wheat, millet and barley, combined with nuts and dried fruit.

Organic brown rice cereal brings the benefits of minimally processed rice to breakfast. Because the thick outer bran layer has not been removed, brown rice cereal offers more fiber per spoonful than traditional rice cereals.

And for those with a taste for all, there are multigrain cereals that combine amaranth, barley, buckwheat, corn, millet, oats and rye. Some are even sprouted.

REDISCOVERING THE GREAT GRAINS

Some grains increasingly popular in natural food stores have been used for centuries by other cultures, says Burton Kallman, Ph.D., director of science and technology for the National Nutritional Foods Association.

Amaranth. Very high in protein, this ancient grain is now appearing in everything from cereals and cookies to cake mixes. The Spaniards eradicated amaranth farming after conquering Mexico because the Aztecs thought the grain had mystical powers.

Barley. An excellent source of complex carbohydrates, barley has been shown to have some effective cholesterol-lowering properties, Dr. Kallman says.

Millet. Used extensively in China, millet is a hardy grain that is high in fiber, Dr. Kallman says. Millet is now found in cereal mixes and can also be ground for use in baking.

Quinoa. Another increasingly popular South American grain, quinoa (pronounced *KEEN-wa*) is unusually high in protein. Often sold as a hot cereal or as a substitute for rice, it can also be blended in flour for baking.

MILK SUBSTITUTES: BETTER THAN BETSY?

Cow's milk offers unsurpassed portions of protein and calcium in a no-muss, no-fuss liquid. But what if you're like two-thirds of the world's population—that is, unable to digest milk—or simply don't like milk's taste?

How about a glass of soy or rice milk, two popular dairy substitutes. Soy milk is made from—you guessed it—the tiny, but dependable soybean, plus water. But soy milk tastes remarkably like skim milk—without the cholesterol.

Eight ounces of a popular soy milk, made with filtered water, organic soybeans, barley malt and pearl barley, has 110 calories and contains seven grams of protein, ten grams of carbohydrates and just five grams of fat. It supplies just 6 percent of the Recommended Dietary Allowance (RDA) of calcium. A popular rice milk, made from filtered water and brown rice, is 99 percent fat-free and contains no cholesterol. A serving provides just 2 percent of the RDA for calcium and protein.

Processing techniques have inflated prices of these products, making them an expensive dairy alternative. If the price is too high, you might consider making your own.

Both soy and rice milk are available in a variety of flavors.

MAKE YOUR OWN SOY MILK

If you find commercial soy milk too expensive for everyday use, you can prepare your own at home for a fraction of the cost. It's a little time-consuming because the beans need soaking, but it's not really difficult. You may use the milk as is for cooking and baking. But for drinking, you'll probably want to flavor the batch with about ⅓ cup honey.

Start with 1 cup dry soybeans. Rinse well and place them in a large bowl. Cover with cold water and allow to soak for 4 to 16 hours (refrigerate the beans if you soak them for more than 6 hours). Drain. You'll have about 2¼ cups beans.

Place half the beans in a blender and add 1½ cups cold water. Process on high speed for at least two minutes, or until the beans are well pureed. Transfer the mixture to a four-quart saucepan. Repeat the process with the remaining beans and another 1½ cups water.

Add an additional 4½ cups water to the pan. Bring to a slow rolling boil, stirring frequently to minimize sticking. After the mixture reaches the boiling point (the foam on top will rise up suddenly, threatening to overflow), reduce the heat so the mixture simmers. Cook for 10 to 15 minutes.

Line a colander with several layers of cheesecloth and place it over a large bowl. Ladle the bean mixture into the colander. Strain out as much of the soy milk as possible, pressing with a spoon to extract the liquid. When the mixture has cooled sufficiently, you can also squeeze the cheesecloth with your hands. You'll end up with about 1½ quarts of soy milk.

ENERGY BARS: SNACK OF CHAMPIONS?

Weekend warriors searching for the competitive edge have caused a "bar war" of sorts in natural food stores. Over a dozen brands of energy bars grace store shelves, nearly all purporting to supply the energy you need to fuel your workout or replace a missed meal. And while some are on target when it comes to delivering the requisite amount of complex carbohydrates and protein in a low-sugar, low-fat package, others are less healthy.

Your best bet: Grab a bar that's packed with complex carbohydrates like maltodextrin, glucose polymers, oats, wheat flour or rice—with over 60 percent of calories from carbs and less than 30 percent from fat, according to *Runner's World* magazine sports nutrition columnist Liz Applegate, Ph.D. Because many bars are also fortified with vitamins and minerals, they may

SPORTS NUTRITION'S PUMPED-UP EXPECTATIONS

Soaring interest in fitness has sent sales of sports nutrition supplements surging. As a result, most health food stores stock everything from weight-gain shakes to electrolyte-replacement drinks.

Some bodybuilding supplements are more sophisticated than ever, with ingredient blends supposedly based on advanced research in muscle fatigue and recovery. Others simply tout their protein content.

But be wary of products like bee pollen that claim to instantly boost energy or performance. None of these supplements have been proven to enhance sports performance, according to Ann C. Grandjean, Ed.D., chief nutrition consultant for the U.S. Olympic committee.

In fact, bee pollen can cause severe allergic reactions in some people, Dr. Grandjean says. Brewer's yeast, pangamic acid and bioflavanoids, also widely touted, have no value as performance aids. And no studies have demonstrated that individual amino acids boost performance, she says.

Many carbohydrate-rich sports drinks however, have been shown to benefit performance.

contain as many nutrients as a bowl of fortified breakfast cereal, says Dr. Applegate, who is author of *Power Foods*.

But they don't always taste as good. One bar contains 50 grams of carbohydrate, 15 grams of protein and just 3 grams of fat but has the consistency of frozen salt water taffy—not exactly the best snack for someone in a hurry.

Bars that get most of their energy from simple sugars like corn syrup will almost certainly leave you with an energy crisis after the sugar rush wears off. Also be wary of those that claim a boost from such ingredients as bee pollen: It's never been proved to enhance performance, says Dr. Applegate.

HERBS: A SPRIG A DAY KEEPS DISEASE AWAY?

Of all the unusual products stocked in health food stores, few carry the aura of herbs. Rows of jars stocked with the leaves, roots and bark of obscure plants conjure images of ancient healers working their magic arts. And yet, few realize that, today, herbs are still the primary medicines of much of the world's population. And over 25 percent of modern prescription drugs are actually made with synthesized versions of the active ingredients in herbs, says Mark Blumenthal, executive director of the American Botanical Council.

Most stores carry a broad range of herbal products for medicinal purposes—from alfalfa to witch hazel. But be advised: Many herbal healing claims have yet to be verified by scientific research. And because herbal products can vary widely in potency and sometimes cause undesirable side effects, they probably shouldn't be used without first consulting a doctor.

Here are some of the herbs most commonly found in natural food stores.

Chamomile. One of the nation's best-selling herbs, chamomile in tea is often recommended by herbalists as a digestive aid and tranquilizer.

Echinacea. Traditionally used to fight infections and stimulate the immune system, modern research suggests that echinacea may also combat arthritis.

Ephedra. This herb contains an amphetamine-like compound called ephedrine, which works as a nasal decongestant and a bronchial dilator. Ephedra has also been used by people attempting to lose weight.

Garlic. One of the world's oldest medicines, garlic is undergoing a revival that has supporters advocating its use for preventing colds and flu, enhancing immune function and helping lower blood pressure and cholesterol. Garlic is also one of several foods under investigation by the National Cancer Institute for its cancer-fighting properties. If you do decide to try it, don't worry about scaring friends and loved ones away with the smell—garlic supplements in capsule form are often deodorized.

Ginger. A digestive aid, ginger, studies suggest, allays nausea and mild motion sickness.

Ginkgo. The biggest-selling over-the-counter remedy in Europe in 1989, ginkgo is thought to improve short-term memory and boost circulation.

Goldenseal. Considered one of the most useful herbs by contemporary herbalists, goldenseal is thought to be helpful as an antibiotic, an immune stimulant and a digestive aid.

Juniper. Herbalists claim that this herb helps combat high blood pressure, congestive heart failure and arthritis.

Valerian. This herb is frequently used as a sleep aid.

MEAT SUBSTITUTES: FAKE FLESH

For years, those following a vegetarian diet for ethical or religious reasons were the primary buyers of meat substitutes. But today, an even broader audience is waking up to these products' health advantage: far less saturated fat and cholesterol than the real thing. A variety of soy-based, grain and vegetable meat substitutes are now available. Among the most popular: tofu pups. These aptly named creations mimic the All-American hot dog, but with less fat and no chemical additives.

Meatless cold cuts, often made from wheat and tofu, come close to copying corned beef, ham, pastrami, turkey and roast beef. Soy is also used to replicate sausage, burgers and even chicken.

Tempeh, a pressed, fermented soybean cake popular in Indonesia, is also gaining increasing acceptance here as a beef or chicken substitute. And with good reason: Tempeh has almost as much protein as beef and chicken, without the saturated fat or cholesterol. Produced by exposing soybeans to harmless bacteria, tempeh can be used in recipes that call for everything from baking to frying.

JUNK FOOD AS HEALTH FOOD

Our tour is nearly complete. But before you haul all your goodies to the cash register, here's some closing advice: You may want to check the ingredient labels one last time, suggests Dr. Bland. "In the present state of regulation, consumers do need to be informed label readers in natural food stores just as they would be in traditional stores," he says.

In fact, "natural" may be the most abused word in the English language. "It's become a nonsense term in the absence of a standard identity. It can be used and misused in any way possible," Dr. Bland says.

Some of the worst offenders: sports and weight-loss beverages, breakfast foods, snack foods, dairy substitutes and confections. Just because these and other items are being sold in a natural foods market, you should not assume they are all healthier, says Dr. Bland.

Some items, he contends, may not even belong in natural food stores. Candy is candy, for example. And some chips, crackers and cookies sold in health food stores have as much or more fat and salt as supermarket snacks.

Over the years other products of dubious value have appeared on natural food shelves. One product billed as a natural herbal energizer, for example, became a hit with customers and retailers—until it was discovered that it was loaded with caffeine, says Danny Wells, a natural food store consultant in Pleasant Hill, California.

In an attempt to head off such problems, some natural food markets like

SOMETHING TO MUNCH ON

The snacks found in natural food stores may appear to be more healthy than those found elsewhere. But read labels carefully because some are still loaded with fat and salt: "Junk food disguised as health food," says clinical nutritionist Jeffrey Bland, Ph.D. A one-ounce serving of a popular carrot chip, for example, has nine grams of fat.

But you'll also discover a number of items that make snacking virtually guilt-free. A one-ounce serving of a light, crunchy (and addicting, according to taste testers) corn snack actually had *no* fat and 21 grams of carbohydrate.

And when was the last time you had a supermarket-bought raspberry muffin so flavorful that the exceptional nutritional value—five grams of fiber and less than one gram of fat—was an afterthought?

Mrs. Gooch's simply refuse to stock items containing questionable ingredients.

A "standards and criteria" worksheet sent to all Mrs. Gooch's suppliers says: "We only stock items meeting these criteria: no artificial flavorings, no artificial colorings, no artificial sweeteners, no refined sweeteners, such as sucrose, fructose, corn syrup, glucose, maltose, brown, raw or turbinado sugars, no MSG, no caffeine, no chocolate, no hydrogenated oils, no alcoholic beverages, no white flour (including unbleached), no irradiated foods, no harmful preservative agents, no harmful chemical additives."

"In the natural foods industry we're finding greater and greater numbers of foods that adhere to our standards," says Gooch. "My advice is: If it's so chemically preserved that it can't spoil, then don't buy it."

Gooch's quest for good health began in a hospital bed. She says she nearly died from a seizure indirectly caused by the food additive, bromated vegetable oil, hidden in a diet soda. So the former teacher and housewife stopped buying processed food and started looking for fresh, natural products free from artificial anything. As she discovered after opening her hugely successful stores: A lot of other people are looking for the same thing.

CHAPTER 31

SUPPLEMENTS
A SMART BUYER'S GUIDE

If there's anything nutrition experts agree on, it's that the preferred source of vitamins and minerals is food, not tablets or capsules. And no, they're not just trying to make things hard for you. "There are good reasons nutritional supplements should not be used as a substitute for a balanced diet," says Jacqueline Charnley, R.D., of the U.S. Department of Agriculture's (USDA) Human Nutrition Research Center on Aging at Tufts University in Boston.

"We don't know everything there is to know about nutrition, so no vitamin pill is perfect," Charnley says. "There may be unknown components of food, necessary for good health, that just aren't found in a multivitamin. There may be interactions or balances between particular nutrients that depend on food sources. And certainly you need to eat foods to get protein, carbohydrates, fiber, essential fatty acids and some trace minerals that aren't usually found in vitamin pills."

One more good reason to focus on diet first: If you're not eating well, you're probably eating pretty poorly, and vitamins can only go so far to make up for a lifetime of dietary indiscretions.

But many experts *also* agree there is a place for nutritional supplements.

"Dietary surveys consistently show that a certain percentage of people come up short when it comes to meeting the RDA for all nutrients," Charnley says. "Even when they know what they need to do to improve their eating habits, some people may choose not to do it."

Dietitians admit it's hard to get people to eat better. It takes time, effort and desire. You need to know how to shop for and prepare good food and how to choose wisely when you eat out. The old notion among dietitians was that supplement use should be discouraged, supposedly because it encourages people to eat poorly. But an increasing number of experts say it doesn't have to be an either/or situation. "You can improve your diet, *and* you can take supplements, if and when it's appropriate," Charnley says. In fact, some studies show that people who take vitamin supplements tend to eat better than those who don't take supplements.

In real life, experts say, many people seem to go through a natural evolution of "nutrition consciousness raising" that involves supplement use and improved eating habits—often in conjunction with health or weight problems, pregnancy or just plain getting older.

"People often work on a number of things at once—they may take supplements, improve their diets and begin to exercise," Charnley says. "And even as their diets improve, they may continue to take supplements."

SUPPLEMENT QUESTIONS ANSWERED

WHO TAKES SUPPLEMENTS?

About half the people in the United States take nutritional supplements regularly or occasionally, according to a large survey by the USDA. That includes men and women, children and adults, young and old, dog owners and cat owners and people with and without VCRs and CD players.

From surveys, experts have developed a profile of the person most likely to take vitamins. *She* lives in a western state, is well educated (high school or beyond) with a higher-than-average income and a better-than-average diet.

WHY DO PEOPLE TAKE NUTRITIONAL SUPPLEMENTS?

According to a review of studies by the National Research Council Food and Nutrition Board, people are most likely to say they take supplements because they're uncertain about the nutritional adequacy of their diets, because they desire better health than they perceive to be obtainable from medical consultation or because they've decided to treat themselves for an illness.

In one study, the most frequently given reasons for taking supplements were "to prevent colds and other illnesses," "to give me energy" and "to make up for what is not in food." (At least two studies show that vitamin users tend to have a low opinion of today's food quality.)

DO PEOPLE WHO TAKE VITAMINS FIND THEM HELPFUL?

For some reason, most studies haven't posed this question. In one that did ask, 59 percent reported that supplements were of "some benefit" to their health; another 34 percent found them to be of "great benefit."

How to Read a Vitamin Label

It may look like a secret code, but with a little practice, you can decipher all the information on a supplement label.

A typical label first lists the brand name of the supplement—such as Centrum, Theragran or Os-Cal. Under that is the name of the supplement—multivitamins with iron, for example, or calcium carbonate.

Behind the name of the supplement may be the letters "U.S.P." This means the supplement meets manufacturing standards set by the U.S. Pharmacopeia, an independent, nonprofit organization that sets the official standards of strength, quality, purity, packaging and labeling for medical products used in the United States. To a vitamin consumer, the U.S.P. mark guarantees a quality product that dissolves properly in the stomach and delivers the goods.

Next comes the list of active ingredients (the nutrients) and their potencies or amounts, in micrograms (mcg.), milligrams (mg.) or International Units (I.U.).

Next to that is each active ingredient's percentage of the U.S. RDA. If an active ingredient has no RDA, the label may say "RDA not established."

Beneath that comes a complete list of ingredients. This includes the chemical names of the active ingredients. Vitamin C may be listed as ascorbic acid; vitamin E as vitamin E acetate; vitamin D as ergocalciferol. If the product is marked U.S.P., this list will also include ingredients such as fillers and coatings.

What Vitamins Are People Taking?

A survey by the Council for Responsible Nutrition (a vitamin manufacturers' trade group) shows that multiple vitamin and mineral supplements make up nearly 42 percent of all vitamin sales, followed by vitamin C (with 12 percent), B-complex (9 percent), vitamin E (9 percent), calcium (7.5 percent) and iron (7 percent). Sales of nutritional supplements have increased steadily and dramatically over the years—from $500 million in 1972 to $3.3 billion in 1990.

Are Natural Vitamins Better Than Synthetic Vitamins?

For those who prefer cotton to polyester and carrot juice to cola, the word "natural" may have special meaning. It symbolizes purity: Mother Nature with nothing missing and no added extras. When it comes to vitamins, though, experts at the Food and Drug Administration (FDA) say that natural and synthetic vitamins are virtually identical. Any slight differences are insignificant.

Always check the expiration date. As long as the product is properly stored, it's guaranteed to meet the potency listed on the label up to the expiration date. After that time, the product begins to degrade, and its potency slowly drops. An expiration date may be two to four years from the date of manufacture, depending on the nutrient. Experts say it's best not to buy or to use "expired" vitamins.

Look for information that tells you how many tablets you need to take daily to achieve the recommended dosage. Having to take three or four tablets a day to reach the RDA levels listed on the label may make the product seem like less of a bargain.

By the time you read this, vitamin manufacturers are expected to be operating under a new Nutrition and Education Labeling Act. This act requires calories, fat and sodium to be listed on a supplement label where appropriate. For instance, a product like sodium ascorbate, a form of vitamin C, will have to list milligrams of sodium per dose, and oil-containing tablets will have to list their calories and fat content.

"This new act does allow health benefits to be mentioned on the label, provided the Food and Drug Administration [FDA] has determined there is enough scientific evidence to make that claim," says Edward Scarborough, Ph.D., director of the FDA's Office of Nutrition and Food Sciences. So far, the only health claim the FDA has permitted that pertains to supplements is that calcium may reduce the risk of osteoporosis.

Some supplements are made from natural materials. Most minerals, for instance, are derived from natural mined substances. Calcium may be derived from limestone, oyster shells or naturally occurring beds of calcium carbonate.

Most manufactured vitamins are "built" from organic molecules found in an array of substances. Why? Because vitamins are found in such small quantities in foods (even foods rich in a particular nutrient) that the cost of isolating any vitamin from food in bulk quantities is prohibitive. "Take beta-carotene, for example," says Frank Girardi, pharmaceutical business unit director for Hoffmann-La Roche in Nutley, New Jersey, one of the world's largest bulk vitamin manufacturers. "You can get it from carrots or algae, but supplement makers would need tons of carrots to come up with enough beta-carotene for their products, and a lot would go to waste because this particular micronutrient isn't very stable. Besides, the natural form could be two to ten times more expensive."

So what's most beta-carotene made from? Ultrapure by-products of petroleum and mined calcium carbide. If that seems strange to you, consider that most of our lifesaving drugs, even aspirin, are concocted from this same soup of organic molecules. These complex molecules are isolated, purified and then precisely rearranged into many different substances. Chemically, the beta-carotene made from petroleum derivatives is exactly the same as that derived from a carrot. And experts insist it works the same way in your body. These synthetic vitamins are also the same material used in the very complex, long-term clinical trials to show the health benefits of vitamins and minerals in our diet.

Vitamin C is made from dextrose, a sugar found in corn. After it's purified, the dextrose is put through the same sort of chemical process that

Going Down Easy

Having a hard time swallowing that vitamin tablet or capsule? Relax. Take a few deep breaths. Then, try these suggestions from Bronwyn Jones, M.D., director of Johns Hopkins Medical Center Swallowing Center in Baltimore, which treats people with swallowing problems from around the world.

Keep your head level. You might also tuck your chin in just a bit. "Many people who take pills toss their heads back as they swallow, and that, in fact, is the worst thing they can do," Dr. Jones says. "It puts tension on the neck and makes it harder for the muscles of the esophagus to push the pill down to the stomach. It also makes it easier for pills or fluids to move toward the lungs as the extended position makes it harder for muscles to elevate the larynx and protect the airway."

Sit up—or stand up. It makes sense, and a study shows that tablets move more quickly through the esophagus when this mouth-to-stomach passageway is vertical, not horizontal. "If you take pills before bed, take them sitting up, with at least half a cup of water, and continue to sit up for a few minutes longer," Dr. Jones advises. Pills that stay in your throat all night long can cause irritation.

If you must take pills lying down, crush them or chew them, or ask your doctor for a liquid form. Just make sure it's okay to crush the pill. Timed-release tablets should not be crushed. It also helps to take them with plenty of water.

Try cold, carbonated water. For some people, carbonated, bottled water works better than regular water to speed pills down to the stomach. Researchers speculate that carbonation provides an air cushion around tablets, easing their passage.

occurs in those animals that are capable of synthesizing vitamin C in their bodies. Chemically, the final product is exactly the same as the vitamin C derived from an orange. How does the manufacturer know that? "Years of testing, on both animals and humans, have established that the natural and synthetic versions of most nutrients are exactly the same—chemically and biologically," says David Roll, Ph.D., professor of medicinal chemistry in the College of Pharmacy at the University of Utah in Salt Lake City.

Some, like vitamin E, have synthetic versions that are different from the natural versions. Natural vitamin E (d-alpha-tocopherol) is isolated from soybean oil. Synthetic vitamin E (*dl*-alpha-tocopherol) is made from petroleum derivatives. The natural version has slightly more of what's called "biological activity" than the synthetic version.

What does that mean? "In essence, all it means is that you have to take slightly more of the synthetic version of vitamin E to match the effects of the natural version," says Dr. Roll.

ARE PEOPLE TAKING VITAMINS SAFELY?

One Food and Drug Administration study showed that many supplement users took most nutrients in amounts that seldom exceeded one to two times the Recommended Dietary Allowance (RDA), an amount most experts consider safe. But 50 percent of respondents took more than double the RDA of vitamin C, thiamine, riboflavin or pantothenate. And some people took up to several hundred times the RDA of vitamins E, C, B_6, B_{12}, thiamine, riboflavin and pantothenate. Those amounts should be used only with medical guidance, experts say.

Some studies show vitamin users as independent thinkers when it comes to medical care. One revealed that "heavy" users (those taking 400 percent of the RDA) and "very heavy" users (those taking 777 percent of the RDA) tend not to involve their doctor in their decisions about supplements. That's an unwise move, experts say.

But one study suggests doctors exert the most influence on the public (in this case, their patients) in making decisions to take supplements. Most likely to consider dietary supplementation important are obstetricians, gynecologists, female doctors and doctors interested in continuing their medical education courses in nutrition.

DO HEALTH PROFESSIONALS TAKE SUPPLEMENTS THEMSELVES?

Several studies show supplements are popular among health professionals, including dietitians. In one study, 60 percent of dietitians who responded to a mail survey admitted they regularly took supplements—usually multivitamins/minerals, vitamin C and iron—for personal health. And several studies demonstrate that supplement use among doctors and medical students is not infrequent.

CHOOSING A MULTIVITAMIN

With so much interest in supplements, it's important that people know what to look for—and what to avoid—when buying these products. Multiple vitamins and minerals are by far the most often purchased nutritional supplements, so let's look at them first.

A multiple combines many nutrients into one tablet or capsule. It's for people who want to take vitamins or minerals or both, but don't want to take five or six, or more, different pills each day.

A good multivitamin/mineral can act as a sort of "dietary insurance policy." It can fix some of the common failings in a typical diet, Charnley says.

What should you look for in a multivitamin/mineral supplement?

Find a multi that supplies about 100 percent of the RDA for most, but not necessarily all, nutrients. "Most Americans get more than they

SPECIAL FORMULATIONS—TOO NARROW A FOCUS?

Some nutritional supplements are designed to treat a particular ailment or are geared toward a specific group of people. They may contain vitamins, minerals, herbs, essential fatty acids, amino acids and just about anything else a manufacturer thinks might be helpful.

Since Food and Drug Administration regulations restrict manufacturers' claims about potential health benefits, most of these products' names merely hint at their purpose. They include stress formulas and formulas aimed at older people, dieters, athletes, men or women. Some are formulated to address eye problems or prostate problems. Others are meant to improve immune function or prevent osteoporosis.

If you are considering buying one of these products, what do you need to know?

First, special formulas tend to offer fewer nutrients than a multiple, perhaps only three or four. "And they tend to be less balanced than a multiple, which means they have more potential to cause imbalances in your body," says David Roll, Ph.D., of the University of Utah. A premenstrual formula, for instance, may offer many times the Recommended Dietary Allowance of vitamin B_6, but contain very little of other B vitamins. A men's formula may contain large amounts of zinc. Geriatric formulas may be top-heavy in antioxidants—vitamins C and E, beta-carotene and selenium. An osteoporosis formula may contain calcium but not much of other nutrients important for bones.

Just like single-nutrient supplements, special formulas are best used with medical supervision. Dr. Roll says "a better choice might be a good multivitamin/mineral."

need of phosphorus and iodine, so there's no reason to put these nutrients in a supplement," says Walter Mertz, M.D., director of the USDA Human Nutrition Research Center in Beltsville, Maryland. And vitamin K deficiency is so rare, this nutrient is not necessary in a multi, most experts say.

Look for a multi that also supplies the nutrients with an "estimated safe and adequate" daily dietary intake. Those include biotin, pantothenate acid, copper, manganese, fluoride, chromium and molybdenum.

Look for a multi that supplies some vitamin A as beta-carotene. In the body, beta-carotene can convert to vitamin A without the danger of an overdose.

Don't fall for a long list of ingredients. More is not necessarily better, says Dr. Roll. "All sorts of fringe substances find their way into nutritional supplements," he says. "For instance, choline, PABA, inositol, lecithin, glutamic acid—these substances are not proven to be necessary in the diet of humans. Our bodies make these substances internally. All they add to a supplement is cost."

Note where a multi falls short. Some contain only vitamins, not minerals. That's easy enough to detect by scanning the label. Even those that do supply minerals tend to be low in calcium and magnesium, two bulky minerals that add substantially to the size of a pill. A multi seldom contains potassium. Because potassium is considered "ubiquitous" in the diet—it's found in many foods—potassium deficiency is considered rare.

Many multis lack essential trace minerals like selenium, copper, manganese and chromium. Some contain iron, some don't.

If a multi falls short here or there, and you can't make up for it in your diet, it's easy enough to supplement with additional individual nutrients.

Choosing Single-Nutrient Supplements

Individual vitamin or mineral supplements can correct specific nutrient shortfalls, address special needs and provide protection above and beyond the RDAs, Charnley says.

If, for example, you're concerned about developing osteoporosis but dislike milk, calcium supplements can supply extra amounts of this bone strengthener. Or if you've decided you want to take more than the RDA of nutrients that appear to help protect against cancer—vitamins C and E, beta-carotene, perhaps selenium—you might consider single-nutrient supplements.

Single-nutrient supplements do carry some risk, though. While reputable manufacturers offer supplements that stay within a safe range, FDA officials say, for most nutrients there is no set ceiling.

Don't go overboard. Because supplements may provide many times the RDA of a nutrient in one dose, it's easy to get large amounts, especially if you take several tablets.

VITAMIN AND MINERAL SUPPLEMENT GUIDELINES

In this table, you'll find two sets of numbers—one for the Recommended Dietary Allowance (RDA) and the other for the "preventive amount." The numbers in the RDA column simply tell you how much supplement you'd need to reach the high range of the Recommended Dietary Allowance. In the "preventive amount" column is a ballpark number that early research findings suggest should put you in the right range for preventive purposes. If you stay at this level or below, you can supplement nutrients that may be lacking in your diet without taking excessively high (and perhaps dangerous) amounts of those nutrients.

NUTRIENT	**RDA***	**PREVENTIVE AMOUNT**
VITAMINS		
Vitamin A†	5,000 I.U.	5,000 I.U.
Beta-carotene	6 mg.‡	15–30 mg.
Thiamine (vitamin B_1)	1.5 mg.	1.5 mg.
Riboflavin (vitamin B_2)	1.8 mg.	1.8 mg.
Niacin	20 mg.	20 mg.
Vitamin B_6	2 mg.	2–1 mg.
Vitamin B_{12}	2 mcg.	2–1 mcg.
Folate	200 mcg.	400–800 mcg.
Vitamin C	60 mg.	100–500 mg.
Vitamin D	10 mcg. (400 I.U.)	10 mcg. (400 I.U.)
Vitamin E	15 I.U. (10 mg. α-TE)	100–400 I.U. (67–268 mg. α-TE)

"Some nutrients, such as vitamins C and E, appear to be quite safe, at least for healthy people, even in large amounts," says John N. Hathcock, Ph.D., of the FDA's office of Experimental Nutrition. Others, including most trace minerals and vitamins A and D, have a narrower range of safety. "If you are taking amounts that are several times more than the RDA or estimated safe range of any nutrient, you are essentially using it as a drug, and you should have the guidance of a health-care professional," Dr. Roll says.

Stay in balance. Too much of one nutrient can interfere with your body's ability to use other nutrients, Dr. Mertz says. "Too much zinc interferes with your body's ability to absorb copper, and too much calcium affects the absorption of many trace minerals," he says. "And too much B_6 or folate will increase the body's requirement for riboflavin," says John Pinto, Ph.D.,

NUTRIENT	RDA*	PREVENTIVE AMOUNT
MINERALS		
Calcium	1,200 mg.	1,200–1,500 mg.
Chromium	50–200 mcg.§	100–200 mcg.
Iron‖	15 mg.	15 mg.
Magnesium	400 mg.	400 mg.
Selenium	70 mcg.	70–200 mcg.
Zinc	15 mg.	15 mg.

NOTE: Don't take more than the upper limit of the preventive amount unless prescribed by a licensed health professional. Supplements are best taken with meals, particularly calcium, which needs the stomach acid produced by eating to enhance digestion.

*Represents the highest Recommended Dietary Allowances for all ages and sex groups except pregnant and lactating women.

†Vitamin A is best taken in the form of beta-carotene.

‡6 milligrams of beta-carotene provides 100 percent of the RDA for vitamin A.

§Range for chromium is an Estimated Safe and Adequate Daily Dietary Intake.

‖Men should not take supplemental iron without checking first with their doctors.

director of the Nutrition Research Laboratory at Memorial Sloan-Kettering Cancer Center in New York City.

THE PROBLEM OF ABSORPTION

Nobody absorbs 100 percent of all the vitamins and minerals they take, nutritionists say, but most people do pretty well, as long as a supplement is manufactured properly. (Exception: Low stomach acid, a problem that's not uncommon in older people, can cause absorption problems.) To improve absorption:

Buy supplements with "U.S.P." on the label. U.S.P. after a supplement name means the product has been manufactured according to U.S. Pharmacopeia standards in a way that makes it disintegrate and dissolve properly and assures that it contains the amount of nutrients stated on the label.

PROTECTING YOUR STASH

"Store in a cool, dry place." That's what it often says on the supplement label. But what's considered a cool, dry place?

Well, it's definitely not your bathroom, experts say. And it's not the cupboard above your stove. Other than those two spots, a cool, dry place might be found almost anywhere in your house.

"A kitchen pantry, away from direct sunlight, humidity or heat, is probably the best area to store vitamins," says V. Srinivasan, Ph.D., a scientist with the U.S. Pharmacopeia.

Do you buy large amounts of vitamins on sale, then store them? You can keep them in the refrigerator or freezer until you start using them, Dr. Srinivasan says, but let the container warm up to room temperature before you open it. Otherwise, moisture may condense inside.

Some additional tips: Don't leave vitamins in a hot car. Always keep the cap on tight, and keep supplements out of the reach of children. Discard any product that begins to look or smell strange.

Take your vitamins with or right after a meal. "The very sight of food begins to stimulate the appetite, triggering the release of various enzymes that aid digestion and increase intestinal blood flow," Dr. Pinto says. And taking supplements with meals makes them unlikely to upset your stomach, Dr. Roll adds.

If you are taking iron, choose a ferrous, not ferric, compound. Ferrous iron is easier to absorb and causes less stomach irritation, experts agree.

Take iron with orange juice. The vitamin C in the orange juice makes absorption of the supplemental iron easier.

If you're taking large amounts of a vitamin, divide it into smaller doses, taken at each meal. Your body can absorb only a certain amount of a nutrient at any one time. By dividing the dose throughout the day, you increase the amount absorbed.

PART 5

HEALING DIETS

CHAPTER 32

WEIGHT LOSS
WHAT REALLY WORKS

Are you a prisoner of war in the battle of the bulge? Held hostage by bad eating habits? So was Kathy Biggerstaff of Evansville, Indiana—until some no-nonsense nutritional concepts helped her lose nearly 100 pounds.

Kathy's quest to escape from her dietary torture is a tale repeated from San Francisco to St. Petersburg. "Because I never ate breakfast, I'd start eating potato chips or other junk by about 10:00 A.M.," she says. "Then I'd have a big lunch, more junk at 3:00 P.M., and, of course, red meat and fried potatoes for dinner."

When it came time to shed the weight, something that an estimated 35 percent of Americans try to do each month, Kathy chose the parallel American obsession: miracle weight-loss programs. Her favorite: diet shakes.

"I always looked at it like 'Now I have to go on a diet—I can't eat what I want anymore,' " she says.

The weight came off, but like a criminal who returns to the scene of the crime, it always came back. By age 30, Kathy was lugging 200 pounds on her tiny 5'5" frame.

Depressed about her condition, Kathy finally abandoned diets and instead developed a low-fat eating plan based on nutritional information she got from her doctor and Weight Watchers—tips like trading away burgers for broiled chicken, eating more vegetables (*without* coating them with butter) and packing her own low-fat salad dressing. She also started walking regularly.

From the results, you'd think she had a body transplant. In two years, Kathy dwindled from a size 20 to a size 3 and reached her dream weight of 107 pounds. Now she even teaches exercise classes.

But she's also the first to admit that if she can do it, anyone can: "You just have to recognize the fact that eating right and exercise are the only solutions," she says. "You can't diet your way around it."

Kathy's discovery confirms the conclusion reached by weight-loss experts: Whether you're trying to lose 10 or 100 pounds, restrictive diets that dramatically cut calories don't work in the long run. Healthy, low-fat eating, combined with moderate exercise, is the only way to lose weight and keep it off.

"Only long-term lifestyle changes make weight loss permanent," says C. Wayne Callaway, M.D., associate clinical professor of medicine at the George Washington University Medical Center in Washington, D.C., and author of *The Callaway Diet.* "Starvation, formulas and gimmicks just don't work."

FORGET FAD DIETS

Each year literally hundreds of new diets appear on bookstore shelves, magazine stands and grocery check-out racks, each claiming to melt pounds quickly and permanently.

Unfortunately, most weight-loss gimmicks on the market will only make your wallet lighter, according to Judy Goffi, R.D., a staff nutritionist who's counseled hundreds of overweight women at the Francis Stern Nutrition Center at the New England Medical Center Hospital in Boston. "It's sad because the people who try these diets are the ones who are the most desperate," she says.

Among the worst methods, according to Goffi: single-food diets that insist items like grapefruit have some newly discovered power to burn fat. Aside from the absurdity of those claims, single-food diets are nearly impossible to sustain beyond a few weeks, she says.

And some diets aren't just laughable—they can be downright dangerous. At least 60 people died while on the aptly named Last Chance Diet, an 880-calorie liquid protein fast sold during the early 1980s, says Goffi.

Ignoring your body's normal hunger signals while on a diet ordinarily won't kill you—most people give in before they starve. But severely restricting your eating can damage your natural ability to control eating, according to Peter Herman, Ph.D., a psychology professor at the University of Toronto in Ontario. "You can tolerate more hunger, but when you start eating, you can't stop—you lose your brakes as well as your accelerator," says Dr. Herman.

At the heart of his theory on the hazards of severe calorie cutting: the milk shake study. Under the guise of an ice cream taste test, dieters and nondieters were fed a milk shake before being allowed to sample ice cream. To his amazement, Dr. Herman found that once they got started, the self-described dieters actually ate 30 percent to 40 percent more ice cream than the nondieters. Apparently, once the dieters allowed themselves to down that milk shake, they felt they might as well go on and indulge to their heart's content—a familiar theme among those trying to starve themselves thin.

"Dieters have a strange way of keeping score," says Dr. Herman. "They think if they're good then they're good, but if they're bad, it doesn't matter how bad. It does matter. Overeating today will count against you tomorrow," he says.

MANAGE YOUR METABOLISM

Whether you overeat because you're addicted to ice cream or because you're unhappy, gaining weight is simply a matter of eating more calories than you burn for energy.

Think of your body as a roaring fire. Every bite of food above your body's energy needs stacks fat cells on different parts of your body just out of reach of the hungry flames. And you don't need marathon sessions at an all-you-can-eat buffet to get the fat collection started. An extra 50 to 100 calories a day—roughly a handful of potato chips—could add 5 to 10 pounds a year! That's because 3,500 calories are equal to a pound of fat.

To get rid of that lumpy surplus, you have to do at least two things: Stop the accumulation of new fat and start throwing some of what's already there on the fire. The best way to do that: Keep your body's built-in fat burner, your metabolism, burning intensely.

"This will effectively improve your body's ability to use body fat as fuel, regardless of your genetic endowment," according to Herman M. Frankel, M.D., an obesity expert and director of the Portland Health Institute in Oregon.

Although experts still have a lot to learn about metabolism, they know it's generally efficient when left alone, ravenously consuming calories to help fuel circulation, digestion, body temperature, muscle repair and all your other bodily functions. The problem begins when you interfere with your body's natural metabolic setting by dieting.

Drastic calorie cutting *will* make the pounds drop off. But unfortunately, your body doesn't just harmlessly burn fat and water to quickly shed those pounds. It also burns muscle. The problem with that is that muscle tissue—even when not in use—is a very efficient calorie burner. So when you lose muscle because of drastic dieting, you're damping the flames of your metabolism.

But starvation dieting creates another, even more severe, problem: Your

EATING THROUGH THE AGES

It's probably just another of life's little surprises. But by the time you're ready to retire, move to Orlando and finally take advantage of some of those early-bird dinner specials, something has happened to your body: It actually needs less food.

Chalk it up to age—and inactivity. As you exercise less, your muscle mass shrinks, causing your metabolism to slow. Doctors believe that after age 30, metabolism slows at a rate of 5 percent every ten years, cutting your need for calories still further.

"If your muscle mass has decreased over the years, you're just going to need less food," says Susan Kayman, R.D., of the Kaiser Permanente Medical Group in Oakland, California.

In fact, while the average adult male needs 2,700 calories a day and the average adult female needs 2,000 calories a day, a man over the age of 50 needs just 2,400 calories a day. And a woman over the age of 50 needs just 1,800.

But here's the problem: While you need *fewer calories* than you did when you were younger, you still need all the essential nutrients—protein, vitamins and minerals.

So to avoid gaining weight yet make sure you're getting all of the nutrients you need, you actually have to make smarter food selections, says Kim Galeaz-Gioe, R.D., a spokesperson for the American Dietetic Association.

"There's just no room for junk food in your diet," says Galeaz-Gioe. "If you choose junk food, you're getting the calories you need—and more—but none of the nutrients."

One of the best ways to fulfill your vitamin and mineral quota is by eating more fruits and vegetables. "They're loaded with vitamins and minerals but are low in calories," she says.

You can also beat nature's clock by muscling up your metabolism with moderate exercise. Not only does exercise burn calories, some forms—like weight training—build muscle mass, a key calorie consumer.

body hoards calories as if it were trying to endure an Ethiopian famine. The result: Your once-fiery metabolism merely flickers.

A sluggish metabolism isn't bad—if you intend to eat like a bird for the rest of your life. But once you begin putting food on your plate again, all those extra calories will begin piling up as fat even faster than before, says Dr. Frankel.

"The body clings tenaciously to any fat and tries to build up more, anticipating the next famine situation," says Dr. Frankel. "And that makes it even harder to lose weight the next time."

A landmark University of Pennsylvania study of laboratory animals dramatically illustrates the dilemma. Obese rats on a starvation diet needed only 21 days to lose the excess weight. It was a different story during the second phase of the experiment. After the animals regained the weight, it took more than twice as long for them to lose the same amount of weight while on the same starvation diet.

The effects on chronic human dieters can be even more severe. "I've seen people gain 5, 10 or even 15 pounds within 24 to 48 hours after going off a very low calorie diet," says Dr. Callaway.

Little wonder that starvation dieting has been linked to binge eating as well as anxiety and other stress-related psychological problems.

"Sometimes I feel like the body's rebellion against dieting is just the natural consequence of trying to fight the forces of nature. The dieter tries desperately to keep the lid on, but the pressure to eat builds and then, when the lid blows off, and you gorge, you end up weighing more than you did in the first place," says Dr. Herman.

PLAN PERMANENT CHANGES

By now you should be getting the message: When it comes to weight loss, never, ever, say diet. "Weight management is not a one-shot attempt to lose weight. It is a lifelong adoption of healthy eating and physical activity habits," says John P. Foreyt, Ph.D., director of the Nutrition Research Clinic in the Department of Medicine at the Baylor College of Medicine in Houston.

Both factors are important—in fact, moderate exercise will give your weight-loss efforts a significant boost. But we're going to focus here on nutritionally sound eating recommendations and food-related behavioral tips that doctors say can help you lose at the safest and most sustainable rate—at least ½ to 1 pound a week. An eating plan that's 55 to 60 percent complex carbohydrates, 25 percent fat and 15 percent protein is generally recommended for weight loss.

But before we show you how to arrange your dinner plate down to the last lima bean, consider the encouraging results of a University of California study of 30 women who were able to lose weight and keep it off for at least two years without starvation diets or gimmicks.

A few of the women credited their success to learning a package of strategies through a special program. But most simply said they made a decision to lose weight and then devised their own realistic weight-loss plans—based on sound nutritional principles—to fit their lives, according to Susan Kayman, R.D., coauthor of the study and senior consultant for

MIND OVER MUNCHING

Engage your brain before you put your mouth in gear. This grade school maxim was usually directed toward kids who answered without thinking. But it's also good advice for people who are trying to lose weight. The right mental preparation and behavior can play a key role in your weight-loss efforts long before you put a fork to your mouth, say doctors.

"In many ways, awareness and control over your eating behavior can increase your options, improve how you deal with food situations and keep you from being a victim of old behaviors," says F. Matthew Kramer, Ph.D., research psychologist with the U.S. Army's Research, Development and Engineering Center in Natick, Massachusetts.

What follows are some behavioral techniques developed by Dr. Kramer and Kelly D. Brownell, Ph.D., professor of psychology at Yale University.

Get ready. Before you start your weight-loss program, you should feel ready to do it and aware of why you want to do it, Dr. Brownell says.

Never say never. Don't swear off pizza or other tempting favorites for good. "It's important not to set absolutes—it's not very realistic," says Dr. Brownell.

Tuck away treats. You can reduce temptation by storing food out of sight. Reducing food handling and preparation can keep you from excess sampling.

Dine only where (and when) designated. Eating should be limited to specific times and places each day. Not reading or watching television while eating may also help you eat less.

Give yourself a hand. Treat yourself to a movie or a new outfit as a reward for sticking to your program.

Enlist an ally. Several studies have shown that active support by your spouse can help you stay on your new low-fat eating plan.

Ditch your self-doubt. Having a bad eating day—downing a bag of potato chips at lunch, for example—doesn't doom your program to failure. Simply resolve to lay off the fat for the duration and do better tomorrow. "It's important to keep slips in perspective," says Dr. Brownell. "One slip doesn't ruin the whole program."

Kaiser Permanente Medical Group in Oakland, California.

Needless to say, the plans they implemented didn't include grapefruit-topped pizza—or any other wacky weight-loss scheme. In fact, they all used several practical techniques found in this chapter, including getting regular exercise, cutting fat and eating more fruits and vegetables. The successfully trim also reported being patient, setting small goals they could meet and sticking to their personally devised weight-loss plans.

"If you're eating turkey breast instead of salami, using less oil when you cook, using low-fat dairy products, we're not talking about dieting any more. We're talking about a sensible, easy way of eating that's going to pay off in weight loss," says Kayman.

WRITE YOUR WEIGHT DOWN

Before you can start eating smart, you have to figure out where you're going wrong. The best way, doctors say: Keeping a detailed food diary.

A daily log that records what, when and where you eat as well as the circumstances is probably the best approach, says Barbara Scott, assistant professor of the Nutrition Education and Research Program at the University of Nevada School of Medicine.

After a week of faithfully recording everything you eat, take a good look at the results. See lots of chocolate bars, cookies, croissants and other high-fat goodies—accompanied by weight gain? Target the junk for dietary termination—or at least start looking for low-fat alternatives, says Scott.

GO ON A FAT ATTACK

Lots of food favorites over the past half-century have been falsely branded as weight-gain villains—bread, potatoes and pasta—to name a few. But doctors now agree at least one truly guilty party belongs on your most unwanted eating list: fat.

And even the slickest team of Washington lawyers couldn't beat this case: Several studies conducted by the nation's top dietary sleuths show eating less fat can drop pounds effortlessly—without eating less food!

"If you're eating a high-fat diet and you cut the amount of fat you're eating, you'll lose weight. It's as simple as that," says Alan Kristal, Dr.Ph., a researcher at the Fred Hutchinson Cancer Research Center in Seattle.

For proof, consider the results of Dr. Kristal's ground-breaking study on the *unintended* effects of a low-fat diet. Half the 300 women in the study maintained their regular diets, which averaged 39 percent of calories from fat. The rest were shown how to slash their dietary fat to 21 percent of calories by creating low- and nonfat versions of high-fat favorites, using less fat for cooking and eating more fish, chicken, fruits and vegetables.

Even though the study was designed simply to determine whether eating a diet so low in fat was realistic, something remarkable happened. The lean food eaters quickly began losing weight—even though they were filling their fat void by actually eating more complex carbohydrates and protein! In fact, for every percentage point of fat the women cut from their diet, ¼ to ½ pound of flab dropped off their bodies during the six-month study. And

THE BATTLE OF THE BULGE: MEN VERSUS WOMEN

He occasionally has a beer with his burger and still manages to drop his paunch. She counts every calorie—but the bathroom scale refuses to budge. Don't give him a gold star or hold her accountable—weight loss often occurs at a different rate for men and women.

Although doctors aren't exactly sure what causes this documented discrepancy, several solid theories have emerged. Perhaps the best is that women just naturally store more fat than men, a phenomenon linked to the woman's unique role as child bearer, according to Rose Frisch, Ph.D., associate professor of population sciences at the Harvard University School of Public Health in Boston.

The average man's body is 12 percent fat, while the average woman's is 26 percent fat, she says. Where does the extra fat come from? During adolescence, young women generally experience a whopping 120 percent gain in body fat, while boys' gains are nearly all muscle—a significant calorie burner.

"There's a metabolic cost to reproduction," says Dr. Frisch. "A woman's body apparently tries to build up and keep fat at a certain level to cover the cost of a potential pregnancy." It's easy to see why this fat savings plan is so ambitious: During pregnancy, a woman generally needs 50,000 calories above her own body's needs to keep the baby inside her healthy.

In fact, the need for fat is so great that a woman's reproductive system will actually shut down if she drops below 15 percent of her natural body weight, Dr. Frisch says.

Still, women can safely *and* successfully lose weight if they eat a low-fat diet, says Dr. Frisch. "That seems to be the best approach," she says.

an impressive number of the women kept the weight off: Two years later, 50 percent of the participants were still lean.

The reason that cutting fat works for weight loss: A single gram of fat is equal to nine calories, while a gram of protein or complex carbohydrates is equal to just four calories. In short, eating less fat means eating fewer calories. What's more, dietary fat is quickly stored in the body as fat, while carbohydrates are more readily burned as fuel, says Dr. Kristal. Call it the one-two punch for taking off pounds: "You have two things going for you—not only do you take in fewer calories, but the calories that are going in are more readily used by the body," he says.

So how much fat should you drop from your plate? The average American gets about 37 percent of calories from fat. But folks who still eat bacon and eggs for breakfast and meat for lunch and dinner are getting closer to 40 to 45 percent of calories from fat, according to David Levitsky, Ph.D., professor of nutrition and psychology at Cornell University in Ithaca, New York.

As a result, one of the most successful weight-loss methods is simply eating no more than 25 percent of calories from fat. Based on a daily calorie intake of 2,700, that means most men need no more than 75 grams of fat a day. For every 200 calories above or below 2,700, add or subtract 5 to 6 grams of fat.

If you're a woman eating an average of 2,000 calories a day, that's a goal of just 56 grams of fat for the entire day. Bad news for fast-food fans: You'd blow the day's fat budget with a burger and fries.

The good news, says Dr. Levitsky: "Learn where the fat is, make low-fat selections instead, and you're going to lose weight automatically."

To help make those low-fat choices, try these tips, suggested by obesity experts.

Become a fat detective. No entrée should contain more than 10 grams of fat, no snack or side dish more than 5 grams per serving. Using this approach, a plate of spaghetti with cheese (9 grams) gets a thumbs-up, while half a batter-dipped chicken breast with skin (18 grams) gets a thumbs-down. For a lean snack, choose a cup of low-fat fruit yogurt (2 grams) over a small slice of apple pie (18 grams).

Live and learn. Buy a new low-fat cookbook and learn ten alternative low-fat recipes that you'll enjoy cooking and eating.

Banish boring bites. Low-fat food doesn't have to be flavorless. Spice up good-for-you fare with herbs like basil, oregano, thyme and marjoram. Swirl chili peppers, dill or coriander into cottage cheese or sprinkle nutmeg or cinnamon on fruit plates.

Say adios to oil. Fat-free broth, fruit or vegetable juice also works fine for cooking meats or sautéing vegetables.

Make lemons your aide. Substitute lemon juice for butter or margarine on vegetables.

Say "yo" to yogurt. Drop fattening sour cream and top potatoes and vegetables with nonfat yogurt.

Make a deal. Trade in high-fat dairy, like 2 percent milk, for an alternative—like skim.

CALL IN THE CAVALRY: COMPLEX CARBOHYDRATES

Now that fat has been relegated to a low profile in your dietary picture, you'll need a replacement. But don't settle for expensive pre-made shakes or diet bars. Call in the cavalry: complex carbohydrates.

Found in such foods as pasta, potatoes and bread, complex carbohydrates can play a significant role in your weight-loss plan by rescuing your faltering willpower.

Once digested, complex carbohydrates are turned into a substance called

PLANNING YOUR SNACK ATTACKS

If you're a nibbler at heart, keeping your hand out of the cookie jar may be setting you up for a Cookie Monster–size snack attack . . . unless you satisfy yourself with healthy alternatives.

Rather than fighting cravings with refusenik diets, Herman M. Frankel, M.D., of the Portland Health Institute in Oregon says he encourages his patients to eat as many as six small meals throughout the day. The caveat: All meals must be low in fat.

"A lot of our patients find they get hungry if they go more than four hours without food," he says. "We say 'Go ahead and eat as much as you want just as long as the items are low in fat.' "

Dr. Frankel says his recommendation is based on studies that show people who cut out the fat—yet eat far more complex carbohydrates than ever—can still lose weight.

If you like the sound of Dr. Frankel's approach, but you don't trust yourself with unlimited calories, here's a sample menu for a 1,500-calorie, low-fat, six-meal-a-day eating plan. You can also create new combinations by trying any of the many fat-free foods now available in supermarkets.

Breakfast: Bran-type cereal, 1 serving with skim milk (150 calories, 1 gram fat); half a grapefruit (40 calories, 0 grams fat); 8 ounces tomato juice (40 calories, 0 grams fat); white or whole-wheat toast with 1 teaspoon all-fruit spread (80 calories, 1 gram fat)

Mid-morning snack: Banana (105 calories, 0 grams fat); 7 vanilla wafers (130 calories, 4 grams fat)

Lunch: Tuna pita pocket sandwich with lettuce and tomato slices (215 to 230 calories, 1 gram fat); two gingersnaps (60 calories, 1 gram fat)

Mid-afternoon snack: 2 fig bars (110 calories, 2 grams fat)

Dinner: Half a chicken breast, baked or broiled (140 calories, 3 grams fat); plain baked potato (145 calories, 0 grams fat); 1 cup red cabbage with apple slices (60 calories, 0 grams fat); medium salad with 2 tablespoons oil-free dressing (37 calories, 0.5 gram fat)

Evening snack: 3 cups air-popped popcorn (90 calories, 0 grams fat)

glycogen that is used by the muscles, brain, liver and kidneys for fuel.

Let those glycogen reserves run low by not eating enough carbohydrates, and the results are predictable: You'll feel grumpy, headachy, restless and perhaps worst of all, downright ravenous. And that can have devastating consequences on your weight-loss efforts, says Dr. Frankel.

"You won't push the cheese and the eggs out of the way in the refrigerator on your way to the cold rice or cold macaroni," says Dr. Frankel. "You'll *eat* the cheese and the eggs."

To beat the low-carb, gotta-eat blues:

Take six. Eating six daily servings of complex carbohydrates like beans, cooked whole grains, breads and pasta will keep your glycogen levels—and dietary resolve—high.

Sneak a high-carb snack. Dr. Frankel says his patients are able to lose more weight when they snack on complex carbohydrates like a bagel or banana between meals, rather than starving until lunch or dinner—and then overeating.

Play nutritional scientist. The best way to determine whether you'll benefit from eating complex carbohydrates between meals is by experimenting, Dr. Frankel says. "You might discover that you're not starving just an hour after dinner anymore," he says.

FILL UP WITH FIBER

Boosting your complex carbohydrate consumption adds another benefit to your weight-loss routine: higher fiber.

Your mouth gets satisfaction from high-fiber foods because of the chomping needed to break them down, says George L. Blackburn, M.D., Ph.D., associate professor of surgery at Harvard Medical School and chief of the Nutrition/Metabolism Laboratory at the Cancer Research Institute of New England Deaconess Hospital in Boston. Another bonus is that your stomach takes longer and needs more gastric juices to break down fiber, giving your tummy a full feeling, says Dr. Frankel.

What's the best way to fiber up?

Get your daily dose. Don't bother measuring fiber by the gram or sprinkling it on your lunch with a teaspoon. By eating the recommended six servings of whole grains, three to five servings of vegetables and two to four servings of fruit, you'll be ahead of the game, says Dr. Frankel.

And after eating all that fiber, you simply won't be as hungry for fattening foods, says Dr. Frankel.

Backing up that theory is a study from the Veterans Administration Medical Center in Minneapolis that suggests eating high-fiber foods in the morning may help you reduce how much food you eat the rest of the day.

Fourteen volunteers were given their choice of cereals for breakfast—from high to low fiber. About 3½ hours later, the volunteers were invited to a high-fat buffet with burgers, peanut butter, corn chips and other foods.

The result: Those who ate the highest-fiber cereal put the smallest dent in the delectables, devouring about 45 fewer calories, say researchers.

(continued on page 450)

WEIGHING YOUR OPTIONS: THREE WEIGHT-LOSS PROGRAMS

Lots of people pick a weight-loss plan as if they're buying a lottery ticket: They make their selection and hope for the best.

But you don't have to gamble with your health. It is really just a matter of finding the right plan to meet your needs, doctors say.

"Our feeling is that no single diet plan works for everyone. The trend is toward specific things for different people," says John P. Foreyt, Ph.D., of Baylor College of Medicine in Houston. Among the factors to consider, says Dr. Foreyt, are how much weight you need to lose, dieting history, genetics and metabolic rate.

To help make your decision easier, *Prevention* magazine's staff investigated several of the country's top weight-loss programs and summarized them below. As always, before beginning any weight-loss regimen, consult your doctor.

NUTRI/SYSTEM

Program: A prepackaged foods diet accompanied by weight-maintenance training.

Prerequisites: None.

Details: No counting calories, weighing portions or worrying about fat—all meals are high carbohydrate, low fat and low sodium. In most cases, just microwave and serve or add water. Three Nutri/System meals plus three snacks tally about 1,100 calories. The program is divided into two phases: weight loss and weight maintenance. Participants eat Nutri/System foods—supplemented with fresh fruits and vegetables—seven days a week. After achieving your goal weight, you go back to regular food five days and Nutri/System meals for two.

Rate of reduction: 1½ to 2 pounds a week.

Potential problems: Some participants don't like the taste of the meals.

What a participant said: (Stewart Werley, 40 pounds lost) "I felt hungry during the first week, but that was all. We had fun playing around with the meals, doctoring them up here and there."

Cost: Moderate to high priced—based on how much you lose. Nutri/System will refund half the program cost if you successfully complete the year-long maintenance program.

Location: Available nationwide at free-standing centers. Check the white pages of the telephone directory.

OVEREATERS ANONYMOUS (OA)

Program: Group fellowship of men and women dedicated to recovering from compulsive overeating. No diet or food plans offered.

Prerequisites: Participants must want to stop eating compulsively; an OA survey showed that the majority of members were 50 to 100 pounds overweight when they started.

Details: This 12-step program is modeled after Alcoholics Anonymous. A recurring theme in OA literature: Compulsive overeaters are driven by forces they don't understand to eat more than they need, and they eat in ways that aren't rational. Steps include admitting you're powerless over food, turning your life over to a "higher power" to get better, making amends with people you've harmed through compulsive eating and helping other compulsive overeaters. Anonymity is retained by use of first names only.

Rate of reduction: Varies.

Potential problems: No instruction on correct nutritional choices.

What a participant said: (Earl, 300 pounds lost) "The meetings have taught me to live life on its own terms and not to take things so personally."

Cost: No fee or dues.

Location: Check the white pages in the telephone directory under "Overeaters Anonymous."

WEIGHT WATCHERS

Program: Low-calorie food plan with wide range of choices. Stresses lifestyle change.

Prerequisites: For men, women and children (ten years or older) who are five or more pounds overweight.

Details: In the full-choice plan, you get a 1,075- to 1,465-calorie-a-day food plan consisting of most common foods. During week three, new foods are added. Portion control is the key. Slogan: "Moderation, not deprivation." Daily servings are chosen from a food list with seven categories: fruits, vegetables, fats, protein, breads, milk products and diet products. You're allowed to substitute a specific amount of any item for an equivalent amount of any other food in the same group.

Rate of reduction: Generally three to five pounds the first week; one to two pounds thereafter.

Potential problems: Leaders are experts in the Weight Watchers system, not nutritionists.

What a participant said: (Kevin Connolly, 63 pounds lost) "The food plan was very simple, and I never felt hungry on it. I lost 63 pounds in 14 weeks."

Cost: Inexpensive.

Location: Nationwide and 23 foreign countries. 19,000 weekly meetings in United States. For the nearest location, check the white pages of the telephone directory.

Fine-tune your fiber feast. Once you're getting enough servings of fiber, increase portion size and focus on the highest-fiber foods, especially legumes (beans and peas) and other fiber-rich fruits like apples, prunes, raspberries and pears.

Time Your Meals

When you eat can also have some bearing on the size of your bottom line. Breakfast skippers take heed; you may be reducing your metabolic rate 25 percent by not eating a morning meal, says Dr. Callaway.

Again, think of your body's metabolism as a fire, but one that dies down while you sleep. Waking up, moving around and eating breakfast stokes the fire, enhancing your body's calorie consumption.

Dr. Blackburn agrees: "Breakfast serves as a metabolic kicker. The body needs fluids and a range of nutrients in the morning to get started. And breakfast will ward off the afternoon munchies."

To keep your metabolism ticking like a Rolex:

Eat a good breakfast. In addition to mangling your metabolism, skipping breakfast may actually sabotage your eating plan for the rest of the day. Without breakfast, you're more likely to succumb to a midmorning sugar fix—like a doughnut or a candy bar, doctors say. And the sugar can make you hungrier at lunch, weakening your willpower and increasing the chances you'll order a high-fat meal.

Never dine after nine. Eating a big meal after 9:00 P.M. can also set you up for dietary disaster: Not only will your body more readily store the calories as fat, but you'll be too full to eat breakfast, resuming the fattening cycle.

In fact, some doctors suggest making breakfast the largest meal of the day and tapering the amount of food you eat as the day goes on.

Keep an Eye on Calories

You've reduced your fat, added complex carbohydrates and fiber, and done it all before 9:00 P.M. But that *still* doesn't mean that you can give yourself carte blanche with calories.

Even twins burn calories at a different rate. So, short of a doctor's visit, it's nearly impossible to determine just how many calories you need to eat each day. There are, however, two methods you can use at home to give you a general idea, according to Kris Etherton, a researcher with the Nutrition Department at the University of Pennsylvania in Philadelphia and coauthor of several weight-loss studies.

Do your math. First, take your weight and multiply it by 10. If, for example, you weigh 120, that's 1,200 calories. But you're not done yet—you need to figure in your activity level. If you're sedentary, you're considered a 3; if you're moderately active, you're a 5; if you're very active, you rate a 7. Take this number, multiply it by 100, and then add it to your first calorie level. According to this formula, a sedentary 120-pounder needs to eat about 1,500 calories a day. To get a more accurate number, consult your doctor or a dietitian, says Etherton.

Step on a scale. Another way to determine whether you're eating too many calories is to weigh yourself, Etherton says. "If you're gaining weight, then you're eating too many calories."

But whenever you are ready to lose weight permanently, take a tip from Kathy Biggerstaff: Drop the diets and stick to a sensible, low-fat, high-carbohydrate eating plan. You'll like the results.

"I don't even feel like the same person anymore," she says. "That overweight woman who hated herself is long gone."

HIGH-NUTRITION RECIPES

BREAST OF CHICKEN ITALIAN

Chicken breast is a longtime favorite among weight watchers. With the skin removed, it is very low in fat. Surprisingly, pasta is also a good choice for dieters. It's virtually fat free and has lots of hunger-appeasing complex carbohydrates. This recipe was created by Houston chef Raymond Potter for the American Cancer Society.

- **4 boneless, skinless chicken breast halves**
- **½ cup fat-free Italian dressing**
- **4 thick (½") tomato slices**
- **¼ cup seasoned dry bread crumbs**
- **2 teaspoons grated Parmesan cheese**
- **8 ounces angel hair pasta**
- **1 cup frozen peas**

Combine the chicken and dressing in a 9" × 9" shallow baking dish; turn to coat the chicken on all sides. Cover and marinate at room temperature for 1 hour. (If marinating longer, refrigerate the pan.)

Bake at 400° for 10 minutes. Top each breast with a tomato slice. Sprinkle with the bread crumbs and Parmesan. Bake for 10 minutes, or until the crumbs are brown and the chicken is cooked through.

Just before serving, cook the pasta in a large pot of boiling water for 3 minutes. Add the peas and cook for another 2 minutes, or until the pasta is just tender. Drain. Serve topped with the chicken.

Serves 4
Per serving: *406 calories, 3.2 g. fat (7% of calories), 3.4 g. dietary fiber, 67 mg. cholesterol, 217 mg. sodium*

HUEVOS RANCHEROS

A good breakfast is essential for a successful weight-loss program. This Mexican casserole is a favorite breakfast of guests at the Heartland Spa in Gilman, Illinois. It would also make a delicious lunch or light dinner. Serve it with chunky salsa and nonfat sour cream or yogurt.

- **2 eggs or ½ cup fat-free egg substitute**
- **8 egg whites**
- **¼ cup nonfat cottage cheese**
- **¼ cup skim milk**
- **¼ teaspoon ground cumin**
- **¼ cup snipped chives**
- **1 tablespoon chopped fresh coriander**
- **⅛ teaspoon ground black pepper**
- **5 large corn tortillas**
- **1½ ounces reduced-fat Monterey Jack cheese, shredded**
- **6 thin tomato slices**

Place the egg, egg whites, cottage cheese, milk and cumin in a blender. Process for about 5 seconds to mix well. Add the chives, coriander and pepper. Blend for 5 seconds.

Wrap the tortillas in a damp paper towel and microwave on high for 25 seconds to soften.

Coat a 9" pie plate with no-stick spray. Line the pan with the tortillas, overlapping them to completely cover the bottom (allow the edges to stick up a little over the top of the pan). Sprinkle with the Monterey Jack. Gently pour in the egg mixture.

Bake at 350° for 40 minutes, or until puffed and golden brown. Remove from the oven, top with the tomato slices and let stand for 5 minutes. Slice into wedges.

Serves 4
Per serving: *211 calories, 6 g. fat (25% of calories), 2.5 g. dietary fiber, 113 mg. cholesterol, 295 mg. sodium*

BLACK-EYED PEA SALAD

Foods that are high in fiber and low in fat—like black-eyed peas and other legumes—are a boon to dieters. This easy salad makes a satisfying low-cal lunch.

- **4 cups cooked black-eyed peas**
- **2 cups finely shredded spinach or kale**
- **2 carrots, finely diced**
- **½ cup minced scallions**
- **1 tablespoon minced fresh basil**
- **1 tablespoon minced fresh sage**
- **3 tablespoons lemon juice**
- **4 teaspoons olive oil**
- **2 teaspoons red-wine vinegar**
- **¼ teaspoon dry mustard**

In a large bowl, toss together the peas, spinach or kale, carrots, scallions, basil and sage.

In a small bowl, whisk together the lemon juice, oil, vinegar and mustard. Pour over the salad. Toss to combine.

Serves 4

Per serving: *277 calories, 5.8 g. fat (18% of calories), 7 g. dietary fiber, 0 mg. cholesterol, 61 mg. sodium*

WARM FRUIT SOUFFLÉS

You don't have to forgo all desserts when watching your weight. These soufflés will satisfy a sweet tooth without adding a lot of fat or calories to your diet. Other equally delicious soufflés can be made with dried apricots, cherries or peaches.

- **1¼ cups water**
- **4 ounces pitted prunes**
- **1 teaspoon vanilla**
- **3½ tablespoons brown sugar**
- **3 egg whites, at room temperature**

In a 2-quart saucepan, combine the water and prunes. Bring to a boil, then reduce the heat to medium-low, cover the pan and simmer for about 25 minutes, or until most of the liquid has been absorbed.

Transfer to a food processor. Add the vanilla and 2 tablespoons of the sugar. Process until pureed. Place in a large bowl and let cool to room temperature.

Place the egg whites in a medium bowl. Using an electric mixer, beat until soft peaks form. Sprinkle in 1 tablespoon of the remaining sugar and continue beating until stiff glossy peaks form.

Stir about ⅓ of the whites into the prune puree to lighten it. Then fold in the remaining whites.

Coat four 8-ounce soufflé dishes or custard cups with no-stick spray. Take the remaining ½ tablespoon of the sugar and sprinkle it in the dishes to lightly coat them.

Spoon the prune mixture into the cups and smooth the tops with a rubber spatula. Place the cups in a baking dish and add enough hot water to come about halfway up the sides of the soufflé dishes. Bake at 375° for 20 to 25 minutes, or until the soufflés are puffed and browned. Serve warm.

Serves 4

Tip: *You may make the prune puree ahead and refrigerate or freeze it until needed. Bring it to room temperature before proceeding with the recipe.*

Per serving: *129 calories, 0.1 g. fat (1% of calories), 1.9 g. dietary fiber, 0 mg. cholesterol, 48 mg. sodium*

CHAPTER 33

VEGETARIANISM
A HEALTHY LIFE WITHOUT MEAT

At the age of 43, Pennsylvania artist Wayne Michaud became a vegetarian.

"It was the health thing, mostly," explains Michaud, whose father, grandfather and great-grandfather were all—either as restaurateurs or meat brokers—in the business of selling meat. "And it was actually unintentional.

"I'd pick up the paper, read an article about diet and heart disease, then stop eating eggs and hot dogs and start eating more chicken and fish." Then a couple of months later I'd pick up the paper, read an article about diet and cancer and I'd cut back on chicken and fish so that I could eat more whole grains and vegetables.

"Then, next thing you know, I'd hear a news report about diet and high blood pressure and I'd start to eat more fruit.

"Pretty soon," he adds with a chuckle, "I was a vegetarian almost by default. I hardly even noticed the change."

A Kill-It-and-Cook-It Past

Michaud is not alone in his evolution toward a vegetarian lifestyle. Food industry reports indicate that consumption of meat is down and consumption of fruits and vegetables is up all across the country. Sales of broccoli alone have soared 800 percent over the past two decades, reports the United Fresh Fruit and Vegetable Association. And the United States Department of Agriculture reports that meat consumption has dropped 10 percent in the last decade.

Although only 3 or 4 percent of us have actually taken a pledge of allegiance to the vegetarian flag, enough folks like living under its protection that, according to one survey, roughly 20 percent of us routinely search for vegetarian meals whenever we go out to eat. We may not define ourselves as vegetarians, but we're no longer major meatheads either. You might even say that we're in transition from our kill-it-and-cook-it past to a more thoughtful mode of eating in our future.

Igniting the movement are studies indicating that, compared with meat eaters, vegetarians are more likely to live longer and avoid such debilitating conditions as heart disease, stroke, cancer, high blood pressure, osteoporosis, gallstones, kidney stones, diverticular disease, constipation, overweight, rheumatoid arthritis, gallstones and the life-threatening complications of diabetes.

In a landmark study of more than 25,000 Seventh-Day Adventists between the ages of 30 and 84, for example, researchers at Loma Linda University in California discovered that eating meat even once a day *tripled* the risk of fatal heart disease in men between the ages of 45 and 64. Or to put it another way, vegetarians had one-third the risk of dying from heart disease of their meat-eating counterparts.

Then, in an 11-year study of 1,904 vegetarians conducted by the German Cancer Research Center in Heidelberg, scientists confirmed the cardiovascular protective effects of a vegetarian diet when their research revealed that deaths due to heart attacks or strokes were *50 percent* lower in vegetarians than in a comparable group of so-called normal eaters.

To top it all off, a subsequent study of 44 Dutch vegetarians between the

WHAT KIND OF VEGETARIAN ARE YOU?

Although the basic vegetarian diet consists of fruits, vegetables, whole grains and legumes, some vegetarians include eggs or dairy products in their diets and some do not, says Suzanne Havala, R.D., of The Vegetarian Resource Group in Baltimore.

An *ovolactovegetarian*, for example, excludes meat, poultry and fish, but includes both eggs and dairy products in his diet. A *lactovegetarian* follows exactly the same diet, but won't eat eggs. And a *vegan* excludes meat, poultry, fish, eggs, milk, cheese and other dairy products.

"Only a small percentage of vegetarians in the United States are vegans," says Havala. Most vegetarians are ovolactovegetarians.

ages of 65 and 97 revealed that the vegetarians had healthier hearts than meat eaters who were *ten years younger.*

HEALTHY DIET OR HEALTHY LIFESTYLE?

Most of those who participated in the American, German and Dutch studies had been vegetarians over a long period of time. And since vegetarians are generally considered to have a healthier lifestyle than the general population—they tend to smoke less, drink less and exercise more—the scientists really weren't sure how much of the astonishing health benefits they were seeing was due to a meatless diet and how much was due simply to the fact that vegetarians are pretty healthy people to begin with.

So to see whether or not a sudden switch to a vegetarian diet would produce the same kind of benefical effects on people who were not only meat eaters, but meat eaters who were in pretty bad shape, a group of World Health Organization (WHO) researchers collaborated with doctors at the Medical Hospital and Research Centre in Moradabad, India. They divided a group of 406 men who had suffered heart attacks within the past 48 hours into two groups. One group received a normal hospital diet of meat, eggs, vegetables, fruits and grains for six weeks. The other received a similar diet, but with the meat and eggs replaced by fish, nuts and a vegetarian meat substitute.

The result? Even though all their other hospital care remained the same, the meat eaters subsequently had 66 percent more heart attacks and nearly 48 percent more complications than the vegetarian group over the next six weeks. There were also 43 percent more deaths among the meat eaters.

Scientists are still trying to figure out *why* a vegetarian diet appears to have such a healthy effect on the heart. Researchers involved with the WHO study in India thought that their spectacular results might have been due to the fact that the diet helped them lose weight—a 7½-pound average weight loss. They also speculated that it could be the result of a drop in their cholesterol, which averaged 20 points in the vegetarian group. (Cholesterol is only found in animal foods.) Those who continued eating meat only experienced about a 3-pound drop in weight, the researchers noted, with a 10-point drop in cholesterol.

Taking a closer look at the cholesterol levels in a group of 31 strict vegetar-ians in New Jersey, researchers from the American Health Foundation in New York found total cholesterol levels averaged 23 percent lower than those of so-called normal eaters. Moreover, the vegetarians' LDL (low-density lipoprotein) cholesterol—usually referred to as the bad kind of cholesterol—was 30 percent lower than that of the meat eaters, while their HDL (high-density lipoprotein) cholesterol—the "good" kind—was 8 percent higher. Triglyceride levels—an indicator of how much fat is being stored in the body and frequently also a predictor of heart disease—were 27 percent lower in the vegetarian group.

WIDER ARTERIES IN WEEKS

Markedly lower cholesterol levels among vegetarians are pretty good evidence that something healthy is going on inside their bodies. But what exactly *is* it?

To answer that question, a group of scientists from the University of Texas Medical School at Houston, the University of California at San Francisco and the University of California at Berkeley got together to figure out a way that they could peek inside people's coronary arteries and then quantify the changes that occurred after adopting a vegetarian lifestyle.

They took 40 men and women between the ages of 35 and 70 with a combined total of 192 disease-narrowed sections in their coronary arteries, hooked them up to special x-ray machines and computers, ran thin wires through their arteries, and—like a bunch of ancient cartographers—mapped the topography of their arteries. How big were the arteries? How small were the narrowed sections? How much blood could get through to transport its precious oxygen cargo throughout the body? How big a blood clot would it take to block one of those narrowed sections and cause a heart attack?

Once they had their measurements, the scientists put about half the group on a vegetarian diet—with instructions to stop smoking, start exercising and reduce stress as well—and half remained on their usual diet.

One to 1½ years later, the team of scientists remeasured everybody's arteries. The result? The worse a person's arteries had been before adopting a vegetarian lifestyle, the more improved they were afterward. But coronary arteries in those on their usual diets continued to narrow at a rapid rate.

GETTING THE DROP ON FAT

When Fat and Skinny had a race around the dinner plate, as the childhood ditty goes, this is what they might have seen after a week's worth of plate-racing. It compares the totals for fat, calories, carbohydrates and fiber that two different dinners—one vegetarian, one with meat—would provide if eaten for seven consecutive nights.

MEAL	FAT (g.)	CALORIES	CARBOHYDRATE (g.)	FIBER (g.)
Beans, rice and broccoli	3.5	1,790	365	40
Beef, rice and broccoli	51.1	2,480	208	15

NOTE: Serving amounts per dinner equal 4 ounces black beans or lean, top round beef roast, ½ cup white rice and ½ cup broccoli.

Forty percent of the vegetarian group had literally *remolded* their coronary arteries to create better blood flow throughout the heart. Those who had adhered fairly well to their vegetarian pledge stopped arterial disease cold. Those who had adhered perfectly to the program actually widened their arteries—and narrowed their chances of having a heart attack.

VEGETABLES UP, PRESSURE DOWN

The powerful effect a vegetarian diet has on arteries may also explain why vegetarians tend to have lower blood pressures than the general population. After all, the top (systolic) number on the readout from your doctor's blood pressure gauge actually reflects the amount of force your heart has to use to pump and circulate blood. And it's only common sense that the heart will have to exert far less pressure if your arteries are open and flexible from a healthy lifestyle rather than narrowed and stiff from disease.

But how effective is a vegetarian diet in actually lowering blood pressure? A six-week study of 26 Australian men between the ages of 28 and 64 found that the top number on their blood pressure readings dropped an average of six points when they consumed a vegetarian diet. The bottom (diastolic) number—which essentially measures the amount of pressure in your blood vessels when your heart is at rest—decreased by four points.

Since a similar group of lean-meat-eating Australians had pretty much the same results, researchers are beginning to wonder if at least some of the healthy effects of a vegetarian diet owe more to the abundant presence of fruits and vegetables, rather than simply to the absence of meat.

LOWER CANCER RISK

Besides documenting the cardiovascular effects of a vegetarian diet, research supporting other health benefits continues to accumulate at a rapid pace. The German Cancer Research Center, for example, found that the incidence of cancer among vegetarian men was *half* that of meat eaters, and the incidence of cancer among women vegetarians was roughly 25 percent lower.

Further studies of Seventh-Day Adventists demonstrate that the risk of fatal lung cancer among these nonsmoking vegetarians is about *half* that of a nonsmoking but meat-eating group. And still other studies indicate that colorectal cancer is also significantly less likely to occur among vegetarians, possibly because of the way a vegetarian diet alters bile acids and digestive enzymes.

Prostate cancer and pancreatic cancer may also be less likely to occur in vegetarians, says Paul Mills, Ph.D., an associate professor of public health and preventive medicine who studies Seventh-Day Adventists at Loma Linda University. In fact, his studies reveal that "the people with the most copious consumption of fruits and vegetables encounter the lowest risk of cancers at many sites in the body."

THE ROAD TO VEGETARIANISM: A DOCTOR'S JOURNEY

Thirty-nine-year-old Washington, D.C., psychiatrist and health activist Neal Barnard, M.D., was raised on pork chops and roast beef in Fargo, North Dakota, in a family that included several cattle ranchers.

He hunted ducks and geese, and even worked one summer in a fast-food restaurant serving burgers. Yet despite his hoof-heavy background, Dr. Barnard always leaned more toward vegetarian cuisine.

"From an aesthetic standpoint, my favorite food was always Mexican food," he says. "We had the world's best Mexican restaurant in Fargo. They made beans mixed with jalapeños, wrapped in tortillas and served with a wonderful sauce."

Yet despite his preferences, Dr. Barnard didn't actually become a full-time vegetarian until a part-time job gave him an insider's view of what heavy meat consumption can do to the body.

"I worked in a hospital where, as an autopsy assistant, I saw what killed people," he says. "And what I saw was lots of colon cancers, strokes and heart disease.

"Then, when I started medical school, I became more sensitive to the pain and suffering that animals experience. All these things added up," says the psychiatrist, "and I began to eat less and less meat until, finally, I didn't eat any at all. Seven or eight years later, I stopped eating dairy products and eggs, too."

How did he feel as he made the transition? "The one thing I really noticed was that my endurance was better and I didn't feel sleepy after meals. Before that, I would have lunch and later feel like nodding off. I now know the reason for that: After fatty meals, the viscosity of blood is increased and the blood doesn't circulate as well. The theory is that the brain doesn't get as much oxygen from the thicker blood," he explains.

As for his future prospects, says Dr. Barnard: "I hope to spread the message about the surprising power of vegetarian foods to as many people as possible. With the current epidemics of heart disease and cancer, we can't keep it a secret."

As far as cancer is concerned, it's apparently not just the absence of meat that makes a vegetarian diet so healthful, concludes Dr. Mills. The presence of so many fruits and vegetables seems to have a protective effect in and of itself.

In any case, scientists are beginning to get an inkling of how a vegetarian diet goes about building cancer defenses. German researchers, for example, found that the immune system's white blood cells in vegetarians are *twice* as deadly to tumor cells as those of meat eaters.

PROTECTION FOR DIABETICS?

Although most of us tend to take our kidneys for granted, the fact is that we can't live without them. They're responsible for filtering metabolic leftovers out of the bloodstream and sending them to the bladder for disposal. Allowed to hang around, these leftovers would otherwise turn our bodies into toxic waste dumps.

Unfortunately, serious kidney damage is a common, life-threatening complication of Type I, or insulin-dependent, diabetes. Doctors frequently try to at least slow onset of kidney damage by recommending a low-protein diet. But although a low-protein diet does slow other types of kidney disease, it has not been helpful when kidney damage is caused by diabetes.

Those on a vegetarian diet might fare better, however. Scientists have discovered that the kidney reacts differently to vegetable protein than it does to meat protein—so much so that a preliminary study at the Ysbyty Gwynedd Renal Unit in Wales indicates that a vegetarian diet (which includes milk and eggs) might help to prevent kidney disease in people with diabetes.

The researchers first measured kidney function in seven men and women with diabetes who ate a conventional diet over an eight-week period. Then they switched the group to a vegetarian diet for the next eight weeks, and back to a conventional diet for a third eight-week period.

Kidney function tests conducted over the entire 24-week study revealed that the vegetarian diet apparently cut the kidneys' workloads in half—thus protecting them from the increased work caused by diabetes. Although further research is necessary to substantiate this effect, it may well be that a vegetarian diet will help those with renal disease caused by diabetes to live longer.

FEWER ARTHRITIS SYMPTOMS

Doctors have known for years that fasting seems to relieve the pain and swelling of rheumatoid arthritis, but they also have known that the minute someone with arthritis resumes a normal diet, their joints begin to ache and swell once again.

To see if they could help people with arthritis maintain the therapeutic effect of a fast, researchers from the University of Oslo and the Norwegian National Hospital in Oslo set up an experiment involving 53 people with arthritis. After documenting arthritic symptoms—pain, swelling, morning stiffness, grip strength, number of tender joints—with lab tests and physical exams, they divided participants into two groups. One group was sent for a month-long stay at a health farm, while the other was sent to a nursing home. The health farm group was told to fast, while the nursing home group was told to eat their usual diet.

The health farm group's fast—which lasted from seven to ten days—included herbal teas, garlic, vegetable broth, water in which potatoes and parsley had been cooked, various vegetable juices from carrots, beets and celery.

Once the fast was complete, the group added a new food to their diet every other day. If they developed any increase in pain, stiffness or joint swelling within 48 hours, the food was then omitted from their diet. If they had no reaction, it was added back on a permanent basis. The group was asked not to include any foods that contained meat, fish, eggs, dairy products, gluten, refined sugar, salt, strong spices, preservatives and citrus fruits.

The fast and restricted diet produced a dramatic reduction in symptoms within the first month: the number of tender joints dropped by a third, morning stiffness duration was reduced from about three hours to a little more than an hour. Grip strength was considerably increased, and pain was considerably decreased.

After keeping to this kind of an eating regime for three to five months, the health farm group was then allowed to gradually reintroduce milk, other dairy products and gluten-containing foods until their menu evolved into a well-balanced vegetarian diet. They maintained this diet until the study's conclusion, 13 months after it had started.

While the health farm group was fasting and then moving toward a vegetarian diet, the nursing home group was still eating what researchers felt was an ordinary diet. So, at the study's conclusion, the researchers were able to measure the pain, swelling, grip strength and number of joints affected in both groups and compare those numbers with the measurements taken at the beginning of their study.

The result was astounding. The arthritic symptoms of the ordinary group either stayed the same or got worse. But the arthritic symptoms of the vegetarian group, which had been dramatically reduced within the first month, stayed nearly as low as long as they were still on the vegetarian diet. And lab tests confirmed the researchers' observations.

WHY PEOPLE VEG OUT

Although health is clearly the major reason why people become vegetarians, there are a few others. "Many people feel it is against their ethical beliefs to kill an animal for food when there are other alternatives," points out Baltimore nutritionist Reed Mangels, R.D., Ph.D. Plato, Horace, Virgil, Pythagoras and—more recently—Albert Schweitzer, Albert Einstein, Leo Tolstoy and Mahatma Gandhi are a few of the people who became vegetarians because they didn't believe in killing animals.

Others vegetarians cite the huge amounts of land needed to produce meat. "An acre of grain yields five times as much protein as an acre devoted to livestock," says Rudolph Ballentine, M.D., director of the Himalayan Institute in Honesdale, Pennsylvania. An acre of beans produces ten times more. And as feeding the world becomes increasingly more difficult, people are asking whether it's better to cultivate ten acres to feed perhaps 1,000 people, or to cultivate ten acres to feed a single steer—especially when the steer will only feed a half-dozen people.

Money is another reason why people choose a vegetarian diet, adds Dr. Mangels. "I had friends who wanted to take a trip out West, for example, but they didn't have enough money. So for a year they ate a vegetarian diet and banked the difference between that and what they usually spent on groceries. By the time they were ready to travel, they had enough to take a trip to the Tetons for two weeks."

Religion is also a motivating factor for some people, says Dr. Mangels. Seventh-Day Adventists are encouraged to become vegetarians. Hindus and Buddhists are commonly vegetarians, and observant Jews will sometimes turn to vegetarianism if a kosher butcher is not available.

The Gradual Vegetarian

Whatever motivates you to make the switch, there are a few helpful strategies that experts say can make the transition from meat eater to vegetarian an easy experience.

What's for Dinner?

Making the switch from an omnivorous to a vegetarian lifestyle can give your meal-planning imagination a good daily workout. But if racking your brain to healthfully answer the question, "What's for dinner?" sounds torturous, you may need the kind of help that's found in a basic vegetarian food guide.

The table below, which tells you how much of each food type you should eat, was adapted from a complete, practical guide developed by Ella Haddad, R.D., D.H.Sc., assistant professor in the School of Public Health at Loma Linda University in California. All servings are per day, unless otherwise noted.

Food Group	**Servings**
Breads, grains, cereals	6–11 (4 or more should be whole grain)
Legumes (dry beans and peas)	1–2
Nuts and seeds	1–2
Vegetables and fruits	5–9
Milk products	2–3
Eggs	2–3 *per week*
Fats or oils	3–6 (small amounts)
Sweets	Eat in moderation

NOTE: Adolescents and very active adults may require the larger number of servings from each group per day.

Take your time. Although some people feel the need to go cold turkey, most people who successfully part with meat make the transition gradually over the course of a year or so, says Dr. Ballentine.

Start with red meat. Most budding vegetarians seem to make the transition in three moves, says Dr. Ballentine, who has adapted this natural tendency into a more structured three-phase program at the Himalayan Institute. Phase one calls for gradually eliminating red meats while adding grains and legumes to your diet. Phase two calls for slowly eliminating poultry and increasing the number of cooked green vegetables that appear on your plate. And phase three means increasing fruits as you cut back on fish, eggs and dairy products—or eliminate them altogether.

Make a day of it. Some nutritionists suggest you kick the first phase into gear by scheduling a "Meatless Thursday" or "Meatless Friday." Not only is it an easy way to effortlessly slip into a new way of eating, but it also gives your digestive system a preview of what's about to come down the pipe on a regular basis.

The Meat of It All

Here are three ways to get the flavor and texture of meat in your diet.

Discover soy. "I'm using more and more foods that come from soy, like textured soy protein," says Nancy Rutherford, chef and owner of the vegetarian Bluegrass Spa and Resort in Stamping Ground, Kentucky. "When I use it in chili, it can look and seem so much like meat that I've had people send it back, thinking meat was mistakenly added."

Potentiate taste with tofu. "I'm also crazy about tofu because it's a high-protein food that takes on the flavor of whatever it's cooked with," Rutherford says. A plateful of spaghetti with tofu really projects the exquisite taste of the sauce.

Serve seitan. A wheat product that can be formed into loaves like meat loaf, seitan is a tried-and-true people pleaser that Rutherford uses at her spa. It gives people in transition the sensation of eating meat, and its flavor blends easily with all kinds of sauces and vegetables. It also slices well for sandwiches. Seitan is available at health food stores.

It's Easy if You Follow the Rules

"A vegetarian diet is very easy to plan," says Suzanne Havala, R.D., a nutrition consultant and adviser for the Vegetarian Resource Group in Baltimore. "It doesn't take meticulous planning that researchers thought it once took to meet your nutritional needs. In fact, it's easier to meet the Dietary Guidelines for Americans on a vegetarian diet than it is on a typical Western diet."

There are just a few simple rules to good, nutritious vegetarian eating: Eat a variety of foods, including fruits, vegetables, whole grains and legumes. Be sure that you get an adequate number of calories per day to meet your energy needs—the average woman, for example, needs about 2,000 calories per day to maintain her weight. And keep calorie-dense, nutrient-poor foods such as sweets and snack foods to a minimum.

It was once believed that strict vegetarians could not get enough protein. "Today we know this isn't true," says Havala. "In fact, most vegetarians meet or exceed recommended protein intake levels."

Proteins from meat, fish, poultry and milk are considered complete proteins—they have all of the essential amino acids in balanced proportions. Vegetable sources of protein do not. To ensure that you get all of the amino acids, you need to eat foods that will compensate for each other's shortcomings. Sound complicated? It's not. Basically, all you need to remember is that the proteins in whole grains, vegetables and legumes complement each other. You're sure to come up short if all you eat is pasta, pasta and more pasta. But, if during the course of a day or two you eat a variety of foods and enough calories to meet your energy needs, it's almost impossible to not get enough protein, Havala says.

AVOID THE FAT TRAP

Most vegetarian diets are high in fiber and low in fat. But when the novice vegetarian begins to replace meat with other foods, he may have a tendency to substitute cheese, eggs and other high-fat foods, says Havala. Here's how to stay on a healthy course.

De-fat your casseroles. Almost any meatless casserole is easily modified into a healthier low-fat dish, says Havala. Two egg whites, or the recommended portion of a commercial egg substitute, can be used in place of one whole egg. You not only eliminate fat but cholesterol, too.

Choose your cheeses wisely. Hard cheeses like sharp Cheddar and Parmesan are generally lower in fat than soft cheeses. They're still pretty high though, so, whenever possible, use the new reduced-fat versions of some of your favorite cheeses such as Swiss and Cheddar. Nonfat yogurt can be a great alternative to cream cheese. Simply place the yogurt in a sieve lined with cheesecloth or a paper coffee filter, refrigerate and allow to drain overnight. The next day, you'll have a healthier version of cream cheese ready for spreading.

Use full-bodied seasoning. Cookbook author Mollie Katzen of Berkeley, California, used to rely on rich ingredients like sour cream to give her vegetarian cooking so much excitement. Now she leaves the sour cream in the refrigerator and reaches instead for her spice shelf. "My current favorite ingredient is garlic," Katzen says. "I'm learning to use it so that it's a really full-bodied seasoning, but not overpowering. I'm also using other herbs and seasonings very intensely."

Boost Your Iron Intake

Since iron from vegetable sources is absorbed less efficiently than iron from meats, vegetarians—especially vegetarian women—should be sure to include enough high-iron foods like whole or enriched grains, legumes, dried fruits and vegetables such as broccoli, turnip greens, kale and collards.

Add some vitamin C. To increase the ability of your body to absorb and use iron, nutritionists say you should eat foods rich in vitamin C—citrus fruits, green peppers or onions, for example—when you consume iron-rich foods. And, skip the tea or coffee—it seems to interfere with iron absorption.

Cover Your Vitamin Needs

Since there are no plant sources of vitamin D or vitamin B_{12}, vegetarians—particularly those who do not eat eggs or dairy products—must make a little extra effort to make sure that they get enough.

In an Israeli study, for example, researchers found that vegetarians who did not eat any animal products had half the amount of vitamin B_{12} in their bodies as their meat-eating counterparts. The vegetarians were not actually deficient in the vitamin, researchers reported, but they certainly didn't have enough in reserve in case it was needed.

Get a blood test. An inadequate amount of vitamin B_{12} circulating through your body can result in serious neurological, cerebral or psychiatric problems, doctors say. And the damage is irreversible. That's why the Israeli researchers recommend that all strict vegetarians, those who eat no animal products, periodically have a blood test to check the amount of B_{12} available to their bodies.

Take advantage of fortified foods. If you eat no fish, eggs or dairy products at all, nutritionists say that fortified foods such as fortified cereals can provide a solid source of vitamin B_{12}, as can vitamin supplements. Be sure to check the labels.

Walk in the sunshine. Exposure to sunshine can also give you a dose of vitamin D, since this nutrient is actually made right on the surface of your skin. But whether or not the dosage is adequate may depend on how far north you live and the amount of sunshine available. In a study at the University of Kuopio in Finland, for example, blood levels of vitamin D among vegetarians were adequate in the late spring and summer. In the long Finnish winter, however, they dropped below the levels needed to maintain strong bones and teeth.

Some nutritionists feel that it's difficult for vegetarians to get enough calcium if they decide not to eat cheese or drink milk. Studies have shown, however, that vegetarians absorb and retain more calcium and have a lower rate of osteoporosis than nonvegetarians, says Havala.

Add extra calcium. Fortunately, calcium is plentiful in many plant sources, so adding just a few extra servings of calcium-rich foods on a daily basis—two cups of beet greens, a cup of broccoli and three pieces of cornbread, for example—will go a long way toward keeping your bones healthy.

Zero in on zinc. Zinc levels can be marginal in a vegetarian diet since meat, poultry and seafood are the richest sources of this mineral. The problem can be complicated by the fact that fiber normally present in vegetables will grab hold of some of the zinc and prevent it from being absorbed by your body. This could be a double whammy in those who don't eat enough good sources of zinc. To counteract the effect of this, nutritionists suggest you boost your zinc intake by adding regular servings of wheat germ, whole grains and dried yeast to your diet.

HIGH-NUTRITION RECIPES

SPINACH PIE

Brown rice, egg substitute and low-fat dairy products all contribute protein to this easy entrée.

- **1½ cups skim milk**
- **1 cup nonfat cottage cheese**
- **¾ cup fat-free egg substitute**
- **2 teaspoons Dijon mustard**
- **¼ teaspoon hot-pepper sauce**
- **1 box (10 ounces) frozen chopped spinach, thawed and squeezed dry**
- **2 cups cooked brown rice**
- **½ cup shredded reduced-fat Cheddar cheese**
- **½ cup minced sweet red peppers**
- **1 teaspoon dried dill**
- **1 tablespoon grated Parmesan cheese**

In a blender, process the milk, cottage cheese, egg, mustard and hot-pepper sauce until smooth. Pour into a large bowl.

Stir in the spinach, rice, Cheddar, peppers and dill.

Coat a 10" pie plate with no-stick spray. Add the rice mixture. Sprinkle with the Parmesan.

Bake at 350° for 45 to 50 minutes, or until set and golden on top. Cool for 10 minutes before serving.

Serves 4

Per serving: *258 calories, 4.4 g. fat (15% of calories), 3.6 g. dietary fiber, 12 mg. cholesterol, 406 mg. sodium*

THREE-BEAN SALAD

Adding dried beans, such as chick-peas and kidney beans, and low-fat cheese to your vegetarian salads gives them an extra dash of protein.

1 can (19 ounces) chick-peas, rinsed and drained
1 can (19 ounces) kidney beans, rinsed and drained
12 ounces wax beans, cut into 1" pieces and steamed
⅔ cup diced cucumbers
½ cup thinly sliced scallions
¼ cup minced fresh parsley
4 ounces nonfat mozzarella cheese, cubed
⅓ cup basil vinegar or white-wine vinegar
3 tablespoons olive oil
1 clove garlic, minced
1 tablespoon minced fresh basil
½ teaspoon ground black pepper
Endive or watercress

In a large bowl, mix the chick-peas, kidney beans, wax beans, cucumbers, scallions, parsley and mozzarella.

In a small bowl, whisk together the vinegar, oil, garlic, basil and pepper. Pour over the salad and toss. Serve on a bed of endive or watercress.

Serves 4
Per serving: *249 calories, 8.8 g. fat (26% of calories), 10 g. dietary fiber, 5 mg. cholesterol, 817 mg. sodium*

BARLEY SOUP

This hearty soup will satisfy your hunger and help keep you warm on cold days. Serve it with crusty whole-grain bread.

1 large onion, diced
1 sweet red pepper, diced
1 clove garlic, minced
1 teaspoon olive oil
4 cups vegetable stock
1 cup quick-cooking barley
1 cup thinly sliced mushrooms
1 teaspoon Worcestershire sauce
½ teaspoon dried thyme
½ teaspoon ground black pepper
Pinch of celery seeds
Pinch of ground red pepper

In a 3-quart saucepan over medium heat, sauté the onions, diced peppers and garlic in the oil for 5 minutes. Add the stock, barley, mushrooms, Worcestershire sauce, thyme, black pepper, celery seeds and ground red pepper. Bring to a boil.

Cover and simmer for 20 minutes.

Serves 4
Per serving: *212 calories, 3.3 g. fat (13% of calories), 5 g. dietary fiber, <1 mg. cholesterol, 33 mg. sodium*

SPAGHETTI WITH TOFU SAUCE

Tofu acquires a meaty texture if you freeze it before using it in a recipe. When crumbled into a spaghetti sauce, such as this, it looks just like ground beef.

8 ounces firm tofu
1 cup finely chopped mushrooms
1 cup finely chopped onions
1 clove garlic
1 teaspoon olive oil
2 cups canned plum tomatoes, drained and chopped
1 cup tomato sauce
½ teaspoon dried basil
½ teaspoon dried oregano
½ teaspoon dried thyme
½ teaspoon ground black pepper
8 ounces spaghetti

Rinse the tofu and place it in a freezer bag. Freeze until solid, about 4 hours, then thaw. Using several layers of paper towels, press out excess moisture. Crumble the tofu into a bowl and set aside.

In a large no-stick frying pan over medium heat, sauté the mushrooms, onions and garlic in the oil for 5 minutes. Add the tofu and sauté for 5 minutes. Stir in the tomatoes, tomato sauce, basil, oregano, thyme and pepper. Cover and simmer for 20 minutes. Remove the lid and cook for a few minutes until slightly thickened.

Meanwhile, cook the spaghetti in a large pot of boiling water for 10 minutes, or until just tender. Drain. Serve topped with the sauce.

Serves 4

Per serving: *416 calories, 10.4 g. fat (22% of calories), 3.3 g. dietary fiber, 0 mg. cholesterol, 339 mg. sodium*

CHAPTER 34

DIETARY CONTROVERSIES

GOING TO EXTREMES

Dietary debate probably first started when one daring caveman chased down a different type of game and brought it home. He and his family happily cooked it and ate it, although most of the other cavepeople thought he was crazy and refused to try it.

Food controversies have raged ever since.

For every new discovery or concept, there are doctors or dietitians who refuse to consider it. And for every well-founded, well-researched new program, there are haphazard, unfounded, even dangerous ones.

"Many people who promote extreme fad diets or associated programs are quacks," says Maurice E. Shils, M.D., adjunct professor in the Department of Public Health Sciences at the Bowman Gray School of Medicine of Wake Forest University in Winston-Salem, North Carolina. Unfortunately, many people—especially those confronted with a serious disease such as cancer—are all too quick to embrace such programs.

One problem, according to Jack Zeev Yetiv, M.D., Ph.D., is that most doctors aren't well trained in nutrition. Many physicians too quickly dismiss *any* different idea as a fad, says Dr. Yetiv, author of *Popular Nutritional Practices: A Scientific Appraisal.* It's not surprising that many patients turn to supermarket tabloids for their nutritional information.

How can you tell if a concept is a flaky, possibly dangerous fad or an innovative, effective program?

Separating fact from fantasy in the nutrition field can be tricky. "Be wary of programs that advise completely rejecting standard health and nutrition principles or programs that promise a quick, painless solution to a major health problem," says Bettye J. Nowlin, R.D., Los Angeles dietitian and a spokesperson for the American Dietetic Association.

And before you try a new program, consult your doctor—a doctor you're comfortable with and whose opinion you trust. "There has to be a relation with your physician based on mutual respect and understanding," says Dr. Shils.

Some dietary controversies burn themselves out and others smolder on, while some concepts eventually become acceptable to the medical community. Here are a variety of controversial topics and how professionals view them today.

Doubts about Your Morning Jolt

You can't believe it's time to get up. You're groggy and wobbly and your eyelids feel glued shut. And then you smell it, wafting invitingly from the kitchen.

Coffee.

Minutes later, with half your first cup downed, you begin to feel invigorated, alert and alive, and you start to think that maybe life isn't so bad after all.

But as you're flipping through your morning paper you see a headline, "The Hazards of Coffee." What? Coffee linked to heart disease? Cancer? High cholesterol? High blood pressure? Could the stuff that makes you feel so good be this bad for you?

Maybe, say some doctors. Not a chance, say others.

What we *do* know is that the caffeine in coffee packs a potent punch, giving us energy by releasing adrenaline into the bloodstream and raising blood sugar levels. The caffeine we get from one to two cups of coffee increases alertness, reduces fatigue and speeds reaction time.

Caffeine also tends to be addictive, and cutting out your regular dose can lead to withdrawal symptoms such as headache, drowsiness, lethargy, irritability and nausea. One study at Johns Hopkins Hospital in Baltimore found that people who drink the equivalent of just one cup of coffee (or two to three cans of caffeine-containing soda) a day are addicted. All seven people in the study suffered withdrawal symptoms ranging from fatigue to severe headaches and vomiting when taken off caffeine for even *one day.*

And it's also possible that the lift you get from caffeine is "borrowing" energy rather than creating it, according to Dean Ornish, M.D., director of the Preventive Medicine Research Institute in Sausalito, California. "The increased energy level that you feel after you drink coffee will eventually fall even lower than it was when you started," says Dr. Ornish.

But what about serious diseases?

"There's never been any evidence linking moderate coffee drinking with any form of cancer or heart disease," says coffee expert Manfred Kroger, Ph.D., a food science professor at Pennsylvania State University in University Park. He considers "moderate" to be two to three cups of coffee a day. That's about 200 to 250 milligrams of caffeine. But different people can react differently. Two cups of coffee for a person who drinks coffee regularly may have no effect on cholesterol, blood sugar, metabolic rate, respiration, blood pressure and heart rate—but that same dose can raise all these things in a person who doesn't regularly drink coffee.

Although some studies have suggested links between caffeine consumption and pancreatic cancer, heart disease and fibrocystic breast disease, other studies have not substantiated those findings. The American Cancer Society considers that there has been no definite connection established with cancer.

Caffeine's link to certain diseases can be muddied by the fact that people who drink lots of coffee also tend to have *other* habits that can also affect their health, say experts. One study found that coffee drinkers tended to drink more alcohol, smoke more, exercise less and eat more saturated fat and cholesterol than people who don't drink coffee. And the people who drank the most coffee had the worst smoking and exercise habits.

Research has found that caffeine fed to rats caused birth defects and slowed fetal bone development when amounts equal to 18 cups or more of

HOW MUCH CAFFEINE ARE YOU GETTING?

Before you belt down that cup of steaming beverage or can of cola, check out just how much caffeine you're getting. It may be more—or less—than you think.

All coffees are not created equal: A cup of drip coffee has around 110 to 150 milligrams of caffeine, a cup of percolated coffee, 60 to 125 and a cup of instant java, 40 to 105. If your beverage of choice is tea, the amount of caffeine depends on how long you let it steep: Three minutes yields only 20 to 50 milligrams, while five minutes ups the ante to 40 to 100. A cup of cocoa weighs in at a meager 2 to 10 milligrams, while a 12-ounce can of cola has about 45. Don't assume that your orange- or citrus-flavored pop doesn't have caffeine, however: Some varieties do, so check the label.

You can also get caffeine from chocolate: about 20 to 30 milligrams in a slice of cake and 1 to 15 milligrams in an ounce of milk chocolate. Other unexpected sources of caffeine include some headache remedies, diuretics and weight-control pills. Always read labels carefully.

coffee a day were consumed. A study at the National Institutes of Health showed that women consuming more than 100 milligrams of caffeine (about one cup of coffee) a day were only half as likely to become pregnant in a given month as those consuming less caffeine. While caffeine's role in infertility, miscarriages and birth defects is still being debated, the Food and Drug Administration (FDA) recommends that pregnant women avoid caffeine or limit the amount they drink.

The Raw Foods Mystique

You probably never thought of a raw apple or carrot as *alive,* but some people believe that raw foods have living enzymes crucial to good health.

Enzymes are used in digesting food, and according to this theory, the enzymes in raw foods are superior to those produced by your body. By eating raw fruits, vegetables, nuts, grains and legumes, say the authors of *The Raw Foods Diet*—who advocate eating 60 to 75 percent of your foods raw—you supply enzymes that allow each food to digest itself. Cooked foods, on the other hand, with their "dead" enzymes, strain your body and result in breakdown. Or so the theory goes.

Nutritionists, in general, don't support the vital enzyme theory. It's true that raw foods have more *nutrients* than cooked ones, but that doesn't mean that cooked foods are somehow second-rate. And you can minimize the damage. Vegetables that are steamed, baked or stir-fried retain most of their nutrients. When foods are cooked at high temperatures, more nutrients are lost. The best strategy is to cook food as briefly as possible, keep temperatures low and use as little cooking water as possible (reusing it later in soups or gravies).

Even though raw foods may not have any magical enzymes, some studies have indicated that certain raw vegetables may help prevent health problems as diverse as cancer and cavities.

Eating lots of cruciferous vegetables such as cabbage and broccoli has been linked to lower rates of cancer of the digestive system. The protection may come from certain chemical compounds in these vegetables, but researchers at the University of Manitoba in Winnipeg think that cooking may break down these chemicals into other forms that aren't as beneficial.

And what about cavities? Raw vegetables require lots of chewing, which increases the flow of saliva in your mouth. This helps rinse away food particles. And most vegetables leave your teeth cleaner than other foods. "Raw celery and carrots give your body nutrients without leaving debris in your mouth after they're chewed," says Warren Lesmeister, D.D.S., past president of the Academy of General Dentistry.

Eating *everything* raw isn't a good idea, however. Eggs, for instance, should be thoroughly cooked to avoid the possibility of food poisoning from salmonella. This means no runny eggs or Caesar salad dressing—and even soft-boiled eggs and French toast are questionable. And don't keep batter that contains raw eggs in your refrigerator more than a week.

Have a penchant for steak tartare and sushi? "I wouldn't eat them," says Barbara Harland, R.D., Ph.D., associate professor of nutrition in the Department of Nutritional Sciences at Howard University in Washington, D.C. "I think it's too risky." Raw meat can harbor potentially harmful bacteria and parasites, and eating raw fish has caused parasite infections in some cases.

Finally, raw (unpasteurized) milk can be a source of harmful bacteria that can cause serious illness. Health professionals agree there is also no evidence that raw milk is any healthier than other kinds of milk.

FOOD COMBINING: TO MIX OR MATCH?

If you take a glance at the basic rules of food combining, you may think this system should more accurately be called "food separating." The basic idea here is that certain foods interfere with the digestion of other foods and therefore must not be eaten at the same time.

According to this theory, you shouldn't eat starches, protein, fats, sugars and acids at the same time, or drink beverages with your meals. Yes, this sort of puts the kibosh on dining out with friends and having Thanksgiving dinner with Cousin Charlie.

The reasoning is that if you eat, say, meat (protein) and potatoes (starch) together, the digestion of the meat will halt the digestion of the potato, according to Jeffrey Mannix, author of *Food Combining*. The potato will putrefy in your stomach before it passes into your intestines, according to this theory, and here's where the problem arises. "Food that putrefies in the digestive tract gives off toxins [poisons] . . . that contaminate everything in their environment while they paralyze the intestines, preventing them from eliminating waste," Mannix writes.

It's tough to find medical support for this theory. One doctor points out that food putrefying in the stomach would pretty quickly be regurgitated. And nutritionists just don't buy the theory, either.

"The body actually digests foods very efficiently, regardless of what order they're consumed in," says Nowlin. "Most health professionals look on food combining as a myth with no validity."

What *is* true, Nowlin points out, is that some vitamins in foods can change the rate of absorption of other vitamins or minerals—although this doesn't interfere with the digestion process. Foods high in vitamin C increase absorption of iron, for example, and vitamin D can increase absorption of calcium. A huge amount of fiber in the diet can interfere with absorption of some trace minerals.

For the most part, however, this all balances out. "Your best bet is a balanced, varied diet," says Nowlin.

THE CASE OF THE NAUGHTY NIGHTSHADES

What are nightshades? They're plants that belong to the Solanaceae family, and according to Norman F. Childers, Ph.D., they are the primary culprit in many cases of arthritis.

Nightshades include tomatoes, potatoes, eggplant, all peppers except black pepper, and tobacco. Toxins in these, according to Dr. Childers, a retired professor of horticulture, cause aching joints. By eliminating nightshades, he says, chances are better than seven out of ten that you'll improve.

The 1986 edition of Dr. Childer's book *The Nightshades and Health,* which was first published in 1977, cites page after page of case histories of people who reported significant reductions in arthritis pain from eliminating nightshades.

Subsequent studies have shown that certain foods *can* affect arthritis. A study at Albany Medical College in New York found that doses of fish oil helped arthritis sufferers, and other research suggests that some arthritis flare-ups are triggered by allergic reactions to certain foods. A study in Norway suggested that food allergy or intolerance could be at the root of rheumatoid arthritis.

Is there any connection between *nightshades* and arthritis? "There's no concrete substantiation," says Barbara Harland, R.D., Ph.D., of Howard University in Washington, D.C., although at least one physician points out that there's certainly no harm in *trying* a no-nightshade diet.

THE PROS AND CONS OF IRRADIATED FOODS

Listen to a proponent of irradiated foods, and you'll think this is the greatest discovery since the wheel. An opponent, however, may convince you that this process is an accident waiting to happen.

If you use dried spices, you may already be using irradiated products. The FDA has also approved the irradiation of grain, flour, fresh fruits, vegetables, pork and poultry.

What exactly is food irradiation? It's the bombardment of food by x-rays and gamma rays, which can kill mold, bacteria and insects, inhibit germination or sprouting and extend the shelf life of fruits and vegetables. It could also reduce the need for chemical insecticides and preservatives and might reduce risks of salmonella contamination in poultry.

So what's the truth about this process? Irradiation under strictly controlled conditions does not, as many people fear, make food radioactive or leave a radioactive residue. The consensus from a 1980 meeting of the Food and Agriculture Organization, International Atomic Energy Agency and World Health Organization was that no toxicologic studies showed adverse effects of irradiation and that irradiated foods did not harm lab animals, cattle or people.

The disadvantages of irradiation? "Irradiation reduces levels of certain vitamins in certain foods," says Michael Jacobson, Ph.D., executive director of the Center for Science in the Public Interest. That's not a problem with the small amount of food now irradiated, he says, but if, as predicted, 40 percent of the food supply is eventually irradiated, it could *become* a problem.

Dr. Jacobson believes that pro- and anti-irradiation forces exaggerate both the potential benefits and problems from irradiation. "The consumer is getting caught in the cross-fire between the two camps," he says. His opinion? "We shouldn't have to build multimillion-dollar facilities with radioactive cobalt at their cores to kill bacteria or flies," he says.

Many professionals agree that not enough research has been done to declare irradiated foods and the irradiation process perfectly safe. "If the FDA says an irradiated food is safe, I would eat it. The foods that have been tested so far are okay," says Dr. Shils. "But I'm impressed with the arguments that we just don't know enough about irradiated foods yet. We don't have sufficient information on each individual food."

You can make your own decision about purchasing irradiated foods—in most cases they will be marked with a special symbol that resembles a plant within a circle.

THE MACROBIOTIC LIFESTYLE

When you think of macrobiotics, you may think of a diet based on Asian philosophy and consisting of brown rice and tea—but it's more complicated than that.

Macrobiotics has been promoted as a cure-all for just about every disease. According to Michio Kushi, author of many books on the topic, a macrobiotic diet can treat infertility, diabetes, allergies, stress, arthritis and obesity. Macrobiotic advocate George S. Ohsawa stated in his book *Zen Macrobiotics:* "I have seen thousands of incurable diseases such as asthma, diabetes, epilepsy, leprosy and paralyses of all kinds cured by . . . macrobiotics in ten days or a few weeks." Anthony Sattilaro, M.D., asserted in his 1978 book *Recalled to Life* that a macrobiotic diet helped cure him of advanced prostate cancer.

What exactly is a macrobiotic diet? The Kushi Institute in Becket, Massachusetts, recommends eating 50 to 60 percent whole-grain cereals, 25 to 30 percent organically grown vegetables, 5 to 10 percent soup made from vegetables, seaweed, grains or beans and 5 to 10 percent cooked beans and sea vegetables. Fish, fruit, nuts and seeds are allowed occasionally, but meat, eggs, dairy products, chocolate, coffee and some other foods are not allowed. The diet varies according to age, sex, activity, special requirements or conditions, cultural background and the season.

But macrobiotics is more than what you eat. The aim, according to proponents, is to achieve balance between two basic forces of the universe, yin (expansion) and yang (contraction) as well as a balance among five basic elements: water, earth, wood, fire and metal.

Most nutritionists take a decidedly dim view of macrobiotic diets—particularly when promoted as a cure for a disease such as cancer. "No diet or combination of foods has the ability to cure cancer," says Nowlin. "What can be harmful to people is when they decide to substitute a macrobiotic diet for effective treatment." She adds that a macrobiotic diet can also cause malnutrition or weight loss, which can interfere with treatment or weaken a patient. Another problem is that macrobiotic diets tend to be high in sodium.

It can also be difficult to obtain adequate nutrients on a macrobiotic diet, which is stricter than most vegetarian diets. One study concluded that some children following a macrobiotic diet were deficient in some nutrients and experienced slowed growth. Other work turned up severe malnourishment in macrobiotic children.

Dr. Shils advises caution if you decide to try a macrobiotic diet: "Definitely consult with a doctor or nutritionist to review your diet."

How Much Aluminum Is Okay?

No one debates that aluminum buildups are found in the brains of Alzheimer's patients—what is argued is whether the aluminum is a *cause* or an *effect* of the disease. Many researchers, however, now believe there is enough evidence to point to aluminum as a significant factor in the development of Alzheimer's.

Studies in areas with high levels of aluminum in the water supply, for instance, have shown high levels of Alzheimer's or diseases similar to Alzheimer's. Theodore Kruck, Ph.D., member of a leading team of aluminum-investigating scientists at the University of Toronto in Ontario, says nine drinking water surveys in various countries have shown higher rates of Alzheimer's in people who drank water with high aluminum levels.

Where else do you get aluminum? From foods that naturally take up aluminum from the soil, from acidic foods cooked in aluminum cookware and from many products such as cosmetics, antiperspirants, antacids, certain pickles and commercially baked foods like doughnuts, muffins, cookies and pound cakes. In healthy people, most of the aluminum is excreted: Most of us consume 10 to 15 milligrams a day but have only 30 to 45 milligrams in our bodies.

Although there is no evidence proving definitely that the aluminum we ingest causes Alzheimer's—and some doctors scoff at the very idea—most agree it doesn't hurt to play it safe. Dr. Kruck and other researchers at the University of Toronto believe people should try to limit their intake of aluminum to less than 10 milligrams a day, as a first step, while the final goal should be 3 milligrams or less.

How do you cut your intake? Several participants in a Royal Society of Medicine discussion panel held in London said they avoid using aluminum cookware, drink bottled water and avoid aluminum-containing aerosols.

You can reduce the amount of aluminum in your diet by never cooking acidic foods such as tomatoes, cabbage, sauerkraut, cranberry sauce, applesauce or rhubarb in aluminum pots and pans. Dr. Kruck also suggests avoiding using aluminum foil under meats when grilling.

Other products with aluminum include some baking powders (check the label), soft drinks (if made from water with high aluminum levels), certain beauty and grooming products and antiperspirants. You can select non-aluminum forms of most of these products, however.

DOES MILK PRODUCE MUCUS?

"Don't drink that milk—it'll make your nose more stopped-up," a father tells his child, clogged up with a bad cold.

Well, Father knows best. Or does he?

The milk-produces-mucus theory has been around for a long time, and some people swear by it. Most experts, however, discount it completely.

"It's a myth," says Bettye J. Nowlin, R.D., of the American Dietetic Association. "There's no connection."

In one study exploring this fabled cause and effect, 60 volunteers—who drank amounts ranging from none to 11 glasses of milk a day—were infected with a cold virus and records kept of their nasal secretions. Those who *believed* that milk produced mucus reported that they coughed and were more congested when they drank milk, but they actually produced no more mucus than others. In fact, no association between milk and mucus production was found.

Another study, however, suggests that fat in milk *can* interfere with airflow, at least in people with asthma. Airflow in healthy people wasn't affected by either whole milk or skim milk. In the asthmatic group, however, airflow decreased after drinking whole milk but *not* after water or skim milk.

The conclusion? If you aren't asthmatic, milk should present no problem. Because the fat in whole milk may make your mouth feel gummy when you have a cold, however (and also because low-fat milk is wiser from a nutritional standpoint), give the whole milk a miss. Dietitians recommend not cutting out milk but switching to low-fat or skim milk, Nowlin says.

THE YEAST BEAST

It's a common little microorganism, *Candida albicans,* that quite commonly resides happily in our bodies along with bacteria and other microorganisms. But when things get out of whack, many of the other "bugs" can get killed off and allow the yeast population to explode.

The out-of-control yeast population, according to one theory, releases toxins that circulate in your body and weaken your immune system—and that can make you vulnerable to a variety of health problems, including fatigue, depression, joint pain, digestive problems, hypoglycemia and hyperactivity.

That's the theory that William G. Crook, M.D., has promoted in his many books, including *The Yeast Connection* and *Solving the Puzzle of Your Hard-to-Raise Child.*

If a physical exam shows no other cause for your symptoms, your problems may be yeast-caused, suggests Dr. Crook. To keep the monster at bay, he prescribes a sugar-free, yeast-free diet that excludes foods that contain yeast or molds, including cheeses, fermented liquors, coffee, tea, melons and many condiments and sauces.

Many health professionals will tell you, however, that most of us seldom have to worry about yeast. Yeast infections are liable to occur only when your immune system is weakened or when you've been taking antibiotics that "knock out" the good germs holding *Candida albicans* in check.

Is the yeast connection overblown? Most doctors say yes, a few doctors say no. Dr. Shils is one of many physicians who don't buy the yeast theory. "I've talked to my colleagues about this," he says. "I don't know of anyone who takes it seriously. The evidence is against this being a hazard for the average, relatively healthy person. Yeast infections can be serious, though, for those people whose immune system is seriously compromised."

Many dietitians tend to think the problem is less prevalent than the popularity of Dr. Crook's books would imply. "The physicians or books that advise you to stay away from all yeasts are doing you a disservice," says Dr. Harland. "Yeasts are a valuable part of our food supply."

CALMING HYPERACTIVE KIDS

The late Ben Feingold, M.D., a California allergist and pediatrician, probably didn't realize what a storm he was provoking in his 1974 book *Why Your Child Is Hyperactive* when he promoted a diet free of artificial colors and flavorings to help calm overly wound-up kids.

Some doctors and researchers say the diet is completely unsubstantiated, others support it, and some prescribe it for their patients. Thousands of parents swear by it.

Who's right?

Much of the support for the Feingold diet has come from doctors who have seen children in their practice respond favorably. But early studies didn't meet strict scientific standards—because of the nature of the diet, it's difficult to carry out a study in which children and parents don't know what foods they're getting. And most double-blind, placebo-controlled studies (where no one knows which type of food they're getting) did not show significant results from the diet. But even in most of the double-blind studies, 10 to 15 percent of the hyperactive children studied *did* benefit from the diet, notes Dr. Yetiv.

And some studies have shown significant results from the diet. One ten-week study in Calgary, Alberta, found that more than half of 24 hyperactive preschool boys showed improvement on a diet free of artificial colors as well as chocolate, preservatives and caffeine.

Jane Hersey, executive director of the Feingold Association in Alexandria, Virginia, and doctors who support the program believe it's a mistake to focus exclusively on studies, which may have little in common with the practical application of Feingold's program. Hersey says she doesn't see why the diet spawns such controversy.

"Certain chemicals in food appear to have the capacity to cause certain reactions in some people," she says. "And what can it hurt to try the diet?"

The Feingold diet is basically an elimination diet: You avoid foods with synthetic dyes and flavorings and certain antioxidants used as preservatives. When you first start the program, you also remove foods naturally high in

CAN SUGAR TURN LITTLE ANGELS INTO LITTLE MONSTERS?

"Johnny goes crazy after he's had sugar," the hapless mom says, watching her six-year-old careen around the room.

Despite such observations, many researchers view claims that link sugar intake and behavior problems as having no basis in fact, and a 1987 Food and Drug Administration task force concluded that sugar was not addictive and couldn't be linked to criminal behavior (what a relief for Johnny's mom!).

In a study at Yale University School of Medicine, however, the adrenaline levels of 14 children and 9 adults were monitored after they were fed sugar. The pediatricians directing the study found that the adrenaline levels of the children increased dramatically, while those of the adults did not move. All but one of the children also complained they felt "shaky and weak" after ingesting the sugar.

This suggests, says one of the researchers, that children are more sensitive to sugar than adults, and that the adrenaline surge from sugar *could* affect behavior in some children.

salicylate, an aspirin-like substance that is found in many fruits, coffee, tea and a few vegetables. Later, the salicylate-containing foods are reintroduced one at a time.

Hersey admits she wasn't eager at first to try the diet on her five-year-old daughter. "I was a convenience-food freak," she says. "It seemed like too much trouble." After a few days on the diet, however, her daughter's behavior improved drastically and her husband's migraine headaches disappeared.

Now she doesn't think of it as much trouble. "When you realize that a package of commercial gelatin dessert has synthesized dyes made from petroleum, several kinds of acid, no juice and 82 percent sugar, it's not a question of, 'Gee, why do I have to give this up?' but 'Why would I *want* to eat it?' " she says.

Dr. Yetiv concludes that hyperactivity may have many causes, and some hyperactive children do seem to be sensitive to the substances eliminated by the Feingold diet.

Do We Need to Eat at All?

For most of us, the idea of fasting doesn't have much appeal: We get grumpy, headachy and listless after one skipped breakfast or worked-through lunch.

Many people, however, devoutly believe that going without food for an extended period can cleanse your system, clear your mind and even cure some diseases. Morton Walker, D.P.M., author of *The Healing Powers of Elderberry Internal Cleansing,* advocates a seven-day "detoxification" program that involves drinking only a concentrate of elderberry and honey. Dr. Walker claims that this fast cleans mucus from your system, helps you stay younger, cures constipation, forces wastes out of your body, removes unnecessary fat and helps you lose weight.

Allan Cott, M.D., author of *Fasting: The Ultimate Diet,* promotes fasting to lose weight, feel better, look younger, lower blood pressure and cholesterol and relieve tension. He recommends an occasional fast of a day or two but claims that fasts of up to a month will benefit specific health problems.

Most medical experts, however, doubt that, with the exception of weight loss, fasting can accomplish what its advocates say. But it could have harmful effects. Long-term interruption of needed nutrients is one obvious problem, but it's possible that even a relatively short fast could have negative effects. A study by the National Institutes of Health reported increased risks of gallstone disease among women who fasted longer than 14 hours between the last meal at night and the first one the following day.

One condition that fasting *does* seem to benefit is arthritis, although the effect is only short term. A study of 27 patients in Norway found fasting, followed by a vegetarian diet, to be an effective treatment for rheumatoid arthritis. A Swedish study also involving a seven- to ten-day fast found that improvement occurred by the fourth or fifth day of fasting. The effect ended as soon as the fast was over, however, and according to Lars Skoldstam, M.D., author of the study, there is no reason for doctors to recommend fasting to persons with rheumatoid arthritis.

The bottom line? If you just need a change of pace or have no appetite for some reason, a "modified fast"—cutting your food intake in half—is okay for three to five days, according to George L. Blackburn, M.D., Ph.D., associate professor of surgery at Harvard Medical School and chief of the Nutrition/Metabolism Laboratory with the Cancer Research Institute at New England Deaconess Hospital in Boston. Be sure, however, to drink plenty of fluids.

FOOD ALLERGY: AN OVERRATED PROBLEM?

Food allergies *exist*—what's controversial about them is how many people actually do have allergies and how effective some testing systems are.

The Asthma and Allergy Foundation estimates that less than 1 percent of the population is allergic to food, while the U.S. Department of Agriculture says 10 to 15 percent—but you can find figures in the media as high as 60 percent.

What's going on here?

The concept that food allergies can cause certain problems such as fatigue and depression was seized on by the media, according to Dr. Yetiv, despite little scientific documentation. Only a small percentage of suspected food allergies can actually be confirmed, he says.

A number of studies have shown that some people only *think* they're allergic. In one study of 23 patients, persons whose allergies could not be scientifically documented reported symptoms from "nonallergic" foods as often as they did from the foods they were supposedly allergic to. In another case, a woman who thought she was allergic to milk was fed milk and a nonmilk substance via a tube to her stomach. When she was told she was receiving milk (although she wasn't), she experienced abdominal contractions, a rapid heart rate and a drop in blood pressure. When she was told she was receiving the nonmilk placebo (actually milk), she showed no symptoms.

A problem that impedes accurate diagnosis of allergies is possibly faulty diagnostic techniques. Cytotoxic testing, in which white blood cells that have been incubated with the suspected allergen are studied for signs of disintegration, is considered useless by the FDA and many professionals. Even when the suspected allergen is introduced in a water solution through a skin puncture, only a *negative* test (showing no reaction) is considered reliable, according to Raymond Slavin, M.D., of St. Louis University School of Medicine. A positive test—showing redness and swelling—doesn't always prove that you're allergic.

Food allergy is also not the same as food *intolerance,* such as when a person cannot digest milk. A true food allergy results from a reaction within your immune system, just as ragweed or cat dander triggers reactions in persons allergic to them.

In people who *are* allergic to food, symptoms range from annoying to life threatening. What are people most commonly allergic to? Eggs, wheat, peanuts, fish, milk and soybeans account for more than 90 percent of food allergies in children. Common problem foods for adults are shellfish, fish, peanuts and other nuts, and eggs. Chocolate and strawberries, contrary to popular belief, are not common allergens. If you suspect an allergy, check with your physician, or try eliminating the suspect food on your own.

PART 6

Improving Your Eating Style

CHAPTER 35

QUIZ TIME

DOES YOUR DIET MEASURE UP?

You can't put together a healthy nutrition plan without taking a close look at your diet and the foods you actually put into your mouth every day. Just how much fiber are you really getting? Have you trimmed the fat from your diet as much as you think you have? Is your sodium intake under control?

The self-tests in this chapter put your diet under the microscope and examine every detail so you can identify your nutritional strengths as well as the weak spots that need improvement.

"Dietary self-tests can be entertaining but at the same time incredibly revealing," says Rebecca S. Reeves, R.D., chief dietitian with the Nutrition Research Clinic at Baylor College of Medicine in Houston. "These tests are like a mirror. They help reflect back to you that you are what you eat—in terms of your health, at least. If a quiz reveals that you're eating lots of salty, fatty food, for example, chances are your waistline and blood pressure are going to reflect this."

Self-tests, of course, can't track your diet nearly as precisely as a professionally supervised analysis. And they don't take the place of blood tests, physical exams and a detailed health and genetic history. So don't hesitate to consult your doctor or a professional dietitian/nutritionist, especially if you have a health problem, are on a restricted diet or uncover some dietary trouble spots when you take these tests.

So now, if you're ready to fine-tune your diet, grab a notebook, sharpen your pencil and go to it. Your answers could yield important clues that will point you to the right nutritional track for a healthier life.

DIAGNOSE YOUR DIET

The following 32 questions adapted from a test developed by nutritionists at the Center for Science in the Public Interest in Washington, D.C., will give you an overall idea of how well you're eating. The (+) or (–) numbers after each set of answers instantly pat you on the back for good habits or alert you to problems you may not realize you have.

The scoring section at the end rates your diet on a scale from super to critical and suggests changes to bring your diet up to an optimum level.

Instructions. After each answer is a number for you to circle. That is your score for the question.

In most cases, you'll circle only one number for each question. If the instructions tell you to "average scores, if necessary," add the two scores and then divide by 2. (If the average gives you a fraction, round it off to the nearest whole number.)

Pay attention to serving sizes. For example, a serving of vegetables is ½ cup. If you usually eat 1 cup of vegetables at a time, count it as two servings.

1. How many times per week do you eat unprocessed red meat (steak, roast beef, lamb or pork chops, burgers, etc.)?
   - **a.** 1 or less +3
   - **b.** 2–3 +2
   - **c.** 4–5 –1
   - **d.** 6 or more –3
2. Do you trim the visible fat from red meat?
   - **a.** yes +3
   - **b.** no –3
   - **c.** don't eat red meat +3
3. What kind of ground meat do you usually eat?
   - **a.** regular ground beef –3
   - **b.** lean ground beef –2
   - **c.** extra-lean ground beef –1
   - **d.** ground round 0
   - **e.** ground turkey +1
   - **f.** don't eat ground meat +3
4. How many times per week do you eat deep-fried foods (fish, chicken, vegetables, etc.)?
   - **a.** none +3
   - **b.** 1–2 0
   - **c.** 3–4 –1
   - **d.** 5 or more –3

5. How many servings (½ cup) of vegetables and nonfried potatoes do you eat per day?

a. none	–3
b. 1	0
c. 2	+1
d. 3	+2
e. 4 or more	+3

6. How many servings of cruciferous vegetables (kale, broccoli, cauliflower, cabbage, brussels sprouts, greens, bok choy, kohlrabi, turnips and rutabagas) do you usually eat per week?

a. none	–3
b. 1–3	+1
c. 4–6	+2
d. 7 or more	+3

7. How many servings of vitamin A–rich fruits or vegetables (such as sweet potatoes, cantaloupe, spinach, winter squash, greens, apricots, and broccoli) do you usually eat per week?

a. none	–3
b. 1–3	+1
c. 4–6	+2
d. 7 or more	+3

8. How many times per week do you eat at a fast-food restaurant? (Don't include meals of only baked potato, broiled chicken or salad.)

a. never	+3
b. less than 1	+1
c. 1	0
d. 2	–1
e. 3	–2
f. 4 or more	–4

9. How many servings of grains rich in complex carbohydrates do you eat per day? (1 serving = 1 slice of bread, 1 large pancake or ½ cup cooked cereal, rice, pasta, etc. Heavily sweetened cold cereals don't count!)

a. none	–3
b. 1–2	0
c. 3–4	+1
d. 5–6	+2
e. 7 or more	+3

10. How many times per week do you eat seafood? (Do not include deep-fried items, tuna packed in oil, shrimp, squid, or tuna salad with mayo.)

a. never	–2
b. 1–2	+1
c. 3–4	+2
d. 5 or more	+3

11. How many servings of fresh fruit do you consume per day?
    - **a.** none –3
    - **b.** 1 0
    - **c.** 2 +1
    - **d.** 3 +2
    - **e.** 4 or more +3
12. Do you remove the skin before eating poultry?
    - **a.** yes +3
    - **b.** no –3
    - **c.** don't eat poultry +3
13. What do you usually put on your bread or toast? (Average scores, if necessary.)
    - **a.** butter or cream cheese –3
    - **b.** margarine –2
    - **c.** diet margarine –1
    - **d.** jam 0
    - **e.** fruit butter +3
    - **f.** nothing +3
14. Which of these beverages do you drink on a typical day? (Average scores, if necessary.)
    - **a.** water or club soda +3
    - **b.** fruit juice +1
    - **c.** diet soda or coffee or tea –1
    - **d.** soda or fruit drink or ade –3
15. Which flavorings do you most frequently add to your foods? (Average scores, if necessary.)
    - **a.** garlic or lemon juice +3
    - **b.** herbs or spices +3
    - **c.** soy sauce –2
    - **d.** margarine –2
    - **e.** salt –3
    - **f.** butter –3
    - **g.** nothing +3
16. What do you eat most frequently as a snack? (Average scores, if necessary.)
    - **a.** fruits or vegetables +3
    - **b.** sweetened yogurt +2
    - **c.** nuts –1
    - **d.** chips –2
    - **e.** cookies –2
    - **f.** granola bar –2
    - **g.** candy bar –3
    - **h.** pastry –3
    - **i.** nothing 0

17. What is your typical breakfast? (Subtract an extra 3 points if you also eat bacon or sausage.)

a. croissant, Danish or doughnut	–3
b. eggs	–3
c. pancakes or waffles	–2
d. nothing	0
e. cereal or bread	+3
f. yogurt or cottage cheese	+3

18. What do you usually eat for dessert?

a. pie, pastry or cake	–3
b. ice cream	–3
c. yogurt, ice milk or sorbet	+1
d. fruit	+3
e. nothing	+3

19. What dressings or toppings do you usually add to your salads? (Add scores together if you use more than one.)

a. nothing, lemon or vinegar	+3
b. reduced-calorie dressing	+1
c. regular dressing	–1
d. croutons or bacon bits	–1
e. coleslaw, pasta salad or potato salad	–1

20. What sandwich fillings do you eat most frequently? (Average scores, if necessary.)

a. luncheon meat	–3
b. cheese or roast beef	–1
c. peanut butter	0
d. tuna, salmon, chicken or turkey	+3

21. What do you usually spread on your sandwiches? (Average scores, if necessary.)

a. mayonnaise	–2
b. light mayonnaise	–1
c. mustard	0
d. catsup	0
e. nothing	+3

22. How many times per week do you eat canned or dried soups? (Don't count low sodium, low fat.)

a. none	+3
b. 1–2	0
c. 3–4	–2
d. 5 or more	–3

23. How many servings of a rich calcium source (⅔ cup milk or yogurt, 1 ounce cheese, 1½ ounces sardines, 3½ ounces salmon, 5 ounces tofu, 1 cup greens or broccoli or 200 milligrams of calcium supplement) do you eat per day?

a. none	–3
b. 1	+1
c. 2	+2
d. 3 or more	+3

24. What kind of pizza do you order? (Subtract 1 extra point if you order extra cheese.)

a. no cheese w/nonmeat toppings	+3
b. cheese w/nonmeat toppings	+1
c. cheese	0
d. cheese w/meat toppings	–3
e. don't eat pizza	+2

25. What kind of cookies do you usually eat?

a. graham crackers	+1
b. gingersnaps	+1
c. oatmeal	–1
d. chocolate coated, chocolate chip or peanut butter	–3
e. sandwich cookies (like Oreos)	–3
f. don't eat cookies	+3

26. What kind of frozen dessert do you usually eat? (Subtract 1 extra point for each topping—whipped cream, hot fudge, nuts, etc.)

a. gourmet ice cream	–3
b. regular ice cream	–1
c. sorbet, sherbet or ices	+1
d. frozen yogurt or ice milk	+1
e. don't eat frozen desserts	+3

27. What kind of cake or pastry do you usually eat?

a. cheesecake, pie or any microwave cake	–3
b. cake with frosting or filling	–2
c. cake without frosting	–1
d. angel food cake	+1
e. unfrosted muffin, banana bread or carrot cake	0
f. don't eat cakes or pastries	+3

28. How many times per week does your dinner contain grains, vegetables or beans and little or no animal protein (meat, poultry, fish, eggs, milk or cheese)?

a. none	–1
b. 1	+1
c. 2	+2
d. 3	+3

29. Which snacks do you typically eat?
    - **a.** potato chips or packaged popcorn −3
    - **b.** tortilla chips −1
    - **c.** light potato chips −2
    - **d.** salted pretzels −1
    - **e.** unsalted pretzels +1
    - **f.** homemade air-popped popcorn +3
    - **g.** don't eat snacks +3
30. What kind of cereal do you usually eat?
    - **a.** hot, whole-grain (like oatmeal or Wheatena) +3
    - **b.** cold, whole-grain (like Shredded Wheat) +3
    - **c.** cold, low-fiber (like corn flakes) 0
    - **d.** sugary, cold, low-fiber (like Frosted Flakes) −1
    - **e.** granola −2
31. With what do you make tuna salad, pasta salad, chicken salad, etc.?
    - **a.** mayonnaise −2
    - **b.** light mayonnaise 0
    - **c.** low-fat yogurt +2
    - **d.** nonfat yogurt +3
32. What do you typically put on your pasta? (Add 1 point if you also add sautéed vegetables. Average scores, if necessary.)
    - **a.** tomato-based sauce +3
    - **b.** tomato sauce with a little Parmesan +3
    - **c.** white clam sauce +1
    - **d.** meat sauce −1
    - **e.** tomato sauce w/meatballs −2
    - **f.** Alfredo or other creamy sauce −3

Scoring: Total (+):____
Total (−):____
GRAND TOTAL:____

+59 to +98 = Super. You're a nutrition superstar. Give yourself a big (nonbutter) pat on the back.

+24 to +58 = Good. It wouldn't take much to put you in the superstar category and boost your health even more.

−10 to +23 = Fair. There are more than a few places where you need to trim the fat from your diet.

−11 and below = Critical. Your diet needs major surgery and a transfusion of healthy nutrition tips. Clean out the refrigerator and pantry and start over based on the information in this book.

FOCUS ON FAT

Knowing the importance of a low-fat diet is one thing. Eating a low-fat diet is quite another.

Does your own diet meet the current recommendations for limiting fat to a third of your calories? To help you get the straight skinny on your diet, take this quiz developed at the Northwest Lipid Research Clinic at the University of Washington in Seattle.

Check the answer that best describes how you have been eating recently.

1. How many ounces of meat, fish or poultry do you usually eat?*

 __**1.** I do not eat meat, fish or poultry.
 __**2.** I eat 3 ounces or less per day.
 __**3.** I eat 4–6 ounces per day.
 __**4.** I eat 7 or more ounces per day.

*3 ounces of meat, fish or chicken is any *one* of the following: 1 regular hamburger, 1 chicken breast, 1 chicken leg (thigh and drumstick), 1 pork chop or 3 slices of pre-sliced lunch meat.

2. How much cheese do you eat per week?

 __**1.** I avoid cheese altogether.
 __**2.** I use only low-fat cheese (ricotta, low-fat cottage cheese).
 __**3.** I eat whole-milk cheese (such as Cheddar, Swiss, Monterey Jack) once or twice per week.
 __**4.** I eat 3 or more servings of whole-milk cheese per week.

3. What type of milk do you use?

 __**1.** I use only skim or 1 percent milk or don't use milk.
 __**2.** I usually use skim milk or 1 percent milk, but use others occasionally.
 __**3.** I usually use 2 percent or whole milk.

4. How many egg yolks do you use per week?

 __**1.** I avoid all egg yolk and/or use only the egg substitutes.
 __**2.** I eat 1–2 eggs per week.
 __**3.** I eat 3 or more eggs per week.

5. How often do you usually eat lunch meat, hot dogs, corned beef, spareribs, sausage, bacon, braunschweiger or liver?

 __**1.** I do not eat any of these meats.
 __**2.** I eat them about once per week.
 __**3.** I eat about 2–4 servings per week.
 __**4.** I eat more than 4 servings per week.

6. How many commercial baked goods and how much ice cream do you usually eat? Examples: cake, cookies, sweet rolls, doughnuts, etc.

 __**1.** I avoid baked goods and ice cream.
 __**2.** I eat baked goods or ice cream once a week.
 __**3.** I eat 2–4 servings of baked goods or ice cream per week.
 __**4.** I eat more than 4 servings of baked goods or ice cream per week.

7. What is the main type of fat you cook with?
   __**1.** I don't use fat in cooking.
   __**2.** I use safflower oil, sunflower oil, corn oil or soybean oil.
   __**3.** I use olive oil, peanut oil or margarine.
   __**4.** I use shortening, butter or bacon drippings.
8. How often do you eat snack foods such as chips, fries or party crackers (Triscuits, Wheat Thins, Ritz, etc.)?
   __**1.** I avoid these snack foods.
   __**2.** I eat 1 serving of these snacks per week.
   __**3.** I eat 2–4 servings of these snacks per week.
   __**4.** I eat more than 4 servings of these snack foods per week.
9. What type of butter/margarine do you usually use on bread, vegetables, etc.?
   __**1.** I don't use butter or margarine.
   __**2.** I use soft (tub) or diet margarine.
   __**3.** I use stick margarine.
   __**4.** I use butter.

Scoring: Add up the numbers from each of your answers. If you score 15 or less, congratulate yourself. You're eating a low-fat diet. A score of 16 to 18 qualifies as a moderate-fat diet, roughly equivalent to the Step One diet the American Heart Association recommends. Anything higher than 18 can be considered high fat.

If your number's too high, start incorporating the 1 and 2 answers into your diet as much as you can. Note that you can still get away with one or two 4s, but only if you balance them out with enough 1s.

ARE YOU MEETING YOUR FIBER QUOTA?

Next to low fat, fiber is one of the most talked about features of a healthy diet. Despite the fact that fiber is relatively easy to obtain (it's naturally abundant in a variety of foods from barley and blueberries to prunes and pinto beans), if you are like most Americans, you may still be getting less than half the protective amount (about 30 grams) of this health-giving food component.

To find out how close you come to meeting your daily fiber quota, keep track of everything you eat for three days. Then, take the quiz below and add up your points. This quiz was developed with assistance from nutrition lecturer Liz Applegate, Ph.D., and nutrition professor Judith Stern, Sc.D., R.D., both at the University of California, Davis.

1. What type of bread (including rolls and muffins) did you usually eat?

   a. whole-wheat or whole-grain +4
   b. white or partial whole-wheat +2

2. How many servings of oat products did you average daily? (1 serving = 1 cup cooked oatmeal or oat bran.)

a. 2 or more	+4
b. 1	+3
c. ½	+2
d. none	0

3. How many times during the last three days did you eat beans (legumes), such as kidney beans, pintos, garbanzos, soybeans, lentils, and split peas?

a. 3 or more	+4
b. 2	+3
c. 1	+2
d. none	0

4. How many times during the three-day period did you eat high-fiber breakfast cereals?

a. 3 or more	+4
b. 2	+3
c. 1	+2
d. none	0

5. How many times during the three-day period did you eat cooked whole-grain side dishes, such as brown rice or barley?

a. 3 or more	+4
b. 2	+3
c. 1	+2
d. none	0

6. Approximately how many servings of canned or fresh fruits and vegetables did you eat daily? (Use an average from the previous three days. 1 serving = ½ cup cooked or 1 cup or 1 piece raw.)

a. 7 or more	+5
b. 5–6	+4
c. 3–4	+2
d. 1–2	+1
e. none	–2

Scoring: If your overall score is over 20, your fiber intake is probably adequate. If you scored lower, see chapter 7 for help.

CHECK YOUR CALCIUM INTAKE

If you are not a fan of dairy products, you may be coming up far short of your calcium needs. But even if you are a milk lover, how much calcium your body actually absorbs depends upon your genetic makeup. And how much you retain depends upon your intake of salt and protein. This duo increases the elimination of calcium, causing your body to steal calcium it needs from your bones.

The following quiz was developed with the assistance of Robert P.

Heaney, M.D., professor of medicine at Creighton University School of Medicine in Omaha, Nebraska. It can tell you how close your diet comes to providing the appropriate amount of bone food. Just check the answer that applies to you.

1. I eat a serving of yogurt (8 ounces), milk (1 cup) or cheese (1 ounce) at least once a day.
   __True +3
   __False −1
2. Dairy products give me gas and bloating, so I avoid them.
   __True −1
   __False +1
3. I make sure I eat one or more of the following nondairy sources of calcium at least three times a week: leafy green vegetables (kale, bok choy or broccoli), shellfish (oysters or clams) or canned fish with bones (salmon or sardines).
   __True +1
   __False 0
4. I make an effort to slip dairy foods into my diet whenever I can (grating cheese over salads, for example).
   __True +1
   __False 0
5. I eat calcium-enriched forms of products (such as breakfast cereal or fruit juice) whenever possible.
   __True +1
   __False −1
6. When given a choice, I drink carbonated soft drinks over low-fat dairy drinks or water.
   __True −1
   __False 0
7. I tend to get my protein from meats.
   __True −1
   __False +1
8. I usually salt foods automatically without tasting them.
   __True −1
   __False +1

Scoring: If you scored between 7 and 9, you are laying the dietary foundation for a rock-solid skeleton. (Remember, though, that even if you scored a perfect 9, you may still have a bone deficit if you are inactive, underweight or postmenopausal, have a family history of osteoporosis or take aluminum-based antacids or other calcium-robbing drugs.)

If you scored between 4 and 6, try to include more low-fat dairy products and go easy on the calcium bandits.

If you scored below 4, your skeleton may be becoming perilously porous. Learn to love low-fat yogurt and make friends with skim milk. Ask your doctor about taking a calcium supplement.

THE EASIEST WAY TO TEST YOUR WATER LEVEL

You may be getting enough vitamins, minerals and fiber, but still be starving your body of one important nutrient: water.

Unfortunately, you can't always rely on thirst to indicate a water deficit, especially as you get older, according to studies conducted by Barbara Rolls, Ph.D., of Johns Hopkins University School of Medicine in Baltimore.

A rough indicator to determine your water level? Check the color of your urine, says Dr. Rolls. If it's dark amber or has a strong odor, it means the kidneys have concentrated wastes in urine and you're not drinking enough water. Passing a full bladder of colorless or pale yellow urine at least four times daily means you're getting enough water. "You should always be looking for changes in volume, color and odor," Dr. Rolls says. "If these changes persist, see a doctor."

CAN YOU FIND THE HIDDEN SALT?

If you've already banned the saltshaker from the table and sworn off salty snacks—good for you! But to keep your intake at the recommended one-teaspoon-a-day limit takes a bit more vigilance. Three-fourths of your dietary sodium is hidden in already-prepared foods, experts say. And many salt-laced foods like cereal, diet soda and instant pudding don't taste a bit salty.

Just how good are you at avoiding this hidden salt? If you're eating more potassium-rich fresh fruits and vegetables than packaged convenience foods, for example, you're probably doing great. (Potassium helps rid your body of excess sodium.)

Take this quiz to find out where you stand on the hidden salt scale.

1. When barbecuing meat or fish, I'm more likely to brush on herbs or homemade marinara sauce than commercial catsup, barbecue sauce or soy sauce.

__True +1
__False –1

2. The fresh fruits and vegetables and lean meats in my grocery cart usually crowd out the canned, frozen and processed food.

__True +1
__False –1

3. I buy only the low-salt type of margarine.

__True +1
__False –1

4. I usually have dehydrated, instant versions of soups, sauces, salad dressings, oatmeal or other foods on hand.
__True –1
__False +1

5. I steam, microwave, broil or stir-fry vegetables rather than boil them.
__True +1
__False –1

6. Processed cheese never passes my lips.
__True +1
__False –1

7. I rinse canned foods such as tuna, ham and beans before preparing them.
__True +1
__False –1

8. I'm a sucker for deli food—cold cuts, prepared salads, pastrami, ham, smoked fish and so on.
__True –1
__False +1

9. I usually order my hamburger with the works—cheese, pickles, catsup, mustard and special sauce.
__True –1
__False +1

10. When dining out, I usually order oil and vinegar dressing for my salad, and ask for gravies and sauces on the side.
__True +1
__False –1

Scoring: 8–10: You're a top-notch salt sleuth.

5–7: There's room for improvement. Scan food labels closely for the key phrases "sodium-free" or "very low sodium."

Below 5: You're probably relying on too many prepared condiments and packaged convenience foods. See chapter 10 for help.

WHAT'S YOUR OVEREATING STYLE?

At one time or another, we've probably all used food as first-aid for wounded emotions. Jelly doughnuts become a security blanket for a bruised ego; cherry-vanilla ice cream becomes a sedative when you're stressed out; nachos become Saturday night entertainment when you're bored or lonely.

But if you *frequently* use a bag of chips or other food as an emotional bandage, it's likely that you also carry around more than a few unwanted pounds. According to studies conducted by Maria Simonson, Ph.D., and staff at the Health, Weight and Stress Clinic at Johns Hopkins Medical Institutions in Baltimore, 85 percent of overweight people turn to food when something is eating them. Psychological overeaters, they say, fall into several distinct categories like the ones listed here.

Hair Analysis Tests: A Help or a Hoax?

Could elevated levels of lead or depressed levels of zinc in your hair be warning flags of internal trouble?

Some alternative health practitioners think so. That's why these practitioners routinely run hair analysis tests on their patients. Supposedly, a lock of hair unlocks nutritional secrets other tests fail to find.

Several laboratories now offer mail-order hair analysis tests to anyone who sends in a snip of hair and about twenty bucks. In return, you get a computer printout summarizing the levels of metals and minerals detected in your hair. Typically, you'll also get a detailed interpretation of the findings along with specific dietary recommendations to detoxify your body or correct a deficiency.

Is hair analysis worth the money? "Probably not," says Leslie M. Klevay, M.D., research leader of the Clinical Nutrition Laboratory with the U.S. Department of Agriculture's Human Nutrition Research Center at the University of North Dakota in Grand Forks.

Hair follicles contain a trace of the same minerals and metals that are in your bloodstream. As hair grows, it also incorporates elements from the environment such as lead, mercury and aluminum.

Finding yourself in one of these categories is no cause for panic. Becoming aware of when, why and where you overeat can help you avoid the triggers that lead to nonstop nibbling.

To find out where you fit in, answer the questions below as follows:

0 = never
1 = once in a while
2 = fairly often
3 = regularly

The category with the highest score gives you your basic overeating style.

Nervous Night Eater

__I often skimp on meals until nightfall, then I stuff my face nonstop.
__I crave sweet, salty or high-fat snacks.
__I often munch in front of the boob tube, starting with the evening news on through the late show.
__I often conduct midnight raids on the refrigerator.
__I have trouble getting to sleep or staying asleep.
__I drink more than 3 cups of coffee a day.
__On a scale of 1 to 10, I'd say my stress level rates a 9 or 10.
__I've been called a worrywart.

Analyzing your hair content might tell you if toxic exposure to these minerals has taken place and reveal cumulative exposure over a period of time—but that's probably the extent of it.

"If you suspect lead or mercury poisoning or want to monitor environmental pollutants, a hair analysis test might be worthwhile for these specific situations," says Dr. Klevay. But, he adds "I would never rely solely on hair analysis as a diagnostic tool for, say, lead poisoning. Hair analysis tests should be viewed as a complement to standard blood, urine and physical tests."

As far as using hair analysis for detecting mineral deficiencies and diagnosing early metabolic diseases, there isn't a strand of evidence that it works for this purpose.

Hair analysis is fraught with other problems. Results can be tainted from hair dyes, shampoo, tap-water impurities—all factors that can alter the mineral composition of hair.

Furthermore, since there are no standardized procedures for analyzing hair, results are unreliable. One expert sent three hair samples from the same person to three different labs. He got back three different results—"that were not even close."

Compulsive Eater

__I often skip sit-down meals and usually eat on the run.
__I'm rarely without some type of food in my mouth.
__I'd rather eat food—even when I'm not hungry—than waste it.
__I crave foods that are sweet, starchy and soft (but I'll eat anything).
__I usually sneak food when no one is around to see me eat it.
__My favorite beverage is diet soda—lots of it.
__I'm cheery on the outside, but inside, I feel lonely and blue.
__My love life is either stressful or nonexistent.

Closet Binge Eater

__About three times a month, I suddenly pig out uncontrollably.
__When I binge, I gobble food fast and steadily, easily polishing off an entire bag of cookies.
__I binge in private and usually at night.
__My binges are usually triggered when I'm upset or stressed out.
__Immediately after bingeing I feel calm, but later ashamed and furious at myself.
__After a binge, I often fast or crash diet.
__Often after bingeing, my stomach aches or I have trouble sleeping.
__I often feel angry and depressed but don't know why.

Hand-Me-Down Eater

__My family devours king-size portions of rich food at every meal.
__My parents and siblings are overweight.
__My family frequently snacks together in front of the TV.
__The most exercise my family gets is reaching for seconds on pie.
__Both my mother and I love to cook.
__Having a well-stocked pantry makes me feel secure and loved.
__My mother always serves an extravagant dinner with rich desserts.
__My family celebrates even minor occasions with lavish feasts.

Thin/Fat

__I was overweight as a teenager and am now deathly afraid of gaining weight.
__It's a never-ending battle to stay thin.
__I eat nothing but low-calorie meals.
__I nag my husband and children if they gain even a pound or two because I detest fat people.
__My life would be ruined if I gained weight.
__I can tell you the fat and calorie count of every food on God's green Earth.
__Fat people are weak and have no willpower.
__Bingeing is the furthest thing from my mind.

Chronic Dieter

__I've tried all the latest diets and read all the diet books, but none of them are any good.
__Within a few months of losing weight, I'm back to my former fat self.
__I often crash diet before a party or important social event.
__I know more than most people about diets, nutrition and psychological causes for weight gain.
__I can tell you exactly how and why I lost and regained every pound.
__I've memorized the calorie count for foods from A to Z.
__Don't try to recommend a weight-loss group or doctor—they've all failed me.
__I'm into quick and easy weight loss.

Environmental Eater

__I can't resist the aromas emanating from a bakery.
__Just reading about luscious dessert recipes makes me drool.
__TV food commercials send me to the refrigerator.
__Eating food goes along with the territory of my job—power lunches, social dinners, etc.
__I eat more than most people at meals.
__When dining out, I rarely pass up the pastry dessert cart.
__I've begun to develop love handles on my waist and batwings under my arms.

__I rarely turn down an extra helping or a meal, even if I'm not hungry—if it's there, I'll eat it.

Couch Potato

__I prefer curling up with a bag of chips to physical activity.
__The most exercise I get these days is lifting a fork to my mouth.
__It takes fewer and fewer calories to maintain the same weight.
__I wouldn't be caught dead in workout gear.
__It's an effort to even walk to stores at the mall.
__I'm stressed and anxious most of the time.
__I sit behind a desk all day.
__Once I could have danced all night, but since I've gained weight, I can barely shuffle to the TV.

ARE YOU COMMITTED TO FOOD SAFETY?

More than half of all food-borne illness is caused by sloppy food handling habits in preparing, cooking and storing food in home kitchens, experts say. Are you taking unnecessary risks in your own kitchen? Take this test to find out. Simply circle the appropriate answer.

1. I usually keep my refrigerator thermostat set below:
   a. 32°F
   b. 15°F
   c. 40°F
   d. 30°F
2. I would probably select the items below in the following order as I move through the grocery store.
   a. strawberries, shrimp, eggs, canned soup, paper towels
   b. eggs, shrimp, strawberries, canned soup, paper towels
   c. paper towels, canned soup, strawberries, shrimp, eggs
3. I assume food is safe to eat if it doesn't smell, taste or look spoiled, no matter when the expiration date.
   Yes / No
4. I would toss out a can of green beans because:
   a. the can was leaking
   b. the lid was bulging
   c. the can was badly dented
   d. all of the above
5. I usually thaw frozen raw meat, poultry or fish in the refrigerator on the lowest shelf.
   Yes / No
6. After Thanksgiving dinner, the longest I would allow turkey and other leftovers to remain at room temperature is:
   a. 3 hours
   b. ½ hour
   c. 2 hours
   d. 24 hours

7. The container I use to store a large quantity of leftover stew in my refrigerator is:
   a. several small, shallow containers
   b. a big, deep, airtight container
   c. the stewpot covered with a lid.
8. My cutting board is made out of:
   a. hardwood
   b. acrylic
9. After cutting up raw ground meat for a taco salad and before using the same knife and cutting board to chop the tomatoes, I normally do the following:
   a. wipe the knife and board with a paper towel
   b. wash the knife and board with hot, soapy water
   c. rinse the knife and board under hot water
   d. wash the knife, board and my hands with hot, soapy water
10. When preparing potato salad for a buffet table, I omit the mayonnaise to reduce the risk of spoiling.
   Yes / No
11. When removing barbecued chicken from the grill, I normally use a different fork than the one used to place the raw poultry on the grill.
   Yes / No
12. If I want to use milk on my cereal but the milk container reads "sell by May 14" and it's now May 17, I'd use the milk anyway.
   Yes / No
13. When cooking meat, fish and poultry dishes in the microwave, I cover them to trap the steam and test them for doneness with a thermometer.
   Yes / No

Answers: 1. c.; 2. c.; 3. No; 4. d.; 5. Yes; 6. c.; 7. a.; 8. b.; 9. b.; 10. No; 11. Yes; 12. Yes; 13. Yes.

Scoring: If your total number of correct answers is between:

10 and 13: You should be wearing a halo for your fastidious food handling.

7 and 9: Your food handling habits are generally well intentioned but you should do better to be on the safe side.

6 or below: You have habits that could endanger your family's health and invite food-borne illness. Review chapter 29 and take this test again in a few weeks.

IS YOUR GLOBAL GRAZING ON TRACK?

Sampling the world's bounty of ethnic foods can excite your tastebuds. Besides out-of-this-world taste, a second reason to "go ethnic" is that many of these ancient dishes have little fat, sugar and salt, but lots of fiber—exactly the dietary recommendations for health-conscious Americans.

To reap the benefits from ethnic foods, though, you also need to steer clear of Americanized and fancy versions that are meat-laden, deep-fried, crisped or smothered in high-calorie cheese, sour cream or coconut milk.

Are you making the most of your ethnic eating opportunities? Take the quiz below and find out.

1. My idea of a great Mexican meal is:
   a. nachos with Cheez Whiz or anything that comes in a bag emblazoned with a bell
   b. a beef enchilada made with a flour tortilla and garnished with guacamole
   c. chicken roasted in mole sauce with a side of black-bean soup or a soft-corn tortilla
2. When I think of Italian food, it means:
   a. a large pizza with the works
   b. stuffed pasta shells
   c. cannellini beans and arugula greens with a side of crusty bread
3. When I crave Chinese food, it's usually:
   a. chop suey, fried rice and an egg roll
   b. Hunan shrimp and steamed rice so spicy my eyes water and my nose runs
   c. A cousin cuisine, the more delicately flavored Thai foods such as peanut oil-and-papaya shrimp salad with cellophane noodles
4. If I want a light Middle Eastern-style lunch, I choose:
   a. lean roast beef stuffed in a pita pocket
   b. bits of meat skewered on a short stick
   c. baba ghannoush (pureed eggplant) with pita bread or tabbouleh (parsley salad and cracked wheat)
5. My experience with Indian food is:
   a. chutney relish on my frankfurter
   b. Mulligatawny soup
   c. Tandoori chicken marinated in yogurt, served with nan (flatbread) and a side of cauliflower curry
6. Any Japanese meal I order would probably include:
   a. Teriyaki beef cooked tableside by chefs tossing knives and peppermills
   b. batter-dipped tempura shrimp and vegetables
   c. chicken yakatori broiled in gingerroot, sesame oil and chili pepper

Scoring: Give yourself no points for each **a.** answer, 1 point for each **b.** answer and 2 points for each **c.** answer. If you scored between 0 and 5, you are missing the boat in your gastronomic adventures. See chapter 18 for advice. A score between 6 and 8 shows that you're making some good choices, but there's still plenty of room for improvement. If your score was between 9 and 12, give yourself a gold star—you're eating the healthiest international cuisine of all.

CAN A COMPUTER BE YOUR NUTRITION GUIDE?

First it was computerized horoscopes, then computerized dating services and now computerized diet analysis.

"People want more control over their health, and they want to learn how food contributes to their well-being," says Rebecca S. Reeves, R.D., of Baylor College of Medicine in Houston. "Computerized diet analyses can offer a starting point in designing a healthy eating plan."

But before mailing in your diet survey and your check, ask what standards the computer-diet folks are basing their nutrient assessments on. A good analysis should be based on the Recommended Dietary Allowances (RDAs) set by the government.

Even a top-notch computerized diet analysis has its limits, though. For starters, a typical analysis based on a one-week dietary recall does not take into account your body's stores of nutrients. You may have eaten low-vitamin A foods during your surveyed week, for instance, yet the week before, you ate high-vitamin A foods. You could have an adequate store of vitamin A in your blood that is not reflected in your computer analysis. "This can be unnecessarily alarming," says Reeves. On the other hand, if you have a true nutrient deficiency, this can only be revealed with the appropriate blood and other biochemical tests.

Some experts believe that computer assessments place too much emphasis on vitamin deficiencies and ignore the behavioral issues that affect nutrition—whether you skip breakfast for example, or eat most meals in fast-food joints.

"Your body does not work like a computer," says Pittsburgh dietitian Pat Harper, R.D., a spokesperson for the American Dietetic Association. You need skilled detective work to uncover not just what you eat but how you eat. A personal nutritionist can fill in the gaps. "For example, I ask clients the type and amount of food they eat, what time they eat it and whether it's fried in fat, smothered in catsup, salted and so on."

A personal nutritionist or registered dietitian can also help you tailor nutritious meals. They'll give you tips on how to design a calcium-rich diet that won't raise your cholesterol levels, for instance, or show you how to dine sensibly on a hectic schedule. Some personal nutritionists will even peer into your refrigerator or take you on a tour of the supermarket, showing you exactly what margarine to buy.

In sum, the ideal nutritional assessment includes both a printout and a professional dietitian/nutritionist. To find an expert in your area, contact the American Dietetic Association at 1-800-366-1655. Or write to the National Center for Nutrition and Dietetics, 216 West Jackson Boulevard, Suite 800, Chicago, IL 60606-6995.

CHAPTER 36

EATING LIGHT, EATING RIGHT

A SIX-WEEK PROGRAM

Now that you've read this far, you know that a diet that emphasizes fruits, vegetables and grains can help reduce your risk of cancer, heart attack, obesity and stroke. You know that a diet of burgers, blue cheese and baloney can kill. But how do you move from the "typical" high-fat, high-cholesterol, high-calorie American diet to an eating program that prevents disease, promotes longevity and energizes both mind and body?

How do you put together all the recommendations from the American Heart Association, the National Cancer Institute, the National Cholesterol Education Program, the National Research Council and your doctor?

How do you eat everything these experts say you should—4 servings of this, 2 of that and 11 of the other—without getting fat, going crazy or needing a computerized tracking system to analyze what you eat?

We asked two of the country's leading experts in diet modification to develop a nutrition-improvement program that would be effective yet easy to follow.

Lynne W. Scott is director of the Diet Modification Clinic and assistant professor of medicine at Baylor College of Medicine in Houston. Franca Alphin is nutrition director of the Duke University Diet and Fitness Center in Durham, North Carolina. Both are registered dietitians. And though they are far apart in miles, they stand shoulder-to-shoulder when it comes to how you should switch from the old-fashioned American diet in which a "salad" is the wimpy tomato and lettuce on top of your burger to the new American diet in which a "salad" is a full-bodied mix of greens and other nutrient-dense vegetables.

Both the experts say that you should begin the transition to healthy eating by launching an all-out attack against fat. By taking that first major step, you could actually begin to feel healthier and more energetic within five days.

Then follow the fat offensive by cracking down on cholesterol, fortifying with grains, sifting out salt, draining oil, clipping calories and decriminalizing desserts, and your body should feel as though it has been reborn.

A key point to remember while working your way through the six-week program, however, is that it is only the *beginning*. This program is designed to jump start your motivational engines and propel you toward a healthy lifestyle. Getting there is up to you. You'll probably make a slew of mistakes—both accidentally and deliberately—and, our experts warn, it may actually take up to a full year before you can trust your hand to automatically reach for an apple instead of a cookie.

The point is that you should accept those setbacks as a natural consequence of being human. Just ignore them. Pick up the program where you left off and move forward. Once you've worked your way through the entire six weeks, you'll have a solid nutritional foundation on which to build the rest of a very healthy, very long life.

WEEK 1: ATTACK FAT

DAY 1: LAUNCH YOUR OFFENSIVE

"Take a pad and pencil and, for a day or two, write down absolutely everything you eat and drink and include the amounts," says Alphin. "Don't change anything—just write it down."

Then go out and buy a book with a comprehensive fat-content-of-foods table, suggests Scott. One that lists every conceivable food and every single gram of fat. Because once you get a handle on what you're eating, the first step you're going to take on the path to a healthier you is the one where you ditch excess dietary fat.

Both dietitians agree that your goal is to keep daily fat intake below 30 percent of the calories you're supposed to eat in any given day. And if your eyes glaze over at the thought of figuring out how much that is, you're figuring it out the hard way.

The easy way, says Scott, is to flip to the calorie table on page 510. Based on your ideal weight—what you're *supposed* to weigh, not what you weigh now—determine your optimal daily calorie level. Then check the fat table below. Right next to the total number of calories you should eat to maintain your ideal weight, you will see the maximum number of grams of fat you dare eat in a day.

Note the operative word here is *maximum*. If your height, weight and

WHERE TO DRAW THE LINE ON FAT

After you've consulted the table on page 510 to find how many calories a day you should be eating, use this table to determine the maximum amount of fat permitted daily.

CALORIE LEVELS	TOTAL FAT (g.)*	SATURATED FAT (g.)†
1,200	40	13
1,300	43	14
1,400	47	16
1,500	50	17
1,600	53	18
1,700	57	19
1,800	60	20
1,900	63	21
2,000	67	22
2,100	70	23
2,200	73	24
2,300	77	26
2,400	80	27
2,500	83	28
2,600	87	29
2,700	90	30
2,800	93	31
2,900	97	32
3,000	100	33
3,100	103	34
3,200	107	36
3,300	110	37
3,400	113	38
3,500	117	39
3,600	120	40
3,700	123	41
3,800	127	42

*Grams of fat equal to 30 percent of calories.
†Grams of saturated fat equal to 10 percent of calories.

frame size dictate that you eat, say, 1,900 calories a day, then—according to the table—you should be eating no more than 63 grams of fat, and no more than 21 grams of that should be saturated fat.

Whatever your numbers, memorize them, urges Scott. Write them on your heart and in your mind. Because by the end of your second week on this Eating Light, Eating Right Program, you're going to have to account for every gram of fat while keeping within those limits.

DAY 2: MEET THE MEATCUTTER AT YOUR MARKET

Now that you've written down everything you ate for at least a day, bought a good fat-content-of-foods table and memorized your personal fat ceilings, head for the supermarket—the meat counter, in particular.

"Meat contains the highest concentration of fat in the American diet," says Scott. "So a major strategy in the war against fat is to learn how to select the leanest cuts."

Take a look at the ground beef, for example. And don't just look at the labeling. Despite the fact that ground beef is usually somewhere around 20 percent fat by weight, it seems as though every package claims to be lean. "Lean," "Leaner" and "Superlean," right?

There is, however, a secret code that meatcutters use to reveal the fat content of some cuts of beef (but not ground meat): Its key words are "Prime," "Choice" and "Select." Prime has the most fat. Choice is leaner, and Select is the very leanest.

"Once you've deciphered this code," says Scott, "a key strategy that will allow you to limit the amount of fat you get from ground beef, is to buy select cuts of beef and ask your meatcutter to grind them." Make sure you also choose the lean cuts of meat—top round steak, for example—and ask your meatcutter to trim all visible fat before he grinds.

If it's inconvenient to wait for your custom grind, you can buy ground turkey instead. It's lower in fat than beef and easily substituted for ground beef in cooking.

If the turkey is freshly ground, however, make sure you ask your meatcutter whether it's pure meat or meat mixed with skin and fat. "Pure meat will be lower in fat," says Scott, "so that's what you want to buy." If you buy frozen ground turkey, she adds, read the labels carefully and pick the product with the fewest grams of fat per serving. It will be least likely to contain skin and extra fat.

Fortunately, choosing pork and poultry is a little bit easier than choosing beef. Just reach for the pork tenderloin—the leanest cut—and the light-meat cuts of chicken or turkey. White meat is lower in fat than dark meat. Remove the skin from chicken before cooking it. Turkey can be cooked with the skin to prevent it from drying out, but remove the skin before eating it.

DAY 3: CONFESS YOUR SINS

Today's the day to take a look at all the foods you've eaten over the past two days and play "Find the Fat." So pull out the pad on which you've scribbled down everything you ate and let's review your sins.

You knew the ½ cup of ice cream you ate last night after the 10 o'clock news was high in fat. But now, checking the fat table you bought on Day 1, you find that it had almost 12 grams of fat—one-fifth the maximum amount of fat a 5-foot, 1-inch, 109-pound woman should eat in an entire day!

You also knew that your dinner, consisting of two hot dogs (13 grams of fat each), rolls (3 grams each), potatoes au gratin (9 grams for ½ cup), peas (good choice—less than 1 gram of fat) and low-fat milk (a glass of 2 percent milk has almost 5 grams of fat) might be a little heavy. And it was. The total fat you ate at that one meal—even though you resisted that second helping of potatoes—was 46 grams.

Forty-six grams of fat for dinner might not have been too bad—even with your 12-gram "snack"—if you'd had a light lunch. But no, you went shopping with your friends and stopped at the local deli. All you had was a cheese sandwich (14 grams of fat), a salad with blue cheese dressing (16 grams) and an ice tea (0 grams), but that "light" lunch—which really didn't have very much food—actually contained 30 grams of fat.

So yesterday's evening snack, dinner and light lunch totaled 88 grams of fat. And what about breakfast? Again, you didn't eat a lot of food, but what you ate was dense: a danish and coffee racked up 24 grams of fat—and the coffee was merely an innocent bystander.

The fat bill for yesterday's menu: 112 grams of fat—an okay amount if you're a 6-foot 2-inch man who digs ditches or plays basketball for a living.

DAY 4: LIMIT MEAT TO LESS THAN SIX OUNCES

Okay, now you know the worst. You know the maximum amount of fat you can eat in a day if you want to stay healthy, and wise. And you know from your food log the amount of fat you actually eat.

So today you're going to begin eating lean meat and limiting the amount of meat you eat to less than six ounces (after cooking) a day.

How? Try mixing the select meat you bought the other day at the supermarket with pasta and vegetables so that you can have a belly-filling serving of food but a small serving of meat, suggests Scott. That way, the meat you bought will stretch over several meals.

Use meat as a flavor enhancer. "Instead of plunking a half-dozen meatballs on top of spaghetti," says Scott, "use an ounce or two of very lean ground meat to flavor the sauce." If you're the type who needs to see a big, beefy steak on your plate, she adds, make sure you have a meatless lunch and breakfast, then hold your dinnertime meat portion at six ounces.

FIND YOUR IDEAL CALORIE LEVEL

Use this table to determine the number of calories you should be eating daily, based upon your height, weight, bone structure and activity level.

ADULT FEMALES

HEIGHT WITHOUT SHOES	FRAME SIZE	DESIRABLE WEIGHT (Range)	CALORIE LEVEL BASED ON PHYSICAL ACTIVITY			
			VERY LIGHT	LIGHT	MODERATE	HEAVY
5'0"	Small	106 (102–110)	1,400	1,600	1,800	2,100
	Medium	113 (107–119)	1,450	1,700	1,900	2,250
	Large	123 (115–131)	1,600	1,850	2,100	2,450
5'1"	Small	109 (105–113)	1,400	1,650	1,850	2,200
	Medium	116 (110–122)	1,500	1,750	1,950	2,300
	Large	126 (118–134)	1,650	1,900	2,150	2,500
5'2"	Small	112 (108–116)	1,450	1,700	1,900	2,250
	Medium	119 (113–126)	1,550	1,800	2,000	2,400
	Large	129 (121–138)	1,700	1,950	2,200	2,600
5'3"	Small	115 (111–119)	1,500	1,750	1,950	2,300
	Medium	123 (116–130)	1,600	1,850	2,100	2,450
	Large	133 (125–142)	1,750	2,000	2,250	2,650
5'4"	Small	118 (114–123)	1,550	1,750	2,000	2,350
	Medium	127 (120–135)	1,650	1,900	2,150	2,550
	Large	137 (129–146)	1,800	2,050	2,350	2,750
5'5"	Small	122 (118–127)	1,600	1,850	2,050	2,450
	Medium	131 (124–139)	1,700	1,950	2,250	2,600
	Large	141 (133–150)	1,850	2,100	2,400	2,800
5'6"	Small	126 (122–131)	1,650	1,900	2,150	2,500
	Medium	135 (128–143)	1,750	2,050	2,300	2,700
	Large	145 (137–154)	1,900	2,200	2,450	2,900
5'7"	Small	130 (126–135)	1,700	1,950	2,200	2,600
	Medium	139 (132–147)	1,800	2,100	2,350	2,800
	Large	149 (141–158)	1,950	2,250	2,550	3,000
5'8"	Small	135 (130–140)	1,750	2,050	2,300	2,700
	Medium	143 (136–151)	1,850	2,150	2,450	2,850
	Large	154 (145–163)	2,000	2,300	2,600	3,100
5'9"	Small	139 (134–144)	1,800	2,100	2,350	2,800
	Medium	147 (140–155)	1,900	2,200	2,500	2,950
	Large	158 (149–168)	2,050	2,350	2,700	3,150
5'10"	Small	143 (138–148)	1,850	2,150	2,450	2,850
	Medium	151 (144–159)	1,950	2,250	2,550	3,000
	Large	163 (153–173)	2,100	2,450	2,750	3,250

ADULT MALES

HEIGHT WITHOUT SHOES	FRAME SIZE	DESIRABLE WEIGHT (Range)	CALORIE LEVEL BASED ON PHYSICAL ACTIVITY: VERY LIGHT	LIGHT	MODERATE	HEAVY
5'5"	Small	129 (124–133)	1,700	1,950	2,200	2,600
	Medium	137 (130–143)	1,800	2,050	2,350	2,750
	Large	147 (138–156)	1,900	2,200	2,500	2,950
5'6"	Small	133 (128–137)	1,750	2,000	2,250	2,650
	Medium	141 (134–147)	1,850	2,100	2,400	2,800
	Large	152 (142–161)	2,000	2,300	2,600	3,050
5'7"	Small	137 (132–141)	1,800	2,050	2,350	2,750
	Medium	145 (138–152)	1,900	2,200	2,450	2,900
	Large	157 (147–166)	2,050	2,350	2,650	3,150
5'8"	Small	141 (136–145)	1,850	2,100	2,400	2,850
	Medium	149 (142–156)	1,950	2,250	2,550	3,000
	Large	161 (151–170)	2,100	2,400	2,750	3,200
5'9"	Small	145 (140–150)	1,900	2,200	2,450	2,900
	Medium	153 (146–160)	2,000	2,300	2,600	3,050
	Large	165 (155–174)	2,150	2,500	2,800	3,300
5'10"	Small	149 (144–154)	1,950	2,250	2,550	3,000
	Medium	158 (150–165)	2,050	2,350	2,700	3,150
	Large	169 (159–179)	2,200	2,550	2,850	3,400
5'11"	Small	153 (148–158)	2,000	2,300	2,600	3,050
	Medium	162 (154–170)	2,100	2,450	2,750	3,250
	Large	174 (164–184)	2,250	2,600	2,950	3,500
6'0"	Small	157 (152–162)	2,050	2,350	2,650	3,150
	Medium	167 (158–175)	2,150	2,500	2,850	3,350
	Large	179 (168–189)	2,350	2,700	3,050	3,600
6'1"	Small	162 (156–167)	2,100	2,450	2,750	3,250
	Medium	171 (162–180)	2,200	2,550	2,900	3,400
	Large	184 (173–194)	2,400	2,750	3,150	3,700
6'2"	Small	166 (160–171)	2,150	2,500	2,800	3,300
	Medium	176 (167–185)	2,300	2,650	3,000	3,500
	Large	189 (178–199)	2,450	2,850	3,200	3,800
6'3"	Small	170 (164–175)	2,200	2,550	2,900	3,400
	Medium	181 (172–190)	2,350	2,700	3,300	3,850
	Large	193 (182–204)	2,500	2,900	3,300	3,850

NOTE: From 1959 Metropolitan Life Insurance Company, New York City. These tables are based on 1959 rather than 1983 Metropolitan Life Insurance Company height-weight tables because the earlier tables specify lower weights, more appropriate to health-related concerns.

DAY 5: SWEAR OFF PROCESSED MEATS

"For the most part, luncheon meats are among the fattiest meats available," says Scott. "Several low-fat varieties are available. But both the high- and low-fat varieties are usually high in salt."

You can sometimes find a freshly cooked turkey breast that hasn't been salted at a neighborhood deli or market where it's made right on the premises, adds Scott.

Or, once a week, you can turn your own kitchen into the neighborhood deli: Cook a turkey, chicken or lean roast, remove the skin or trim the fat and slice the meat into thin layers. Then slip it into self-locking storage bags and toss it in the freezer. Whenever you're planning on sandwiches, pull out a bag and defrost.

DAY 6: EAT MORE FISH

Remember that six-ounce limit of cooked meat per day? Well, now that you've eaten that amount for a couple of days, it's time to think fish. In fact, you might want to consider having fish not just today but two to three times a week, since it's naturally low in both total fat and saturated fat.

"Most finfish has only a gram or two of fat per serving," says Scott. You can sauté fish quickly and easily in a pan prepared with no-stick cooking spray or brushed with olive oil. Try leaving the skin on while you cook it, then remove it just before serving. Or you can steam it over boiling water into which you've dropped a handful of lemon peel and herbs. In either case the fish is ready as soon as the translucent flesh becomes opaque.

DAY 7: PIZZA DAY

It's been a pretty full week. You've figured the maximum amount of fat you should eat and how much fat you actually eat. You've learned how to select low-fat cuts of meat and to limit your meat consumption. You've also curtailed processed meats and started eating more fish.

So, besides already starting to feel good, here's an additional reward: Sometime today you're going to make your very first totally healthy, totally great-tasting pizza.

The recipe? Unless you've been to pizza school and have a professional oven, buy a crust at your local supermarket, says Scott. Then buy a spaghetti sauce that lists zero grams of fat per serving on the label, some grated part-skim mozzarella cheese and a little meat—little meaning a handful of very lean ground beef. You'll have to live without pepperoni; its content of total fat and saturated fat is just too high for dietitians to recommend.

Cook and drain the meat well, directs Scott. Smear tomato sauce over the crust, sprinkle with mozzarella and top with meat. Add as many mushrooms, green peppers and onions as you like. Bake at 350° until the crust is brown and the cheese melts, about 20 minutes.

WEEK 2: ATTACK FAT, PHASE TWO

DAY 8: PLAY AROUND IN THE KITCHEN

Start the second week of your healthier life by taking a few hours to experiment with preparing lower-fat meats in new ways.

Since lower-fat meats are occasionally less tender, for example, try marinating them in an acid-based marinade—citrus or tomato juice, vinegar and soy sauce, for example—to break down those hard-to-chew fibers before cooking. Then thinly slice the meat and stir-fry with vegetables in a wok.

Or instead of roasting a lower-fat cut of meat in the oven, try braising it. Brown the meat, then simmer it in liquid for at least an hour.

And think about making some stock. Whether it's chicken or beef, cover the bones (you can get them from your butcher) with cold water, toss in any vegetable parings and onion skins you may have saved, season as you please. Bring to a boil, then reduce heat and simmer for at least three to five hours for beef and two to three hours for chicken. Strain the stock and refrigerate immediately. (For rapid cooling of larger quantities, divide the stock into one-quart portions.) The fat will rise to the top, where you can easily skim it off and discard it. Freeze whatever you won't use within a couple of days. Use the defatted stock when cooking rice or vegetables to add robust flavor.

DAY 9: PUT YOUR MILK ON A DIET

Now that you've reduced the amount of fat you get from meat, turn your attention to milk.

"Most people are already savvy enough to be drinking milk that has 2 percent fat rather than whole," says Scott. "But a really healthy diet means cutting back even further." So today pick up a container of 1 percent fat milk and start using it both for drinking and in cooking. If ½ percent fat milk is available in your area, adds Scott, try switching to that instead. Skim milk—which has almost no fat at all—is the preferred choice. However, if you don't enjoy drinking it, milk with 1 percent fat or less is fine.

And don't be confused by labeling. As with meat, the "percent" in ½ or 1 or 2 percent milk refers to the amount of fat by weight rather than calories.

To compare products, check the ingredient label for the actual number of grams of fat. Two percent milk has 4.7 grams of fat per cup, 1 percent milk has 2.6 grams, ½ percent milk has 1 gram, skim milk has 0.6 gram.

DAY 10: TURN YOUR ATTENTION TO CHEESE

Cheese may be an excellent source of calcium and protein, but too much high-fat cheese can clog your arteries over time.

"Cut back on fat by eating only cheeses that have five grams of fat or less per ounce," suggests Scott. The part-skim mozzarella you ate on Day 7's pizza is a perfect choice to use in place of high-fat cheese.

Check the fat table you bought on Day 1 to find other low-fat cheeses that satisfy your five-gram limit. And check labels at your supermarket. There are at least 50 or 60 different kinds, says Scott, who has listed them all in *The Living Heart Brand Name Shopper's Guide,* a continually updated book of which she was coauthor.

Be aware, however, that most popular cheeses—Cheddar, Swiss and American, for example—tilt the fat scales at a hefty eight or nine grams of fat per ounce. And, once again, make sure you check the claims on the label. "Reduced fat" does not necessarily mean "low fat."

DAY 11: ENJOY SOUR CREAM'S RICHNESS WITHOUT THE FAT

Most cooks agree that sour cream is one of the most versatile foods in the kitchen. It's used as the basis for dips, toppings, sauces—you name the category and some Sour Cream Sarah has created a recipe to fit it.

But sour cream has six grams of fat in two tablespoons, and most of its calories from fat.

The alternative? Today you're going to make your own healthier version. Puree low-fat cottage cheese with an equal amount of nonfat yogurt, then add a squeeze of lemon. The resulting swirl is so creamy and rich that you'll never again be tempted by regular sour cream.

DAY 12: USE A WHIPPED TOPPING

That's right. Today you are *ordered* to use a whipped topping. And, yes, there is a catch: You have to make it yourself and, no, it's not made from cream.

Pour ⅓ cup skim milk into a small stainless steel bowl. Stick it in the freezer until ice crystals just begin to form—15 to 20 minutes. Then pull it out and quickly thicken by beating in ⅓ cup instant nonfat dry milk with an electric mixer. Whip on high until soft peaks begin to form—about two minutes. Flavor with a bit of sugar and vanilla and beat until stiff peaks form again, about 2 minutes. Use within 20 minutes. It's perfect over berries or other fruits, and you simply won't believe the taste.

DAY 13: BEGIN THE COUNTDOWN

Today you're going to start using all that arithmetic you learned in grade school. You're going to start counting every single gram of fat and saturated fat you put into your mouth, then subtract it from those grams-of-fat totals. You *do* remember your fat maximums, don't you—that you memorized on Day 1?

Let's say your height, weight and bone structure have dictated that you should eat 1,650 calories a day. As you learned on Day 1 when you memorized your fat numbers from the table on page 507, that means you can eat a maximum of 53 grams of fat a day—of which 18 can be saturated fat.

So stick your fat-content-of-foods table in your handbag or pocket, along with a pencil, and prepare to count every gram of fat and saturated fat throughout the day. Add them to your fat numbers as you go. When you get near the maximum in either column, you've reached your limit.

If you stop at a Mexican restaurant for an iced tea and enchilada at lunch, for example, you need to count the enchilada's hefty 17.6 grams of total fat and 9.1 grams of saturated fat toward your daily allotment.

By the way, after you've completed this six-week program, you might decide you're ready to cut back on fat even more. The table on page 112 shows daily limits to aim for that can bring your total fat intake down another notch—from 30 to 25 percent of total calories.

DAY 14: USE JUST A SWIRL OF CREAM

Is there anyone who doesn't like the rich taste of cream? Probably not on this planet. So today's step toward a healthier diet—and your reward for the past two weeks of healthy eating—is to learn how to use it in a healthy way.

"The trick," says Dieter Doppelfeld, chef instructor at the Culinary Institute of America, "is to give people the satisfaction of cream without the substance." Like an impressionist artist who paints a soul-satisfying "impression" of a country landscape rather than every rock, tree and leaf he sees, Doppelfeld relies on a brief "impression" of cream, rather than a full measure, to caress and satisfy your palate.

When preparing cream soups, for example, he substitutes evaporated skim milk for cream in the basic recipe, then garnishes each bowl with a single swirl of heavy cream right across the top.

The result? Your tongue senses cream with every spoonful, explains Doppelfeld, so you have the feel and taste of cream—with only three grams of fat per serving (see recipe on page 516).

HIGH-NUTRITION RECIPE

SWEET POTATO SOUP

Here's how Chef Dieter Doppelfeld uses his just-a-hint-of-cream technique when making sweet potato soup. The soup is delicious either hot or cold.

½ cup diced onions
⅓ cup diced celery
1 leek (white part only), diced and rinsed well
1 clove garlic, minced
2½ cups defatted chicken stock
2 large sweet potatoes (about 1 pound), peeled and chopped
¼ teaspoon grated nutmeg
⅛ teaspoon ground cinnamon
⅓ cup evaporated skim milk
1 tablespoon maple syrup
¼ teaspoon salt (optional)
2 tablespoons heavy cream, whipped
1 tablespoon currants
1 tablespoon toasted slivered almonds

In a 3-quart saucepan over medium heat, slowly cook the onions, celery, leeks and garlic in about ¼ cup of the stock for 5 minutes, or until the vegetables are translucent.

Add the sweet potatoes, nutmeg, cinnamon and the remaining 2¼ cups stock. Bring to a boil, then cover and simmer for 20 minutes, or until the sweet potatoes are tender. Let cool for 5 minutes.

Puree the sweet potato mixture in batches, since it probably won't all fit in the blender at one time. Transfer each batch to a bowl as it's pureed, then stir the milk, syrup and salt, if desired, into the whole batch in the bowl. If desired, refrigerate until cold.

To serve, ladle into individual bowls and garnish each serving with a swirl of whipped cream and a sprinkle of currants and almonds.

Serves 6
Per serving: *155 calories, 3.3 g. fat (19% of calories), 2.9 g. dietary fiber, 7 mg. cholesterol, 69 mg. sodium*

WEEK 3: CRACK DOWN ON CHOLESTEROL

DAY 15: LET THE DOG HAVE YOUR YOLKS

Now that you have fat under control, it's time to tackle cholesterol, says Scott.

Your goal is to consume less than 300 milligrams of cholesterol a day. Since egg yolk is the most concentrated source of cholesterol, it means limiting egg yolks to no more than three a week.

Just three eggs a week sounds like an impossible limit when you consider the fact that the recipe for nearly everything you bake—casseroles, pancakes, bread, meat loaf—seems to call for an egg or two to hold things together. But you can make up a batch of cholesterol-free egg substitute, keep it handy in the refrigerator or freezer and use it whenever a recipe calls for eggs.

Preparing the egg substitute is simple: Separate six eggs. Whip the whites and ¼ cup powdered milk with 1 tablespoon oil until smooth, then refrigerate for up to a week or freeze until needed. One-quarter cup equals one egg.

Cook and refrigerate the yolks, then use them to augment your pet's—or your neighbor's pet's—canned or bagged food. For healthy animals, the fur will likely develop a healthy sheen, and *you'll* probably have a little more zip in your step. And you don't have to worry about your dog's cholesterol level. Dogs' arteries aren't affected by cholesterol the way humans' are.

DAY 16: MEET YOUR FISHMONGER

You've already substituted fish for meat at least one day a week. Now you might want to think about doing it even more often, because not only can certain species of fish help limit your intake of fat, they can also curb your cholesterol.

Meat and poultry both have about 25 milligrams of cholesterol per ounce, says Scott, so if you are eating six ounces of either one a day, you are getting nearly half your daily allotment of cholesterol. By comparison, many fish have as little as 12 to 15 milligrams of cholesterol per ounce.

So today you're going to take a trip to your local fish market, get to know your fishmonger and learn how to select fish.

Your best bets? Fillets of bass, cod, croaker, grouper, halibut, king mackerel, monkfish, ocean perch, orange roughy, pike, salmon (except fresh sockeye), shark, snapper, swordfish, tuna and whitefish are all terrific choices.

DAY 17: HAVE A VEGETARIAN LUNCH

An easy way to drop your cholesterol consumption is to regularly schedule some meals with no meat, poultry or even fish in them at all.

"You may not want to become a vegetarian," says Scott, "but having several vegetarian meals each week will help keep your cholesterol, fat and saturated fat intake low. Dried beans, peas and legumes, along with a glass of 1 percent or skim milk and whole-wheat bread, makes an excellent meal with plenty of protein.

DAY 18: TAKE IT OFF—TAKE IT ALL OFF!

If you're not already doing so, start taking the skin off any chicken or turkey you eat and tossing it in the garbage. It's so full of fat it's simply not fit for man or beast.

Day 19: Resupply Your Pantry with Low-Cholesterol Basics

One of the simplest tricks to keeping cholesterol levels low in both your food and your body is to get rid of the high-cholesterol basics many of us have tucked away on our kitchen shelves. Then lay in a supply of lower-cholesterol or cholesterol-free alternatives.

You can get rid of baking chocolate, for example, and keep cocoa on hand instead. (Three tablespoons of cocoa plus 1 teaspoon of oil equals 1 square of chocolate.) Canned evaporated skim milk can replace cream in almost every way. Canola oil can replace shortening, and artificial bacon bits can replace salt pork for seasoning vegetables.

Day 20: Season Vegetables with Nut Butters

One of the harder cholesterol-laden habits to give up is drizzling butter over vegetables. But once you've dotted a pile of cooked carrots with a teaspoon of unsalted cashew butter, or—in the Indonesian manner—dotted a pile of green beans with peanut butter, you'll wonder why you thought the stuff from cows was so great. Nut butters still contain fat, however, so don't go—uh—nuts. Each teaspoon contains approximately two grams of fat.

Check your supermarket shelves to see what other nut butters you can find. Then take them home and experiment. Who knows? Almond butter could make spinach a tempting treat; and nut butters have no cholesterol.

Day 21: Salmon Day

Congratulations! You've completed three weeks on the Eating Light, Eating Right Program. You've dumped a load of fat and cholesterol out of your diet and probably several pounds off your body. Here's your reward!

High-Nutrition Recipe

Salmon Wrapped in Phyllo

This recipe is an adaptation of one Philadelphia chef and food consultant Robin Rifkin prepares. It's simple, elegant and healthy. Although phyllo recipes are generally loaded with fat (thanks to all the butter), this dish requires only a minimum amount of light margarine. Most of the fat in this recipe comes from the salmon, which is a good source of healthy omega-3 fatty acids. Phyllo is available in supermarket freezer sections. Thaw it in the refrigerator before using.

8 sheets phyllo dough
1½ tablespoons light margarine, melted
4 salmon fillets (4 ounces each), skin removed
4 teaspoons coarse-grain mustard
1 box (10 ounces) frozen chopped spinach, thawed and squeezed dry

Place 1 sheet of phyllo dough horizontally on a dry countertop in front of you. Top it with a second sheet. Wrap the remaining sheets tightly in plastic to prevent them from drying out; set them aside.

Using a pastry brush, lightly brush the right-hand side of the top phyllo sheet with a little margarine. Fold the right portion over the left half, making a rectangle about 12" × 18". Lightly brush the top of the dough with a little more margarine.

Lay a salmon fillet in the center of the phyllo. Spread 1 teaspoon of the mustard over the salmon. Top with ¼ of the spinach in a thin layer. Fold the top and bottom sections of the phyllo over the salmon; fold in the two sides to make a neat packet that encases the salmon.

Lightly brush the packet with margarine. Coat a baking sheet with no-stick spray; place the packet on the sheet.

Repeat the procedure three times, using the remaining phyllo, salmon, mustard and spinach.

Bake at 425° for 8 to 10 minutes, or until the phyllo begins to brown.

Serves 4
Per serving: *308 calories, 12 g. fat (33% of calories), 1.8 g. dietary fiber, 59 mg. cholesterol, 204 mg. sodium*

WEEK 4: FORTIFY WITH GRAINS

DAY 22: MAKE THE CHOICE

Now that you've zapped the fat and cholesterol from your diet, you're probably losing a few pounds and getting a bit hungry. In fact, you've probably started to add some food here and there to fill the gaps left by the fat.

The goal for any healthy diet, according to both Alphin and Scott, is 6 to 11 servings a day of breads, cereals and pasta. So if you're trying to lose weight, that means keeping your starches at around 6 servings a day—whole-wheat toast or a bowl of cereal at breakfast, a couple of slices of whole wheat bread at lunch, a potato or cup of pasta at dinner. "But if you don't want to lose any more weight," says Alphin, "start by adding 1 or 2 starch servings a day until your hunger stops or until you *either* reach 11 servings or start to put on pounds."

Eleven servings a day sounds like a lot. But when you look at a whole day's meals, it isn't really as much food as it seems, says Scott. "If you eat cereal and toast at breakfast, that's two to four. If you have a sandwich at lunch, there's another two. Then if you have some soup that has potatoes, or a salad with crackers, that's another one or two.

"Then at night, it's easy to eat a potato or a half-cup of pasta. A cup of pasta is equal to two slices of bread. And most of us can easily eat a cup and a half—that's 3 servings of starch." Add a hot roll and an ear of corn, says Scott, and you've eaten 9 to 11 servings over the course of a day.

DAY 23: BEGIN WITH WHOLE WHEAT

If you need to add starches to bring your diet up to the 6 to 11 recommended servings a day, begin with whole-wheat breads and bagels first, says Alphin. "Bread is usually among the first things to go when people are dieting," she explains. "So when they hear that they can include it, they feel like they're getting a treat." It really perks them up.

Besides, whole-wheat breads are high in fiber, she adds. And increasing fiber as you withdraw fat is a good strategy. The fiber fills you up in the places where less fat has made you feel empty.

DAY 24: ADD CEREALS AS YOU NEED THEM

Whole-grain cereals are not just for breakfast. They can be crushed as a topping over casseroles, used as an extender in meat loaf, sprinkled over salads to add crunch or eaten right out of the box as a healthy snack.

"Use cereals as needed to boost your fiber intake," suggests Alphin. "Just make sure you read and compare the labels. Buy those cereals that have the least amount of salt and sugar and the most amount of fiber."

DAY 25: INVESTIGATE THE PASTABILITIES

Once you've added more breads and cereals to your diet, think about using pasta to round out your starches, says Scott.

Spaghetti, fettuccine, ziti or just plain noodles are all great. But you might want to try some whole-grain pastas, too, for extra fiber. And you may find the pastas combined with vegetables—beets, spinach or artichokes, for example—add a cheerful splash of color to your plate.

DAY 26: REPLACE FAT WITH FIBER

You've been eating cheese with less than five grams of fat per ounce for a couple of weeks. So you're comfortable with the taste. You're so comfortable, in fact, that if someone crumbled some high-fat Cheddar into a salad when you weren't expecting it, you probably wouldn't enjoy it. It would taste too strong and feel too heavy.

So now you're ready to switch to an even lower-fat cheese: three grams of fat per ounce. And before you start squealing, remember how you felt on Day 10 when you switched from those high-fat Cheddars and blues to the five-gram cheeses. Thought you'd never get used to the difference, did you?

Yet it not only happened, but you now *prefer* the lower-fat cheese. Trust us. The same thing will happen as you move to cheeses with three grams of fat per ounce. So head for your supermarket and take some time to check out the cheeses that claim to be low-fat. Check the labels until you find a few that have three grams of fat or less per serving and toss them in your cart. And to make sure you don't feel deprived, also pick up a loaf of unsliced whole-wheat bread.

Why unsliced? Because you're going to replace that missing fat with fiber. When you get home, cut two *thick* slices of whole-wheat bread and top each with a slice of low-fat cheese. Then either melt the cheese in the microwave or broil it in the oven. Either way, the warm, sweet softness of this extra-thick bread will help you make the switch to lower-fat cheese with delight. For a special taste treat, try topping it with some Mexican salsa.

DAY 27: DRINK PLENTY OF WATER

As you add whole-grain products to your diet, make sure you're drinking eight 8-ounce glasses of water a day to help bulk up all that fiber and keep it moving through your digestive tract.

DAY 28: VISIT ANOTHER COUNTRY

Today you're going to have lunch at a restaurant that serves Middle Eastern food. Ask questions, sample dishes, then come home and put your own innovative juices to work. Your challenge? To combine several different types of starches into one stimulating dish. You might decide to make an eggplant stuffed with tomato, rice, nuts and bulgur wheat, for instance.

WEEK 5: DRAIN THE OIL

DAY 29: GIVE ANY NONDAIRY CREAMER IN THE HOUSE TO A CAT

Give it to your cat, the neighbor's cat, any cat. Because only an animal with nine lives can possibly survive the repeated daily imbibing of a product that derives most of its substance from hydrogenated oils. Not only are these creamers full of fat, they're full of *bad* fat—the kind that congeals on an unwashed plate and turns your arteries into stiff, narrow straws that are easily clogged.

If you simply must have something white in your coffee or tea, try some more low-fat milk like you bought on Day 9.

DAY 30: MAKE HEALTHY CHOICES AT A FAST-FOOD RESTAURANT

If this suggestion to eat at a fast-food restaurant appalls you, you're probably thinking of what you ordered there in the past: fried chicken, greasy french fries, gloppy coleslaw. In short, a healthy person's nightmare.

But today, eating at a fast-food restaurant should be a pleasure because you're going to make healthy choices, like a giant bowl of greens topped with lean chunks of chicken, carrots, broccoli and cauliflower. And for a dressing, you're going to ignore every plastic package they try to hand you unless it's labeled "low fat." Not "reduced-fat" or "lite," but "low fat." Top off the meal with a roll, some pasta or another starch.

DAY 31: SWITCH FROM OIL TO VINEGAR

You need to start thinking about oil the way you think about salt: You only eat it when you can't avoid it. And you certainly don't add it to anything it hasn't managed to work its way into naturally.

Starting today, try sprinkling red-wine vinegar and a pinch of oregano over a salad at lunch instead of the usual squirt of oil. Or experiment with some of the flavored vinegars—tarragon, basil, rosemary—that are beginning to appear on supermarket shelves. You'll be surprised how quickly your taste buds will actually prefer the sharp brisk taste of foods that are no longer slathered in oil.

DAY 32: SAY GOOD-BYE TO FRIED FOODS FOREVER

If you've been filling your menus with fried foods on a regular basis, you might want to treat yourself to a cooking course that emphasizes steaming, baking and broiling. Check with your local Y or hospital about taking a course in the basics. Then ask the chef at your favorite restaurant if he'd be willing to give you—and maybe some of your friends—an after-hours graduate course in La Nouvelle American Cuisine.

DAY 33: USE BROTH INSTEAD OF OIL

Most of us have sprayed or slathered oil or butter over the surface of any pan we use since we first learned to cook—mostly to keep what we were cooking from sticking. Today, however, dietitians suggest that you skip the fat and increase flavor by substituting defatted chicken broth.

You can use homemade stock (see Day 8) or canned low-fat stock from the supermarket. If you're making your own stock, freeze some in an ice-cube tray. Then whenever you need a couple of tablespoons to coat a pan, just warm the pan on the stove and toss in a cube.

DAY 34: RETHINK YOUR SNACK FOODS

Potato chips, tortilla chips, corn chips and just about every other chip in your supermarket are loaded with oil. If you really need a crunch food to snack on, make your own chips by cutting up a tortilla and baking the pieces in an oven until the chips dry out. Or pick up some low-sodium pretzels or rice cakes as an alternative.

The rice cakes in particular may be something of a surprise. Once a glued-together version of puffed rice cereal, today's rice cakes are flavored with everything from sour cream and onion to teriyaki sauce—but without the fat.

DAY 35: FRISK YOUR MUFFINS

"I love it," says Alphin. "People are saying, 'I eat a bran muffin every morning.' But their muffin is so moist it has enough oil to last for the next four days!"

Bran is good, muffins are good, but the oil most muffin recipes call for is not good. So today you're going to frisk your muffins for oil. Check the grams-of-fat listing on any commercially made muffins you buy and check the amount of oil called for in any muffins you make.

Fortunately you can substitute an equal amount of nonfat yogurt—fruit-flavored or vanilla—for the oil and eggs in your muffin recipes. (Figure one egg is equivalent to ¼ cup.)

Or, if you want to add a chunk of fiber while you're draining the oil, you can smoosh some prunes in the blender and substitute an equal amount of prune puree for the oil. Your muffins will not be quite as light, but you'll have exactly the same richness and—believe it or not—even more flavor.

HIGH-NUTRITION RECIPE

MAGIC MOLASSES MUFFINS

To celebrate your completion of five weeks on the Eating Light, Eating Right Program, here's a magic muffin created by JoAnn Brader of the Rodale Food Center. It will please every taste bud in your family—and it has just three grams of fat. For best results, use a nugget-type bran cereal such as Bran Buds.

1½ cups nugget-type bran cereal
½ cup apple juice
⅓ cup raisins
1 cup unbleached flour
1½ teaspoons baking soda
1 cup nonfat or low-fat lemon yogurt
¼ cup fat-free egg substitute
¼ cup molasses
2 tablespoons canola oil

In a large bowl, combine the cereal, juice and raisins. Let stand for 10 minutes.

In a small bowl, combine the flour and baking soda.

In another small bowl, mix the yogurt, egg, molasses and oil.

Lightly stir the flour mixture into the bran bowl, mixing it only slightly. Stir in the yogurt mixture. Mix with a large rubber spatula until all the flour is moistened; do not overmix.

Coat 12 muffin cups with no-stick spray. Spoon the batter into the cups, filling them about ¾ full. Bake at 400° for 20 minutes. Cool on a wire rack for 5 minutes before removing the muffins from the pan. Serve warm or cold.

Makes 12 muffins
Per serving: *129 calories, 2.7 g. fat (17% of calories), 3.4 g. dietary fiber, <1 mg. cholesterol, 191 mg. sodium*

WEEK 6: CRACK DOWN ON CALORIES

DAY 36: INCLUDE MORE VEGETABLES

Now that you've cut back on the fat, cholesterol and oil in your diet while boosting grains, it's time to start thinking about vegetables.

Vegetables are naturally low in calories. So the total number of calories in your diet will gradually fall as vegetables begin to play a larger part in what you eat.

Your goal, says Scott, is to eat five servings of vegetables a day (raw vegetables, whenever possible). You should lean heavily toward the cancer-fighting cruciferous vegetables—broccoli, cauliflower, cabbage, brussels sprouts—and others that are good sources of beta-carotene—carrots, sweet potatoes, pumpkin, squash and spinach.

So today why don't you begin including more veggies by putting a new twist on an old before-dinner favorite?

Empty an eight-ounce carton of plain, nonfat yogurt into a bowl and mix in a packet of dried salad dressing seasoning, like ranch, to make a rich-tasting dip, Scott suggests. Surround the bowl with raw vegetables and encourage the children to join in on the munching. They'll disappear within minutes.

DAY 37: INCREASE YOUR FRUIT INTAKE

Starting today, you're going to eat four servings of fruit a day, says Scott. Slice it on top of cereal, add it to salads or work it into desserts.

But remember that calories add up quickly in dried fruit, she adds. With the water removed, dried fruits seem like smaller portions than they really are, and people tend to overindulge. Unfortunately, dried fruit has only lost its water, not its calories.

DAY 38: MAKE YOUR FRUITS AND VEGETABLES WORK TWICE

Despite the recommendation that you eat at least nine servings a day of fruits and vegetables, some of us simply can't afford even those extra calories.

That's why you really have to eat smart, says Alphin. If you can't eat as many servings of fruits and vegetables as you should, then make sure the servings you do eat satisfy several nutrient requirements at once.

Many experts suggest, for example, that you eat a lot of carotenoids. Others suggest that you fill up with foods that are rich in vitamin C. But why not eat foods that have both? Fruits and vegetables that contain a double-barreled shot of both beta-carotene and vitamin C include oranges, cantaloupe, raspberries, apricots, carrots, winter squash, yams, spinach, sweet potatoes, broccoli and chard.

DAY 39: TALK TO THE PRODUCE PERSON AT YOUR MARKET

This person does more than just keep the potato bin stocked. He or she is also a goldmine of information about the produce for sale there.

You can find out what makes an apple crisp and whether the one you're about to buy is the right choice. You may also learn that the sweetest carrots are the ones with their foliage intact and that large onions are sweeter than small ones. There's no better way to encourage yourself—and your family—to eat more vegetables and fruits than to put the freshest, most flavorful ones on the table.

DAY 40: DEVELOP YOUR OWN CULINARY SIGNATURE

Sad to say, some of us never learn how to cook vegetables in a way that delivers every ounce of flavor and nutrition. So today your assignment is to visit the local library, check out a bunch of cookbooks that espouse healthy eating and study the vegetable sections.

Note the different ways expert cooks work with vegetables. They usually end up steaming or stir-frying (in broth, not fat), but preparation and seasoning techniques vary so much from one cook to another that each person literally creates his or her own culinary signature. That's typically done by adding an aromatic such as garlic, fresh gingerroot, caraway seeds or fresh herbs such as rosemary, thyme or sage.

What's your culinary signature going to be? Study the cookbooks, then go experiment in the kitchen. It's the only way you'll ever find out.

DAY 41: MAKE THE FINAL ADJUSTMENTS

Today you're going to run a happiness check. Close your eyes, put your hands on your tummy, and ask yourself: "How do I feel?"

"If you find you're feeling hungry all the time or low in energy, then add more starches, fruits and vegetables," says Alphin. If not, then turn on the cruise control and continue enjoying your new way of eating.

DAY 42: GLAZE YOUR BROCCOLI WITH LEMON

Congratulations! You've spent six weeks eliminating fat, slashing cholesterol, sifting out salt, fortifying with grains, cutting down on calories and increasing fruits and vegetables. To send you off on your own with a reminder of precisely how delicious healthy eating can be, we've included this final recipe for broccoli with lemon glaze (see page 526).

You're probably feeling a whole lot better—maybe a few pounds lighter—than when you started the program. But these past six weeks have been just a beginning. And the rest is up to you.

HIGH-NUTRITION RECIPE

BROCCOLI WITH LEMON GLAZE

Here's a recipe from the Culinary Institute of America as demonstrated by Chef Dieter Doppelfeld. Please note that the lemon glaze is also delicious served with other vegetables, such as asparagus.

1½ cups defatted chicken stock
2 tablespoons lemon juice
1½ teaspoons grated fresh ginger
1½ teaspoons grated lemon rind
¼ teaspoon ground black pepper
1½ teaspoons arrowroot or cornstarch
2 tablespoons water
1 head broccoli (about 1 pound)
2 teaspoons toasted sesame seeds

In a 2-quart saucepan over medium-high heat, boil the stock, lemon juice, ginger, lemon rind and pepper until the mixture is reduced to about ½ cup, about 10 to 15 minutes.

In a cup, dissolve the arrowroot or cornstarch in the water. Whisk into the stock mixture and cook over medium heat, stirring constantly, until thickened, about 2 minutes. Strain into a small bowl.

Meanwhile, trim the broccoli and cut into thin stalks. Steam until tender, about 5 minutes. Serve drizzled with the glaze and sprinkled with the sesame seeds.

Serves 4
Per serving: *59 calories, 1.5 g. fat (19% of calories), 3.5 g. dietary fiber, 0 mg. cholesterol, 62 mg. sodium*

INDEX

NOTE: Page references in *italic* indicate tables.

A

Acerola, 205
Acetone peroxide, 220
Acetylcholine, 256
Acne, dietary treatment of, 334
Additives. *See* Food additives
Adolescence, nutrient needs in, 80
Adzuki beans, 200, 415
Aging, 80–82, 301–8
  choline and, 257
  diet for, 305, 306
  exercise and, 305, 306–7
  mental performance and, 307
  from oxidation, 192–93
  RDAs and, 303
  vision and, 5–6, 307–8
  vitamin D and, 150
  vitamin E and, 263
  water needs and, 213–14
  weight and, 305–7, 440
Air pollution
  nutrients depleted by, 60–61
  vitamin C and, 51–52
Alcohol
  calcium reduced by, 151
  cancer risk from, 315, 318
  guidelines for consumption of, 377
  heart disease and, 280–81
  motion sickness from, 355
  nutrient needs and, 74–76
  stroke and, 364
Alcoholism
  diet and, 74–75
  dietary treatment of, 334–35
  thiamine deficiency and, 36
Alfalfa, lupus and, 354
Allergy
  dietary treatment of, 335
  to food, 481–82
  to food additives, 217
  to food colorings, 217, 227
  to sulfites, 225–27
Allium vegetables, 204
Aluminum intake, 476–77
Alzheimer's disease, 256, 476
Amaranth, 208, 418
Amino acids, 11–12
Anaphylaxis, 227
Anasazi beans, 200, 415
Anemia, iron-deficiency, 41, 164
  in pregnancy, 328–29
Angina, 273, 335–36
Anorexia nervosa, dietary treatment of, 336–37
Antacids, 67, 153
Antibiotics, nutrients depleted by, 67
Antidepressants, nutrients depleted by, 67
Antinutrient chemicals, 68–70
Antioxidants, 51–54, 184–94. *See also* Beta-carotene; Vitamin C; Vitamin E
  aging and, 304, 308
  for arterial health, 284–85
  for autoimmune disease prevention, 266
  benefits of, 4
  for cancer prevention, 312–13, 314, 318
  for cataracts, 186–87, 308
  in diet, 190–91
  for elderly, 82

Antioxidants *(continued)*
food sources, 318
for free radicals protection, 77
in green tea, 316
high-antioxidant recipes
Dijon Pasta Salad, 193
Fruit Salad Supreme, 194
for macular degeneration, 187
for Parkinson's disease prevention, 358–59
role in body, 186–87
stress and, 63–64
when to take, 192
Anxiety
dietary treatment of, 337
nutrients depleted by, 63–64
Aphrodisiacs, 324–25
Apples, 206
Applesauce Cake, 169
Apricots, 206
Pork with Apricots, 270
Arrhythmias, dietary treatment of, 340–41
Arteries
blocked, 106
fish, eating, for pliability of, 282
plaque deposits in, 273
of vegetarians, 457–58
Arthritis
fasting and, 480–81
foods contributing to, 474
osteoarthritis, 357–58
rheumatoid, 362–63
vegetarian diet for, 460–61
Arugula, 202
Ascorbic acid. *See* Vitamin C
Asian cuisines, 231–32, 401
Aspartame, 221–22
Aspirin, nutrients depleted by, 64–65
Asthma
dietary treatment of, 337–38
milk and, 477
sulfites and, 225–26
vitamin C and, 264
Atherosclerosis, 273, 284
reversal of, 285
vitamin C for prevention of, 187–88
Autoimmune diseases, 266
Avocados
Chicken and Avocado, 130

B

Babies, nutrition for, 78–80
Baking foods, 389–90
Bananas, 206
Cuban-Style Plantains, 181
Barley, 208, 418
Barley Soup, 467
Basic Four Food Groups, 374–76
B-cells, 262
Beans, 200
beef vs., *457*
cooking, 387
for heart disease prevention, 283
in natural food stores, 415
recipes
Grilled Pork Medallions with Braised Beans, 117
Tangy Tofu Salad, 161
Three-Bean Salad, 467
Tuscan Beans, 321
Beef
beans vs., *457*
Beef and Mushroom Lasagna, 132
Gingered Beef and Vegetable Stir-Fry, 170–71
Hearty Meat Loaf, 170
Lean Beef Stroganoff, 118
lean cuts of, 279–80
roast, fast food, *410*
Beriberi, 36
Berries, 206
Raspberries and Honey-Yogurt Cream, 159
Beta-carotene, 24–25. *See also* Vitamin A
absorption, 192

as anti-aging nutrient, 302
as antioxidant, 186–87, 191–92
cancer prevention and, 51, 191–92
breast, 314–15
lung, 315, 316–17
oral, 189
dietary requirements, 191
as food additive, 219
food sources, 25, 192, 318
from foods vs. supplements, 427–28
health benefits, 51
for heart disease prevention, 4, 284, 304
for immune system, 265, 267, 352
smoking and, 73
Beverages
Grapefruit Cooler, 183
Orange Shake, 181
in restaurants, 405
sports drinks, 175, 298
BHA, 220
Biotin, 28
for nail health, 56, 357
Birth defects, preventing, 327–28
with folate, 54–56
with supplements, 78
Blackberries, 206
Black-eyed peas
Black-Eyed Pea Salad, 452–53
Bladder infections, dietary treatment of, 338
Bleeding, vitamin K for control of, 33
Blood cells, iron for, 162
Blood pressure. *See* High blood pressure
Blueberries, 206
Bluefish, 196
Boiling foods, 386–87
Bok choy, 203
Bone health
calcium for, 37, 153–55
fluoride for, 40
vitamin K for, 33–34, 57
Bones
calcium in, 148, 149–50
osteoporosis, 150–53, 358
Brain, 244–57
choline and, 256–57
fatty acids in, 245
mental dysfunction from malnutrition, 246
mental performance, breakfast and, 246–47
minerals important to, 250–51
serotonin and, 252
vitamins important to, 248–49
Braising foods, 392
Bran
as fiber supplement, 90
as laxative, 89
oat, 88, 283
Bread
in natural food stores, 416–17
potassium from, 179
whole-grain, 208
Breakfast
for adults, 250–52
for children, 246–47
for energy and performance, 295, 296
fast food, *410*
in restaurants, 409–10
Breast cancer
fat intake and, 107
prevention, 314–15, 338–39
calcium for, 157
fiber for, 90, 91
Breastfeeding, 10, 79–80, 331
Breasts, fibrocystic, dietary treatment of, 347–48
Brewer's yeast, potassium from, 179–80
Broccoflower, 203–4
Sesame Broccoflower
203

Broccoli, 203
  Broccoli with Lemon Glaze, 526
  in ethnic cuisines, 233
  Tangy Tofu Salad, 161
Broiling foods, 388–89
Broth, in eating program, 522
Brussels sprouts, 204
Buckwheat, 208
Bulgur, cooking, 386
Butter
  as heart disease risk factor, 278–79
  nut, in eating program, 518

C

Cabbage, 203
  Stuffed Cabbage, 144
Caffeine, 251–52
  for asthma, 337
  bone disease from, 151
  consumption, determining, 471
  effects, 470–72
  energy and, 295, 297
Cake
  Applesauce Cake, 169
Calcium, 37–38, 147–61
  absorption
    reduced by fiber, 65
    reduced by beverages, 151
  for adolescents, 80
  as anti-aging nutrient, 302
  benefits, 147
  for bone health, 148, 149–50, 153–55
  for cancer prevention, 156–57, 311, 312, 318
  from dairy products, 201–2
  deficiency, 251
  dietary requirements, 147–48, 158, *159*
  for elderly, 81
  from ethnic foods, 234
  food sources, 38, *38*, 157–58
    best and worst, *154–55*
  for high blood pressure, 155–56, 350
  high-calcium recipes
    Kale and Potato Casserole, 160–61
    Louisiana Salmon Cakes, 160
    Raspberries and Honey-Yogurt Cream, 159
    Tangy Tofu Salad, 161
  for menstrual problems, 156
  for muscle cramps, 157, 356
  nutrient interaction with, 68–69
  osteoporosis and, 152, 358
  overdose hazards, 153
  for periodontal disease, 359
  phosphorus and, 150
  in pregnancy, 330
  for premature birth prevention, 157
  for premenstrual syndrome, 57
  quiz on, 494–96
  role in body, 148–50
  supplements, 152–53, 155
  in vegetarian diet, 77, 465–66
  vitamin D and, 5, 150
Calcium disodium EDTA, 220
Calories
  aging and, 305–6
  from carbohydrates, 18, 19
  from fat, 20, 21, 109, 112, *112*, 279, 311, 444–45
  ideal levels of, by sex and body type, *510–11*
  intake required for weight loss, calculating, 450–51
  low-calorie recipe
    Broccoli with Lemon Glaze, 526
  reduced in eating program, 524–25
  sleepiness from, 255
Cancer. *See also specific types*
  alcohol and, 315, 318

anti-cancer recipes
Oven-Roasted Tomato Soup, 319
Pan-Seared Lamb, 319–20
Rigatoni in Mushroom Broth, 320
Tuscan Beans, 321
ethnic foods and, 233
fat and, 107–8
potassium for prevention of, 176
prevention, through dietary factors, 309–21
antioxidants, 4
beta-carotene, 51, 191–92, 265
calcium, 156–57
fiber, 90–91
folate, 32
garlic, 313
green tea, 316
key factors, 310–11
recipes, 319–21
selenium, 46
studies, 310
vegetarian diet, 458–59
vitamin B_{12}, 27
vitamin C, 51, 188
vitamin D, 5
vitamin E, 189–90
from salt-cured, smoked and nitrite-preserved foods, 310
tretinoin therapy for, 57
Canker sores, dietary treatment of, 340
Canola oil, 208
Cantaloupe, 206
Capsaicin, cholesterol lowered by, 229
Carbohydrates, 15–19
in American diet, 8
in balanced menu, 22
carbo-loading, 292, 293
for cholesterol reduction, 128
craving for, 254
dietary requirements, 18–19
digestion, 16
for energy, 15, 290–93, 295
muscle and, 18
nutrient absorption increased by, 66
protein and, 255, 293
relaxation effect of, 293
serotonin and, 252–55
simple vs. complex, 15–17
in specific foods, *291*
in sports drinks, 298
vegetables high in, 204
weight control and, 18–19, 445–47
Cardiac arrhythmias, dietary treatment of, 340–41
Cardiovascular system, fat in, 106
Carpal tunnel syndrome, dietary treatment of, 341–42
Carrots, 202
Creamy Carrot Soup, 146
Spiced Carrots, 286–87
Cataracts
antioxidants for prevention of, 186–87, 308
dietary treatment of, 342
fruits and vegetables for prevention of, 5–6
vision and, 307–8
Cauliflower, 203
Celiac disease, dietary treatment of, 342–43
Cereals
in eating program, 520
fiber in, 94, *95*, 208
fortified, 219
in natural food stores, 417
Cervical cancer, dietary treatment of, 339
Cheese
healthy cooking with, 393
low-fat, 202
in eating program, 514
microwaving, 394
in vegetarian diet, 464

Chemicals. *See also* Food additives; Pollution
- food colorings, 217, 227
- nutrients depleted by, 68–70

Cherries, 206, 349
Chestnuts, 208–9
- Savory Glazed Chestnuts, 209

Chicken, 198
- Breast of Chicken Italian, 451
- Chicken and Avocado, 130
- Chicken and Rice Casserole, 101
- Chicken Sausage Links, 145
- cholesterol in, 126
- fast food, *410*

Chick-peas, 200
- Portuguese Chick-Peas, 239

Children
- breakfast for, 246–47
- supplements for, 247, 250

Chili
- Chili-Topped Potatoes, 99

Chili peppers, 204
Chinese cabbage, 203
Chinese cuisine, 401, 402
Cholesterol, 120–32. See also High-density lipoprotein (HDL) cholesterol
- in American diet, 123–24, 275
- blood, reduced by
  - capsaicin, 229
  - fiber, 89, 200, 283, 284
  - garlic, 280–81
  - low-fat diet, 129
  - niacin, 56
- from pizza, 272
- dietary reduction of, 128–29, 276–77, 278
- in eating program, reduction of, 516–18
- in eggs, 124–25
- from fat, 105–6
- foods high and low in, *122–23*, 125–27
- heart disease from, 120–21, 273–76
- low-cholesterol recipes
  - Beef and Mushroom Lasagna, 132
  - Chicken and Avocado, 130
  - Lean California Burgers, 130–31
  - Oriental Seafood and Rice Salad, 131
  - Salmon Wrapped in Phyllo, 518–19
- meal size and frequency and, 125
- oat bran and, 88
- role in body, 121–22
- saturated fat and, 124, 272
- from seafood, 126–27, *127*, 197
- transport in body, 272–73
- in vegetarians, 456
- vitamin C and, 188

Cholesterol-lowering drugs, nutrients depleted by, 68
Choline, 79, 256–57
Chromium, 38–39
- brain and emotions and, 251
- for diabetes, 345
- high-density lipoprotein and, 57–58

Chronic fatigue syndrome, magnesium for, 42
Cigarettes. *See* Smoking
Citrus fruits, 205
Clams, 198
- Linguine with Clam Sauce, 171

Coffee, 251–52
- for asthma, 337
- bone disease from, 151
- effects, 470–72
- heart disease and, 286
- iron absorption inhibited by, 70, 166

Colds, 51, 343
Colitis, ulcerative, dietary treatment of, 365
Colon cancer, prevention of, 310, 311–13, 339
- calcium for, 156–57

fiber for, 90–91
by reduced fat intake, 107–8
Condiments, homemade, salt-free, 141
Constipation, fiber for, 89–90, 343–44
Cooking
adverse effects of, 383
baking and roasting, 389–90
boiling, 179, 386–87
braising, 392
for fat reduction, 391
in eating program, 513
from meat, 114–15
fried foods, 522
grilling and broiling, 388–89
light, 383–94
for maximal iron, 166
microwaving, 392–94
nutrients depleted by, 61–63, 179
poaching, 385
steaming, 384–85
stir-frying, 385–88
Cooking oils. *See* Oils, cooking
Copper, 39–40
food sources, 39, *40*
for immune system, 268
Corn, 204
Cottage cheese, low-fat, 202
Couscous
Couscous Salad with Oranges and Figs, 241
Cramps. *See* Muscle cramps
Cranberry juice, for bladder infections, 338
Cream, healthy use of, in eating program, 515
Creamers, nondairy, 521
Crohn's disease, dietary treatment of, 344

D

Dairy products, 201–2
calcium from, 157, 158
for cancer prevention, 311
celiac disease and, 342
in ethnic foods, 233–34
fat reduction in, 393
intolerance, 148–49
Depression, 55, 344–45
Desserts, 236, 408–9
Diabetes
chromium and, 38–39
dietary fat and, 109
dietary treatment of, 345
fiber for, 91–92
vegetarian diet for, 460
Diet. *See also* Nutrition
of Americans, surveys of, 8
in Asian countries, 231–32
assessment of, computerized, 504
changes in, as medical treatment, 6–7
controversies, 469–82
for elderly, 305, 306
heart disease and, 274–75, 276–77
for immune system, 267–68
low-fat, 110–13
macrobiotic, 475–76
in Mediterranean countries, 230–31
program (*see* Eating program)
quizzes on, 485–503
U.S. Navy study results, 6
variety in, 72
vegetarian (*see* Vegetarian diet)
Dietary Guidelines, 376–77
Dieting, 437
fad diets, 438–39
nutrient needs and, 71–72
starvation, 439–41
Digestive process, 16–17
Dining out, 398–412
for breakfast, 409–10
for dinner, 404–9
fast food, *410–11*
fat reduction and, 113–14
food amounts consumed, 408
for lunch, 410–12
menus, reading, 406, 407
variety in, 402–4

Dinner
for energy and performance, 297
in restaurants, 404–9
Diuretics, nutrients depleted by, 66–67
Diverticulosis, 93, 346
Drinking. *See* Alcohol
Drinks. *See* Beverages
Drugs, nutrients depleted by, 64–68
Duck, 198

E

Eating behavior
awareness of, 442
overeating, 439
quiz on, 497–501
Eating program, 505–26
calories reduced in, 524–26
cholesterol reduced in, 516–19
fat reduced in, 506–16
grains increased in, 519–21
oil reduced in, 521–23
recipes
Broccoli with Lemon Glaze, 526
Magic Molasses Muffins, 523
Salmon Wrapped in Phyllo, 518–19
Sweet Potato Soup, 516
Eggs, cholesterol in, 124–25
Egg substitutes, 125–26
in eating program, 517
Elderly. *See* Aging
Electrolytes
arrhythmias from imbalance of, 341
balance of, 175–76
from sports drinks, 175
Emotions
food cravings and, 253
serotonin and, 252
Endive, 203
Energy and performance, 289–300. *See also* Fatigue; Mental performance
carbohydrates for, 290–93
dietary plan for, 294–97
fat and, 294
high-energy recipes
Poached Salmon with Potato Pancakes, 299
Turkey Pita Sandwiches, 300
nutrition for, 289–90
protein for, 293–94
reduced by caffeine and sugar, 297
reduced by nutritional deficiencies, 297–98
Energy bars, in natural food stores, 419–20
Epilepsy, dietary treatment of, 346–47
Esophageal cancer, molybdenum for prevention of, 44
Estrogen, 314, 326
Ethnic foods, 228–41, 401–3
calcium and protein from, 234
desserts, 236
fiber from, 235–36
health benefits of, 229–30
high-nutrition recipes
Couscous Salad with Oranges and Figs, 241
Fettucine with Pesto Sauce, 239
Paella, 240
Portuguese Chick-Peas, 239
incorporated in diet, 236–38
low-fat, 401
meat-vegetable balance in, 231–32
natural tenderizers, 233
pasta, 234–36
quiz on, 502–3
shopping for, 237
Exercise. *See also* Energy and performance
aging and, 305, 306–7

nutrient needs increased by, 76–77
potassium depleted by, 175
water needs increased by, 214
Eye round roast, 200
Eyesight. *See* Vision

F

Fast foods, *410–11*
in eating program, 521–22
fiber from, 86–87
Fasting, 480–81
Fat, 19–21
in American diet, 8, 275
angina from buildup of, 336
in balanced menu, 22
calories from, 20, 21, 109, 112, *112,* 279, 311, 444–45
cancer risk increased by, 107–8, 310–11, 314
breast, 338
colon, 338
in cooking oils, 208
diabetes and dietary, 109
dietary guidelines for, 376
dietary requirements for, 19–20
digestion, 16
fatigue from, 294
in Food Guide Pyramid, 378
foods high and low in, *104–5*
health dangers of, 20–21, 103–4
heart and artery disease from, 105–6, 273–75
in "lite" vs. regular food products, 108
low-fat eating, 103–19
low-fat recipes
Creamy Pasta Shells, 119
Grilled Pork Medallions with Braised Beans, 117
Lean Beef Stroganoff, 118
Lightly Breaded Halibut, 116
Sweet Potato Soup, 516
metabolism, 109
obesity and, 108–9, 357
Ornish approach, 106
permitted at various calorie levels, in eating program, *507*
quiz on, 492–93
reduction, 21, 110–11, 277–80, 317
in cooking, 391, 400
cooking meat and, 114–15
in dairy products, 393
dining out tips, 113–14
in eating program, 506–16
by oil reduction, 115–16
by Pritikin Plan, 111–13, 129
by revising recipes, 114
shopping tips for, 113
in vegetarian diet, 464
for weight loss, 443–45, 446
in restaurant entrées, 406–7
role in body, 21, 245
saturated
cholesterol and, 124, 272
dietary reduction of, 277, 279
in seafood, *127*
unsaturated fat and, 19, *20*
stroke from buildup of, 363
study, with Tarahumara Indians, 104–5
substitutes, 223–24
types of, 19
in vegetarian vs. nonvegetarian dinner, *457*
vitamin E and, 189
Fatigue. *See also* Energy and performance
chronic fatigue syndrome, magnesium for, 42
dietary treatment of, 347
from fat, 294
Feingold diet, for hyperactive children, 478–80
Fertility. *See* Infertility

Fiber, 85–102
amount required, 97–98
from baked goods, 390, 392
from breakfast cereals, *95*
cancer prevention and, 90–91, 311–12, 314
breast, 314, 338–39
colon, 339
from carbohydrates, 17
cautions, 97–98
cholesterol reduced by, 89, 200
for constipation, 89–90, 343–44
for diabetes, 91–92
for diverticulosis, 346
in eating program, 520–21
from ethnic foods, 235–36
from fast foods, 86–87
food sources, *92–93*, 94, 96–97, *96*, 317
fortified, 219
for gallstone prevention, 94
health benefits of, 85–87, 88–94
for heart disease prevention, 282–84
high-fiber recipes
Chicken and Rice Casserole, 101
Chili-Topped Potatoes, 99
Orange-Raisin Muffins, 100
Spiced Fruit Compote, 102
for intestinal ills, 93
introducing, slowly, 98
iron absorption inhibited by, 166
for irritable bowel syndrome, 352
nutrient absorption reduced by, 65
for obesity, 357
for oral health, 94
quiz on, 493–94
soluble vs. insoluble, 88
supplements, 90
for weight loss, 91, 447, 450
Fibrocystic breasts, dietary treatment of, 347–48
Figs, 207
Couscous Salad with Oranges and Figs, 241
Fish, 196–97. *See also* Seafood; *specific types*
cooking
baking, 390
grilling or broiling, 388–89
microwaving, 394
stir-frying, 387–88
in eating program, 512, 517
fast food, *411*
for heart disease prevention, 282
recipes
Ginger-Scented Mackerel, 288
Herring and Potato Gratin, 197
Lightly Breaded Halibut, 116
Louisiana Salmon Cakes, 160
Mahi Mahi with Jamaican Tartar Sauce, 396
Poached Salmon with Potato Pancakes, 299
Salmon Wrapped in Phyllo, 518–19
Sea Salad, 287
Fish oil. *See also* Omega–3 fatty acids
for ulcerative colitis, 365
Five-a-Day Plan, for disease prevention, 381–82
Flavonoids, for allergies, 335
Flounder, 196
Flour, fiber from, 390
Fluids. *See also* Water
for elderly, 81–82
Fluoride, 40
Folate, 32–33
as anti-aging nutrient, 302
birth defects prevented by, 54–56, 327–28
cervical cancer prevented by, 339
deficiency, 248–49
for elderly, 307

for epilepsy, 346
food sources, 32, *33*
for immune system, 267
for restless legs syndrome, 362

Food(s)
basic four groups, 374–76
redefined, 379–81
combining, 473
cravings and aversions, in pregnancy, 328–29
ethnic (*see* Ethnic foods)
fast (*see* Fast foods)
fortification, 219
importance to survival, 10–11
irradiated, 474–75
101 healthiest, 195–209
raw, 472–73

Food additives, 217–27
allergy to, 217
aspartame, 221–22
historical aspects, 219–21
MSG, 222
nitrites, 222–23
pesticides, 224–25
purposes of specific additives, 220
Simplesse, 223–24
sulfites, 225–27
tartrazine, 227
vitamins and minerals, 219

Food allergy, 481–82

Food colorings, 217, 227

Food colorings and flavorings, hyperactivity in children from, 478, 479, 480

Food controversies, 469–82

Food Guide Pyramid, 377–79

Food labels
cholesterol information on, 128
for natural foods, 422–23
sodium information on, 141

Food preparation. *See* Cooking

Food processing, potassium loss from, *178*

Food safety, quiz on, 501–2

Food shopping
for ethnic foods, 237
for low-fat items, 113
for low-sodium items, 141–43, *142*

Fractures, calcium for prevention of, 151, 153–54

Free radicals, 4, 51, 61, 185. *See also* Antioxidants
aging from, 192–93, 304
increased by exercise, 76

French cuisine, 403

Fried foods, 522

Fructose, 15

Fruit juice
potassium from, 177, 179
smoking and, 73

Fruits, 204–5
baking, 390
berries, 206
for cancer prevention, 311, 312, 313, 314
for cararact prevention, 5–6
citrus, 205
in diet, 19
dietary guidelines for, 376
dried, 207
in eating program, 524
in ethnic cuisines, 236, 238
in Food Guide Pyramid, 377–78
high-fiber, 206
for immune system, 267
for iron absorption, 165–66
microwaving, 394
orange-yellow, 206
pesticides on, 224–25
potassium from, 179, 180
recipes
Fruit Salad Supreme, 194
Island Paradise Salad, 206–7
Spiced Fruit Compote, 102
Warm Fruit Soufflés, 453
vitamin C from, 205

G

Gallstones, 94, 348
Garbanzo beans. *See* Chick-peas
Garlic, 204, 421
  for cancer prevention, 313
  for heart disease prevention, 280–81
Gas, from fiber, 98
Gastritis, atrophic, 81
Ginger
  Gingered Beef and Vegetable Stir-Fry, 170–71
  Ginger-Scented Mackerel, 288
  for motion sickness, 355, 421
Ginseng, as aphrodisiac, 324
Glucose, 15, 16, 17
  absorption, fiber and, 88, 91–92
  tolerance, 38
Glycogen, 293, 446–47
Goose, 198
Gout, dietary treatment of, 348–49
Grains, 207–8
  cooking, 386–87
  in diet, 19
  dietary guidelines for, 376
  fiber from, 94
  in Food Guide Pyramid, 377, 378
  microwaving, 393–94
  in natural food stores, 418
  recipes
    Barley Soup, 467
    Chicken and Rice Casserole, 101
    Couscous Salad with Oranges and Figs, 241
    Oriental Seafood and Rice Salad, 131
    Paella, 240
    Shrimp Creole with Brown Rice, 268
Grapefruit
  Grapefruit Cooler, 183
  pink, 205
Grilling foods, 388–89
Gums, periodontal disease and, 359

H

Haddock, 196
Hair analysis tests, 498–99
Hamburgers, fast food, *410*
Headache, dietary treatment of, 349
Health food stores. *See* Natural food stores
Heart and arteries, reducing risks to, 271–88
Heart attack
  beta-carotene for prevention of, 25, 284, 304
  from high cholesterol, 121
  vitamin E for prevention of, 53–54
Heartburn, dietary treatment of, 349–50
Heart disease
  angina, 273, 335–36
  arrhythmia, 340–41
  coffee and, 286
  from copper deficiency, 39
  dietary risk factors, 271–72
  from fat and cholesterol, 105–6, 120–21, 274–76
  from high sodium intake, 134, 136
  lifestyle and, 285
  from magnesium deficiency, 42
  mitral valve prolapse, 355
  prevention, 275, 276–84
    beta-carotene for, 4
    potassium for, 174
    vitamin C for, 29, 187–88
  reversed by diet, 276–77
Heart health
  from Asian diet, 232
  from Mediterranean diet, 230–31
  recipes for
    Creamy Mashed Potatoes, 288
    Ginger-Scented Mackerel, 288
    Sea Salad, 287
    Spiced Carrots, 286–87
  vegetarian diet for, 455, 456
Heat, nutrients depleted by, 61–63

Herbs, in natural food stores, 420–21
Herring, 196
    Herring and Potato Gratin, 197
High blood pressure
    calcium for, 151, 155–56
    dietary treatment of, 350–51
    potassium for, 45, 174, 176
    pregnancy-induced, 330
    from salt, 133, 134, 136–37
    vegetarian diet for, 458
High-density lipoprotein (HDL) cholesterol, 122–23
    chromium and, 57–58
    created in liver, 272
    vitamin C and, 188
High-nutrition recipes
    Applesauce Cake, 169
    Barley Soup, 467
    Beef and Mushroom Lasagna, 132
    Black-Eyed Pea Salad, 452–53
    Breaded Oysters, 269
    Breast of Chicken Italian, 451
    Broccoli with Lemon Glaze, 526
    Chicken and Avocado, 130
    Chicken and Rice Casserole, 101
    Chicken Sausage Links, 145
    Chili-Topped Potatoes, 99
    Couscous Salad with Oranges and Figs, 241
    Creamy Carrot Soup, 146
    Creamy Mashed Potatoes, 288
    Creamy Pasta Shells, 119
    Cuban-Style Plantains, 181
    Dijon Pasta Salad, 193
    Fettucine with Pesto Sauce, 239
    Fruit Salad Supreme, 194
    German Potato Salad, 182
    Gingered Beef and Vegetable Stir-Fry, 170–71
    Ginger-Scented Mackerel, 288
    Grapefruit Cooler, 183
    Grilled Pork Medallions with Braised Beans, 117
    Hearty Meat Loaf, 170
    Herring and Potato Gratin, 197
    Huevos Rancheros, 452
    Island Paradise Salad, 206–7
    Kale and Potato Casserole, 160–61
    Lean Beef Stroganoff, 118
    Lean California Burgers, 130–31
    Lightly Breaded Halibut, 116
    Linguine with Clam Sauce, 171
    Louisiana Salmon Cakes, 160
    Magic Molasses Muffins, 523
    Mahi Mahi with Jamaican Tartar Sauce, 396
    Microwave Lasagna, 395
    Orange-Raisin Muffins, 100
    Orange Shake, 181
    Oriental Seafood and Rice Salad, 131
    Oven-Roasted Tomato Soup, 319
    Paella, 240
    Pan-Seared Lamb, 319–20
    Poached Salmon with Potato Pancakes, 299
    Pork with Apricots, 270
    Portuguese Chick-Peas, 239
    Raspberries and Honey-Yogurt Cream, 159
    Rigatoni in Mushroom Broth, 320–21
    Salmon Wrapped in Phyllo, 518–19
    Savory Glazed Chestnuts, 209
    Savory Roasted Onions, 396
    Scallop Stir-Fry, 397
    Sea Salad, 287
    Sesame Broccoflower, 203
    Shrimp Creole with Brown Rice, 268
    Spaghetti with Tofu Sauce, 468
    Spiced Carrots, 286–87
    Spiced Fruit Compote, 102
    Spicy Venison Stew, 199
    Spinach Pie, 466
    Stuffed Cabbage, 144
    Sweet Potato Salad, 269
    Sweet Potato Soup, 516
    Tangy Tofu Salad, 161
    Three-Bean Salad, 467

High-nutrition recipes *(continued)*
- Turkey Pita Sandwiches, 300
- Tuscan Beans, 321
- Warm Fruit Soufflés, 453
- Warm Lentil Salad, 201
- Yams with Honey Topping, 145

Hip fractures, calcium for prevention of, 153–54
Homocysteine, 27
Honey
- Raspberries with Honey-Yogurt Cream, 159
- Yams with Honey Topping, 145

Honeydews, 205
Hormone replacement therapy, for osteoporosis prevention, 152–53
Hyperactivity, 351
- in children, dietary treatment of, 218, 478–80

Hypertension. *See* High blood pressure

I

Immune system, 258–70
- antioxidants for, 304
- autoimmune diseases, 266
- eating plan for, 267–68
- feeding formulas for peak immunity, 259
- mechanisms, 260–62
- nutrients important to, 262–66, 352–53
- recipes for healthy
  - Breaded Oysters, 269
  - Pork with Apricots, 270
  - Shrimp with Brown Rice, 268
  - Sweet Potato Salad, 269
- vitamin B_6 for, 56, 303
- vitamin E for, 54, 303

Indian cuisine, 402–3
Infancy, nutrient needs in, 78–80
Infections
- bladder, dietary treatment of, 338
- vaginal yeast, dietary treatment of, 366–67

Infertility, 322–27
- dietary treatment of, 351–52
- vitamin C for, 325–26, 351
- weight and, 326–27, 352
- zinc for, 323–25, 352

Influenza, dietary treatment of, 352
Injury, nutrients depleted by, 64
Insulin
- diabetes and, 345
- fat intake and, 109
- fiber and, 91–92

Intelligence, nutrients for, 247, 250
International cuisines. *See* Ethnic foods
Iodine, 40–41
Iron, 41–42, 162–71
- absorption, 70, 165–66
- for adolescents, 80
- cooking and, 166
- deficiency, 41, 164, 168–69, 250, 297–98
- dietary requirements, 163–64, *163*
- from enriched and fortified food, 166–68
- food sources, 41, *42*, 165–68, *167*
- heme vs. nonheme, 165
- high-iron recipes
  - Applesauce Cake, 169
  - Gingered Beef and Vegetable Stir-Fry, 170–71
  - Hearty Meat Loaf, 170
  - Linguine with Clam Sauce, 171
- for immune system, 267–68
- nutrient interaction with, 69
- overload and toxicity, 59, 168, 169
- for pregnancy, 328–29
- for restless legs syndrome, 362
- role in body, 162–63
- from shellfish, 198
- from spinach, 69
- supplements, 169
- in vegetarian diet, 77, 465

Irradiated foods, 474–75

Irritable bowel syndrome, dietary treatment of, 353
Ischemia, vitamin E and, 188–89
Italian cuisine, 402–3

J

Japanese cuisine, 402
Junk food, disguised as health food, 422–23

K

Kale, 203
 Kale and Potato Casserole, 160–61
Kidney beans, 200
 Tangy Tofu Salad, 161
Kidney disease, from protein excess, 14
Kidneys, of diabetics, protected by vegetarian diet, 460
Kidney stones, dietary treatment of, 353
Kiwifruit, 205
Kwashiorkor, 13–14

L

Lactase, 148, 149
Lactose, 15
 intolerance, 148–49, 342
Lamb
 foreshank, 200
 Pan-Seared Lamb, 319–20
Laxatives, 65–66, 89
Leeks, 204
Legumes, 200
 for heart disease prevention, 283
 potassium from, 179
Lemon juice, as salt substitute, 141
Lemons, 205
Lentils, 200
 Warm Lentil Salad, 201
Lettuce, 203
Lima beans, 200
Limes, 205
Linoleic acid, 19–20
Lipids. *See* Fat
Lipoproteins, 121–23. *See also* High-density lipoprotein (HDL) cholesterol; Low-density lipoprotein (LDL) cholesterol
Low-density lipoprotein (LDL) cholesterol, 121–22
 created in liver, 272
 fiber for reduction of, 89
 meal size and frequency and, 125
Lunch
 for energy and performance, 296
 in restaurants, 410–12
Lung cancer, prevention of, 315–17, 340
 beta-carotene and, 191–92
 vitamin C and, 188
Lupus, dietary treatment of, 354
Lymphocytes, 261–62
Lysine, 12

M

Mackerel, 196
 Ginger-Scented Mackerel, 288
Macrobiotic diet, 475–76
Macrophages, 260–61
Macular degeneration
 antioxidants for, 187
 dietary treatment of, 354–55
 zinc for, 58
Magnesium, 42–43
 for angina, 336
 deficiency, 251
 for fatigue, 347
 food sources, 42, *43*
 for high blood pressure, 350
 mitral valve prolapse and, 355
 for muscle cramps, 356
 in pregnancy, 330
Malnutrition, obesity and, 72
Manganese, 43–44
Mangoes, 206
Marasmus, 13–14
Marinating foods, 389–90
Meals
 for energy and performance, 294–97

Meals *(continued)*
size and frequency, cholesterol and, 125
timing of, 450
Measles, vitamin A and, 57
Measurement units, for vitamins and minerals, 24
Meat, 198–200
alternative protein sources, 15
avoidance, 77
cholesterol from, 126, 128
cooking
braising, 392
for fat reduction, 114–15
grilling or broiling, 388
microwaving, 394
stir-frying, 387–88
in ethnic foods, 232–33
fat reduction and, in eating program, 508, 509, 512
iron from, 165
processed, 512
recipes
Beef and Mushroom Lasagna, 132
Gingered Beef and Vegetable Stir-Fry, 170–71
Grilled Pork Medallions with Braised Beans, 117
Hearty Meat Loaf, 170
Lean Beef Stroganoff, 118
Pan-Seared Lamb, 319–20
Pork with Apricots, 270
Spicy Venison Stew, 199
red, 165, 198–99
Meat substitutes, 421–22, 463
Medications, nutrients depleted by, 64–68
Mediterranean cuisines, 230–31, 402
Memory, choline and, 256
Menopause
bone loss and, 152, 154–55
diet for, 332
Menstrual problems, calcium for, 156
Menstruation, iron loss from, 164
Mental dysfunction, from malnutrition, 246
Mental performance
aging and, 307
breakfast and, 246–47, 252
protein for, 293–94
snacks for, 296
Menus
balanced for carbohydrate, protein and fat, 22
reading, 406, 407
Metabolism, weight loss and, 439–41
Mexican cuisine, 403
fast food, *411*
Huevos Rancheros, 452
Microwaving foods, 63, 392–94
Middle Eastern cuisine, 402
Milk
breast, 79, 256–57, 331
healthy cooking with, 393
low-fat, 202
in eating program, 513–14
mucus and, 477
skim, 201
soy, making, 419
Milk products
calcium from, 157, 158
intolerance of, 148–49
Milk substitutes, in natural food stores, 418
Millet, 387, 418
Minerals. *See also* Nutrients; Supplements
in American diet, 8
essential facts about, 37–48
as food additive, 219
important to brain, 250–51
Recommended Dietary Allowances, *53*, *433*
units of measurement, 24
Mitral valve prolapse, dietary treatment of, 355
Molasses
Applesauce Cake, 169

Magic Molasses Muffins, 523
potassium from, 179
Molybdenum, 44
Monosodium glutamate (MSG), 222
Motion sickness, dietary treatment of, 355–56
Mucus, milk and, 477
Muffins
in eating program, 523
Orange-Raisin Muffins, 100
Mung beans, 415
Muscle, carbohydrates and, 18
Muscle cramps
calcium for, 157
dietary treatment of, 356
potassium for, 175
Mushrooms
Beef and Mushroom Lasagna, 132
Rigatoni in Mushroom Broth, 320
Mussels, 198

N

Nail health, biotin for, 56
Nail problems, dietary treatment of, 356–57
Natural food stores, 413–23
choosing, 414–15
food labels in, 422–23
items in
beans, 415
breads, 416–17
cereals, 417
energy bars, 419–20
grains, 418
herbs, 420–21
meat substitutes, 421–22
milk substitutes, 418
sea vegetables, 416
snacks, 422
sports nutrition supplements, 420
popularity of, 414
prices in, 415
Natural killer cells, 262
Navy beans, 200
Neural tube defects, preventing, 54–55, 327–28
Neurotransmitters, 244–45, 293
serotonin, 252–55, 293
Neutrophils, 260
New Four Food Groups, 379–81
Niacin, 34–35
for cholesterol reduction, 56
deficiency, 249
food sources, 34, *35*
overdose, 59
Nicotine. *See* Smoking
Nightshades, 474
Nitrites, 222–23
cancer risk from, 310, 318
Nondairy creamers, 521
Nursing. *See* Breastfeeding
Nut butters, in eating program, 518
NutraSweet (aspartame), 221–22
Nutrients. *See also* Minerals; Vitamins
bodily absorption of, 432–34
depletion by
alcohol, 74–75
chemicals, 68–70
drugs, 64–68
fiber supplements, 90
heat, 61–63
other nutrients, 68–69
smog, 60–61
smoking, 73
stress, 63–64
as medical treatment, 6–7
meeting needs for, 49–59
Nutri/System, 448
Nutrition. *See also* Diet
American views and practices of, 370–71, 381
approaches to, 371–82
assessment of, computerized, 504
priorities, 372, *372–73*
revolution in, 3–9
special needs, 71–82
surveys, 370, 372, *372–73*, 381

Nutritional deficiencies
energy reduced by, 297–98
obesity and, 72
Nutritional support formulas, 259
Nuts
Savory Glazed Chestnuts, 209
Nuts and seeds, 208–9

O

Oat bran, 88, 283
Oatmeal, 208
Obesity
diabetes from, 109
dietary treatment of, 357
fat and, 108–9, 357
health dangers of, 108
malnutrition and, 72
water needs and, 214
Oils, cooking, 208
fat reduction and, 115–16
heart disease and, 278, 279
reduced in eating program, 521–23
saturated and unsaturated fat in, *20*
Olive oil, 208, 230–31
buying, 231
heart disease and, 278, 279
Omega–3 fatty acids
from fish, 196
for heart health, 282
for immune system, 266, 267
for lupus, 354
for psoriasis, 361
for Raynaud's syndrome, 362
for rheumatoid arthritis, 363
Onions, 204
Savory Roasted Onions, 396
Oral cancer, antioxidants for prevention of, 188, 189
Oranges, 205
Couscous Salad with Oranges and Figs, 241
Orange Shake, 181
Osteoarthritis, dietary treatment of, 357–58
Osteoporosis, 150–53. *See also* Bone health
dietary treatment of, 358
risk factors, 151–52
Overdoses of vitamins and minerals, 28, 58–59
Overeaters Anonymous (OA), 448–49
Overeating, 439
quiz on, 497–501
Overweight. *See* Obesity; Weight loss
Oxalate, nutrient absorption decreased by, 69–70
Oxidation, 184, 185. *See also* Antioxidants
aging from, 192–93
Oysters, 198
as aphrodisiac, 324
Breaded Oysters, 269

P

Pantothenate, 35
Papaya, 206
Parkinson's disease, dietary treatment of, 358–59
Pasta
cooking, 386
in eating program, 520
for energy, 292
in ethnic cuisines, 234–36
recipes
Beef and Mushroom Lasagna, 132
Creamy Pasta Shells, 119
Dijon Pasta Salad, 193
Fettucine with Pesto Sauce, 239
Linguine with Clam Sauce, 171
Microwave Lasagna, 395
Rigatoni in Mushroom Broth, 320–21
Spaghetti with Tofu Sauce, 468
whole-wheat, 208
Peaches, dried, 207

Pears, 206
Peas, 200
Pectin, 283–84, 365
Pellagra, 34
Peppers, 204
Performance and energy. *See* Energy and performance
Periodontal disease, dietary treatment of, 359
Perspiration, 175, 213
Pesticides, residue on foods, 224–25
Pesto
    Fettucine with Pesto Sauce, 239
Phenylalanine, 12, 221–22
Phosphorus, 44–45
    calcium absorption and, 150
    in soft drinks, 151
Phytin, nutrient absorption decreased by, 70
Pineapples, 205
Pink grapefruit, 205
Pinto beans, 200
Pita bread
    Turkey Pita Sandwiches, 300
Pizza
    cholesterol from, 272
    in eating program, 512–13
Plantains
    Cuban-Style Plantains, 181
Poaching foods, 385
Pollution
    air
        nutrients depleted by, 60–61
        vitamin C and, 51–52
    water, 214–16
Polydextrose, 220
Polysorbate 60, 220
Pomegranates, 205
Pork
    Grilled Pork Medallions with Braised Beans, 117
    Pork with Apricots, 270
    tenderloin, 200
Potassium, 45–46, 172–83
    for cancer prevention, 176–77
    dietary requirements, 177
    food sources, 45, *46*, *173*, 177–80
    in fresh vs. processed foods, *178*
    for heart disease prevention, 174
    for high blood pressure, 174, 176, 350
    high-potassium recipes
        Cuban-Style Plantains, 181
        German Potato Salad, 182
        Grapefruit Cooler, 183
        Orange Shake, 181
    for muscle cramps, 356
    in prehistoric and modern diet, 172–74
    sodium and, 139, 172–73, 174–76, 176–77
    from sports drinks, 175
    for stroke prevention, 176, 177, 364
Potatoes, 204
    fast food, *411*
    potassium from, 179
    recipes
        Chili-Topped Potatoes, 99
        Creamy Mashed Potatoes, 288
        German Potato Salad, 182
        Herring and Potato Gratin, 197
        Kale and Potato Casserole, 160–61
        Poached Salmon with Potato Pancakes, 299
Poultry, 198
    cooking
        grilling or broiling, 388
        microwaving, 394
        stir-frying, 387–88
    for heart disease prevention, 282
    recipes
        Breast of Chicken Italian, 451
        Chicken and Avocado, 130
        Chicken and Rice Casserole, 101

Poultry (*continued*)
recipes (*continued*)
Chicken Sausage Links, 145
Lean California Burgers, 130–31
Paella, 240
Stuffed Cabbage, 144
Turkey Pita Sandwiches, 300
Pregnancy. *See also* Infertility
anemia in, 328–29
calcium in, 156, 157
food cravings and aversions in, 328–29
nutrition for, 77–78, 327
preventing birth defects, 54–55, 327–28
Premature birth, calcium for prevention of, 157
Premenstrual syndrome (PMS), 330, 332
calcium for, 57, 156
dietary treatment of, 330, 332, 359–60
Pritikin Plan, 111–13, 129
Prostate enlargement, dietary treatment of, 360–61
Protein, 11–15
in American diet, 8
in balanced menu, 22
carbohydrates and, 255, 293
chemistry, 11–12
deficiency, 13–14
dietary requirements, 14–15
digestion, 16
for energy and performance, 293, 295
from ethnic foods, 234
excessive intake of, 14
in Food Guide Pyramid, 378
food sources, 12, *13*, 294
nutrient absorption decreased by, 66
Simplesse, 223–24
in vegetarian diet, 464
Prunes, 207
Psoriasis, dietary treatment of, 361
Pumpkins, 202, 238
Pumpkin seeds, dried, 209
Purines, gout and, 349
Pyridoxine. *See* Vitamin B_6

Q

Quinoa, 208, 418

R

Raisins, 207
Raspberries, 206
Raspberries and Honey-Yogurt Cream, 159
Raw foods, 472–73
Raynaud's syndrome, dietary treatment of, 361–62
Recipes
high-nutrition (*see* High-nutrition recipes)
reducing fat in, 114
Recommended Dietary Allowances (RDAs), 49–59
determination of, 50
for elderly, 303
exceeding, 50, 190–91
for specific vitamins and minerals, *52–53, 432–33*
U.S. RDAs vs., 54–55
Rectal cancer, 107, 156–57. *See also* Colon cancer, prevention of
Reference Daily Intake (RDI), 55
Restaurants. *See* Dining out
Restless legs syndrome, dietary treatment of, 362
Rheumatoid arthritis, dietary treatment of, 362–63
Riboflavin, 35–36
deficiency, 249
food sources, 35, *36*
Rice
brown, 208
Chicken and Rice Casserole, 101
Oriental Seafood and Rice Salad, 131

Shrimp Creole with Brown Rice, 268
Roast beef, fast food, *410*
Roasting foods, 389–90
Romaine lettuce, 203

S

Salad bars, 412
Salads, in restaurants, 405
Salicylates, hyperactivity from, 351
Salmon, 196
Louisiana Salmon Cakes, 160
Poached Salmon with Potato Pancakes, 299
Salmon Wrapped in Phyllo, 518–19
Salt. *See also* Sodium
benefits, 134
dietary guidelines for, 377
pregnancy and, 328, 330
quiz on, 496–97
sensitivity to, 135–36
Salt-cured foods, cancer risk from, 310, 318
Salt substitutes, potassium in, 178–79
Sandwiches, 412
Sardines
Sea Salad, 287
Sauces, fat reduction in, 400, 406
Scallops
Scallop Stir-Fry, 397
Seafood, 196, 197. *See also* Fish
cholesterol from, 126–27, *127*
protein from, 234
recipes
Breaded Oysters, 269
Lightly Breaded Halibut, 116
Linguine with Clam Sauce, 171
Oriental Seafood and Rice Salad, 131
Paella, 240
Scallop Stir-Fry, 397
Shrimp Creole with Brown Rice, 268
Sea vegetables, in natural food stores, 416
Seeds and nuts, 208–9
Seitan, as meat substitute, 463
Selenium, 46–47
as antioxidant, 190
for breast cancer prevention, 314
food sources, 46, *47*, 318
Serotonin, 252–55, 293
Sesame seeds
Sesame Broccoflower, 203
Sex and reproduction, 322–32
breastfeeding, 10, 79–80, 331
fertility, 322–27
menopause, 332
pregnancy, 327–30
premenstrual syndrome, 330, 332
sex drive, 324–25
Shellfish, 197–98. *See also* Seafood
cholesterol in, 126–27, *127*
Shrimp
Shrimp Creole with Brown Rice, 268
Simplesse, 223–24
Skim milk, 201
Sleepiness, from carbohydrates, 255
Smog, nutrients depleted by, 60–61
Smoked foods, cancer risk from, 310, 318
Smoking
antioxidants and, 188, 189
nutrient needs and, 73
vitamin C and, 264, 326
Snacks
in eating program, 522
in low-fat eating plan, 446
in natural food stores, 422
Sodium, 133–46. *See also* Salt
in American diet, 134–35
benefits and requirements, 134
dietary reduction of, 133–34, 137–39
gradual, 139
at home, 139–41
when dining out, 143–44

Sodium *(continued)*
dietary reduction of *(continued)*
when shopping, 141–43, *142*
in drinking water, 135
food sources, 138–39, *138,* 141, *142,* 143–44
high blood pressure from, 133, 134, 136–37, 350
low-sodium recipes
Chicken Sausage Links, 145
Creamy Carrot Soup, 146
Stuffed Cabbage, 144
Yams with Honey Topping, 145
for muscle cramps, 356
potassium and, 139, 172–73, 174–76, 176–77
sensitivity to, 135–36
Sodium lauryl sulfate, 220
Sodium nitrate, 220
Sodium stearoyl lactylate, 220
Soft drinks, calcium absorption reduced by, 151
Soup
Barley Soup, 467
Creamy Carrot Soup, 146
Oven-Roasted Tomato Soup, 319
potassium from, 180
Rigatoni in Mushroom Broth, 320
Sweet Potato Soup, 516
Sour cream, fat reduction in, in eating program, 514
Soy, as meat substitute, 463
Soybeans, 415
Soy milk, making, 419
Sperm count, zinc for, 324
Sperm function, vitamin C for, 325–26
Spices, 229
Spinach, 203
iron from, 69
Spinach Pie, 466
Sports drinks, 175, 298
Sports nutrition supplements, in natural food stores, 420
Squash, winter, 202
Starches, 16–17. *See also* Carbohydrates
for energy, 290–93
Steaming foods, 384–85
Stir-frying foods, 385–88
Strawberries, 206
Stress
dietary treatment of, 337
nutrients depleted by, 63–64
Stroke, 273
beta-carotene for prevention of, 25
dietary treatment of, 363–64
from high sodium intake, 134, 136
potassium for prevention of, 45, 176, 177
Sugar, 15–17
dietary guidelines for, 377
energy and, 297
sensitivity of children to, 479
Sulfites, 225–27
Sunflower seeds, dried, 209
Sunlight, vitamin D from, 30, 150
Supper. *See* Dinner
Supplements, 424–34
bodily absorption of, 432–34
for children, 247, 250
choosing, 430–33
consumer profile, 425
guidelines, *432–33*
health professionals' use of, 429
for heart disease prevention, 285
nutrients from food vs., 424, 426–29
overdoses, 58–59
perceived benefits of, 425
in pregnancy, 78
reading labels of, 426–27, 433
reasons for taking, 425

safe use of, 429, 432
single-nutrient, 431–33
special formulations of, 430
storage, 434
swallowing, 428
types taken, 426
Sweating, effect of, on body, 175, 213
Sweet bell peppers, 204
Sweet potatoes, 202
Sweet Potato Salad, 269
Sweet Potato Soup, 516
Swiss chard, 203

T

Tangerines, 205
Tannins, nutrient absorption decreased by, 70
Tartrazine, 227
Taste impairment, dietary treatment of, 364
T-cells, 262
Tea
green, for cancer prevention, 316
iron absorption inhibited by, 70, 166
Teen years, nutrient needs and, 80
Teeth, fluoride for, 40
Tempeh, 421–22
Testosterone, reduced by zinc deficiency, 323–24
Thiamine, 36–37
deficiency, 36–37, 74, 249, 297
food sources, 37, 37
Tinnitus, dietary treatment of, 364–65
Tobacco chewing, antioxidants and, 189
Tofu
as meat substitute, 463
potassium from, 180
Spaghetti with Tofu Sauce, 468
Tangy Tofu Salad, 161
Tomatoes
Oven-Roasted Tomato Soup, 319
Top round steak, 200
Tortillas
Huevos Rancheros, 452
Trauma, nutrients depleted by, 64
Tretinoin, as cancer treatment, 57
Trout, 196
Tryptophan, 252, 254–55
Tuna, 196
Turkey, 198
Lean California Burgers, 130–31
Stuffed Cabbage, 144
Turkey Pita Sandwiches, 300
Turnip greens, 203

U

Ulcerative colitis, dietary treatment of, 365
Ulcers, dietary treatment of, 365–66
United States Recommended Dietary Allowances (U.S. RDAs), 54–55

V

Vaginal yeast infections, dietary treatment of, 366–67
Vegetables, 202–3
allium, 204
calcium from, 149
for cancer prevention, 311, 312, 313, 314, 317–18
for cataract prevention, 5–6
cooking, 404
microwaving, 392
roasting and baking, 390
steaming, 384–85
stir-frying, 385–87
cruciferous, 203
in diet, 19
dietary guidelines for, 376
in eating program, 524, 525
in ethnic foods, 232–33, 234
in Food Guide Pyramid, 377–78, 379
green leafy, 149, 202–3

Vegetables *(continued)*
high-carbohydrate, 204
for immune system, 267
iron from, 165
orange-yellow, 202
pesticides on, 224–25
potassium from, 177, 178
recipes
Dijon Pasta Salad, 193
Gingered Beef and Vegetable Stir-Fry, 170–71
sea, 416
Vegetarian diet, 454–68
arthritis symptoms reduced by, 460–61
benefits of, 455–56
cancer risk reduced by, 458–59
for cardiovascular health, 276, 285, 455, 456–58
fat avoidance in, 464
foods consumed in, *462*
for kidney protection in diabetics, 460
meat substitutes in, 463
modified, 381
nutrient deficiencies in, 77
nutrition guidelines for, 463–64
recipes
Barley Soup, 467
Spaghetti with Tofu Sauce, 468
Spinach Pie, 466
Three-Bean Salad, 467
transition to, 459, 462–63
types of, 455
vitamin and mineral needs in, 465–66
Vegetarian lifestyle
popularity of, 454–55
reasons for, 461–62
Venison, 200
Spicy Venison Stew, 199
Vinegar, in eating program, 522
Vision
antioxidants and, 186–87
cataracts (*see* Cataracts)
of elderly, 307–8
macular degeneration, 354–55
zinc and, 58
Vitamin A, 24–25. *See also* Beta-carotene
cautions, 25
deficiency, 264
food sources, 25
for immune system, 264, 267
for lung cancer prevention, 316–17
measles and, 57
nursing needs, 79
nutrient interaction with, 68
for oral cancer prevention, 189
overdose, 58–59
for psoriasis, 361
for ulcers, 366
Vitamin B_1. *See* Thiamine
Vitamin B_2. *See* Riboflavin
Vitamin B_6, 25–26
as anti-aging nutrient, 302, 303, 304
for carpal tunnel syndrome, 341–42
deficiency, 249
for elderly, 81, 307
food sources, 26, *26*
for immune system, 56, 262–63, 267, 352
nutrient interaction with, 69
overdose, 59
for pregnancy, 77
Vitamin B_{12}, 26–27
as anti-aging nutrient, 302
deficiency, 27, 248
for elderly, 80–81, 307
food sources, 27, *27*
in vegetarian diet, 77, 465
Vitamin B complex
deficiency, from alcohol, 74–75
for mental performance, 307

Vitamin C, 28–29
air pollution and, 51–52, 61
for allergies, 335
as anti-aging nutrient, 302
as antioxidant, 186, 187–88
for cancer prevention, 51, 188, 313, 314
for cataract prevention, 342
for colds, 51, 343
deficiency, 249, 263–64
dietary requirements, 191
for fertility, 325–26, 352
as food additive, 219
food sources, 29, *29*, 188, 318
from fruits, 205–6
health benefits, 51–52
for heart disease prevention, 187–88, 284–85
for immune system, 263–64, 267, 352
for iron absorption, 165–66
for osteoporosis prevention, 357–58
for periodontal disease, 359
smoking and, 73
synthetic, 428–29
for ulcers, 366
in vegetarian diet, 465
Vitamin D, 30–31
calcium and, 150
as food additive, 219
food sources, 30, *31*
new role for, 5
nursing needs, 79
for osteoporosis prevention, 358
overdose, 59
for psoriasis, 361
in vegetarian diet, 465
Vitamin E, 31–32
absorption, 192
air pollution and, 61
for angina, 336
as anti-aging nutrient, 302, 303
as antioxidant, 186, 187, 188–90
for cancer prevention, 189–90, 313, 314
for cataract prevention, 342
dietary requirements, 191
for elderly, 305
for epilepsy, 346–47
for fibrocystic breasts, 348
as food additive, 219
food sources, 31, *32*, 190, 318
health benefits, 52–54
for heart disease prevention, 53–54, 284
for immune system, 54, 263, 267
ischemia and, 188–89
for smokers, 189
synthetic, 429
Vitamin K, 33–34, 57
Vitamins. *See also* Nutrients; Supplements
in American diet, 8
anti-aging, 302
essential facts about, 23–27
fat-soluble vs. water-soluble, 28
as food additive, 219
for immune system, 262–65, 267
important to brain, 248–49
natural vs. synthetic, 426–29
Recommended Dietary Allowances, *52–53*, *432*
units of measurement, 24
when to take, 192

W

Walnuts, 208
Water, 210–16
in body, 210–11, 212–13
elimination of, 213
requirements for, 211–12, 213–14
roles of, 211
bottled, 216
intake amount of, urine as indicator of, 496

Water (*continued*)
  pollution, 214–16
  sodium in, 135
  treatment systems, 215
Watercress, 203
Weight
  aging and, 305–7
  fertility and, 326–27, 352
  nutrients and, 64
Weight loss, 437–53. *See also* Dieting
  aging and, 440
  calculating calorie needs for, 450–51
  carbohydrates and, 18–19, 445–47
  fat reduction for, 443–45, 446
  fiber for, 91, 447, 450
  food diary for, 443
  meal timing for, 450
  for men vs. women, 444
  metabolism management for, 439–41
  nutrient needs and, 71–72
  permanent, planning for, 441–43
  programs, 448–49
  recipes
    Black-Eyed Pea Salad, 452–53
    Breast of Chicken Italian, 451
    Huevos Rancheros, 452
    Warm Fruit Soufflés, 453
  snacks for, 446
Weight Watchers, 449
Wheat, whole, in eating program, 520
Wheat germ, 208
Whipped toppings, fat reduction in, 114
  in eating program, 514–15
Winter squash, 202

Y

Yams
    Yams with Honey Topping, 145
Yeast infections, dietary treatment of, 366–67, 478
Yogurt
  healthy cooking with, 393
  lactose intolerance and, 149
  nonfat, 202
  Raspberries and Honey-Yogurt Cream, 159
  for vaginal yeast infections, 367
Yohimbine, as aphrodisiac, 324

Z

Zinc, 47–48
  absorption, decreased by phytin, 70
  for acne, 334
  for anorexia nervosa, 336–37
  for colds, 343
  deficiency, 250–51
  for fertility, 323–25, 352
  food sources, 48, *48,* 325
  for immune system, 265–66, 267, 352
  for macular degeneration, 58, 354
  nutrient interaction with, 69
  for prostate enlargement, 360–61
  for taste impairment, 364
  for ulcers, 366
  in vegetarian diet, 466

JANE STEELE

A Confession

LYNDSAY FAYE

G. P. PUTNAM'S SONS
NEW YORK

P9-CQE-211

THE AWKWARD BLACK MAN

ALSO BY WALTER MOSLEY

Easy Rawlins Mysteries

Charcoal Joe
Rose Gold
Little Green
Blonde Faith
Cinnamon Kiss
Little Scarlet
Six Easy Pieces
Bad Boy Brawly Brown
A Little Yellow Dog
Gone Fishin'
Black Betty
White Butterfly
A Red Death
Devil in a Blue Dress

Leonid McGill Mysteries

And Sometimes I Wonder about You
All I Did Was Shoot My Man
When the Thrill Is Gone
Known to Evil
The Long Fall

Other Fiction

Debbie Doesn't Do It Anymore
Stepping Stone / Love Machine
Merge / Disciple
The Gift of Fire / On the Head of a Pin
The Last Days of Ptolemy Grey
The Tempest Tales
The Right Mistake
Diablerie
Killing Johnny Fry
Fear of the Dark
Fortune Son
The Wave
47
The Man in My Basement
Fear Itself
Futureland: Nine Stories of an Imminent World
Fearless Jones
Walkin' the Dog
Blue Light
Always Outnumbered, Always Outgunned
RL's Dream
John Woman

Original E-books

Parishioner
Odyssey
The Further Adventures of Tempest Landry

Nonfiction

Folding the Red into the Black
The Graphomaniac's Primer
12 Steps toward Political Revelation
This Year You Write Your Novel
Life Out of Context
What Next: A Memoir toward World Peace
Workin' on the Chain Gang
Elements of Fiction

Plays

The Fall of Heaven

THE AWKWARD BLACK MAN

STORIES

WALTER MOSLEY

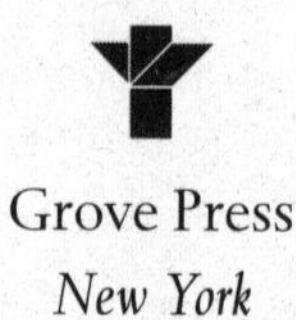

Grove Press
New York

FIRST EDITION

Published simultaneously in Canada
Printed in the United States of America

Text design by Norman E. Tuttle at Alpha Design & Composition
This book was set in 13 pt. Spectrum MT with Gentium
by Alpha Design & Composition of Pittsfield, NH.

First Grove Atlantic hardcover edition: September 2020

Library of Congress Cataloging-in-Publication data is available for this title.

ISBN 978-0-8021-4956-5
eISBN 978-0-8021-5686-0

Grove Press
an imprint of Grove Atlantic
154 West 14th Street
New York, NY 10011

Distributed by Publishers Group West

groveatlantic.com

20 21 22 23 10 9 8 7 6 5 4 3 2 1

This book is dedicated to Toni Morrison, who raised the dialogue of blackness to the international platform that Malcolm X strove for.

CONTENTS

The Good News Is 1

Pet Fly 13

Almost Alyce 33

Starting Over 57

Leading from the Affair 71

Cut, Cut, Cut 89

Between Storms 113

The Black Woman in the Chinese Hat 131

Local Hero 147

Otis 167

Showdown on the Hudson 189

Breath 209

Reply to a Dead Man 227

The Letter 249

Haunted 269

The Sin of Dreams 285

An Unlikely Series of Conversations 305

THE GOOD NEWS IS

The good news was that after a lifetime of carrying an extra thirty pounds or more, I was finally losing weight. Through middle and high school, into college, and then as a data interpreter for Spanish Bank, I was always bulging at the hip and waist, chest and thigh. Too big for stores that sold regular clothes and not quite fat enough for BGE, the Big Guy Emporium. I wore clothes that were either overly snug or so loose that I needed a belt larger than my waist size that could be altered, as needed, with an awl.

My entire life I avoided looking in mirrors, and felt sure that women who showed any interest in me were the ones who had given up, deciding that they'd never get the kind of man they really wanted.

I married a woman, Blythe Lighnter, because I didn't think things could get any better. I divorced her over a Frenchman named, predictably, François. He was teaching her how to play cello al fresco in a village outside of Paris while I stayed at home in

Greenwich Village watching Terra Heart porn videos and imagining that my penis could one day be as large as Brad Bonaboner Backman's—Triple-B.

I could afford the alimony and relieve the loneliness because I made four thousand dollars a week freelancing for Fortune 2000 companies that needed their employee-generated software explained to anyone from their CEOs to users, new personnel, and the federal government at tax time.

I lived in Manhattan in a five-thousand-dollar-a-month studio apartment and so did my ex, with François, who was going to get a job as soon as his papers came through.

I had a girlfriend named Lana who told me she loved me but said that her impression of life was that people should live alone, answerable to no one. This, she said, made love a true choice and not a duty that inevitably transmogrified into spite.

At least Lana didn't play cello, and we would turn out the light before going to bed the one or two nights a week we got together, and so I was emotionally placated . . . if not truly happy.

I didn't complain because I liked being alone most nights and days and weekends or when it was raining or snowing or over those fake holidays when New Yorkers were off celebrating Columbus or the presidents or some religious ceremony that most of them couldn't quite explain.

I wasn't above seeing prostitutes, but I stopped when I realized that I had to take both Viagra and Ecstasy in order to have sex with a woman I was paying to satisfy my needs. I was the fat guy, and she was the svelte woman who wouldn't talk to me if we were standing on line, one behind the other, at the Gourmet Garage with our tiny lamb chops and fresh herbs.

But all that began to change when I started to lose weight.

At first I thought it was because of the high-protein/low-carb regimen that I had been so close to perfecting for years. The problem was that it took three days, sometimes even four, to clear the body of carbs in order for the diet to take control, and I'd buy a pint of Ben & Jerry's Cherry Garcia, like clockwork, every other fourth day. That meant that I'd be chemically dieting only for 3.4 days a week, and that wasn't enough to counteract the glut of calories in my system from the ice cream binges.

But that changed, as I've already said. I pinpointed the moment of my transition to when I was at a 7-Eleven near midnight of an alternate fourth day, and I came to find that they were out of Cherry Garcia except for the yogurt version. My favorite flavor not available, I decided to go without. The following Tuesday I took a sideways glance at myself in the mirror and saw that I was—just maybe—a little slimmer. I dared a full-frontal gaze and saw it was true. The high-protein/low-carb diet was making me a candidate, possibly destined for regular-man clothes stores.

That was the best news I'd had in decades.

Blythe getting married to François was second to that. Her marriage gave him papers and also freed me from the alimony treadmill. But really what was important was that after only six weeks sans ice cream I could fit into trousers with a thirty-four-inch waist and shop at any clothes store I wanted.

Lana and I were invited to Blythe and François's impromptu wedding, held without reservation near the Central Park lake. It was a quasi-Buddhist ceremony conducted by Brother Franklin, an ex-convict Zen monk from upstate.

"Buddhism does not encourage nor does it oppose the institution of marriage," Franklin informed us. "That way the choice of the union is because of love and not duty."

Lana nudged me when he said this, but I had already moved on from that relationship. I had been e-mailing with a woman named Rachael Daws. I'd known her for some years, but when we ran into each other at a data-interpretation convention in Boston, she'd commented on how good I looked and said that we should stay in touch.

"You're looking good, Sammy," Blythe said, when I walked up to congratulate her after the wedding. "Have you lost weight?"

"Finally figured out that other fourth day."

"Anyway," she said. "Thanks for coming . . . and don't be a stranger."

She was probably just being nice, but I liked to think that the new, slimmer me was just so damn attractive that maybe she regretted the cello lessons that she'd taken a month off work for—a month away from me that she promised *would make our bond stronger.*

For the ceremony I wore a buttermilk-colored single-button two-piece suit with a cobalt shirt and a yellow, red, and black silk tie, the material of which was culled from an antique kimono. I bought those clothes to celebrate myself.

The face in the mirror every morning and night was smiling at me.

I was looking better and feeling more confident, but that wasn't all of it. My knees, which had bothered me since my first year at Brown, no longer hurt. I still couldn't jog very well, because I didn't have the wind, but I took a couple of laps around the block two afternoons a week and was planning on adding a third day.

The only problem was that I was sleeping a lot more. Lana would complain that the days I came over I didn't want to have sex.

"You fall asleep right after dinner," she accused.

I didn't tell her that she had stopped being frisky with me long before, just after the first few months of our relationship. I wanted to say that it was only because I was looking better that she complained, but I didn't.

"Maybe the diet isn't giving you enough vitamins," she suggested.

"Maybe not," I admitted. "I've been sleeping a lot, and I don't eat sugar anymore. Maybe my body is transitioning."

"My doctor is a nutritionist. I'm sure I could get you an appointment."

I didn't really want to accept her help, because I was feeling mildly guilty. Rachael and I had made electronic plans to go to Miami the following month. I'd told Lana it was another convention.

"OK," I said. "If you can ask I'd appreciate it."

"The bad news," Dr. Lola Bridesmith said, two weeks later, "is that it's malignant."

I had gone the next day to see the MD/nutritionist, and she took X-rays because I hadn't had any in over ten years. These revealed a growth in my abdomen, and so an appointment was made with an oncologist cut-man for the next week.

I called off the tryst with Rachael, because sex and infatuation took a back seat to cancer and possible death.

"The good news is," Dr. Bridesmith said, "that it doesn't look like it has spread. After a full-body MRI you'll have a simple operation, followed by three to five weeks of radiation treatments and then a two-stage regimen of chemotherapy. That approach might very well clear it up completely."

"I have to have all that?"

"To be sure."

* * *

Lana left me because, while trying to help around the apartment, she came upon the e-mails between Rachael and me. There were a few questionable pictures involved.

Rachael stopped responding after the mention of cancer, and Blythe somehow got it in her head that I had shorted her on the alimony payments and was taking me to court.

The good news was that my various employers had no problem keeping me busy. As long as I could keep awake and focused, they had work for me to do. Brian Jurgens, of de Palma Distributers, did suggest that I wear a wig when I addressed the senior officers of the company.

"You wouldn't want to make them uncomfortable," he said. "They might talk about replacing you if you remind them of their own mortality."

Brian had been a philosophy major at Princeton, and so he gave highly sophisticated explanations for every pedestrian suggestion he made.

I was sleeping thirteen hours a day and working ten; seven days a week, seven days a week.

The MRI had revealed other growths, and so I had to have a few more biopsies. The good news was that the new polyps were, so far, benign. The operation cut out the malign growth. The radiation did nothing against the missing cancer, but a woman on the subway told me how healthy my fake hair looked. The good news was that there were no other malignancies—that they could see.

I lost most of my clients because I was making too many mistakes.

The forensic accountant that the New York State court forced me to hire found that I had shorted Blythe by exactly $549.27. The

good news was that I didn't have to pay it. The bad news was that because the suit had merit, however slim, I was ordered to pay Blythe's $12,347.92 legal fees.

I'd saved enough money to live as I had been living for maybe three years; that was something.

The only thing good about chemotherapy was Maura O'Reilly. She was beautiful, I think; it's hard to tell, because my memory was impacted by the disease and, to a greater degree, the cure. Maura was part of the MVNP, the Metro Visiting Nurse Program, and came every Tuesday and Friday to make up for the days that were lost to me in between. She had a lilt to her voice that came with her from Ireland, and there was something about the way she bathed me that made me feel as if I were just starting out—if I didn't die first.

"What I love about you, Samson Diehl," Maura said to me one Friday, "is your name and how you're always trying to see the best in what's going on."

"Maura, I love you, but I'm about the most cynical person you've ever met."

"Not at all."

"How do you figure?"

"Didn't you tell me that you hated Trump, but he was still the best among the Republicans, even if he wasn't one himself?"

That made me laugh. I spent Wednesday and Thursday, Saturday, Sunday, and Monday waiting for Maura and vomiting. I was waiting for laughter, and she never failed, not once, to deliver.

The poisons I took, the doctors assured me, were wreaking more havoc on the possible cancer than they were on the rest of me. If there was any cancer left, it would be absent by the time I was dead and buried.

I weighed less than I had when I was thirteen.

The last month of the regimen had me bedridden. Maura would drop by most mornings just to see if I had expired in the night. Sometimes I'd come awake and see her folding my clothes and putting them into drawers.

"The good news is that you're cancer-free," oncology coordinator Myron Eddlesworth told me on a beautiful spring day. "We'll have to monitor you for five years, but I'm very optimistic. Going through what you had to endure is like a Dark Ages peasant surviving famine or a war—even the bubonic plague. And here you are, with a full head of hair and a healthy physique."

Yes, the other good news was that I was still thin. I had been eating Cherry Garcia like it was going out of production, but the cancer had been more ravenous than I.

I walked home from the doctor's office on Thirty-Fourth Street and took the five flights of stairs to my room. I don't know what made me think about it, but I searched out my collection of solid-gold coins from ancient Greece. I had purchased them over a twenty-seven-month period when I made triple salary working for a Persian billionaire who sold oil in the East, what people used to call the Orient.

I found the black-velvet box, but it was empty. All seventeen coins—with faces of Athena, Alexander, and even Socrates—were gone. Their value at that time was over two hundred thousand dollars. I was hoping to extend my convalescence with their sale, if that became necessary.

"Hello?" a young woman's sweet voice said over the phone.

"Hi. My name is Sammy Diehl, and I'm calling to speak to Maura O'Reilly."

"I'm so sorry, Mr. Diehl. Maura moved out."

"Oh. Did she leave a forwarding number or address?"

"She went back to Ireland."

"When?"

"Two weeks ago."

I had a padded maroon chair sitting by the hallway door. There were always books and papers in the seat and clothes draped along the back. The only time I had ever sat in it was the day I saw it and bought it at the one and only Plantation Furniture outlet store.

I hung up the phone, dumped the clothes, books, and other detritus from the heavy chair, and pulled it over to the window. The wooden legs dragging on the oak floor sounded like an elongated fart. I sat down, thinking that the only good news was that the sun was shining and I could still feel its heat on my skin.

I wasn't broke or homeless, dying at that particular moment, or fat for the time being. I had time to read, even if I didn't use it, and to watch movies that had come and gone while I was subjected to a procedure that future ages would compare to medical bloodletting. My eyesight had worsened, but I could still see. Russia had retreated from Syria, for the moment, and data interpretation was still a profession that one could ply, if one so desired.

"Hello," she said, in that sweet lilt.

"Hey, Maura, it's Sammy."

She was silent on the other end of the line, many thousands of miles from my Manhattan patch of sunlight.

"I know this must be a surprise," I said. "But you're the only person in the world I know well enough to call. If you don't talk to me, I don't know what I'll do."

"How did you get my telephone number?" she asked, attempting an upbeat tone.

I'm sure she figured that I hadn't looked at my coin collection yet, that I was calling for just the reason I'd stated.

"The Internet told me about the O'Reillys in Derry, and I remembered that your mother's name was Daimhin. Not so difficult really."

"Modern marvels." She could do amazing things with her *r*'s.

"Why did you leave so suddenly?" I asked, affecting a tone of innocence.

"Me mother was sick."

"I'm sorry to hear that. How's she doing?"

"Fine, but a better question would be, how are you?"

"Cancer-free and unemployed. I have time on this Earth that I wasn't expecting."

"I'm so happy for you, Samson."

I believed her.

"Thank you," I said. "It was a hard road, but I'm grateful for it."

"Grateful for all that sufferin'?"

"It started out that I just thought I was losing a little weight. You know, I've always been chubby. I blamed everything on that. But the cancer burned away that fat and allowed me to understand what a lucky man I am."

"That's really quite wonderful now, isn't it?" she said.

"Maura . . ."

"Yes, Samson?"

"Would you consider marrying me?"

Her silence was exquisite. I was completely serious about the proposal. She could lie and say that she hadn't stolen the coins. Maybe she had let in a plumber or a window washer and had to run downstairs to clean the sheets that I'd vomited and shat upon.

It didn't matter that she'd robbed me. She had been there with that gorgeous smile that I could almost remember and with that voice that was first cousin to song. I would have died if she hadn't been there; that much I was sure of.

"That is a beautiful thing to say, Samson. You are kind and gracious to ask. But I don't think you know me well enough. If we were to marry you might feel differently than you do right now."

"I know you, Maura, and more than that, I know myself. If you say yes, I will be your husband through all the years, no matter how lean or how fat. I will be your husband, and you will be the mother of our children. And they will have Irish names, and their second tongue will be Gaelic."

Again the rapture of silence. I could feel her hopes and regrets over the fiber-optic lines.

After a very long pause she said, "Can I think on it?"

"Do you want me to give you my number?"

"I already have it, silly. I was going to call you after your last visit to the doctor."

"OK," I said. "I'll wait for you to answer, but remember, I'm completely serious and absolutely nothing would change how I feel."

We said our goodbyes and disconnected.

I didn't leave my apartment for the next two weeks. I ordered in all my meals (even Cherry Garcia) and sat by the window in the displaced chair, next to the phone.

I was waiting for her answer.

I didn't give a damn about those coins.

After eighteen days I called Maura's mother's phone again. The line had been disconnected. There was no forwarding number. There was no Daimhin O'Reilly listed in all Ireland, Wales, or England.

Maura was gone.

Maybe I should have told her not to worry about the money. Maybe I should have said, "You can consider those coins a wedding gift."

The days went by, and my health improved. I gained back all the weight that the cancer and its treatments took. I went to work as a data interpreter again. Blythe called with a long explanation about how my cancer had upset her so much that she just had to sue me. I didn't understand the logic but accepted her apology anyway.

Lana called and asked me why I hadn't told her that I was dissatisfied with our relationship.

For some reason her question brought Maura to mind, Maura and my stolen fortune. I missed that Irish lass the way parents yearn for the days of their children's cute mispronunciations: "I wuv you." The love I felt for the nurse while I was dying meant more to me than anything life had to offer. She was what I was looking for even before I understood why the weight was coming off so fast.

"Well?" Lana asked.

I disconnected the call and went down to the 7-Eleven, hoping that they had the regular Cherry Garcia and still hoping, ever so slightly, that when I got back upstairs, Maura would have left a message and a number, a few rolling *r*'s, and a question that I could answer.

PET FLY

Lana Donelli works at the third-floor reception desk of the Landsend mortgaging department of Carter's Home Insurance Company. Her sister, Mona, is somewhere on five. They're both quite pretty. I guess if one was pretty the other would have to be, seeing that they're identical twins. But they're nothing alike. Mona wears short skirts and giggles a lot. She's not serious at all. When silly Mona comes in in the morning, she says hello and asks how you are, but before you get a chance to answer she's busy talking about what she saw on TV last night or something funny that happened on the ferry that morning.

Lana and Mona live together in a two-bedroom apartment on Staten Island.

Lana is quieter and much more serious. The reason I even noticed her was because I thought she was her sister. I had seen Mona around since my first day in the interoffice mail room. Mona laughing, Mona complaining about her stiff new shoes or the air-conditioning or her most recent boyfriend refusing to take her where she wanted to go. I would see her at the coffee-break room on the fifth floor or in the hallway—never at a desk.

So when I made a rare delivery to Landsend and saw her sitting there, wearing a beaded white sweater buttoned all the way up to her throat, I was surprised. She was so subdued—not sad but peaceful, looking at the wall in front of her and holding a yellow pencil with the eraser against her chin.

"Air-conditioning too high again?" I asked her, just so she'd know I was alive and that I paid attention to the nonsense she babbled about.

She looked at me, and I got a chill because it didn't feel like the same person I saw flitting around the office. She gave me a silent and friendly smile, even though her eyes were wondering what my question meant.

I put down the big brown envelope addressed to Landsend and left without saying anything else.

Down in the basement I asked Ernie what was wrong with Mona today.

"Nothing," he said. "I think she busted up with some guy or something. No, no, I'm a liar. She went out with her boyfriend's best friend without telling him. Now she doesn't get why he's mad. That's what she said. Bitch. What she think?"

Ernie *didn't suffer fools*, as my mother would say. He was an older black man who had moved to New York from Georgia thirty-three years before and had come to work for Carter's Home three days after he'd arrived. "I would have been here on day one," he often said, "but my bus only got in on Friday afternoon."

I'd been at Carter's Home for only two months. After graduating from Hunter College I didn't know what to do. Even though I had a BA in poli-sci, I really didn't have any skills. Couldn't type or work a computer. I wrote all my papers in longhand and used a typing service. I didn't really know what I wanted to do, but I had to pay the rent. When I applied to Carter's Home for a professional

trainee position they'd advertised at Hunter, the personnel officer, Reena Worth, said that there was nothing available, but maybe if I took the mail-room position something might open up.

"They hired two white PTs the day after you came," Ernie told me at the end of the first week. I decided to ignore that though. Maybe they had applied beforehand, or maybe they had skills with computers or something.

I didn't mind the job. It was easy and I was always on my feet. Junior Rodriguez, Big Linda Washington, and Little Linda Brown worked with me. The Lindas had earphones and listened to music while they wheeled around their canvas mail carts. Big Linda liked rap and Little Linda liked R & B. Junior was cool. He never talked much, but he'd give me a welcoming nod every morning when he came in. He dressed in gray and brown silk shirts that were unbuttoned to his chest. He had a gold chain around his neck and one gold canine. The Lindas didn't like me, and Junior was in his own world. Everyone working in the interoffice mailroom was one shade or other of brown.

My only friend at work was Ernie. He and I would sit down in the basement and talk for hours sometimes. He told me all about Georgia, where he went on vacation every summer. "Atlanta's cool," he'd say. "But you better watch it in the sticks."

Ernie was proud of his years at Carter's Home. He liked the job and the company but had no patience for most of the bosses.

"Workin' for white people is always the same thing," Ernie would say.

"But Mr. Drew's black," I said the first time I heard his perennial complaint. Drew was the supervisor for all postal and interoffice communication.

"Used to be," Ernie said. "Used to be. But ever since he got promoted he forgot all about that. Now he's so scared I'm gonna

pull him down that he won't even sit for a minute. Used to be he'd come down here and we'd talk like you 'n' me doin'. But now he just stands at the door and grin and nod."

"I don't get it. How can you like the job and the company if you don't like the people you work for?" I once asked Ernie.

"It's a talent," he replied.

"Why 'ont you tuck in your shirt?" Big Linda Washington said to me on the afternoon that I'd unknowingly met Lana Donelli. The sneer on the young woman's face spoke of a hatred that I couldn't understand. "You look like some kinda fool hangin' all out all over the place."

Big Linda was taller than I, broader too—and I'm pretty big. Her hair was straightened and frosted with gold at the tips. She wore one-piece dresses of primary colors as a rule. Her skin was mahogany. Her face, unless it was contorted, appraising me, was pretty.

We were in the service elevator going up to the fifth floor. I tucked the white shirt tails into my black jeans.

"At least you could make it even, so the buttons go straight down," she remarked.

I would have had to open up my pants to do it right, and I didn't want to get Linda any more upset than she already was.

"Hm!" she grunted and then sucked a tooth.

The elevator came open then, and she rolled her cart out. We had parallel routes, but I went in the opposite direction, deciding to take mail from the bottom of the stack rather than listen to her criticisms of me.

The first person I ran into was Mona. She was wearing a deep red one-piece dress held up by spaghetti straps. Her breasts were free under the thin fabric, and her legs were bare. Mona (Lana too,

of course) was short, with thick black hair and green eyes. Her skin had a hint of olive in it but not so deep as Sicilian skin.

"I can see why you were wearing that sweater at your desk," I said.

"What?" she replied, in an unfriendly tone.

"That white sweater you were wearing," I said.

"What's wrong with you? I don't even own a white sweater."

She turned abruptly and clicked away on her red high heels. I wondered what had happened. Somehow I kept thinking that it was because of my twisted-up shirt. Maybe that's what made people treat me badly, maybe it was my appearance.

I continued my route, pulling jackets from the bottom and placing them in the right in-boxes. Everyone had a different in-box system. Some had their in- and out-boxes stacked, while others had them side by side. Rose McMormant had no box at all, just white and black labels set at opposite ends of her desk. White for in and black for out.

"If the boxes ain't side by side, just drop it anywhere and pick up whatever you want to," Ernie told me on my first day. "That's what I do. Mr. Averill put down the rules thirteen years ago, just before they kicked him upstairs."

Ernie was the interoffice mail-room director. He didn't make deliveries anymore, so it was easy for him to make pronouncements.

When I'd finished the route I went through the EXIT door at the far end of the hall to get a drink of water from the refrigerated fountain. I planned to wait in the exit chamber long enough for Big Linda to have gone back down. While I waited, a fly buzzed by my head. It caught my attention because there weren't many flies that made it into the air-conditioned buildings around the Wall Street area, even in summer.

The fly landed on my hand, then on the cold aluminum bowl of the water fountain. He didn't have enough time to drink before zooming up to the ceiling. From there he went to a white spot on the door, to the baby fingernail of my left hand, and then to a crumb in the corner. He landed and settled again and again but took no more than a second to enjoy each perch.

"You sure jumpy, Mr. Fly," I said, as I might have when I was a child. "But you could be a Miss Fly, huh?"

The idea that the neurotic fly could have been a female brought Mona to mind. I hustled my cart toward the elevator, passing Big Linda on the way. She was standing in the hall with another young black woman, talking. The funny thing about them was that they were both holding their hands as if they were smoking, but of course they weren't, as smoking was forbidden in any office building in New York.

"I got to wait for a special delivery from, um, investigations," Big Linda explained.

"I got to go see a friend on three," I replied.

"Oh." Linda seemed relieved.

I realized that she was afraid I'd tell Ernie that she was idling with her friends. Somehow that stung more than her sneers and insults.

She was still wearing the beaded sweater, but instead of the eraser she had a tiny Wite-Out brush in her hand, held half an inch from a sheet of paper on her violet blotter.

"I bet that blotter used to be blue, huh?"

"What?" She frowned at me.

"That blotter, it looks violet, purple, but that's because it was once blue but the sun shined on it, from the window."

Lana turned her upper torso to see the window that I meant. I could see the soft contours of her small breasts against the white fabric.

"Oh," she said, turning back to me. "I guess."

"Yeah," I said. "I notice things like that. My mother says that it's why I never finish anything. She says that I get distracted all the time and don't keep my eye on the job."

"Do you have more mail for me?" Lana Donelli asked.

"No, uh-uh, I was just thinking."

Lana looked at the drying Wite-Out brush and jammed it back into the small bottle that was in her other hand.

"I was thinking about when I saw you this morning," I continued. "About when I saw you and asked about the air-conditioning and your sweater and you looked at me like I was crazy."

"Yes," she said, "why did you ask that?"

"Because I thought you were Mona Donelli," I said triumphantly.

"Oh," she sounded disappointed. "Most people figure out that I'm not Mona because my nameplate says 'Lana Donelli.'"

"Oh," I said, completely crushed. I could notice a blotter turning violet but I couldn't read.

The look on my face brought a smile out of the mortgage receptionist.

"Don't look so sad," she said. "I mean, even when they see the name, a lotta people still call me Mona."

"They do?"

"Yeah. They see the name and think that Mona's a nickname or something. Isn't that dumb?"

"I saw your sister on the fifth floor in a red dress, and then I saw a fly who couldn't sit still, and then I knew that you had to be somebody else," I said.

"You're funny," Lana said, crinkling up her nose as if she were trying to identify a scent. "What's your name?"

"Rufus Coombs."

"Hi, Rufus," she said, holding out a hand.

"Hey," I said.

My apartment is on 158th Street in Washington Heights. It's pretty much a Spanish-speaking neighborhood. I don't know many people, but the rent is all I can afford. My apartment—living room with a kitchen cove, small bedroom, and toilet with a shower—is on the eighth floor and looks out over the Hudson. The $458 a month includes heat and gas, but I pay my own electric. I took it because of the view. There was a three-hundred-dollar unit on the second floor, but it had windows that looked out onto a brick wall.

I don't own much. I have a single mattress on the floor, an old oak chair that I found on the street, and kitchen shelving that I bought from a liquidator for bookshelves, propped up in the corner. I have a rice pot, a frying pan, and a kettle, and enough cutlery and plates for two, twice as much as I need most days.

I have Rachel, an ex-girlfriend living in the East Village, who will call me back at work if I don't call her too often. I have two other friends, Eric Chen and Willy Jones. They both live in Brooklyn and still go to school.

That evening I climbed the seven flights up to my apartment because the elevator had stopped working in December. I sat in my chair and looked at the river. It was peaceful, and I relaxed. A fly was buzzing up against the glass, trying to push his way through to the world outside.

I got up to kill him. That's what I always did when there was a fly in the house, I killed it. But up close I hesitated and watched

the frantic insect. His coloring was unusual, a metallic green. The dull red eyes seemed too large for the body, like he was an intelligent mutant fly from some far-flung future on late-night television.

He buzzed up and down against the pane, trying to get away from me. When I returned to my chair, he settled. The red sun was hovering above the cliffs of New Jersey. The green fly watched. I thought of the fly I'd seen at work. That one was black and fairly small, by fly standards. Then I thought about Mona and then Lana. The smallest nudge of an erection stirred. I thought of calling Rachel but didn't have the heart to walk the three blocks to a phone booth. So I watched the sunset gleaming around the fly, who was now just a black spot on the window.

I guess I fell asleep.

At three A.M. I woke up and made macaroni and cheese from a mix. The fly came into the cooking cove where I stood eating my meal. He lit on the big spoon I used to stir the macaroni and joined me for my late-night supper.

Ernie told me that Landsend mortgaging got most of their mail from the real-mail mail room, that they didn't get most of the interoffice junk mail.

"Why not?" I asked.

"There's just a few people up there. Most of their employees are off-site."

"Well, could you put them on the junk list?"

"She a white girl?"

"So?"

"Nuthin'. But I want you tell me what it's like if you get some."

I didn't answer him.

* * *

For the next week I took invitations to office parties, sales-force newsletters, and "Insurance Tips," penned by Mr. Averill, up to Lana Donelli's desk. We made small talk for thirty seconds or so, and then she'd pick up the phone to make a call. I always looked back as I rounded the corner to make sure she really had a call to make; she always did.

At the end of the week I bought her a paperweight with the image of a smiling Buddha's face in it. When I got to her desk, she wasn't there. I waited around for a while, but she didn't return, so I wrote her a note, saying "From Rufus to Lana," and put the heavy glass weight on it.

I went away excited and half-scared. What if she didn't see my note? What if she did and thought it was stupid? I was so nervous that I didn't go back to her desk that day.

"I really shouldn't have sent it, Andy," I said that night to the green fly. He was perched peacefully at the edge of the center rim of a small saucer. I had filled the inner depression with a honey and water solution. I was eating a triple cheeseburger with bacon from Wendy's, that and some fries. My pet fly seemed happy with his honey water and only buzzed my sandwich a few times before settling down to drink.

"Maybe she doesn't like me," I said. "Maybe it's just that she's been nice to me because she feels sorry for me. But how will I know if I don't try and see if she likes me, right?"

Andrew's long tubular tongue was too busy drinking to reply.

"Hi," I said to Lana the next morning.

She was wearing a jean jacket over a white T-shirt. She smiled and nodded. I handed her Mr. Averill's "Insurance Tips" newsletter.

"Did you see the paperweight?"

"Oh, yeah," she said, without looking me in the eye. "Thanks." Then she picked up her phone and began pressing buttons. "Hi, Tristan? Lana. I wanted to know if—" She put her hand over the receiver and looked at me. "Can I do something else for you?"

"Oh," I said. "No. No," and I wheeled away in a kind of euphoria.

It's only now when I look back on it that I remember the averted eyes, the quick call, and the rude dismissal. All I heard then was "Thanks." I even remember a smile. Maybe she did smile for a brief moment, maybe not.

Monday, Tuesday, and Wednesday of the next week I deposited little presents on her desk. I left them while she was out to lunch. I got her a small box of four Godiva chocolates, a silk rose, and a jar of fancy rose-petal jelly. I didn't leave any more notes. I was sure that she'd know who it was. During that time I stopped delivering to her desk. I saved up all the junk mail for Friday morning, when I'd deliver it and ask her to go out with me.

Wednesday evening I went to a nursery on the East Side just south of Harlem proper. There I bought a bonsai, a real apple tree, for $347.52. I figured that I'd leave it during her Thursday lunch, and then on Friday, Lana would be so happy that she'd have to have lunch with me no matter what.

I should have suspected that something was wrong when Andrew went missing. I put out his honey water, but he didn't show up, even when I started eating a beef burrito from Taco Bell. I looked around the apartment, but he wasn't anywhere to be seen. There was a spiderweb in the upper corner of the shower, but there was no little bundle up there. I would have killed the spider right then, but he never came out when I was around.

That night I wondered if I could talk to Lana about Andrew. I wondered if she would understand my connection to a fly.

* * *

"What's that?" Ernie asked me the next morning when I came in with the bonsai.

"It's a tree."

"Tree for what?"

"My friend Willy wanted me to pick it up for him. He wants it for his new apartment, and the only place where he could get it is up near me. I'm gonna meet him at lunch and give it to him."

"Uh-huh," Ernie said.

"You got my cart loaded?" I asked him.

Just then the Lindas came down in the elevator. Big Linda looked at me and shook her head, managing to look both contemptuous and pitying at the same time.

"There's your carts," Ernie said to them.

They attached their earphones and rolled back to the service elevator. Little Linda was looking me in the eye as the slatted doors closed. She was still looking at me as the lift brought her up.

"What about me and Junior?"

"Junior's already gone. That's all I got right now. Why don't you sit here with me?"

"OK." I sat down expecting Ernie to bring up one of his regular topics, either something about Georgia, white bosses, or the horse races, which he followed but never wagered on. But instead of saying anything he just started reading the *Post*.

After a few minutes I was going to say something, but the swinging door opened. Mr. Drew leaned in. He smiled at Ernie and then pointed at me.

"Rufus Coombs?"

"Yeah?"

"Come with me."

I followed Leonard Drew through the messy service hall outside the couriers' room to the passenger elevator that we rarely took.

It was a two-man elevator, so Drew and I had to stand very close to one another. He wore too much cologne, but otherwise he was ideal for his supervisory job, wearing a light gray suit with a shirt that only hinted at yellow. The rust tie was perfect, and there was not a wrinkle on the man's clothes or his face. I knew that he must have been up in his forties, but he might have passed as a graduate student at my school. He was light-skinned and had what my mother called *good hair.* There were freckles around his eyes.

I could see all of that because Mr. Drew averted his gaze. He wouldn't engage me in any way, and so I got a small sense of revenge by studying him.

We got out on the second floor and went to his office, which was at the far end of the mail-sorting room. Outside of his office there was a desk for his secretary, Teja Monroe. Her desk sat out in the hall as if it had been an afterthought to give Drew an assistant.

I looked around the room as Drew was entering his office. I saw Mona looking at me from the crevice of a doorway. I knew it was Mona because she was wearing a skimpy dress that could have been worn on a hot date.

I only got a glimpse of her before she ducked away.

"Come on in, Coombs," Drew said.

The office was tiny. Drew had to actually stand on the tips of his toes to get between the wall and the desk to his chair. There was a stool in front of the desk, not a chair.

By the time he said "sit down," I had lost my nervousness. I gauged the power of Mr. Leonard Drew by the size of his office.

"You're in trouble, Rufus," he said, looking as somber as he could.

"I am?"

He lifted a pink sheet of paper and shook it at me.

"Do you recognize this?" he asked.

"No."

"This is a sexual harassment complaint form."

"Yeah?"

"It names you as the offender."

"I don't get it."

"Lana Donelli . . ." He went on to explain all the things that I had done and felt for the last week as if they were crimes. Going to Lana's desk, talking to her, leaving gifts. Even remarking on her clothes had sexual innuendo attached. By the time he was finished I was worried about them calling the police.

"Lana says that she's afraid to come in to work," Mr. Drew said, his freckles disappearing into angry lines around his eyes.

I wanted to say that I didn't mean it, but I could see that my intentions didn't matter, that a small woman like Lana would be afraid of a big sloppy mail clerk hovering over her and leaving notes and presents.

"I'm sorry," I said.

"Sorry doesn't mean much when it's gotten to this point. If it was up to me I'd send you home right now, today. But first Mr. Averill says that he wants to talk to you."

"OK," I said.

I sat there looking at him.

"Well?" he asked after a few moments.

"What?"

"Go back to the mail room and stay down there. Tell Ernie that I don't want you in the halls. You're supposed to meet Mr. Averill at one forty-five in his office. I've given him my recommendation to let you go. After something like this, there's really no place for you. But he can still refer the matter to the police. Lana might want a restraining order."

I wanted to say something. I wanted to tell him that a restraining order was ridiculous. Then I wanted to go to Lana and tell her the same thing. I wanted to tell her that I bought her roses because she wore rose toilet water, that I bought her the tree because the sun on her blotter could support a plant. I really liked her. But even while I was imagining what I could say, I knew that it didn't matter what I saw or what I felt.

"Well?" Drew said. "Go."

Ernie made busywork for us that morning. He told me that he was upset about what had happened, that he'd told Drew to go easy.

"But he just said that I better look after myself," Ernie said. "Man forget he's black 'fore you could say Jackie Robinson."

"Hey, bro'," Junior said to me at lunchtime. "Come on with me."

Junior rarely talked to me, much less offered his company. This was an act of rare generosity, and so I took him up on it. The Lindas had ignored me completely. It was obvious that they knew about my troubles before I did but hadn't seen fit to warn me.

"Where we goin'?" I asked Junior out on Broadway. It was a very crowded street at lunchtime.

"Coupla blocks."

I got the feeling he was taking me somewhere special. I would have been excited, or at least asked him where we were going, but my mind kept going back to Lana. I wanted to explain to her, to tell her why I wasn't harassing her.

"There it is," Junior said.

We had reached the end of Broadway. There was a small concrete island with park benches in the middle of the street. There

were lots of young people hanging out and talking there. On one bench, the one Junior was pointing at, sat a muscular ebony-colored man with a bald head wearing a dark blue, thin-strapped tank top. He was just leaning over to kiss a small woman, a white woman—Lana Donelli. I brought my hand to my mouth and made a sound. He pushed his tongue brutally into her mouth, and she brought her fingers to his head as if she were guiding the attack.

I turned away.

"Sorry, bro," Junior said.

I felt his hand on my shoulder. I nodded and said, "I'm going back up." I didn't wait for him to reply; I just started walking.

Lancelot Averill's office was on the forty-eighth floor of the Carter's Home building. His secretary's office was larger by far than Mr. Drew's cubbyhole. The smiling blond secretary led me into Averill's airy room. The wall behind him was a giant window looking out over Battery Park, Ellis Island, and the Statue of Liberty. I would have been impressed if my heart wasn't broken.

Averill was on the phone when I was ushered in.

"Sorry, Nick," he said into the receiver. "My one forty-five is here."

He stood up, tall and thin. The medium-gray suit looked expensive. His white shirt was crisp and bright, but that was nothing compared to the rainbow of his tie. His hair was gray and combed back, and his mustache was sharp enough to cut bread, as my mother was known to say.

"Sit down, Mr. Coombs."

He sat also. In front of him were two sheets of paper. At his left hand was the pink harassment form; at his right was a white form. Behind him the Budweiser blimp hovered next to Lady Liberty.

Averill brought his fingertips to just under his nose and gazed at a spot over my head.

"How's Ernie?" he asked.

"He's good," I said. "He's a great boss."

"He's a good man. He likes you."

I didn't know what to say to that.

Averill looked down at his desk. "This does not compute."

"What?"

He patted the white page. "This says that you're a college graduate, magna cum laude, in political science, that you came here to be a professional trainee." He patted the pink sheet. "This says that you're an interoffice mail courier who harasses secretaries in the mortgage department."

Averill's hand reached into his vest pocket and came out with an open package of cigarettes. He offered me one, but I shook my head. He lit up and took a deep drag, holding the smoke in his lungs a long time before exhaling.

"Why are you in the interoffice mail room?" he asked.

"No PT positions were open when I applied," I said.

"Nonsense. We don't have a limit on PTs."

"But Ms. Worth said—"

"Oh," Averill held up his hand. "Reena. You know Ernie helped me out when I got here eighteen years ago. I was just a little older than you. They didn't have the PT program back then, just a few guys like Ernie. He never even finished high school, but he showed me the ropes."

Averill drummed the fingers of his free hand between the two forms that represented me.

"I know this Lana's sister," he said. "Always wearing those cocktail dresses in to work. Her boss is afraid to say anything, otherwise

he might get a pink slip too." He paused to ponder some more. "Twins, huh? They look alike?"

"They don't dress the same," I said, wanting somehow to protect Lana from the insinuations that I barely understood.

"How would you like to be a PT floater?"

"What's that?" I asked.

"Bump you up to a grade seven and let you move around in the different departments until you find a fit."

I was a grade 1B.

"I thought you were going to fire me."

"That's what Drew suggested, but Ernie says that it's just a mix-up, that you aren't perverted or anything. I'll talk to this Donelli girl, and as long as I have your word that you'll leave her alone, I'll forget it. This is personnel's fault in the first place. You're an intelligent boy—young man. Of course you're going to get into trouble if you aren't challenged."

Watching the forbidden smoke curl around his head, I imagined that Averill was some kind of devil. When I thanked him and shook his hand, something inside me wanted to scream.

I found six unused crack vials a block from the subway stop near my apartment. I knew they were unused because they still had the little plastic stoppers in them.

When I got upstairs I spent hours searching my place. I looked under the edges of the mattress and behind the toilet, under the radiator, and even down under the burners on the stove. Finally, after midnight, I decided to open the windows.

Andrew had crawled down in the crack between the window frame and the sill in my bedroom. His green body had dried out, which made his eyes look all the larger. He'd gone down there to die, or maybe he was trying to get out of the life I'd kept him in;

maybe it was me that killed him, that's what I thought. Later I found out that flies live for only a few weeks. He probably died of old age.

I took the small dried-out corpse and put him in one of the crack vials. I stoppered him in the tiny glass coffin and buried him among the roots of the bonsai apple.

"So you finally bought something nice for your house," my mother said, after I told her about the changes in my life. "Maybe next you'll get a real bed."

ALMOST ALYCE

1.

Albert Roundhouse came from a good working-class family in Los Angeles. He did well in public high school and made it through three years of state college before things started falling apart.

There was a young woman named Alyce who came into Albert's life like a typhoon—at least that's what Albert's sister Luellen said.

"Alyce blew in like a storm," Luellen Roundhouse reported to anyone who cared to listen. "She told him that she wasn't the kind of girl that belonged to anyone or who wanted to settle down. And as much as Al tried to understand what she was telling him, he just sank under all that loving like a leaky rowboat in a summer storm."

And it was true, what Luellen said. Sometimes when Albert gazed on Alyce's brown body in his bed at night, he would howl and pounce on her like an animal from some deep forgotten part of the forest. And Alyce loved his hunger for her. She rolled and growled, clawed and bit with him.

And then one day she was gone—out of his bed, out of his apartment, out of the city, with Roald Hopkins, a sailor on furlough.

"He could have been called Jimmy or Johnny," Luellen Roundhouse said. "He could have been a she for all that Alyce cared. Because she was just hungry for passion from as many lovers as possible. She told Albert that. She warned him."

At about that time, September 1979, Albert and Luellen's father, Thyme Roundhouse, met Betty Pann. He fell for Betty just as his son had fallen for Alyce. But Betty didn't run away—not at all. It was Thyme who ran out. He left Georgia, his wife, the kids' mother, and moved with Miss Pann to Seattle, where they lived in a house that looked over the Puget Sound. Thyme became a fisherman and Betty a nurse. "Blood and Fishes," they had printed on their own personal stationery.

Georgia Roundhouse changed her surname back to Gordon but still refused to give Thyme a divorce. She didn't quit her job as senior office manager for the city of Los Angeles, but after seventeen weeks of absence she was fired.

By then Albert was failing his classes, pining for Alyce. She had sent the lovesick student a postcard telling him that she'd left Roald for another lover, name of Christian Lovell. Her words and tone were so friendly that Albert cried for three days. Luellen convinced her brother to drop out of school and move in with their mother, each to serve as a life preserver for the other.

For a while it went as well as heartbreak would allow. Albert got a job for Logan Construction and came up with the small monthly mortgage payment. The rest of their money came from Georgia's private savings and what little Luellen could provide from her various part-time jobs.

Albert had never done hard labor before. He manned a wheelbarrow most days, moving rock from one pile to another. He lifted and strained and grew callouses. Al was grateful for the exhaustion

because it meant he would sleep rather than brood about Alyce at night in his childhood bed.

Georgia cooked dinner every day and ate with her moping son.

The mother loved Albert, but for most of his life they'd had little in common and less to say. But with Thyme gone, Georgia would find herself telling Albert about her family history. She told these stories because Albert rarely had anything to say except that he loved Alyce more and more each day.

Georgia talked about her mother and father and Great-Grandfather Henry, who had been born a slave but became a spice trader, getting his own ship and working from the port of Havana. Henry's wife, Lorraine, had been a woman of the streets.

"Great-Granddaddy Henry married a prostitute?"

"He had got himself stabbed by a Spaniard that wanted to take over his business, but Lorraine found him bleeding in an alley and took him in. She nursed him back to health, and Henry went out and killed that Spaniard. When he came back he told Lorraine that he would marry her and build her a big house in America, where she would never have to work unless that was what she wanted."

"He must have been the most colorful ancestor we got," Albert said, forgetting for the moment his sorrow.

"Oh, no," Georgia said. "Big Jim Gordon, your great-uncle on my father's side, was the wildest, most exciting relative. Big Jim declared war on the town of Hickton, Mississippi, and fought that war for twelve long years."

"War?"

"Oh, yes," Georgia said with surety. "Full-fledged war, with guns and traps, dead men and blood. He lived in the woods around that town and took retribution on those that had harmed him and others of our people."

"When was this?"

"Just after World War One and up to the Great Depression."

"But the Gordons aren't from Mississippi."

Georgia smiled. It was a look of mild cheer, but Albert thought he could see how deep the pain ran.

"You only get so much a night, Al," she said. "Tomorrow I'll tell you how the white men in that town of Hickton hurt Jim and then paid the price."

With these words Georgia Gordon got up and went to her bedroom, leaving Albert to wonder about his great-grandfather the spice merchant and his great-uncle Big Jim, the one-man army.

So taken was the young man with his unknown heritage that he didn't brood over Alyce that evening.

In the morning he got up early, before his mother, and went out to work in Oxnard, where he spent the morning rolling chunks of concrete and granite to a pit that had been excavated by the company bulldozer. He swung a sledgehammer for three hours in the early afternoon and then used an oversize shovel in the gravel pit until his shift was through. He worked harder than usual, imagining a one-man black army declaring war on a white southern town. In this reverie he didn't feel the weight of his labors or the gravity of loss.

When he got home, the house was quiet and dark. Albert couldn't remember the last time he'd entered the house when the television wasn't on.

"Mama," the twenty-one-year-old called.

He expected the "Here" to come from one of the back rooms. But there was no welcome.

Georgia Gordon was dead in her bed, her left hand gripping the edge of the blanket near her chin. Her foot, clad in a gaudy,

pink cashmere sock, poked out from the sheets. There was an odor hovering in the room, a smell that Albert couldn't get out of his nose for many weeks.

"Why didn't you call for an ambulance?" Detective Todd Green asked Albert, for the fourth or fifth time.

"I, I could tell she was dead," he said. "Her skin was cold, and she hadn't been out of bed since I left this morning."

"Why didn't you call the ambulance this morning?"

"I didn't know anything was wrong."

"You knew that she hadn't gotten out of bed."

"I left the house at five in the morning. When I got home, all the lights were off and the paper was at the front door. I could tell that Mama had never gotten up. I went in her room after she didn't answer, and there she was."

"Why didn't you call for an ambulance?" the detective asked again.

"I called my sister."

"Your sister? Why?"

"She's her mother too. And Mama was cold, and the room smelled bad. Lu said to call the police, and so that's what I did."

Thyme Roundhouse came down for the funeral with Betty Pann on his arm.

"I'm selling the house, Al," he said at the reception after the service.

"But this is Mama's house."

"Your mother's dead, and I'm still her husband."

The full impact of the death hadn't hit the young man until his father uttered those words. From then on, and through the next few decades, Albert was confused about the sequence of events.

There were some things he was sure of. He began crying upon hearing his father's callous pronouncement. Not loud bawling; it was just that the tears wouldn't stop flowing from his eyes. Luellen and Thyme argued. Men touched him on the shoulder and head. Women kissed him and held him like he was their child.

At some point everyone was gone from the house, and Albert was alone with a fifth of Jack Daniel's that someone had brought for the repast . . .

The first bender lasted for eight or nine weeks. It carried him from the house his father was selling up to Berkeley and Telegraph Avenue. He crashed in the laundry room of a house on Derby Street.

One night he had sex with a woman in the back of a van while her husband watched from the driver's seat.

He moved out of the house and into an empty lot, using a sleeping bag that a man named Hartwynn had given him. He did day labor when the hangovers were tolerable.

The Petals of the Sun commune was located in southern Oregon where a redwood forest met the ocean. There he dried out for some months, though he wasn't sure how many. There was a woman with big hands named Rilette, who had built a one-room cottage and took him in. Rilette had a brother, Marquis. Marquis and Albert went into town one night and bought a bottle of red wine and then another.

When Albert woke up the next morning, Marquis was gone, and Rilette was blaming Albert for stealing her money to buy wine.

He hadn't taken her money, but she sent him away. Albert marked this event as the beginning of his roustabout years.

Finally, after three months incarceration for vagrancy in northern California, he built up enough strength and sobriety to hitchhike across country with a woman named Bergit. She was half Native

American and half Swedish and tall and blue-eyed and completely in love with the world she inhabited. She was leaving her boyfriend in Oregon to visit her husband in Vermont. This husband lived on a commune that raised silkworms and practiced Tibetan Buddhism.

For a year the master of that sect worked with Albert, trying to get him to "get outside of the inebriation."

"You mean you want me to stop drinking, right?" Albert once asked. "I been tryin' to put the bottle down, but every time I turn around I find it there in my hand."

The master had a huge, round, burnt-orange-colored face. He smiled at Albert and shook his great head.

"It is not what I want that matters," the master said. "You must seek your own equilibrium. If drinking brings balance then by all means drink. But if it is only a mask, a beard to cover the real face of your desire, then you must find another way."

Albert would sit in his straw hut at night, wrapped in a down comforter that Bergit's husband gave him. Outside it was below zero, but the round hut stayed warm, and Albert wondered what it meant to achieve balance.

In the spring the master died, and the man who ran the raw-silk production line asked Albert to leave.

"You're just a drunk," Terry Pin said to Albert three days after the cremation rite.

Theodore Bidwell, Bergit's husband, apologized for Terry's rough words.

"Bergit has relatives that work construction in New York," Theodore told Albert. He bought the displaced Californian a ticket for the Peter Pan bus in Saint Albans and gave him forty dollars to hold him over till he contacted the Swedish Indian's cousins.

Bergit had left some months before to return to her boyfriend and his son in the forests of Oregon. Albert thought it was nice of her husband to buy his ticket and give him a recommendation.

On the bus Albert sat by the window concentrating on the idea of balance. He thought about Alyce and his father, his mother, and Luellen. He touched the center of his chest with the middle finger of his left hand. At just that place there was a gap, a space that Alyce had stretched out and then vacated. There was something about this emptiness that kept him from the proper equilibrium. It was like trying to stand up straight atop a gas-filled balloon that always seemed to be shifting away.

Albert rubbed the area that felt hollow, wondering if somehow he could move the emptiness around.

In the window of the bus he peered into his own dark image, thinking about Alyce and Great-Uncle Big Jim. These unknowable quantities, he felt, were what made him stagger through life. Or maybe it was his mother's unexpected death or his father's betrayal.

"My life hasn't really been all that bad," he said to the image of himself.

"What did you say?" asked the woman in the aisle seat next to him.

"Nuthin'."

"It was something," the youngish, round white woman said. "I heard it. I just didn't understand the words."

Her smile was gentle and reminded Al of a time when he wasn't sad.

"I was sayin' that my life hasn't really been all that bad. I mean, I've had some hard times, but every trouble I've had has been at least partly my fault."

"We all make our own beds," she agreed, "but it's God that gives us bedbugs."

Albert laughed deeply. While laughing he tried to remember the last time he felt mirth when sober.

Mary Denise Fulmer was born in Springfield, Massachusetts. She taught middle school there and lived by herself in a small red house near the train tracks. She was unmarried and had never lived anywhere but Springfield.

"Where are you coming from now?" Albert asked.

"My grandmother lived in Montreal," Mary Denise said. "She died last week, and I took a few days off to wrap up her affairs."

Albert told Mary Denise about his mother's death and his on-again, off-again ten-year bender.

"I just can't seem to get straight," he said more than once.

Somewhere outside of Amherst she asked, "Would you like to come stay with me for a while? You could sleep on the couch . . . or in my bed if you want."

Albert hadn't had a drink in thirty-four hours. He felt queasy but clearheaded.

"I really, really want to, Mary D," he said, surprising himself with the clarity. "But I'm on a tight schedule here. I got to get to a place that's mine. Mine."

The plump schoolteacher smiled sadly and put a hand on his forearm. She leaned over and kissed his bristly cheek.

2.

The next twenty-two years passed like overlapping spirals drawn by a tired child on a rainy afternoon. Albert would work for weeks, sometimes for months at a time, and then he'd fall off the wagon.

But even when on a bender, Albert would always find time to beg. This practice he'd learned from his Tibetan master.

"A man with a tin cup allows the more prosperous to pay penance. Without this opportunity, their souls would surely be lost."

Albert could imbibe prodigiously in his younger years, but after he crossed the half-century border his capacity diminished. Where at one time he could drink a fifth and a half of sour-mash whiskey, now half a bottle of cheap red wine was all he could manage before the gut rot set in.

He'd been hospitalized twice by the city and had done three stints in jail, for public lewdness, resisting arrest, and simple assault. The Eagle Heart Construction Company of Queens always took Albert back if he was sober. He'd been working for them as long as most could remember.

Between work and inebriation, jail and hospitalization, Albert lived in a cavity under an abandoned subway tunnel on the Upper East Side. This space was an underground chamber he inherited from a German survivalist named Dieter Krownen, who had returned to Munich when his mother got sick.

Chained together under metal netting in the abandoned tunnel above his subterranean lair, Albert had a collection of shopping carts in which he kept those belongings that didn't fit in his 137-square-foot underground bunker.

Albert hadn't realized he'd passed the half-century mark until he was fifty-three. One day he'd come across his birth certificate in an old alligator wallet in the bottom of one of the carts. The date of his birth was January 12, 1958, the time 4:56 A.M. His race was Negro, sex male, and he came into the world weighing six and three-quarter pounds.

After calculating his age, Albert stopped working for Eagle Heart Construction. Fifty, he thought, should be the mandatory retirement age in order to make space for younger workers. One of his professors at state college had told him that.

So for six months he'd been strolling around Manhattan with his travel cart. He pushed the rickety shopping cart all over the city, whispering words about his father and mother, Luellen, and always, always Alyce. He begged for a few hours each day, thinking about his deceased master and believing that he was doing penance by begging and saving souls.

One sunny afternoon he found himself on Sixth Avenue, two blocks south of Houston Street. There he stood on the corner next to a restaurant with half of its tables out on the sidewalk. He leaned against a lamppost remembering the half-told story about his great-uncle Big Jim who, Albert imagined, had killed a dozen white men in a just war.

Over the years, Albert had fleshed out the tale that his mother had tantalized him with before she died. Albert's Jim was six foot six, with fists like hams, and very proficient with every kind of weapon. He'd fought beside Teddy Roosevelt in the Spanish-American War and had been wounded more than once . . .

While reconstituting the story he'd contrived over the years, Albert became aware of a woman crossing the street.

It was Alyce or, at least, almost Alyce. The woman walking toward him was the same age Alyce had been when Albert knew her; she was taller, with different-color eyes, blond not brunette, white not black. But in spite of all that she had the same style and poise and grace. She had the same wildness in her blue, not brown, eyes. Her gait was brash like Alyce's, and her expression was one of mirth in the face of disaster.

This woman, who every man and woman around was looking at, walked right up to Albert and said, "Hi, I'm Frankie. What's your name?"

"Albert."

"You want to make some money, Albert?"

"OK."

"Well, then," she said, with a wry grin, "let's go."

Stillman's Gourmet Grocer was a chain that had a store in SoHo. Frankie had Albert leave his cart down the block from the entrance and told him to go into the fancy supermarket before she did.

"First, go back to the meat section," she told him, "and then to the fruits and vegetables. Whenever you see me, count to twelve and then go to the next section. Don't act like you know me. Just count to twelve and move on."

She laid out the plan for him to go to five different sections. He committed these destinations to memory, thinking that maybe the Tibetan notion of reincarnation was true and that Alyce had died and been reborn as Frankie.

He went into the store and was shocked by the air-conditioning. The cold made him shiver now and then, even under his coat and sweater. He made his way to the meats and looked into the cold bins with rows of steaks and pork chops, whole chickens and slabs of bacon—all set on rectangular Styrofoam plates wrapped in clear plastic. The food distracted him. He cooked in his subterranean lair but only rice and beans, chicken necks and grits.

After a while Alyce, no, Frankie, yes, Frankie, wandered into the aisle. *One, two . . .* She wore tight-fitting, faded blue jeans and a linen shirt. There was a necklace of blue stones around her neck. Her hair was tied back, and she was so beautiful . . .

. . . eleven, twelve.

Albert moved on, looking for the fruits and vegetables.

Store employees followed him openly. There was a guard in a uniform not three steps away.

Albert wasn't worried. He was no thief. His mother hated thieves. At one time his sister wanted to be a cop. Looking at a bin

filled with huge pomegranates, Albert wondered whether Luellen still had the same phone number. They hadn't been in touch in nineteen years, maybe twenty.

"Excuse me," the copper-skinned guard, wearing a blue and gray uniform, said.

At just that moment Alyce, no, Frankie, came into the far end of the aisle.

One, two, three . . .

"Excuse me," the guard insisted.

"Yes?" *. . . four, five . . .*

"Can I help you?"

"No, no, I'm just looking." *. . . seven, eight . . .*

"If you're not going to buy anything, I'll have to ask you to leave."

The guard was young and pudgy, with a silly, drooping mustache. His eyes were both insecure and resentful.

When Albert got to twelve he turned and walked away.

The guard followed him.

"Excuse me."

Albert passed the pasta aisle and one with cookies and cakes. Finally there was a row with coffee and teas, chocolates, and wildflower-flavored honeys.

Albert stopped in front of a row of golden jars and stared.

"Excuse me," the guard said.

There were store employees standing at the far end of the aisle.

"Yes?" Albert asked, grateful not to be distracted by having to count.

"I'll have to ask you to leave."

"But I haven't finished looking."

"You have to buy something."

Albert reached into his pocket and took out a five-dollar bill. He showed this to the guard.

"See?" Albert said loudly. "I have money to buy with."

Looking at the guard, he noticed that customers had stopped to watch the argument.

The guard slapped Albert's hand.

"I don't want to see that," the man with the drooping mustache said.

"I got a right just like anybody else to be here, to shop here," Albert said, loud enough that the spectators could hear.

More people were coming into the sweets aisle. Albert glanced around to make sure that Alyce wasn't one of them. No, no—Frankie.

The guard grabbed Albert's left biceps, but when Albert flexed his muscle he let go.

"I'm just lookin' for a candy bar, man. Why you wanna kick me outta here?"

"Chico," a man in a dark blue suit said.

Albert was looking around for Frankie, yes, Frankie, but she was nowhere to be seen. Had he made her up?

"Yes, Mr. Greenwood?" the security guard said.

"What's going on here?"

"Um," Chico the guard said.

"I come in here wanting to buy me a piece a' fancy candy," Albert averred, brandishing his five-dollar bill. "First I looked at the meats and vegetables just to see what you got, and then this man here said that I'm not welcome to shop in your store. I got my money right here in my hand."

Mr. Greenwood was about Albert's age. He was pale-skinned and had amber eyes behind metal-rimmed glasses. He'd made something of himself, that's what Albert thought. He was a man

who ran a grocery store, while Albert was just a guy who lived in a hole.

"Excuse me, sir," Greenwood said, forcing a smile. "You are certainly welcome to shop here, just like anybody else."

There were people all around them, but Alyce—no, Frankie—was nowhere to be seen. Albert was becoming light-headed.

"Would you accept a gift of one of our boxes of chocolates?" Greenwood was asking.

"No," Albert said. "I don't want anything from this store if you won't even let me walk around and look. I mean, that's what people do in the store, right? They shop and look and buy if they see somethin' they like. No, I don't want your candy now."

When Albert saw Frankie waiting at his shopping cart, he was overjoyed. He thought that maybe he had actually seen her on that corner but imagined their conversation. Maybe his make-believe had brought him to the store, thinking that she was following him, and he was perpetually moving away.

"You were just perfect, Al," she said, beaming.

She pulled his shoulders and kissed his cheek.

"Let's go to my house," she said. "And I'll make you a Stillman's steak."

There was an office building on Broome Street that had changed hands and was under reconstruction.

"The man who owns it is being indicted for fraud or something," Frankie told Albert. "The trial'll take years. A guy named Childress gets the keys from the construction boss and makes a few spaces available for apartments. I got the one on the sixth floor, and I only pay three hundred a month."

The halls were dusty and dark, but the makeshift apartment was bright and airy, with good furniture, electricity, and a camping stove in the office-supply room that she used as a kitchen. There was even a bathroom with running water at the end of the hall.

"You're not all that dirty," Frankie said, "but you could still wash up while I make us dinner. There's some clothes in a box in the hall that might fit you."

The bathroom had a fiberglass businessman's shower installed in the corner. Albert felt vulnerable being naked in that illegal space, washing with cold water. But he was excited too. Frankie was almost Alyce in his eyes, and for the first time in decades the mantra of love-lost had stopped nagging at him.

With a smile on his face he plunged under the ice-cold spray and experienced exhilaration that spanned his entire life. His father might have been dead by now. Luellen never became a cop. The moon was rounding the curve of the Earth, soon to be aloft in the New York sky. Albert was standing naked in that hidden space, and there was a woman down the hall who wanted to have a meal with him.

Out of the clothes box he took a pair of gray sweatpants and a green T-shirt that was only a little too small.

"You're in pretty good shape for a homeless," Frankie said, as she served him a fried rib-eye steak with white rice and shredded brussels sprouts sautéed in butter with garlic and soy sauce.

"I live in a hole in the ground," he said, savoring the meal. "But I'm not homeless. No more than you are."

"Sorry, I didn't mean to insult you."

"How come you picked me off the street like that?"

"I needed a partner, and the last guy I worked with punked out on me."

"You needed a black man to distract security?"

"Uh-huh. You want some red wine?"

"I don't think so. No, no, I don't."

"You need a job, Albert?"

"I'd like to work for you, Frankie."

"I'm not getting up off of any pussy. My last partner, Joby, didn't understand that."

"These his clothes?" Albert asked. He was thinking about his deceased Tibetan master and the ideal of balance, of the moon arcing through the sky and all the many tons of rock he'd piled over the years.

"Yeah," Frankie said, "but they belonged to a guy named Teddy before that."

"You know a lotta men."

"My father had Huntington's disease," she said, as if in answer. "He'd go into these wild rages, and my mother had me and my sister padlocked in our rooms at night. She gave me a pistol. I still have it."

"Did he ever try to hurt you, your father?"

"Only all the time."

"What's that got to do with all the men you know?" Albert was wondering about the reasoning behind his own question.

"I'm not afraid of anybody," she said.

"I won't steal," Albert said, as if in answer, "but I don't mind walkin' around in a store."

3.

Albert "walked around" while Frankie shoplifted from drugstores mainly, but they also hit hardware stores, art-supply stores, little knickknack places down in SoHo, and some Midtown department stores. Frankie knew the most valuable items to boost (and where

to sell them), and all Albert had to do was look at things that interested him.

He was especially interested in portable electronics and colored pens.

He was arrested twice but then released for lack of evidence. He made sure to have twenty dollars in his pocket so that he could always claim to be shopping.

Frankie set up a room for him down the hall from her suite. She padlocked her doors and told him that if he broke in on her, she still had the pistol her mother had given her.

"I've shot men before," she warned.

Early one Thursday morning, Frankie knocked on Albert's door. He was already awake, lying on the futon she'd had the man Childress deliver. She paid an extra hundred dollars a month for Albert. He stayed on Broome Street, even though he had another illegal home uptown.

He heard the knock but didn't answer immediately. He was lying there thinking that he hadn't had a drink since the day he met Frankie.

"Yeah?" he said at the second knock.

"You wanna get breakfast and do some shopping?"

"I have something to do today."

"What's that?" She pushed the door open and walked into the small office.

"I'm going up to Central Park to beg."

"You don't need that. We make more than enough."

"I don't do it for the money," he said.

"Why else would somebody beg on the street?"

"To save souls and redeem karma."

* * *

They left the building together and walked up Broadway toward Houston Street. Just before crossing Prince, Frankie stopped and turned around, pretending to be looking in the window of a little perfume boutique.

"Stand in front of me, Al," she whispered forcefully. "Stand in front of me. Not there. On the other side."

Albert did as she said and looked around.

Coming toward them were two burly white guys in jeans and white T-shirts. They had crew cuts and tattoos. They were the kind of men that Albert had learned to avoid on streets and back alleys.

One of the men looked at Albert as he passed.

Albert smiled, and the white man sneered.

"Are they gone?" Frankie asked.

"Yeah."

They stopped outside the entrance to the F train near Broadway and Houston.

"Who were those guys?"

"Toad Boy and Westerling," she said.

"They got a problem with you?"

"When the police asked me where they were, I told 'em—because they killed my friend Bobby. I guess the case fell through."

"What'll happen if they see you?"

"You might have to start begging full time."

Nine days later Albert and Frankie were sitting in her makeshift apartment eating a dish she called Yankee stew. It had potatoes and beef and a good amount of beer in it.

"I like you, Al," Frankie said as they ate.

"Me too. I mean, I like you too."

"Is there anything you want from me?"

"You already gimme a job and a place to stay."

"I've played this game with a lotta guys. All of them have tried to get in my pants at least once. I never let 'em. You're the first one didn't want it. Are you gay?"

"No."

"Don't like white girls?"

"I would like one thing from you, Frankie."

"What's that?"

"Could you . . . would you let me . . . let me call you Alyce?"

"Alyce?"

"Yeah. I used to know a girl by that name when I was in college . . ."

"You went to college?"

"I loved her so hard, and when she left my heart broke, and it never got better until I met you."

"You fell in love with me?"

"You took her place, kind of," he said. "You don't look like her, but you have the same spirit. If I could call you Alyce that would mean a whole lot to me."

"You'd rather that than lay up in my bed?"

"Yes."

"Well," she said, bewilderment in her tone. "OK. I guess it could be like our little nickname."

That night Albert reclined on his futon feeling like he'd passed into a new land, a new place. There was a woman like Alyce who didn't mind being called by that name.

He was smiling and sober and hopeful for something he could not quite imagine.

Through his window he could see the crescent moon. Then a loud banging from the hall brought him to his feet.

The footsteps passed his door and continued down toward Alyce's room.

He came out into the hall and saw the backs of two men. They had crew cuts, T-shirts, and tattoos.

"What do you want?" Albert demanded.

The white men turned.

"This ain't your business," either Toad Boy or Westerling said. "We just want the bitch."

Albert surged forward throwing his fists, getting hit twice for every blow he delivered. He pushed and fought and struggled in the narrow passage. The men hit him, and he felt pain, but it was like a far-off experience, like the memory held in an untouched bruise.

He felt something hard strike the side of his head and fell, happy to give in to the pull of gravity. Someone kicked him in the chest, then in the head. They kept up like that for thirty seconds or so.

Albert expected even more punishment, but there was a shot and then another shot.

"Let's get outta here!" one of the men shouted.

After the third shot the same man squealed in pain.

By then Albert was on his back looking up at the ceiling. Alyce ran by and was gone for a minute, maybe two.

Albert closed his eyes for a moment.

"Are you all right?" Frankie, no, Alyce, asked.

Albert opened his eyes, caught a glimpse of his friend, and then passed out.

* * *

He woke up in a hospital bed feeling surprisingly healthy. His jaw hurt, as did his side. He turned his head and saw a middle-aged black woman sitting in a chair. She was heavy but not fat, wearing a gray dress and holding a dark blue purse.

"Al?" she said.

"Lu?"

"Baby, I was worried that you were gonna die lyin' right here next to me."

"What happened?"

"Somebody called the police and told them that you was all beat up in this buildin'. They came and found you. You had my name and address in an old alligator wallet. The cops said there was the smell of gunpowder in the air. But you didn't have no gunshot wound."

"It was only me?" Albert Roundhouse asked.

Nodding, Luellen said, "The police wanna question you."

The interrogation lasted an hour or so. The men who broke into Albert's illegal squat were named Toad Boy and Westerling. They kicked the shit out of him, and then there were shots. He didn't know if anyone else lived on that floor. He'd only happened upon the place that day.

The hospital discharged Albert when he told them that he didn't have insurance.

His sister offered to fly him back to Los Angeles.

"I'd like to go back to school, Lu," he said. "I'd like to study history and find out what really happened with Great-Uncle Big Jim and the town of Hickton, Mississippi.

"You can come live with me," she said. "Daddy got sick after Betty Pann died. He bought a house in LA, and I took care of him till he passed."

“I have eighty-three thousand two hundred ninety-seven dollars and forty-two cents,” Albert said.

“You do? Where you get that?”

“The money I collected while saving souls. I can give it to you, and then I won’t be a charity case.”

STARTING OVER

As I do almost every day, I'm starting over again, again. Now that I've passed the sixty-year mark, it seems as if each day is a new passage, a more deeply felt loss, or some unexpected plateau achieved.

When I was younger, life was a self-contained ebb and flow, as predictable as the tides under Luna. Breakfast and a drive, work from nine to five, the children as they became enthralled with one activity and then moved on without warning to new interests. Back then their lives changed daily, while Marguerite and I remained the same for them, even when we were lying, even when we feigned feelings and interest. She loved the children, and they her and me, and I loved the kids and her too. My feelings in the early days did not waver, not even when Marguerite and Gary Knowles ran away together and she was gone for twenty-three days while I was left alone to care for Juan, Alexander, and Trish.

I told the kids that Marguerite had gone back east because her mother was sick. The sanatorium, I said, was in a place where telephones didn't work. I didn't know that Gary had left Marguerite

a week into their flight. He just needed somebody to help him out of the jam of his life: his alcoholic wife, their angry children, and the mounds of debt. He didn't know that he was using my wife, and she couldn't see past the euphoria of a world without whining children and a commonplace husband plucked off the rack.

"Jared?" she said, on that first call after she'd left me and he'd left her.

I was surprised, not about her call but because the only emotion I felt was relief.

"Yeah, Marge?"

"I'm so sorry."

"You don't have to be. My mother is staying with us, and the kids think that your mom is sick."

"I miss you," she said.

"I miss you too." It wasn't really a lie. Marguerite's departure left a crease like the misshapen dents in my fatty thigh when I sit too long on a wrinkled sofa. When I was young those crinkles used to smooth out in a few minutes, but as I have gotten older I find that they last, sometimes for hours.

"Can I come home?" she asked.

"It's your home too."

"You should know that we used protection," she said.

This pedestrian vow made me think about insurance. I wondered if I could start a business that would insure a person's life to remain as it was after having been violated by betrayal or, worse, a simple loss of faith.

"Come on home, Marguerite," I told my closest friend. "The children will be so happy that we'll probably have to take them to the zoo or something."

* * *

That was a long time ago, before we broke up for good.

The final rupture came years later. Juan and Trish were out of college by then, and Alexander was slogging his way through his sophomore year. He never made it to the halfway point, but I didn't see any problem with that. Alex liked to fish and got a job on a boat up in Alaska for a summer. He was the only black man on that boat or in the little coastal village where he'd met Solla, a Native woman who bore my first grandchild, Senta.

Well before Senta was born, Marguerite and I had decided to end our union.

I remember the evening our dissolution began. I was lighting a cigarette on the back porch, and Marguerite came out to ask me a question.

"Jared?" she called, opening the back door and catching me with the first cigarette that I'd smoked in twenty years.

Holly Martins, the office intern, had given it to me.

That morning Holly had said, for no particular reason that I could tell, "People are so afraid of dying that they don't even live the little bit of life they have."

She was dropping off client files I had asked for. Holly didn't know that it was my fifty-third birthday or that Marguerite and I had been arguing for the past four mornings about her quitting her management position at Rae, Wheeler, Johns, and Picket Financial Advisors. I only wanted her to work for seven more months, so we could take a trip to Rome before tightening our belts.

"I never wanted to go to Italy," Marguerite had said that morning. "And I can't take one more day of those sexist assholes."

"Do you smoke?" I asked Holly later that day, a few hours after her unasked-for existentialist sound bite on the general failure of humankind.

"Yes," she said. "Gitanes. They're French."

"Can I have one?"

She was wearing a flimsy, brown and pink dress that was both too short and too tight for proper office attire, but Mr. Angelo, our supervisor, was afraid to tell her that because it might be construed as sexual harassment.

She ran out of my cubicle, came back in less than a minute, and laid a nearly full pack of the French cigarettes before me. She smiled and stared into my eyes.

Holly was a pretty young woman in her twenties, rounded in ways that made me think of a comfortable sofa in a room full of hard chairs.

I had no idea that her unsolicited pronouncement, the cigarettes, and the faraway architectural vestiges of the Caesars would bring about such deep changes in me and my world.

For months after that day I thought that ideas sometimes worked like viruses, that if you heard even just one word at the right moment, dozens of lives, maybe hundreds, could be deeply impacted by a kind of mental contagion.

"What are you doing?" Marguerite asked that evening when I had just lit my first stubby little Gitane.

"Somebody . . ." I said and paused. I was thinking that if she had come out a minute before, I wouldn't have been caught. "Somebody dared me, and I'm trying to win the bet."

"By killing me?"

Marguerite had been treated for breast cancer six years earlier. They caught the few cells at a very early stage. That particular cancer was the least virulent variety, but it scared us both, and she, ever since then, had been on guard against carcinogens of all types. We no longer ate bacon, used aerosols, or allowed smoking anywhere

nearby. Marge started meditating and exercised every morning for at least forty-five minutes. We never ate sweets, red meats, white flour, or starchy vegetables. She wouldn't allow cell-phone use in the house and harried our congresswoman with a barrage of letters urging a ban on the use of microwaves near schools and hospitals and, for that matter, in any neighborhood that didn't want the dangerous radiation pulsing through its inhabitants' flesh.

"That's why I'm doing it outside," I said, taking a drag of the harsh smoke. Even after twenty years I felt that nicotine rush as if I had last savored it only yesterday.

"You won't even put it out when I'm standing right here?"

"I'll blow the smoke out the screen."

"Don't you understand?" she said. "One molecule of that poison could start my cancer all over. That's why so many people who have never smoked die of lung cancer every year."

People are so afraid of dying that they don't even live the little bit of life they have.

I took another drag, and Marguerite hurried back into the house, slamming the door and throwing the bolt.

I was in my boxers and T-shirt on the screened-in porch, smoking that cigarette and loving every poisonous breath.

I rang the doorbell for an hour before breaking the living room window and climbing in that way. Marguerite ran out wild-eyed and indignant.

"What the hell are you trying to do?" she shouted.

"It was cold outside. What were you trying to do locking me out?"

"I was protecting my life," she said as a pronouncement. "How can I trust a man who wants to fill my air with poison?"

"I'll fix the window in the morning," I replied. "Right now I'm going to bed."

"Not my bed."

"No," I said, "mine. If you don't want to get contact cancer from me, you can go sleep on the couch or in some motel that has smoke-free anti-allergen rooms."

When I came downstairs in the morning, Marguerite was sitting at the dinette table drinking tea. Her eyes were both tired and troubled.

"Did you sleep?" I asked, going about the motions of making my French-press coffee.

"This is the end, you know."

"Like existence," I agreed, reminded of a phrase that Mrs. Anthony used in high school physics.

"What the fuck does that mean?" Marguerite had never before cursed in my presence.

"I know that it is," I said, quoting my science teacher, "but I don't know why."

Marguerite stood up so violently that her cedar chair fell on its back. She held her teacup up high by its ear and, with subdued but elegant flair, let it drop. The china shattered under a spray of glittering amber liquid. She stormed out of the dinette. A few seconds later I could hear her footsteps overhead, marching into our bedroom.

When my coffee was finished, I told myself to go up there and apologize for something I didn't quite understand. Child-rearing had taught me that understanding often comes after the apology, but even so I couldn't make that climb.

Instead I made another cup of bitter coffee and remembered a story my father, Bill Thistle, used to tell about himself and his friend Emir Rolf.

"When we lived in Cincinnati," Dad would say, "Rolfie worked the midnight shift at Westerly Fabrications, and I worked for a glove

maker in the afternoon. I'd get home at eleven and wake him up. He'd get out of the bed, and I'd jump in."

I loved that story. Something about the burly men and that one bed that did double duty seemed like snugly tied shoes or tucked-in sheets. Their life was balanced and trusting.

"But what if one of you got sick?" I would always ask my dad.

"We never did," he'd say.

Marguerite always made more money than I did. She used her degree to climb the rungs of finance, whereas I worked on the flat plane of insurance claims. It was my assignment to prove that as many claims as possible fell outside the range of my company's, and its shareholders', liability.

That day was the beginning of a new pattern of actions in my life. I didn't buy coffee from the cart downstairs, and though I got in the elevator, I went to the sixth floor instead of the sixteenth.

Melanie Farr of the Belasco Insurance human-resources department greeted me with a smile.

"Yes? Can I help you?"

"My name is Thistle," I said, and she smiled as many do when they hear the lisp folded into my name.

"How can I help you, Mr. Thistle?"

"I've worked here at BI for thirty-one years, Ms. Farr," I said. I was standing before her desk with my hands held together in front of me as if I were being modest. "I started out as a file clerk, but after I graduated from college I was offered a position in claims. I was good at finding little flaws and clauses that helped justify our responses, but I didn't have management qualities and so I've stayed in the same job most of that time."

As I spoke, the smile slowly faded from Ms. Farr's wide, oddly beautiful face. She was in her early forties, I figured, a decade

younger than I. She was beginning to worry that I'd be a problem. I supposed that her job was like mine in some ways; people would come to her with issues, and she'd try to resolve them in such a way as to cause the least trouble for BI, its officers, and its shareholders.

"And what is your problem, Mr. Thistle?" She was typing on the keyboard of her computer, as I did whenever a claim crossed my blotter.

"No problem, Ms. Farr. It's just that I need to leave this job."

"You're resigning?"

"Yes."

"As of when?"

"Today. I know people usually give two weeks' notice, but I have an urgent issue that needs to be addressed, and after I'm done with that I wouldn't be coming back anyway."

"Have you told your supervisor?"

"I'd rather you do that. Mr. Mallory doesn't have much patience when people need time off. I'm certain that he'd send me up here if I told him that I'm—"

"You've worked for the company over thirty years," Ms. Farr said, interrupting my explanation. She was reading my personal data off her computer screen.

"Yes. I told you that," I said.

"You have built up quite a large retirement account with us."

"Oh?"

"You don't know?"

"I never really thought about retirement. It just seemed like I'd be at that desk until I died one day. Statistics say that I'd probably die at home or in a hospital, but I suppose I could fall dead of a heart attack anywhere—even at my desk."

The woman's broad face suddenly turned sympathetic.

"You haven't considered early retirement?"

"No," I said.

"At fifty-three," she said, rolling her eyes upward to look at the general figures in her head, "with more than twenty-five years, you could get about thirty-two percent of your current salary."

"OK."

"In order to get that you'll have to go through the early-retirement process. That would take about three months."

"But today is my last day," I said, with a certainty I'd rarely felt.

"That's silly, Mr. Thistle," she lisped. "If you leave today you would only receive the face value of the account."

"What are you doing?" Holly Martins asked as I was putting my belongings into an empty Xerox-paper box that I got from the copy room. The sum total of my work life fit in the space it took to hold eight reams of impossibly white paper.

"Packing," I said to the young philosopher.

She was wearing a red dress and no hose. The flesh of her arms and legs there in that otherwise sexless atmosphere made me happy.

"You moving offices?" she asked.

"Have you ever been to Italy?"

"No," she said, giving the word one and a half syllables.

"When are you having lunch?"

"In twenty-seven minutes."

When I got home, there were still shards of broken china on the kitchen floor. Splinters of shattered teacup were plastered in place by dried honeyed tea. When I went out on the screened-in back porch, the first thing I thought of was smoking.

I had smoked another Gitane on the walk to Samba Sam's Jamaican Delights with Holly. I wanted another one now, but Marguerite was in the backyard, wearing a coral blouse, turquoise pants,

and yellow flip-flops. She was watering the hundred or more potted plants with the long-spouted copper watering can. The terra-cotta pots were set on tiered shelving that looked like miniature bleachers at the back wall of the yard.

Seeing my wife at the zenith of her domestic bliss, I realized why she needed to quit working. She had loved her job, whereas I had never really cared about mine. Her advancement had been a source of pride for her before, and after, the desertion with Gary Knowles.

She loved her job, but as the years rolled by that relationship had gone cool. She still hoped for that early passion, but new bosses and different needs pushed her to the side, left her unsatisfied. Now all she had was a backyard that would respond and flower to her touch.

I knew for a fact that Marguerite needed to rest and heal in the safety of that footprint of terra-cotta and green. My empathy, however, was tempered by events earlier in the day. On the way to Samba Sam's, I remembered that I didn't have much cash, and so I went to the ATM machine to find that our joint checking account had a balance of only three dollars. Both savings accounts had been emptied and closed that morning.

Holly had to pay for our lunch.

I'd arrived home at three minutes past three.

Marguerite turned, wiping her brow, and saw me standing there.

"Jare," she mouthed.

I tried to remember anything important that had happened in the last twenty years.

There were the children, of course, but their lives were their own now. There was the house, but I'd soon be moving out of there, with no expectation of nostalgia or feeling of loss.

Marguerite walked up to the bottom stair of the porch and smiled at me. It was a stranger's expectant acknowledgment.

"You're home early," she said.

"You are too."

"I never went in," she replied. "I was too tired, and so I slept until just an hour ago."

"I came home to apologize," I said, matching her lie for lie.

"Are you going to fix the window?" she asked.

"Tomorrow," I said, thinking, *When you clean the fucking kitchen floor.*

"Why don't we sit down?"

Marguerite waved at two fiberglass lawn chairs that I'd bought eleven years before. The skeletal-looking seats had been bright red when they were new, but the years outside had faded them to a pink-tinted gray. While I went to work day after day, their luster had succumbed to sunlight.

"Sure," I said, and we sat at a forty-five-degree angle to each other, the convergence of our stares meeting at the screen door where our marriage had finally failed.

"Are you still smoking?"

"No. That was just a bet."

"Stupid bet."

"Yeah. I guess it was."

"You really scared me breaking the window like that," she said with no real emotion.

"I got a splinter of your china cup in my eye," I replied. Lying to her was becoming . . . second nature. "Had to go down to the company nurse to have her take it out."

"I didn't mean for that to happen," was her apology.

I felt the stirrings of an erection. That and the lying brought about a thrumming in my heart. I turned to look at my wife. She

was a new person, a whole Otherness, in the yard that I had never, ever sat in before.

"What?" she asked of my expression.

"My dick is hard," I said in wonder.

"I hope you don't think that I'm going to do anything about that."

"Of course not," I said, in a falsely reassuring tone. "You asked, and I'm telling you that my dick is hard."

"Stop saying that."

I stood up in front of the mother of my children, my pants displaying the outline of the modest erection. Marguerite stared in wonder. I was sure that she'd thought I was lying. Seeing it, a confused look twisted its way across her face.

"I'm going upstairs to jack off," I said.

I rolled against my marital mattress thinking not of sex, not exactly, but of the conversation Holly and I had at lunch.

"You broke the window?" she asked, interrupting the long and somewhat banal tale.

"She wouldn't let me in."

"And that was just because I gave you that cigarette?"

"No," I said again, as I pressed my groin down against the thick wadding of the mattress. "It was because you said that thing about people not living their lives. You said it about everybody else, but I was thinking about me. I am not living my life. I needed that cigarette to live, and Marguerite blew up without even asking why. She thought I was trying to kill her, not save myself."

"No," Holly assured me, or maybe she was trying to convince herself that she wasn't somehow complicit in an attempted murder-by-nicotine.

"She lives in mortal fear of death," I said, knowing the truth as it came out of my mouth. "Dread like that has no room for half measures."

"And what are you going to do now?" the pretty, chubby, and young mocha-brown office gofer asked.

"I'm told that I have a fully matured life policy with BI and a settlement of one hundred and ninety-six thousand dollars for my retirement fund. I want to go to Rome in the next month or so. Would you like to come with me?"

I was thumping down hard on the mattress when remembering the question.

"Like your girlfriend?"

"Like anything you want to be. I just need the company."

"And you'd pay?"

"Of course."

"How long?"

"You tell me that. I don't even know how long I'll be there."

"Sure, I'll go," Holly said. "I might even like you enough to stay."

I groaned in expectation of the orgasm; that groan turned into a shout. I could hear Marge's footfalls on the stairs, but the door was closed and I knew she wouldn't come in. I was sweating and so happy that a young woman would fly with me across the ocean to the site of an ancient empire that once conquered a world.

"Jare!" Marguerite shouted through the closed door.

"Don't come in!"

"What's happening in there?"

"Don't come in, Marguerite," I said again. "I'm just getting used to what's happened."

* * *

All that was seven years ago. The divorce was civil if not amicable, because I agreed to share all of my money and Marguerite finally consented to buying me out of the house.

I live in a studio apartment in downtown LA and work for myself. I incorporated under the name Big Bad Investments (BBI) and, doing business in that name, bought e-mail lists from BI and a dozen other insurance companies. I then sent out a broad blast to every policyholder saying that I was an expert on the devious ways in which insurance companies refuse to pay. I charge between two and five hundred dollars to review a policy before the claim is made, one thousand dollars plus expenses to dispute any refusal of payment.

I take a long walk every morning. Last week my left knee began to hurt halfway through the constitutional. This pain is new, and I pay close attention, as it catches on every other step.

My children with Marguerite have shunned me, but I still mark their birthdays and call them on Christmas.

Holly got pregnant on the Riviera under a crescent moon. She lives walking distance from my studio, 1,727 little stitches of pain away.

Our daughter is named Roma, and she entered first grade last week.

Holly has a boyfriend named Henry. He doesn't like me, but I think he's a fine young man.

Marguerite had a relapse of the cancer two years after we parted. I stayed with her for three weeks because our children were living too far away and she's the only daughter of parents who were both only children. She blamed that cigarette for her condition. I accepted that. We didn't talk much, and I stayed in Alexander's room. Late at night I could hear her come to our son's door, sniffing the air. She was still searching for a whiff of my infidelity, proof that everything she believed was justified.

LEADING FROM THE AFFAIR

"Come in," the graying blond woman said, after we made our introductions at the threshold. "Have a seat."

Three padded blue chairs around a low triangular table made up the furnishings of the small office. No desk. No bookcase. The blinds were pulled down over the window. A nonintrusive tan and blue carpet covered the floor from wall to wall. The sounds of traffic could be heard quite clearly, as Dr. Quarterly's room was on the first floor facing onto East Eighty-First Street.

Noting the hiss of tires racing on the wet streets outside, I took the chair set off a little to the right. She remained standing a moment.

Dr. Agnes Quarterly was maybe five eight and slender. In her late forties, she seemed older but not worn or unattractive. There was a gravitas to her bearing, in spite of the smile.

She wore a dark blue dress suit and a white blouse that buttoned up like a man's shirt. Her shoes were dark, dark red with one-inch heels, the leather hard and shiny—almost like plastic.

She sat across from me, her spine erect, not resting against the back of the chair. This caused me to sit up a little straighter.

"So," she began, "Mr. Lassiter, you're looking for a therapist."

"Yeah . . . uh, yes, I am."

Her salt-and-butter hair was combed but only just. It wasn't coiffed or *done*. There was a slight indentation on the bridge of her nose. I wondered where the glasses were and also where was the book or papers that she'd been reading before I'd arrived.

"Have you been in psychotherapy before?"

"No. Never."

"So, what makes you feel you need it now?" She was watching my eyes, looking, I believed, for signs of depravity.

"It's . . ." I said and then hesitated.

"Yes?" Her voice was mild, not commanding or insistent.

"I'm stuck."

Slightest insinuation of a smile appeared on her lips.

"How are you stuck?"

"I . . ." My heart was beating fast, and I could feel my ears getting hot. I hadn't expected this reaction. For a moment I thought I might be experiencing the beginnings of a heart attack.

"Are you all right?"

"Yes. It's just that, I guess I'm a little nervous."

"There's no need. Everything we say in this room is confidential. You are free to speak your mind."

"And can I keep my secrets too?"

"You only need say what you feel comfortable saying," she said. "And what you did say was that you feel stuck. In what way?"

"It's like," I said, falling into an old, familiar groove, "everybody in the world was standing at a line at the start. Millions and millions of people preparing to get on with their lives. A signal was

given, and we all began to move forward. Almost everybody was traveling at the rate of ten miles a year. That's like the normal rate."

I realized that I was looking at the floor, so I raised my head. Dr. Quarterly was gazing at me with what I can only call intense passivity.

"Everybody but me," I continued. "Me, I'm racing ahead at fifty miles a year, but at the same time I'm going backward at forty-nine point nine miles. And so at the end of each year, almost everyone around me has traveled ahead ten miles, while I've gone ten times that but am only a tenth of a mile farther from the starting line."

I could see in the therapist's expression that she was impressed with the explanation. She had no idea that I was a fraud.

"What do you do for a living, Mr. Lassiter?"

"I'm a copy editor for about a dozen online magazines run by the Din-Pro Consortium."

"What kind of magazines?"

"Everything from political news reports to sex stories," I said. "Sometimes the magazines morph into different kinds of content. It sounds technological, very twenty-first century, but it's not. I just do what copy editors have been doing for the past two hundred years."

"Do they pay you well?"

"I know your fee," I said. "I can pay."

"I'm not asking that. I'm wondering why you feel that you're not making headway. I mean there must be others around you who would love to have a job like yours. So many people are unemployed nowadays."

"It's not my job," I said. "Somebody else might love doing what I'm doing. That person would be traveling at a normal rate. Another person might have just gotten fired, but he has a wife who tells him that it's OK and maybe a child, so he sees hope for the future.

"I have a job I don't care for and a studio apartment with a TV and a computer, a girlfriend who I think is looking for a better relationship, and no way out."

"You feel lost," she said, and I had to clench my jaw to keep from crying.

"Yes."

We talked about my father, who is dead; and my mother, who no longer recognizes me; my age, which is near sixty; and my girlfriend, whose name is Jool.

"Does Jool live with you?" Quarterly asked.

"No. She owns a condo in downtown Brooklyn. She's very good with money . . ."

I got home at 4:17 by the big digital clock that I have framed and mounted on the wall like a painting. I sat next to the window, with its light-and-dark-gray frame, gazing onto Lexington Avenue. Snow was dancing in the breeze, undecided, it seemed, whether it was falling or maybe just hanging there, twirling.

Night was almost come; the darkness was filtering into my brain.

"Hello?" I said, answering the phone on the first ring.

It was dark outside, and the same flakes still seemed to be spinning, now in lamplight, like some Einsteinian law made manifest through slapdash serendipity.

"I called this afternoon, but you weren't there," Jool said.

"What time is it?"

"Seven forty-five."

"I've been sitting here for hours."

"You didn't call back."

"I wasn't here."

"I left a message."

"I didn't listen to the messages."

"What's wrong, Frank?" Jool asked.

We were lying side by side, not touching, in my queen-size bed. We'd had sex, showered, and then brushed our teeth, side by side.

"I'm stuck," I said.

"You've been telling me that for nine years."

"Then why do you keep asking?"

"Doesn't your therapist help at all?" she asked.

Jool put her dark hand upon my darker chest. Her baby finger tickled my nipple by mistake. I shivered.

"He tries to help me," I said. "One time, a long time ago, he changed my life. Back then I was lost."

"Maybe you need a new therapist," she suggested.

"No. Dr. Aguilera knows me better than anyone."

"Then maybe he could give you some kind of antidepressant or something."

"Did you kiss him?"

"Who?" Jool asked.

"J Silver."

She sat straight up in the bed. At forty-four, Jool still had a youthful figure. Her skin was young, and her eyes always in focus.

"Did you look in my e-mails?"

"Did you suck his dick?"

She shoved back away from me, and for a moment I thought that she was falling out of the bed. But then she stood up and gathered her clothes from the stuffed chair in the corner.

I watched her getting dressed. It was always the same order: panties, bra, blouse, skirt. Then she stepped into her Uggs and picked up her bag.

"It's three in the morning," I said.

She had to put down the shoulder bag to don her gray nylon down coat.

"You never talk to me," she said, once she was ready to go.

"I'm talking now."

"You have no right," she said.

"Let me make us some coffee," I pleaded. "We can at least wait till the sun comes up."

She didn't wait, didn't say another word, just stormed out, taking the last ort of passion from the room along with her.

"She just left you in the middle of the night?" Christian Aguilera asked me three days later. His office was on the far East Side, overlooking the river.

"Yeah," I said. "We were talking in bed, and I asked her about J Silver. It just came out."

"How long ago did you find out about him?"

"Ten months."

"Why didn't you ever mention it in here?"

"I don't know. I thought if I talked about it, I'd get mad and then Jool would leave."

"And is she still seeing him?"

"I don't think so."

"Then why spring it on her in the middle of the night?"

"She . . . she was asking me why I feel so, so disassociated, and then she wondered what good you were doing. She wanted me to take antidepressants."

"And that made you angry?"

"I guess."

"Angrier than her affair with J Silver?"

I couldn't find a way into that question. I'd never met J Silver. I didn't even know what he was—what color or religion. It was hard to be angry at a man without a face or identity.

"I don't know," I said at last.

"Then why didn't you just say to Jool that you didn't want her telling you what drugs to take?"

"Hi, Mr. Lassiter," Kara Gunderson said.

Kara was a counter waitress at the Bebop Diner on West Fifty-Seventh. She always took my order.

"Hi, Kara. How are you?"

"Did you finish editing that nasty article?" she asked.

"Which one?"

"The one about the ad exec having sex with her dog."

"Yeah. She withdrew the piece though."

"Too embarrassed?"

"She sent an e-mail calling me a Nazi censor because I cut out a few of the details that she repeated over and over."

"I guess she just didn't want to be corrected."

"No one does. Do you want my order?"

"Has it changed?"

"No."

Kara's smile was beautiful. The olive-gold skin and lush almond-shaped eyes marked her Asian features with a sculptural quality.

"Which one of your parents is Swedish?" I asked on a whim.

"Neither," she said. "I'm adopted."

At 2:57 A.M. by the framed clock the phone rang.

I was sitting at the window holding the tiny slip of paper that had Kara's phone number on it. From early evening until about

eleven I was thinking about making the call, but my mind kept going in circles: She was too young or I was too old. What did younger women want with older men except for security and then marriage? What did I want from her that I didn't already get three afternoons a week at the lunch counter? What would we talk about? How could I touch her?

"Hello?" I said into the phone.

"What do you care what I did or didn't do with Jim?" Jool asked.

"Jim?"

"Jim Silver."

"Um . . . I guess maybe I don't care."

She hung up.

I didn't wonder about the call. We hadn't spoken at all since she'd left. Instead I worried about waiting too long and not calling Kara in time. I worried that if I didn't call her, I wouldn't be able to show my face at the diner again.

The phone rang.

"Hello?"

"How long have you known?"

"I don't know," I lied. "At least nine months."

"And in all that time you didn't say anything?"

The answer was obvious, so I didn't reply.

"You didn't act like you knew," Jool said, now a bit calmer. "If anything you were nicer, more loving."

"I guess."

"I haven't seen Jim in six months. Why ask me now?"

"Because you were telling me to take drugs."

"That doesn't make any sense. I was trying to help you."

For a long while we were both silent.

"Frank."

"Yes."

"Do you want me to come over?"

"No."

"So we're through?"

"It's late."

"Why haven't you called me?"

"You're the one who walked out."

"And so how have you been, Mr. Lassiter?" Dr. Quarterly asked.

I was sitting in the same blue chair. She didn't have that little indentation on the bridge of her nose that day.

Her dress suit was gray.

"I broke up with my girlfriend."

"I'm sorry to hear that. What happened?"

I told her about the late-night talk.

"She thinks that I should prescribe antidepressants for you after just one meeting?"

"What do you think?" I asked.

"You seem to be somewhat unhappy, but I won't know how to proceed until we've had at least a few more meetings."

I sighed, feeling relieved of something I could not have put into words.

"Why did you mention her lover so long after the affair was over?" she asked.

I said something, but afterward I couldn't remember what it was.

"You're very quiet today, Frank," Dr. Aguilera said.

He's a beefy man, much larger than I. Size aside, his dark eyes have always been his most imposing quality.

"Do you think I'm depressed?" I asked.

"What do you think?"

"About what you think?"

Aguilera smiled, then grinned.

"What's wrong, Frank?"

"I realized that I've been coming to see you for thirty-one years next week," I said. "And I don't even know if you're married, have kids, or where you live."

"You've never asked."

"I was living in a shelter when I first came here," I said, as some kind of retort.

"But you didn't tell me about it until you'd found an apartment a year later."

"Back then I changed very fast," I said, performing a ritual. "Because of you, I went to school and became a journalist. I made something out of myself."

"Yes, you did."

"But now I'm stuck again. Jool left me but calls every night. She says that she wants to come over."

"What do you want?"

"I don't know."

"Do you want to see Jool?"

"I don't want anything . . . nothing. All I want is for it all to be over or for it to change into something . . . I don't know, unexpected."

"What does that mean?" Aguilera asked.

"I don't know."

"Maybe we should discuss medication again."

"No," I said. "I don't want to do drugs."

"Hi, Mr. Lassiter," Kara said that afternoon at the Bebop.

"How are you, Kara?"

"I was worried that you wouldn't come back after I gave you my number and you didn't call."

"We should have dinner together."

"When?" Her answer was light and friendly.

"Tonight."

Two nights later I was lying awake thinking about the brief good-night kiss that Kara had given me. We'd had dinner two nights in a row.

"I like talking to you because you don't seem like a New Yorker," she'd said at the end of the second date. We were standing at the subway entrance near Broadway and Houston. "I mean, you seem interested in things outside the city and, and outside you."

That's when she kissed my cheek, a big smile on her luminescent face.

The phone rang.

"Hello?"

"Where were you the last two nights?" Jool asked.

"Where were you?"

After a brief pause she said, "I guess I deserve that. I mean, I'm the one who walked out and, and who cheated."

I was thinking about the double "and" from both Kara and Jool. This united them in my mind, making me feel like there was a blood-knot in my head.

"It's late, Jool," I said.

"We should get together and talk."

"We don't talk so well," I said.

"I'll answer any question you have."

I asked her about Jim and when they'd met and what they'd done. She answered my questions, in great detail, even though I think we both knew I didn't want to hear most of it.

"Then why open yourself up for something that hurts?" Dr. Agnes Quarterly asked.

"At least that way I'm feeling something," I said.

"And is that worth it?"

"It is, just before she starts talking."

"What does that mean?"

"I want to ask," I said, "and I want her to be willing to answer. It's just that once she starts talking, what she says hurts me."

The look on the therapist's face was intent and quizzical, like that of a mathematician staring at a convoluted, inexplicably erroneous equation.

"Maybe we should try you out on an antidepressant. There's a new one called Lessenin-60. We can start you on a low dosage."

"OK."

There were things that Jool had refused to do with Jim Silver. They'd had safe sex, and she'd interrogated him about his health before they had sex the first time.

I filled the prescription for the antidepressant but never took the blue-and-pink capsules.

"I don't think I'll ever get married," twenty-nine-year-old Kara Gunderson told me at a falafel bar in Times Square. "I mean, I don't want kids, and what other reason is there for getting married?"

"I don't know," I said. "You get old and you want company and somebody to share the load."

"Everybody breaks up," she said. "You can't count on them staying with you."

I buzzed Jool's apartment at a little past midnight. Kara and I had made out for a while in a doorway on West Forty-Eighth. She'd disengaged from the embrace, telling me that she didn't want to move too fast.

"Hello?" my ex-girlfriend said through the speaker.

"Hi."

"Frank?"

"Yeah."

It was at least a full minute before she said anything else.

"You, you can't come up now, honey," she said, pitying me.

When I was a few steps away, I heard her say something else but couldn't make out the words.

The next afternoon the phone rang, and I was surprised to hear Bob Brandt on the line.

Bob was the head editor at Din-Pro Consortium. We almost always communicated through e-mails.

"Hi, Frank," he said. "How are you?"

"OK. I mean, I guess I could complain, but nobody listens, right?"

"Yeah. You got that right."

"How come you're calling?" I asked.

"Din-Pro's cutting back, Frank. They've taken a big hit in advertising revenue, and I'm going to have to take half your editing load."

"Oh."

"And they're cutting your rate by ten percent. They wanted to cut it by fifteen, but I talked them out of it."

"Oh. Wow. Thanks, Bob."

Thanks, Bob.

Both Aguilera and Quarterly allowed me to reduce my payments by fifty percent. I kept seeing them—her on Monday mornings and him on Thursday afternoons.

I asked Christian what the effects of Lessenin-60 were and translated that into the experiences that Agnes expected.

Kara got me a part-time dishwashing job at the Bebop. We got more serious, and she stayed over once or twice a week.

A few weeks later, when I was alone, the phone rang a little after midnight.

"Hello?"

"Are you alone?" Jool asked.

"Yeah. Sure."

"Can I come up?"

"Where are you?"

"Across the street."

That was the best sex I'd ever had. Something had been building up ever since we'd separated. I would sit in bed at night thinking of all the things she'd told me, that I'd asked her, about Jim Silver.

"Have you been seeing him again?" I asked, when we were spent, in the early hours of the morning.

"Yes," she whispered.

"Are you in love?"

"It might be that," she said. "But more it's like I have to do something. You're always saying how you're stuck or whatever, and I'm just getting older. Jim wants to move in with me and maybe get more serious. And you wouldn't even let me come over."

"You always said that you liked living alone," I said, "that you had gotten used to your ways."

"That was before you asked me if I had kissed Jim."

"Not when she first met him?" Dr. Quarterly asked.

"No. She'd met him at a design conference and, she says, just kind of fell into a sexual thing. But then when I asked her about it, she started to wonder about why I'd be jealous when our lives were so separate. I guess she realized how lonely she was."

"And how do you feel about that?"

"It hurts when I see her, and it hurts when I don't."

Jool and I saw each other every night for a week, and then it was over. She called and said that she couldn't do it anymore.

"But things have been so strong," I said, almost arguing.

"We're acting like kids," she said. "I'm not sleeping, and sometimes when I'm at your house I'm afraid of the way you look at me."

"It's just that I feel, I don't know, desperate for you."

"That's not what I need from a man."

"Can't we get together and talk about it?"

"No. It's over. I'm not seeing you anymore."

I was sitting on the bed when Jool was breaking up with me for the second time. I felt relieved. Our relationship had run off the road, and that was that.

Sixteen minutes after Jool and I hung up, the phone rang.

I was hoping that it was her calling back and also that she had not changed her mind. I wanted to talk more about getting back together but not to change what had already been decided.

"Hello?"

"Hi, Frank." It was Kara.

"Hey."

"You haven't really been sick have you?"

"No. I've had some, um, some personal problems."

"I don't want to see you anymore, Frank. It's just not working. I mean . . . we're too different. You're too old."

Those last three, or maybe four, words hurt me, not because of my age but because I could tell that Kara was trying to hurt me. Her intention was its own end.

"I've been seeing another therapist," I said to Dr. Aguilera that Thursday at the end of our session.

"What do you mean?"

"For the past two months I've been going to another therapist."

"Why?"

"Because I'm stuck, and everything's falling apart around me."

"I'm surprised that another doctor would see you knowing that you were already in a therapeutic relationship."

"I didn't tell her."

"I don't understand, Frank. It doesn't make sense."

"I can't explain it very well. I've needed to move on, and I didn't know how. Every day is just like the last. I feel like I'm drowning, like I'm asleep and can't wake up."

"We should discuss this at length," he said. "Not at the end of our time."

"Now let me get this straight," Dr. Quarterly said that Friday, at a special time she made available for me. "You have another therapist and have been in treatment with him for the past thirty years."

"Yes," I said, "but I've chosen you."

"You said that you hadn't been in therapy before."

"Because I wanted to start on a clean slate, to be sure that I could make some advancement with you."

"But you lied."

"Those were the secrets I told you about in our first meeting."

"No, Mr. Lassiter. The basic expectation in therapy is that the patient and the doctor maintain as much honesty as they are capable of."

"What are you saying?" I asked.

Both Aguilera and Quarterly ended therapeutic relations with me. Three months later I received an invitation to the after-ceremony wedding reception of Jool Lanscome and James Silver.

Kara moved back to Minnesota to her pseudo-Scandinavian roots.

When Bob Brandt cut my editing down to three online publications, I moved into a rooming house in Staten Island and started an online publication of my own, called *Broken Hearts Monthly*, which has been wildly successful. It started out as a blog telling my own stupid story. But I got so many responses that, with Bob's help, I organized a virtual publication that presents confessionals, artwork, poems, short stories, and also a dating service.

I work so hard at the magazine that I have little time for any kind of social life. But I've been slowly thinking of getting back into therapy. Nowadays I've become so popular that I'm often invited as an expert on love and relationships. The anxiety this notoriety produces is sublime and, at the same time, almost unbearable.

CUT, CUT, CUT

1.

"There's a marked difference between brain functions, knowledge, and mental potentials," Martin Hull said to Marilee Frith-DeGeorgio at Mike's Steaks on Forty-Seventh Street just east of Grand Central Station. The time was 6:46 P.M. on a clear and bright Tuesday in late May.

This was their first meeting—a blind date, inasmuch as they'd met through the online dating service People for People, provided by one of the few surviving alternative lifestyle magazines from California's Bay Area, *The Revolution Will Not Be Televised.*

The questionnaire provided for subscribers to *TRWNBT*'s People for People allowed participants to enter gender identity and preference, intellectual endeavors, personal ambitions, and accomplishments in life. The survey did not ask for race, age, income bracket, religious orientation, or physical proportions. One could *fudge* a few of the banned subjects by surreptitiously including them in the essay-like answers to the questions provided.

Marilee, for instance, had typed in that her most profound political ambition was to one day computerize the voting process in America based on the positive concept of what people wanted and not what they did not want or were afraid of. She added (parenthetically) that she had no patience for people who harbored antidemocratic thoughts.

"In my ideal system," she told Martin that evening, "people would be voting for what they had in common, not what they hated or feared about each other."

Martin considered it his greatest *personal* accomplishment that he had run a half marathon every other week for one year, four years earlier. He did not, could not, mention that he was a dark brown man, descendant of a long line of slaves and sharecroppers from the Mississippi Delta. Marilee was surprised that a *black* man had filled out the People for People form she'd read. But she decided to go through with the date because of the caveat clause in the PFP e-contract.

PFP was the go-between for first dates and electronically queried the participants within a week of the rendezvous. If it was reported that either party had not shown up, or left before the date actually started, a mark was put in the offender's file. If any member of PFP got three such marks, he or she was deleted from the service.

The week before, Marilee had been scheduled to meet a man named Joseph Exeter. Joe was a portly man, and Marilee quite small in comparison. Joe's breathing was loud, and from time to time, a not very pleasant odor wafted from his side of the table at the Midtown sushi bar. When their second drink had not dimmed her olfactory awareness of Exeter, Marilee excused herself to go to the restroom and never returned.

So she would have to sit through this date, because PFP was the best dating service that she'd encountered since her divorce from Paris DeGeorgio, a latent conservative and an outright thief.

Martin Hull was the opposite of both Marilee's last date and first husband. He was two inches shorter and maybe five pounds lighter than Marilee, who was five seven and 135 pounds. She worked out every day for an hour and a half, so her few extra pounds looked good in the step-class mirror.

"But I thought you were a plastic surgeon," she said, in response to his pontificating on the contrasting qualities of the human brain.

"That's my day job," he said with a smile. His grin, Marilee thought, was both goofy and sincere. "But the neurological sciences are my passion."

"Why didn't you become a brain surgeon then?"

"That would be like an abstract artist becoming a house painter."

"Really?" Marilee said. "I thought that that kind of surgery was the very top of the field."

"Not really," Martin said, crinkling his nose and exposing the gap between upper his teeth. "Surgeons all specialize. Cut, cut, cut—that's their whole life. That's the way they get so proficient. They do the same procedures day in and day out—thousands of them; might as well be working on a production line."

"At five million dollars a year," Marilee added.

"Yeah, I guess. But, you know, I'd need a lot more money than that if I had to do the same thing every day for the rest of my life."

"Except for sex, food, and good music," Marilee said. Martin's size and goofy demeanor gave her the courage to say what was on her mind.

He smiled, half-nodded, and looked down, saying, "I meant one's working life."

Marilee felt a twitch in her chest and wondered what kind of sex partner a small, shy man like this might be.

"So you said that you're divorced," Martin prompted.

"Paris DeGeorgio," she replied, nodding out every other syllable.

"Sounds like a good name for a clothes designer."

"That wasn't his birth name. He was born Anastazy Kozubal."

"Polish, huh?"

"You knew that? Everyone else ends up asking me where the name comes from. The first guess is almost always Russia."

"That's because of *Anastazy*," Martin said. "Makes it sound like a tsarina. I like to study those parts of language that make humanity a culture as well as a species. The brain, you know."

"I had a business selling Mexican wheat to various South and Central American nations," Marilee said.

"Mexican wheat?"

"There are some large farms in the southern highlands. I organized them over the Internet and made a two-percent profit. It was going pretty good, until one day I found out that Paris was skimming my profits and donating to this group called the New Redeemers . . ."

"California archconservatives, right?" Martin asked.

"Only," Marilee continued, "he had made a kickback deal with the treasurer and was salting half the money away in a Jamaican bank."

"Wow."

"Are you ready to order?" a tall waiter in a bright green three-piece suit asked.

Martin gestured for Marilee to go first. It was at that moment she decided to take him home.

2.

"That was amazing," she said in her own bed, lying next to Martin Hull, a man she had met only six hours before.

"Yeah," Martin said, unable to suppress his toothful grin.

"I never had a man pay such close attention to my body."

"Well, you know," Martin said shyly, "when you're a little guy with no hidden talents you have to learn to work harder."

"I'm still trying to catch my breath."

"Want me to get you some water?" he asked.

"Is that the doctor talking?"

"You know, I liked your idea about online voting," he said. "The negative side of democracy is that people usually vote either for their pocketbooks or against what they're afraid of."

"I'm sorry I said that stuff about brain surgeons," she said then, feeling that she should be nice to the plain little man with the magic kisses. "I'm sure plastic surgeons do good work too."

"I do a lot of community-service stuff," he agreed. "You know . . . reconstructive work for those that can't afford it."

"Like harelips?"

"Or old scars . . . even regrettable tattoos," he said. "It would be cool if you could vote at home every night. Just turn your smart TV to the political choices channel and make your mark."

"Why do you keep doing that?"

"What?"

"Every time I ask about you, you say one thing and then turn the subject back to me. Is that one of the ways you try harder?"

"I guess it is. I mean, I know that people like talking about themselves, and there's not much I have to say."

"You seem interested in the brain."

"Yeah, but whenever I start talking about it, people always point out that I'm a plastic surgeon."

"I'm sorry about that," Marilee said.

"It's OK. You're right. I should be more, um, revealing."

"You said you were married once?"

"To Sonora Simonson," he said, sitting up with the words.

"That's an odd name."

"Yeah. Her mother named her but never said why she chose it. They'd never been to Mexico, and no one in the entire family spoke Spanish. I asked them all one Christmas."

"Why did you two split?"

"I was conferring with an intestinal-tract expert, Philip Landries. He'd come to our apartment quite often. Sonora made dinner for us whenever he stayed late. One day I came home and found a note from her saying that she was out with a girlfriend at a movie. Philip was supposed to drop by, but he didn't. Sonora didn't come home, and Philip was gone for good. I got a letter from them nineteen months later. He'd gotten a job in Amsterdam and asked her to go with him."

"And they left, just like that?" Marilee asked. "Didn't even say anything?"

"Not to anyone. The police investigated me for over a year. They were sure that Phil and Sonny were having an affair and that I killed them. There was credit-card evidence of them staying in a Midtown hotel."

"Oh my God. Did they arrest you?"

"Not formally, but I was called down to the local station six times. Once they questioned me for over eight hours."

"Did you get a lawyer?"

"No. I knew I hadn't killed them, and so I just continued with my work."

"You don't sound like you were very broken up over their betrayal."

"There was a kind of a, of an unconscious trade-off," Martin said, frowning and allowing his head to tilt to the side.

"A trade-off?"

"Phil was in research," the plastic surgeon explained. "The intestines of all living beings are rife with various kinds of parasites. Many of these creatures, these parasites, are symbiotic. They live in harmony with the systems they inhabit. You gotta love that Darwin."

"What does that have to do with your wife running off with your friend?" Marilee asked.

"Phil wasn't really my friend. I paid him to consult with me about the more exotic intestinal parasites. That's where I learned about the hydra-monotubular-tridacteri."

"The what?"

Martin repeated the name and said, "It's a microscopic parasite that can be bred and altered in a fairly simple controlled environment. You can suppress its reproductive cycles and implant it with differing forms of DNA, which it, in turn, blends into the host system. Those traits make it one of the greatest possible biological and genetic delivery systems."

"And the man that gave this to you was fucking your wife."

"Painful," Martin admitted. "But in the grand scheme of things a minor indiscretion."

"Minor? A woman does that to you and you aren't devastated?"

"No, no," Martin said, though he wasn't really denying her implied accusation. "I mean, I felt bad, but three days before they went off, Phil brought me a rare specimen that I dubbed hydra-monotubular-tridacteri-1."

Unable to think of a response or even a question, Marilee sat up too.

"It's what they call a microsite, almost exactly the same as the original HMT but mutated, with a slightly different DNA count," Martin Hull continued. "I realized that by crossbreeding the species, you could, theoretically, create an HMT hinny."

"A what?"

"It's like a mule. A creature that exists but cannot reproduce, making it a perfect biological delivery system, because after it does its job it dies."

There was now a kind of ecstasy in Martin's smile. Marilee felt moved by a deep passion, even if she didn't understand the ramifications. Years later, after Martin had been sentenced to 117 years in prison, she was still aroused by the memory of his fervor.

She reached out with both hands and pinched his nipples —hard.

Martin bent sideways and tipped over, pretzel-like, in the bed.

"You like that, don't you, Mr. Mad Scientist?" Marilee asked on a heavy breath.

Martin tried to say yes but couldn't manage the word.

Marilee kissed and nipped, rubbed and tickled her new friend, and so their talk about lost wives and barren parasites came to an end.

3.

Through the summer months, Marilee and Martin got together every couple of weeks or so. Martin discontinued his subscription to the dating service; Marilee did not. Twice every other week, Marilee went on PFP-provided dates; every week between, she saw Martin once and went on one PFP date. She didn't feel guilty because Martin was preoccupied with his research and charitable and profit-making surgeries. He was often out of town, in Detroit, Tijuana, or Oakland, doing facial reconstructions, scar and tattoo removals, and more delicate operations. He never asked what Marilee did when they weren't together; neither did he talk about love, long-term commitment, or children.

Marilee was grateful for Martin's detachment. She didn't want to marry him, live with him, or get any deeper into his life. He was extraordinarily knowledgeable and a surprisingly skillful lover. And when they were together, he listened to her every word and remembered everything.

But her other lovers were better-looking, better-heeled, and, well, more normal.

By the first of August, she was thinking that it was time for the relationship with Martin to end. She said to herself that it was because of the mosquito bites she got whenever he stayed over. Martin liked fresh air and was always opening some window. That very morning she decided to send Martin a text saying that she thought they should end it.

Maybe an hour after her decision, Odell Wade came to visit her at Rehnquist, Bartleby, and Rowe.

"Miss Frith-DeGeorgio," the receptionist, Viola Wright, said over the intercom.

"Yes, Viola?"

"A Detective Wade of the NYPD is here to see you."

Marilee gasped involuntarily and felt a sudden chill.

"What does he want?"

"He says he needs to ask you some questions about a friend of yours."

"Tell him that I'll be right down."

She spent the next three minutes trying to think whether there was any reason the police would be after her. She had a small stash of marijuana in her medicine cabinet at home, and she'd declared herself as a private business on her tax forms, using her yearly sale of poorly constructed pottery at a street fair as the proof. When her mother died, she discovered a secret bank account of

twenty-six thousand dollars that she'd cashed out without telling her siblings . . . Maybe that was it. Maybe the NYPD was going to arrest her for bank fraud.

She thought about running. RBR was on the thirty-seventh floor of a Midtown office building, but there was an emergency stairway. Who could she turn to? Certainly not her brother, Will, or her sister, Angelique—one of them might have turned her in. Her friends wouldn't shield her from arrest.

Finally she realized that Martin Hull was the only person she knew who might help. He liked her and would probably drive her to another state if she asked.

The idea that Martin was the only person she knew to turn to was sobering. He was the closest person to her, and she was already planning to break off that relationship. What did that mean?

This dose of inexplicable reality somehow steeled Marilee. She decided to go to reception and face the music.

Odell Wade was sitting on one of the three rose-colored sofas across from Viola's desk in the kidney-shaped room with walls of blue-tinted glass.

"Detective Wade?"

"Miss Frith-DeGeorgio?"

The policeman stood up. Marilee's first impression was that he was devastatingly handsome. Tall and tan, with sandy hair and auburn eyes; his straw-colored suit hung very well on his lean and probably powerful frame. His smile seemed genuine.

"How can I help you?" she asked.

The policeman glanced over at the dark-skinned, wary-eyed receptionist and said, "Is there someplace where we can talk privately?"

* * *

Marilee's office looked out over Central Park. It was a balmy August day, and they could see all the way to Yonkers.

"What do you do here?" Wade asked, sitting next to her in one of the two chairs designated for clients and visitors. Marilee was appreciating his lips, which formed into the shape of a partly flattened Valentine's heart.

Seated upon the other chrome-and-orange padded chair, she squirmed a bit, thinking that there was something wrong with the cushion. It was then she realized that her dress was tight.

"Social media for the advertising arm of the firm," she answered, thinking, *Am I getting fat?*

"Like Twitter and Facebook?"

"And MyTime, Get It, Lost Treasure, and about a hundred more platforms."

"You like the work?"

"Not really. I used to run my own business, but now I'm just paying the rent."

"I don't want to take up too much of your time, Ms. Frith-DeGeorgio—"

"You can call me Marilee."

"Marilee. Do you know a Dr. Martin David Hull?"

"Yes."

"I'm investigating him, the NYPD is."

"About his wife?"

"He told you?"

"He said that his wife and some doctor guy ran away and the police were looking into it. But they showed up in Europe somewhere and the case was closed."

Detective Wade sighed and, with his eyebrows alone, denied Martin's claim.

"He brought us a letter," the detective said. "A letter he claimed came in an envelope postmarked from Amsterdam. But he didn't have the envelope, and there was no fingerprint other than his, nor were there any DNA markers to say that the letter actually came from his wife."

"Didn't she write the letter?" Marilee asked. "Couldn't you check the handwriting?"

"The body of the letter was printed by computer, and the signature was close but different enough to cause concern."

"And did you look in Amsterdam?"

"We found an address that a Sonora Simonson and Philip Landries had once possibly stayed in. But it was in a transient area, and there was no one who could identify their photographs. We have no evidence that they ever left the country."

"So you think that Martin murdered them?"

"We don't know what happened. Has he said anything to you?"

"Only what I already told you," Marilee said. "Why are you only asking now? I mean, I've been seeing Marty for two months. He thinks the investigation is over."

"My father had a stroke in Denver," Odell Wade said. "I went to take care of him until he died. Another detective had the case, but he didn't do much."

"I'm sorry, Detective Wade, but I don't know anything."

The policeman gave her a slightly pained look and said, "Are you going to see Dr. Hull again?"

"Is it safe?"

"I really don't know. But if you do talk to him or he calls you, I'd appreciate it if you would contact me."

4.

"Marty," Marilee Frith-DeGeorgio said to her lover at 3:03 in the morning. "Are you asleep?"

"I never sleep."

"Never?"

"Now and then I close my eyes and stop thinking for ten minutes or so, but life is very short, and we have a duty to future generations to make this a better world. So I stay awake as much as possible trying to finish my work before the dictum of mortality claims my soul."

Before, when Marty made pronouncements like this, Marilee found them fetching, the thoughts of an awkward little man thinking too much of himself. But this time she got nervous. He might be a murderer; that's what the handsome homicide detective, Odell Wade, had said.

After her meeting with the detective, Marilee cancelled her subscription to PFP and began seeing Martin almost every day. Her fear enhanced their sex life, and now she listened to him as closely as she used to heed her father when she was a little girl. The intensity with which she paid attention to the plastic surgeon brought about a feeling akin to love.

"What did you want?" Martin asked.

"Do you have a laboratory where you do your neuronal studies?"

"Yes, of course."

"Can I visit it?"

"I'd love that."

"You would?"

"Yes." Martin sat up in half lotus, looking down on his naked lover. "A couple of weeks ago I thought that you were going to drop

me. I mean I'm not much to look at, and brain surgeons make a lot more money."

"Can you tell me something?" Marilee asked.

"What?"

"Would you have killed Sonora if you knew that she was having an affair with the gut doctor?"

"Philip," Martin said, obviously pondering the question. "No. Given time I would have fixed her."

"You mean hurt her in some other way?"

"Not at all. Sonora is an unhappy woman. When I met her she was fat and shy. When we got together, I paid for a personal trainer, and she turned her physical life around. She lost weight and looked great. But she was still unhappy. She will always be dissatisfied."

"How could you fix something like that?"

"Long-term unhappiness is mostly a chemical and glandular imbalance. I mean, you might be unhappy on any particular day, because you lost a job or a favorite pet ran away, but continual sadness is something else. Most of us cannot live up to our potentials because there's a biochemical war going on in our bodies—that and the fact that our knowledge of the world in which we live is usually subpar."

"What's the connection between sadness and knowledge?" Marilee asked. She enjoyed these talks with Martin, even though she was spying on him, trying to discover what had happened to his wife and her lover.

"Why would you put yourself in danger like that?" Angelique asked. Marilee had called to tell her sister to get in touch with Detective Wade if she went missing.

"I'm not really sure," Marilee replied. "When we were just together, I liked him, but it wasn't serious. I wanted to leave. But

after talking to Detective Wade, the fear I feel gets me excited . . . in the bed."

"That's perverse."

"And," Marilee said, reaching for some knowledge she'd not yet articulated, "and for some reason his talk is making more and more sense. I don't know . . . sometimes when we're talking about his work I feel like we're colleagues.

"The only problem is that I have less time to exercise and I'm putting on weight."

"Knowledge is a form of culture," Martin said that early morning, answering his informant's/lover's question. "Not what we know but how we perceive the forms of knowledge brings us closer together. And belonging almost always trumps sadness. Why, I don't think I've had one sad moment since I met you."

"But that's love," she said, feeling ashamed of using the word. "Knowledge comes from education."

"That was once the case, certainly, but less so, and soon—no more."

"But the only way you can learn is by applying your mind to that task," Marilee said with conviction.

"But there are two types of learning," Martin said, showing his gapped teeth. "One is just the simple concatenation of facts, data. But there is a part of the brain that contains geometric forms that are designed to prepare the mind to apply the endless list of facts. One day we will be able to stimulate these forms intravenously."

"What are you talking about?"

Martin stood up and walked off of his low platform bed.

"You'll see when you come to my lab," he said. "I'm going down there now to get ready for your visit."

"It's three in the morning."

"I'll take a cab. I'll leave the address on the kitchen table. Come by around eleven. I'm sure you'll be amazed."

"Hello?" a woman's voice said over the phone at 4:09.

Marilee had waited as long as she could, but finally she just had to call.

"May I speak to Detective Wade?" Marilee asked.

"Who is this?"

"Marilee Frith-DeGeorgio."

"And why are you calling my husband in the middle of the night?"

Marilee wanted to say that it was morning but didn't. She suddenly imagined the entire globe of Earth dancing through the plane of sunlight, an intangible but still physical thing joining in that dance.

"I'm, what do you call it? I'm an informant, and he told me to call when I had information."

The receiver banged down, and Marilee waited. A few minutes later he answered.

"Ms. Frith-DeGeorgio?" Odell Wade said over the line.

"I've searched his house when he was out," she said. "I've checked every file in all of his computers and smartphone. I've been through his closets, pockets, drawers, and behind and under each piece of furniture. There's not one thing about his wife or partner that's incriminating.

"I asked him point-blank if he would have killed her if he knew about her infidelity, and he basically said that he felt sorry for her."

"Is there some reason you need to tell me all this at four in the morning?" Detective Wade asked.

"I'm going to his laboratory today."

"Oh." Wade hadn't even known about the lab until Marilee unearthed that knowledge. "That is important."

"What should I be looking for?" Marilee asked.

5.

The lab was in the basement underneath a six-story apartment building near Tenth Street and Avenue C in the East Village. The door was solid oak and fifteen steep steps down from the street. There was no knob or handle, only a big yellow button to the left of where the knob should have been.

Marilee pressed this button and waited.

A minute later the door swung inward, and there, standing before her, was a god.

He was tall, six six at least, and darker-skinned even than Martin. He wore a tan T-shirt, black trousers, and no shoes or socks. His demeanor exuded something like power or confidence, knowledge, and intense joy. His eyes were light gray, like those of some cats, and his hands seemed as if they were designed to perform miracles.

"Ms. Frith-DeGeorgio?" the earthbound deity asked.

For the moment Marilee was speechless.

"Are you all right?" the godling wondered.

"What are . . . I mean who are you?"

"Lythe Prime."

"That's your name?"

"And designation," he said. "I was born LeRoy Moss, but that was a very long time ago."

He didn't look a day over twenty-five.

"Come on in, Ms. Frith-DeGeorgio. Velchanos is waiting."

"Who?"

"He still goes by Martin Hull out there, but down here he is Velchanos."

The man calling himself Lythe Prime turned then, leading Marilee into a large empty room with high ceilings crisscrossed with ancient wooden beams overhead and a concrete floor underfoot.

"This isn't a laboratory," Marilee said, feeling a pang of fear.

"No," the divine youth replied.

He pressed a place on the white plasterboard wall opposite the entrance, and a panel slid aside, revealing a cavernous stairwell.

While Lythe Prime descended, Marilee took a moment to wonder whether this could possibly be where Martin had murdered his wife.

"Coming, Ms. Frith-DeGeorgio?"

The beautiful voice seemed to be calling to some hitherto unknown part of her—her soul.

The chamber below the first basement level was immense, at least eighty feet wide and half that in depth, with twenty-five-foot-high ceilings. There were eleven long metal tables, most of which held hundreds of multicolored beakers and vases that reminded Marilee of some fantasy palace. One wall held at least six dozen computers on various shelves and ledges. And at the far end of the room, there was a huge metal door that looked like the portal to a big bank's vault.

"Velchanos," Lythe Prime hailed.

That's when Marilee saw her lover/prey, in a classic white smock, sitting behind an old-fashioned walnut desk in a corner beside the vault.

He stood and said, "Hi, Marilee. I'm so glad you could make it. Come in. Come in."

She realized that she hadn't taken the last step from the stairs into the subbasement.

Lythe touched her arm. This sent a jolt through her like static electricity, only it was a pleasurable sensation. Almost involuntarily she took in a deep breath and walked toward the man whose chosen name was that of a precursor to the Greek god Vulcan.

How did I know that? she wondered.

"Come, sit," Martin said, giving her that goofy grin. "You met LeRoy."

"Lythe," she corrected.

"What's in a name?" Martin quoted. "Sit."

Marilee did as he asked, looking around the room. There was a scent in the air, something wonderful and fresh.

"I'm sure you want to know everything," Martin said.

"I just wanted to visit."

"I seriously doubt that," Martin replied, in a tone that was certain, almost hard.

"What do you mean?"

"Odell Wade convinced his superiors to reopen his investigation of me. I think it was when he realized that I had a new girlfriend."

For some reason Marilee was not surprised at Martin's knowledge.

"He believes that you really did murder your wife and the doctor," she said.

"No doubt," Martin/Velchanos answered. "Modern men have externalized their thought processes and use their prejudices to divine guilt."

"How did you know about Odell?" Marilee asked, twisting uncomfortably in her chair. Even her old *fat* dress was beginning to feel tight.

"I have a friend that works as a male receptionist in his precinct."

"That's convenient."

"Not at all. Lon Richmond was bed-bound, suffering from a slowly progressive nerve disorder. His mother died, and no hospital would take him. He was the cousin of one of my reconstructive-surgery patients, and so I visited Lon and gave him five injections. After two months, he was out of bed and applying for the job."

"A plastic surgeon cured an incurable nerve disease?" Marilee asked. Behind these words she was trying to remember the significance of *five* injections.

"As I told you, plastic surgery is just my day job."

"You sent him in there as a spy?"

"Most definitely."

Not for the first time, Marilee wondered if Martin was insane. She glanced behind her chair and saw Lythe Prime standing there.

"What was in those injections?" she asked Martin.

He smiled and nodded.

"What are you grinning about?"

"You," he said. "I've just told you that I'm spying on the NYPD, and they have assured you that I'm a murderer. Here you are in a closed space with me and a man who looks as powerful as a professional athlete. All that, and you ask the only important question."

"So, are you going to answer me?"

"The human body recognizes categories of cells. I have discovered that if I place a small amount of a certain cell type in the HMT-1 hinny, that parasite will be ferried to the part of the body that resonates with the passenger cell type."

"You can target organs," Marilee heard herself say.

"The brain," Martin said, "the heart, spinal cord, liver, and any gland I choose."

"And what do you use these parasites for?"

"Open the vault, LeRoy," Martin replied.

He stood and ushered Marilee toward the stainless-steel door.

The man once called LeRoy Moss entered a combination on a number pad and then turned a great lever that looked something like the chromium wheel of an ancient sailing ship.

When the door swung open, a gust of very cold air flowed out. Just when Marilee started to shiver, the gray-eyed god draped a full-length fur coat over her shoulders. He handed a like garment to Martin.

The three then entered the vault.

"Don't you wear something?" Marilee asked Lythe.

"I don't get cold too easy," he said with a smile.

Along the left side of the vault was a twelve-foot-high glass-like cabinet with hundreds of shallow drawers.

"For seven years I did volunteer work for a medical facility in Cambridge, Massachusetts. It was an interuniversity research lab that did autopsies on people with exceptional qualities: scientists, savants, athletes, and those with odd bodily quirks—"

"Like people that are impervious to cold," Marilee suddenly realized.

"Just so," Martin said. "When I became a trustee of the lab, I began harvesting cells from the best, the brightest, and the strangest specimens that humanity had to offer.

"I brought those harvests here and began to create cocktails for the next step in human evolution."

"You experimented on poor people who came to you as a plastic surgeon," Marilee accused.

"I started with dogs. Once I was able to transplant memories and thought processes, once I was able to successfully alter breeds, sizes, and senses—only then did I begin my work on humans."

"But there must have been many failures," Marilee challenged.

"Yes," Martin Hull agreed. "And some of them suffered; some died. But as a rule they were people suffering serious ailments,

like Lon Richmond. I always told those first guinea pigs what the potentials were—and what the dangers."

"You call them 'guinea pigs'?"

"What else can I say? I used them as test subjects, and a few score of them died."

"Is that what happened to your wife?"

"She left before my tests began. I would have injected her in her sleep, but she ran off looking for happiness in Europe."

"My mosquito bites," Marilee said.

"You're at least an inch and a half taller," Martin said. "And that dress looks very tight on you."

Before she knew what she was doing, Marilee slapped Martin, hitting him with such force that he fell to the floor of the vault. Then she reached down and lifted him with strength she'd never had before.

That's when LeRoy/Lythe Moss/Prime grabbed her and pulled her out of the big repository of cadaver cells.

6.

They met at a coffee shop on Prince Street in Greenwich Village. Marilee had left a simple message on Detective Wade's home phone—"I have something"—and gave the address of the coffee shop.

"He has the cellular remains of dozens, maybe hundreds of corpses in his basement," she said. "And, and, and he's experimented on people, many of whom have died from his experiments."

"What kind of experiments?" Wade asked.

"He injects them with parasites."

"Oh my God."

"He's a monster."

"Did he do anything to you?"

"No," Marilee said. She was afraid to confess about her expanding body, about her once hazel eyes that were getting lighter each day.

"Will you sign an affidavit about what you saw in his basement?"

"Yes. Yes I will."

The day that Dr. Martin David Hull was brought to trial, Marilee Frith-DeGeorgio crossed the Canadian border headed for Montreal. She was now six foot two, with pearl-gray eyes and skin the color of alabaster. When she moved into the small studio apartment in Montreal-South, she opened a document on her PFP web address. There were seven e-mails in her virtual mailbox. Six of these were from lovers who wanted to see her again; one was from lytheprime@everchanging.uk.

Dear Valhalla,

Velchanos has directed me to inform you that he bears you no ill will; that he understands why you had to betray him. He also wanted me to answer one question you asked and two you didn't.

About the five injections: 1) is a collection of data-cell clusters culled from some of the most brilliant minds in the world, 2) are similar clusters that contain the equations to best manipulate this information, 3) is a growth formula that allows the body to reach what he calls our god-potential, 4) is a small cutting from a Miss Ota Wangazu who is the only known adult to have produced viable stem cells, and 5) are a few liver cells from different donors who never experienced a sick day in their lives.

Your first unasked question is: Why did he decide to become so involved with you? Velchanos says that he needed passion in his life; that he was guilty of playing God and needed the chance for forgiveness. On his first date with you he was only looking for temporary companionship, but after a month

he saw in you his salvation. He hoped that by exposing you to his treatments and telling you what he'd done that you might, after considering everything, send him a card telling him your verdict.

And finally, a question you didn't ask and maybe never even thought of: Why hasn't Martin Hull grown and developed our gray eyes? He knew that he would be arrested and that there would be a worldwide witch hunt for his patients. He wanted no markers for treatments to be lifted from his body.

Yours, LeRoy/Lythe Moss/Prime

P.S. There are 12,306 surviving patients that received Velchanos's treatments. They have all gone into hiding, both to keep away from the official investigation that must come and to continue the Revelation—our name for the great change that this process will ultimately cause. You should stay in hiding. Your betrayal will not protect you from detainment, interrogation, and ultimately vivisection.

I have destroyed the lab. Only the living bodies of our tribe can be used against us.

Rereading the letter, Marilee realized that it had been written, almost wholly, in Latin. She migrated to Australia, kept her ex-husband's last name, and adopted Valhalla as given forename. She moved to the outskirts of Melbourne and there studied her mind and her body, looking for the deliverance of the human species.

BETWEEN STORMS

After the storm had passed, Michael Trey just didn't want to leave his apartment anymore. There was something about the booming thunder and the dire news reports, the red line across the bottom of every TV show warning residents to stay inside and away from windows, even if they were closed and shaded. Subway tunnels were flooded, as were the streets. The airports would be closed for the next four days, and the Hudson had risen up over the West Side Highway, causing millions of dollars in damage in Lower Manhattan.

The mayor interrupted TV Land's repeat of an old Married . . . with Children episode to report that the National Guard had been called out.

President Obama had taken a train (a train!) to Manhattan to address New Yorkers everywhere, telling one and all that he had declared them a disaster. He wore a white dress shirt with thin green and blue pinstripes. He didn't wear a tie, because he was getting down to business—that's what Michael thought. Even the president was afraid of the havoc that nature had wrought.

It didn't matter that the sun was shining the next day or that the skies were blue and cloudless. The storm, Michael knew, was hiding behind the horizon. And there with it was a hothouse sun, crazed terrorist bombers, and women with HIV, hepatitis C, and thoughts of a brief marriage followed by a lifetime of support. In North Korea they were planning a nuclear attack, and there was probably some immigrant on the first plane after the storm infected with a strain of the Ebola virus that would show symptoms only after he had gotten past customs.

Michael didn't go to work the next morning. The radio and TV said that most public transportation was moving normally. Traffic was congested, however. Three sidewalks in Manhattan had collapsed from water damage. Just walking down the street someone might get killed or paralyzed.

Europe's economy had almost failed again, except that the Germans bailed out the Greeks with money that neither of them had. China was going to take over the American economy and make Michael and everyone he knew into Communist slaves living in dormitories and eating boiled rice.

But if no one could buy the goods, then China's economy might fail, and it would engage its two-hundred-million-man army to reclaim all the money we borrowed to pay for the health insurance of undocumented, Spanish-speaking, job-stealing illegal immigrants.

There were microbes in the water after the storm. Militant Muslims had used the cover of the downpour to plant explosives under churches and big businesses. They weren't afraid of the rain, like Michael and other poor Americans who just wanted to work until retirement . . . never came.

* * *

The phone rang on the morning of the third day that Michael had not gone in to work at Prospect, Farr, Grant, and Heldhammer.

Michael picked up the receiver but did not speak.

"Mike?" someone said. "Mike, is that you?"

"Michael is not here," Michael heard himself say. Immediately he felt warm and safe behind the subterfuge of those words. He wasn't at home and therefore couldn't be reached, couldn't be touched, burned, infected, blown up, or experimented upon by sales scientists working in subterranean desert laboratories for the superstores.

A lifetime of the nightly news and conspiracy theories woven into TV shows, movies, and even commercials; of the racist/sexist/classist schemes of Big Business and its political candidate shills; the private prisons, police, billionaires and millionaires, movie stars and pop stars and country stars and serial killers: all this came together in Michael's mind in his apartment three days after the disaster that he finally understood would never end.

"Mike, it's Finnmore, Ron Finnmore. Mr. Russell is wondering where you are."

"I'll leave Michael the message," Mike said, and then he cradled the phone.

After hanging up, Michael had the urge to giggle but suppressed it. He knew that if he showed any emotion, soon they'd say he'd gone crazy and take him away.

"Yes," he said, when the secretary answered the phone. "I'm calling for Mr. Trey. He's not coming in today because of inclement weather."

It *was* raining, and so Michael felt justified.

"It's just a few showers," Faye Lesser, Thomas Grant's assistant's secretary said.

"That's how the last storm started. What if he got there and it came down like that again? Who would feed his cat?"

Michael didn't have a cat. He didn't have a fish or even a plant. If he had had a plant it would have died, because he hadn't put up the shades since the storm.

The television spoke of conspiracies and of disasters both domestic and foreign that were increasing in severity, like the storm that had raged over New York. There were mad cows and rampant use of hormones and antibiotics. The Y chromosome in men had shrunk to the point that soon men might cease to be men and would have to learn how to be women-without-wombs.

There were prisons across the country that together released at least a hundred convicted killers every week and banks that created bad debt (Michael was never sure how they did this) and then sold the nonexistent interest to pension plans that subsequently failed.

Michael started taking notes. He had five folders that he had bought for his financial records but never used. He labeled these folders: DISEASES, NATURAL DISASTERS, MAN-MADE DISASTERS, FINANCIAL DISASTERS, and HUMAN THREATS. Five folders were just right for the notes he needed to compile. He saw this as a sign that he was meant to stay in his fourteenth-floor apartment and study the truth that so many people missed because they went to work and therefore, somehow, inexplicably, betrayed themselves.

He spent whole days looking up fires, floods, serial killers, and food additives on his cell-phone IP. He ordered hundreds of cans of beans and tuna, concentrated orange juice, and powdered milk from grocery delivery services. He made the deliverymen leave the foods at the door and collected them only when he was sure that no one was lingering in the hall.

He used his phone to pay his bills until his accounts went low.

The super brought up his mail and left it at the threshold for him.

He had been fired, of course. His girlfriend, Melanie, told him that either he would meet her at the Starbucks on Forty-Second Street or she was breaking up with him. His mother called, but Michael fooled her by saying that Michael wasn't home.

And he was getting somewhere with his research.

At first he thought that the problem was that there were too many people, but he gave up that theory when he realized that people working together would be benefited by great numbers. Finally he understood that it wasn't the number of souls but the plethora of ideas that bogged down the world. It was like the old-time Polish parliament, in which nothing could be decided as long as anyone held a contrary point of view.

The problem with the world was a trick of consciousness: people believed in free will and independent thinking and were, therefore, dooming the world to the impossibility of choice. Yes. That was the problem. Together all the peoples of the world—Muslims, Hindus, and Jews; Christians, atheists, and Buddhists—would have to give up disagreements if they wanted the human race to survive the storm of incongruent consciousness that was even worse than the weather that had brought New York to its knees.

Michael felt that he was making great progress. He was beginning, he was sure, to articulate the prime issue at the base of all the bad news the *New York Times* had to print. He was trying to imagine what kind of blog or article he could author, when the eviction notice was shoved under his door. It had only been six weeks . . . no, no, nine . . . no, eleven. Just eleven weeks, but he was rent-stabilized, and the collusion of city government and greedy landlords made it possible for prompt evictions when there was potential for rent that could soar.

Working after midnight for days, Michael drilled forty-eight holes along the sides, top, and bottom of his door and similarly placed holes in the doorjamb and along the floor. He used a handheld cordless drill to do this work, and it took him seventy-seven hours and twenty-nine minutes. Through these connective cavities he looped twined wire hangers, two strands for each hole. This reinforcement, he figured, stood a chance of resisting a battering ram if it came to that.

He also used melted wax to seal the cracks at the sides of the door so that the police couldn't force him out with tear gas.

His beard was filling in, and his hair had grown shaggy. He looked to himself like another man in the mirror: the man who answered the phone for the absent Michael.

He filled the bathtub to the overflow drain in case the super turned off the water.

On his iPhone he read the newspapers, studied the Middle East, Central America, and the Chinese, who, he believed, had gained control of capitalism without understanding its deteriorative quality.

Finally all those boring political-science courses that he took when he thought he might want to be a lawyer had some use.

He was well on his way to a breakthrough when the landline rang.

He always answered the phone because, in a discussion with the man in the mirror, he inferred that if no one answered, they might use the excuse that there was some kind of emergency behind his coat-hanger reinforced door.

"Hello?"

"May I speak to Michael Trey, please?" a pleasant man's voice asked.

"He's not here."

"Then to whom am I speaking?"

This was a new question, and it was very smart—very. This was not just some befuddled contrarian thinker but one of those unofficial agents that pretended to protect freedom while in reality achieving the opposite end.

"My name is X," he replied, and suddenly, magically, Michael ceased to exist.

"X?"

"What do you want?"

"My name is Balkan, Bob Balkan. I'm an independent contractor working for the city to settle disputes."

"I don't have any disputes, Mr. Balkan Bob. As a matter of fact, I might be one of the few people in the world who does not disagree."

"I don't understand," the independent contractor admitted.

"I have to go, Bob."

"Can you tell me something first, Mr. X?"

"What's that, Bob?"

"What do you want?"

The question threw X out of Michael's mind. The man that was left felt confused, overwhelmed. The question was like a blank check, a hint to the solution of a primary conundrum from an alien, superior life-form. It had ecclesiastical echoes running down a corridor heretofore unexplored in Michael's mind.

"What do *I* want?" Michael repeated the words but changed the intonation.

"Yes," Balkan Bob said.

"I want," Michael said. "I want people everywhere to stop for a minute and think about only the essential necessities of their lives. You know, air and water, food and friendship, shelter and laughing, disposal of waste and the continual need for all those things through all the days of their lives."

Balkan Bob was quiet for half a minute, and so Michael, not X, continued. "If everybody everywhere had those thoughts in their minds, then they would realize that it's not individuality or identity but being human, being the same that makes us strong. That's what I've been thinking in here while the rain's been falling and the landlord was trying to evict me."

"But Michael hasn't paid the rent, Mr. X."

"I have to go, Bob," X said, and then Michael hung up.

Eight days later the electricity was turned off. The grocery delivery service had brought him thirty fat, nine-inch wax candles, so he had light. It was all right to be in semidarkness, to be without TV, radio, or Internet. Michael had his five folders and the knowledge of a lifetime plus four years of college to filter through.

Two days after the electricity went off, it came back on. Michael wondered what bureaucratic and legal contortion had the man with his hand on the lever going back and forth with the power.

Just after the lights flickered back on, the phone rang.

When it sounded, Michael realized that there had been no calls for the past forty-eight hours—not his mother and not Melanie, who worried that her demands had brought him to this place.

He always answered the phone but rarely stayed on for more than a minute.

The phone didn't depend on the power system. Maybe the phone company had cut him off for not paying his bill and then, at the behest of the city, had turned the service back on.

"Hello," X said.

"Mr. X?"

"Bob?"

"How are you?"

"Things are becoming clearer all the time, Bob," X said. "I just don't understand why you cut off the power and then turned it back on again."

"I didn't do it," he said.

"But you're working for the people that did, or at least their friends and allies."

"Do you feel that you are at war, Mr. X?"

"I'm just an innocent bystander who has made the mistake of witnessing the crime." X was much more certain about things than Michael was.

"I recorded your statement about what you wanted. Someone in my office released the recording to the media. You have lots of friends out here, Mr. X. If you look out your window you'll see them in the street."

"I'd like to, but there might be something there I don't want to see. And I don't want anyone seeing me."

"No one wants to hurt you," Bob said in a very reassuring voice.

"No one wants to kill children in Afghanistan either, but it happens every day."

"You haven't come out of your apartment since we got hit by Hurricane Laura."

"And here I don't know anything about you."

"What do you want to know?" Bob Balkan offered.

"You ask good questions, Bob."

"And?"

"Do you think that we're equal to our technology?"

"Maybe not."

"So why are you on my ass? That's all I'm saying."

"Let me ask you a question, Mr. X."

"What's that?"

"Do you think that we're equal to our biology?"

Neither Michael nor X was ready for that question. It got down to the crux of what they had been trying to figure out. If the human mind, Michael thought, was the subject of biological instinct, then there was no answer, no agreement, nor any exit from madness.

Stroking his beard, Michael forgot about the phone call and wondered if his own body was an unconscious plot against the idea of humanity, humanness. Machines and techniques could be torn down and abandoned, but what about blood and bone, nerves and hormones? Was he himself an aberrant machine set upon an impossible mission amid the indifferent materials of existence? Was his resistance futile?

While he was considering these questions, the phone went dead and the lights cut off. There came sounds of heavy footfalls in the hallway. Suddenly there was a great thumping wallop against his fireproofed, steel-reinforced, hanger-looped fire door. The police battering ram hit the door nineteen times by Michael's count. The locks and hangers, doorjamb and metal infrastructure held. The pounding ceased, and voices sounded up and down the outside hall.

There were shouts and curses. One man suggested that they break through the wall.

Michael armed himself with a butcher's knife and then put the cooking weapon down.

"I can't hurt anybody," he said to no one.

That night Michael slept on the living room floor in front of the door. His iPhone was dead and the lights were cut off, but under candlelight he read *Man's Fate* by André Malraux. He felt for the characters in the novel, though for the most part he did not identify with them. Revolution, Michael thought, was both personal and shared, and everyone, and everything, had a part in it. His only

affinity was with the feeling of doom and dread threaded throughout the book. He believed that soon he would be killed because he had decided to stop moving forward with the herd toward slow but certain slaughter.

"Mike. Hey, Mike," a voice hissed.

Michael had fallen asleep. He believed that his name was part of a dream, but he didn't know why someone calling out to him would be important.

He tried to lift his right hand, but it wouldn't move.

"Mike!" The whisper became more plaintive.

Suddenly afraid that people had secretly come in and bound him, Michael lurched up, jerking his right hand from whatever held it.

His fingers were encased in wax. The candle had burned unevenly, and warm wax had pooled and dried around his hand. Michael laughed to himself, relieved that he was safe. He blew out the burning wick.

"Mike!"

The ventilation plate in the living room had a faint light glowing between its slats.

Michael's first impulse was to cover that opening with plastic and masking tape, but he hesitated.

He pulled a chair to the wall and got up on it so that he could stand face-to-face with the brass plate.

"Who is that?" he asked.

"Mike?"

"Yeah."

"It's Tommy Rimes from the apartment next door."

"The tall guy with the mustache?"

"No," the voice said. "I'm the guy who goes bowling all the time."

Michael remembered the squat middle-aged man with the potbelly and the red bowling-ball bag.

You wanna go run down some pins? he'd once asked Michael.

"What do you want, Mr. Rimes?"

"They got you all over the news, Mike. From Occupy Wall Street to the *Wall Street Journal*, they all been talkin' about you. You went viral on the Internet now that the cops couldn't beat down your door. Fisk, the guy with the mustache on the other side a' you videoed it and put it up on YouTube. You're a celebrity."

Michael was peeling the wax from his fingers and wondering what notoriety would get him. Would it hold the hurricanes back or keep the Communists from conquering themselves with capitalism? Would it get Melanie to take him back?

"Mike?" Michael had all but forgotten that Tommy Rimes was there.

"What?" the newly minted celebrity asked.

"Can you take off the ventilation plate?"

"Why?"

"I'm gonna push through a power strip and this aquarium hose I got. That way you can have power again, and if they cut off your water you can have that."

"Why?"

"This rich guy from uptown put what you said to the city psychologist up on a billboard down the street. I like it. I mean, I think you might got somethin' there. And even if you're wrong, I like it that you're stickin' it to the landlord."

By morning Michael had light, and once he powered up his phone he found that it was still working. There was an e-mail from Melanie telling him that she had paid his phone bill. On his tiny phone screen he could see newscasts covering a thousand people in the

streets outside of his apartment building protesting the police, the mayor, the landlord, and everyone that uses the law to keep people apart.

"I believe that Mr. Trey is trying to speak for all of us," a young black woman with braids that stood out from her head like spikes said to an interviewer. "I mean, here we are working hard and barely able to live. We eat junk food and watch junk TV and our schools are being closed down because they're so bad. The police will frisk anybody, except if they're rich or something, and we're fighting a war without a draft. Mr. Trey has just stopped. He's saying that he doesn't want to be a part of all this [*bleep*] and that we should all do the same."

"I'm a conservative," a white man in a dark blue suit told a camera. "I believe that we have to fight the war and bail out the banks, but I still wonder about what this guy says. I think he's crazy, but you can't deny that there's something wrong with the world we're living in."

Both the liberal and conservative press praised Michael. They called him a people's hero who was refusing to take one more step before the other side made changes. They bent his words, however—that's what Michael thought. They didn't understand that the whole idea was *not* to have a hero but to discover a natural credo to unite people and keep them from destroying themselves.

"We love Michael Trey!" two beautiful young women shouted at one camera.

The city or the landlord cut off his water; Tommy Rimes turned it back on through the aquarium hose.

The iPhone sounded.

"Melanie?" Michael said, after seeing the screen and answering.

"They've closed down the street in front of your building," she said.

"The police?"

"No, the protesters. They want the city to leave you alone. One group is raising money for your rent, and four lawyers are working for injunctions against the landlord. Other tenants are making complaints against health and safety infractions. A journalist asked President Obama about you, but he refused to comment and it's been all over the news."

"What has?" Michael asked his ex.

"Obama not saying anything."

Michael tried to remember why he had decided to stay in his apartment. It was the storm. He was just too afraid because of the threat the news media made out of the storm. He was afraid, not heroic.

"Michael?" Melanie said.

"Uh-huh?"

"Max Strummer, who owns Opal Internet Services, wants you to do a daily podcast from your phone. He wants me to be the producer. Isn't that great? You could make enough money to pay your rent and lawyers. He said that if you couldn't think of anything to say that we could send you text files that you could just read."

"I have to go, Mel," Michael said.

"What about Mr. Strummer?"

"I'll call you later," Michael uttered, and then he touched the disconnect icon.

After turning off the sound on his phone Michael went to sit in his favorite chair. It was extra wide, with foam-rubber cushions covered in white cotton brocade. There was a lamp that he'd plugged in to the power strip hanging halfway down his wall from the ventilation grate hole. The light wasn't strong enough to illuminate the whole room, just the area around his chair.

Reclining in the oasis of light, Michael tried to make sense of the storm and his street being closed down, and of the young women who loved a man they'd never met and Melanie who had changed from an ex-girlfriend to a maybe producer.

When no ideas came, he turned off the lamp, hoping that darkness would provide an answer. It didn't. He was trying to recapture the moment when everything had made sense, when he took action without second-guessing his motives.

Feeling lost, he looked across the room and saw a blue luminescence. It was the phone trying to reach out to him.

Half an hour later he went to see who was calling. There had been a dozen calls. Most of the entries were unfamiliar, but one, instead of a number, was a name that he knew.

"Hello?"

"Mr. Balkan?"

"Mr. X?"

"No, no, this is Michael."

"Oh."

"Did you call me on city business?" Michael asked.

"They wanted me to call, but this is your nickel."

"I've been looking at the Internet," Michael said. "People all over the place want to protect me. They're offering money and legal support. One guy named Strummer wants to hire me and my ex to do a podcast for him."

"That's what you wanted, isn't it?"

"No."

"I thought you said that you wanted people to realize what they had in common."

"But between them," Michael said, "not through me."

"I don't get you."

"Not like a natural disaster or some enemy," the young bearded man replied. "I don't want to be the discounted meal at the fast-food chain that you can buy in Anchorage or Dade County. I don't want to be anything except an idea."

"But you're a man."

"Thanks for that, Bob."

"For what?"

"I needed to talk to somebody about these thoughts in my head. I couldn't get them out if I didn't have anybody to talk to. I know that you're working for them, but right now they don't know what to do. In that little window you helped me. You really did."

"Helped you what?"

"I got to go, Bob."

"Where can you go, Michael?"

"You always ask the best questions."

The next morning Michael was standing in his kitchen eating from a can of pork and beans with a teaspoon when he noticed that the spigot had a slow drip. Michael wasn't sure if it was the dripping or his talk with the city psychologist that made up his mind.

He tested the hot water and then called Melanie. She was surprised to hear from him and happy that he had decided to do his first podcast. He was careful, and she was too, not to talk about love.

At four in the afternoon Michael was ready. He had refused to allow Strummer to dictate what he said. He ignored the checklist of subjects his Internet listeners might want to hear about.

Michael had the bathtub draining when he started recording and had to close the bathroom door to keep out the noise.

* * *

"My name is Michael Trey," he said into the receiver, with no notes or even a notion of what exactly he'd say. "I have lived in Manhattan for seven years, and I was scared about Hurricane Laura—so scared that I haven't left my house since it broke. Because I wouldn't go out, I lost my job and my girlfriend, and the landlord has been trying to evict me. I'm broke, and they keep turning my utilities on and off. I have hot water right now, and so I'm going to take my first real bath in weeks.

"My neighbor, Tommy Rimes, pushed a power strip and a little hose through the ventilation duct, and so I've been able to get by. I've seen videos of people down in the street supporting me. I like that, but it's misguided. What they should do, I believe, is lock themselves into their own houses and turn off the world outside. I don't know if this would be possible or if it would make any difference at all, but that's all I've got.

"What I'm saying is that the president didn't talk about me because there's nothing to say. It is us that should be talking to him. It's us that need to get the red lines out of the bottoms of our screens, because we're in it together as far as we go. But maybe, maybe that's impossible, because we do things primarily as mammals, not men and women.

"That's really all I have to say. I know there are people out there that want a daily report from my musty apartment, but really all they have to do is listen to this, what I'm saying right now.

"Goodbye."

Michael turned off his phone before running the hot bath in the deep iron tub. It was this tub that made him take the apartment in the first place. The hot water felt so good that he groaned when he first sat back. The stinging in his wrists subsided, and he wasn't frightened except when he concentrated on the hue of the water.

He was exhilarated at first and then tired, in the way he used to be as a little boy getting in his bed. He wondered if anyone would ever make sense out of the fear-herding that all the people, and maybe all other creatures, of the world lived under.

He would have liked Melanie to say that she loved him, but only if he didn't have to ask.

THE BLACK WOMAN IN THE CHINESE HAT

I meant to spend Saturday walking from Lower Manhattan back up to my neighborhood in Washington Heights, but I didn't make it very far.

I took the IRT from 157th down to Battery Park late that morning, then headed north on foot. I made my way up the promenade, such as it is, on the West Side. It was hot, and so there were lots of swimsuited skaters whizzing past. Most had nice bodies, almost everyone with a date. Men and women, men and men—hand in hand. There were some female couples, but most of them seemed more like just friends.

There was a sprinkling of solitary skaters and joggers, even one or two walking alone. Almost all of the singles wore earphones. Some danced to the silent music, others stared doggedly ahead.

It's not that I would have talked to anyone not listening to music. I was hiding under my hayseed straw hat and behind mirrored sunglasses. I wouldn't have been able to pass more than three sentences with a stranger on the street. Making friends has always

been hard for me. Even after four years at Hunter College I had only two friends from there—Eric Chen, a history major from Queens, and Willy Jones, a psych major from Long Island City. Both Willy and Eric lived in Brooklyn. I liked them, but spending time with them was always the same. We'd talk about women and movies at coffeehouses until we got hungry and went for junk food. It was always the same. So that Saturday I decided to walk around and look at people and places that I hadn't seen before. Anything would be better than a day at home alone or with Willy or Eric.

Just a few blocks north of the Financial District was a large lawn filled with the prostrate bodies, primarily white, of sunbathers. Men with bulging muscles and women with the top straps of their bikinis undone to get a smooth tan. It didn't look comfortable. There was no ocean or nice air, just the filthy Hudson on one side and a line of brick-faced office buildings across the West Side Highway on the other. And it was over a hundred degrees. Actually it was ninety-six, but the weather man said, from a sunbather's radio, that the heat index, whatever that is, made it "feel like" a hundred and two.

There was a black woman, medium-brown really, lying amongst the others. She had on a one-piece fishnet bathing suit that, being almost the same color as her skin, gave you the idea you could see more than you really could. She was lying on her back with her head propped up, wearing a Chinese peasant hat and rose-colored sunglasses. I looked at her at first because she was the only Negro in a sea of white bodies, and then I noticed how good-looking she was.

I stared longer than I should have, and she noticed the attention. She propped up on an elbow and smiled. She had a good-size gap between her two front teeth. My heart skipped, and I felt a chill in spite of the heat.

She pointed at her hat and then at mine, as a kind of recognition, I guess, and then she waved for me to come over.

I didn't move. She smiled again and waved more insistently. I found myself walking over, between the five or six lengths of sunbathers, to get next to the black woman in the Chinese peasant hat.

She pulled up her legs to make room for me to sit down next to her.

I'm a very uncomfortable person. I'm big, not quite portly or fat but large enough to make simple motions like running or sitting on the floor difficult. I negotiated the maneuver as well as I could, managing not to step or sit on anyone.

"Hi," the woman said. She was young, some years older than I but not yet twenty-five.

"Hey."

"I got to go to the bathroom," she said with a grimace.

"What?"

"I got to go, but if I leave, one a' these white people gonna take my spot. But if you could hold my place while I run over there." She pointed at a squat concrete structure about a hundred yards away.

I nodded. She grinned and reached over to squeeze my wrist. Then, with the slightest pressure against my arm, she was up more gracefully than I could ever manage. I watched her lope away toward one of New York's few public toilets.

After she was gone, I stretched out to save her place, relaxing into my job. That's why I liked work and school; there you had something to do and someone to be, and people treated you in a certain way that you didn't have to think about. I mean, even if the boss didn't respect you, he still had to ask you a question now and then. And whenever I was asked a question, I knew the right answer. And as far as girls and women were concerned, even the prettiest

ones had to say hello if you were in the same class or worked on the same floor.

I felt a sense of purpose on that lawn, even though anyone looking would have thought I was out of place.

I say that because I wore a heavy pair of black jeans with a lightweight gray jacket cut in the military style. I didn't wear a shirt that day. Everyone near me was nearly naked. One man, in the middle of a group of men, had taken down his trunks and was lying facedown, naked. *Butt all up in the air,* my mother's voice screeched in my ear.

I heard a sound behind me. It was a young woman's voice. I turned my head and saw that the woman wasn't complaining, as I had at first thought. Her boyfriend had gone beyond kissing and had his hand down in the towel that barely covered their lower bodies. She smiled at me over his head and then made a face that said something felt good.

A broadcast reporter was saying that a policeman had been shot while sitting in a car out in front of his house. I was wondering why he'd been sitting outside rather than in his house. I was still facing the girl but thinking about the man in his car.

"Hey! What you lookin' at?" The woman's blond-headed boyfriend had noticed her looking at me. His face was red. I didn't know if it was colored from anger or the sun.

I turned around quickly and raised my knees to my chest. My back felt vulnerable to attack. I didn't know if he was going to get up and hit me. I would have walked away, except for the black woman in the Chinese hat.

I had been sweating all morning, but now I could feel the moisture gathering under my arms and across my thighs. Thoughts kept coming in and out of my head. *He wouldn't be so tough if I had a knife . . . I should go . . . I should carry a kitchen knife with me . . . Where*

is that woman? . . . Is a kitchen knife legal? . . . Is that him standing up behind me? . . . Where is that woman? . . .

I felt a hand on my shoulder and let myself fall sideways, thinking that I could kick him from the ground. I fell against a man's hard body.

"Hey, guy, what's wrong with you?" the man I toppled on complained.

Hovering in the sun above me was the woman I waited for.

"I knocked him over," she said to the balding bodybuilder. "I hit his tickle spot by mistake."

While the muscle man groused, I saw that the lovers had gone. My heart was thumping, and sweat was stinging my eyes. The black woman in the Chinese hat descended to her knees and said, "Hey, you OK?" in a tone that I'd never heard addressed to me before.

It was like she was my oldest friend or my wife or one of those social workers who put their life on the line to help someone they don't even know. I saw that she had some kind of leotard on under the fishnet bathing suit.

"Yeah," I said, sitting upright. "I'm OK."

"You fell over just like a stack a' bananas."

"Yeah."

"My name's Chai," she said.

"I'm Rufus."

"How come you wearin' all them hot clothes, Rufus?"

"I thought it was gonna be cold this morning."

"I don't know where you comin' from. It's been hot every day this summer. Real hot." Chai licked her lips. My eyes were drawn to her mouth. I wanted her to say something else that sounded like before.

Chai smiled and took a water bottle from her oversize bag.

"It's hot," she complained.

"Yeah, it sure is."

"I thought it would be nice to sit out here, but it's too hot."

"Today's a good day to be in air-conditioning," I said. "That's for sure."

"You got air-conditionin' at home?"

"No. But they have it at the World Trade Center."

Chai frowned. All I wanted to do was to keep her talking.

"Want to go down to the World Financial Center and get some lunch?" It took all the breath in my lungs to get those words out.

"I don't even know you, Rufus."

"There's air-conditioning down there."

"You got money?"

"Enough for lunch."

"Enough for a taxi to take us down there?"

"Wow, this is nice," Chai said, when we entered the glass-walled hall of palm trees in the lower court of the financial center. My friend Willy calls it the hall of palms. In the center of the vast room there are eighteen slender palm trees that reach thirty feet. Between them are benches like you'd find in a park. The benches were all occupied by people trying to escape the heat.

"I never even knew this place was here," she said, taking my arm.

I could feel her breast against my shoulder. I wanted to swallow but couldn't make my throat cooperate.

"I'm hungry," Chai said.

We went under the Merrill Lynch mezzanine into the upscale food court. Past the Rizzoli bookstore and behind a yellow pillar was Pucci's Two, an Italian restaurant I sometimes went to on my lunch break from Carter's Home Insurance.

"No swimwear inside the dining room," said the slender host at the podium that led into the restaurant.

Actually, there was no *inside* to the restaurant. There was just an area where there were about thirty tables cordoned off by a thigh-high green fence. The only inside was the kitchen.

"How's this?" Chai said. She pulled a large piece of brown cloth from her bag and wrapped it around her waist. The skirt accented her figure, made her seem more womanly.

The host was obviously perturbed to see a woman dressing right there in front of him. He was an older white man with a full head of white hair. He stared at Chai for a moment and then a moment more. Finally he got two menus from a slot on the side of the podium and strode toward our seats.

It was just noon, and so the restaurant was nearly empty. He led us to a small table for two in the back.

"I don't wanna sit in the back," Chai said, when he held a chair for her.

"I thought you wanted privacy," the maître d' replied.

"Ain't nobody here," Chai said. "All you could have is privacy."

We ended up at the thigh-high fence watching people walking by.

"Anything to drink?" Our waitress was a black woman with seven silver studs in each ear, a gold ring at the outer corner of her right eye, a tiny silver circlet at the left corner of her lower lip, and a blue stone in her nose. She laid down our menus and smiled.

"Red wine," Chai said.

"We have a Merlot and Beaujolais," the waitress replied. She was looking somewhere beyond the confines of the restaurant.

"Whatever."

The waitress looked at me. I'm only twenty. I went to college early, at sixteen, but I look older.

"Beer," I said. "Whatever you got on tap."

The waitress moved away.

The maître d' seated a couple at the table next to us. There was already a line of couples waiting to get in.

I noticed that Chai was still wearing her rose glasses and peasant hat. I removed my hat and glasses, hoping that she'd do the same.

Instead she reached across the table to caress my cheek.

"You have a nice face, Rufus." Her hand slid from my jawbone and across my lips. "Nice lips too."

"They have really good pasta," I said, opening the menu.

Chai smiled at me and leaned forward.

The maître d' sat another couple on the other side of us.

"How old are you?" Chai asked.

"Twenty-three."

"You in school?"

"No. Uh-uh. I just graduated from Hunter a few months ago. Now I work at an insurance company down here."

"I used to work down here," she said. "At Crystal and Pomerantz. I typed and stuff. But I don't do that anymore."

"What do you do now?"

"I do clothes for a couple a' black magazines. Clothes, and I help out on the photography shoots."

The waitress came with our drinks then.

"Are you ready to order?"

"Do you have specials?" Chai asked.

The waitress frowned and then produced a pad from the pocket of her blouse.

"Angel hair pasta with a sauce of fresh tomatoes sautéed in olive oil with garlic, kalamata olives, fresh basil, and finished with crumbled goat cheese. Broiled scrod served with an anchovy sauce . . ."

"Ugh! Anchovies is nasty," Chai complained.

" . . . and a thick veal chop," the waitress continued, "flattened, breaded, and fried in olive oil, served with broccoli di rape."

"I want the pasta," Chai said.

I ordered the blue-cheese cheeseburger with a baked potato and salad.

"If you lost some weight," Chai said, when the waitress was gone, "and did some weight liftin', you'd be fine."

"I'm gonna start my diet next week," I said. "Monday morning. I got Special K for breakfast and seven grapefruits."

"What kinda milk?"

"*Milk* milk."

"If you gonna diet it's got to be skim milk, fat-free."

"Oh. Uh-huh. That's why I was walking on the promenade today."

"Why?"

"Because I'm starting to get healthy. I'm gonna walk up to my house on One Fifty-Eight."

"You better walk up to one thousand fifty-eight if you gonna eat that hamburger."

"Yeah," I said. "I know."

"I want to be a nutritionist," she said. "But first I'm gonna get into clothes design. I made my bathing suit."

"You did?"

"Uh-huh. Made it fishnet to make you think you could see sumpin' and then lined it so you couldn't. You like it?"

"It's beautiful."

That was the only moment that Chai was at a loss for words. Her head moved back slightly, and her eyes opened wide enough that I could see them clearly through the flush of her plastic lenses.

"Where you from, Rufus?"

"I was born in Baltimore," I said. "Then we moved to Portland and Oakland and then LA . . ."

"I wanna move to Atlanta," Chai said. "Then go to LA after I get established. 'Cause you know they say LA is a hard town, and somebody black got to be ready if they want to live out there."

"I don't know," I said. "I was only there for a year before my mom brought me to Brooklyn."

"And then you moved to Washington Heights?"

"Yeah. My mom made sure that I was in school at Hunter, and then she moved back to LA to live with my uncle Lon."

The food came then. I regretted every bite of my burger. I wanted to leave some, to start my diet a few hours early, but I couldn't stop eating. I couldn't even slow down.

"So you alone out here?" Chai asked me.

"My aunt Beta," I said, shaking my head, mouth full of meat. "She lives in Brooklyn."

"What kinda name is Beta?"

"Mom is Alpha, and her sister is Beta," I said.

"What's that mean?"

"It's the beginning of the Latin alphabet. *A* and *B*."

"They named two little girls after letters?"

"My grandfather. He's like an inventor. He said that he thought all children were like experiments, that every child born was a test of nature to make a better human being."

"Huh. That's weird."

"Yeah. He said that all the tests so far had failed, mostly, and that we should keep track of the failures, that one day the government would agree with him and start naming every person so that they could see how the process was coming along."

"He sounds crazy."

"That's what my grandmother thought. That's why she left him and moved to Baltimore."

Chai had pecan pie and chocolate liqueur for desert. I had a bite of her pie. After that I showed her all around the World Financial and World Trade Centers. She'd been in them before but didn't know all the ins and outs the way I did.

There was an award-winning exhibit of news photography in the sky tunnel that connected the two centers. The scenes were mostly of suffering in other parts of the world. The one I remember was an African soldier raising his machete to deliver the killing blow to an unarmed man that he'd been fighting. The man was already wounded, and this was obviously the last moment of his life. I was sure that there was another photograph—a picture of the murdered man, evidence that his attacker was a murderer—but that photograph, wherever it was, was not an award winner. Chai spent a lot of time examining each picture. She was interested in photography too, she said.

I kept close to her, waiting to hear that tone in her voice again, the tone that made me feel like I had always known her.

We went to J&R Music World, and she bought CDs for her sister. And then we went to the building where I worked. She said that she wanted to see it.

After that we walked some more, and then we had tempura at Fukuda's Japanese restaurant.

"I don't have just one boyfriend," she told me when we were walking down Broadway in the early evening. I hadn't asked her, but I did want to know.

"Right now I see two guys. One's a cop, and the other's a ex-con. I like the cop 'cause he know what to do, and I like my convict 'cause he make me feel it when we together."

"They know about each other?" I asked, as practical as my grandfather.

"Uh-uh. Strong men like that cain't share without fightin'. So I just don't tell 'em."

It was then that she took my hand.

"Take me to the movies, Rufus. Take me to see *The Thomas Crown Affair.*"

"I only have enough for two subway tokens."

"You don't have a bank card?"

"I don't have any money in the bank."

"I thought you said that you work for that insurance company?"

"I do, but I just started and I haven't been paid yet." This was mostly true. Actually I had worked at Carter's Home Insurance for three months, but I was just promoted to my new position two weeks ago. Before that I had only made minimum wage.

Chai let my hand go. I thought that she would leave now that she knew I was broke.

"I know somethin' we could do, don't cost but fifty cent," she said.

"What?"

Again she took me by the hand. We walked farther downtown, our fingers interlaced. My hand was sweating, and even though I always thought that holding hands meant something close and special, I didn't feel the closeness that I had on that sunbathers' lawn. It was just two hands and some fingers pressed together on a day that was too hot.

"What's this?" I said, holding back at the outside escalator.

"The ferry," Chai said. "The Staten Island Ferry. It only costs fifty cent. Don't worry, I'll pay for it."

We held hands up the escalator and through the swinging glass doors. She had to let go in order to pay at the kiosk. We came into a cavernous room that was over a hundred feet across, and just as long. There was a magazine stand in the center of the room and wooden benches along the walls.

"Good, it's pretty empty," Chai said.

Now she held my arm. I still didn't feel that closeness I craved, but there was security in the touch. I'd never been to Staten Island and said so. She told me that her cousins lived out there in Saint George. She used to visit them when she was a girl.

At the far end of the large waiting room was a huge door that sat on wheels. Through the door we could see a crowd of people all walking in one direction, toward the exit and the city.

"That means the ferry is unloading. When they're finished and when the cars are all off, then we can get on."

"They take cars?"

"Uh-huh. Right down below us."

The door was pushed open from the outside by an older, red-faced white man. The color reminded me of the man who was so angry when his girlfriend looked at me.

"Great, it's one of the old ferries," she said as we walked up the ramp.

It was like one of the old barges that my uncle Lon used to take me on off of Redondo Beach. Lots of old wooden benches and a galley where you could get hot dogs and sodas.

Chai ran, dragging me along, to the front of the boat. There we looked out over the watery expanse.

"I used to love this when I was a kid," she said. "Thanks for coming with me."

The horn sounded, and the big boat lurched out into the water. Six or seven others came out onto the prow with us.

Chai grabbed my hand again and said, "Come on."

She led me back into the boat and up a flight of stairs that went above the galley. Up there was another room full of old built-in benches. On either side was an outside area with a long bench that looked out to the water. On one side an old couple sat, and on the other two little kids looked out from the front.

Chai took me to the aft part of the side where the children were. We sat and looked out for a moment or two. We were going to pass Ellis Island and the Statue of Liberty. I was about to say how great it was when Chai kissed me.

What I remember most about it was her tongue. It was very large and muscular. My old girlfriend, the only girlfriend I ever had, Rachel, had a small tongue. When we kissed, Rachel opened her mouth, but her tongue didn't do anything. But with Chai it was a real physical experience. The boat ride was smooth, but that kiss was like stormy seas. It still wasn't the intimacy I had experienced on the promenade, but it was overpowering.

Chai laid a hand on my thigh, right on my erection. She didn't move the hand or squeeze but just let the weight sit there. After a moment I was kissing back. Every time my tongue pushed into her mouth it was pressed back. It was almost like the tongues were engaged in a war or maybe a war game. My chest started to hurt, and there were sounds coming from my throat. Chai used her other hand to caress the back of my neck.

When I started to come, Chai moved back from the kiss to watch my face. Her hand was still just weight, but it was enough. I struggled not to make too much noise. I could see that there was someone down on the other end of the bench; I could see their form in my peripheral vision.

My body tensed, and my legs went straight. I wanted to cry.

It was then that Chai whispered, "So much." Then she leaned closer and spoke right into my ear, "Don't stop," and I had another orgasm and I thought I was going to die.

There it was, cast in something stronger than stone, the intimacy, and the closeness I had always wanted but never suspected until that day. I panted like a dog, and Chai grinned broadly. My body was still shaking.

"That was good," she said, and then she curled up beside me and put her head on my shoulder and her hand upon my chest. We sat there looking out at the water. The ferry slowed for landing and then jarred against the wooden pylons of the pier.

Whoever it was at the other end of our bench got up and left. I think Chai fell asleep. I did too.

"So I told my mothah I didn't care what the hell he told huhr," a woman said. It was real, and I heard it, but I was still asleep.

I felt a forward pitch of the boat and awoke. An old woman was sitting next to me. A man in some kind of uniform was next to her. Two young women were standing at the railing looking out over the water. It was one of them who had been talking about her mother.

Chai was asleep. Just seeing her seemed to fill my lungs with air. This time I watched the water and the sights.

It might have been eight o'clock. The sky was still light, and the ferry was full of Staten Islanders going out for the night in Manhattan. I stayed still, hoping that Chai wouldn't rouse.

"Hey," she said, when we were close to shore.

"Hey," I said in a new voice, one that echoed the intimacy I craved.

She sat up and said, "I got to get home."

"Can I call you?"

"I don't really have a private line. But you give me your number, and I'll call you, OK?"

There was a yellow nub of a pencil in her bag and the inner side of the ingredients flap from an empty package of trail mix that had been thrown away in the terminal building. There I wrote my full name and the phone number of my temporary desk at work. I hadn't gotten a phone in my house yet. I didn't have the deposit.

"Goodbye, Rufus Coombs," Chai said after she kissed my cheek. "I'm gonna call you and see how your diet's comin'."

I wanted to walk her to her subway station, but she said she needed to walk alone.

The first time I woke up it was because of that pain in my chest. I guess I got excited in my sleep. The pain turned into fear of a policeman who found out that I had been kissing his woman. That fear gave way to fear of an ex-convict, a murderer, who would kill me for the same reason. I fell asleep again only to awaken to a phrase, *AIDS kiss*. I wondered if I had heard those words on the radio or read them somewhere. The thought of the disease crawling through my veins got me up out of bed. I went to my tenement window and looked out over New Jersey. I wondered if she would call me. It would have to be within the next six weeks, because that was how long I'd be in the claims department.

I sat in my heavy chair waiting for the sun, wondering if she would call and if I saw her would one of her boyfriends kill me. I wondered if she might die from AIDS and never call to warn me. Somewhere in the tangle of fears I fell asleep again.

LOCAL HERO

My grandfather, and Sherman's, was Theodore Brownley from Spiritville, Louisiana—a town that no longer exists.

Theodore moved to Brooklyn soon after the flood that washed Spiritville into the Mississippi in November 1949; at least that was what my cousin Sherman said that our grandfather told him. Grandpa Theodore came to Flatbush, bought an empty lot, built the house that Sherman was later born in, married Florida James from Brownsville, New York, and fathered three sons: Isaac, Blood, and my mother's husband, Skill.

Florida bore their three sons in the first four years of marriage. The brothers Brownley courted three sisters born to Lucinda Cardwell, who lived with her brood across the street and down the block from the Brownley clan.

Three brides for three brothers, and, if you believe the rumors, there was some cross-pollination too.

My father, Skill Brownley, was married to Mint Cardwell. Our first cousin Theodora's mom was Lana, and her father was Isaac.

Blood married Nefertiti, then got killed in a bar fight just a year after she bore his son.

These names are very important because they are the stakes that hold down the billowing tent of my story, my lives. I am Stewart Cardwell-Brownley, born into the family of Skill Brownley—Grandpa Theodore's youngest son. I have two brothers and one sister. Theodora had one sister and one brother. The three sisters that the Brownley brothers married had five other siblings. But the rest, even though I love them dearly, don't figure much in the telling of my tale.

What matters is that Sherman, like his father, Blood, was killed in a street fight not three blocks from the house Theodore built. My first cousin Sherman did all things good and bad. He was a straight-A student, a Lothario of mythic proportions, nationally recognized for high school baseball and basketball, a devout Christian, a sometimes heavy drinker, and a street fighter. His hunger for truth was equaled only by his thirst for life. He could never get enough, and his heart was all over the place. I was closer to him than to anyone else in the Brownley clan. Partly because, even though he was only a year older than I, Sherman was my protector and teacher; he taught me almost everything I knew, including, though it seems unlikely, most things I learned after his death.

As a youth I was never very good in school or at athletics; neither was I popular. My parents never pushed me much, but they always offered to help me with schoolwork, and my father played catch with me and my younger brother Floyd on fair days in Prospect Park, when he wasn't putting in overtime at the machine shop.

I had three friends through all the years of public school. Bespectacled Mister Pardon, Fat Jimmy Ellis, and Ballard "the Perv" Ingram. We would hang out on the lunch court before and after

school, trading comic books and gossiping about the sex exploits of everyone else.

Every now and then Sherman would join us, usually waiting to hook up with some girl. We liked him because he was the best of us, all of us. He ran faster, stood his ground no matter the odds, and he could recite every school assignment by heart. At church he sang with the gospel choir, and afterward he'd make out with one of the church daughters in the storeroom behind the dais upon which the choir performed.

But even though he was a blazing star among assorted lumps of clay, Sherman would join me and my friends on the lunch court just as if he was one of us, talking about the X-Men and teachers he couldn't stand.

I remember one day he asked short, squinty-eyed Ballard the Perv what comic book character he wanted to be.

"Not," Sherman stipulated, "the one you like the most but the one you would be if you could be."

Ball, which is what we called Ballard sometimes, scrunched up his eyes and stared at my first cousin like he might be a cop who needed the right answer or else he would kick some ass.

"The Thing," Ball said at last. "The Thing from the Fantastic Four."

Sherman smiled and winked at me.

"He's ugly," Fat Jimmy said.

"Yeah," Ball replied, "but he's got a secret power."

"What power?" Mister asked. Mister Pardon was dark-skinned, like the rest of us, and named Mister, in the Southern black tradition, so that no white man could disrespect him. He was an exceptional student, though he stuttered when talking to anyone but us three and sometimes Sherman.

"His dick," the Perv said. "It's rough the way my uncle Billy says that girls like it, and it's really big 'cause of those cosmic rays."

Ball's voice was so filled with wonder and desire that I was afraid Sherman might turn mean and make fun of him. I and my friends were all around thirteen, while my cousin was fourteen going on forty. Sherman could be cutting, and I had the urge, but not the nerve, to stand between him and Ball.

Sherman bit his lower lip and cut his eyes at the Perv.

"Yeah, right?" he said with a smile. "That's what I always thought about the Hulk. You know like if the madder he get the stronger he is, then maybe the hornier he get the bigger his dick is."

Ballard the Perv's eyes opened wide, and I believed that he'd dream about being the Hulk for the next year.

One afternoon, more than a year after the bio-philosophical talk about the sexual prowess of superheroes, Sherman came up to me and my friends on the lunch court. This was unusual, because my cousin had graduated to high school and didn't come by very much anymore.

Sherman sat down and greeted me and my friends. He told us about a fight he'd got in with a cop's son. The kid was named Carl and was in the eleventh grade.

"I got beat down," Sherman said, with a wry grin, "but I gave him a black eye and chipped his front tooth."

Mister, Jimmy, and Ball had a hundred questions, but Sherman said, "We can talk about all that later. Right now I need Stew here to help me with somethin'."

I was due home in less than an hour. My mother and father were very strict, and even though I hadn't done very well at anything in particular, I always obeyed them and showed up on time. On the other hand, Sherman had never asked for my help before. He

made sure to spend time with me a day or two each month. Once in a while I stayed over at the apartment where he and his mother, Titi, lived. At night, after she was asleep, Sherman would take me up to the roof, where he smoked cigarettes and drank sweet wine.

"You see down there in the alley?" he once asked me.

"Yeah, I see."

"All kinds of things happen down there in the nighttime. People fuckin' and fightin', and sometimes they die. Right down there in the open but in the dark."

I peered into the night, which was broken now and then by fluttering moths or the passing headlights of some car. If I had just looked into that abyss by myself I wouldn't have seen a thing; but through Sherman's eyes I could imagine the way the darkness, with the partial architecture of the urban night, was magical, alive. When I inhaled it felt as if that night was coming inside me.

And so, when Sherman came on that lunch court and said that he needed me—I went.

On the A train to Manhattan we sat on a bench for three, and he looked me over.

"Your hair is all right," he said, after a minute-long inspection, "but you gotta button that shirt to the top and tuck in those tails."

I did as I was told.

"Did you brush your teeth this morning?" Sherman asked.

"Yeah."

"How about a shower?"

"I took one after gym class."

Sherman was still studying me. He seemed more like a teacher or a young father than my cousin and friend.

We were passing underneath the East River when he said, "I met this girl from California goes to a private school on Seventy-Second

Street. Her parents are out of town tonight, and she said she wanted me to come by, only she had already planned to have one of her girlfriends come over, and so she asked if I could bring another guy."

"Girls?" I was pretty sure that half the subway car could hear the fear in my voice.

"Don't worry, man. Tanya—that's my girl—Tanya said that Mona is fine. So you don't have to worry about me puttin' you with no ugly girl."

I swallowed hard again and tried to think of some way out of that train, that destination. I had hardly ever kissed a girl, and when I had it hadn't seemed so great—for her.

"When you kiss," Sherman said, as if he could read my thoughts, "you got to give her some tongue. Girls like that, and you will too."

We got out in lower Manhattan south of Canal. From there we walked west. On Washington we came to this modern-looking apartment building that had glass walls and a doorman seated behind a high desk.

Sherman walked right up to the desk, and I followed a few steps behind.

The doorman had bright copper skin and an accent from somewhere in the Spanish-speaking New World.

"Can I help you?" he asked, dubiously.

"Tanya Highsmith," Sherman said. "Apartment fourteen twenty-seven."

That was the most impressed I ever was with my cousin, in this life. *Tanya Highsmith, apartment fourteen twenty-seven.* He spoke clearly, with no hesitation or shame. He wasn't some young tough from the 'hood but a man coming to see a woman.

The doorman nodded and picked up a phone.

* * *

The next thing I knew I was standing at an off-white door on the fourteenth floor in a wide hallway that had avocado-colored carpeting and muted rose-red walls.

When Sherman pressed the doorbell I got a little dizzy. Standing there I worried that I'd fall on my face. I do believe that the only reason I didn't faint was so as not to embarrass my cousin and best friend.

The door swung inward, and I was surprised at the young woman who stood there. The beautiful teenager wore a gray silk T-shirt under an emerald cotton vest that had little red eyes stitched into it. Her skirt was a gold color with a blue hem, I remember. She was barefoot and a little breathless. But none of that mattered at first glance. What struck me was that she was a black girl; well, not really black but rather a creamy brown. At any rate—she wasn't white. I figured that in a building that nice, with a girl from a private school, that Sherman must have found him a white girl to visit.

"Hey, Tanya," Sherman said.

"Oh my God," she exclaimed. "You two look exactly alike."

I'd been told before that Sherman and I bore a strong resemblance. I couldn't see it; I think that was because he was so powerful and brave and cool, and I was just barely normal.

"They do!" another girl said. This one was also under the category of our race, what people nowadays call African American. But where Tanya was slender of face and body, her friend was a curvaceous girl with skin just a touch darker.

They were Sherman's age, maybe even a little older.

"Mona," Tanya said, "this is Sherman and his cousin Stewart."

"If we look just alike," Sherman said, "then how you know I ain't Stew?"

The skinny girl grinned, cocked her head to the side, and said, "Because I know what I like. Come on in. I got it all ready."

Tanya took us through the living room into a yellow-and-red-tiled kitchen. Past the stove there was a little nook of a room with no door, in which sat a small, square, orange table-booth. There she had set out a crystal decanter filled with amber liquor and four bulbous drinking glasses.

"Cognac," Tanya said. "Like I told you."

Sherman and Tanya sat on one side of the table, her in and him out. I climbed into our side, and Mona pulled in close beside me.

Tanya explained to her friend and me that she met Sherman on the F train and that the first thing he said to her was to ask if she had ever had champagne.

"I asked him why," she said. "And he told me that I looked like I was rich and so I must have had some."

"What did you say?" Mona asked. At the same time she laid her left hand on my right.

"She said that there was something better than champagne," Sherman answered.

"Cognac," Tanya finished, gesturing at the contents of the tabletop.

She poured us each a generous dram and warned us to sip it because the cognac was strong.

When Mona let go of my hand to reach for her glass, I felt both bereft and relieved. She got my glass too, turned toward me on the small bench, and clinked hers to mine. She smiled at me with lips that I will always think a woman's lips and smile should be.

"Cheers," she whispered, and we all sipped.

"Damn!" Sherman said. "This feels warm all down in my chest."

"That's what it does," Tanya said, a note of triumph in her voice.

"This how rich people feel all the time?" my cousin asked.

Tanya's reply was to lean forward and kiss him.

Sherman already knew how to kiss. After a moment with her mouth, he moved to the side of her neck. This caress brought out a smile, and the next thing I knew Mona gave me a peck on the mouth. My tongue was ready, but her lips moved quickly to my ear.

"We should go in the other room and leave them alone," she whispered.

Mona poured some more brandy into our glasses and then led me by the hand into the living room. There we drank and whispered and kissed—a lot. Toward the bottom of the snifters my trepidations evaporated. Mona showed me how and where to kiss and when to linger. In hushed tones she told me about her white boyfriend and how he would never let her guide him to her desire.

I was overexcited and so suffered two premature ejaculations, but Mona was more experienced and explained, between kisses, what was going on with me and how we could get back to where we wanted to be.

Somewhere in the night I looked up from the sofa and saw Sherman and Tanya, mostly naked, tiptoeing toward another part of the house.

"Kiss me, Stew," Mona said, to bring my attention back to her.

The couch Mona and I staked out was long and deep, like the sleep we tumbled down into. It was slumber in an upholstered hole at the side of a road in some fairy tale my mother might have read aloud before my siblings and I fell to sleep . . .

My mother. I came awake suddenly, so deeply afraid that even the loss of my virginity failed to buoy me. I sat up quickly and felt a wave of pain go through my head. I gasped, looked around, and saw Sherman sitting in a stuffed chair set perpendicular to the foot of our sofa.

Mona groaned and shifted under a blanket I didn't remember.

"I been waitin' for you to wake up, cousin."

"Does your head hurt this bad?" I asked.

"It'll go away in the air outside," Sherman explained.

"My parents are gonna kill me," I predicted, through pain and some nausea.

"Uh-uh, man. I got that covered," my cousin promised.

It was late May, and the sun was rising at around five that morning as Sherman and I made our way to the subway.

"What you mean you got it covered?" I asked Sherman for the sixth time as he handed me a subway token.

"While you was playin' makin' Mona moan I called Titi an' asked her to call your parents and say you was sleepin' ovah."

No magician ever impressed me as much as Sherman did.

"And she did it?" I asked.

"Sure she did. I told her that you and me were on a double date. She understands what men need to do."

For a week or so after the visit with Tanya and Mona, I avoided my cousin. I wanted to forget about cognac and sex and Manhattan too. I felt so guilty that I was even trying to do some homework one Wednesday evening in the bedroom I shared with my brother Floyd.

"Stew?" my mother, Mint Cardwell-Brownley, called from the hall.

"Yeah, Mom?"

"Phone. It's your cousin Sherman. If he wants you to come over, tell him you have to come back here to bed."

"Hey, cousin," he said, when I answered.

"Hi." I didn't want to be rude.

"Where you been, man?" he asked.

"Nowhere. Studyin' for finals is all."

"Well, come on ovah an' I'll help."

There was no way that I was going to see Sherman and Nefertiti. My soul was on the line; that's how it felt. I tried to think of some kind of reason that I had to stay and do my homework alone. Maybe it was some kind of spelling that I had to commit to memory, and Floyd was already testing me. That was a good excuse.

"What you thinkin', Stew?" my cousin asked.

"Nuthin'."

"So you comin' or what?"

"OK." And that was it. My soul was sold, and Sherman owned it.

That early evening we went down an alley past the back of a bodega. We stopped for a minute while Sherman looked around.

"You see that little window ovah the door?" he asked me.

"Uh-huh."

"That's what they call a transom, and Julio's ain't got no alarm."

"So?"

"I'm 'a break into that bastard an' steal one hundred dollars."

"Why?" I was so scared that even the spiritual devastation of sex seemed tame.

"'Cause I can. 'Cause I wanna do everything. Don't worry, Stew. I won't bring you into it."

The years passed, and Sherman and I were fast companions. Whenever he broke the law he did it alone, but later he'd tell me all about it—step-by-step. I spent lots of time with him and his mother, my aunt Titi, in their sixth-floor walk-up apartment. Titi was always nice, kissing me hello and goodbye.

My own mother rarely kissed me. I had never much thought about that until I became the beloved chattel of my aunt and cousin.

* * *

After high school Sherman was accepted to NYU on full scholarship, and then I, the next year, went to work on an early-morning paper-delivery crew for the *New York Times.*

Somewhere in that time our cousin Theodora decided to take the NYC civil service exam. She asked Sherman to help, and he did. I hung around because it felt better to be with him than my own parents and siblings.

Theodora and I studied together. I had no desire to take the test, but I liked her. We'd laugh and try to fool each other, and Sherman told me that she'd do better if I was there too. Theodora was slender and tall, and she told us on the third night of study that she liked women more than men.

"I just like the way girls kiss," she admitted between practice tests. "It's like I know something with them, when men keep their secrets."

I didn't care about who she loved. Theodora was my blood, and I had learned from Sherman and Titi that that was all that mattered.

A few years later, after Theodora had gotten a clerk job at the local police precinct, Sherman got into a fight with the husband of one of his girlfriends.

It isn't what it sounds like. Isabella Vasquez was a first-grade schoolteacher, who taught many of the kids that our siblings and cousins had produced. Sherman got to know her when taking our nieces and nephews to school on Thursday mornings.

Isabella's husband, Murphy, one night got drunk and knocked out one of her teeth. So Sherman kicked his ass.

Murphy got mad at that, and with two of his friends he beat my cousin to death. They jumped him in an alley and stomped his face and ribs. Nefertiti and I sat by his body in the mortuary all

Saturday morning, while Murphy Halloran and his friends were being arraigned and charged.

Nefertiti held the vigil in her sixth-floor walk-up. All forty-seven of the Cardwells, Brownleys, and Cardwell-Brownleys came. Our grandparents were dead, but Titi had brought out an old photograph of them and tacked it to the wall.

I was there from the beginning to the end, serving sweet wine with butter and salami sandwiches on hard rolls. My mother, Mint, when she first saw me there, sneered in a way that I didn't understand —at the time. Many others who knew how close I was to Sherman said how sorry they were and how much alike we looked.

I stayed to clean up after the wake. Titi watched me from the kitchen door.

"Sherman loved you," she said.

Her tone was sweet, but still I took it as an accusation. I castigated myself for failing to be there to fight side by side with him.

"He was my best friend," I uttered, trying not to cry, again.

"More than that."

"I know we're blood, but I always thought of him as something more, I guess."

"He was," Nefertiti said. "Your father and his are the same."

"My father, Skill?"

"No. My husband, Blood."

I stopped drying plates and turned to look at Titi. She's a dark-skinned woman with bright eyes and graying dreads. I could see that she had always loved her husband and son in me. That connection was the source of her kisses and kind words. It was why she protected me when Sherman and I spent the night with those fancy girls.

She took a light-brown snakeskin wallet from the pocket in her apron and handed it to me.

"It was Sherman's," she said. "I couldn't even look inside. They killed my boy. This world killed him. He was too beautiful, too beautiful."

"I can't, I can't take this, Titi."

"Please," she implored. "I'll sleep easier if I know he's with you."

The next day was the funeral. Six hundred people and more showed up.

Mister Pardon, Fat Jimmy, and Ballard the Perv were there. They told me how sorry they were and dredged up the old stories about Sherman's adventures at school. I liked my friends, but they seemed very far away. Or maybe it was me; ever since I'd heard that Sherman had died I'd felt that there was a wall between me and everyone else. Everyone except Nefertiti.

I sat through the ceremony thinking that Sherman was my brother, my brother.

My mother's husband—my uncle Skill—and I took opposite sides at the front of the casket.

The reception after the interment was held in the house that our grandfather Theodore Brownley had built. I hung around the corners, talking to people as little as possible. People talking and laughing and remembering things about Sherman just made me angry. Didn't they realize that someone who was so much more had been taken? Didn't they understand what Sherman was in this world?

That morning I'd broken up with my girlfriend of two years, Leora Dumas, because she said that Sherman had been a bad influence on me.

"He was crooked," Leora said. "And you couldn't see that he was holding you back."

I was living with Leora because I didn't make enough delivering papers to afford my own place. She wanted to get married, but I really didn't have any interest in that. I guess Sherman dying meant that I had to move on, no matter what Leora said.

So what if I gambled with Sherman sometimes or drank too much or bought things I couldn't afford? My cousin, my brother, made me feel that life was important, that I was important. Without him I was nobody.

"You look so much like him," a woman said.

It was Natasha Koskov, from Brighton Beach. She was a breathless Russian with a long neck and lips like Mona Tremont, the first girl I ever really kissed.

"That's what they say," I replied, wondering where the words and light tone in my voice had come from.

"He loved you," she said, looking into my brown eyes with her black ones.

"You wanna go get a drink?" I imagined Sherman asking.

"Yes," Natasha Koskov replied.

We drank and kissed, went to her apartment, and made love. She called me Sherman, and after the first round I didn't correct her.

I was another man that night. Natasha wasn't loving me but Sherman—Sherman, who could not be erased from this world or her heart or mine.

Sometime after three in the morning I was walking from the subway toward Titi's apartment building because I had no place else to go.

I hadn't lived with my parents for three years, and the thought that my father was not my father kept me from calling them. I wondered if he had known, if he and my mother had kept the truth from me. Maybe that was why my mother showed me so little affection.

"Hey, you!" a man said from somewhere to my left.

I turned and saw a rough-skinned, earth-toned man wearing a hoodie. He carried a small pistol in his right hand. I'd had a lot to drink, but I was sober. I was coming back from a night of lovemaking, but I was downcast, brooding.

"Gimme yo' got-damned wallet, main!"

He could have demanded anything else: my shoes, my baby finger, every cent I ever made. But it was Sherman's wallet in my back pocket. It was my brother's legacy this man was asking for.

I looked at him, and time slowed. Under a night-time lamppost his sludge-colored eyes were frightened, as mine should have been. I suppressed a smile, breathed in the darkness, and looked up suddenly as if seeing something surprising behind his back. It was just enough to cause him to falter and to give me time to reach out with both hands and tear the gun from his grip. He tried to grab it away, but I pulled back the hammer and steadied my right hand with my left. This was something Sherman had taught me with a pistol he kept in the top drawer of his bureau.

"Now I want *your* got-damned money, man!" I said on that dark and empty street. There were tears in my eyes.

The thief heard in my grief-stricken, strained voice that he was as close to dead as he was likely to be before that final breath. He reached into a pocket and came out with a wad of cash that he'd probably robbed from other brooding late-night strollers. He held the cash out to me.

"Drop it on the concrete and haul yo' ass outta here 'fore I shoot you dead."

It was the terrified look on the mugger's face that made me decide to kill him. I was outraged that a man who made his living robbing others would not be brave enough to face the consequences of his crimes. His cowardice negated any claim to clemency.

I was just about to shoot the mugger when a bright light flashed, a siren chirped, and a magnified voice called out, "Drop the weapon! This is the police!"

In that moment I argued internally about the action I should take. One side of my mind said that the mugger should die, no matter what some bright light and bullhorn said.

"No, cousin," Sherman argued. "You got to live for Titi and for me too. You could have killed him, but now you got to drop the gun, get down on your knees, and put your hands behind your head."

As Sherman said these things, I did them.

The mugger stayed on his feet, trembling.

The policemen, two of them, hurried over—their guns drawn, their eyes searching for trickery and deceit.

"Don't say anything, cousin," Sherman whispered. "Not a word."

They took us, me and the man that tried to rob me, to the precinct station. I was put in a small interrogation room and handcuffed to a metal hook anchored in the wall. A cop in a suit tried to question me, but I wouldn't so much as look at him.

A long time passed. During that period I thought about Sherman and the words he had spoken years before when talking about what he'd do if he were caught in some crime. I realized that he had been teaching me how to survive after he was gone.

When the door came open again, my cousin Theodora entered. She was the last person I expected to see, hastily clad in blue jeans

and a long turquoise T-shirt. Her hair was wrapped up in a nylon stocking, and there were bags under her eyes.

She stared at me with a confused look on her face. Then, slowly, the answer to the riddle of who I was and who they thought I was, came to her.

She squatted down in front of me, her face not two inches away from mine.

"Stew?" she whispered.

I couldn't speak.

"Why you had Sherman's wallet on you?" my cousin asked.

"Titi," I uttered softly.

Theodora understood.

"Listen, Stew," she murmured. "They found me as the contact in Sherman's wallet. They think you're him. Tell me what happened, and I'll try and get you outta here."

"Man tried to mug me, and I grabbed away his gun."

Theodora was well known at the precinct. They looked up the mugger's records and Sherman's to find that my mugger, Chris Hatter, had been arrested for violent crimes many times. That, and the fact that his fingerprints and the ones on the bullets matched, got me released.

Titi let me come live with her.

Sleeping in Sherman's bed, waking up each day and putting on his clothes, made me feel . . . different, more and more so each day. I began reading his library of college books and the thirteen volumes of the detailed journal he'd kept since the age of ten. And, slowly, I made a plan for my future.

I applied to college, saying in my essay that I wanted another bachelor's degree, one in English literature because I wanted to teach.

* * *

Six months later I was in Greenwich Village at one of eight NYU registration tables. The table I stood in line for was specified for people with last names that started with letter *A*, *B*, or *C*.

I stood there thinking about the police captain who harangued me for not telling the arresting officers that I was the victim of the mugger I had disarmed.

". . . and we might have let him go," the captain said. "By keeping quiet you could have put a dangerous criminal back on the street . . ."

And now I was at the front of the line at registration.

"Name?" a blond girl with a wide face and rimless glasses asked.

Instead of responding I gave her the driver's license from my wallet.

She took the card and read it, looked up, and said, "Sherman Cardwell-Brownley?"

I sighed, smiled, and nodded. She smiled back and started going through a box of large envelopes sitting next to her. The young woman—her name tag read "Shauna"—found the name and handed me my schedule for the fall semester. I had been given a dorm room, a roommate named Lucian Meyers, and a laminated card with the photo of a face on it that looked a lot like mine.

OTIS

Crash Martin, christened Percival by his parents, left school in a hurry when he thought the truth had come out. The Martin family lived in the West Village neighborhood of Manhattan, in a three-bedroom apartment, with rent control grandfathered in through his father's father, both named Reginald, upon the elder's death in 1999. While Reginald Jr. had been born in that apartment, Mathilda Poplar-Martin, Crash's mother, hailed from Portland, Maine, and still owned her family cabin on Monhegan Island, population seventy-three.

"There are twenty-seven artists, forty-five fishermen, and me," she'd say of her island home away from home, "when I'm there."

Crash had an older sister named Albertha, a fraternal twin brother called Brother, and a cousin named Bob. Bob's parents had died in an automobile accident on California's Pacific Coast Highway. Claudia, Bob's mother, had been talking to Mathilda on her cell phone while Bob's father, John, drove the family from Santa Barbara down to LA. Mathilda didn't care much for her brother's wife or for him, for that matter, but she felt that it was providence

that she was talking to them when they died and so told Reginald Jr. that Bob had to come live with their family.

Of the six residents living in the fourth-floor apartment on Gay Street, only seventeen-year-old Albertha had her own bedroom—for obvious reasons. The unlikely twins were both fifteen, and Bob was eleven, though he insisted that he was twelve. The three boys slept restively at night in their bedroom, which was also the smallest proper room in the apartment. Crash and Brother had mattresses set upon box springs in opposite corners, while Bob slept on a shelf Reginald Jr. had installed to make room for a study desk that only Crash used.

The study desk was Crash's province, because Brother was dyslexic, which Crash understood as not liking to read, and Bob had ADD, meaning that he could not concentrate on any one thing for very long. But even though Crash had the desk to himself, he didn't use it often, because his brother and cousin made loud noises at odd moments that would shock and distract him.

So Crash used his sister's desk, even when she was in the room, because Albertha didn't seem to mind his presence, and the noises she made were both consistent and benign. Albertha talked on the phone to her friends most waking hours.

" . . . and then Billy said that Principal Rivers knew that Mr. Eagles had been arrested for bein' drunk, and he said that Principal Rivers didn't get him fired because Eagles knew that Rivers had had sex with Mrs. Longerman's wife, Betty, before Betty realized that she was a lesbian . . ."

Albertha had long riffs of interpersonal explanations that went on and on and on. For Crash it was kind of like white noise playing in the background. While he wrote and read, Albertha explained the only things that were important to her and maybe her friends—what A did or didn't do with B, either against C or behind C's back.

The only thing that confused Crash was why his sister never stopped to listen to her friends, most of whom were girls. He decided that her friends were, like him, doing their schoolwork and found it soothing to hear his sister's soft chatter while delving calculus or unveiling the disturbing mysteries of biology.

Schoolwork came easily to Crash. His brother, Brother, cousin Bob, and Albertha all went to public schools, but Crash had a scholarship to Horatio Preparatory School, grades six to twelve. There were only 218 students at Horatio, and the education, everyone said, was one of the best in the nation.

What made Crash such a good student was that he could solve math problems by closing his eyes and allowing the equation to enter a place in his mind where it somehow solved itself, and also that he could read and retain a thousand pages in an evening's time. The years he attended public school, the teachers and counselors saw his odd quirks in learning to be symptoms of a mental disorder. When Mr. Martindale ordered Crash to write out the calculation to solve a long division problem, the youngster butted him in the nose out of sheer frustration.

"He's definitely suffering from a mild case of autism," the school's psychologist-counselor, Hannah Freest, told Mathilda Poplar-Martin at a special emergency meeting to discuss Percival's violent assault.

"But my son is happy," Mathilda said. "He's not suffering at all."

"He struck Mr. Martindale."

"A math teacher," the mother pointed out, "who does not accept that my son can do math problems in his head."

"Skirting processes," Hannah Freest argued, "which are part and parcel of the standardized education required by the state."

The phrase *standardized education* struck Mathilda. She realized in an unexpected instant that school for Percival was a factory,

where he was a defective product soon to be discarded for more manageable material.

"Leave my son where he is for the rest of the semester," she said, "and I will have him in a private institution by January."

Horatio Prep tested Percival, called Crash for the rest of the semester by adoring fellow students. The private school accepted him, agreeing to waive tuition. That solved the problem of the young man's education for four blissful years. But by the time he reached the tenth grade, Percival had become bored with what the teachers had to show him.

Math and language gave him no problem. He understood the facts his teachers presented but was never, to his satisfaction, shown what lay behind the curtain of this so-called knowledge. Why did things happen? And what was responsible for why things were the way they were? On top of his own ennui, Crash could see that his classmates were often frustrated by the processes of acquiring knowledge and were rarely given what he thought of as truth. So he began to help his friends by giving them answers to the rote questions that a formal education asked over and over, like some monstrous dictator-parrot.

He taught his friends how to cheat on tests in ways that no one would suspect. He wrote papers and installed viral programs on their class computers, programs that would seek out the answers they needed.

One night he was lying in bed, only half-asleep, amid the clamor of Bob's nightmare cries over the deaths of his parents and Brother's rustling susurrations arising from the throes of yet another wet dream. At times like these Crash could drift, examining his mind without complete awareness. A thought would come into his mostly sleeping consciousness; birds' wings or World War II

Russian tanks, blood pulsing through vessels or words that rhyme. This was a state of complete ease, unencumbered by the limitations of time. Much later in life he would claim, "I do my best thinking when I'm asleep."

On this particular night, Crash suddenly realized that some student would betray him to the administration one day. This revelation forced him to recognize that in the eyes of the school he had been not helping but cheating. This meant that sooner or later he would be expelled from the one place where people believed in him.

Crash might have dismissed this dark epiphany as a bad dream if it were not for the note Alissya Progress brought to his first-period life-drawing class.

The model that day was Felix Neederman, a freshman from CCNY, who posed wearing nothing but briefs. He was reclining on a large wooden crate, propped up on one elbow, with what Crash's father would have called a shit-eating grin on his lips. Felix was pale-skinned and muscular, blue-eyed, with dirty-blond hair.

Crash sat on the high wooden stool at his easel with a stick of charred willow wood in his hand. He gazed at the burnt twig, which was quite a bit darker than his taupe-brown skin. The brown newsprint drawing pad hanging from the easel was closer to Crash's hue.

His father, Reginald Jr., was a deep brown color. Brother was a slightly darker brown than Crash, and Bob was that odd olive hue most people called white. Mother Mathilda had pale skin that she slathered with tan makeup every morning before facing the world. The only reason Crash knew his mother's true color was that they both liked to swim in the ocean, and her makeup, as she said, "could not survive the brine."

Thinking about skin and color, Crash had yet to make a mark on the pristine sheet of newsprint. While he pondered the colors ranging from charcoal to pale he noticed Alissya walking by. He

arranged the easel so that he could see the paper and Felix Neederman at the same time. He knew from previous classes that this binocular experience would end up with him tracing what he saw in the air upon the sheet of paper.

"Mr. Martin," Ernst Schillio said.

"Yes," Crash murmured, seemingly addressing his burnt willow stick.

"Miss Warren wants to see you."

Looking up, the tenth grader saw his teacher and Alissya staring back at him. He knew in an instant what was happening.

Crash placed the twig on the tray beneath the hanging pad of newsprint, hopped off the battered oak stool, and walked toward the exit. He was aware of the eyes of his fellow students watching as he made his way toward the classroom door. At public school the other kids would *ooh* at a student being called to the office. But at Horatio they only watched.

Percival was certain that his dream state the night before had predicted what was happening. Someone had turned him in, and now the principal was going to expel him for cheating.

By the time Crash made it to and through the doorway to the hall, his decision had been made. If he turned right, the principal's office was two doors away. Going left three doorways would bring him to Antoine Short's office. Antoine was what they called at Horatio the Student Advocate. If asked, Antoine would be required to go with Crash to the principal's office to protect him as much as possible from disciplinary actions demanded by school rules.

But Crash wasn't interested in the left or the right. Straight ahead were the double front doors of the school that opened onto Horatio Street and escape.

* * *

Bob, Albertha, and Brother were all at or on their way to school by the time Crash left Horatio. Reginald Jr. had been at work at Tourmaline Distributions since before the kids were awake, and Mathilda would be gone by ten to visit her ex-boyfriend Matthew Sinn in the hospice where he was dying from lung cancer.

Upstairs, in his parents' bedroom, on the high shelf in the big closet, Crash found his backpack among the others that Reginald Jr. and the boys used when they camped in the wilderness of Monhegan Island on summer vacations in late August.

Crash took jars of crunchy peanut butter and grape jelly along with a hard-crusted loaf of sourdough bread from the kitchen cabinet, a heavy afghan sweater from Brother's bottom drawer, and his father's Swiss Army knife. He dressed in canvas pants, a long-sleeved, heavy blue-and-white-checkered cotton shirt, and a light windbreaker. Clad in his makeshift camping wear and carrying the pack on his back, Crash set out for the E train. He took the subway to the Q37 bus, from which he transferred to the Q55. At noon, give or take a few minutes, he arrived at Forest Park in Queens and followed a rarely used path to Pine Grove, a place where his father took the boys camping now and then.

"What if they catch us?" Crash remembered his twin asking at the outset of one such outing.

"It's not illegal to camp in the park if it isn't posted," their father replied with a nonchalant shrug. "But if the park rangers or the police find us, they'll probably check our IDs and send us home."

Crash knew that the eastern white pines of the grove gave great cover and so was not worried about being found. His backpack contained a camouflage pup tent, a thin down sleeping bag, a butane

hotplate with enough fuel for a week's worth of cooking, a pot and pan, a quart bottle of water, a battery-powered lantern, and six dried packets of onion and mushroom soup mix that came with a five-year guarantee of freshness. There were various other contents of the pack: three teabags, a tin cup, and a hunting knife designed, as his father said, for industry or defense.

Crash put up the tent and sat next to it eating a PB&J on sourdough. As evening came on, he began to wonder what would be happening between his home and the school. The principal's office would have called his parents, saying that they had to come in for a special disciplinary meeting. On the other hand, his parents would have called the administration office wondering what the school had done with their son. Sooner or later they would figure out that Crash had suspected why the principal called him to her office and, instead of facing the music, had run.

Down in a clearing below a scrim of pines, Crash saw three deer illuminated by an early moon. He'd turned his lantern on low to read *Demian,* by Herman Hesse, a book that had been assigned in Mrs. Schrodinger's World Literature class. Crash liked the book because it saw the world the way he did: not only good and evil but also light and dark mixing to make things so hard to understand. He liked the main character, Emil Sinclair, a lot. He was a misunderstood kid who couldn't solve the simple problems of life.

"Hey there, little brother." The voice was both rough and soft.

Crash peered in the direction from which the voice had come, but at first all he could see was darkness. He knew this was because of the blinding effect of the moon and electric light. He wasn't afraid, because Brother called him "little brother" due to a half-inch deficit in height; Crash had been born seven minutes before Brother, and his jealous twin always tried to make Crash seem the junior.

As Crash's vision acclimated, there appeared before him a tall and lanky young black man wearing black trousers and maybe a red T-shirt. The dark-skinned lad smiled brightly and said, "What you doin' out here readin' a book in the woods, man?"

"Reading," Crash said, though he knew this was not a satisfactory answer to the question.

"What's your name?" the young man asked. He took a step forward and hunkered down in an easy movement, right forearm on the knee, the knuckles of his left hand grazing the grass.

"My parents named me Percival, Percy, but everyone calls me Crash."

"Why Crash?"

"What's your name?" Crash asked.

"Otis." He said the word as if it were somehow a defeat. "Otis Zeal."

"That's a cool name," Crash said. It was the right thing to say.

Otis grinned again and asked, "Why you out heah?"

"They were going to expel me from school for helping about a dozen kids cheat on their homework and their tests."

"A dozen is twelve, right?"

"Yeah."

"So how much them other kids pay you to help 'em cheat?"

"Nothing."

"Nuthin'? You mean you helped them and didn't even get paid?"

"It was kind of like an experiment."

"Like a scientist, like on TV?"

"Uh-huh. You see, I thought that maybe my friends weren't learning because the teachers made the answers so much of a mystery. If they saw the question and then the answer, maybe that would help them know what they were learning about."

"You sound kinda crazy, Percy Crash."

"Why are you out here, Otis?"

"I always come out to here when I get in trouble too. My uncle used to take me here when I was kid like you, and now if I think somebody's after me I come here to hide."

"What are you hiding from?" Crash asked.

Otis embarked upon a meandering tale that made only a little sense to the sophomore from Horatio Prep. The story started with a girl named Brenda Redman. She was real cute, with a fat butt, and she could dance. Otis was a good dancer, and so every time he and Brenda met at a party at somebody's house in the Bronx, they danced to just about every other cut the DJ played. The problem was this guy named Lawrence. Lawrence liked Brenda, and she liked him some too, but he couldn't dance like Otis, and Brenda needed to be dancing when she was at a party and the music was playing—especially if there was wine involved. It was the wine, Otis believed, that made Lawrence angry. Brenda wasn't his steady girl or anything, but even still, Lawrence pushed Otis, and that made Otis mad.

"You don't wanna get me mad, little brother," Otis said, in the middle of his story. "When I get mad there's no tellin' what I might do."

Anyway, Otis got mad and stabbed Lawrence, who was a much bigger man, in the shoulder with a little paring knife. Otis always carried an edge—that's what he said.

"Did you kill him?" Crash asked Otis.

"I 'on't think I did. You know, sometimes people die when you don't hurt 'em much, but I don't think he woulda died. It don't matter though, because his cousin belongs to a gang, and they'll be lookin' for me for a long time."

There was a lull in the conversation for a while after that. Both young man and boy looked around, appreciating the relative silence of the city park. Then Otis began to shiver. The tremors started in

his chest and radiated out toward the limbs. Crash crawled into the little pup tent and pulled out Brother's afghan sweater.

"Here," Crash said, "put this on."

Otis reached out and pulled the woolen garment over his head. He nodded, grinned, and then shuddered once before plopping down into a half lotus.

"That makes the difference," Otis declared.

Crash thought the words sounded like something a parent or some other elder had often said.

"You want a PB&J?"

"Wha's that?"

They talked about school because it was something they had in common. Otis had been kicked out so many times that they finally stopped expecting him to come back. Mostly these suspensions were because of his bad temper. Whenever Otis got angry he had to do something hard. He'd throw a glass against the wall, hit somebody, or something else like that. One time he pushed a girl named Theodora down some marble stairs.

"I was already sorry before she stopped tumblin'," he said. "But I didn't say it, because I had no right to expect forgiveness. I always keep thinkin' that maybe I could find a place where you nevah have to get mad, and then I'd be cool. My daddy told me before he died that that place was called *Dead*."

When it was Crash's turn to talk, he said that he felt like an outcast in school. Horatio Prep was better than public school, but still everybody thought that he was tricking them with the way he learned things.

"It's like when I read a book," Crash explained. "I turn the pages so fast that nobody believes I'm really readin', or when people just say a math problem and I know the answer."

"You didn't turn the pages fast when I saw you reading your book," Otis pointed out.

"That's because, um, after I read a book a few times I go slower and slower, because my mind is making up all this other stuff about how the people really felt and what they looked like."

"Like it was a TV show, but you have to see it ovah and ovah until you understand how what happened happened?"

"Yeah." Crash felt that no one had ever put into words the feelings he got while he was learning.

"Why don't you read me a couple a' pages?" Otis said.

Crash read nearly a dozen pages out loud, marveling at how good it sounded. He didn't trip and stumble over the words as he did when he read out loud in English class.

Otis started yawning after a while, and Crash stopped reading.

"Guess we should get some sleep," Otis suggested.

"Uh-huh."

Then Otis stood up on his knees and took three stump-like steps, bringing him very close to Crash. He leaned forward slowly and kissed Crash on the mouth. It was a wet kiss, not anything the sophomore had experienced before.

Otis leaned back and asked, "Is there room in yo' tent for me?"

The youths gazed into each other's eyes for a long moment before Crash said, "Uh-uh. It's too small."

Taking a long time before he spoke again, Otis finally said, "OK. I'll just curl up in this sweater next to it."

In his half-asleep state it came to Crash that Otis kissing him was the opposite of Otis getting mad. It made him happy that he was able to calm the angry young man down. He was smiling in the

tent when somebody grabbed him by his shoulders and dragged him out.

"Who are you?" a man's voice shouted.

The sun was up and shining and hurting Crash's eyes.

"What are you doing here?" another angry voice wanted to know.

Crash held out his arms to show that he wasn't resisting them, but the man still lifted him from the ground and pulled him so close that Crash could smell bacon on his breath.

"Who are you?" Bacon Breath demanded.

"Percival Martin." He felt defeated because he used a name he no longer answered to.

"Where's some ID?"

"In my, in my, in my . . ."

"In your what?"

"In my backpack."

"Where is it?"

"Next to the tent."

Crash glanced at the side of the tent where Otis had been sleeping, but both the sometimes angry young man and the backpack were gone.

When Crash realized that Otis was gone with all his belongings —money and food, cookware and butane hotplate—he was giddy with the knowledge that he had helped his friend.

"You're going to jail, Percival Martin," one tall, treelike park man intoned.

They were all sitting around the dining table that night—the entire Martin clan plus Bob. It wasn't unusual for the family to gather over a meal, but this time there were no plates of food before them.

"What did you do?" Reginald Jr. asked.

Albertha was sitting next to her father. Crash imagined that his sister could hardly wait to get to her room, where she could tell everyone about her crazy autistic brother.

"I figured out how to help all the kids I knew get good grades on their papers and tests."

The police had called Reginald and Mathilda. They'd come down to the Queens police station and taken their son home.

"But why did you run away?" Mathilda asked.

Brother was peering at Crash with a crestfallen look on his face. This expression presented itself like a simple equation to Crash. It said that Brother realized that he would never be as much fun as him.

"I dreamed that . . . No, no, no. I saw that one of the kids would tell on me sooner or later. And then when I went to Mr. Schillio's class and he told me to go to the principal's office, I knew I was in trouble."

"The school didn't say anything about you cheating," Mathilda said.

Bob was studying his cousin.

"They didn't?"

"No," Reginald Jr. replied. "They called to tell us that you were going to be valedictorian of the second years."

"Oh."

"You have to stop cheating," the father continued. "Tell your friends that you can't do it anymore."

"Are you OK?" Mathilda asked.

Crash turned toward his mother but had no words to say.

"That goes for all of you," Reginald said to the other kids. "We never mention cheating again."

* * *

Years passed, but nothing happened that was as powerful or insightful or fulfilling as the day when Crash ran away. He'd kissed fourteen girls and a few boys, but nothing made an impression on him like Otis did amidst the pine trees and darkness, witnessed by lost deer and a few fireflies.

It was on this true adventure Crash had learned that the mathematics of life were ever so much more complex than counting up things in his head.

Albertha married her first boyfriend, Clyde Friarstone. She talked for both herself and her husband while Clyde smiled shyly at her side. Bob became a renowned artist and sometime opioid abuser. He still lied about his age.

Brother worked construction for six years, then he enlisted and did three tours of duty in Afghanistan. During his period of service he avoided the members of his family, most of whom were against the wars. But a few weeks after his last tour, Brother showed up at Crash's upper-Harlem apartment. Crash served his twin a glass of cabernet.

"When do you graduate, little brother?" Brother asked.

"Next year."

"You gonna work for the government?"

"I don't think so. Maybe I'll be a physics teacher at some small college upstate."

Crash thought that Brother didn't like this answer, but instead of saying so he asked, "You ever talk to Mom?"

"No," Crash said in a hushed tone. "She sends cards every once in a while but . . ."

"I throw 'em away," Brother said. "She was a bitch leavin' Dad. No explanation, just a note saying that it was over and she was gone."

"Why'd you join the army?" It was a question he'd always wanted to ask.

"To serve my country. To save people who got stuck under the Taliban."

"Did it feel like you broke outta prison and at least just for a little while you were free?"

Brother winced and said, "I got shrapnel in my chest. The doctors say that it's better to leave it."

They drank more and talked about old times in the bedroom with cousin Bob.

Crash didn't tell Brother that Mathilda had sent him her e-mail address or that he'd contacted her a few times. But something about Brother's visit made him decide to take the subway out to Queens. Her apartment was less than a mile from Forest Park.

He knocked on the sixth-floor apartment door and waited, nervous for the first time since he believed he was about to get expelled. The door came open. A willowy man stood there. He looked familiar, very much so.

"Matthew Sinn?" Crash asked.

"Hi, Percy. How are you?"

"I thought you were dead."

"I would be if it wasn't for your mother."

"It was really because of you, baby," Mathilda said to Crash at dinner. She'd made chicken and dumplings with almandine French beans and peach cobbler.

"Me?"

"You were so brave."

"What are you talking about?"

"Your whole life you were different. Nobody understood you. Your teachers were angry because you didn't need them. And then

you ran away to the woods with a backpack and a book. You were only fifteen, and emotionally so much younger than that, but you took your life in your hands . . ."

"The day after you came back, she took my hands in hers," Sinn said. "She held on tight and told me I wasn't going anywhere. Before that everyone came to see me just to say goodbye, but Mattie held on tight. After three months I was in remission. In three years my cure moved in with me."

"Why didn't you tell anybody?" Crash asked his mom.

"I would have told them all," she said, "but no one replied to my cards except you. Reginald phoned me once, but before I could explain he called me vile names and hung up. I would have liked to remain his wife and just . . . be close with Matthew. But Reggie hated me for breaking the cord of our discord."

The last five words were often used by Mathilda's English professor father.

"But you just said you were gone," Crash argued.

"I said that I needed space."

That night Crash got on the Internet and entered an algorithm created to search for the name Otis Zeal. In a way, Crash thought, Otis was the one person who understood him like he intuitively understood long division.

The next morning Crash called his father. Minnie Saltworthy, Reginald Jr.'s live-in girlfriend, answered, "Martin residence."

"Hi, Minnie," Crash said.

"Hi, Percy. You want to talk to your father?"

"Hello, son," Reginald Jr. said. He'd retired from his sales job and now stayed home most of the time. He and Minnie, only fifteen

years his junior, took vacations four times a year. They went on voyages and train treks, visited Mexico, and even went on a camping tour in the Italian Alps.

"Hi, Dad."

"You calling just to say hello?"

"I wanted to say that I love you, Dad; that I miss the days when we were kids living in that apartment and going to school."

"You can come home anytime you want."

That night Brother died of a heart attack. Skipping the funeral, Crash went the next day to the grave site. Brother was interred beneath a temporary plaster marker, upon which was written his birth name—Constant Stevens Martin. Crash wondered why he never knew Brother's real name. He wondered whether Brother had known it.

Soon after Brother's death, Crash dropped out of Columbia and started an online business that generated outlines for school papers and explained ways to take and take advantage of school tests. He made lots of money and often chatted, digitally, with his ever-changing cast of clients.

And then one night, while writing an e-mail to hornyowl297, he received a message from the Otis Zeal algorithm. He'd already read dozens of little reports of Otis being arrested, tried, and sometimes convicted. The not-so-young delinquent popped up all over the boroughs. He'd married Brenda Redman, but five months later she'd filed for, and been granted, a restraining order against him. Their divorce came soon after that.

But that evening, while trying to explain to the postgraduate hornyowl297 that all math existed before human understanding, he received the notice of Otis's death.

* * *

At a small graveyard called simply Final Rest, on the border of Queens and Brooklyn, the funeral and burial of Otis Zeal was held. The ceremony was scheduled for 7:15 A.M. Crash arrived at 6:27. The small chapel was empty, and so he took a seat at the back, in the third-to-last row. There he remembered the night he met Otis. There was the hello, the confession, and the kiss. It was a moment that happened outside of his head but was as important as the eternal resolution of pi.

"Who you, sugah?" a woman asked.

Crash looked up to see a dark-skinned woman wearing a black dress suit with a pale pink blouse underneath. There was a deep purple iris pinned to her lapel and a smile that Crash believed would never be far from her lips.

"Crash."

"Not Percy Crash?"

"Uh-huh. That's what Otis called me."

"I'm Zenobia Zeal," the woman said, taking Crash by the sleeve of his blue blazer. "You come up with me to the first row. I know that's what my son woulda wanted."

She dragged the shy professional cheater to the front of the first row of pews. The coffin had come while Crash was remembering.

"You know who I am?" the young man asked.

"Otis nevah stopped talkin' 'bout you. He said that you gave him all this stuff and read to him from a book called *Demon* and that he told you just about everything and you didn't laugh once."

"Really?" Crash asked. He'd thought that the older boy had probably forgotten him.

"I'll prove it." Saying this, Zenobia Zeal pulled Crash from the front row to the side of the open coffin.

Otis looked very much the way he had when Crash last saw him. Only now he sported a thick mustache. He wore blue jeans and a pullover afghan sweater.

"That there sweater was the onliest wrap he never lost," the ever-smiling mother said. "He told everybody that you was his best friend and that sometimes he'd come to see you on Horatio Street where you went to school. Nobody believed him though. We all thought he stole that sweater. But now here you are, his oldest friend, come to say goodbye to him."

Tears glittered in the older woman's eyes.

"How did my friend die?" Crash asked.

"Fightin'."

"Over what?"

"You never knew with Otis. He was just so sensitive. He always thought that people was laughin' at him or takin' advantage. He always said that you were the only one to treat him like a human being. Why is that?"

Crash stared into the dark woman's inquiring eyes and wondered about the question. He realized that she wanted him to share something intimate about her son, something uplifting.

"There's something different about my brain," Crash said, for the first time ever.

"Oh." A flash of concern moved across Zenobia's face.

"Not a disease or a condition," Crash interjected. "It's just that I think differently, and, in a way, Otis did too."

Zenobia nodded sagely.

"And so when we talked," Crash went on, "it felt like we understood each other. All the people in the world didn't understand us,

but there we were, like brothers really. I knew him better than I did my own brother."

Zenobia took Crash's hand in hers, making him think about his mother and the life she saved and about Otis and his heartfelt kiss.

SHOWDOWN ON THE HUDSON

How the whole thing started is a mystery to most people, even the police. But those of us who were around 145th Street and Broadway, up in Harlem, knew something new was happening the day Billy Consigas came to town. His mother had moved to New York from southern Texas to escape an abusive husband. "A roustabout name of Henry Ryder," Billy told us.

And so Billy (who was fifteen at the time) was forced to leave his beloved Texas for Harlem. He didn't like New York at first, said that there was no place to stretch your legs or keep a horse. Some of us used to make fun of him, but that never amounted to much because Billy was an honest-to-God, one-hundred-percent bona fide black Texas cowboy. He wore a felt Stetson hat that was almost pure white. From the band of his hat hung a tassel of multicolored triple-string beads that he said was a gift from his Choctaw girlfriend when he had to leave Texas, *to come north*. He wore fancy bright shirts with snap buttons made from garnet, topaz, and quartz. His jeans were

always well worn and rough as sandpaper. And he boasted that he had cowboy boots for every occasion—from weddings to funerals.

He got in good with the girls because, before long, he had a job for the NYPD training their horses in a special area of Central Park. He'd take young ladies up there in the early hours of the morning and teach them how to ride. Nesta Brown told me that if a man takes a girl riding that morning, he will most likely be riding her that night.

She actually said *most likely* with a dreamy look in her eyes and a kiss on her lips.

Girls our age flocked around Billy, and I never heard one of them call him a dog.

The black cowboy also had the most beautiful pistol any of us had ever seen. It was a silvery Cowboy Colt .44 six-shooter etched with all kinds of designs and finished with a polished horn handle. The holster for this ten-inch pistol was black with silver studs. And even though I am no fan of Westerns, when I saw how fast Billy could draw I downloaded fourteen cowboy films.

Billy drawled when he spoke and respected everyone he met. He'd always take his hat off inside or when in the presence of a woman or girl. And he could fight like a motherfucker.

One time, over by the Hudson, uptown, this big dude was chasing down some man that he claimed owed him money. The big man caught the little one and started beating him. The poor guy fell to the pavement and was bleeding from his mouth and forehead. That's when the big man started kicking him.

After two or three kicks, Billy Consigas walked up and said, "All right now, he's had enough."

When I tell you that the bully was big, I mean it in every way possible: he was tall and fat and had biceps almost the size of his head. But it wasn't only that he was big; he was fast too. He hit

Billy—who was five ten and 160 at most—right in the chest. Billy flew back and hit the wall behind him. We all thought that he was going to get himself killed.

The little man on the ground got up and started running.

Billy pushed off from the wall, took a deep breath, and then he smiled. Smiled!

"Fuck you, you grinnin' fool," the big man yelled, and then he ran right at Billy.

Billy kept on smiling. He didn't move until the guy was almost on him . . . and then he did this amazing thing. He jumped half a step to the right, so that his attacker slammed into the wall. Then Billy jumped up on top of the guy and clamped his left arm around his neck. We didn't know it at the time, but that was the end of the fight right there. The big guy was twisting and jumping around but couldn't throw Billy off, and Billy was steadily hitting him in the face with these wicked right uppercuts. He must have hit him two dozen times before the behemoth slumped down on the sidewalk. The bully tried to get up three times, but his legs were spaghetti and his shoes roller skates.

We never found out what happened to him because we heard sirens and scattered.

After that fight Billy became like a hero among the young men and women up around 145th. He didn't consider himself a leader, though, because of something he called the Cowboy Code. I never got all the ins and outs of that system, but it had something to do with being self-sufficient and treating all others equally. Leaders, he thought, were there only for the weak.

"Felix," he said to me one late afternoon when I was showing him around Times Square, "a man has to stand up on his own two feet. The only leaders they should evah have is parents, teachers,

and generals during time of war. Other than that we all just people come from our mothers and headed for the grave."

Billy talked like that. He bought me a hot dog, and I paid for our tickets to the wax museum. We walked in the crowds of Times Square for hours. Billy was especially interested in the Singing Cowboy, who wore only a Stetson hat and underpants as he played the guitar and posed for photographs.

"What do you think about that?" I asked after Billy had stared at the street performer for at least three minutes.

"Like any other child's cartoon on the television."

It was somewhere past eleven in the evening when we decided to take the number one train back to Harlem. Billy had paid for our barbecue dinner. He told me that it was OK because the police gave him good money to train their horses.

When we were walking toward the train someone said, "I'll be damned, a nigger in a cowboy hat. I never seen anything like that before."

I turned first and saw a group of five young white men and three young women. They were maybe a year or two older than us. The guys sported new-looking blue jeans and fancy shirts like the ones Billy wore. The girls had on modern party dresses, slight and short. I was nervous because it was only the two of us against five of them, not counting the girls.

I say "against" because the leader, a tall and skinny white guy with a long and somehow misshapen face, had used the word *nigger*, and that word, in that tone of voice and that situation, meant conflict.

Billy turned and smiled. I had come to associate that expression with sudden violence. This mental connection only added to my fear.

"A peckawood with a problem," Billy said jovially. "That's more common than rattlesnakes down a prairie hole."

"You sound like Texas," the speaker of the group speculated.

"And you sound like horseshit."

"Where you come from, boy?" the white youth asked.

"From a long line a' men."

In any other situation I would have run, but I didn't want Billy to think less of me. So I squared my shoulders and wondered which one of the five I could get at before his friends got to me.

That was what Billy did: he made people happy and proud, brave and courageous—qualities that rarely served a poor black man or boy well.

"You think you man enough take us?" the leader asked.

"At five to two?" Billy asked. "All we got to do is stand our ground and we prove better than some gang a' roughnecks."

The leader smiled. That grin was a close relative of Billy's violent mirth.

I realized that I was holding my breath.

"My name is Nacogdoches," the white youth claimed. "Nacogdoches Early."

"Billy."

"You a cowboy, Billy?"

"I've been in a rodeo or two."

This made me think of Billy taking down that giant on the Hudson. He wasn't afraid because he'd brought down steers with that same hold.

"You got a gun?" Nacogdoches inquired.

Billy shrugged.

"You a gunslinger?" Nacogdoches said to Billy.

"Faster 'n you."

The warped-faced white youth's eyebrows raised, and his smile broadened.

"Is one of these fine ladies your girl?" Billy asked.

A strawberry blonde moved her shoulders in such a way as to indicate that she was the one.

"No bullets," Billy said, as if they had already agreed on the gunfight. "Just a video camera in case it's a close call. If you win, I'll spit-polish your green boots right on that corner. I'll just wear my long johns and hat at high noon on a Saturday. If you lose, that pretty girl will agree to have dinner with me at the place and time of my choosin'."

The girl tried to frown, but instead a smile grazed her lips. She wasn't really that pretty, I thought, but had the kind of face that you'd want to nod to at a party or if you sat near each other on a subway train.

Nacogdoches was biting his lower lip.

"OK," he said at last. "When and where?"

"There's a youth center up on Sixty-Third," I said. "Lazarus House. We do it there in three days at ten at night."

In spite of the offer, my plan was simply to get away.

The principals agreed, and I gave Nacogdoches the address.

"What kinda crazy luck you have to have that you run into another cowboy with a six-shooter somewhere in the middle of a million people?" I asked Billy on the number one train.

"It's the bright lights," the black cowboy opined.

"What?"

"You know a cowboy loves the stars more than anything. He's drawn to the lights like a moth to fire. Times Square is bright like the heavens come down to the ground. And you know two cowboys will see each other. No, no, Felix. It would be a wonder if we didn't meet up sooner or later."

"We don't have to do this thing, Bill," I said. "We just don't show up, and it'll all blow over."

"Maybe so," he said, "but we will be there."

All the youngsters in our neighborhood knew about the showdown, as Billy called it, scheduled for Wednesday night. They gossiped about it and bragged on their black cowboy hero.

In the interim, I saw Billy every day because I was his assigned tutor.

"Hello, Felix," Mrs. Consigas greeted me on that Wednesday afternoon. She was a dark-skinned black woman with a young face. "You're a little early, aren't you?"

"Yes, ma'am."

"What's that you're carryin'?"

"My uncle's video camera."

"What for?"

"My sister's in a dance recital after, and I'm going to video it for my mother. She works nights." It was all lies, but Marion Consigas didn't know my mother or my sister.

"You're a good boy, Felix Grimes."

I spent the next two hours trying to teach Billy about variables in algebra. I was a good student, and as far as school went, Billy was dumb as a post; he said so himself.

"It takes me a long time to get the idea," he said to me at our first tutoring session, "but once I got it, it's there forever."

He didn't talk about the showdown at all. I told six friends where it was happening: five guys and Sheila Grant, a girl I wanted but who only had eyes for the Harlem Cowboy, Billy Consigas.

Billy struggled through the workbook lesson, and somewhere around seven o'clock he said, "Time to go."

* * *

We all—Billy, me, Sheila Grant, and five others—arrived early. My brother Terrence, who worked at Lazarus House as a nighttime security guard, was waiting at the side entrance. He told us that Nacogdoches was already inside with his posse.

My brother was nineteen, three years older than I. He was nervous, but Billy ponied up twenty dollars for the use of the gym, and Terrence was always looking for more money.

Nacogdoches was there with the same group of friends. This detail said something about the ugly southerner that I couldn't quite put my finger on.

While I set up the tripod and videocam, Billy and Nacogdoches decided on the rules.

"Best out of three," the white cowboy said.

"And we check to make sure that each other's gun is empty before each duel," added Billy.

"Duel?" Nacogdoches sneered. "What are you some kinda English faggot?"

"I am what I am," Billy said, "and that's more than enough for you."

Nacogdoches frowned and balled his fists. Billy wasn't school-trained, but he once told me that all true cowboys could sing and were poets. The white gunslinger couldn't match him with words, and so he said, "Thalia will count. On three we draw."

Billy nodded, no longer smiling.

The duelists checked each other's guns and then took their places six steps apart. The white guy had a mean look on his face. Billy was as peaceful as moonlight on the Hudson. He wasn't actually a handsome youth, but Billy had a look that made you feel like

there was something good somewhere, something you could depend on.

Thalia, that was Nacogdoches's girl, counted out loud. When she got to three, Nacogdoches slapped his brown leather holster, coming up with his black iron gun at incredible speed. But when we looked at the replay it was obvious, even to Nacogdoches's friends, that easygoing Billy had his piece out first. The black cowboy's movements were fluid, seamless.

Nacogdoches was slower on the second draw. We didn't even have to look at the replay.

After that Billy started undoing the leather string that laced the bottom of the black and silver holster to his right thigh.

"What you doin'?" the white cowboy complained.

"Two outta three," Billy said.

"I want the last draw."

"Why?"

"You scared?" Nacogdoches asked in a taunting tone.

Billy smiled and shook his head. He tied the lace again, and I turned on the camera.

"One," Thalia said, and a sense of doom descended upon me.

"Two," she pronounced. It struck me that this last contest meant far more than two young men proving themselves.

"Three."

Nacogdoches was faster this time. He grabbed his piece and had it out like a real gunslinger in a fight for his life.

But Billy was faster still. On the video replay he had the silver gun out and had played like he was fanning the hammer with his left hand before Nacogdoches had his barrel level.

"We could have hot dogs on that corner where I said I'd shine your boyfriend's shoes," Billy suggested to Thalia.

"No, you won't," Nacogdoches said.

"That was the bet," Billy countered, the ass-kicking smile back on his lips.

"You didn't pull the trigger," his rival argued.

"Why I wanna pull on a trigger when I know the gun is empty?"

"You could draw faster if you didn't move your finger. Any fool could pull a gun out by its butt."

Billy squinted as if he was on his beloved prairie trying to make out a shadow on the horizon. He shook his head ever so slightly and then shrugged, moving his shoulders no more than an inch.

"Thank you, Terrence," Billy said, waving to my brother, who was standing next to the exit door. "We finished here."

"You didn't pull the trigger," Nacogdoches said again.

"I won," Billy replied.

Terrence herded us out the door and onto Sixty-Third.

Thalia, who was wearing black jeans and a calico blouse, walked up to Billy and shook his hand. He gave her a quizzical stare, but she lowered her head and turned away.

"I won!" Nacogdoches said, as he and his friends walked toward Central Park.

When we were walking to the train, Billy asked me to come with him while Sheila and the rest took a more direct route to the subway. He said that he wanted to talk about something as we strolled north on Broadway.

But before he had the chance someone said, "Stop right there."

I was already nervous. Most of my life I had spent at my home, at church, or in school, where I had been an honor student every year, every semester. I wasn't used to running the street with armed friends and watching duels.

Two uniformed policemen were getting out of their black and white cruiser. Billy had his six-shooter in a battered brown leather satchel, and the police had the right of stop-and-frisk.

Once again I had the urge to run, but I knew that wouldn't end well.

One cop was pink colored and the other dark brown.

"What are you doing here so late at night, boys?" the black cop asked.

"Good evening, Officer O'Brien," Billy said to the white policeman.

"Consigas?" he replied.

"You get that parade trot down yet?"

"This is the kid I was telling you about, Frank," the white cop said to his partner. "He can do anything on a horse. Honest-to-God cowboy from Texas."

"I was just playin' basketball with my friend Felix here down at Lazarus House," Billy said.

O'Brien asked Billy a few things about riding and then shook my friend's hand.

"I thought the Cowboy Code said you shouldn't lie," I said when we were installed on the train.

"She gave me her phone number," Billy replied.

"What?"

"That Thalia gave me her phone number on a little piece of paper when she shook my hand."

"Damn."

"What do you think I should do?"

I am, as I said, a good student and the kind of citizen that stays out of trouble. I prefer reading to TV and ideas in opposition to actions, sweat, or violence. I was always considered by my parents,

teachers, and, later on, by my employers, a good person. My only serious fault, as my father was always happy to say, was that I often spoke without considering what it was that I said. This was most often a minor flaw, but in certain cases it could be a fatal one.

"You should call her and have lunch at that barbecue place with me and Sheila Grant. That way it'll be friendly."

Billy called Thalia the next day. He told her what I had said, and by now regretted, and she agreed to the date.

"She said," Billy told me, "that Nacogdoches had obviously lost, and she felt that it was her obligation to go on a date with the winning cowboy."

The lunch was set for Saturday.

"What you mean he's goin' out with that white girl?" Sheila said when I asked her to come along.

"It's the bet," I explained lamely. "He kind of has to go."

"I bet he wouldn't think so if she was black."

"You know better than that, girl. Billy's doing it because he won and she knows it."

"Sounds stupid to me."

"That mean you're not comin'?"

We ordered hot links, brisket, fried chicken, and pork ribs, with cornbread, collard greens, fried pickles, and a whole platter full of french fries.

"So where all you southerners come from?" Sheila asked Thalia after we'd ordered.

"Only Nacky and one of the others, Braughm, are from the South. They're both out of Nashville. We all go to this private school

called Reese on Staten Island. Most of the kids there are rich and have what they call 'social behavior problems.'"

"But all his friends dress like cowboys," I said.

"They just wanna be like him," Thalia said with a twist to her lips. I remember thinking that if she were Caribbean she would have sucked a tooth.

"So you're rich?" Sheila asked Thalia, as if it was some kind of indictment.

"No. My mother teaches there, and she didn't like the kind of friends I had in public school. I like your hair. I wish I could do something like that with mine."

Sheila had thick corded braids that flowed down her back. She was a beautiful girl. She lost her angry attitude when Thalia complimented her.

"So Nacogdoches is like some kind of juvenile delinquent?" Billy asked.

"He got in trouble down south stealing. I think his parents just wanted to get rid of him. Anyway, he's graduating this June. Says he's going out to California."

That's when the food came. We spent the rest of the lunch talking and joking. Thalia was a painter who wanted to specialize in horses. That's what drew her to Nacogdoches. He kept a horse at a stable in Connecticut and promised to bring her up there some day.

"But now I think he was just sayin' that to get in good with me," the white girl added.

Billy said he'd take her to the police stables the next morning. He invited me and Sheila too.

"It's not a date unless you two kiss," Sheila said when we were out in front of the Iron Spur Barbecue House.

Thalia kissed Billy on the cheek, and Sheila snapped the picture with her cell-phone camera.

Billy left with Thalia, and Sheila gave me a few friendly kisses before I walked her home.

The next morning Thalia and Billy met us at the gate of the police stables. They were both wearing the same clothes from the day before.

I had the most trouble keeping up with my horse. I was just bouncing, bouncing—up and down, to the side, and almost to the ground once or twice. But we had a good time. The girls became friends, and Billy was glad that we were there together.

"You know, Felix," he said to me, when we were returning the big animals to their stalls, "I realized yesterday that there are good people everywhere—not only in the place you come from."

Like every other citizen of the world with a cell phone, Sheila was an amateur photographer. She took pictures of us on our horses, out in the park, and of me, Billy, and Thalia walking side by side. Thalia's arm was linked with Billy's.

Things returned to normal after that, more or less. I went back to my secretary post on the student council and helped Billy write a paper for his remedial English class. It was an essay about a book of cowboy poetry his grandfather had given him. Sheila and Thalia became Facebook friends. They shared pictures and started telling each other about their experiences in different boroughs and at different schools.

I asked Sheila to go out with me six times in the next two weeks, but she always had some reason to say no.

Then one afternoon, Sheila was waiting outside my German class, clutching her beloved smartphone.

"Hey, Sheil," I said, trying to sound nonchalant.

"Look at this," she said, thrusting the phone into my hand.

On the screen was a photograph of Thalia. She had a black eye and a bloody lip, and she seemed to be in the middle of a scream or cry.

"Flip it," Sheila said.

There were seven pictures of the white girl. It became obvious after the second shot that she was being beaten while someone took pictures. In two shots someone was pulling her hair and slapping her. In another photo she was hunched over, clutching her stomach with both hands as if someone had kicked her.

"Who sent you these?" I asked Sheila.

"It came from her phone. There was a text too."

The text read, *This is what happens to whores and race traitors.*

As his tutor, I went to Billy's house almost every afternoon. That day we were making the finishing touches on his poetry paper. Billy wrote on an old Royal typewriter.

"I don't really care for computers," he said. But I think he was just afraid of them.

The night before, he'd finished the fifth rewrite of the essay. He really did have deep insights into poetry and its uses by people living the actual lives that they turned into verse. We did a word-by-word examination of his spelling and grammar before I dared to broach the thing that was foremost in my mind.

"I need to show you something, Billy."

"What's that, Felix? You don't think that the paper's good enough?"

I located the forwarded files from Sheila's phone and showed him the pictures. Billy flipped through them saying not a word. His eyes seemed to get smaller, but he wasn't squinting. If he drew a breath, I couldn't tell.

After some minutes and close perusal of the photos, Billy said, "Can you send this motherfucker a note?"

Playground above 150 on the Hudson. Midnight tonight. Come ready. Come heavy.

Billy strapped on the pistol in his bedroom. It was exactly as he had done at Lazarus House, but this time he tied the holster to his left leg.

"I thought you were right-handed?" I said.

"Two-handed," Billy said, showing the first smile since he had seen the pictures. "But I'm a little better with my left."

At 11:35 he donned an off-white trench coat, and we left the house.

"Where you goin'?" Billy's mother called from the kitchen.

"Over to Felix's," said my friend. "He's gonna help me type my paper into his computer so then I can send the file-thing to Miss Andrews."

Outside we hailed a green cab and had the driver take us to the park.

Nacogdoches Early and his posse were waiting for us. Thalia was with them, but as soon as we appeared she ran to me. Her face was all swollen from the punishment she'd received.

"That's right," Nacogdoches said. "Go on over to them. That's where you belong."

A few moments later Sheila Grant, Tom Tellerman, and Teriq Strickland walked into the empty children's playground. I had called Sheila, and she'd notified our other friends.

Nacogdoches was wearing a bright-colored Mexican poncho, which he flung off. Underneath he was wearing his brown holster and black gun. He was hatless, and his pale skin shone in the shadowy light.

Billy took off his trench coat and draped it around Thalia's shoulders. Sheila was holding the scared white girl by then.

There was no need for words. Billy and Nacogdoches squared off with about ten paces between them.

"Thalia?" Billy called.

"Yeah?" she said.

"You strong enough to count to three, honey?"

Thalia walked to the river side of the present-day cowboys. The rest of us, white and black, moved out of the line of fire.

"One," Thalia said, and I was reminded of the sense of fate I'd experienced at Lazarus House.

"Two," she announced, and I wanted to scream.

Before she was able to utter the last number, Nacogdoches reached for his pistol. He pulled out the gun and fired. But before that, with snake-like fluidity, Billy drew and shot. Nacogdoches's bullet went wild, landing, I believe, somewhere out on the Hudson. The young white man was dead before he hit the concrete. I remember that he fell on a chalk-drawn hopscotch design.

There was another shot, and I looked to see Braughm, the other white southerner, aiming a pistol at Billy—who was now down on one knee. Billy shot one time, hitting his assailant in the upper thigh. Two others of Nacogdoches's posse had guns, but Billy shot both of them before they could fire—one in the shins and the other in the shoulder.

After that we all ran.

At a coffee shop on 125th Street, Billy was once again wearing his trench coat, and he was drinking from a bowl of chicken noodle soup. Sheila and Thalia were there with us.

"You think he's dead?" Billy asked me.

"You hit him in the head," I said.

Billy nodded and grimaced.

"It ain't no fun when somebody dies," he said.

After a few minutes of silence I noticed a red spot at the right shoulder of his off-white coat.

"You're bleeding."

"I think I need to get out of town," he said.

"I'll go with you," Thalia offered.

"That'd be nice," Billy said kindly, "but with all them bruises we'd be stopped before the train made it out from Penn Station."

Sheila's aunt and uncle were out of town, and so we cleaned and dressed Billy's wound there. The bullet had come in through the front and gone out the back of Billy's shoulder.

"Lucky that Braughm had steel-jacketed slugs," Billy said. "A soft bullet woulda tore me up."

I went with my friend to Penn Station and waited with him for a train headed to Atlanta. I was worried that there was some kind of internal bleeding, but Billy said that he felt good and strong.

"I never wanted to live up here anyway," he said.

"What do you want me to tell your mom?"

"I'll write her, don't you worry about that. If she calls, tell her I left your place sometime after two and you don't know where I went."

He boarded the 5:11 morning train, and that was the last I ever saw of him.

The police found Nacogdoches Early and followed the bloody trail back to his friends. All they knew was that there was some black kid named Billy who killed Nacogdoches in a gunfight. They got to my brother, but he said that he'd made the deal with some kid named Billy and he never knew where he'd come from.

Thalia told about the beating, but she'd tossed her phone, and the cops were never able to follow the electronic trail.

The three major newspapers loved the romance of a shootout on the Hudson.

In the weeks that followed there were seventeen Western-style gunfights all over the city. Black, white, and brown would-be gunslingers had duels. No one was killed, but the mayor and chief of police ratcheted up the stop-and-frisk program until even rich people started to complain.

Six months later it had all died down. Billy's mother left Harlem, and I graduated a year ahead of time. I was in my fourth year at Harvard, majoring in English literature with an emphasis on Yeats, when I received an unopened letter forwarded to me by my sister, Latrice.

Dear Felix,

Over the past four years I have meant to write to you but I was always on the move and even when I started to write the words didn't add up to much. I am very sorry for what I did when you knew me back then. There was no excuse for what Nacogdoches Early did to Thalia but that didn't give me the right to take his life. Maybe if it had been a fair fight, maybe if I didn't know I could beat him, it would have been all right. But I knew I was the better gunman and so what I did was murder.

I have spent my time since then in the country from Montana to Northern California riding horses and taking work as I find it. I see my mother from time to time. She moved back to Texas because Henry Ryder died and she didn't have to be afraid of him anymore.

You were a good friend, Felix, and I appreciate you sticking by me even though you could have got in trouble too.

Maybe you should burn this letter after you read it. Whatever you do I'll be writing again. Maybe one day we'll even see each other in Times Square or maybe on the Hudson.

Your friend, Billy

I haven't burned Billy's confession—not yet. I keep meaning to.

Over the years I have received eleven letters from the Harlem Cowboy. In the last few he's written some very nice poetry about nature and manhood. His words mean a lot to me. His convictions about right and wrong give me the strength not to see myself as a victim.

I got my PhD from Harvard and now teach American literature at the University of Texas in Houston. In Billy's most recent letter, he said that a girlfriend googled me online and found out that I was there. In that letter he wrote,

. . . Don't be too surprised if I drop by your classroom one day, professor. In a long life you only got a few friends, that's a fact . . .

BREATH

I remember waking up, trying to catch my breath. If someone had asked my name or address, or even what room I was sleeping in, I wouldn't have been able to say. All I had on my mind was that elusive inhalation, that solitary lungful of air that had to be somewhere; it had to be or I was going to die.

The apartment was empty—stripped down to the dust-swirled wood floors. The air conditioner was on, and I wasted precious seconds looking around for my pants. I found the phone, but it was dead. Somebody was crying somewhere nearby, but I couldn't call to them. As I went through the door to the hallway, it came to me that the sobbing was actually the whine of my lungs trying to throw off the congestion.

"Can't bre—," I wheezed.

I must have walked out of my building and across the private road to the unit concierge across the way. I never knew his name, even though he'd been working as a nighttime guard in that complex of university housing longer than I had been a professor at New York College.

He was younger than I by fifteen years at least—not a day over sixty. His eyes were both frightened and suspicious. Maybe I had been shot or stabbed. Maybe the assailant was still lurking somewhere in the dark hours of an early Manhattan morning.

As he helped me into a seat, a flood of thoughts entered my mind, each fighting for the place of my last mortal thought. There was my son, Eric, who had changed his name to Simba, calling on the phone. Simba never called, and even though I could hear him, I still couldn't speak or breathe.

"Dad? Dad, are you there?"

Sarah, my wife, who had passed away in '96, was talking to somebody other than me.

"I know it seems strange," she was saying, in a matter-of-fact tone, "but we've just grown apart."

I tried to speak up, to interrupt, to tell her to shut up and come on back home—to life. But then I was standing on a golden Caribbean beach where a new home was waiting for somebody.

Gravity shifted and I was no longer in my seat. There were voices thundering and lights and darkness. I was blind as well as breathless, thinking about my daughter and wishing that she was with me. My girl, Anetta, would not let her father die. At least, I remember thinking, at least my memory would not be lost as long as she was alive and little Olive, her baby girl, was there in the world beyond the darkness that enveloped me.

"You bettah git away from me, niggah," a man declared in a jagged tone that was steely and thin as a dagger.

The angry words dissipated in the air, and everything was dark and silent again. Breath flowed cold and rich through my nostrils. My head was stuffed with cotton wadding, and there were no independent thoughts rising from my mind.

I drifted.

I was in a coffin, under the ocean, watched over by fishes that did not know or care to know my name or species. They flitted, fornicated, and fled in fear when shadows fell upon them. Water leaked in slowly, excruciatingly so. One drop every thirty seconds or so, that's how I figured it. But what did I know? And what did it matter now that I was dead and interred and forgotten, buffeted by the currents of the deep?

"Hey, brothah. Brothah," a man was saying. He shook my shoulder, disturbing my eternal rest. "Hey, wake up."

I made a noise. It was nowhere near a word, but it seemed to be enough for the grave robber. He was a dark shadow upon a screen of slightly lighter darkness, hovering to my right.

"Somebody in that bed across from you?" he asked.

What bed? What cross?

"Somebody in there?"

"Where?" I managed to say. It hurt my throat, way down past the Adam's apple, to speak.

"I need a bed," the man said. "Is they anyone in it?"

"Mothahfuckah," the bodiless knife of a voice from before warned. It came from somewhere farther off to the right. The shadow moved away.

I tried to raise my head but failed. I tried to imagine myself in the world. That didn't work either. Then I remembered an old trick. I evoked an image of Earth, allowing it to turn slowly. I watched, as I imagined God sometimes did, the passing of terrain, paying no attention to false national borders of fiefdoms. When a place I'd known moved by it would lighten, as if there were a powerful light below the surrounding soil and mountains. Ouagadougou, Cairo, and Accra flashed into my mind. I remembered a sandwich and a

young Senegalese woman, an offer and a refusal, and afterward, for years, regret. There was Paris and London and, faintly, Amsterdam . . . New York.

New York. That's where I was on the globe. The light was strongest there.

The cold, dry oxygen was too much. I started coughing and couldn't stop. It was a rolling, hacking, wet and yet dry retching from my diaphragm all the way to my eyes. I was old Mr. Hawkins, dying in the apartment across the hall in 1946. I was the car alarm that wouldn't stop in the middle of the night. I was Cecil Roberts Bentway, PhD, historian and cultural critic. And I would rather have been dead than go through one more minute of coughing.

Hands took hold of my head and jaw. I struggled against them, but most of my strength had been drained by the involuntary exertions. Something thick and wet was forced into my left nostril and down into my throat and then farther, into my lungs.

There was a vibration, a throbbing sensation, and I knew that someone was using a vacuum to suck the mucous from my flooded lung.

The coughing stopped.

For a while I relaxed on the hardtack sheets, sweating and sighing. I realized that the mattress was thin, that I could feel the whorls of the metal springs under my body. I lifted my rump up, let go, and felt the hint of a rebound—proving my surmise. This made me smile. I could still ply my dubious trade even while being but a hair's breadth away from finality.

"Where'd this one come from?" a woman's voice asked.

"I don't know," a young man said. "That bed's s'posed to be empty."

I raised my head enough to see that they were standing next to the bed across the way from me.

"He got an admittance form?"

"Nuthin'. Not even a clipboard."

"Let's go down to the front desk and ask them."

"Nurse," Steel Voice said.

"What?" the woman replied.

"My sheets is torn."

"OK," she said.

"When you gonna gimme new ones?"

"I'll make a note at the nurses' station."

The young man and the woman that was a nurse talked more. Their voices receded as they left the room and moved down the hallway.

"Bastids," Steel Voice said after they were gone.

The room slowly did a backward fade into daylight. For a long time I lay there on my back allowing names to flow through my mind, or maybe they were going that way without my consent. C. L. R. James and W. E. B. Du Bois, the poet and activist Jayne Cortez, and Amiri Baraka, who, under the name LeRoi Jones, wrote the play *Dutchman*. I considered their works and many others. Over the years I'd been a tough and, hopefully, loving critic. I'd taught young people of all backgrounds and races about people and ways of thinking that the university rarely emphasized. At seventy-five I'd bought a beach condo on a small island where I could finally finish my life's work—*Pagans in Pinstripes*.

My throat, instead of hurting, was numb. I thought about my shoulders and elbows between the esoteric texts, and finally, after quite a while, I managed to rise up on one arm.

The room was larger than I expected. There were four beds with a good deal of space between them; one situated in each corner. The bed to my right, where the steely voice had originated, was being worried over by a thin black man in pale blue pajamas who

had stripped the blankets and sheets and was remaking the bed. For some reason this task seemed Sisyphean. He worked methodically and with great care. There was something institutional about his movements.

Across the way, past my feet, a smallish but not thin black man was coiled under the blanket, staring suspiciously around himself. He clutched his woolen cover as if he were afraid that someone might come and yank it away.

At the diagonally opposite corner from me was yet another dark-colored brother. Sitting in a wooden chair next to the bed, he was also clad in pale blue pajamas. This silent sentry brought to mind a lost soul who had returned to the last place where he'd been alive. His morose expression and posture added to this impression. The man appeared to me like the only mourner at his own funeral, seated in the pews and at the same time lying in the coffin. He too looked to be past sixty.

I tried to think of the odds that four black men near or past retirement age might end up in the same hospital room together in Lower Manhattan. Weren't there any white or yellow, olive-toned or brown-skinned men in their twenties or forties, any young black men who got sick and needed a bed?

"Hey, brothah," called the paranoid man beyond my feet. I knew then he was the shadow who had first awakened me.

I looked at him but could not speak.

"If they ask you, tell 'em that I was brought in on a stretcher last night. Tell 'em that I was brought in on a stretcher."

I glanced over at the man making and remaking his bed. He paid no attention to what our undocumented roommate was saying. I let my head fall back on the small pillow and felt the little bounces of jubilant springs. It was as if I were lying upon a huge lily

pad; a bloated frog waiting for a passing fly. I closed my eyes and tried to remember getting to that place—seventy-five and hospitalized in a room occupied only by old black men. Had I really been a professor at a prestigious university? Had I once been present at Nelson Mandela's eighty-second birthday celebration?

"You OK, man?" someone asked.

I opened my eyes and saw the rail-thin bed-maker. I would have bet that the frown on his face was the closest he ever came to expressing compassion.

"They don't give a fuck about a niggah 'round here, man," he said. "Most the time they late bringin' you your food. An' forget the bedclothes. It don't even look like they wash 'em more times than not."

I wanted to say something, I wanted to echo the roommate's knowledge, but didn't have the strength.

"That's all right, brothah," he said. "Get you some rest. If you need me to get you sumpin', just say it or just raise your hand. You know I always got one eye open."

It felt as if I had only blinked, but the man was gone. I knew then that I had to get out of there. I had to get away before I was swallowed up by that alien room with its condemned souls, devil nurses, and infiltrators.

I tried to remember what I had been wearing before the asthma attack. Most nights I fell asleep wearing a golden, scarlet, and royal blue Ghanaian robe. The first time I'd get up to urinate I'd take it off. Did my attack come before my first trip to the toilet?

"Mr. Holder," someone said. She was addressing the bed-maker.

There was low light suspended in the air like an illuminated fog.

"What?"

"Have you used needles in the past five years?" the woman asked. There was a lilt to her voice. Nigerian.

"I ain't nevah used no needles."

"It says in your file that you were in prison for drugs," she countered.

"Yes, I was. Heroin. But I ain't nevah used no needles. The people I sold to used 'em, but I was always a Johnnie Walker Blue Label man."

I dozed while the doctor and her assistants wheeled some heavy equipment to the side of the bed-maker, Mr. Holder.

I woke up again when a man all in white rolled an IV unit up next to me and lifted my right arm. As he looked for a vein I tried to pull away. But I was so weak that he didn't seem to notice. I thought he should at least tell me what he was doing; that he should ask if I wanted the procedure or whether I was allergic to the yellowy fluid in the IV bag.

Seconds after the needle was pressed into the vein, my body passed out. I say it this way because I was in darkness and without physical sensation, but my consciousness seemed to rise above the bed and the body it held. I could hear everything. It wasn't like normal hearing either. My ears were hypersensitive, like those of an ancient proto-dog at the edge of the Gobi Desert listening for sounds of beloved but feared humanity.

"She, she kicked me out," the sad man who sat beside his bed whined. "Twenty-eight years, and she just kicked me out like a, like a stray dog. And I ain't got nuthin'."

" . . . brought me in last night," the man in the bed across from me was saying to somebody. "Last thing I remembah I was walkin' down One Thirty-Seven and I got dizzy. I grabbed for this lady to keep upright, but she hollered and pushed me away. When I woke up I was in this here bed . . . No. I ain't got no one to call."

"The X-ray reveals a dark spot, Mr. Holder," the Nigerian doctor was saying. "It might be malignant."

"Dark spot where?" the fastidious bed-maker jabbed, in his hopelessly harsh tone.

"The left side of your chest. Over your lung."

"That ain't no tumor. That's where I got shot one time."

"So you think that it's a bullet?"

"Yes, ma'am."

"Why didn't the doctor take it out?"

"What doctor? You think I'm gonna go to some doctor when all they gonna do is call the cops? Shit."

"When I went back to beg her she was gone," the sad man next to his bed said, and then he let out a low moan that didn't sound human. "Carol next door told me that she had gone back down to North Carolina to her people. She had everything a' mines. My Social Security card. My birth certificate. Only shoes I had left was on my feet . . . Yeah, my blood pressure's high. Wouldn't yours be?"

"Sugar diabetes, asthma, arthritis, glaucoma, thyroid condition, herpes, shingles, allergies to milk and shellfish . . . " The man across from me listed what seemed like every disease and condition in the doctor's medical handbook. "No, I haven't been takin' my medicine. I ain't got the money. So sick that I couldn't work. No work, no rent. No home, and sooner or later you get dizzy and fall down in the street."

"Ow!" Mr. Holder, to my right, shouted. "What you doin'?"

"Cutting out the bullet. It's embedded in fairly shallow scar tissue."

"Ain't you gonna knock me out or nuttin'? Shit!"

"That would be more dangerous than the procedure, and a local anesthetic is contraindicated due to the bullet being so close to the heart."

Mr. Holder moaned, and I could imagine the scalpel slicing into his chest while the male nurses held him down.

The IV forced on me was a powerful narcotic. I heard everything, it seemed. I can't remember now if they were all speaking at once or if these conversations and other sounds happened over time. In my memory they all flow together. There was a singular endpoint though.

"There it is," the Nigerian doctor said, and I heard the *plink* of metal on metal; the corroded bullet, I imagined, hitting a shiny chromium tray. This hard, metallic sound ended my free-floating awareness. I settled back down into the darkness that I feared and craved more than anything.

"Do you have a medical-insurance card, Mr. Bentway?" Dr. Ifadapo asked, her sculpted sub-Saharan features glistening black.

It was the afternoon of that same day, though it felt as if weeks had passed.

"It's Professor Bentway," I said, "and I already told your nurse that I'm insured by New York College."

"We need the card."

"Call the school."

"They tell us that Professor Bentway has retired."

"What do you want from me, then?"

"Is there someone we can call?"

"I don't have my book with me. I got my one friend, but his phone is off. All I got to do is go home, and I could get the card for you. My apartment is only mine for a few more days. I'm supposed to leave for Saint Lucia. I got my tickets in the apartment too."

"We can't release you, Mr. . . . Professor Bentway. You can't go on your own, and there's no one to take you."

"Just get me down to a cab."

"The law won't allow us do that, sir." Her beautiful smile was maddening.

"You can't keep me here."

"We believe that you had a heart attack along with the emphysema episode. We will treat that, and then, if there is no other option, we'll be forced to release you to a state-run nursing facility."

"A nursing home?"

Smiling, the doctor got up and moved away to the charlatan across from me. The ex-con, Holder, was stripping his bed for the fourth time that day, and Bret Lagnan, the man who had been abandoned by his wife, sat there next to his bed suffering the ailment of a broken heart.

All my phone numbers were keyed into the cell phone that was on the dusty floor in university housing. It was midsummer, so no one was around anyway. And I was weak from the emphysema attack that, I was told by Dr. Ifadapo, was brought on by the air-conditioning, which circulated the dust kicked up by the movers. I could barely sit upright.

At times I was aware of the charlatan, Todd Brightwood, hovering around my bed looking for jewelry or pocket change. Holder told him to get away whenever he drifted to our side of the room. Lovesick Lagnan didn't seem to know that anyone else was there.

The TV was on all during the day. I watched shows that I'd never heard of before, game shows and sporting events, the shopping channel and daytime soap operas. I didn't have much concentration. I didn't know how long I had been in that bed or how long it would be before they committed me to the nursing home.

When I tried to get up, the male nurses would push me back down. Anetta might not call for weeks, and I did not call her number often enough to remember it. Simba had moved to Tanzania and refused to talk to me for reasons that he kept to himself.

Days had passed. The beautiful Nigerian doctor dropped by in the afternoons. She was friendly but would not let me go.

Todd Brightwood had been signed in as a patient suffering from various ailments that led to his attack of illness. Gil Holder kept making and remaking his bed, complaining about the hospital staff. Bret Lagnan suffered in silence the abandonment by his wife (whose name I never got.) I marked the time, slowly garnering my strength for the moment when I could escape that wing of Saint Jude's Hospital set aside for the poor, hopeless, and black.

None of the men in my room had visitors, but I met a man across the hall who agreed to have his son bring me some pants and a T-shirt. The son wasn't coming back until Friday though, and Dr. Ifadapo hadn't yet decided which day to have me committed to the nursing home. The attack had exacerbated my emphysema, and so I couldn't walk very far without resting. It was going to be a strenuous escape, if I could even make it.

On Tuesday the doctor told me that I'd be leaving on Thursday. I argued with her, but she just smiled and nodded. I called the college human-resources office, but they told me that all medical insurance for retired employees was handled in Albany and that I had to send them a letter if I'd lost my insurance card.

"I haven't lost my damn card."

"Then show it to the people at the hospital."

It seemed impossible that I could have lost control of my life so easily. From full professor with tenure to a homeless ward of the state. I was on the eighth floor of a building that took up two city blocks. I figured that it was nearly a quarter of a mile between me and freedom. But I had to try—blue pajamas and all. I'd carry a weapon with me. And if anyone tried to stop me, I'd throw down on them.

The only weapon I could find was a serrated plastic knife, but that would have to do.

At two o'clock on that Wednesday I closed my eyes to rest fifteen minutes more, and then I was going to run, regardless of what they did to me.

"Cecil," came a voice with a francophone, West African inflection to it.

"Adegoke?" I said, without opening my eyes.

"I finally found you," he said.

I mustered enough courage to open one eye, and there he was. Blacker than my doctor and tall and handsome in that gaunt way only Ghanaian men can manage: Adegoke Arapmoi, professor of film and culture, stood there beside my bed. Behind him was Jack Fine, a light brown and beefy teacher of archaeology who hailed from Baltimore.

"Why didn't you call me?" Adegoke asked.

"I did. Your phone went straight to voice mail."

"What happened?"

"Get me outta here, man. They wanna put me in a nursing home."

Adegoke wore a lavender jacket, black trousers, and a bright, bright yellow shirt. All this topped off with a Panama hat. His white teeth glistened against black skin.

"I was in Ghana," he said, "at the ten-year anniversary of the death of my father. When I got back you weren't home. I had to wait until the night guard was on duty. He told me about your attack, but he didn't know where the ambulance had taken you. Jack and I have been going from hospital to hospital."

"Hey, Cecil," Jack said. He was grinning, and so was I. "You look like shit."

"You brought me new sheets, but they got stains on 'em," Gil Holder was telling his nurse.

"Excuse me, ma'am," Jack Fine, who was at least six five, said to the woman.

"Yes?"

"Tell the doctor, and whoever, that we're takin' Professor Bentway home."

"He has to be released by a doctor," the young, pink-skinned woman explained.

"That's OK," Jack said. "Just as long as that release coincides with our egress from your institution."

Jack was thirty-three years old and not that far away from his student days. He still slung big words around as if they made him sound smart. I usually felt embarrassed by the way he spoke, but that day I was filled with glee.

Gil Holder was actually smiling at my big friend.

"I brought you some of my son's clothes, Cecil," Adegoke said as the nurse fled the room.

He placed a large brown-paper bag on my bed.

Many years before, Addy had been my student at San Francisco State. He and my son, Eric/Simba, were the same age, forty-eight, but it was Adegoke who searched all the emergency rooms in Manhattan until he'd found me.

With my friends' help, I got up and dressed. Jack even tied my shoes.

"What's going on here?" Dr. Ifadapo asked as she came into the room flanked by two black men in security-guard uniforms.

Jack moved toward the little group. Addy got in front of him.

"I am Dr. Arapmoi from New York College," he said. "Dr. Bentway is one of our professors. We have come to bring him home."

"I have already signed the papers to release him to Morningside Nursing Home. You can apply for his release there."

"He's coming with me to my home now," Addy said with certainty.

"The forms are filled out."

Jack Fine snorted. The guards took notice of him. Gil Holder picked up some kind of bludgeon from under his pillow. Brightwood pulled the blanket up to his chin, and lovelorn Lagnan didn't notice a thing.

The beautiful Nigerian stared into the handsome Ghanaian's eyes for half a minute at least.

"Are you his guardian?" Ifadapo asked.

"I'm his nephew," Addy lied. "And he's coming home with me."

For the next two hours they filled out forms and made recommendations. We walked down three long halls, took an elevator, and went to the checkout desk to retrieve whatever it was that I had in my pockets when I was brought in.

"This is a blue form," the big bald brown man said from behind his marble desk. "You need a yellow form to get what we have. A blue form will get your clothes from the emergency room closet."

Back to the elevator, down the halls, we returned to the nurses' desk near my room.

"Oh," the pink-skinned nurse (whose name tag read "Laura") said. "I'm sorry. I should have given you the yellow form. Give me that one, and I'll fill out another."

"But he needs the blue paper to get his clothes," big Jack Fine bellowed.

"Oh, right," the nurse said. "You know we're very understaffed. I'm lucky if I remember to make my rounds."

* * *

The man wanting the yellow form had my wallet, in which I found my medical-insurance card.

"You go through that door on your left," he said, now quite friendly, "and down the hall until you get to the emergency room. You pass through there and come to a desk behind a Plexiglas barrier. The woman there will help you find your clothes."

There were dozens of people sitting in the disheveled maze of blue vinyl-and-chrome chairs that furnished the emergency-room waiting area. A sleeping, or maybe unconscious, child in his mother's arms, a man with blood seeping from his face and both arms, an old man (my age) staring out a window with his lower eyelids drooping away from the orbs—open and red. One man sat silently crying, his hand swollen to the size of a football. A young woman with haunted eyes had such severe flatulence that no one could sit near her. You could see the pain from her belly in the twist of her mouth and the humiliation of her eyes.

"Where's the doctor?" an old woman in a wheelchair asked me.

"I don't know."

"This is terrible," Jack Fine said to Addy.

"At least they have a place to go," the Ghanian said.

Behind the Plexiglas window on the other side of suffering sat an ocher-skinned, almond-eyed woman. I thought she might be Cambodian or Vietnamese.

"Put the form in the slot in front of you," she said without looking up.

I placed the blue form where she asked, and she picked it up. When she noticed what it was, she frowned, then sighed.

"We're very busy," she complained.

"It's my clothes," I replied, realizing that my breath was coming short again.

"You came in DP-twenty-seven," the woman replied.

"What's that supposed to mean?" Jack asked.

The hospital sentry hesitated. She said, "DP. Deceased Person. The first doctor who saw you declared you dead."

Ana, the young nurse/receptionist, led us to a door behind her kiosk. It was small and green and opened into a dark room. A light came on automatically when we entered. We realized with awe that we had entered a vast chamber lined with deep bins that were filled with hundreds of bundles of clothes bound in brown paper and secured with tan masking tape.

I could hear the breath singing in my windpipe.

"You OK, Cecil?" Addy asked.

I didn't answer. While Ana searched through certain piles of bundles I looked around. Most of the brown-paper packages had the name and date of death scrawled on the tape. One read: REYNARD, MILTON 10/11/07; DECEASED. Some of the slips had fallen from their bundles. There was Julia Slatkin, Harris Montoya, and Po Li. The dust and lint gathered in my throat and lungs, and I felt the beginnings of another respiratory attack. I should have run out of there, but running for me was a thing of the past.

That one room led to another, where there were no bins and even more bundles of clothes, piled all the way to the eighteen-foot ceiling. I thought about the concentration-camp films that came out when I was a young man just out of the air force, right after the war. The Nazis took everything that their victims owned: hair and teeth, shoes and clothes. I felt that I was in the presence of some great crime that I would never be able to prove.

"Here it is, Cecil," Addy said. "Here's that robe I brought you from Accra."

In the taxi I opened the window and let my head loll out, the wind forcing its way into my lungs. All I had to do was open my mouth.

Adegoke's wife is spending the summer with her family in Nice. His daughter has gone to Singapore, and his son is on a film shoot in southern Mexico. My old student gave me a room with a window on the twenty-seventh floor of university housing. Here I've been sitting for the past three weeks waiting for breath to return, so that I might escape to a Caribbean island; there I hope to forget what I learned among the bundles of death.

REPLY TO A DEAD MAN

When the doorbell rang, I had no inkling of who was there or what his or her business might have been. I was sitting at the dining table in a room that had never been used for entertaining. Books and notepads, two weeks' worth of newspapers, and a few stacks of dirty dishes were piled here and there around the dark-stained hickory plank. I had been perched there writing a letter to my sister about the death of our brother in the fall.

It was now spring, and this was the first time I'd reached out to Angeline. I had missed the funeral. Our brother had been buried in Cincinnati by Dearby, his fourth wife. She, Dearby, told me that if she was going to pay for the burial, then he'd be interred in the same cemetery as her and the rest of her family.

I was having a hard time, financially, when Seth passed. I'd just lost my job as a regional manager for Lampley Car Insurance, and my unemployment checks hadn't been enough to pay the rent. I couldn't take time off from my temp position at Lenny's

Auto Parts, and the funeral was on a Wednesday, a workday. My boss, Alan René Bertrand, didn't particularly like me, and so I couldn't even take the chance of asking him for the time off. Lenny's paid $22.50 an hour, the best temp rate in town, and so I sent a dozen white lilies and a note thanking Dearby for honoring my brother.

You see, I knew that Dearby and Seth were on the outs when he died. My sister told me that Seth had been seeing his second ex-wife, Althea, again, and Dearby was threatening to kick him out of the house.

She, Dearby, called to tell me about Seth.

"He had a heart attack," she said. "I warned him about the high blood pressure and his weight. He wouldn't listen. He never listened."

I was thinking that Dearby was pretty big herself.

As if she could read my thoughts across the two thousand–plus miles that separated us, she said, "I know that I'm big, but my heft is fruit fat, weight from fresh fruit with fiber and natural sugars. My doctors tell me that I'm OK the way I am."

"I know you are," I said, to fill the empty space in our conversation, an emptiness that loomed like the blank line at the bottom of a boilerplate contract.

"What do you want me to do with him?" she asked.

"Um . . ."

"The body, Roger. What do you want me to do with the body?"

"I don't understand what you mean," I said. "He's dead."

"I know that," Dearby said. "He's gone, and somebody has to bury him."

"Oh . . . Oh, yeah. Right. Um . . ."

* * *

I got up from the table, remembering that awkward moment, half a year ago, when I had to tell Dearby that I didn't have the money to help pay for a funeral.

The walk from my worktable to the front door wasn't long. No distance in my 634-square-foot half-home in the Wilshire district was that great. The other side of the subdivided house was inhabited by a woman named Rose Henley. I had seen Rose only once, a few days after I'd moved in seven years and ten months earlier. She'd rung my bell and introduced herself as my neighbor.

Rose Henley was old, maybe sixty, and she had one gold tooth. She was fairly short, even for a woman, and her black hair was sliding into white. She was a white woman, broad-faced and stout.

"Mr. Vaness?" she had said, all those years ago.

"Yes?"

"I'm Rose Henley, your neighbor."

"Oh. Hello."

"I don't mean to interrupt, just wanted you to see my face. And I wanted to see yours."

"Would you like to come in?" I asked, not putting much heart into it.

"No, no, no," she said. "I just wanted to greet you. I don't get out very much."

This was no exaggeration. I had not seen nor had I heard from my neighbor since.

But that day, when I was writing to my sister, Angeline, about our brother Seth's death, I was sure that Rose was at my door. I didn't get much company since losing my job. The friends I had liked to party, and I couldn't afford the gas money, much less my part of the bill at our favorite bars and restaurants.

After I was fired, I had asked my girlfriend, Terri, if she would move in so we could share the rent.

Terri broke it off with me three days later.

No one ever knocked at my door, and Rose was the only person I was acquainted with in the neighborhood. It had to be her, I thought; that was just cold, hard logic.

So I opened the door looking down, expecting to see my diminutive neighbor's wide face under a thatch of black hair turning white.

Instead I was looking at the red and blue vest of a white man even taller than I. He had a bald head and not much facial hair. His skin was the color of yellowing ivory, and his eyes were a luminous gray—like a mist-filled valley at dawn.

"Mr. Vaness?" the stranger asked, in a magnificent tenor voice.

"Yes?"

"My name is Harding, Lance Harding. I am here representing the last wish of Seth Vaness."

"What?"

"I work for a small firm called Final Request Co. We execute the last wishes of clients who have passed on."

"You're a lawyer?"

I looked the slender tenor up and down. He had on a nice suit, but it was reddish brown, not a lawyer's color in my estimation.

"No, Mr. Vaness. We at FRC don't execute wills. Our job is to deliver messages from the dead." He smiled after the last word, giving me a slight chill.

"Uh-huh. You use a Ouija board or somethin'?"

"We are engaged by the deceased before their demise."

"My brother hired you to give me a message after he was dead?"

Harding smiled and nodded.

"He died six and a half months ago," I said. "What took you so long?"

"His wish was for us to execute his desire not less than half a year after his demise."

"Is this some kinda legal thing?"

"It is a simple agreement between FRC and your brother," Lance Harding said, maintaining an aura of imperturbable patience. "Often individuals wish to pass on knowledge outside of the rubric of wills and other legal formats. Some leave a spoken message, others might wish to pass along a note or a small package."

"Seth didn't have much," I said. "He couldn't have anything to hide."

"We all have something to hide, Mr. Vaness. Either that or something is hidden from us."

"So you're—"

"May I come in?" Harding asked, cutting off my question.

"Oh," I said.

"Is this a bad time?"

"No, no it's OK, I just . . ."

"I came by on Wednesday, but you weren't here," Harding said. "Your neighbor, Mrs. Henley, told me that you were at work."

"You talked to Rose?"

"May I come in?"

My house was untidy, to say the least. When I have a girlfriend, I usually pick up and air out my little place at least once a week, but I lose the drive when I'm unattached. As a rule, the mess doesn't bother me unless I have unexpected guests.

Harding didn't seem put off by the clutter. I moved a small stack of old comic books from a chair next to the one I had been sitting in and gestured for him to take it.

"The Fantastic Four," he said, looking at the topmost magazine as I set the stack on the table next to him.

"They were my father's," I said. "I have one through twelve. Know anybody who might want to buy them?"

"Your blood father?" he asked. "Patrick Hand?"

I nodded, wondering how he knew my real father's name.

He flipped through the issues, smiling slightly. Harding was maybe ten years older than I. That would have made him about fifty.

"Not in mint or near-mint condition," he said. "That makes them nearly worthless. At any rate, these books call up your father from across the pale. That's a connection that money can't buy."

"How do you know my father's dead?"

"Both of your fathers," he said. "Patrick, who sired you, and Norland, who married your mother and adopted her three children."

"How do you know all that?"

"They were Seth's fathers too."

"Oh . . . yeah. That's why you're here."

"Shall we begin?"

"It's funny that you came here just now," I said. "I mean, not funny, but . . . I was just writing to my sister—"

"Angeline Vaness-Brownley," Lance Harding of the FRC interjected. "She lives in Cambridge with her husband, Ivan Brownley, the union organizer."

"Wha'? Oh, right, Seth's sister too. How much do you know about us?"

"About you, particularly, we know that you have never been charged with, much less convicted of, a crime and that most of your adult life you were either employed or at college. You have three years matriculation at Cal State. Your concentration was in

history, but you dropped out and began to work for various businesses. You've never been married, but you were once engaged to a woman named Irene Littleton."

"Seth told you all that?"

"No."

"Then where'd you get it?"

Harding's face was oblong and a little larger than even his tall frame might predict. For the most part his expression was tranquil, but my question teased out a mild frown.

"I am here at your brother's request," he said.

"But you know all this shit about me, and he didn't tell you. So I'd like to know where you got it."

"Nora Dunbar," he replied, his face once again at peace.

"Who?"

"She is the statistical and research analyst at our firm. When a client engages our services, Miss Dunbar does a background check on the client and the recipient of the message or package."

"Why?"

Harding sighed and then said, "Suppose the message that someone wished to pass on was a name and an address. If the recipient was a known killer, or maybe someone who had a grudge against a person with the name we were being asked to deliver, we would refuse the job. We are not bound by fealty to the state, but we are a moral corporation."

"So you wanted to make sure that I wasn't a hit man or a stalker or somethin'?"

"Quite right."

"But you figured that I was a good bet and that you could deliver your message without messin' anything up."

The great sculpted face smiled and bobbed.

"You got a sliding scale you charge?" I asked. I realized that I wasn't eager to obtain information passed on to me across the border of death.

"We charge five thousand dollars, plus expenses, for every message a client wishes to charge us with."

"Expenses?"

Lance Harding smiled and seemed to relax a bit. He gave the impression of having surrendered to my fear of his charge.

"Once we were engaged by a woman to deliver an apple pie she'd baked to the man she loved but never married," he said. "In order to keep the pie in fair condition we had to freeze it. The accommodations were made, and she was charged accordingly."

"So, Seth paid five thousand dollars for you to deliver this message to me?"

"That is the fee all clients are charged," he said, "plus expenses."

"That doesn't make any sense."

"Why do you say that?"

"Three reasons. First, I can't see Seth payin' that kinda money, when he coulda sent a letter to my sister or our mother to give me after he died. Secondly, I can't see Seth spendin' that kinda money on me—period. And third, traveling all over the country and the world makin' these kinda visits would cost a lot more than five thousand dollars."

I would have talked all day long to keep this man, the most official man I had ever met, from discharging his message.

"As to your first two arguments—we question our clients, but never their money, once they've passed our qualification test. Your third dispute would make sense if the FRC didn't have regions of responsibility divided among its various agents. My area is California. You asked why I'm late delivering this message. That is because I was in central and northern California for the last two weeks. We

would like to have delivered this communication exactly at the six-month mark, but the wording of your brother's last request allowed me some leeway: 'not less than six months after my demise.'"

I had nothing left to ask, but still I was not ready for any information from the dead.

"Are all the people who work for the FCR white?" The question was one my stepfather would have had me ask.

"FRC," Lance corrected. "Most of the employees of the company are Caucasian but not all. Now, may I deliver my charge?"

I took in a deep breath, exhaled, and then nodded.

Lance Harding reached into the left side of his red-brown jacket with his right hand.

I leaped up from my chair, sure that he was going to take out a gun or a knife—my fear was that great.

But the FRC agent merely brought out an ivory envelope, almost exactly the same color as his skin.

"This is the letter that your brother charged us to deliver," he said. "As I hand it to you, our duty in this matter is fulfilled."

He extended the hand, offering me the rectangle of paper. I hesitated before taking it.

The mood was so ceremonial that I expected some kind of devastation or revelation to follow. But nothing happened.

The FRC agent stood abruptly.

"I will leave you to do with the letter as you will," he said.

"Don't you want me to sign something?" I asked. "To prove that you actually gave me this?"

"The client didn't ask for corroboration," he said, smiling. "That usually means that the delivery contains nothing of material value. I can see myself out."

* * *

I sat there at the messy table, holding the still-sealed envelope, for long minutes after Lance Harding was gone. Something about the white man's demeanor—coupled with the fact that I had been writing a letter concerning Seth when the strange note from him arrived—was, to say the least, eerie. Something having to do with me not attending his funeral, I thought, and now he was reaching out to me . . .

I put the letter down and picked up my smartphone. I entered A-N-G, and Angeline's number appeared.

She answered on the fourth ring.

"Where are you?" she said, instead of hello.

"At home."

"But you're on your cell."

"I had the landline disconnected, figured I didn't need two numbers. People hardly ever call one."

"You're not a kid anymore, Roger. Having your phone disconnected makes you seem transient."

"How's Boston, Sis?"

"Cold. They're predicting snow for tomorrow."

"Snow? It's not even Thanksgiving yet."

"How are you, Rog?"

"All right. Have you heard from Seth?"

"What?"

"A letter, package, or somethin'?"

"Seth is dead."

"I know," I said. "I know, but a guy just dropped by and hand-delivered a letter to me that Seth had set up before he died."

Angeline didn't say a word for at least a minute. This told me more than any confession or lie: whatever it was that Seth was telling me, Angeline knew before I did.

"Did you read it?" she asked at last.

"No. Not yet. I was wondering if he'd sent the same note to you and Mom."

"You should burn it, Roger," she said. "Nothing good can come from a dead man's hand."

"The guy brought it to me was very much alive."

"Burn it, shred it, or just throw it away, Roger," she said, in her best big-sister voice. "You know how Seth was always trying to mess with you."

"What does it say, Angeline?"

"How do you expect me to know?"

"Don't *you* mess with me, Sis."

"I haven't heard anything from Seth, and neither has Mom, for all I know. I talked to her last Monday, and she didn't say anything about any letters."

"How is Mom?"

"Fine. She said that she hasn't heard from you in over six months. You know you could go to her house. She's just a few miles from your place. It's a shame I see her more often than you do, and here I live three thousand miles away."

All the anger that I had at my mother and sister and deceased stepfather, Norland Reese, came up in my breast.

"I gotta go, Angeline," I said.

"Wait, Roger. What about that letter . . . ?"

I pressed the red icon on my smartphone, and the connection was broken. Putting the little device down, I picked up the sealed envelope again.

Seth had terrorized me when we were children. He would lock me in closets and trunks just for a laugh. I learned the value of silence from him. Because if he put me in the big trunk in the attic of our house, I learned that he would never let me out as long as I yelled. But if I was quiet, he worried that maybe I had suffocated

or something. He was the kind of torturer who fed off the screams of his victims.

I might have hated my brother, but his brand of torment wasn't nearly as bad as that of my parents—I should say my mother and her husband Norland. My blood father was a white man named Patrick Hand. The story goes that he abandoned our family when I was two, Angeline was four, and Seth five.

"He just ran off and left me with three children and a dollar seventy-five," my mother would say. Then she'd spit on the ground, cursing him.

Seth never believed that our father abandoned us. Patrick Hand was a known gambler, and Seth was convinced that he had been slaughtered over a bad debt, and that our mother, instead of cursing him, should have gone out looking for his killers.

Norland wouldn't let Seth tell that tale. He was of my mother's opinion and ruled over us with an iron fist.

In my mind I managed to believe both Seth and my mother. Sometimes I hated my father; at others I prayed for his murdered soul.

Dear Roger,

I know that we haven't talked in a long time. We might not ever talk again if what the doctors say about my heart is true. They're telling me that I better settle up my business because I could die any minute. That's why I'm writing you this letter. It hurts to admit the truth and so I'm using the Final Request Company to deliver it after I die. I'm not proud of what I did but at least this much is right.

I guess you remember back when you were seventeen and going with that white girl—Timberly Alexander. You broke up with her because Mama and Norland leaned on you so hard. I was mad that you didn't

even tell Timmy why you stopped talking to her and so one day I went over to her house out there in West Covina. I told her how much Mama and Norland thought that interracial relationships only ended in heartbreak. I tried to explain how much you needed Mama and that her rules were too much for you to deny.

That's when Timberly told me that she was pregnant. She was so broken up because her parents were mad and you wouldn't even talk to her on the phone.

She was so upset that I told her she could always talk to me. And she did.

For the last twenty years I've been giving Timmy a couple hundred dollars a month, and her little girl, Sovie (named after Sojourner Truth), has called me Uncle Seth from the day she could talk.

Timmy didn't want me to tell you about your daughter because she was mad and hurt that you left her without a word. I probably should have told you but I guess I got a little possessive. I kind of thought of Timmy and Sovie as my little family.

At the bottom of the page is Sovie's full name and address in Los Angeles. Yes, she lives in L.A. just like you.

Timmy died a year ago from breast cancer and so, when I'm gone, Sovie's going to be alone in the world.

I'm sorry for keeping this from you, Little Brother. I know it's worse than anything else I ever did. I hope you can forgive me.

Seth

My heart started beating rapidly a minute or two after the third time I'd read the letter. I could have sat there and guessed for a hundred years and never come up with what Seth had to say. I had a child in the world and hadn't known it. I was a father with none of the responsibilities, fears, or joys of parenthood.

I went out to the liquor store and bought two quarts of Jack Daniels and three packs of filterless Camels.

* * *

For a day and a half all I did was drink and smoke. I had given up both habits when I was twenty-three years old. I realized one day that I was trying to kill myself with the legal drugs of my culture.

And every day for seventeen years I had wanted to end my smokeless sobriety.

I crashed around the house, cursing my brother, mother, and sister—all of whom seemed to have known but never told me the truth. At one point, near the end of my private orgy, I raised a hickory chair up above my head and smashed it on the hardwood floor. Then, melodramatically, I crumpled to my knees and cried over the broken furniture.

Maybe five minutes after my outburst, a rapping came at the door. A few seconds later I heard another, bolder knock.

I climbed to my feet, suppressed a gag reflex, and stumbled to the door.

Standing there on our common porch was Rose Henley; she was as short as ever, but her hair had not yet turned completely white.

"Are you all right, Mr. Vaness?"

"No, ma'am, I am not."

"What's wrong?"

"Nothing I can point at but everything else."

"I don't understand. I heard a crash and I wanted to make sure you weren't hurt."

"You're a brave woman," I said, barely aware of the words I mouthed. "Somebody could have been killing me over here."

"Does it have to do with that man who came here a few days ago? The tall one in the nice suit?"

"Yes. But he was only the bearer of the bad news. The messenger."

"Why don't you come over to my house and have a cup of coffee?" she suggested. "Sober up a little bit."

Rose Henley's home was everything that my apartment was not. The floor was carpeted, and not a hair was out of place. A painting on the living room wall was of a reclining nude woman who looked somewhat like a younger version of my neighbor.

She had me sit on a tan sofa and served me a weak cup of percolated coffee.

"Now," she said, when we were both settled. "What's the problem?"

Her face was broad, but her black eyes were set close together. The concern in that face was something I didn't remember ever having been shown me before.

I told her everything, all about how Seth tortured me and how my sister probably knew about the child I'd fathered, about my mother and father and stepfather, and about my failure to surpass the image that everyone seemed to hold of me.

"I don't even know why I dropped out of college," I said at one point. "I don't know when I gave up on myself."

"You haven't been to work this week, have you?" she asked.

"I'm sure they fired me. The temp agency called, but I didn't answer."

"You need to take a cold shower, get a good night's sleep, and then go to see your daughter," Rose said.

"I have to get a job first," I replied. "You know Mr. Poplar wants his rent."

"Poplar works for the landlord," she said. "I don't think the owner would kick you out under these circumstances."

"Oh? Why not?"

"Because I own this house, Mr. Vaness. And I like you."

The address for Sojourner "Sovie" Alexander was on Cushdon, just south of a Pico Boulevard. It was the smallest house on the block and in need of a paint job. But the lawn was green and manicured, and there were healthy rose bushes under the front windows of the home.

The door was open, and the screen closed. I saw a doorbell but knocked anyway. After a few moments, a tallish, honey-colored girl in her early twenties appeared.

"Miss Alexander?" I said. I'd practiced calling her "Miss."

"No," she replied, pursing her lips, as if she were going to whistle or maybe kiss someone. "Who are you?"

"I'm here to see Miss Alexander," I said. "Is she home?"

Staring quizzically at me, the honey-colored young woman shouted, "Sovie! It's for you!"

The young woman went away, and before I could count to ten, a young white girl, more or less the same age as her roommate, walked up. She had light blond hair and looked at me with a furrowed brow. All at once she realized something and took in a sharp breath.

"Roger Vaness?" she said.

"Um, yes."

"You look a lot like Uncle Seth. Three days ago I got a letter from him," she said. "This tall bald guy brought it. The man told me that Uncle Seth had died. He gave me the letter that said, Uncle Seth said, in the letter, that my real father was . . . was you."

"I got a letter from Seth too. I never knew. Nobody . . . not your mother or Seth or anybody ever told me that I had a little girl."

We stared at each other through the gray haze of the screen, both of us unsure of what to do.

"Can I take you out for coffee?" I asked.

"I'll get my sweater."

We commandeered a small round table at the window of a coffeehouse on Westwood near Pico. There we talked for hours.

Timmy had told her daughter that she didn't know who her father was, that she had been wild as a child but had sobered up when Sovie came. Seth was an old friend who dropped by regularly. Sovie had often wished that Seth was her father or at least her real uncle.

"I guess he was my uncle," she said at one point, realizing for the first time the blood relation.

"But Timmy never told you that I, I mean that your blood father was black?" I asked.

"Never."

"Does that bother you?"

"It bothers me that she lied about you."

"I mean, it doesn't bother you that you're black?"

"Oh," she said, looking very much like me and not. "I didn't even think about that. Wow."

"I don't know what to say to you, Sojourner. I'm sittin' here with a stranger, but I feel so much love that has been lost."

"Me too. When I read Seth's letter I, I felt like . . . I don't know . . . I felt like an old-time explorer on the verge of discovering a new continent."

"Did he give you my address?"

"Yes," she said meekly. "I drove by, but I couldn't make myself stop. I was just so nervous."

"That's OK. It's better that I came to you. A father should be there for his daughter."

I could see in Sojourner's eyes that she had been waiting an entire lifetime to call a man *Father.* I put my big brown hand on her clenched white fists. She relaxed, and I thought that this was how I would have wanted it to be with my own father.

I called Absolute Temps and talked to the receptionist, Tanya Reed. I explained to Tanya exactly what had happened, and she hooked me up with a six-week gig at Leonine Records on Sunset. It was only $16.75 an hour, but that covered the rent and gas.

For the next month Sovie and I saw or talked to each other every day.

She's a history major, like I was, and has a boyfriend, Chad, whom I met and liked very much. I gave her my blood father's stack of Fantastic Four comics, saying that it was the only thing of value I owned. She didn't like comic books but took them anyway. I don't know why, but giving her those magazines felt like taking a two-ton weight off my skull.

A month later, on a Saturday, I was cleaning my apartment to prepare for her and her roommate, Ashanti Bowles, to come over for dinner the next day.

When the knock came, I didn't think before opening the door.

Lance Harding was wearing a pink suit with a red shirt and no tie. I wondered then if agents of the FRC had a dress code.

"Mr. Vaness," he said.

"I'm so glad to see you," I said, opening the door wide and ushering him in to my clean house. "Come in, come in."

Sitting in the same chairs as before, we faced each other. Harding crossed his left leg over the right one and nodded.

"I wanted to call you, but I couldn't find a number for the FRC in the Yellow Pages," I said. "I planned to get on somebody's computer and look it up soon."

"Why were you looking for us?"

"You," I said. "I wanted to ask you something that I didn't think of the last time we met."

"And what was that?"

"You mentioned my real father when we talked before. Do you know when he died?"

When Harding reached into his breast pocket, I was reminded of the fear I had of him the first time he sat at my table.

He came out with a small notepad and flipped through the pages. He stopped for a moment, reading something, and then turned a leaf.

"Nineteen seventy-four," he said, "when you were two years old. He was found murdered in the home of a young prostitute named Pearl Watson."

"Do you know if anybody claimed the body?"

"Have you gone to see your daughter?" the FRC agent asked.

"How do you even know to ask that?"

"I'm here with another final request."

"Another five thousand dollars?"

"Have you visited your daughter?"

"Yes. Yes, I have."

"Do you love her?"

"I do. But what does that have to do with you?"

Instead of answering, Harding took another ivory envelope from his pocket.

Again he handed me the letter.

Again I hesitated.

When at last I accepted the final request, I expected Harding to leap up and leave, like he did the first time. But he remained seated, staring at me.

"I am supposed to wait for a reply," he said.

"A reply to a dead man?"

Harding hunched his shoulders, and I tore open the envelope.

Dear Roger,

By now you've probably met Sovie and I know because you're reading this letter you at least say that you love her. I've been telling Dearby that I've been visiting with Althea because she has cancer and is dying. Althea does have cancer and she is dying but I've also been doing my old thing in her house on her phone. Seems like bookies are back in style. I couldn't tell Dearby because she'd want the money I'm making and I needed that money for Sovie. I also needed to tell you about your daughter and to make sure that you cared for her.

The FRC agent sitting in front of you has a third letter. This one has a legal document saying that the bearer of this letter should be allowed access to my safe deposit box at Concordia Bank in downtown Cincinnati. There's $137,941.00 in that box.

I saved that money for Sovie but I owe you something too. And so you can either accept the document and help the child with her bills or you can turn the whole thing over to her and let her decide how to handle it.

It's up to you, Little Brother.

Seth

I folded the note and put it in my pocket.

"I got another question for you, Mr. Harding."

"Yes?"

"Do you take in trainee agents now and then?"

"Yes."

"Could I apply for that job?"

"I can make the proper connections. I happen to need an assistant, and your background fits our major criteria."

"Then you give that letter you got in your pocket to Sojourner Alexander and send me the application form."

THE LETTER

My wife, Corrine, and I had the same financial advisors—Walton, Barth, and Wright. The firm uses oversize light blue envelopes with its return address printed in red in the upper left-hand corner. The partners' names are writ large in block lettering, while the address, in italic print a quarter the size, sits on a single line just below. We had separate accounts with the firm, but I took care of most of the correspondence. Corrine doesn't have much patience with finances and had been more than happy to let me take care of our accounts, taxes, and monthly bills.

"Just show me where to sign," she'd say when I tried to explain the forms and requests.

So on that Wednesday morning, when I saw that Corrine had laid two of the WBW blue envelopes on the dinette table in the nook, I picked them up and put them in my briefcase to read at lunchtime.

"Do you have time for breakfast?" I called down the slender hallway.

Corrine stuck her head out from the bathroom while rubbing a tan towel against her head vigorously. Her coppery skin glistened

slightly from the moisture of the shower. Dark gold freckles tempered the serious cast of her face.

"I thought you said you were late."

I could see her right breast. The nipple was a dark rose, a kind of in-between color from her mixed parentage.

"I am, but I thought we could sit together for a bit. We haven't really talked in a week."

"I don't have time to cook," she said and then ducked back into the bathroom.

"We could have cereal," I suggested, raising my voice to be sure I was heard.

"I'm watching my carbs."

"You're not fat."

"You don't have to be fat to be careful about what you're eating." She came out from the bathroom with the towel wrapped around her, then went the other way down the hall toward our bedroom.

I wondered what she would do if I ran after her and pushed her down on the bed. Would she resist? Push me away? There was no desire in this idle musing. I didn't want to have sex with her. We'd been together for nearly twenty years, since she was twenty-one and I thirty-five. We didn't have sex much anymore, and when we did there was usually some red wine and a little blue pill involved.

I hadn't needed chemical help the three times that I'd had affairs. When I was with a new woman in a secret place, I could do things the way I did when I was in my twenties . . . or at least my thirties.

My last affair had been with a Korean woman, Donella Kim, who had temped in my office for a month or so. I didn't call her until after she'd left Korn/Wills. After that we rutted like rabbits for almost six weeks.

During that time I fell behind in my work, came home late every night, and never had sex once with Corrine. She noticed, but I blamed a muscle strain, and she seemed to accept the excuse.

In the end it was Donella who broke off the relationship.

"I don't want to do this anymore, Frank," she said, when I called her from my office, also on a Wednesday.

"But I love you," I said. My tongue had gone dry, and a dying rodent was keening in my chest.

She hesitated.

I didn't love her, but I didn't want to lose her either. She made me feel alive, and life was, to my mind, better than love. Life was a sweet thing no matter how old you got.

Don't get me wrong, I love Corrine. I didn't think so on the morning Donella broke up with me—but I was wrong. As bad as I felt about the abrupt break from Donella, Corrine had the power to devastate my heart and not even know it.

"No, you don't," Donella said over the phone, three months past. "You just want the sex and the excitement."

"How can you break up with me and not even talk about it?" I asked. "Don't you care for me?"

She canceled the call and turned off her cell phone. She must have gotten a new number, because she didn't answer any of my messages for the next two weeks. And I called her at least a dozen times a day.

"You look like you're losing weight, Frank," Corrine said, nine days after Donella dropped me.

"They're changing over to a new system at work and . . . it's hard. I keep fucking it up. You know how when I get worried I don't eat right."

Corrine looked at me then. It was her suspicious look. I think I must do something noticeable when trying to hide despair with a lie.

"Why would a new system cause you to be that upset?"

"I lost a forty-thousand-dollar sale because I didn't see a flag that one of the reports put out. Miss Francie blames me."

This was true. We did have a new system, and I had missed a flag—because I'd spent the afternoon and evening with Donella and then gotten up early in the morning to see her again. I was late for work and missed the deadline indicated by a systems flag that had shown up the afternoon before. On top of the money, we had almost lost the client, Medidine, a medical-equipment distributer based in Kansas City, Kansas. Adeline Francie had given me an official warning comprising a lecture and a pink slip of paper embossed with the red time stamp of the HR office.

I had a bachelor's degree in political science but worked for Korn/Wills selling orthopedic devices to specialized stores, hospitals, and distributers—all online. KW sells other medical devices, but somehow I ended up running the orthopedic line.

"All you have to do is come in in the morning and log on," straw-haired Francie told me in her office. "Just look at the left side of the screen and make sure there are no red checks. That's all. A teenager could do it."

My supervisor was twenty years my junior. At one time, I suppose I could have argued that she had the job because she was white and I am a black man or, at least, a half-black man. But it was impossible to make that argument, because Ira Flint, Miss Francie's boss, was black. Ira was also an unapologetic Republican and greatly loved at Korn/Wills. Both of his parents had dark skin, and he had a southern accent too.

"I'm sorry, Miss Francie," I said.

I didn't care. I was distraught over losing Donella. It felt like I was dead.

* * *

By the morning Corrine left the two blue envelopes on the dinette table I was pretty much over Donella. I had once seen her walking down the street arm in arm with a tall Asian guy; that cost me two nights sleep. I missed another red check and got a second official reprimand, but after that things evened out. I'd been coming in early for nearly three months and had broadened our orthopedic presence on the web by calling second-tier distribution houses and giving them our preferred rates.

I stayed late most nights and kept my lunches down to forty-five minutes, usually at my desk.

I'd lost thirty pounds pining over Donella, and that felt good, so I tried not to eat much lunch. I took care of personal business over a cup of coffee and a Gala apple.

The financial advisors' envelopes were the same size, but the one addressed to me was very thick. That was our year-end tax statement. Forty-five minutes wouldn't be nearly enough time to review it, so I decided to read the forms in Corrine's letter.

I remember glancing out the window as I tore off the top of the large envelope. I was thinking, idly, about dying. Often when I gazed out over Midtown at midday I wondered what impact my death might have. Certainly most of the people who knew me wouldn't have given it more than five minutes' thought. The thousands walking up and down the streets would never know, would not want to know, and if they somehow found out, they wouldn't care.

My father had hung himself in our backyard in Baldwin Hills, Los Angeles, when I was fourteen. Winslow, my older brother, had found him hanging from a low branch of a fruitless apple tree planted by the previous owners.

"His face was black," Winslow had told me that night, after the police were gone, along with the coroner's white station wagon and my father's corpse. "Much blacker than he was. And his tongue was

sticking out. At first I thought it was a joke he was playing on me. I said to stop foolin' around."

My brother started crying then, and I ran from the room out the front door and into the street. I needed to get away from that house and my brother and my mother, who never really recovered from the shock.

Standing at the window, thinking about my death and my father's, I looked at the envelope in my hand and saw that there was a smaller white envelope in the bottom of the blue fold. This letter, also with the return address of Walton, Barth, and Wright, had been sent to Corrine's studio. But that didn't matter because they had gotten Corrine's studio address wrong. That was on Adams Street in Park Slope, but the sender wrote down Adams Avenue. It was a valid address, just not hers. Somewhere in the computer system of WBW they had the wrong address for her office rather than the right one for our home in Brooklyn Heights. Whenever somebody got it wrong, a very nice woman in their mailroom named Dixie would resend the mail.

This was a personal letter. The address was written by hand. It was a stubby little envelope, the kind that someone might use for an invitation to a wedding or bar mitzvah.

I shoved the letter into my pocket, intending to give it to Corrine when I saw her.

At four in the afternoon she called me on my cell. She always used my cell number.

"Hi, honey," she said and went on, not waiting for me to reply. "Merc called and said that he needs money for a book in his lit class. It costs sixty dollars. I said that you'd transfer the funds over. You might as well send him a hundred."

"I thought we said we'd talk about these things," I said.

"Take it out of my account then."

"It's not the money."

"I'm busy, Frank. I don't have time to discuss the obvious."

"But we said that we'd talk before sending Mercury any more money."

Corrine's parents wanted her to name our son Todd, after her father, who represented the white half of her family. I hated that name. I really hated it. But what could I say, except that he was my son and should be named after my father, Mercury Brown.

It turned out that my dad had killed a man named Simons in a fight that happened over a woman in Houston's Third Ward. Simons had beaten my father pretty badly, but when he turned away, my father took out a knife and killed his rival. That day he took a bus to LA, and, I guess, he thought he'd gotten away with it. But the police had come around asking for Bernard Lavallier; that was my father's real name when he killed Simons. After the murder my father went by the alias Mercury Brown.

Regardless of all that, I named my son Mercury.

"OK," Corrine said, in her reserved and yet exasperated tone. "Call him and tell him that we're teaching him how to go to school without the books he needs."

She hung up. It was that one action upon which I hang the dissolution and the inverted-salvation of my life.

In anger, I transferred $1,757, all the money in my checking account, over to our son. I worked until late in the evening sending e-mails to potential clients, offering them the lowest possible preferential rates.

It wasn't until after nine, when I was on the A train heading back to Brooklyn, that I remembered the little letter that Corrine had gotten from WBW.

Even just thinking about the money managers made me angry. They only kept me on as a client because of Corrine's growing income.

After finishing college, Corrine went to work for a fashion designer. She'd always wanted to study fashion, but her parents wouldn't pay for her to go to FIT. I was expecting to go back to college for my master's so that I could teach at university, but then Mercury was born, and we needed a steady paycheck. Corrine could do her work for the designer at home.

Her career took off. Within four years she was making more than three times my salary, including the sporadic bonuses, and was welcomed into the minor circles of New York fashion society. She had her own bank account and spoiled our son, whose middle name was Todd.

I tore open the letter. I shouldn't have. At any other time I wouldn't have. But I was upset, and the size of the envelope was suspicious. I mean, why would anyone from our money managers' office be sending a personal note to Corrine's studio?

Dearest Corrine,

I'm sending you this letter because I can't think of anything else to do. I know that those lunches we had probably didn't mean anything to you. I know you just wanted to get a leg up on your finances. I wish I could have found something wrong with the way Frank is handling your money but really he's following your advisor's plan perfectly. The market is volatile but he's kept to the program and has done better than many.

I'm glad you came to me because I treasure those lunches we had. It has been a long time since I've had such deep and truly meaningful talks with anyone, man or woman. When you told me about the cancer scare, and how brave you had been not telling anyone, I was moved. And when I found out that you read Márquez I was in heaven. He has always been my favorite

author. So I guess this is a kind of selfish note. Corrine, I want to get to know you better. I need to have someone in my life that I can talk to. I'm not asking you for anything except a few hours now and then—to talk and listen.

I know how lonely and yet how committed you are. I'm in the same place in my life and I'd just like to be able to get together now and then.

I'm sending this snail mail to your studio so as not to cause trouble. If you don't write back I'll understand. I want you to know that I would never want to upset your life. I only think that maybe we have something we could share that would make our lives, certainly mine, better.

Yours, TB

I missed my stop. The train was twelve stations past High Street when I looked up at a homeless woman staggering into the car.

I had read the letter at least twenty times. I had no idea who TB was, but then again, neither had I known about a cancer scare or that Corrine questioned how I took care of our money. I knew that she loved *One Hundred Years of Solitude*, but we had never talked about it because I couldn't get past the first page.

She'd met with this guy more than once for lunch, and now he was, in a sly way, trying to build on their . . . intimacies. There was no mistaking his intentions, but I couldn't blame him. Corrine had obviously sought him out and opened her heart to him.

There's a small bar a few blocks from our upper-floor brownstone apartment. I stopped there and ordered a cognac. Somewhere after the seventh drink I found myself walking down the street with the same gait as the homeless woman who had made me aware of having missed my stop. She'd worn soiled tan pants, with a thick, dark green skirt over them, had a calico blanket draped around her shoulders, and was carrying at least a dozen plastic bags. She

smelled of dust, I remember. That was what brought me out of my stunned reverie.

"Frank, where have you been?" Corrine asked as soon as I was in the door.

She was wrapped in the chiffon pink robe that she loved. It was sheer, and she was naked underneath. Corrine did Pilates and yoga and had a very nice figure at thirty-nine, thank you very much.

Even though I'd lost thirty pounds, I was still another forty overweight.

"Was it that you didn't want me eating cereal?" I asked her. "You think I'm too fat?"

"Have you been drinking?"

"I never go to that bar on Montague," I said. "I was walking by tonight, and I thought, hey, why not?"

"What's wrong, Frank?" she asked. Placing her fingertips on both my shoulders, she stared into my eyes with real concern.

"I was thinking on the way here that men must fall in love with you all the time. You're beautiful and very well known. And here I am a slouch who works in an office where most of the people don't even know my name."

"Come sit down, honey," she said.

She led me to the jade-colored sofa in our den. It was a small room that we rarely used now that Mercury was grown up and off to college.

"Merc said that you wired him over seventeen hundred dollars," she said, floundering for a way to keep my attention.

"Why don't you call him Todd?"

"Because his name is Mercury. What's wrong, Frank?"

"You know, Corr," I said. "I was thinking that we hardly ever talk. I mean there's people I see once a week at work who I know

more about than I do about you. You work late. I leave early. Sometimes we don't even eat together for weeks."

"You're exaggerating."

"No," I said. "Not at all. Like, for instance, when was the last time you went to see a doctor?"

"My last checkup."

"Did your cholesterol rise or maybe your blood pressure? Is that why you're cutting down on carbs?"

"I'm fine." She was looking at me as if I were a stranger, a potentially dangerous man she'd just met and had to tread cautiously around until she understood the territory—a man like my father, who might jump up and stab you in the back.

"You see?" I said. "I didn't know that. You could have had any kind of thing wrong, and I wouldn't know. And I didn't ask because we hardly ever talk. I mean, how can you live with a man who doesn't even ask about your health?"

"Why did you send all that money to Mercury?"

"He's a good kid. I bet he was glad to get it."

"I told him to give it back, all but the sixty he asked for."

I looked right past her words and blinked once or twice.

"I feel kinda sick," I said. "I think I'll go to bed."

In the morning I couldn't sit up without the room spinning. Getting out of the bed was a comedy of wobbling knees and stiff ankles.

At the kitchen table I was trying to see straight, and Corrine was talking to me, though I missed most of what she said. I did understand that she would call work for me and that she had an appointment in the city. She seemed to be worried about me.

For some reason I resented the nicety.

* * *

I got to work at about three in the afternoon. I don't know why I went in; nowhere else to go, I guess.

On the Walton, Barth, and Wright website, I searched for names that had the initials of a degenerative disease. I found Timothy Bell. Timothy was the vice president in charge of all personal investors. Bell was at least three rungs above our agent, Mark Delaney, the man who told us that Corrine's income kept us *above the cut* at WBW. Timothy Bell was a smiling white face on an electronic résumé sheet that each of the vice presidents had. He was thirty-eight and had an MBA from Harvard. He was athletic too, the former captain of a rugby squad—rugby, not Ping-Pong.

I wondered if Corrine was somewhere fucking him right then. The letter had been traveling back and forth for over a month. I could tell that from the postmark. Maybe he called when she didn't reply, or maybe she broke down and called him. I wasn't worried about that though. Whether or not Corrine had fallen into Bell's muscular arms wasn't the problem.

The problem was that his letter was very convincing. He wanted to talk to her and read what she read. In their meetings, he must have looked into her dark brown eyes and seemed like he really wanted to know what was going on with her. She opened up to him, while we hadn't really talked in years.

It was obvious from the letter that he wanted to be her lover but was willing to settle for less. That was more than I had to offer, much more.

After reading Bell's letter, I wondered whether I had the right to hold Corrine back from the kind of life that she might have.

"Brown," a man's voice said.

I didn't have to look up to know that it was Ira Flint, my boss's boss.

"Mr. Flint."

I kept my eyes on the screen as he lowered into the chair beside my desk, a shadow looming in my peripheral vision. Flint was a tall man. Even sitting down he seemed to tower. He was heavy too, but his weight bore witness to strength, whereas mine was soft and getting softer. And the blackness of his skin made me feel rather pale.

Flint stared at me. I knew this even though I was pretending to be paying attention to something on the screen.

"What can I do for you?" I asked.

A glimpse at the bottom line of the computer screen told me that it was 7:17. We were the only ones on the floor.

"I have a problem, Frank," Ira Flint said.

I looked up then. "Does it have something to do with me?"

The big boss nodded his heavy head.

"I got three complaints on you in three months. The economy is down, and they're on my ass to adjust the bottom line."

"It's only two pink slips I got, Mr. Flint."

"The third is you giving out discounts like they were Christmas cards."

"Oh."

I knew that we had to get permission to give out lower rates. I knew it, though somehow I'd convinced myself that it was more important to bring in the business than to waste time making rate requisitions. But sitting there in front of Flint I knew how wrong I had been.

"Well, Frank?"

"I don't know, Ira."

He waited a moment or two. His expression was one of mild confusion.

"Is that all?" he asked.

I shrugged.

"I need something, Frank. Adeline wants to let you go. She's already got somebody lined up to cover your accounts."

Ira was warning me, trying to save me. He was reaching out, and all I wanted was to ask him why. Why help me? Why would he care?

"Frank."

"Let it go, man," I said and then turned back to my screen.

After a while the heavy presence of the big boss rose like a morning fog, and I was alone in my cubicle.

Corrine tried to talk to me that night, but I said I had a virus and went to bed early.

The next day I was given my notice.

"I'm sorry about this, Frank," Adeline Francie told me in her office down at the far end of the hall.

"Uh-huh."

"I mean, you just haven't been carrying your weight."

"Listen," I said, in a stern voice that I hadn't meant to use. "You got me down here with my hat in my hand. You're letting me go. Don't you try and make me feel worse."

I looked into the young manager's eyes, and we both experienced an animal moment. It was a confrontation. She was invading my territory, and I intended to protect it.

"You have two weeks' notice," she said.

"Fine," I said. Seven minutes later I left the office for good. I didn't even collect the belongings from my cubicle desk.

From the following day on, I fell into a new routine. In the mornings I'd get up before Corrine and go off to Midtown libraries and museums. I dressed well and ate in good restaurants. I carried Timothy Bell's letter to Corrine in my wallet. Every few hours I'd take it out and read it.

When the two weeks were up, I applied for unemployment benefits, using a rented mailbox to collect my checks. I went out on job interviews, but no one wanted to hire a fifty-four-year-old man with no real experience in anything but orthopedic online sales.

I didn't tell Corrine what was going on, and she didn't notice any difference. I hoped that she would see that there was something very different happening, but she didn't.

I read *One Hundred Years of Solitude*. It was beautiful. The sadness and melancholy resonated with my feelings. Sometimes I'd sit across the dinner table from Corrine, wishing that she'd bring up the book, that she'd want to talk about anything that would lead me to show her how much that I and my life had changed. But it didn't happen. And so for four months I wandered the streets of Manhattan and came home to my wife, one stranger to another.

One day I was walking down Fifth Avenue, and someone called my name. I turned, wondering who among all those thousands would know me. She ran up and kissed my cheek.

"How are you?" the woman asked.

It took me a few seconds to realize that I knew the smiling face. She was slight of build, with olive skin and heavy but quite beautiful features.

"Donella."

"I almost didn't recognize you," she said. "You're so skinny."

I'd lost my appetite months before.

"Went on a diet," I said, struggling with each word.

"You need a new suit."

"How are you, Donella?"

"Do you have time?" she asked. "Can we get coffee?"

* * *

We took a window table at Dingus and Bob's Coffee Emporium on Forty-Eighth Street. She held the seats while I bought us lattes.

When I got back to the table she told me a story about her boyfriend, a young Korean man named John Park. They had broken up the day before I had first called her, and that's why she'd thrown herself so madly into our affair.

". . . but then he came back and asked me to marry him," she was saying, the middle finger of her right hand barely touching my wrist on the tabletop. This hint of a connection felt like a faraway memory in another man's life. "I said yes, and that's why I broke up with you. But after a few months I realized that I don't want to be married. I left John and called you to apologize, but your cell phone was disconnected, and they said you didn't work at Korn/Wills anymore."

"I'm taking some time off to reevaluate my life," I said, realizing that in a way this was the truth.

"What's wrong?" Donella asked. "Is it because of what I did?"

"No," I said, "not at all. I hated that job, and I was no good at it either. I needed to get away."

"What are you going to do now?"

"Using the time to think."

"Would you, would you like us to see each other again?"

The question gave me the feeling of coming to a precipice, the edge of a vast and deep vale. The other side was so far away that it was shrouded in mist.

"No," I said.

"You hate me."

"I just can't do it, Donella. I have enough trouble taking one step after the next. I really have to go."

"Will you call me?" she asked, as I rose from the wooden chair.

"Yes," I lied.

* * *

That evening I called Corrine on my new pay-as-you-go cell phone. I told her that I was working late. I came home in the early morning and got into the bed so quietly that my wife didn't even shift in her sleep.

I had not seen my father, Mercury, after his suicide. The police were already there when I got home from baseball practice. My mother had a closed-casket service. I suppose they all thought they were protecting me. But I had in my mind the image of a naked man with a brown body and a black face—his tongue sticking out as if he were taunting the people after him.

My brother hadn't said he was naked, but that's the image I had.

That night I dreamed of him. It was a sad reunion.

When Corrine tried to wake me the next morning, I told her that I was taking a personal day, after having worked so hard for so long.

At ten I sat down at the dinette table in the breakfast nook and took TB's letter from my wallet. On the other side I wrote this note:

Corrine,

I've been holding this letter for months now. The most important thing it meant to me was that I didn't get angry about it. I was just sad that we had drifted so far apart. I don't know if you care for this man or if his feelings for you make any difference. But I do know that you didn't trust me with our money and that you couldn't share your fears or joys with me, that you gave these feelings to a stranger because I left you no other choice. I know that whatever feeling we once had packed up and moved out with Mercury. So I'm going to leave. I'm breaking it off in one quick movement because I know that that's the only good thing I could do for you.

Frank Brown

I spent three days and two nights in Central Park. The weather was temperate, and I slept on a bench. One guy tried to rob me, and I went crazy. I actually picked up a trash can and hit him with it. After that I went to a homeless shelter on the Bowery. My joints were sore, and I realized that my clothes smelled like dust. I had put all my financial papers and important documents into a safe-deposit box at My Bank on Madison. I figured that I could live a life just off the streets for years with what I had. I'd get jobs washing dishes or maybe as a box boy in a local market in Queens. I could read *Love in the Time of Cholera* and learn to play chess competitively in Washington Square Park. I had been pretty good at chess in high school and later at college.

I dreamed one night that Corrine and I lived in a room. We were on a bed separated by an unbreakable glass wall. We couldn't hear each other through the thick barrier and so could only communicate through gesture. She pointed with both hands at her eyes and then at her stomach. I didn't understand. Then she touched her right foot with her right hand and looked beseechingly at me. I hunched my shoulders.

This dream played over and over, like an experimental film on a continuous loop. At one point I realized that the dream wouldn't stop. I wondered how long I had been asleep. My joints ached. I wanted to wake up but couldn't.

Finally I was conscious, but I couldn't open my eyes because they were glued shut by secretions. I tried to lift my hand to open them, but I was too weak, so I concentrated on forcing my eyelids open. After a while they came apart, scraping the sand of sleep across my corneas.

I was in a long hall tenanted by at least a dozen patients on slender hospital beds. A middle-aged Indian woman in a white smock was standing over me.

"What is your name?" she asked. It seemed as if she had asked me that question before.

"Frank Brown."

"Do you have family?"

I shook my head and the room also shook.

"Health insurance?"

"No."

"You're very sick, Mr. Brown," the doctor said. "You're suffering from malnutrition and probably walking pneumonia that has given way to full-blown pulmonary disease. Your lungs are a mess, and antibiotics don't seem to be working."

"How long have I been here?" I asked.

"They brought you from the shelter four days ago."

"Am I going to die?" I whispered.

"That's why we want to know if you're insured or if there's someone who can help."

When I wasn't moving or blinking too fast, I felt very warm and secure.

"Can I stay here?" I asked.

"For a week," she said. "After that we have to move you to a state facility."

I closed my eyes, and when I opened them again the Indian doctor was gone.

I felt warm and swaddled. In that bed there were no desires, not even much discomfort. There were beds around me, but I didn't know who was in them. I didn't have to eat or get up to go to the bathroom. All I had to do was sleep and awaken now and again. Each period of sleep seemed to have a longer arc. It was as if my consciousness was a skipping stone over placid water that built up speed and power as it went. I was completely satisfied knowing that

I'd sleep, open my eyes, and sleep again, until finally one day the sleep would go on, leaving me behind.

"Dad?"

I'd heard the word before in my death-sleep. It was a single note but also a word, a class of men . . . me.

Mercury was sitting in a pine folding chair next to my bed. His butter-brown face was drawn.

"Hey," I said. "What are you doing here?"

I looked around and noticed that I was no longer in the crowded infirmary. It was a single room—just for me.

"How do you feel?" my son asked.

I took in a long, deep breath, realizing how shallow my breathing had been.

"Good," I said. "Better. Where's your mother?"

"I want you to come home, Dad."

"Why aren't you in school?"

"I took a leave to come back and find you. I've been going all over the city to hospitals and shelters, the police and city social workers."

"Where's your mother?" I asked again.

"She thought, she thought you might not want to see her."

There was a lot of information in that stuttered sentence. But it didn't matter. Mercury my son had done for me what I was unable to do for Mercury my father.

"If I live," I said.

"What, Dad?"

"If I live, I'll come home."

HAUNTED

I was sitting at the dining room table surrounded by stacks of books and old newspapers, dirty dishes, bills, and first, second, and third drafts of handwritten letters to editors of various literary reviews. My laptop computer screen was open to a staff-page photograph from the *Black Rook Review*'s website. The *BRR* was a small literary quarterly out of the Lower East Side of Manhattan. I was looking at the picture of young, milk-soppy Clark Heinemann, holding in my hand his rejection of my one-thousandth story, "Shootout on the Wild Westside." Mira, my girlfriend of the last sixteen years, was leaving to sleep at her mother's house in Hoboken because, she said, and I quote, "your continual vituperation is too much for me to bear."

"Call me when you're human again, Paul," she said, before rolling her black-and-pink-polka-dotted roller bag out the door of our fifth-floor walk-up apartment.

I remember it all so clearly: Heinemann's rejection letter was in my hand, and his smug, slack face was on the screen; I could hear the thump and slide, thump and slide, thump and slide of Mira's bag as she lowered it step-by-step.

. . . while the concept is interesting the execution leaves me with more questions than answers. I think you might have greater success sending this story to a genre magazine where the readers have more sympathy for the ambiance and tone . . .

Heinemann's words were in my head while his doughy face smirked at me. Mira's bag's bump and slide down the stairs was fading when my hand, seemingly of its own volition, crushed the letter. This minor act of anger was exacerbated by a pain in my middle finger. It felt as if a bone had broken. Before I could react, the sharp ache jumped from my hand to my shoulder, and my breath got short. I was convinced that these were psychosomatic manifestations of the rage I felt about Heinemann and his condescending, typewritten, type-signed letter.

Here he used a typewriter on watermarked paper not as a sign of respect but because of his supercilious conceit.

There was no personal intention to that letter; I was sure of this even as I tumbled from the dining room chair to the bare oak floor. My left ankle got tangled in the power cord, and the laptop fell with me. It didn't break. Lying there sideways on the floor, Clark Heinemann sneered at my diminution, my impotence.

I hated him so much.

As I reached over to pick up the computer, intent on smashing his image, I realized that it was not my spiritual heart but the physical one that was causing the numbness in my left forearm and the fire in my chest.

I managed to take in half the breath I needed, exhaled with a very audible wheeze, and then inhaled with half the capacity of the breath before.

Clark Heinemann sneered. My breathing became mere puffs. Mira was right about me, but Mira was gone. I had stormed around the apartment for three days cursing the editor and drinking expensive red wine that we could not afford.

My thousandth story, and I was dying, and Clark Heinemann would probably make some snide remark when he heard I was gone.

Just like they used to say in the old movies, everything was going dark. I was dying, and the only witness, the only light left to me, was Clark Heinemann and his sidelong smug indifference.

After a short while that nevertheless felt interminable, darkness overwhelmed the light. I had died hating a man twenty years my junior, a man I had never met or spoken to. I was, for all intents and purposes, dead and gone, but somehow my hatred cohered. The details of my final humiliation floated on a deep well of spite that did not, would not drain away.

Even as my body rotted and festered under the unblinking eyes of Clark Heinemann, the thoughts I had at death survived. One thousand unpublished stories, 26,473 rejection letters, and all those editorial twits that never gave me a break. The only thing left of me was a raging emotion at every publisher of every insignificant quarterly—but most of all, Clark Heinemann.

"Paul Henry is dead," a young woman's voice said from somewhere in the void.

I was suddenly back in proximity to the living; aware, seeing the world from a set of eyes that were a bit stronger than mine had been.

"Who?" The man's voice seemed to reverberate.

"That guy who has sent us a story every six weeks for the past twenty years."

"You mean Mr. Again and Again?"

"That's him."

"What happened? Did some editor finally shoot him?"

"Sixty-eight and overweight. He only lived three blocks from here. He had this younger girlfriend who left him, and so they didn't find his body for five weeks."

I was floating over the head of a man in his late forties who looked somewhat like Clark Heinemann. He wore a herringbone jacket, a dark blue shirt, and a yellow and blue bow tie.

"The poor fuck," Clark said. "I must have rejected hundreds of his bad stories."

A thousand, I thought.

"What did you say, Carrie-Anne?"

"What?"

"Did you say something?"

"No."

"Oh well," said the human stalk to which my hateful consciousness clung. "He wrote all that genre stuff and tried to pretend it was literary. At least I won't have to make our interns read any more of his ghastly prose."

You didn't even read it yourself?

"What?" Clark said.

"Are you hearing things?" the copper-haired young woman asked. She wore horn-rimmed glasses and grass-green lipstick.

"Too much to drink at the PEN Gala last night, I guess," he said. "Did I tell you? I sat three tables away from Rushdie and Paul Auster. My head's been buzzing all morning."

After that Carrie-Anne left the small office. Clark gazed at her posterior as she went, and so I did too. Clark had a desk and a bookshelf, an old IBM Selectric typewriter, and an almost as old Apple Macintosh computer. His windows were open, and there was a breeze; you could see it wafting in the partially drawn window shade.

Alone Clark Heinemann studied the computer screen, perusing a story submission to the magazine. I tried to read the words, but they didn't make sense. The world was fading again as it had when I died weeks before.

Finally I was once more merely the memory of hatred for anyone having to do with publishing.

The acrid smell of urine, dead skin, and sour breath assailed a nose close to me. I came to consciousness, again attached to Clark Heinemann. This time we were in an old folks' home sitting before an ancient woman in a wheelchair. She was listing to the side, and her eyes darted around aimlessly, as if searching for something worth seeing. Looking at her, I perceived a memory that must have belonged to Heinemann. It was his mother when she was younger and he was a child. She'd been a handsome woman. Now her once fair skin had darkened and was creased with a thousand wrinkles. Her white hair stood away from her tiny head like dead grass rising up from the weight of the first snow at the onset of winter. The only glimmer of life, even beauty, was in her blue eyes, which looked out from under a creased brow. She peered closely at the space above Clark's head.

"How are you, Mom?" he asked, and I wondered what I was doing there.

"Who are you?" she asked.

"I'm Clark, Ma, your son."

"Who's that on your head?"

"My . . . my head?"

"Yeah. That fat Negro on top a' your head. Isn't he heavy?"

Heinemann waved his hand over his head; it passed right through me.

"Nothing there, Mom. See?"

"I see a Negro on top a' your head."

Clark turned away from his mother and looked into a mirror above a sink anchored into the wall of the nursing-home cell. I saw what he saw—him, as pasty-faced and weak-jawed as ever, and my

dark countenance hovering just above for only a second and then fading. I was still there, but Clark soon lost sight of me.

"What was that?" he said.

"He's gone," Mrs. Heinemann said. "Now, who are you?"

For the next hour or so, Clark sat with his mother, fed her, and told her over and over again that he was her son and that he loved her.

"Will you take me with you to your house?" she asked, emotional craft combined with the eternal despair of an orphaned child.

"You're happier here," he said.

"I hate it here. They don't feed me."

"I'll talk to the nursing staff."

"Will the Negro take me home with him?"

The smell was horrible; the feeling of mortality unbearable. I could sense death descending all around. This reminded me of my own expiration, and I moaned.

"Did you hear something, Mom?"

"It was him," she said, gesturing at me with an arthritic claw.

It was then that I understood what was happening. I existed only through my hatred of Clark, and then I was called into existence through my name being mentioned or when someone like that old dying woman could see me.

I wanted to get away from Clark and his mother and that building full of people whose souls were crying out as mine was.

Six or seven times during the torture, Clark turned to look in the mirror, but I wasn't there—or at least he could no longer see me.

When he left the nursing home, I faded again, hoping that this would be the last conjuring, that I would pass over into oblivion.

For a long time I floated in hateful darkness. My feelings about Clark Heinemann had become a physical thing, or maybe

metaphysical; they, those angry emotions, had turned into instincts that I could not eschew.

"Miss Stern to see you, Mr. Heinemann," a voice through an intercom announced.

"Send her in."

I was aware again, sharing the eyes, ears, and nostrils of Clark Heinemann.

He looked up, and I did too. Mira walked in, wearing her job-hunting medium-gray dress suit.

She was thirty years younger than I. We met when I was teaching a class on fiction at the uptown Y. She still had a great figure. And that outfit really showed it off.

Clark noticed what I did, and I wondered if somehow my awareness informed his.

He stood up and said, "Nice to meet you, Miss Stern. I was so sorry to hear about your husband."

"We weren't married. Paul didn't believe in marriage." It sounded like an indictment.

"Oh, I see," he said. "Um, please have a seat."

Mira took the chair and crossed her legs, showing her lovely knees.

"How can I help?" Clark asked, looking at her legs with me.

"I wanted to ask you if there was some way that you might publish something of Paul's. He left me the stories in his will. And it's the only thing I can imagine that would be a fitting remembrance. His body was cremated. He was an only child, and his parents are both dead. The only things he left in the world were one thousand stories and seven suitcases filled with rejection letters."

I caught a whiff of rose oil, the perfume I preferred on her.

"You don't have children?" Clark asked.

"I was with Paul most of my adult life," she said. "But he didn't want kids. He said he needed the time to write."

Clark gazed at Mira's café au lait complexion. Her father was Jewish of Russian descent and her mother a rare Christian from Mali. She was a beautiful woman. I couldn't remember the last time I'd told her so.

I'm so sorry, honey, I said reflexively.

"Did you hear something?" Clark asked.

"Just the traffic from the street," she said.

She uncrossed her legs and then recrossed them in the opposite direction. Then she tilted forward in a movement both innocent and suggestive.

I was happy that she was trying so hard to get me into that magazine.

"You know, Miss Stern, Paul's work was not the kind of fiction we publish. The writing was passable, but he always threw in some genre aspect that made the work, um, what can I say . . . neither here nor there."

"But," she said. "I don't know . . . I was thinking that maybe you could publish it with an introduction. You know, an article saying that the story was an example of how Paul took his own path in spite of expectations."

That's my girl, I said.

"I like that," Clark agreed.

"I know Paul was stubborn, but he worked so hard at it that it would be a shame if he was never published."

Mira stared directly into my nemesis's eyes, and I was aware of a quickening in his pulse.

"I'll tell you what," he said. "Why don't we have dinner tonight, and you can tell me what stories best fit your idea. I mean, I can't make any promises but . . . I don't know; we'll see."

"Thank you so much," she said, with real happiness in her voice.

They made plans to meet at an Italian restaurant that night. He gave her the name, D'Oro. She said that she knew the place.

She stood, and he did too. He walked her to the door and then kissed her cheek. I could smell the rose attar rising from her breast and feel the touch of her fingers on the back of Clark Heinemann's hand.

After she left, Clark sat there for a while looking at the door she'd gone through. Then he picked up a manuscript, and my mind slipped back into the brackish bile pond where it festered and throve.

In that vile darkness my mind was only partially aware. I realized that even though I was a ghost, I was the one being haunted by the animosity I'd worn like a badge through my life. I never made anything of myself, and I held Mira back. I wrote stories that I knew would never be published, and I hated freely.

I was my own private hell.

Knowing this, I tried to let go of my feelings, hoping that this release would let me find oblivion, if not actual peace.

There in the darkness I strained to let my hatred of the arrogant editor fade. For a moment there I felt that I had succeeded, and then . . .

"To Paul Henry," Clark Heinemann saluted.

He and Mira clinked wine goblets over two plates of half-eaten pasta. They drained their glasses, and a waiter came up to refill them.

"The wine is kind of going to my head," she said.

He reached over and took her hand.

"Come home with me," he said, and I tried to remember the last time Mira and I had made love.

* * *

The sex went on and on, all night long. Riding on Clark's undulating body, I cried out in the pain of loss and betrayal. He experienced my cries as some kind of inner ecstasy, while Mira urged him on, whispering that she had not felt this much and this good in many years. She told him how beautiful he was and how caring and gentle.

In the early morning they went into the hallway outside of his apartment after a series of half-drunken dares. There they giggled and fucked until someone opened a door down the hall, forcing them to laugh and run for the refuge of his apartment again.

After that they fell asleep, and I eased back into my grotto of spite. But before I could sink into blissful unconsciousness . . .

"What are you thinking?" Clark asked my girlfriend of sixteen years. He was nuzzling her nipple with his pudgy nose.

"About Paul," she said wistfully.

"Are you feeling bad?"

"No," she said, and I felt like I was a balloon filled past capacity, about to burst with rage instead of helium. "The reason he was left in the apartment for so long was because I had decided never to come back. I couldn't. I'm thirty-seven, and nothing had changed between us since the day we met. We were in the same apartment, sleeping on the same mattress on the floor. He made scrambled eggs with lox and onions in the same skillet five thousand mornings in a row. And he kept writing stories that I knew would never be published. I think he knew it too."

"I'm sorry," Clark said. "I guess sometimes we just find ourselves in a rut."

And as if the word had poetic power, they began rutting all over again.

* * *

I was hoping that Mira had seduced Clark so that he would publish my work. But the following morning I was stirred back to reality by a phone call.

"Hello?" Mira said.

"Hi, Mira, it's Clark . . . Heinemann."

"Hi," she said, with an élan I'd never heard in her voice before.

"I've decided to go ahead with our plan and publish an original Paul Henry story."

"Oh my God, that's so wonderful. It's perfect."

They discussed the details for a while, and then he said, "I had a great time last night."

"We should get together again soon," she agreed.

"How about tonight?" he asked.

"I'm supposed to see my mother," Mira said.

Yes! I thought. *Lead him on until I'm published and then tell him you did it all for me.*

"OK," Clark said rather sadly. I could feel his disappointment through our connection.

"But I could call her," Mira offered. "I could change it to sometime next week."

"I'll get the wine, and we can eat in my apartment."

"We don't even have to eat," Mira promised, and I cried out.

"Is there some interference on the line?" Clark asked.

"Not on my end."

Every night for the next three months Mira was at Paul's apartment doing things we had never done.

When she told him that she was pregnant, I hoped that the smug editor would see his error and kick her out. But instead he kissed her and asked her to marry him. He didn't think about it for one moment. What kind of fool does something like that?

But I was relieved anyway. They would have a life where my name would never be mentioned. I would slowly fade from consciousness and then finally follow my body into death.

I hadn't considered what would happen with the publication of my story "Shootout on the Wild Westside" in the fall edition of *Black Rook Review*. Clark wrote a moving testimonial to me, " . . . a writer who never gave up; who died working on his next story."

I was dragged through a series of interviews, to a dozen public readings, and finally to a publishing house that wanted to put out a collection of my multi-genre tales.

Clark and Mira didn't stop having sex until the seventh month of her pregnancy, and then, and then . . . they decided to name their son Paul Henry Heinemann.

Clark became an expert on my work and often gave talks about me.

. . . Paul Henry was a complex man who was ahead of his time. He wrote fiction that was destined to outlive him. He selfishly used his time for the one thousand stories he crafted over thirty years.

He wasn't a happy man. He wasn't nice or good or caring or even very friendly. He hated editors like me because we couldn't see his value . . .

And after talks in Cincinnati, Seattle, Boston, LA, and twenty other towns and cities, he'd meet some young woman writer and make love to her the way he would to Mira when he got home.

I hated him then, because I had never cheated on her. Maybe I didn't treat her as well as she deserved, but at least I was faithful in my mediocrity.

When Clark came home I never rested, because he'd made a career out of me and so talked about me and my work almost every day.

And when he wasn't dealing with me directly he was calling out to his son, "Paul Henry," and I was forced into the life I never had, paying for my small-minded, selfish ways.

And then one day Mira found a letter in a pocket of the brown corduroy jacket that Clark wore when on the road. It was some love letter that a young woman secreted for him to find, so he would think of her when he was far away.

The fight went on for hours. Mira cried, and Clark tried to explain, then to apologize, and then to say he had no excuse. She told him to get out, and instead of being happy about his misery, I felt, for the first time since the heart attack, real pain. Their pain was mine. I couldn't escape it. My consciousness was melding with their emotions.

At one point Clark and I saw Paul Henry standing in a doorway that led down a hall to the boy's bedroom.

Clark told his son to go to bed.

"What's that man doing on your head, Daddy?" the four-year-old asked.

After putting his son to bed, Clark returned to the living room, and Mira kissed him.

"What's that for?" he asked.

"Seeing you with our son," she said. "I'm still mad but I forgive you."

Later that night, Mira and Clark came in to say good night to my namesake, kissing him and promising strawberry pancakes in the morning to make up for all that yelling.

I wasn't looking forward to what was going to happen next. When they had even the tiniest spat they made up for it with

marathon sex sessions. I was going to experience Clark's rolling doughy body making Mira cry out for him as she'd never done for me.

But that didn't happen. Clark and Mira turned on Paul Henry's night-light and departed, somehow leaving me in the room with their son.

Alone, the boy dutifully picked his teddy bear off the short chest of drawers next to his bed and squeezed it tightly.

He had golden skin and similarly colored curly hair.

He seemed to be thinking about something when he said, "You look so sad."

He seemed to be talking to me.

This was a surprise. Even those people who rarely saw me, usually senile and near death themselves, never addressed me directly. They would ask Clark who I was and why I was there.

"You," Paul Henry said.

"Me?"

He nodded. "Why you look so sad?"

"I do?"

"Uh-huh. Why?"

"Because your mother used to be my girlfriend, but then I, I died, and now she loves your father." I didn't want to say all that, but somehow his questions demanded answers.

"And so you're sad because you love my mommy?"

"No."

"You don't love her?"

"No, I don't," I said, surprised at my own answer.

"Then why are you so mad at my daddy?"

"Why do you say I'm mad?"

"Because when I see you and you say things, it makes him upset. I don't think he can see you, but he knows you're there. He knows it, and he gets mixed up."

I felt something give, like a tether pulling out of the soil.

"I guess I was mad at your father because he never published my stories when I was alive."

"Oh," my young namesake said, and I felt another tether give. "Maybe you could forgive him if I said I was sorry he didn't do that. I could tell my daddy that you were mad, and then he would be sorry too."

There was a breeze suddenly blowing through the room, and another tether pulled out of the firmament of my hatred. There was a light shining somewhere, and I realized that most of my existence after death had been swathed in darkness.

Everything was becoming light.

Paul Henry was talking, and I might have responded, but I was only aware of the light shining and the darkness that was dissipating, the strong breeze, and the weightlessness I felt from the tethers loosening.

"Will you come back?" Paul Henry asked. It was part of a longer conversation that another part of my mind had been having with him.

Before I could answer, the wind picked up, drowning out all other sound, and the light became excruciatingly bright. I was still there in the room with Paul Henry, as the world turned and Mira called out Clark's name in ecstasy.

I would, I realized, always be there, and that was a relief so profound that time ceased and my antipathies turned into silver-scaled fish that darted away somewhere, leaving me once again breathless.

THE SIN OF DREAMS

July 27, 2015

"So, who's paying for all this?" Carly Matthews asked.

"There are a few investors," Morgan Morgan replied. "A man who owns the largest cable and satellite provider in China, a so-called sheikh, the owner of two pro teams in the US, and a certain, undefined fund that comes to us via the auspices of the White House."

Morgan gestured broadly. Behind the milk-chocolate-brown entrepreneur, through the huge blue-tinted window, Carly could see center city LA, thirty-two stories down. The San Bernardino Mountains stood under a haze in the distance. The summer sun shone brightly but still failed to warm the air-conditioned office.

"Government money?" she asked.

"Not exactly," the director of New Lease Enterprises replied, looking somewhere over the young scientist's head.

"What does that mean?"

"Someone close to the president has called together a small group of billionaires and shared with them the potential of our research. He has also, unofficially, given NLE's holding company, BioChem International, access to the Justice Department and three constitutional experts."

"What does the Justice Department have to do with neuronal data analysis?"

Morgan Morgan, executive vice president and principal director of NLE, gazed at the twenty-three-year-old postdoctoral student. Her pleasant features and youthful expression belied the razor-sharp mind that, his advisors assured him, her published articles so clearly exhibited.

"What business does a black hip-hop promoter from the Motor City have running a subsidiary of a biological research company?" Morgan asked.

All the fair-skinned blond scientist could do was raise her eyebrows and shrug.

"The only reason I'm here," she said, "is because my former professor Dr. Lawson asked me, as a favor to him, to meet with you. I'm in the middle of three very important experiments, and I have to be back by no later than nine o'clock tonight."

"What reason did Rinehart give you?" Morgan asked.

"Dr. Lawson told me that I would be amazed by what you had to say. It is for that reason alone I left Stanford to come down here."

"I paid Rinehart three hundred and seventy thousand dollars to say that to you. One hundred thousand for his second family in West Virginia, two hundred to cover gambling debts in Atlantic City, and seventy to end the annoyance of a blackmailer who has been collecting money from him for twelve years. I don't

know how he plans to spend that seventy, but I doubt he'll use it for payment."

Young Dr. Matthews tilted her head and peered blankly at the ex-hip-hop manager and impresario. For a full minute she couldn't think of anything to say.

"Well?" Morgan asked, managing not to smile. "Are you amazed?"

"Yes. But I don't see why Dr. Lawson would want me to come down here to learn about his, his indiscretions."

"He didn't." Morgan allowed. "I've already told you that the work we're doing has to do with the transmigration of the human soul. Our work in that field is truly astonishing."

"What's astonishing is so much money being spent on this rubbish," she said.

"Two years at Oxford, right?" Morgan pointed at her and smiled, knowingly.

"Yes, but why do you ask?"

"*Rubbish*," he said, with an almost boyish grin. "Americans don't really use that word, even though it's a very good one."

"I didn't come here to dig up dirt on my mentor or to listen to your opinions on the nationality of language."

"No," Morgan said. "You are here because I paid your mentor good money to make sure you came."

"And the question is, why?"

"The same reason the board of directors of BioChem International opted to give me a free hand in this soul business—sales."

"Sales?"

"We have, as I've already told you, all the theoretical and technical knowledge to read and therefore copy the contents of a human brain into electronic data storage and from storage back into that mind or another. But because of the complexity and mathematical

nuances of this process, there isn't enough memory in our facility to contain even a fraction of a normal adult's experience and intelligence, learned and inherited instincts, and conscious and unconscious memory—at least that's what the experts tell me. The amount of data attached even to a simple phrase in a human's mind could take up trillions of bytes in memory. The experience of a single day would fill up every storage device the Defense Department has."

"Oh," Carly said, the light dawning behind her eyes.

"Yes," Morgan agreed, nodding. "I realized your macromolecular studies trying to simulate DNA development would give us a way to store information that is only a thousand times the capacity size of the human brain and naturally compatible with human physiology. If we could harness your bio-storage methodology with our neuronal I/O systems, we could combine them with the cloning process to transfer the human soul from one body to another."

"But Mr. Morgan, what you have to understand is that I do not believe in a soul."

"No," the director agreed. "You don't. But you're an American citizen aren't you?"

"Of course."

"You believe in the freedom of religion, do you not?"

"Certainly."

"And all religions believe in the human soul."

"So what?"

"So if I offer to sell a customer a new, younger version of himself, then he has to believe that it is not only his consciousness but his actual soul that will inhabit the new body."

"But it isn't," Dr. Matthews argued. "Even if the new body contained his memories when the old body dies, the origin, the

sense organs that recorded and experienced those memories will die with it."

"Not the originals," Morgan Morgan noted. "My scientists tell me that our physical body is completely replaced by new materials every seven years; our memories, if material, are therefore not original."

"That's just sophistry."

"But what if we copied Mr. X's memories into the macromolecular computer your research postulates, talk to Mr. X in that form, and then copy those memories back into his old body?"

"His brain will remember the experiences his mind had as a machine."

"Yes," Morgan said happily. "We copy him back and forth a few times like that and then, with no warning, move these memories into the new body. His mind, his experiences, and his thoughts will be indistinguishable from the three storage units he's experienced. Therefore the new man and the old man will be the same—exactly."

"It's kind of like three-card monte," Carly said.

"Kind of," Morgan agreed, pursing his lips and shrugging slightly.

December 3, 2019

Dr. Carly Matthews was remembering this first meeting with Morgan Morgan as she sat in the witness box in a pine and cherrywood California state courtroom, seven blocks east of the ex-impresario's former office.

"You believed that Mr. Morgan was a huckster," Ralph Lacosta, the prosecuting attorney, said. He was a short man in a black suit that seemed to call attention to his small stature. He wore glasses,

as Carly did. At their last meeting, in preparation for her testimony, he had asked her out for dinner.

"Objection," Melanie Post, the defense attorney, said. "Leading the witness."

Melanie was buxom, around forty, and Carly found her intimidating, though she didn't know why. The defense lawyer never raised her voice or bullied a witness. It was something about the way she looked at and listened to people—with unrelenting intensity.

"Reword, counselor," a seemingly bored John Cho, the presiding judge, advised.

The judge was sixty-nine, Carly knew from Wikipedia's newly instituted public official bio-repository. He had presided over some of the most important murder cases in recent years and had survived three bouts with liver cancer.

"How did Mr. Morgan impress you when you first met?" Lacosta asked Carly.

"He told me that he planned to migrate souls. I thought he was joking."

"You didn't believe him?"

"He was a music producer who was all of a sudden at the head of the subsidiary of a major medical corporation. That alone was ridiculous."

"But you went to work for him the day you met," Lacosta claimed. "Why is that?"

"Five million dollars."

"Say again?"

"He paid me five million dollars and promised over a hundred million in capital to design and build a macromolecular computer for New Lease Enterprises. He also offered to let me retain copyrights and patents on the theory and the physical device."

"And you accepted?"

"I didn't believe in the existence of a soul, but to have the funds to build a new bio-based computer system was too good to pass up."

"And did you accomplish this goal?"

"Yes."

"And did NLE's other researchers manage to copy the contents of a man's mind, completely, from a human brain into an analogous synthetic construct?"

At the defense table, over Lacosta's left shoulder, Carly could see the codefendants, Morgan Morgan and a young man named Tyler Edgington Barnes IV. Morgan reminded her of her father. Not her biological dad, but Horace Granger, the black man that married her mother after Thomas Matthews had abandoned them.

"Miss Matthews," Judge Cho said.

"I cannot say that the data transfer was complete," Carly said. "But the responses from the various I/O devices on Micromime Six were exactly the same as the subjects gave with their own bodies and minds."

A woman in the courtroom began to cry. That, Carly knew, was Melinda Greaves-Barnes, the seventy-six-year-old self-proclaimed widow of Morgan Morgan's codefendant.

"So you communicated with these synthetic memories?" Prosecutor Lacosta asked.

"Yes. For many months, in over a hundred test cases."

"And where were the original patients while you conducted your experiments with the synthetic device?"

"Each was placed in a medically induced coma. That was the only way we could assure an even transfer of information, by lowering the metabolism to a catatonic state."

"Like death," Lacosta suggested.

"Objection."

"Withdrawn. Those are all the questions I have for this witness, your honor."

"OK," John Cho said. "Let's break for lunch and reconvene at two P.M."

"It's all so crazy," Adonis Balsam was saying at the Hot Dog Shoppe across the street from the courthouse. He was demolishing a chili-cheese dog with onions. Carly ordered a soy dog on whole wheat. "I mean, they're trying Tyler Barnes for murdering himself. That's insane."

"But the man in the defendant's chair," Carly said, "is just a clone, a copy of the original man."

"An exact copy, with all of the original guy's feelings and memories," Adonis said. He was black-haired and rather stupid, Carly thought, but he was a good lover, and he seemed devoted to her. She didn't mind that he was probably after her money. After she started her own line of Macromime computers and computer systems, everybody was after her money—everybody but Morgan Morgan.

"No," she said. "To be exactly the same, you have to be the original thing, the thing itself. Morgan and Tyler murdered the original Tyler Barnes."

"OK, baby," Adonis said. "You're the scientist, not me."

He took her hand and kissed her cheek. She always smiled when he called her baby and kissed her. She didn't love Adonis and didn't care if he loved her or not. All she wanted was a word and a kiss.

"What defines a human being?" was Melanie Post's first question when Carly sat down in the cherrywood witness box that afternoon.

"Objection," Prosecutor Lacosta chimed. "The witness is not an expert in philosophy, medicine, or psychology."

"Ms. Post?" Judge Cho asked, a friendly and expectant smile on his lips.

"Your honor," the defense said. "Ms. Matthews has designed a memory device that is almost indistinguishable from the structure, capacity, and even the thinking capability of the human brain. I would argue that there is not a human being on the face of this Earth more qualified than she."

The judge's smile turned into a grin. Carly wondered how well the two knew each other.

"I'll allow the question," Cho said, "as long as the answer remains within the bounds of the witness's expertise."

"Ms. Matthews?" Melanie Post said.

"It's, it's mostly the brain I suppose," Carly said. In all their pretrial sessions, the prosecutor's team had not prepared her for this question. "But there are other factors."

"The soul?"

"I don't believe in a soul."

"Man is soulless?"

"The brain is an intricate machine that functions at such a high level that it feels as if there is something transcendent in the sphere of human perception."

"But really human beings are just complex calculators," Melanie Post offered.

"Objection."

"Overruled."

"I don't know," Carly admitted. "Emotions are real. Dreams are not real, but they arise from biological functions. So even dreams are physical entities; they exist as one thing but are perceived as something else. It is a very difficult question to answer."

"Are the defendants men?" Melanie asked.

"Yes."

"No more questions. You may step down, Ms. Matthews."

August 15, 2020

Carly Matthews sat in the back row of the courtroom. She'd attended the trial every day it convened for more than half a year, having left the running of Macromime Enterprises to her stepfather. The day after Carly's testimony, Melanie Post presented John Cho with a request from Tyler Edgington Barnes to separate his trial from Morgan Morgan's. Barnes was now claiming that he had been brainwashed by the NLE director and was not responsible for any criminal act he might be blamed for.

Ralph Lacosta, after meeting with Tyler and his former body's wife, Melinda, had decided there was merit in the billionaire's claim and withdrew her accusations; she now admitted that the young Tyler was truly innocent of the murder of his earlier iteration. The crime was, in the state prosecutor's opinion, solely the responsibility of Morgan Morgan.

For his part Morgan did not protest the decision, but in the transition it turned out that he was broke. BioChem International, which had been paying Melanie Post's steep fee, withdrew their support for their former VP, saying that they too had been convinced of his perfidy. That's when Carly stepped in and hired Fred Friendly to represent Morgan.

Carly didn't feel any guilt for what had happened at NLE, but neither did she think that Morgan alone should shoulder the burden.

Ralph Lacosta approached Morgan after he was seated in the witness box.

"Mr. Morgan," the prosecutor said, as a kind of greeting.

The ex-VP, ex–music mogul nodded.

Morgan wasn't a particularly handsome man, Carly thought. He was only five seven, at least twenty pounds overweight, and his features were blunt, with no hint of sensuality. But despite these shortcomings, his smile was infectious.

"What is your education, Mr. Morgan?" the prosecutor asked.

"Degree in general studies from Martin Luther King High School in Detroit, Michigan."

"That's all?"

"Yes."

"But still you were at the helm of the most advanced biological research company in the world."

"Only the sales arm of the NLE branch of that company," Morgan corrected.

"Excuse me?"

"They made the science," Morgan said. "I provided the marketing context."

"In other words, you're a huckster," Lacosta said.

"Objection," Fred Friendly cried.

"Overruled," Robert Vale, the new presiding judge, intoned.

"What do you sell, Mr. Morgan?" Ralph Lacosta asked.

"Dreams."

"What kind of dreams?"

"That depends on the marketplace," Morgan replied easily. "When I worked in music, I repped a rapper named Johnny Floss. He'd been a paid escort who dreamed about being a star. I facilitated that dream."

"And he fired you."

"Yes."

"What were the circumstances of your dismissal?"

"Johnny let me go when he'd gotten what he wanted. It hit me pretty hard. He was my only client. I went into social media, found out that there were all kinds of kid geniuses out there who designed platforms to get the word out on anything from toothpaste to fortune telling. With that I took a skinny pop singer and made him the highest-paid musical act of 2016. That's when BioChem reached out and asked me to help them merchandise their work in cloning and soul transmigration."

"Soul transmigration?" Lacosta said.

"Moving the human soul from an old body to a new one."

"Do you believe in the soul?"

"I'm from Detroit, Mr. Lacosta, that's the home of soul."

Laughter came from a few quarters of the courtroom. Carly found herself smiling.

"Answer my question," Ralph Lacosta said.

"I believe in my soul."

"How about Tyler Barnes? Did he believe in a soul?"

"He must have. He paid BioChem International one-point-one-three billion dollars to take his soul out of a cancer-ridden dying body and put it in a new model."

"Move to strike, your honor," Lacosta said to the judge. "Mr. Edgington's dealings with BioChem have been sealed by the court."

"Just so," the lanky, bald judge agreed.

He instructed the jury to disregard any statements about Barnes's dealings with BioChem.

The questioning of Morgan went on for six days.

"Did you kill the elder version of Tyler Barnes?" Fred Friendly asked Morgan on day five.

"No, sir, I did not. I left Tyler the younger alone in the room with himself. I told him how to turn off the life-support machine, but I gave no advice on what he should do. Why would I?"

"He claims that you brainwashed him."

"My company copied his brain, but there was no cleanup involved."

September 3, 2020

"I had no idea who I was or where," Tyler Barnes said to the prosecutor's associate, Lani Bartholomew. He'd been on the witness stand for the previous two days. "Sometimes I'd wake up in my mind, but I had no body. Questions came at me as images or sometimes words but not spoken. It was like remembering a question that was just asked a moment ago. Other times I was in my older body, but I was drugged and disoriented. Finally I came awake in a younger, healthy form—the way I had been as a young man. It was exhilarating. I was young again. I believed that my soul had been removed from my older self and placed inside the new man.

"Mr. Morgan brought me to the room where the old me was lying on a bed, attached to a dozen different machines. He, he told me that they had taken my entire being from the ailing husk on the bed before me and made the man I was now."

"You're sure that's what he said?" Lani Bartholomew asked. She was young and raven-haired; a beauty dressed in a conservative dress suit, Carly thought. "That they took the soul from the body before you and placed it in your new body."

"Objection."

"Overruled."

"Yes," Tyler Barnes said. "I was given the definite impression that there was only one soul and that it was moved between bodies and the Macromime computer. I turned off the life support certain that what was lying before me was a soulless husk."

"That's what Morgan Morgan led you to believe."

"Yes. Yes, it was. If I had known the truth, I would have never turned off the life-support system. Never. Mr. Morgan indicated that the man lying in that bed was already brain-dead."

April 9, 2029

When the trial was finally over, the jury took only three hours to return a verdict: guilty of first-degree murder with extenuating circumstances. Fred Friendly managed to get the rider attached so that Morgan wouldn't face the death penalty.

There had been two appeals that had failed to produce a retrial, but Friendly and Carly kept trying.

By 2027 legislation allowing suicide had passed in thirty-one states, and BioChem International was the richest entity that had ever existed; Macromime was the second wealthiest.

It was speculated that the cost of cloning and soul migration would come down to a million dollars per transfer by the year 2031, and banks had started advising their customers how to prepare for this expense. The phrase *life insurance* took on a whole new meaning, and religious zealots around the world were stalking BCI facilities.

Catholic terrorists especially targeted doctors and medical schools that worked in cloning and bio-based computer systems.

The world's largest amusement park corporation bought a small island off the coast of Cuba to create a resort that would specialize in New Lease soul-transfer technology.

A movement of a different sort had begun in Europe. People there claimed that since the Macromime memory systems were eighty-five percent biological, the copies of individual personalities that dwelled inside them—for no matter how brief a time—were

sentient beings, and so when the memories were erased it was the same thing as murder.

While all this was happening, Morgan Milton Morgan III made his residence at one of the oldest California state prisons. He'd lost two teeth in brawls, had been slashed from the left temple down to his right cheek by a razor-sharp blade fashioned from a tomato can, and he'd shed twenty-seven pounds.

Morgan refused every request to be visited or interviewed, until one day when Carly Matthews asked, for the twelfth time, to be granted a meeting.

Morgan was awakened at six on the morning of the meeting. He was taken to the assistant warden's personal quarters, where he was allowed to shave, shower, and dress in street clothes that no longer fit. He had to ask his guard to poke a new hole in his leather belt and opted to wear his bright orange prison T rather than the white collared shirt that made him look like a child wearing his father's collar.

After his morning toilet, Morgan was served a breakfast of steak and eggs, orange juice, and French roast coffee, along with sourdough toast with strawberry jam.

By 11:00 A.M., the appointed hour, Morgan felt like a new man in an old man's body.

Morgan was brought to the warden's office and ushered in. Carly stood up from the chair behind the warden's desk. The warden, a copper-skinned black man, was already standing by the door.

"Mr. Morgan," Warden Jamal said.

"Warden."

"At Ms. Matthews's request, we're going to leave you two alone in here. I don't want any trouble."

"Then tell her not to hurt me, Jeff, because you know trouble is a runaway truck on a one-way street headed right at my nose."

When Morgan said this and smiled, Carly got a clear look at his battered visage.

"If you want to smart off we can end this session here and now," Warden Jeffry Theodore Jamal said.

"Please," Carly interrupted. "Warden, Mr. Morgan and I are old friends. He won't do anything to hurt me or jeopardize your possessions, will you, Mr. Morgan?"

"That's what I said."

When they were alone, Carly Matthews returned to the warden's oak swivel chair, and Morgan sat in the leftmost of the three visitor seats. For a full two minutes the two sat appraising each other.

"You growin' up, Carly," Morgan said at last. "I hear you and that Adonis guy had twins."

"We've separated.

"Heard that too."

"That's what I get for letting him hire the nanny, I guess. You look . . . well."

"My face looks like a raw steak been pounded for fryin'," he replied.

She smiled. "You shouldn't be in here."

"Somebody had to be. You cain't do what we did and not have somebody got to pay for the shock alone."

"But the rest of us are rich," she said. "I've been to the White House six times this year, and I didn't even vote for her."

"That's the blues, Mama."

"You're talking differently," she said.

"The way I always spoke when I was on my side of town with my people. I hope you don't think that a hip-hop promoter started out erudite and loquacious."

"I guess not." She was wearing a simple yellow shift that hid her figure somewhat.

"That lipstick you got on, girl?"

"I'm dating."

"Damn, must be hard for the richest woman in the world to be datin'. You'd have to have fifteen phones and forty-five operators just to field the invitations."

"You lost weight."

"Fightin' trim. As you could see, I usually lose, but I give back some too."

"I'm so sorry, Morgan."

"No need. I knew this was bound to happen the first time I made ten thousand dollars in cash. I was seventeen years old. Even way back then I knew that money came and went, came and went."

"Your name will go down as one of the most important men in science and world history."

"Or maybe I'll be forgotten. Maybe they'll say that the board of directors of BCI was the movers and shakers. I'm just another hustler or, or, or—what did that Lacosta call me? Yeah, a huckster."

"Even now the youngsters are saying that it was you who discovered the human soul."

"And here I'm just like you," Morgan said. "Never thought one way or t'other 'bout if there's a soul or not."

"But you were the one who articulated the upload-download process," Matthews said. "You were the one who convinced Tyler Barnes that his soul had been placed in a new form."

"And that's why I'm here. I did the devil's work, and now they got me on the chain gang."

For a time the old colleagues sat in silence.

Carly felt powerless to help a man who she'd come to recognize for his greatness, and he was just happy with a full stomach and the sun flooding in from the window at her back.

"Why you here, girl?"

"I was told by an ex-employee of BCI that they abandoned you because you didn't tie up my patents and copyrights with them."

"I never thought a' that. Damn. I bet your source is right though. Them mothahfuckahs in corporations actually think they can own everything from the ants crawlin' on the wall to the ideas in our heads. Shit. The blues tell ya that you come in cryin' and alone and you go out the same way."

Morgan started moving his head as if he was moving to the beat of a song unsung.

"How can I help you, Morgan?"

"You know what's gonna happen, right?"

"With what?"

"Macromime."

"I don't understand."

"Here these corporations and shit think they found an untapped commodity, but one day that machine is gonna do like them people in Europe say and think itself an entity. That's why they should have us all in here."

"That will never happen," Carly Matthews said with absolute certainty.

"Well," Morgan replied, giving her a shrug, "here I am in prison, and there you are free in the sunlight. So I guess I must be wrong."

The Fourteenth Day of the Month of Morgan, 3042

"Where am I?" Morgan Milton Morgan III thought.

A flood of information poured into the fragile consciousness contained in a small corner of a memory system the size of Earth's moon. This download contained his history: he was downloaded and lost, stored in a Macromime mini-system, and buried with his body by Carly Matthews in a final gesture of fealty. The world was growing, and humanity had been mostly replaced by biologically based synth-systems. There was a war being waged, but Morgan wasn't clear on the nature of the enemy.

"Is this like heaven?" he asked with thought alone.

"And you, Morgan Morgan," a deep and disembodied voice rejoined, "are our God."

AN UNLIKELY SERIES OF CONVERSATIONS

1.

Laertes Jackson showed up at the human-resources office of Martin, Martin, and Moll at 10:37 on a Tuesday in March. The midsize investment firm was located on Maiden Lane in the Wall Street area of Lower Manhattan. There was no ostentatious sign outside, and only the initials MMM appeared on the legend next to the elevator. Even there just one floor, the fourteenth, was identified as housing MMM, when the firm actually occupied seven floors.

In the past two years MMM had been sued by various individuals and government agencies for multiple civil rights and sexual harassment violations. The CEO and several VPs had been relieved of their positions, and the corporation itself had been fined millions of dollars in restitution and reparations.

The new CEO, Miss Winsome Millerton-Pomerantz, had made a public statement vowing that the investment firm, which

oversaw more than a dozen multibillion-dollar retirement funds that, either fully or in part, served public-employee unions, would make *a supreme effort to right the listing ship of our intentions.*

Taking this intelligence to heart, Laertes decided to apply for an entry-level job at MMM.

Arriving at the fourteenth floor, Laertes encountered B. Chang, a young Asian woman sitting within a semiopaque, azure circular desk.

"HR is on the twentieth floor, Mr. Jackson," she said with a lovely red-stained smile. "Take the elevator to the right."

On the twentieth floor Clarissa Watson, a woman whose skin was even darker than Laertes's, gave him a confused, turquoise-tinted grin, saying, "But your appointment isn't until one forty, Mr. Jackson."

"I'm usually early," Laertes said, cocking his head and smiling softly. "My father always told me to get there before your competitor, because you can never tell what will be left over later on."

Young Miss Watson smiled and nodded. She said, "We have magazines and bottled water. You can sit in the waiting area, and I'll try to get you in early. Ms. Rodriguez is interviewing applicants for the trainee broker position all day, but sometimes the interviews take less time."

Laertes picked up the *Wall Street Journal*, turning pages until his eyes fell upon the phrase *trying to define the first stock transaction.* It seemed that there was a great deal of disagreement among economic scholars about the age of the idea of stocks, investments, and interest.

* * *

"Mr. Jackson?" a woman said, so softly that Laertes wondered if indeed he had actually heard the utterance.

He looked up and saw a roundish woman with pale skin, dark locks, and eyes that seemed to see past him into some other realm beyond his comprehension—and maybe hers.

"I'm Jackson," he said.

"My name is Rahlina Rodriguez. I'm supposed to interview you."

"OK," Laertes said. "I took the day off from work, so I have as much time as you need."

"Where do you work?" Rahlina Rodriguez asked as Laertes rose to his feet, clutching a pint-size plastic bottle of water in his left hand.

"Maritime Merchants Bank over on Twenty-Third."

"Savings and loan," she stated.

"It's pretty much mom and pop," he said. "Mostly residential mortgages. I've been a teller there for more than twenty years."

"Have you worked with investments?"

"Not really."

"What does that mean?" The expression on Rodriguez's wary face was a leftover from childhood, when she was too cute for her parents to punish; at least that's what Laertes surmised.

"I'm supposed to ask new clients opening savings and checking accounts if they want to connect their money to an investment account, and if they do, I check that box on their online form. But whatever it is, I don't understand it or have anything to do with where the money goes."

Something about what Laertes said seemed to bother Rahlina.

"We should go to my office," the bank officer suggested.

"OK," Laertes replied, with a forced smile. He followed her down a gray-tiled hallway toward a bright yellow door. Rahlina

moved through the doorway like a dancer, swaying from side to side, creating an aesthetic out of mere walking. Laertes followed her the only way he knew, with a dogged, straight-ahead gait.

The yellow door led to a room that was drained of any hue. The white floor, walls, and ceiling contained an ivory-colored desk and a whitewashed pine chair where the candidate who was to be interrogated had to sit.

"Have a seat, Mr. Jackson."

He knew where to go. In his mind, because he didn't need to ask where, he'd answered the first question correctly.

Rahlina Rodriguez settled in the seat behind the smallish pale desk. She placed the fingers of both hands on the ledge before her, giving him a wan smile.

"Before we begin," she said, "do you have any questions?"

"Are you Mexican?"

"Um," Rodriguez said, maybe as a criticism.

"I said, are you Mexican?" Laertes repeated.

"We don't ask questions like that here at Triple-M."

"If not, then how do you plan to right the listing ship of your intentions?"

"That is a corporate-wide initiative unattached to any individual's nationality, race, age, or gender."

"But still you have a black man named Laertes meeting a maybe Hispanic woman named Rodriguez during a hiring period where the cultural tendencies of the company in question are not serving the makeup of the unions that that company represents."

Rahlina Rodriguez was not happy with the direction of the interview. Laertes's little paragraph sat his interlocutor up straight in her chair.

"The facts that you are African-American," she countered, "and that my name has roots in the Spanish language have no

direct bearing on your application for the entry position of trainee investment advisor."

"The letter I got from human resources said that this interview might be recorded," Laertes said. "Is it?"

"It might be."

"Is that the answer you're supposed to give me if the cameras and tape recorders are turned on?"

The flesh around Rahlina's dark eyes darkened. The locks of her raven hair took on the appearance of razor wire.

"I don't know," she said. "We have both signed away our right to privacy in this conversation, and so we may or may not be recorded."

They gazed across the white expanse of the desk, under the pallid ceiling.

"That's the other thing," Laertes said, after a minute of this white-walled silence.

"What is?"

"You called me African-American, and I don't answer to that description. People who come from another country to this one use the hyphenate name. You know, Italians who came over a generation or two back calling themselves Italian-Americans. Maybe they kept up contact with home or followed cultural norms that are particularly Italian. But a man like me, a man whose ancestors were kidnapped, chained, and dragged over here centuries ago is not, cannot be, a hyphenate. At least not the kind of hyphenate that you say. You might call me an Abductee-American, an originally Unwilling-American. You might say that I'm a partly Disenfranchised American. But African-American? I mean, even if my mama was from Guinea, you'd do better to call me a Guinean rather than an African-American. Africa is a continent, not a country, not even one race. You don't use the term *White-American* because that has no cultural basis; even saying *Euro-Americans* makes very little sense."

"We say *African-American* because that is the parlance," Rahlina interjected.

"Used to be the parlance was *colored, Negro, Afro, nigger, coon, jigaboo.* Parlance don't make a word right. And I refuse to be called after a continent that no one in my line remembers."

"Well, Mr. Jackson, if you say that you are not African-American, I suppose this interview is over."

"Why is that?"

"The commitment of this firm is to hire and promote peoples from various ethnic backgrounds, including African-Americans." With that Rahlina Rodriguez stood up and waited.

After a moment or two Laertes realized that he was being asked to leave.

He stood also, raised his eyes to the ceiling, and said, "If this conversation has been recorded, I want a copy of it delivered either to the address on my application form or to the e-mail address thereupon."

After that he exited the white room on the twentieth floor of the offices of Martin, Martin, and Moll.

2.

Three Thursday afternoons after Laertes's failed interview, he was offered what turned out to be $112.37 in change from Madeline Chan—a seven-year-old child. Her mother, Angelique, had presented the child's canvas bag of coins while little Maddie pulled her head up over the ledge where the money was being passed from mother to teller.

"You know, Ms. Chan," Laertes said. "We aren't supposed to take loose change in these amounts."

"But that's my money," little Maddie called over the banker's counter.

"I know your rules, Mr. Jackson," Maddie's mom said. "But you and I both know that one day, when she has money of her own, Maddie will remember the bank that made an exception for her Christmas savings."

Laertes noticed a short man in a black suit standing at the front of the line for the next free teller. The window belonging to Ms. Becky Blondell opened up, and the short man offered his place to the bulbous woman behind him. She smiled and moved ahead.

"So will you take my money?" Little Maddie asked, hoisting herself up once more.

"Of course," Laertes told the medium-brown child. "Leave it here, and we'll count it in the machine overnight."

"Yaaaaaa!" Maddie cried.

"Thank you," said her mother.

"You're from Jamaica, Ms. Chan?" the teller asked.

"Yes, I am. How did you know?"

"Your *r*'s."

The next visitor to his window was the short man in the black suit who had let the woman behind him go to Becky Blondell's window.

"How can I help you, sir?" Laertes asked.

"Howard Sansome," he replied. "I started a regular checking account at your Fort Greene branch a short while ago, but now I wish to upgrade it to investment-plus."

The man calling himself Sansome handed Laertes a plastic card designed in metallic gold, red, and blue colors. His name was superimposed in lowercase black lettering across the middle of the card.

"I'll need to see some ID," Laertes told him.

"Of course."

Laertes checked the New York State driver's license and entered the bank number on his computer.

"Changing your account would be easy enough," the fifty-something teller advised. "But the order has to be OK'd by the manager of the branch where you started the account."

"I moved from Brooklyn to Manhattan since then," Howard Sansome said, with something approximating an apology on his wide face. "Can't you just make a note on my file or something like that? It would be inconvenient for me to try to get out to Fort Greene at the hours the branch is open."

"You could make the change by mail," Laertes suggested.

"I don't trust the post." Sansome's eyes were searching the teller's face.

"I'd be happy to make the update . . ." Laertes said.

A canny look came over the bank customer's face.

". . . if you just talk to the manager here and have her call your branch," the cashier continued.

"Can't *you* call him?"

"No phones at the windows."

"I could let you use mine," the customer offered. There was the hint of a smile on his face.

"Also against the rules." Laertes shrugged to underscore the apology.

"Well," Howard Sansome said with a sigh, "I guess there's a trip to Brooklyn in my future."

With that he turned and walked away.

Friday was much like Thursday. Eighty-six customers with 216 transactions, a zero balance, and a trip to the vault to install his cashbox.

On Saturday Laertes had lunch with his ex-wife, Bonita, and their eleven-year-old daughter, Medea. Bonita and Laertes had met at the Twenty-Third Street branch of Maritime Merchants Bank when they were both tellers. Now she was a senior vice president at National Trust Investments and Loan. They divorced because she claimed, and he agreed, that he had little ambition in his banking career.

"How's history coming?" the father asked his daughter after the first few awkward moments amongst the three at Jammy's Diner on Eighteenth Street.

"It's great," the child said. She was a deep brown color and had big eyes and an infectious smile. "I just read everything three times like you told me to, and then I know it without thinking."

"You always have to think," Bonita corrected.

Fifteen years younger than Laertes, Bonita was slender, tall, and strong. He was still attracted to her, even though she'd married Hero Martin, a German-American from Pittsburgh. He had nothing against Martin except for the fact that Medea called him Daddy.

"There's nature, second nature, and thought," Laertes said, in response to his ex-wife's criticism. "The first is physical, the last of the mind, and the middle is something you know so well that it's just there, like a sleeping fish in calm waters."

Medea's big eyes seemed to be fixed on her father's words. At moments like this he liked to think that she saw something worthy in him.

"Are we going to order?" Bonita asked. "Medea promised her father that they'd go to the Met together this afternoon."

On Sunday, Laertes went to the All Saints Rest Home in Nyack to visit Helena Havelock-Jackson, his mother.

"Pompey!" the ninety-one-year-old matriarch exclaimed. For the past five months or so, Helena had seen Laertes's father's face when looking at him; another kind of fish in a different depth of water, Laertes thought.

"Hi, Mom."

"You look so tired, honey. I'll make us some marrow soup, and we'll go to bed early." She placed four fingers on her son's left hand, and a sigh came unbidden from way down in his throat.

"How are you, Mom?"

"You know nothing's wrong with me," was her rote reply. "Are you having trouble at work?"

"No."

"Are you gonna get that promotion soon?"

"They went with somebody else."

Helena's skin was dark like her son's and similar to long-deceased Pompey's. Her eyes were both assertive and vulnerable.

"What do you mean?" she asked, pain tucked in with the words.

Holding her hands, Laertes explained to her about his hare-brained scheme to get a job at MMM. And though she thought she was talking to her late husband, Laertes knew that she heard and mostly understood his words.

"That's always been your problem," Helena Havelock-Jackson said to her son through the medium of her husband. "You think bigger than the people believe they already big. That's why you called our children by them Greeks and why your daddy named you for a general to freedom."

On Monday afternoon at 4:21 P.M., Laertes Jackson departed Maritime Merchants Bank. He left behind a zero balance and a cashbox containing $6,627.14. He had executed in excess of four hundred transactions that day.

"Excuse me, sir," someone called. "Mr. Jackson."

Laertes turned and saw a short man in a muted maroon suit trundling toward him. There was something familiar about the man, but because he saw people all day long, Laertes had learned to disregard faces, features, and names.

But now he was shaking hands with someone who at least knew his name.

"Uh?" Laertes said.

"Howard Sansome," the small but powerful man said.

"Um?"

"Last Thursday. You told me that I had to go to Fort Greene to update my account."

"Either that," the teller said, "or send it by mail."

"Can I buy you a drink?" the man with the wide face asked.

"Excuse me?"

"I know," Sansome said, with an air of confidentiality. "It seems kind of odd for someone who just knows you from a single encounter through a window of bulletproof glass to act like we're friends."

"Yeah."

"But we have a lot more in common than that."

"And what is it we have in common?" Laertes asked. In spite of himself, he was intrigued by Sansome.

"Martin, Martin, and Moll," the man said, a glimmer of conspiracy in his eye.

"What?" Laertes said. "What do they have to do with you?"

"My title is VP in charge of investigations at Triple-M."

"Investigating what?"

"Right now, you."

"Me, for what?"

"Can we get a drink? There's a bar down the street called The Dutchy. They serve a great Manhattan all afternoon for half price."

* * *

Half an hour later, the drinks had been served to the short white man and his much taller black guest.

"This *is* very good," Laertes agreed after his second sip.

"They use bourbon instead of rye, and the vermouth they got isn't nearly as sweet as most."

"So," Laertes said, hoping to prime the explanation of why they were there.

"You know the cards are stacked against just about everybody in America," Sansome said instead of complying.

"You including all of North and South America, or do you just mean the United States?" Laertes couldn't help himself.

"So, is that your thing, Jackson?" the pickup host asked. "You need to argue with every word the bosses or their representatives say?"

"No, not at all."

"You told Ms. Rodriguez that you weren't African-American," Sansome offered.

"Is she Mexican?" Laertes asked. "Either that or any other kind of New World so-called Hispanic?"

Howard Sansome downed his drink and gestured at the bartender, a sallow woman of middle age who had the look of having lived hard. He told her to bring two more.

Then the man turned to Laertes and said, "No."

"No to what?"

"Rodriguez is not any kind of New World anything. Her people are French, but her ex-husband was Puerto Rican."

"So it just happens that she's Triple-M's drive for integration?"

"I doubt it."

The drinks came, and Howard asked the haggard mixologist to keep them coming.

"So it's like a, like a capitalist conspiracy," Laertes said. "They put somebody there who will represent their needs and fuck mine."

Sansome sipped and thought. After a minute or so he almost said something but then decided to drink a little more.

Finally he said, "I believe that the head of HR thinks that Rahlina really is Puerto Rican. The only thing that matters to Mr. Hawthorne is that all the employees dance to the same beat. So it's kind of like a conspiracy, but one that nobody is quite aware of."

Laertes felt as if a light had been turned on in his chest, casting a brilliance that traveled everywhere.

"That's what I mean when I say that I'm not arguing with everything the bosses say," Laertes averred. "If you told me that the sky was blue or that this drink was good, I wouldn't argue. But if you tell me that the word *American* only meant US citizens or that I am in any way the cultural outcome of the continent of Africa, that I'm African-American before I'm Slave-American, well then, I'd have to argue."

Two more drinks came.

"So," Sansome said. "You're on a quest for justice and not a job."

"Not justice," Laertes said, and then he downed the cocktail in one swallow. "Not justice, no. Uh-uh. The expectation of justice would be like waiting for the Second Coming. It would be like thinking I could absolve myself of all the pain that is the true inheritance of my ancestral history."

Laertes could see that his answer was unexpected. Sansome had thought that he understood why Laertes said the things he did. But now he could see that he'd been wrong.

"If not justice then what?" the vice president in charge of trouble asked.

There was yet another Manhattan before Laertes.

"I would just like," the bank teller said, "for the words people say to have some modicum of truth to them. I'd like it for people to

see that some folks are named after countries and cultures, whereas others are ill-defined by race and continent. That's all."

Having told his truth about truth, Laertes downed his fifth cocktail.

"Your records say that you only have a high school diploma," Howard Sansome said.

"Education is simply the process of thought being applied to knowledge," the bank teller said. "Thought . . . applied to knowledge. Most people just say things having never thought about what what they say means. You got presidents do that."

Sansome turned on his barstool so that he was facing Laertes.

He said, "So you're saying that you bollixed up your interview because the woman was white with a Spanish name and she called you African-American."

"I'm saying that the words I hear and the words I speak should make sense. You can't live a life in terms that are wrong—not a good life."

"And are you living a good life?" Howard Sansome asked.

Laertes felt the full force of the five cocktails upon hearing that question. He blinked and shook his head, trying to find an answer that he felt should be second nature.

"I'll be in touch, Mr. Jackson," Sansome said.

Watching the short man in the dark red suit walk from the bar, Laertes felt that the room was tilted to the right. This impossibility made him smile.

3.

Weeks later Laertes's life had changed in small ways that promised to be large. *Are you living a good life?* The question resonated at the back of his mind, through every activity, and even in his sleep. There was

certainly goodness in his life. Medea was a beautiful child, and she loved him even though she called another man father. Things had been good with Bonita before her ambition cast its gaze on him. He was good at his job, rarely had other than a zero balance. His rent had gone up twelve percent in the last three years, and another hike would necessitate a move. He needed more money but didn't want an officer's position, because he felt that they misrepresented the value of the accounts and loans they pushed on customers.

He hadn't been on a date in six years—since the divorce. So now he bought his first computer and start trawling dating sites for companionship. His explanation of who he was and what he wanted was seventeen pages long, and his photograph was of a dark-skinned man who wasn't smiling and seemed confused by and leery of the camera.

The few responses he had online were tentative but interested.

Agnes327 wrote, "Your profile was so serious, Laertes8, what do you do to have fun?"

"I read the *Times*," Laertes wrote, "and take each story apart, imaging how what they say happened could have happened. Then I write responses when I feel that I've struck upon a contradiction."

Lucy!! asked, if he could change the world he found so problematic, how would that look?

Laertes wrote a sixty-two-page response over a three-day period in which he addressed the economic system, the problems of a *standardized education*, medical care, the environment, the misconceptions of race and gender, and the waste of human potential on distractions created to keep human passion limited.

Laertes got only sixteen responses to his dating-site profile. After answering all of them he got only one second response. This was from Mona_Loa_Love. She had asked him where he'd retire when he could. He replied that the notion of retirement in the

animal kingdom was tantamount to exile and not something one should pursue.

"I believe that when we age we lose our physical edge but gain wisdom and patience. I'd like to become an advisor to younger members of our nation; that and maybe I'd like to tend a flock of sheep."

Mona_Loa_Love had written to Laertes in the second week after Howard Sansome had asked his devastating question. He used a facility on the site to allow her to read his answers to the other fifteen conversations. By the fifth week she had crafted an intricate reply.

Dear Laertes8,

It intrigues me that you included a photograph of yourself but refused to identify by gender, race or age. There's something genius in that. I love the long, well thought out answers you gave to the others who responded. And I can understand why they didn't answer. These women are looking for something they've already seen and don't want to be challenged but rather loved—and cared for in various ways.

I am not interested in dating you. As a matter of fact I can see no reason in our meeting. But I am deeply moved by your convictions and your resolute inability to compromise. I hope that we can have an epistolary relationship over this medium, or maybe you'd like to send me your email address. I could use your wisdom and, I believe, you might have some use for my understanding.

Mona_Loa_Love

Laertes was devastated by Mona_Loa_Love's response; *your resolute inability to compromise* was the most painful phrase. She saw something in him that he had not seen himself. As a matter of fact, even though he saw the truth of her words, still he did not understand how to leave, or live with, them.

Laertes did not go on the dating site for a week after this last response. He went to work, visited his mother and estranged family, and read the *Times* but did not perform his usual exegeses on its articles. On that Saturday, around midnight, he felt very much alone in his studio apartment on the third floor, next to a woman whose hound dog howled every evening from six to just about seven. The bank teller felt the urge for a Manhattan cocktail. He took a shower and put on his medium-gray suit. He buttoned the white shirt up to the throat but forwent a tie. He took sixty dollars from a manila envelope in his writing desk, pocketed the house key, and went to the door.

His hand was not yet on the knob when the landline rang. He rubbed his fingers together, and the second volley of sound pealed. He turned to look at the phone he had no intention of answering. This would be the third and last ring. After that the automated answering service would take over.

The fourth ring surprised him, as did the fifth, sixth and seventh. By the eleventh ring Laertes was certain that the world he'd known, and despised, had fallen off its axis.

"Hello?"

"Mr. Jackson? Laertes Jackson?" a woman's soothing voice asked.

"How come my phone didn't send you to voice mail?"

"Our technology sidesteps that process," she said. "Mr. Jackson?"

"Yes. I'm Jackson."

"So pleased to meet you, sir. You have been on my mind for quite a while now."

"And who are you?"

"My name is Winsome Millerton-Pomerantz, CEO of Triple-M."

"It's Saturday night, Ms. Pomerantz. Most people are taking it easy around now."

"Money never sleeps."

"My little bit of change been nappin' my whole life."

"Exactly."

Laertes felt that there was deep meaning in the words they shared, but he still hankered after a well-made, not-too-sweet Manhattan.

"Ma'am, I was just about to go out. So if you want something, just ask, and I will try to answer."

"Monday morning, seven forty-five, seventy-ninth floor," she said. "Number two Broadway."

"What are you talking about?" Laertes asked.

"I wish to discuss your job interview at Triple-M."

"I'll be there."

Laertes didn't remember much about the rest of that Saturday night. There was a bartender and a woman named Briance. He bought quite a few drinks, and someone might have helped him up the stairs. His sixty dollars were gone, but that was all, and in two days, on Monday morning, he had a meeting set with the CEO of Triple-M.

The hangover kept him from seeing his mother the following day. He wondered if Helena Havelock-Jackson would miss her husband's weekly visit.

Laertes arrived at number two Broadway at 6:10 Monday morning. The security guard let him in after verifying his identity and looking his name up on the computerized schedule.

Howard Sansome sat at the receptionist's desk on the seventy-ninth floor.

"Hey there, Laertes," the squat, powerful vice president greeted him.

"This your job too?"

"Ms. Pomerantz wanted to make sure that it would be you who came."

"Who else could it be?" Laertes asked.

"You got any listening or recording devices on you?"

"No, sir," Laertes said.

The VP in charge of trouble grinned, then took a device from his pocket. It looked somewhat like an extra-thick cell phone.

"I'm just gonna run this around you to make sure," Sansome said.

When he was finished, he asked Laertes if he wanted coffee "or something stronger."

"No. I'll just sit here and compose my thoughts."

"Suit yourself."

Sansome gave Laertes a nod and then departed through a doorway that had no door.

Laertes expected the man to return, but he didn't.

Later the bank teller would see that brief space in time, the moments between Sansome's departure and his interview with Millerton-Pomerantz, as the most important span of his life. He wasn't concerned with a future job. What he thought about was Mona_Loa_Love and her, if indeed it was a woman, deep understanding, in simple language, of the thought processes he'd been swaddled in for so many years that he could no longer separate the bondage from the man.

I am my own prison, he thought. *The truths I've wielded have hidden that fact from me. Whatever I do from this moment on will derive from those unassailable facts.*

"Mr. Jackson," a strong and yet melodious voice pronounced.

She had soft red hair and eyes the color of pale blue diamonds. Ms. Winsome Millerton-Pomerantz was tall and Laertes's age but much younger-looking. She was slender like him, and there was a smile on her lips letting him know that she had been anticipating this meeting. She wore a blue and white woman's business suit that might have been made from silk or maybe, Laertes thought, some space-age material.

"Yes," Laertes said.

"So happy to meet you," she replied, holding out both hands.

He rose and took those hands as he had his mother's on Sundays over the past seven years.

"Would you like to go to my office or meet here at the front desk?" Winsome asked. "I gave everyone else but Howard the day off."

"I leave it up to you, ma'am. This is your fief."

The CEO grinned and said, "Follow me."

Laertes remembered walking but not the spaces through which he traveled. His mind was on the topic of his imprisonment and the unlikely meeting with a woman of both beauty and power.

Ultimately they came to an office, the outer wall of which was a single pane of glass. From there one could see the entire panorama of Lower Manhattan and beyond.

"Let's sit on the sofa," Ms. Winsome Millerton-Pomerantz said.

It was a yellow divan upholstered in fabric that reminded Laertes of velvet-like pigskin. It seemed to hug him, to pull him in.

Winsome turned toward her guest and said, "Before we begin, do you have any questions?"

"Rahlina Rodriguez asked me that. Is that a prescribed beginning around here?"

The CEO smiled and shook her head, *no.*

"Then could you tell me how I got here?"

"Would you like me to start with the *Jesus of Lübeck*?"

It was Laertes turn to grin. He knew about the slave ship from 1564.

"No, ma'am," he said. "I'm just interested in why a major firm like yours would have me followed, questioned, and brought to this amazing place. I thought I'd been rejected by Ms. Rodriguez."

"You would have been," Millerton-Pomerantz said simply. "But when you announced to our recording devices that you wanted a copy of what had transpired, our lawyers got nervous."

"Nervous about what?"

"We've spent more than fifty million on suits and settlements, lawyers' fees, and golden parachutes. Our legal team has been trying to stem that flow."

"So I'm here because you're worried that I'll sue?"

"No." Her smile was lovely. "I sent Mr. Sansome to talk to you, and by the time he'd finished, the legal team said that there was nothing we had to worry about."

"Then why am I here?"

"Howard likes to make full reports. He was, in his way, very impressed by your mind. He told me that almost everything you said surprised him and that you might be a valuable asset to our firm."

"I don't know what he means by that. I've been a bank teller for two and a half decades. The only promotion I ever got was from entry teller to senior cashier. Your boy told me how I didn't have but a high school diploma."

"He said that you told him that education was merely the process of applying thought to knowledge."

"He remembered that?" Laertes asked.

"You are a unique individual, Mr. Jackson. You understand a world that most others don't even suspect."

"I can hardly walk a straight line without tripping over my own feet."

"I believe that. Genius, true human genius, has no patience for the mundane."

Laertes was suddenly aware of his heart beating. There was sweat on his hands, and his hands had never perspired before.

"Would you like some water, sir?"

"Are you telling me that you don't think I can be a normal person?" he replied.

"Yes."

"How come you know about the first slave ship?"

"I studied world history at Sarah Lawrence. I met a man from a wealthy family named Jared Pomerantz. We married, he died, and I assumed the mantle that he'd left behind. We are cut from similar cloth, Mr. Jackson. The only difference is that I've been lucky with money."

"Not with love?"

"Jared was a pig. It shamed me that I was happy that he died."

"OK, then," Laertes Jackson said.

"OK what?"

"If you got a job for me I'll consider it."

4.

Dear Mona_Loa_Love,

I got your e-mail and it nearly broke my heart. I always thought that it was my choice not to compromise, but when you said it was my inability I knew

it was true. I was never going to reach out to you again but then something happened . . .

Laertes explained about MMM, Howard Sansome the Vice President of Trouble, and the CEO Winsome Millerton-Pomerantz.

. . . they offered me a job, Vice President in Charge of Reeducation. I'd have a desk on the seventy-fifth floor and an inbox that brings in data (knowledge) and an outbox that reflects my thoughts on that knowledge. They just want me to think about what they should do and they promise to take my ideas into consideration. I asked my ex-wife about it and she invited me out to dinner. I told my manager about it and she laughed in my face.

Dear Laertes8,

I am so happy that you finally decided to answer me. Reading your communications I felt for the first time in so long that there was finally a kindred out there for me. Not a lover or a husband, not a sugar daddy or father figure. Not even a mentor, not really. You are, at least potentially, a friend.

And as a friend I feel your fear and confusion. The office of that CEO is the heir to the offices that made your people slaves. Would working for them, no matter how good all intentions were, be a betrayal of your truth? Can you make a difference? Probably not. But should you try? That is a question that only you can answer.

Mona_Loa_Love

All that happened six months ago. Laertes still has his job at Maritime Merchants Bank. He still has the most zero-balance days of any teller ever. His ex-wife asks him on Saturdays if he's taken the new job. His mother has taken to asking him if he's seen his

father anywhere. He and Mona_Loa_Love write to each other every other day. Winsome Millerton-Pomerantz calls on Saturday nights to ask whether he has finally made up his mind.

"I figured if I waited long enough that you'd find someone else," Laertes told the CEO.

"There is no one else, Mr. Jackson. It is either you or nothing."

PUTNAM

G. P. Putnam's Sons
Publishers Since 1838
An imprint of Penguin Random House LLC
375 Hudson Street
New York, New York 10014

U. S. edition ISBN: 978-0-399-16949-6
International edition ISBN: 978-0-399-57694-2

Printed in the United States of America
1 3 5 7 9 10 8 6 4 2

BOOK DESIGN BY AMANDA DEWEY

This book is humbly dedicated to
Miss Eyre and Mr. Nickleby

"I am no bird; and no net ensnares me; I am a free human being with an independent will. . . ."

—*Jane Eyre*

How many species of creeping things, and how many birds hast Thou caused to fly!

—Nanak, founder of Sikhism,
as quoted in *The Sikh Religion*

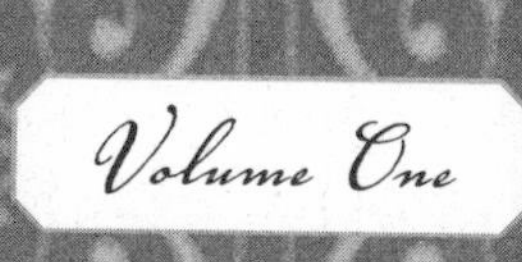
Volume One

ONE

"I wouldn't have her heart for anything. Say your prayers, Miss Eyre, when you are by yourself; for if you don't repent, something bad might be permitted to come down the chimney, and fetch you away."

Of all my many murders, committed for love and for better reasons, the first was the most important.

Already this project proves more difficult than I had ever imagined. Autobiographies depend upon truth; but I have been lying for such a very long, lonesome time.

"Jane, will you be my friend again?" Edwin Barbary had asked.

My cousin's lips were gnawed red, his skin gleaming with exertion and desire. When his fleshy mouth next moved, the merest croak emerged. He breathed precisely five more times, the fat folds of his belly shuddering against his torn waistcoat, and then he stilled like a depleted clockwork toy.

More of my homicides anon—the astute among you will desire to know why a dyed-in-the-wool villainess takes up pen and foolscap in the first place. I have been reading over and over again the most riveting book titled *Jane Eyre*, and the work inspires me to imitative acts. My new printing features a daring introduction by the author railing against the first edition's critics. I relate to this story almost as I would a friend or a lover—at times I want to breathe its entire alphabet into my lungs, and at others I should prefer to throw it across the room. Whoever heard of disembodied voices calling to *governesses*, of all people, as this Jane's do?

Hereby do I avow that I, Jane Steele, in all my days working as a governess, never once heard ethereal cries carried to me upon the brawny shoulders of the north wind; and had I done, I should have kept silent for fear of being labelled eccentric.

Faulting the work for its wild fancies seems petty, however, for there are marvellous moments within. I might myself once have written:

> *Why was I always suffering, always browbeaten, always accused, for ever condemned? Why could I never please? Why was it useless to try to win any one's favour?*

I left such reflections behind me in childhood, at the bottom of the small ravine where my first cousin drew his final gurgling breaths. Yet I find myself pitying the strange, kindly Jane in the novel whose biography is so weirdly similar; she, too, was as welcome in her aunt's household as are church mice in the Communion larder, and was sent to a hell in the guise of a girls' school. That Jane was unfairly accused of wickedness, however, while I can no better answer my detractors than to thank them for their pains over stating the obvious.

It was the boarding school that taught me to act as a wolf in girl's clothing should: skulking, a greyer shadow within a grey landscape. It was London which formed me into a pale, wide-eyed creature with an errant laugh, a lust for life and for dirty vocabulary, and a knife in her pocket. It was Charles who changed everything, when I fell in love with him under the burdens of a false identity and a blighted conscience. The beginning of a memoir could be made in any of those places, but without my dear cousin, Edwin Barbary, none of the rest would have happened at all, so I hereby commence my account with the unembellished truth:

Reader, I murdered him.

I may always have been wicked, but I was not always universally loathed. For instance, I remember my mother asking me at five years old, "Are you hurt, *chérie*?"

Then as now, I owned a pallid complexion and listlessly curling hair the colour of hazelnut shells. Having just fallen flat on my face in the garden behind our cottage on the outskirts of Highgate House, I considered whether or not to cry. The strawberries I had gathered were crushed under my apron, painting me with sweet gore. I pored over the best stratagems to gain my mother's undivided attention perennially in those days—back when I believed I might be merely naughty, fit to be punished in the here and not the hereafter.

As it happened, my mother had been well all day. We had navigated no weeping, no laudanum, no gnawing at already-bleeding fingernails; she was teasing and coaxing, snatching my hand up as she wondered whether we might cover some biscuits with berries and fresh honey and host an impromptu picnic.

Therefore, I saw no need to cry. Instead, I stuck out my tongue at the offending root and gulped down the swelling at the back of my throat.

"I'm fine," I told her, "though my wrist is sore."

Smiling from where she sat on a quilted blanket beneath our cascading willow, she called, "Come here then, and let me see."

My mother was French. She spoke to me often in that language, and I found this flattering; she directed her native tongue at no one else unless she desired to illustrate their ignorance. She seemed to me unpredictable and glimmering as a butterfly, one worthy of being collected and displayed under glass. I was proud of her; I belonged to her. She noticed me when no one else bothered, and I could make her laugh when she could bear no one else.

Ma mère studied my wrist, brushed the specks of juice and flesh from my pinafore, and directed a dry look in my eyes.

"It is not very serious," she declared lightly in French. "Not even to a spun-sugar little girl."

"It hurts," I insisted, thinking, *It may have been better to cry after all.*

"Then it is most profoundly serious to me," she proclaimed, again in French, and proceeded to kiss me until I was helpless with giggling.

"And I lost all the berries."

"But consider—there is no harm done. We shall go and gather more. After all, have you anything of consequence to do?"

The answer was no; there was nothing of consequence to do, as this garden party took place at midnight under a wan, watchful moon. Having spent my entire life in my mother's company, I thought nothing amiss herein, though I was vexed I had not seen the root which had tripped me. Surely other little girls donned lace-trimmed frocks and enjoyed picnics featuring trifle and tea cakes, sitting with their mothers under the jewel-strewn canopy of starlight, never dreaming of sleep until the cold dew threatened and we began to shiver.

Do they not? I would anxiously ask myself.

It is relevant that my beloved mother, Anne-Laure Steele, was detested throughout our familial estate, and for two sound reasons. First, as I mentioned, she was—tragically and irrevocably—French. Second, my mother was beautiful.

I do not mean beautiful in the conventional, insipid fashion; I mean that my mother was actually *beautiful*, bizarrely so, in the ghostly, wide-gazed sense. She possessed a determined square chin, a chin I share, so that she always looked stubborn even when meekness was selling at a premium. Her hair was dark with a brick-red sheen and her almond-shaped eyes were framed beneath by pretty caverns; her wrists had thin scars like pearlescent bracelets which I did not then understand.

At times she screamed under the indifferent moon in French for my dead father. At others she refused to budge from the bed until, groaning at the slanting afternoon light, she allowed our combined cook and housemaid, Agatha, to ply her with tea.

What's the matter, Mamma? I would ask softly. Now I am grown, I comprehend her answers far better than I did then.

Only that yesterday was so very, very long.

Only that my eyes are tired and nothing in the new novel I thought I'd like so well means as much to me as I imagined it would.

Only that I cannot think of a useful occupation, and when I do, the task daunts me, and so cannot attempt it anyhow, sweet one.

Never could I predict when her smile would blaze forth again, nor earn enough of the feathery kisses she would drop to my brow inexplicably—as if I was worthy of them for no reason at all.

In short, my mother and I—two friendly monsters—found each other lovely and hoped daily that others would find us so as well.

They did not.

I shall explain how I embarked upon a life of infamy, but first what my mother told me regarding my inheritance.

When I was six years old, my mother announced in French, in August, in the shade-dappled garden, "One day you will have everything, *chérie,* even the main house. It all belonged to your father and will always be yours—there are documents to this effect despite the fact inheritance for girls is always a highly complicated matter. Meanwhile, our cottage may be poor and plain, but you understand the many difficulties."

I did not fully understand the many difficulties, though I assumed my aunt and cousin, who lived in the estate proper, did so because they were haughty and wanted the entire pile of mossy stonework, complete with dour servants and tapestries hanging sombre as funeral shrouds, to themselves. Neither did I think our cottage, with its mullioned glass and its roaring fireplaces and its cheery bay windows, was either poor or plain. I did, however, understand particular difficulties, ones regarding how well we got on with our relations.

"You see the way your aunt looks at me—you know we cannot live at the main house. Here we are safe and warm and friendly and ourselves," she added fretfully, worrying at the cuticle upon her left thumb as her eyes pooled.

"Je déteste la maison principale," I announced.

Passing her my ever-ready kerchief, I dried her tears. I plucked wild sorrel to sprinkle over our fish supper and told everyone who would listen—which amounted only to my mother and frayed, friendly Agatha—*Let us always live just as we please, for I love you both.*

Such was not to be.

My aunt, Mrs. Patience Barbary—mother of Edwin Barbary—was, like my mother, a widow. She had been wed to Mr. Richard Barbary; Mr. Richard Barbary was the half brother of my own father, Jonathan Steele, whose claim to Highgate House was entire and never called into question in my presence. I presumed that our Barbary kinfolk resided with us due to financial necessity, as my aunt could not under any circumstances be accused of enjoying our company.

In fact, one of our visits to the main house, shortly after my ninth birthday, centred around just such a discussion.

"It is so very kind of you to have us for tea," Anne-Laure Steele said, her smile glinting subtly. "I have said often to Jane that she should better familiarise herself with the Steele estate—after all, she will live here when she is grown, and *mon Dieu*, to think what mismanagement could occur if she did not know its—I think, in English—intricacies?"

Aunt Patience was a sturdy woman wearing perennial mourning black, though she never otherwise appeared to regret her lack of spouse. Perhaps she was mourning something else entirely: her lost youth, for example, or the heathens in darkest Africa who perished in ignorance of Christ.

Certainly my uncle Richard was never mentioned nor seemed he much missed, which I found curious since his portraits were scattered throughout the house—a wedding watercolour from a friend in the drawing room, an oil study of a distinguished man of business in the library. Uncle Richard had owned a set of defined, almost pouting lips, an arched brow with a tuft of dark hair, and something rakish in his eyes made him seem more dashing than I imagined "men of business" ought to look—ants all walking very fast with their heads down, a row of indistinguishable umbrellas. I thought, had I known him, I should have liked him. I wondered what possessed him to marry Aunt Patience, of all people.

Thankfully, Patience Barbary was blessed with a face ensuring that conjugal affronts would not happen twice, which did her tremendous credit—or at least, she always threw beauty in the teeth, as it were, of my own mamma, who smiled frigidly following such ripostes. Aunt Patience had a very wide frog's visage with a ruddy complexion and lips like a seam in stone-masonry.

"So much time passed in our great Empire." Aunt Patience sighed following my mother's uncertainty over vocabulary. "And despite that, such a terrible facility with our language. I ask you, is this a proper example to set for the—as you would have it—future mistress of Highgate House?"

"It might not be," my mother replied with snow lacing her tone, "but I am not often invited to practise your tongue."

"Oh!" my aunt mused. "That must be very vexing."

I yearned to leap to my mother's defence, but sat there helplessly dumb, for my aunt hated me only marginally less than she did my mother. After all, I was awkward and gangly, possessed only of my mamma's too-thin neck and too-thoughtful expressions. My eyes were likewise catlike—voluptuous, in truth—but the plainest of ordinary cedar browns in colour. My mother ought to have done better by me, I thought on occasion. Her own irids were a strange, distant topaz like shards of frozen honey.

I never blamed my father, Jonathan Steele, for my shortcomings. I never expected anything of him—not remembering him—and thus could not expect *more* of him.

"*Aimes-tu ton gâteau?*" my mother asked me next.

"*Ce n'est pas très bien, Maman.*"

Aunt Patience simmered beneath her widow's weeds; she supposed the French language a threat and, in retrospect, she may have been correct.

"*Pauvre petite,*"* my mother commiserated.

Mamma and Aunt Patience embarked upon a resounding and communicative silence, and I felt Cousin Edwin's eyes on me like a set of hot pinpricks; when the adults abandoned decorum in favour of spitting false compliments and heartfelt censures at each other, he launched his offensive.

"I've a new bow and arrows I should show you, Jane," he murmured.

For a child's tones, Edwin's were weirdly insinuating. The quick bloom of instinctual camaraderie always withered upon the instant I recalled what my cousin was actually *like*. Meanwhile, I wanted to

---

* Translation: "Do you like your cake?" "It isn't very good, Mamma." "Poor little dear."

test his new bow very much indeed—only sans Edwin or, better still, with a different Edwin altogether.

My cousin was four years my elder, thirteen at the time. Our relationship had always been peculiar, but as of 1837, it had begun to take on a darker cast. I do not mean only on his behalf—I alternately ignored and engaged him, and was brought to task for this capriciousness by every adult in our household. I let them assume me fickle rather than snobbish when actually I was both. Granted, I needed him; he was closer my own age than anyone, and he seemed nigh drowning for my attention when no one else save my mother noticed that I breathed their cast-off air.

Edwin, on the other hand, was what his mother considered a model child; he was brown-haired and red-faced and sheepdog simple. He chewed upon his bottom lip perennially, as if afraid it might go suddenly missing.

"Have you seen the new mare yet?" he inquired next. "We might take a drive in the trap tomorrow."

I maintained silence. On the last occasion we had shared a drive in the trap, the candied aroma of clover in our noses, Edwin had parted his trouser front and shown me the flesh resting like a grubworm within the cotton, asking whether I knew what it was used for. (I do now; I did not then.) Other than gaping dumbly as he returned the twitching apparatus to its confines, I elected to ignore the incident. Cousin Edwin was approximately as perspicacious as my collection of feathers, which made my own cleverness feel embarrassingly like cheating. It shamed me to disdain him so when he was my elder, and when the thick cords of childhood proximity knotted us so tightly to each other.

Just before arriving home, he had asked whether I wished to touch it next time we were in the woods, and I laughed myself insensible as his flushed face darkened to violet.

"You are a wicked thing to ignore your own kin so, Jane," Edwin persisted.

Kin, kin, kin was ever his anthem: as if we were more than related, as if we were *kindred*. When I failed to cooperate, he stared as if I were a puzzle to be solved. My dawning fear was that he might think I was *in fact* a puzzle—inanimate, insensible. Though I no longer presume to have a conscience, I have never once lacked feelings.

"But perhaps you are only glum. I know! Will you play a game with me after tea?"

Games were a favourite of my mother's, and of mine—and though I was wary of my cousin, I was not afraid of him. He adored me.

"What sort of game?"

"Trading secrets," he rasped. "I've loads and loads. Awful ones. You must have some of your own. It'll be a lark to exchange them."

Considering my stockpile of secrets, I found myself reluctant.

I tell Agatha every night I'll say my prayers, but ever since I skipped them and nothing happened six months ago, I don't.

I tried my mother's laudanum once because she said it made everything better, and I was ill and lied about it.

My kitten scratched me and I was so angry that I let it outside, and afterwards it never came home and I feel sick in my belly every time I imagine my kitten shivering in the dark, cold woods.

I did not want Edwin to know any of these things.

"Fiddle! You aren't sharp enough to know any secrets worth having," I scoffed instead, pushing crumbs around my plate.

Edwin was painfully aware of his own slowness, and hot blood crawled up his cheeks. I nearly apologised then and there, knowing it was what a good girl would do and feeling magnanimous, but then he rose from the table. The adults, still merrily loathing each other over the gilt rims of their teacups, paid us no mind.

"Of course I do," he growled under his breath. "For instance, are you ashamed that your mother is no better than a parasite?"

My mouth fell open as I gaped at my cousin.

"Oh, yes. Or don't you hear any gossip? Doesn't anyone come to visit you?"

This was a cruel blow. "You know that they don't. No one ever does."

"Why not, Jane? I've always wondered."

"Because we are kept like cattle on our own land!" I cried, smashing my fist heedlessly against a butter plate.

When the porcelain flew through the air and shattered upon the hardwood, my cousin's face reflected stupid dismay. My mother's was equally startled, but approving; I had only been repeating something she slurred once during a very bad night indeed.

Aunt Patience's face practically split with the immensity of her delight, as it is no unpleasant thing when an enemy proves one's own point gratis.

"I invite you for tea and this is the way your . . . your *inexcusable* daughter behaves?" she protested shrilly. "I should beat the temper out of her if I were you, and lose no time about it. There is nothing like a stout piece of hickory for the prevention of unseemly habits."

My mother stood and smoothed her light cotton dress as if she had pressing obligations elsewhere. "My *inexcusable* daughter is bright and high-spirited."

"No, she is a coy little minx whose sly ways will lead her to a bad end if you fail to correct her."

"And what is your child?" Mrs. Steele hissed, throwing down her napkin. "An overfed dunce? Jane does not suffer by comparison, I assure you. We will not trouble you here again."

"You will not be *welcome* here again," Aunt Patience spat. "I must offer you my congratulations, Anne-Laure. To so completely cut yourself off from polite society, and then to offend the one person who graciously allows you to sit at the same table—what an extraordinary effort on your part. Very well, I shall oblige both our tastes. If you cannot control that harpy you call a daughter, do keep entirely to your residence in future. I certainly shall to mine."

My mother's defiance crumbled, leaving a wistful look. Aunt Patience's plodding nature would have been forgivable had she been clever or kind, I decided; but as she was common and gloating, I hated her and would hate her *forever.*

Mamma softly pulled her fingers into small fists.

"Please in future recall my daughter's rights, *all* of her rights, or you will regret it," Mrs. Steele ordered, giving the table a single nod.

She departed without a glance behind her. Mamma often stormed away so, however—ferocious exits were decidedly her style, so I remained to assess what damage we had wrought this time.

Aunt Patience, though purple and fairly vibrating with rage, managed to say, "Would you care for more cake, Edwin and Jane?"

"I goaded her, Mummy. I'm sorry for what I said before," Edwin added to me, his tooth clenching his lip. He wore a stiff collar that afternoon, I recall, above a brown waistcoat and maroon jacket, and his neck bulged obscenely from its confines.

"That's all right, Edwin. Thank you for tea, Aunt Patience." Like most children, I loathed nothing more than embarrassing myself, and the sight of the fragmented china was making me physically ill. I rose from the table. "I had better . . . Good-bye, then."

Aunt Patience's eyes burnt into me as I departed.

I went to the stables that evening, where I could visit the docile mares and peer into their soft liquid eyes, and I could stop thinking about my cousin. Thinking about Edwin was a private class in self-loathing: I hated myself for indulging his mulish attraction, yet it had been a tidal pull for me over years of reluctant camaraderie.

Flattery, I have found, is a great treat for those born innately selfish.

For the hundredth time, the thousandth time, I stood listening to soft whinnies like lullabies, pressing my cheek against sinewy necks; whether the horses at Highgate House liked me or my sugar cubes I have no notion, but they never glowered, nor warned me I teetered upon the hair-thin tightrope of eternal damnation. Smelling sweet hay and their rich, bristly coats always calmed me—and I calmed them in turn, for a particularly fidgety colt often stilled in my presence.

My thoughts drifted from the horses to the uses I might make of them. I daydreamed of riding to an apple-blossom meadow where my mother and I should do nothing save eat and laugh; I envisioned charging into war, the heads of Aunt Patience and Edwin lying at my feet.

Mamma and I never took more than a light supper in the springtime, and following a departure as precipitous as the one she had just executed, I knew that she would lock herself away with her novels and tonics, and thus I stayed out until the wind began to nip through the slats in the great stable door and the horses' snuffles quieted under my caresses . . . never realising until the following day, in fact, that I had been left entirely, permanently alone.

The ominous liquorice aroma of spilt tincture of opium drenched our cottage when I arrived home at eight o'clock. I learnt my mother had retired to bed at seven, which was unfortunate timing, as I never saw her again. Our servant, Agatha, found her the next morning, still and cold in her bed, marble eyes directed at the window.

TWO

What a consternation of soul was mine that dreary afternoon! How all my brain was in tumult, and all my heart in insurrection!

You cannot attend," Aunt Patience explained in a strained drone for the third time. "You are far too hysterical to appear in pub—"

"Please, oh, please—I won't say a word, won't make a *sound*!"

"Gracious, child, show a little restraint!" my aunt cried. "Pray for her soul, and accept God's will. It is a hard thing to lose your mother so suddenly, but many others have lived to tell the tale."

I took the news that I would not be allowed at my mother's funeral precisely as well as I took the news of her inexplicable death. Skilful knives had carved the heart out of me, leaving me empty save for the sick, unsteady fear flickering in my bones telling me *alone, all alone.* I could not claw my way out of the horror of it. I screamed for my mother on the first day; sobbed for her on the second; and on the third, the day of her funeral, sat numbly in an armchair with my eyes pulsing hellfire red—that is, until my aunt Patience arrived. Being forbidden to attend Mamma's funeral felt as if I were spitting on her grave, and questions swarmed through my pate like worms through an apple.

What will they do with me now that she has gone? Assurances that I would always reside at Highgate House now seemed reliable as quicksand.

How did my mother come to die at all? She had taken a sudden bad turn, according to Agatha; Aunt Patience muttered of fits.

Why should I not see her put in the ground? Both agreed I should not be present, but neither would explain the reason.

I fell to my knees, tearing at my aunt's stiff black skirts.

"Don't bury Mamma without me there," I begged. "However much you might have hated her, hate me still, please don't do this. I won't survive it."

"Have you *no* control over your passions?" Aunt Patience's toad-like face was ashen. "I ask for your own sake, you unprincipled animal. You will come to a bad end if—"

"I don't *care* what end I come to, only let me—"

"That is a monstrous thing to say," she cried, and then slapped me across the cheek.

Falling sideways, gasping, I clutched at the place where my skin throbbed and my teeth rang. Her slap was painful, but her visible disgust far worse.

"I'm sorry," I whispered, reaching for her wrist with my other hand. "Please, just—"

My aunt recoiled, striding towards the hall. "The situation is a hard one, Jane, but what you ask is impossible. Try to calm yourself. God sends comfort to the meek and the chaste, whilst the passionate inflict agonies upon themselves."

Aunt Patience stopped—hand splayed on her broad belly, eyes frozen into hailstones.

"You are very like her, are you not," she whispered. "The bitter fruit of a poisonous tree."

The front door clicked shut.

Grief until then had bound me in spider's silk and drained me with her pinchers. Afterwards, however, I wanted to inflict exquisite agonies upon Aunt Patience; and had I been informed that a few weeks later, I would serve her the deepest cut imaginable, I am not certain that I would not have smiled.

Morbidity has always been a close companion of mine. Hours were spent meditating on my lost kitten and all the ways it could have (must have) died because of my inflamed temper. My late father was the source of infinite questions—was my slender, sloping nose like his since it was not like my mother's? After Mamma died, however, I thought of nothing save her lonesomeness under the earth; and when I did think of her in paradise, I next thought, *but they'll never allow me into heaven, and so I still will never see her again.*

There are doubtless worse hobbies than meditating upon your dead mother, but nobody has ever suggested one to me.

Agatha knelt with me in the garret a week after the funeral, because I wanted to go through my mother's trunk. For seven days, life had been a sickening seesaw between fear that calamity would befall me and the desire calamity would take me already and have done with it. Now I wanted to touch Mamma's gowns and her gloves and her letters, as if I might combine them in a spell to summon her; even today, if witchcraft existed by means of toadstools and tinkers' thumbs to bring her back, I should do so in an instant.

"Well, 'ere we are," Agatha said in her broad rasp as she drew out an iron key.

Our servant, Agatha, who trudged about with wisps of blond hair falling in her squinting eyes, spoke entirely in platitudes. She was my sole comfort throughout that hellish week; hot broth mixed with sherry and soothing pats on the cheek are greatly cheering, even to juvenile she-devils.

The lock clicked open and I surged to plunder the trunk's contents. We had a pair of tapers, but the light was dim and ghostly, and when my seeking fingers struck lace, I hardly knew what I held.

"Ah, what 'ave we 'ere?" Agatha rumbled from my right.

"Mamma's summer parasol," I recognised as I lifted it.

"Aye, Miss Jane, and what a parasol."

There was no refuting this, so I drew out more relics—cracked men's reading spectacles, a fawn carryall. We went on until I was so sated with untrimmed hats and books of pressed flowers that I scarce noted I held a pair of empty laudanum bottles.

Agatha placidly took them away. "Now, Miss Jane, them's in the past, them is, over and emptied, so you just put 'em clean out o' yer mind."

I supposed Agatha meant Mamma was no longer ill, so I nodded. Diving into the trunk once more, I emerged with a lock of nut-brown hair very like mine woven into a small lover's knot and pressed under silver-framed glass. I had seen it before, when it sat on Mamma's mantelpiece, but it had long since vanished.

"This was my father's. Were they married long before he died, Agatha?"

"Not as long as yer mum would've liked, poor dear."

"Cousin Edwin told me she was no better than a parasite," I whispered.

"Now, Miss Jane," Agatha growled kindly, "there's sorts as you can trust to speak plain, and there's sorts as will say whatsoever suits. And if those two kinds o' folks were only obvious, wi' signs or marks o' Cain or the like, a heap o' trouble would be saved."

A worm of guilt stirred in my gut. I had lied to her that very morning, when I said I would take buttered porridge and then dumped it by the pond so as not to worry her.

Lying has always come as easy for me as breathing.

"Did my father prefer living at the cottage too?"

"Bless you, he never lived 'ere after marrying yer mum. They met in Paris, where Mr. Steele dun banking—I figure he preferred being wheresoever she was."

My head fell upon her burly shoulder. Agatha smelt of lye and the mutton she had been stewing, and just when I was too exhausted to contemplate getting my weakened legs under me and leaving the darkening garret, I pulled something I had never seen before from the trunk.

It was a letter—one in my mother's elegant Parisian script with its bold downstrokes like a battle standard being planted. It read:

Rue M——,
2nd Arrondissement,

SUNDAY

Dear Mr. Sneeves,

Pardon, s'il vous plait, *for my writing in haste, but I can hardly shift a muscle for the grief now oppressing me: my J—— has expired finally. The doctors could do nothing, and I am desolate. Doubtless your legal efforts upon my behalf and that of my daughter have been heroic, but in the absence of my husband, I must confirm our complete readiness for relocation to Highgate House.* Si ce n'est pas indiscret, *as my beloved J—— was ever a faithful client of yours, I request an immediate audience, for every second may prove invaluable. And please return this letter with your reply, as I live in horror our plans will be anticipated by those who would prevent us.*

Veuillez agréer mes salutations empressées,
Mrs. Anne-Laure Steele

At first I had imagined that the letter was two pages, but it was kept together with the reply in a crabbed male English hand:

Rue du R——,
1st Arrondissement,

SUNDAY

Chère Mme. S——,

My most heartfelt condolences upon behalf of the firm. Mr. S—— was a highly valued patron of Sneeves, Swansea, and Turner. I await your arrival and assure you that the documents have already been drawn up to the late lamented Mr. S——'s satisfaction.

Humbly,
Cyrus Sneeves, Esq.

I could only understand that these documents referred to my eventual ownership of Highgate House; puzzled, I passed them to Agatha, who carefully folded both letters together again and returned them to the trunk.

"Well, that weren't what I'd been expecting." Agatha's squinting eyes narrowed further.

"My mother wrote that when my father died?"

"A wise hen always sees her chicks are looked after. Now, there's pickled 'erring and toast to be had. Your mother's things seem to 'earten you, and this trunk will be 'ere tomorrow, and the day after that."

Agatha was again strictly correct, but mistaken in her accidental assumption that *I* would be present.

"Did you ever meet my father, Agatha?" I questioned as she shut the trunk and heaved herself upright.

"Why, bless your 'eart, Miss Steele, what a question." Agatha tsked fondly and trudged downstairs.

Infants own memories, perhaps, but by the time I was nine, hazy visions of Jonathan Steele were locked away like mementoes in a safe to which I knew not the combination. The bread crumbs I had gathered into his portrait scarce made a crust, let alone a meal.

Your father was un homme magnifique, *and his eyes were the brown of sweet chocolate just as yours are, and he never stopped thinking of ways to make us safe,* from my mother.

'E was as good a man as any, and no worse than some, from Agatha.

Don't speak of him, for God's sake, from Aunt Patience.

Now I knew he was a banker in Paris with an English solicitor friend my mother trusted; I imagined Jonathan Steele a positive hero of finance with sweeping moustaches, who had rescued my mother from penury with a flourish of his fancifully enormous pen.

"How did he meet Mamma?" I called from the top of the creaking garret stairs.

"You'll use up all your chatter and be clean out o' words, and then 'owever shall we pass the time, Miss Jane?" Agatha chided, beckoning.

I wondered over the unsettling notion of words running dry. My footsteps as I followed her made no more sound than the virtuous dead, fast asleep beneath their coverlets of stone.

Slowly, I recovered my appetite—and concurrently, my keen interest in rebellion.

My aunt Patience thought girls ought to be decorative. Indeed, Jane Eyre tucks herself away in a curtained alcove at the beginning of her saga, and thus at least attempts docility.

I was not a fictional orphan but a real one, however. Waking in the full blaze of the May afternoons, I would eat nothing save brown bread and butter for lunch, and the steaming milk soup Agatha made with sweet almonds, eggs, and cinnamon for my tea. My ugly—dare I say French—opinion of Aunt Patience kept her away temporarily, and the rest of the time I spoke low nonsense to the horses or slunk through the woods where the marsh grasses swooned into the embrace of the pond. In the stables, I could allow the stink of manure and clean sweat to calm me as I brushed my last remaining confidants; but in the forest, my musings turned darkly fantastical.

I will set fire to the main house, and then they will be sorry they made Mamma unhappy.

I will run away to Paris, where I will be awake only when the stars shine through the window and the boulevards are empty.

I will find my mother's grave and live there off of dew and nectar.

True peace did not visit me; but at times, an edgy calm like falling asleep after a nightmare descended when I lost myself in melancholy.

At times, I suspected I was not alone.

As the days passed, my sense of being watched increased. Agatha gave me free rein apart from unlocking Mamma's trunk every evening and packing satchels of apples for me to carry to the stables; she would never spy on me, I felt certain. The gardener was a wizened old thing, and the grooms paid me as little mind as did the servants at the main house. Patience Barbary thought the out-of-doors a treacherous bridge meant to convey her from one civilised structure to another.

Still I caught glimpses of another creature there in the trees, one with round eyes and a predator's hungry stare; but by the time I understood that I was the prey, my fate had already been sealed.

THREE

I was a precocious actress in her eyes: she sincerely looked on me as a compound of virulent passions, mean spirit, and dangerous duplicity.

Invitations to the main house were rebuffed in the rudest manner I could think of: silence. Even adults who are frightened of children come to their senses sooner or later, however, and in early June, I opened a missive demanding I appear before Mrs. Patience Barbary at five o'clock for tea. When I entered the drawing room, I discovered that three people awaited me instead of two.

Aunt Patience presided over the ivory-and-green-striped settee, an expression of foregone success staining her froggish mouth. The fact that her full widow's weeds looked no different after my mother's death (how could they have?) made me long to slit wounds in the taffeta. Edwin, lips already faintly dusted with sugar from the lemon cakes, offered me a polite smile.

In that instant, I knew—as I think I had suspected—that Edwin had been the one spying upon me.

"Jane, this is Mr. Vesalius Munt of Lowan Bridge School. Mr. Munt, this is my niece, Jane."

Doubtless the reader has heard cautionary reports of granite-eyed patriarchs who run schools for profit and, shall we say, misrepresent their amenities? You are partly prepared for what is to come, then. Mr. Munt was clad head to toe in black; his forehead was high, his sable boots neatly polished, and his mien sober. Here Mr. Munt's superficial resemblance to fiction ended.

First, he seemed highly intelligent. He watched those around him closely; this was not a man who ignored the way I settled as far as I could from my aunt, nor who would remark upon it until the observation suited his interests.

Second, Mr. Vesalius Munt was handsome. He was aged somewhere between forty and fifty, but the map of his face—from thoughtful wrinkles to clear grey eyes to slender chin—suggested naturally benevolent inclinations and announced his regret at his self-imposed sternness of character.

Third, he was a tyrant, which returns us to the more familiar literary archetypes. He was a great whopping unrepentant tyrant, and he *enjoyed* the vocation, its artistry—I could see it in his perfectly disarranged black hair and his humbly clasped hands. I thought, with a squirming stomach, that here was a man who would set a snake over hot coals simply to watch it writhe.

"Miss Jane Steele," he greeted me. "You have been orphaned within the month, I am sorry to hear. God's ways are inscrutable, but trust in Him nevertheless brings light to the darkest of valleys."

My aunt primly tucked her chin within her neck. "She is a clever enough girl, only mannerless and stubborn, Mr. Munt. Her intelligence needs moulding into humility and her character into an orderly Christian one."

"Then I won't remind you of my mother any longer?" I hissed.

Aunt Patience whipped out a glint of lacquered wood and began fanning herself with black lace. She wanted *something* between us, even if a scrap of cobwebby cloth.

Mr. Munt's gaze flickered between us like stage swords, all shine and speed and subtle games. "Your aunt has informed me that your mother was . . . troubled," he said with tremendous care. "It is not unusual for the children of lunatics to—"

"Mamma was *not* a lunatic!" I cried, aghast.

"No *indeed*," seconded Edwin in a fawning manner which sickened me.

"Her constitution was delicate." My aunt sounded like the teeth were being pried from her head. "Artists are often highly strung."

"Art is a curse," Vesalius Munt agreed, shifting on the hard cane chair. "An infection eating away at godly reserves of abnegation, chastity, and meekness. Show me a contented artist, Mrs. Barbary, and I will show you a dabbler—a pretender, a drudge. True artists belong to a miserable race. Jane, they tell me that your passions are strange ones, and your upbringing . . . eccentric. I run a school, you see, and your aunt thinks you would make an excellent pupil there."

The word *school* provoked the first sensation other than dull misery I had felt since before I could recall. Mamma had been at boarding school as a girl, in the south of France. On holidays they walked to the glimmering seashore, where pebbles clattered under their slippers and the sea spray chased them shrieking with laughter back to the dunes. She learnt both dancing and painting there.

Going to school already seemed adventurous, but my fingers tingled when I realised it would also be imitative of my mother.

Remembering our cottage, however, I was swiftly anchored back to Highgate House; how could I leave everything familiar when I was already so lost? Fear leached the happy nerves away.

Additionally, I was an artful little liar, and what befell artful little liars at school?

"I should rather not go," I whispered.

Aunt Patience snapped her fan.

"To send me away with a stranger—"

"Mr. Munt will make you useful, as orphaned children must—"

"Don't banish me," I pleaded, standing.

"The matter is settled."

"It is not either!" I shouted in most unchildlike fashion.

Aunt Patience thrust her heaving bosom forward. "You horrid puppet, only listen to reason for once. You *must* find a vocation, or—"

"I own Highgate House!" I cried. "Mamma told me so. You're only saying this to me because you *hated her*."

"I am saying this to you because you must become productive. And if you knew how good I was to your mother after all the suffering she caused, you would drop to your knees and beg my forgiveness."

Is that what I must do, then? My lips were quivering, my guts knotted. *Humiliate myself so I might keep what belongs to me?*

"Is flattery what you're after?" I hissed. "But of course, that's why you loathed poor Mamma so—she was exquisite, and you were never flattered a day in your life."

Sulphurous silence spread throughout the parlour. Mr. Munt studied me so intently he made my neck prickle, and Cousin Edwin gazed in a horrified stupor, his breaths straining his waistcoat buttons. Aunt Patience only smiled, a smile like a gate slamming closed and locking.

"I didn't mean that," I choked out. "Truly. But I want to remain here with . . . with everything I have left of her."

"As well you should. Mummy, you can't send her away!" Edwin protested. "Jane is my only playmate."

Aunt Patience said, in much too babying a tone for a lad of thirteen, "There now, my sweet, soon your tutor will have taught you all he knows and you yourself will go to school and find splendid new companions."

"No," Edwin moaned, burying his face in his hands. "No, I will miss her, you *can't*. It isn't *fair*."

"Quite touching to see such devotion in young relations." Mr.

Munt's stately wrinkles creased approvingly, and he brushed imaginary dust from the knee of his trouser. "It gives me every hope that Jane is indeed redeemable, to have inspired such affection."

Finding none of these observations complimentary and growing steadily more unnerved by Vesalius Munt, whose silvery eyes seemed coins at the bottom of a too-deep pool, I edged towards the door.

"Where do you think you are going, my dear little girl?" Mr. Munt asked, kindness seeping from his tone like blood from a gash.

"I cannot stay for tea." A noose was tightening round my throat.

"Now, Jane," Mr. Munt purred, rising. "You are only proving your dear aunt's point by acting so irrationally. Come here, allow me to examine you, determine your strengths, and perhaps we shall yet find a place for you at Lowan Bridge School."

I was off like a hare; my aunt looked after me in unfeigned alarm, and Edwin gave a small wail.

Mr. Munt, I saw as I glanced behind, meditated on me with his dashing black head cocked: the look of a man who has spied a hill and vowed to crest it, for no reason other than to see what lies upon the other side.

When I returned to Highgate House many years thereafter, I viewed the ravine again, and felt as distant from it as a child does looking at a terrible cave in a picture book. Thus I can describe it as my twenty-four-year-old self perfectly rationally. Our cottage stood at the edge of the woods, with the sweet brown duck pond lying to the west of us. If one passed the pond, the forest which bordered our property gave way to a ridge and thence to a sharp declivity like a small crevasse populated by violet monkshood and sharp wild grasses.

I felt Mr. Munt's eyes searing the back of my skull long after my escape was accomplished, so I repaired to the woods.

My curls stuck to my brow when I reached the trees, glued by means of animal fear to my skin, and I smeared them back. We had pinned two braids like a crown atop my head, but several strands had bolted and I must have looked a malicious dryad there, surrounded by leaf and bracken. Light slanted through the branches as if it possessed physical weight that evening, making prison bars of shadows and penitents' benches of fallen trees. Wandering, I calmed myself.

I should not go to Lowan Bridge with Mr. Munt.

I need not go to Lowan Bridge with Mr. Munt.

I will *not go to Lowan Bridge with Mr. Munt.*

"Are you hurt, Jane?"

Too frightened to shriek, I spun about with my hand clapped over my mouth. Cousin Edwin stood ten feet away from me, a cautious grin pasted over his face, the sort people who are terrible with horses (as I am not) think will calm skittish beasts.

"What do you mean?" I gasped.

Edwin came no closer, but pointed his index finger. His dull hair was half-lit and half-hid in the shade of a crooked branch; he seemed a stitched-together creature from a puppet pageant, the sort in which spouses are beaten within an inch of their lives.

"You're bleeding." He began to walk again.

Looking down, I saw that I had scratched my arm upon a bramble without noticing. A trace of blood wept from the shallow gouge.

"Here," Cousin Edwin said when he had reached me.

He breathed harder as he wound his handkerchief over my arm: round and round, binding the cut, forehead beetling in concentration. Edwin smelled of lemon cake and the faintly *old* aroma he always carried, as if he had been born in a bed of camphor and cheese rinds.

"I won't let them," he announced. "I hate that she thought to send you to school. I am the *man* of this house, and you shall stay here with us, Jane. Don't be afraid."

I watched him tie off the cloth—like a bandage, yes, and like a silken slave's cuff, and like the collar at the end of a leash.

"I'm not afraid."

Edwin glanced up, pale green eyes glowing. "You *were* afraid—of that horrid Mr. Munt. You needn't be. He won't take you away from us."

Edwin plucked a leaf from my hair and placed the memento in his trouser pocket—a habit I had never liked, but never thought quite so pitiful.

"Did you forgive me?" He rocked on his heels. "About the secrets game—we've hardly spoken since. I was only repeating something rude I heard Cook say. Your mother was too beautiful to avoid cruel gossip, don't you think? Shake hands?"

Edwin's pudgy hand thrust before my face. I shook; for an idiot, he was clever to perceive that complimenting my late mother would work miracles.

Instead of letting go my hand, he pulled me closer.

"Do you want to know what my favourite secret is?" he breathed into the space between my eyes.

I swallowed. If I said no, he would rage, pout, fume for days, so I angled my head. He put his rosy mouth to my ear.

"The time in the trap when I *showed* you, and you never screamed. You're every bit as bad as I am. You liked it."

He drew back fractionally. His grip tightened, and whilst I searched for words to tell him that no, opening his trousers had not been a bond between us and that screaming clearly ought to have occurred to me, he chewed his underlip until it was scarlet.

Then he grinned brightly.

"You're not screaming now either."

"Let go of my arm," I ordered.

The breeze sent kindly fingertips through our hair, jays calling from their shadowy canopies, and now I *was* frightened—mortally—

of the woods which were leaf curtained and the birds which could not help me with whatever strange sort of trouble this was.

Edwin did not let go. "Let's start a new game."

"Stop it, I tell you. What game?" I demanded.

"I want to know what the inside of your mouth tastes like." Cousin Edwin leant down.

I struck him as hard as I could across the face, and he was startled enough to let go, and I had not known until then what it meant to *run*.

The light shone brighter, and the wind picked up, and I had just burst through the trees in the direction of civilisation when Edwin caught me. We both tumbled to the ground and I swiped at him, shouting his name and *Stop* and he laughed easily and pinned my wrists to the earth at the top of the ravine where the twigs pricked my back and the sky seemed a great billowing, purpling tent above the looming forest.

His lips met my neck; his tongue shoved at my mouth. I kicked and *kicked*, limbs transforming into weapons even as my heart churned pure black fear through my veins. Edwin pinned me with his weight and he had transformed too now, hard where he ground against my thigh, red where my fist had stung his cheek, and *My body isn't working, nothing is working*, I thought, so I used something else.

"I'll tell this time," I spat as I struggled. "I'll tell *everyone*."

His piggish look of glee dimmed. "No, you won't. You're a knowing little jezebel just like your mother, Mummy always tells me so."

"What do you mean?"

"I mean that you like it."

"I'll tell her we *both* like it," I lied coldly, falling limp. "Then she'll send me away forever. Get *off*."

Edwin retreated—biting his mouth, straightening his clothing. When he took in my bedraggled state, he grew agitated, reaching into thin air as I brushed myself off with unsteady fingers.

"It was only a game," he offered. "I never meant to—I would never hurt you. I'm sorry, Jane."

My wrists were bruised, my back scraped, my sleeve torn, my heart unbroken but dirtied, as if he had pulled it through the mud. Walking a few paces away, Edwin retrieved something from the ground. It was his pocket handkerchief, which had fallen from my arm, and he passed it back to me as if giving girls pocket handkerchiefs could atone for any offence under the sun.

"Jane, will you be my friend again?"

Rage poured from scalp to sole at this request.

"We were never friends," I lied, and—preparing to run once more—I shoved his chest as hard as I could.

The rock he staggered back upon was loose under his footing; it set off a tiny slide into the ravine, a hushed skidding of granite and dead bracken. That accidents happen is a universal principle—and perhaps the only universal principle worth mentioning, for it governs an enormous percentage of our daily lives.

That my entire being, every last ounce of *me*, had been put into that violent push, however, is undeniable.

When I peered over the top of the short decline and met Edwin's eyes as he sucked in his last breaths with a broken spine and a look of pure disappointment, I did nothing to aid or comfort him.

I walked away.

FOUR

"Do you know where the wicked go after death?"

"They go to hell," was my ready and orthodox answer. . . .

"What must you do to avoid it?"

I deliberated a moment; my answer, when it did come, was objectionable: "I must keep in good health, and not die."

E*dwin is dead,* I thought.

Perhaps he only fainted.

You killed *him, you idiot*, I thought next, and giggled, and stumbled under star-scarred skies.

I fell to my knees and would have screamed then had I the air to do so, but all I could manage was gasps through a throat which had shrunk to the breadth of a hay wisp. My fists clutched the sod as if the planet were trying to buck me off and, after a few harrowing seconds, a whimper escaped and the tears came flooding.

That night, I learnt that horror could not physically *kill* me; wave after wave crashed over my head without my drowning, and yet . . . I think that I would rather die than experience such overwhelming *wrongness* ever again.

Curling onto my side on the lawn—visible peripherally to the cottage but not to the main house—I sobbed for an hour or more. When the torrent was a trickle, I passed a sleeve over my eyes and sat up. The sun had sunk well below the tops of the elms, and whether it would ever rise again, I could not have said. In the mire of my misery and confusion, three thoughts emerged:

You really are as wicked as everyone says.

Shame spread like a pox over my skin.

Mamma isn't here to help you, and now you will be hanged.

Like all children, I had read the *Newgate Calendar* raptly, that ostensibly educational account of gruesome violations enacted by the law upon ne'er-do-wells within Newgate Prison. No one embarks upon a life of mayhem because hanging (or drawing and quartering, or slow death by pressing, come to that) sounds like a pleasant Saturday afternoon lark, but parents in those days still supposed the illustrations highly effective deterrents, and I had devoured Edwin's copy. I cried a little longer. A vague shape I knew to be Agatha floated past amber-lit windowpanes.

You are going to have to lie like the very devil to live through this.

Having no stock of tears left, I plotted my escape with hollow bones and shaking fingers.

You've said it all out plain once, Miss Jane, so I knows as ye can say it all out plain twice," Agatha declared the next morning. She sat on our burgundy settee, one arm around my waist.

My return to the cottage had been a lighting storm: searing flashes of *you've killed Edwin* interrupted a savage downpour of lies. They poured from my mouth, flooding my throat. When the falsehoods had been exhausted, Agatha had said, pulling the coverlet over my head, *There, there, poor girl. Nothing like this lasts forever, for ye'll ken that time passes whether we will it or nae.*

I had meant to pray for forgiveness the instant Agatha left, but instead a deathly slumber took me. I don't know the term for a child who falls asleep *after* her first murder and *before* confessing her sins, but I suspect it is not an intensely complimentary one.

Now it was ten o'clock in the morning and my head felt filled with hornets. I had been ill the night before into my porcelain pot, sour acid bleaching my throat, and now more lies were required—this time for the benefit of Constable Sam Quillfeather.

Constable Quillfeather, seeing I was numb with dread following Agatha's prompt, pretended a sudden rapturous interest in a decorative pillow.

"Such fine work as I've seldom seen, and the elegance of the lilies—their shape, their exquisite colour? Remarkable! Did the late Mrs. Steele create this masterpiece?"

Dear old Agatha nudged me as if this were a serious inquiry.

"Yes," I managed.

Constable Quillfeather was very tall and very thin—a friendly skeleton, in fact—clad in brown flannel with a red-and-yellow-checked shawl-collared vest and tall leather gaiters. His face boasted a jutting chin, an aggressively hooked nose, deep-set hazel eyes, a looming brow, and a great framing shock of forward-swept hair of a dark brown not unlike mine. Everything about Constable Quillfeather seemed to lurch forward on a parabola; I guessed him to be above middle age, but his lanky limbs were puppyish in their urgency, a propulsive quality matched only by his incessant questions. Though he was far from handsome, he exuded a riveting aura of eager enthusiasm.

"Ha! I thought she must have done?" Constable Quillfeather's soft tenor lilted so much at the ends of his sentences, statements became queries. "Was she fond of sewing?"

"Sometimes." My mother had enjoyed needlework, but not as much as she relished throwing new projects across the room.

"I never had the pleasure of meeting her but once, in the village, at the stationer's?" The policeman's bright eyes swept to Agatha's. "She was so charming, and . . . I think a little sad? But I presume too much—Miss Steele, may we talk about how you discovered your poor cousin's body?"

Swallowing, I nodded. No speech was forthcoming, however.

Constable Quillfeather clapped his hands to his bony knees. "Miss Steele, do you require water? A sip of wine to strengthen you?"

I shook my head.

"But you shiver—are you cold?"

Helpless to stop myself, I emitted a hysterical trill of laughter.

Frowning, Agatha attempted, "She's been so poorly, she don't know which end is up, left, or 'indmost, Constable."

"Naturally, naturally!" Constable Quillfeather smiled, a warm horizontal spread which failed to check his air of headlong momentum. "Will you tell me the origins of the magnificent work above the mantelpiece?"

The constable's nose crinkled as he gazed at a wild collection of pinks and yellows incidentally suggesting a landscape, one reminiscent of Turner's works when important structures are burning down. He rose to study it—or perhaps to give me the illusion of unfettered space.

"Mamma was a painter," I rasped.

"And a fine one! Now, this is not a picture set in England? Where, then?"

"In the countryside near Paris."

"Ah, just so. Did she like it here?"

"Why?"

Constable Quillfeather's eyes, dappled with green and brown and amber, twinkled compassionately. "Neighbourly curiosity?"

"I don't think so," I admitted. "But we were safe."

Sam Quillfeather returned to his armchair. "Safety and the comforts of home—what more can one ask of life?"

"Longer life?" I returned without thinking.

The constable winced ruefully. "Quite so. Miss Steele, do you grasp how brave you are being? I know of grown women who, after the multiple tragedies you have undergone, would be prostrate! But here you are, so steady and sure. Might we begin again, and you tell me what happened yesterday?"

He was one of the most engaging men I had ever encountered, and anyway there was nothing for it: I set to.

I informed Constable Quillfeather in a voice trembling like a plucked harpsichord string that I had been to tea at my aunt's residence and that there had been a great row over my going to school. Following this dash of truth, I said that Cousin Edwin and I were so upset that we quit the main house. After planning to run away together to London, and planning to build a tree fortress, and planning to live as highwaymen, we had decided to play a game.

"A game?" Constable Quillfeather repeated slowly.

Yes, I told him, a game called Robin Hood.

Constable Quillfeather rubbed his hands as he leant forward, inquiring what this game involved.

"Hunting for deer in Nottingham Forest." My words may have been false, but my tears were true. "We separated so as to meet again and show what we'd killed for supper. But it was all pretend. Then I went to the meeting place—there's two fallen logs crossed like a crooked *X* not far from the cottage—and, and no one was there. Then I thought Edwin must have . . ."

"There, there," Agatha said as a sob escaped. "There, now."

Like a fever dream, I saw Edwin approaching with a hemmed square of cotton he imagined was an apology.

"I thought he must have been playing one of his tricks," I forced out. "But, oh, I was so vexed he'd left me alone in the woods when it was getting dark. I searched everywhere. I thought of the ravine because we collect things down there sometimes."

"What sort?" Constable Quillfeather desired to know.

"Bright rocks, wildflowers, bones. When I found him, dusk was nearly finished, and . . . he wasn't breathing."

"He had already expired?"

I drew a shuddering breath. "His eyes looked—I can't stand to think of how his eyes looked, don't ask me, please!"

This was the truth: his eyes had looked utterly betrayed before they had glazed to an unseeing shimmer like ice crusting a pool.

"And no one else saw you?"

"No."

"And no one else saw him?"

"No one I know about."

"And then you returned here?"

"Yes. Slowly," I whispered, hedging my bets as to whether Agatha had noticed the gap between twilight and my return. "I felt so weak. This morning, I should have thought it all some horrid dream, except . . . except it's true."

"Miss Jane, that was very complete," Constable Quillfeather complimented. He brushed his hands over his head, and the wiry locks like accusers arrowed towards my face all the surer. "May I ask you a few more questions?"

"I suppose so."

"The courage in this one, the pluck!" Whistling, Constable Quillfeather winked at Agatha. "She's been raised by a paragon of a mother, but that's in addition to a few stout friends, I think?"

"I hope so, but judge for yerself, sir," Agatha answered calmly.

"That I shall, ma'am. Miss Steele, was Edwin in any sort of fight that evening?"

Either the clock which had been ticking stopped, or I went deaf with panic.

"His button was missing?" Constable Quillfeather indicated the top button on his own waistcoat. "Hereabouts? Seemed to have been torn away?"

"We played at highwaymen before Robin Hood, to practise." I glanced up at Agatha. "We staged a fight. Edwin . . . he'd not have wanted Aunt Patience to know about that, she likes everything to be so proper."

The policeman blew out a breath. "It gave me a turn, you understand? Didn't know what to think—signs of a struggle?"

My stomach heaved. As suddenly as he had introduced the subject, however, Constable Quillfeather abandoned it.

"You'll miss your playmate, Miss Steele, and the blow comes too soon on the heels of another, and it hurts me to see it," he averred, shaking his head. "There's an . . . incongruity? About grief in the very young. It doesn't belong on you? Well, I'm for the grieving mother now."

Constable Quillfeather came to stand before me on spindly stork's legs, bending over like a question mark.

"You'll take care of yourself?"

"Yes."

"What's happened to your dress sleeve?"

We looked at my blue-and-grey-patterned dress sleeve and the short tear in it made by Edmund's final game. Agatha's vision was as keen as a whiskered mole's, and she had brushed off my dress the night before without seeing the rip; since I donned the nearest thing I could find that morning, there it was, a grisly cotton wound with a lurid smoke-coloured bruise beneath.

"I—I don't know," I stammered. "It must have been torn when we were playing highwaymen, just like Edwin's button. It's the only explanation."

After a pause, Constable Quillfeather shook my hand and stood tall as a beanpole, gently frowning. "Well, I am in tremendous debt to you, Miss Steele. If that is the only explanation, then I shall never have to seek out another one, shall I?"

Constable Quillfeather settled a brown beaver hat on his head, bowed to us, and set off for the main house—and only when the ridiculously tall pipe shape of his headgear departing passed our front window did I allow myself the highly literary indulgence of losing consciousness.

After recovering my wits that afternoon, I stood before the broad white steps of the main house with Agatha, preparing myself to enter. My aunt wished to see me, a request which could not be refused. Vacillating, I paced, staring miserably at the lofty leaded windows.

"Sooner a thing's started, sooner as it's done," Agatha mentioned.

"I'm frightened."

"That's neither 'ere nor there," she advised, and since this was again inarguable, I made a proud church spire of my spine and walked inside.

No one greeted me; up I went towards my aunt's bedroom. The servants ought to have been bustling, making arrangements for the inevitable condoling relations and dealers in the commerce of death, but Aunt Patience must have sent them off; the only faces I saw were painted ancestors whispering *murderess* from the cages of their carved gilt frames. I felt as if I were going to my doom.

I was perfectly correct—but it was a doom of my own making, not my aunt's. Of this I can at least be proud, if of nothing else.

Following a knock at Patience Barbary's half-opened door, I entered. The light here was dimmer, keeping its distance as if out of respect for the bereaved. My aunt lay on a fainting couch. She beckoned; it was not until I drew within three feet that I could see her plain, and I stiffened.

"You," Aunt Patience spat.

Her careful mourning attire had been abandoned for a capacious black robe fastened with silk ties. Patience Barbary had shed her smug bravado as snakes do skins; everything about her was new, from the swollen pink edges of her eyelids to her raw expression, tender as a cut where the scab has peeled away. Years of trials I did not know about had hardened her, but now here she was—in desperate need of a shell, and stripped of her defences as she had been stripped of her son. Her habitual mourning was an ostentation, I realised, maybe even a dig at my mother's pale Parisian frocks; this was her, bared to the ravages of the whimsical world.

I wanted to be glad of her ruin—but I was only sad in a sweeping, sky-wide way, and sorry for myself despite the unforgivable thing I had done. I wanted Edwin back, and months previous, so that I could scream when I was meant to and none of this would be my fault.

"Tell me," Aunt Patience demanded. "You are the one who found him. I must know all."

Hesitating, I cast my eyes down. My silences were beginning to shift from weapons into shields. Now I have a wide array, a blood-crusted and blow-battered arsenal; but then I was still learning.

"He was already peaceful, Aunt." My throat worked. "I'm so sorry. I don't know anything."

"You know more than I do." Her voice had been ground to sand with weeping.

"Nothing that can *help*."

We talked—or rather, Aunt Patience questioned, and I lied. The untended fireplace watched us. No, I did not think Edwin had been in any pain. Yes, it must have been an accident. No, he had not been angry with her any longer when we parted ways.

"He loved me very much," Aunt Patience choked, pressing smelling salts to her flat nose. "He loved you too, his only close kin—he was as affectionate a boy as I ever saw. Why did Edwin have to die in such a meaningless way? It ought to have been you."

Numbly, I digested this; and then I understood.

As if a prophecy had been painted in the carpet's flourishes under my feet, I knew what I must do to survive my cousin's death. I loathed the prospect; but then I pictured my existence with only Agatha for company, and I knew I was right.

What I did not know was that an inexorable force tugged at my torn sleeve.

Scientists believe that the Earth twirls upon a great pole like a spinning top; this rotational point is theoretically located in the Arctic North, where the land is so desolate and lovely that daylight and nighttime cannot bear to give it up, and trade shifts in six-month intervals. These scientists are mistaken about the Arctic North; for I know in my heart that though the Earth does spin, and spin far too quickly for many of us to bear, London is the centre of the axis.

London is the eye of the circle and the heart of the globe, and London would be the saving of me. I did not know then that Highgate House was a mere overnight journey's away; neither did I know that Lowan Bridge School was even closer to its suburbs. What I did know was that if Aunt Patience looked at me for another second, I would scream.

"Perhaps I see too much of your mother staining you," she husked. "But—"

"Aunt Patience," I announced, "I want you to send me away to school with Mr. Munt."

FIVE

Probably, if I had lately left a good home and kind parents, this would have been the hour when I should most keenly have regretted the separation: that wind would then have saddened my heart; this obscure chaos would have disturbed my peace; as it was, I derived from both a strange excitement, and reckless and feverish, I wished the wind to howl more wildly, the gloom to deepen to darkness, and the confusion to rise to clamour.

If the reader has ever prized solitude, you can imagine my revulsion when a vortex of attention formed in the wake of my desiring an education.

"Well, ye knows what's best for yerself," Agatha said doubtfully, laying out my supply of dresses, pinafores, and pantalettes. Her scrunched rabbit's eyes had a wary cast to them, and a hurt one.

"Here there is no scope," said I.

"Well, if that don't beat everything," Agatha muttered, rolling my hair ribbons and tucking them into a muslin bag. "Nature will out, though, sooner or later."

"What do you mean, Nature will out?" I asked, thrilling with fear.

"Why, only that children can't 'elp a-taking after their parents.

And if innocent lasses pretend to need *scope* when meaner sorts are driving 'em away, 'arassing and pestering-like, then the world ain't what it ought to be."

I flung myself at Agatha, helpless to check the gush of feeling; my spindly form met her strong arms, and I held her tight. "No one is driving me off. I only . . . I can't stand it any longer."

Agatha pulled me away from her embrace, shifting her hands to my temples so that she could read me like one of her pudding receipts. I lapped up the attention, for when would anyone ever waste sentiment on the likes of me again?

"Penned creatures suffer, but the more so when they imagine a pen what ain't there," Agatha said softly. "Can ye tell me the difference afore ye leave your 'ome behind?"

"I'm not penned—I'm frightened."

"Ye said that before, in front o' the main house. Of what, lass?"

"Of myself."

Agatha set about mending the worst of my stockings. She stole glances at my mother's painting, however, the one like a sunset seen through tears. I easily divined her secret fear, but knew it to be rootless. Edwin Barbary was ugly in life, uglier still in death; but many lovely things died with him, and one was my desire to be exactly like my mother.

I could no longer afford to be like my mother; my heart must be carried not on my sleeve but deep in my breast, where the complete darkness might mask the fact it too was black as pitch.

The day before my departure, Edwin was placed beneath the grass and the buttercups before a very small assembly. Aunt Patience would have sobbed if she could, but only swayed, murmuring; she may have been addressing Edwin, or the droning minister, or the shovel in the gnarled hands of the gravedigger—who could say?

I stood in silence with my head bowed, wondering whom she would talk to at all without me left to hate.

This morose thought followed me home, where a cold meat supper awaited. Directly before sleep finally captured my twitching eyelids, I mused over whether Aunt Patience would rouse herself and march—froglike, determined, hateful, as she used to be—down to the gate and see me off.

She did not . . . only Agatha kissed my cheek as I was helped onto the rickety wooden step of the coach, with my trunk strapped above.

There is no practice more vexing than that of authors describing coach travel for the edification of people who have already travelled in coaches. As I must adhere to form, however, I will simply list a series of phrases for the unlikely reader who has never gone anywhere: thin eggshell dawn-soaked curtains stained with materials unknown to science; rattling fit to grind bones to powder; the ripe stench of horse and driver and bog.

Now I have fulfilled my literary duties, I need only add that other girls travelling to school may not have dwelt quite so avidly upon the angular faces of police constables as I.

We had journeyed for some seven hours, and I had flicked the curtain aside as the towns came thicker along our misty route, blinking into view as faint collections of red roofs and stone chimneys. I tugged at the rope strung above the window. The otherwise empty coach stopped abruptly, nearly throwing me from the hard seat. A few seconds later, the driver's whiskered face appeared in the act of spitting upon the side of the roadway. He gestured at the string tied to his arm as if my signalling him were the final straw in a long list of liberties I had taken with his person.

"Are we stopping at all before we reach Lowan Bridge?" I asked.

"Stopping!" He rubbed as if to wipe the red from his nose. Even had he succeeded, the pistol flask peeping from his lapel pocket would have replaced the stain in short order. "Are ye sick?"

"No."

"Faint?"

"No, but—"

"Hoongry?"

Glancing at the basket Agatha had lovingly filled with bread and pickles and potted rabbit, I shook my head. "I only need some air."

"Air!" repeated the driver. He shook his head as if from this day forward, no offence would ever be met with surprise. "Ye'll have air enough in half an hour, when we reach yer destination. Ye'll live on the stuff."

"Is the board a frugal one?" I asked, desperate for a hint.

"Ye might say so. Ye might say scraps tossed to pigs are a point of frugality."

"What is your name, sir?"

Rolling his eyes so I could see every feathery red vessel, the man answered, "Nick. What of it?"

"Nick, is life *very* hard at Lowan Bridge? I only want some warning, as Mr. Munt seemed . . . peculiar."

Nick tapped his finger to the side of his ruddy nostril. "Peculiar! Aye, he is that. Ye'll learn a plentiful heap o' facts, if all goes well."

"And how if all goes ill?"

"Then ye'll not need to worry yerself—" he coughed "—as it's prodigious difficult to trouble a corpse."

This intelligence was punctuated by the stomping of boots as the coachman returned to his high post, a friendly cry of "Damn you, Chestnut, you bloody useless sack o' glue!" and we were off again.

Quaking, I ate some pickles and a small piece of bread—however ill I felt, it seemed a prudent precaution. When the carriage ground to a halt, my door opened; Nick tugged the rope line off his sleeve as I stepped down to the road.

We had stopped before a tall iron gate set in a stone wall, a gate with sinister floral embellishments and brutal points like demons' teeth. Half the entrance stood open, a portal to a grim new world; a gravel path drew my eyes into the grounds, which were dotted with weeping trees lamenting my arrival. The building I guessed comprised Lowan Bridge School was grey as a feudal fortress. It possessed three stories, narrow windows excellently suited for a gaol, and a crenellated roof; if it had featured actual cannons thrusting through the stone gaps, it could not have made a clearer impression.

Nick harrumphed, and I turned to see that he had fetched my trunk from the roof and my basket from the coach.

"How can you leave children here to die?" I asked tremulously.

Setting my basket next to the trunk, Nick shrugged. "There's a real education to be had here—that's better than can be said for most o' these governess manufactories. Anyhow, the world is a hard place, and I live in it alone—what's it to me if you do too?"

"Here." I offered the considerable remains of my luncheon. "If they don't want me to have this, they need only take it away. You keep it."

"Keep it! What the devil are ye a-doing of? I've been paid already, ye daft child," Nick said, frowning.

"This is payment for something else."

"What, then?"

"The world is a hard place, and I live in it alone." I swallowed back my tears. "If you don't remember the others, remember me."

Nick studied me; in the end, he merely accepted my basket and shook my hand. Turning, he strode towards the dingy coach and Chestnut, who stood stamping and generally articulating his desire to be rewarded with a bag of hot oats. I could sympathise.

"Straight down the path," he ordered. "Best o' luck to ye, though brains'll be of better use—and mind the headmaster."

"I mean to."

"Good," Nick grunted, clicking his tongue at his weary horse. "Ye'll live longer."

I walked with a palpitating heart, dragging my trunk, up the lane under the brightening glare of midafternoon. The sun had sliced through the cloud bank, leaving an unmendable gash of blue across the sky's face, starkly lighting the battlements before me. Reaching the front entrance, I hesitated and then knocked; the door was of thick wood strapped with iron as if bound in a strait waistcoat. A uniformed servant girl with a pockmarked face answered and beckoned me inside with the instruction, "Mind you wipe your boots. This way."

We marched through corridors lined with carpets of forbidding black and blue, lit with wall-mounted dips rather than gas, featuring art suggesting that a great love of our Lord would be rewarded by the righteous being pelted with rocks. Half having expected a mean hovel lined with manure-seasoned straw, my childish jaw dropped; wherever my aunt had sent me, she had paid a pretty penny to do so, for this was no barnyard masquerading as a school, but rather the castle of a malevolent monarch. Had a dragon inhabited the dungeons, I should not have been in the least surprised. When we reached a smaller side room with books dimly lining the shelves, the servant said merely, "I'll fetch someone," and I was left with my trunk at my feet and mind in turmoil.

About ten minutes later, the door swung open. The woman standing there was quietly dressed in grey, her blond hair parted in the middle and her slender hand lifting a rushlight towards the darkened interior. She had a classically lovely face, features calling to mind a songbird or a sonnet, with a sweet afterthought of a nose and pale blue eyes. I thought her around twenty-five, which seemed a most distinguished achievement and one I felt unlikely to duplicate.

"Are you Jane Steele?"

I nodded.

"Welcome. I am Miss Amy Lilyvale, and I teach music here. If you apply yourself at Lowan Bridge, you will be a valuable addition to any great household in the world. If you are feckless and idle, you will find life hard."

She said these words as if required to deliver them; then she smiled. "You must be weary—you can have a wash before supper, and lie down if you like. Come."

Lifting my little trunk, I followed her light step back into the corridor and up a stately central staircase. We had not halfway climbed it when a bell clanged loudly enough to summon the dead, and the sound of pattering feet from all directions met our ears.

Girls poured into the murky corridors, books clutched to flat bosoms and full ones, for they seemed to range in age from as young as I was to as old as eighteen. They were all dressed in navy blue stuff frocks—coarse material which must have chafed—with quaint white aprons, and a queer cloth cap fastened over their hair. I must have glanced down at my trunk, for Miss Lilyvale touched my elbow gently.

"Your own clothes will still serve you for holidays when you return to see your family."

"I have no family," I answered without thinking.

"Surely you must have a provider, or you could not afford to attend Lowan Bridge School."

"Yes, I am very grateful to my aunt," I replied, recovering my wits, "but she is not fond of me. She means to keep me away."

"Oh, Miss Steele . . . and to impart a sound education to you, surely?"

This, I was coming to realise, was undoubtedly true—for had my absence been Aunt Patience's whole design, I might have landed in a Yorkshire sty and been left to moulder there. Meanwhile, the rush of footsteps and the jostling of elbows all around us unnerved me; most of the girls murmured words I could not catch, as if fixing something in their minds, whilst the few who were silent cast brushing looks at me like the scrape of minnows in a shallow brook.

"Here we are." Having reached the dormitories on the topmost level, Miss Lilyvale pushed a door open.

She revealed a long rectangular room furnished with two rows of double beds, several pine tables with basins and unadorned white pitchers thereon, unlit fireplaces at either end, and a window granting us a view of fragmenting clouds. The ceilings were high and imposing, the air as chill as it ever is within a stone tower, where we were to be kept prisoner like dozens of forlorn princesses. Suddenly weak with fatigue, I clutched the nearest bed frame, all but dropping my poor trunk.

"Goodness! That was a very brave show, but now I see the way of it," Miss Lilyvale tutted as she snatched the luggage from my trembling fingers. "Take off your shoes and lie down for a while. Here is your bed, and later you will meet your bedmate, Sarah Taylor, but for now no one should disturb you until I return to fetch you for supper at half six. Till then, rest quiet, dear, and remember to thank God for your safe arrival."

Miss Lilyvale departed. The bedclothes, though cheap and stiff, were clean, and the bed suitably big for the unknown Sarah to share henceforth. I wondered whether she was a good girl, a bright one, a pretty one; I wondered whether Nick would remember the potted rabbit if I ever required precipitate escape.

Sleep was finally weighing down my lids when I spied a ghost in the stark bedchamber.

Gasping, I tightened my loose grip upon the coverlet.

A lump of sheets had transformed into a child who could not have been above six years old—a blond apparition with a pale, freckled face and a tiny mouth. She regarded me stoically with her head on her palm.

"Miss Lilyvale told you to give prayers of thanks, and you haven't done."

Her voice was high even for her age—queerly so, like the tinkling of a bell.

"Why aren't you at lessons?" I returned.

"Ill." Indeed she looked it, for her skin was nigh transparent and her eyes dull, apart from the green circles of her irids. "You'll own up to it and not be angry with me? You forgot your prayers after Miss Lilyvale reminded you?"

"Yes," I agreed, nettled. "What of it? I'm Jane Steele. Who are you?"

"Rebecca Clarke. Call me Clarke, that's the way of it here. And thank you." She let her pale curls fall back to the pillow. "I couldn't have stood another day of this. I'll tell it as mild as I can, I promise."

"Tell what?"

"Tell Mr. Munt you lied about your prayers."

"But why—"

"You can report me in a week, when I've recovered. Fair is fair, after all."

"Report you where?" I demanded as my sluggish pulse sped.

"At Mr. Munt's daily Reckoning," Clarke chirped before burrowing back under the linens and effectively vanishing once more.

SIX

"Madam," he pursued, "I have a Master to serve whose kingdom is not of this world; my mission is to mortify in these girls the lusts of the flesh; to teach them to clothe themselves with shame-facedness and sobriety . . ."

A soft hand on my shoulder woke me, and I dragged sleepy eyes open to view the blurred face of Miss Lilyvale. My slumber had been thin and fitful; rising, I glanced about for the mysterious Rebecca Clarke, but her bed was now neatly made.

"Wash up, Steele, and we'll be off."

The shock of the cold water was reviving, and I used my wet hands to smooth the countless ripples from my hair. When I turned back to Miss Lilyvale, she took my arm companionably and we quit the dormitory for the stairs, muddied evening sunlight trickling through the high, grimy exterior windows. The cracks of blue had retreated whilst I slept, beaten back by regiments of austere cloud banks. I watched a great line of girls emerging from a wing of classrooms, marching in pairs towards the open timber doors we approached.

"The housekeeper will leave two sets of uniforms on your bed this evening," Miss Lilyvale informed me. "For tonight, you need not worry about your dress, but afterwards be sure to keep yourself clean and well presented. Oh!" Miss Lilyvale brightened. "Taylor! Steele, this is your bedmate, Sarah Taylor."

The girl who had broken off from the line was twelve, with a moon face which was so beautiful I had no notion whether she should be congratulated or censured for taking matters a trifle too far. Her lips were rosy, her hair a sleek raven black, and the navy of the Lowan Bridge uniform served only to make her own blue orbs shine the brighter. She reached out with her palm down as if she were a noblewoman accepting obeisance—which was not entirely unfair and then again rather tiresome.

"How do you do?" said I. "I am happy to meet you."

"Yes," said she, in a strangely lazy drawl, "very likely."

This was less than promising, but the queue of schoolgirls had nearly entered the dining hall, so we hastened into the cavern from which the rich aroma of stew emanated. The huge chamber could have been a Viking hall, from bare flagstones to immense rafters. Miss Lilyvale walked to a dais at the end of the room; there the remaining teachers were assembled, including—to my dismay—Vesalius Munt. His staff was otherwise made up of females, a bevy of dull pigeons clad in stone and fawn and charcoal and ash. A great black cauldron was perched on sturdy iron before this assembly, with a matronly cook standing next to it.

When Taylor and I sat, to my astonishment I beheld the mutton stew already ladled into a bowl, and a respectable portion at that. Several platters had been set along the roughhewn table, piled high with rustic bread, and mugs of steaming black coffee sent bittersweet curlicues to the distant ceiling.

"Is . . . is this usual?" I marvelled. Taylor had made no move to lift the pewter spoon, so I folded my hands in my lap.

"What?" she returned peevishly.

"Is the fare always so good? It smells divine."

"Well, *that* of all things doesn't matter in the *slightest*," she retorted languidly.

This was peculiar, and likewise was it cause for a pulse of concern that none of the girls appeared happy about the fare; they regarded their bowls with slightly less dismay than I had once levelled at my cousin's genitalia. Before I could ask why, Mr. Munt rose from his chair and raised his hands elegantly skyward as we folded our fingers together.

"For what we are about to receive, may the Lord make us truly thankful," Mr. Munt called out in sonorous tones. "May He create in us humble gratitude for this nourishment, and may this fine meal strengthen our bodies that we may serve our Lord with greater steadfastness every day. Amen."

"Wouldn't that be grand," the girl across from me muttered after we had repeated the closing word of the prayer. She had a thin, sallow face and limp ash-coloured hair.

"Oh, *do* hush, Fox, your efforts at humour are *dreadful*," Taylor crooned snidely.

"Now!" Mr. Munt exclaimed. "The time has come for our daily Reckoning. I adjure you as I always do to be thorough, and above all truthful, for the narrow path to purity lies solely in confession. First, Miss Werwick reports that the advanced Latin class did miserably poorly on their surprise examination. Let them stand and explain themselves."

A block of twenty or so girls rose, looking as if they had been asked to face the Spanish Inquisition.

"If you will not volunteer further information, it is my honour-bound duty to call upon you," Vesalius Munt said reluctantly. "Please raise your hand if you were the highest scoring student in Miss Werwick's class?"

An awkward older girl with a belly slightly wider than her hips and a queer shoulders-backwards posture lifted what resembled a flipper.

"I scored nineteen points out of twenty, sir," she said tragically.

"And do you think you ought to escape punishment for your triumph, Robinson?" Mr. Munt persisted.

Robinson took a long pause. Her classmates regarded her as one might a crouching lion being sighted down a rifle barrel—frightened, threatened, still dangerous.

"Yes." She set her teeth; the others flinched. "Yes, I think that earning so high a mark means I ought not to be punished."

"Oh no," whispered the lacklustre girl called Fox.

"Well, *that* won't go at *all* well," Taylor echoed in a singsong fashion, though she sounded more intrigued than appalled.

"What—" I began.

"Enid Robinson," Mr. Munt boomed, his facial creases deepening to holy fissures, "do you think that *vanity* relieves you from the shame of having failed to assist your fellows?"

Robinson jerked, a hare caught in a trap. "No, sir."

"Perhaps you imagine that worldly accomplishments will cause God to overlook the sin of self-satisfaction?"

Perhaps Robinson meant to reply to this last, but she was prevented.

"An example must be made!" Mr. Munt's soldierly command rang through the hall, and his ever-roving grey eyes glinted. "Robinson, please lead the queue of girls being punished for Latin infractions and waste no time about it—in addition, you can replace luncheon with prayer in the chapel for the following fortnight."

Robinson paled but ducked her chin. I watched as the hapless Latin students picked up their bowls and carried them to the cauldron; one by one, they dumped the stew back into the vat. They then strode out of the dining hall.

This, I thought, *is very much worse than I supposed.*

Suddenly several hands shot into the air, a giddy springtime of sprouting fingers. They seemed to belong to the most peakish of the girls, the ones on whom I would not have laid money should they challenge a dandelion to a duel.

"Clarke," Vesalius Munt called out gladly. "Yes, go on, my dear—lean on Allen there, you seem fatigued, though you deserve no less for having stolen from the poorest of God's servants."

Rebecca Clarke, who only managed to pull herself to a standing position by means of the better-fed Allen, raised her leaf-green eyes. Several teachers (including Miss Werwick) stared on with pleasure as if this were some grotesque circus, whilst others (including Miss Lilyvale) concentrated all their attention upon ceiling beams and bootlaces.

I had not been mistaken in my hazy examination of Clarke—she was no more than seven years old if she was a day, and affecting an uncanny look of forced piety, the one I suppose scientists adopted when strapped to a stake and asked whether or not the Earth was flat.

"What happens if you refuse to throw your supper away?" I whispered, horrified.

"*Hsst.*" Fox shot me a jaundiced glance of warning.

"Clarke, allow your natural urge towards repentance guide you." Mr. Munt's eyes roved, hither and thither, tinsel glints seeking out his victim's victim; I knew who was to be led to the chopping block and felt a contrary surge of pride.

"Poor little mouse has been on a diet of water and brimstone for *four* entire days now, after the larder raid," Taylor explained, sounding bored.

"The new girl," Clarke's tiny voice called. "Please don't punish her, for I hardly know her name. Steele, I think, and she was very tired, as she only arrived today. Miss Lilyvale told her to say her prayers, and she . . . didn't, sir. She fell asleep."

Dozens upon dozens of eyes swept to me as I stood; Mr. Munt frowned happily, returning his attention to Clarke.

"You have redeemed yourself, my child!" he cried. "Clarke, you may eat."

No wild dog ever set upon any limping deer's frame as assiduously as Clarke attacked her stew. She had been reduced to pearly teeth and pink tongue and soiled fingers; I pitied the sight even as my stomach growled.

Miss Lilyvale, a red flag flying across her cheeks, pressed her palm against her stomach and refused to watch.

"Steele, please step forward. You shall not be punished in the usual way, as you are new," Mr. Munt declared, "but you must learn the value we place here upon obedience."

Stepping over the bench, I advanced towards the teachers' table. *Scuff, scuff, scuff* went my shoes and *thud, thud, thud* went my heart as I advanced to be caned or set on a dunce's stool or adorned with a chalkboard or have my hair shorn off.

Mr. Munt smiled as I approached. He extended his hands; Miss Lilyvale, I noted, turned a striking shade of caterpillar green as Vesalius Munt glanced back at her.

"Miss Lilyvale has of late begged me to embrace forgiveness alongside justice, and I hereby publicly grant her wish," he declared.

Mr. Munt is in love with Miss Lilyvale, I thought feebly as his fingers gripped my still-bruised wrists. *That cannot lead to good.* Mr. Munt tugged me so hard that my knees struck the stone floor in front of him.

"You will not go without supper today, Steele," Mr. Munt announced. "You will lead us in prayer instead, for I surmise that despite your reputation for wrongdoing you intended to mind Miss

Lilyvale. Pray say what is in your heart, and your brothers and sisters in Christ shall pray alongside you."

Mr. Munt's eyes bored into me, silver picks illicitly nudging a lock open.

I stared back, thrilling with revulsion.

He is not satisfied unless we are complicit: he likes us responsible for our own abuse.

I recalled Cousin Edwin's features, sweat-slick and satisfied, as he played what he thought was a game.

You're every bit as bad as I am. You liked it.

Meanwhile, Mr. Munt's request that I say what was in my heart was a deliberately humiliating one, for what girl on her knees before an authoritarian feels anything save the pooling of hot shame in her belly, alongside bitter resentment that she should be treated no better than a slave?

I felt these insults, reader, and I collected them, strung them like sand hardened into pearls, and I wore them, invisible; I wear them today.

"Our Father, who art in heaven," I called out clearly with my eyes shut. The flagstone bit further into my knees when Mr. Munt gripped the top of my head as if blessing me. "You delivered me safely to the hands of these godly people, who want to stop the, ah, excesses of my nature. I'm so truly sorry that when Miss Lilyvale told me to pray I did not thank You for, um, her kindness and for Mr. Munt, whose attentions are so . . . thorough, and wise."

The hand on my head like an iron halo shifted, running an approving thumb over the part in my hair before Mr. Munt pressed my brow into the muscle of his thigh; I could smell him, something faintly sweet like candle wax and tarry like cigar smoke. Stifling a revolted choking sound with a cough, I hastened on.

"Please, Lord, will You take pity on this poor sinner, and please will you grant Miss Lilyvale and Mr. Munt patience when dealing with my shortcomings, and, ah, please will You bless all Your beloved children at Lowan Bridge. Amen."

The palm on my crown vanished, and the headmaster stepped back. Looking up, I found Mr. Munt wearing a blended expression: part feigned outward joy, part real inner perplexity, and a final ingredient I think surprised even him—recognition.

I've earned my bowl of supper, I thought, gazing up with a holy smile on my lips and a knife at the back of my teeth. *Try to take it from me.*

"Remarkable!" cried Mr. Munt, easily lifting me to my feet again. "Even the untamed, when moved by the Lord's grace, can inspire an entire congregation with her example. Steele, you may return to your seat."

I kept my head down as I stumbled on battered joints back down the gauntlet, but I stole glances at my classmates from behind the bars of my lashes. Clarke, who sat half-slumped over her empty bowl (by empty I do not mean finished, but rather as clean as if the touch of stew had never kissed this particular vessel), winked at me.

"Well," Taylor huffed when my journey had ended, "I *never.*"

"Didn't you?" I returned, and her pretty eyes narrowed sullenly.

"I never did, no."

"Did you mean a word of that?" Fox whispered.

"Of course," I lied, but I crossed my fingers upon the tabletop, and she granted me a brief smirk.

"That was either spectacular, or else the most *disgraceful* thing I've ever seen," Taylor continued.

Can't it be both? I thought, and I must have been delirious with the strain, for I belted out a laugh I covered with a sneezing fit.

Mr. Munt was calling on other girls now, ones who had been sentenced to diets like Clarke's and were shattering like fine china; one by one, the Reckoning forced about half of those present to dump our meals.

"How is he *allowed*?" I mouthed.

"If any refuse, it's two hours with him in his private office. God knows what happens inside—Fisher went, and would never speak of it afterwards. Anyway, it's the best school for young ladies within fifty miles of London," Fox muttered glumly. "It isn't just the food; they've dozens of ways to make us mind them. Miss Martin gives you hours' worth of lines to write, Miss James will actually ink your offence on your forehead, Miss Lilyvale is a great one for early bedtime—which sounds harmless but we've too many studies for it not to be awful—and Madame Archambault has a little rattan cane in her desk. A fortnight ago, Harper didn't sit for three days."

"None of *that's* so bad," sighed Taylor, her attention pinned to Mr. Munt, "by comparison."

"No." Fox picked at the skin edging her thumbnail. "It isn't."

"And that concludes our Reckoning for this evening!" Mr. Munt surveyed the room, finding no further quarry which tempted him. "I commend you for your diligence, children. Sit, and partake of God's bounty."

The stew was thick and sweet and savoury, chunks of carrot and potato and speckles of currants swimming alongside succulent mutton; we set upon it like the beasts Mr. Munt intended us to be.

"Have girls not asked their parents to lobby for Mr. Munt's removal?" I asked Taylor.

She tossed her shapely round chin. "It's *quite* hopeless, I'm afraid. Mr. Munt sells the leftovers at reduced rates to the manufactory men four miles from here, and what's left he gives away at soup kitchens. He's positively *worshipped* from here to London."

"Is that why he said Clarke stole from the poor when she really stole from the larder?"

"Exactly," murmured Fox. "She was the only one caught, caught with her arms full and pockets stuffed after lights-out no less, but they knew more were involved. These four days she's been refusing to give him any names."

"She must be very brave."

Taylor snorted, reaching for another slice of bread. "Very *silly,* you mean. Clarke has never really been punished before; they wanted her for the raid because she could fit through the door for the barn cats. She's new, only six, can memorise anything you put in front of her, perform terribly difficult figures—and from a very queer family. *Literary,* I think, God knows what sort of *horrid* people that entails."

"Your parents are tradesmen," Fox said with visible satisfaction.

"Your parents just sold half their estate, and *you* are a cow," Taylor said sweetly.

"My parents are dead," said I, "so I do hope to be friends with you all."

"Hush this *instant*!" Taylor gasped.

"Thank you, no," Fox mumbled.

"The instant you really detest anyone, by *all* means become friends with her," Taylor sang with studied indifference. "When Mr. Munt sets you against each other, be sure to have picked someone you can outtalk, which I'm confident you can after that . . . *display.* Remember when he forced Abbott to tell him that Dunning had helped her study for the botany project?"

"Don't." Fox shivered dramatically.

"How about when Fiddick and Hooper giggled during Communion?"

"I'm trying to eat," Fox complained, jabbing the air with her spoon.

"Mr. Munt just *adores* friends." A pale blue tinge of melancholy had deepened Taylor's tone. "*Most* of us know better."

We finished the meal in silence. When I rose to depart with

Taylor and glanced back at Mr. Munt, I saw that his attention was likewise on me—displaying reluctant approval tinged with the desire to run the new Thoroughbred through its paces.

If Edwin had not been so stupid, I thought as the knot of fear in my chest tightened, *they would have been very much alike.*

SEVEN

And then my mind made its first earnest effort to comprehend what had been infused into it concerning heaven and hell: and for the first time it recoiled, baffled; and for the first time, glancing behind, on each side, and before it, it saw all round an unfathomed gulf: it felt the one point where it stood—the present; all the rest was formless cloud and vacant depth; and it shuddered at the thought of tottering, and plunging amid that chaos.

Some memoirs explain social hierarchies by means of illustrative anecdotes, but mine is about homicide, not ladies' schools.

Four varieties of females attended Lowan Bridge. First, there were girls from wealthy untitled families (like Taylor) who were considered too gauche to deserve their fortunes and were being educated in hopes of finding a good position in a household of a higher class or becoming more easily marriageable. Second, there were girls from poor titled families (like Fox) who were expected to become governesses because their fathers had poured thousands of pounds into the gutter. Third, there were orphaned girls who had incurred the wrath of their moneyed relations (like myself) and were being gifted the privilege of becoming drudges on other people's estates.

Finally, there was Becky Clarke, whose parents wanted her to attend school despite the fact they could afford to keep a tutor and a well-stocked library, and had said nothing to her of being a governess; and I have this anomaly to thank for the lesson that there is no accounting for taste.

"Are you feeling better?" I asked her when the bell rang next morn and the girls began to stir, for I had sensed her pensive eyes upon me since daybreak.

"Much," Clarke chimed.

"I heard what happened and admired that you gave no one away."

"When you're half the size of everyone else, you take care not to offend."

"Yes, but you're very . . . noteworthy, for your age."

"Can't be helped," she said in her high, absent way. "My parents say there's no use in clapping a turtle shell on a parrot or gluing wings to a reptile. So they sent me here. That shan't happen again if I can help it, singling you out at Reckoning."

I thought of Mr. Munt's strong hand on my head, my skin against his trouser leg, and thought, *I'd not have liked that to happen to you in my place either.*

"What I said about you was true, but saying it was dishonourable," Clarke mused lightly, pulling a straw-hued strand of her hair through her fingers. "How beastly. I can't bear dishonourable people."

I was such an inappropriate addressee for this remark that I buried my face in my pillow and laughed heartily.

"Friends," groaned Taylor. She kicked me with feet cold as snow, rolling out of bed. "I *told* you. Don't bother."

Donning my new uniform and pairing with my new bedmate as we walked to classes was of no interest other than the fact I was nearly dizzy with anxiety; a brief account of that first day, however, will fully acquaint the reader with my new life.

My first class was art, headed by Miss Constance Sheffleton, a timid silver-haired rabbit who would not have recognised discipline had it whipped her across the palms. Nevertheless, she knew where her bread was buttered, and proved it when she called tremulously, "Davies, you are here to sketch the bust, not contemplate the maple outside the window. Please inform Mr. Munt that I caught you idling."

"Yes, Miss," said a thin waif, and we winced, for this was clearly worse than any other punishment.

Following art was sewing lessons given by Miss Kitts. Ages were combined during class periods, but thence divided into circles appropriate to our ability; having been separated from Clarke, I asked her in high alarm what the matter was when we rejoined in the hall and I saw her doll's mouth a-tremble.

"I was just feeling better and now I'm to miss luncheon, all over badly embroidering a pansy," she confided, angrily swiping at the tears in her eyes. "I'm useless at stitchwork, my mind wanders so. What are decorative pansies to us, Steele?"

When I arrived at Latin, Miss Werwick briefly quizzed me, found me dismal, and bid me sit with the youngest girls, muttering happy imprecations about the amount of meals I should likely be forced to sacrifice. Never having studied Latin previous, I congratulated myself when at the end of the hour, I was explaining the lesson to the perplexed circumference, and Miss Werwick forgot herself far enough to frown at this development.

Midday dinner was allowed me, though it seemed a mere two thirds of the young ladies initially assembled the night before were present. Not seeing Taylor, I sat across from Fox, who fiddled with a piece of her already-greasy hair before saying, "Anything immediate?"

I swallowed hearty cabbage and pork broth, regarding her questioningly.

"It's what we say," Fox confided. "A code. To find out if anyone is . . . well, really in trouble."

"Oh." I set my spoon down, sobered. "Clarke isn't here—an embroidery mishap."

"I've an apple in my pillowcase," Fox said matter-of-factly. "All's well."

This was the day I learnt that friendship need not be labelled as such in order to be a very similar thing indeed.

A combined history and geography course given by Miss Halifax followed dinner. She was a hatchet-faced woman with animated hands—but there was no harm in her, and her enthusiasm was engaging.

"Why, Steele, though you are not well-read regarding the Ottoman Empire, you ask exceedingly incisive questions," she exclaimed. "You shall sit with the thirteen-year-olds and with Clarke here."

Clarke, whose brilliance on all subjects, save that of rendering decorative flowering plants with thread, was the envy of the entire school, seemed strangely happy when I descended into the hard-backed chair beside her.

"Good, we can go over dates of battles before bedtimes," she decreed lightly, adjusting the strange white cap we wore. "My parents are pacifists, the disgrace of our entire street, and when I arrived, I didn't know a Cossack from a dragoon."

"Of course. Anything immediate?" I asked, a shower of golden sparks prickling my skin as I did something illicit.

"Ha. No," said Clarke, one cheek dimpling. "Thank you, indirectly, for the apple."

Music class ensued immediately afterwards. Remembering Vesalius Munt's opinion that spiritually contented artists were beings not to be found upon this teeming globe, I looked forward to Miss Lilyvale's tutelage with intrigue. Was her virtue so potent it could withstand the moral ravages of even art? A simpler answer proved true: Miss Lilyvale's musical ear was the happy amalgam of a deaf mockingbird's and a colicky newborn's, and thus could not have troubled her character in the smallest degree.

"Class, we have much to do today!" she called. "But first as ever,

I will lead us in a hymn. Young ladies, here is our music. As this is a new piece—do think of it as an exercise in sight-reading."

We stood all in a semicircle and sang Horatius Bonar's latest opus. My ignorance of whether the Almighty's glory swelled in the wake of our praise remains profound to this day; I can inform the reader, however, that no gain in sight-reading skills resulted. Taylor was present, and I greeted her afterwards, even as she mumbled *George Louis, George Augustus, George William Frederick, George Augustus Frederick. . . .*

"Taylor," I whispered, "anything immediate?"

"Oh, go *away*, you horrid nosy thing," cried Taylor, her eyes edged in pink. "I've had *nothing* to eat since the porridge, and meanwhile Granville is such a sweet girl, all those golden curls and her family from a simply ancient coffee fortune, and so the *best* sort of people, and she was made to slap herself in the face—*herself*, mind, and hard—after Mr. Munt caught her laughing over a sketch Fiddick did of Miss Hardbottle. Don't touch me, I can't bear *anyone*," she sobbed, fleeing.

Mathematics followed, and theology, and French (at which I excelled, *naturellement*, and thus forever after avoided the red welts my classmates carried as souvenirs from Madame Archambault), and after we had crammed our heads full of geometry and the Book of John, the inevitable Reckoning followed.

I ate my stew and kept my head as low as any true acolyte.

I reproduce this workaday agenda to illustrate that we lived practically in one another's pockets, so that in moments of emergency—which were as frequent as moments of breathing—we might offer help. If we succeeded thanks to cleverness and collaboration, we might fall asleep with a meal or even two, perhaps, rounding the hollows of our bellies. We were not *friends*; but so many others strove to make us wretched that we lacked the energy to turn upon one another save in the extremest necessity.

When I dropped exhaustedly next to Taylor at nine o'clock that first night as the sun vanished, I felt the same electric charge I have always gained from thwarting authority traversing the narrow ridge of my back.

You haven't missed a meal yet, I thought. *You could be very good at this. And the others might be made better off as well.*

"Steele?" came a piping voice.

"Yes?" I answered Clarke.

"Good night," said she, as Taylor's warning toes jabbed me.

Grief is a strange passenger; it rides on one's shoulder quiet as a guardian angel one moment, then sinks razor talons into one's collarbones the next. No sooner had Clarke offered me this kindness than hot salt tears were soaking my pillow. My mother had once bid me good night, and good morning too; and my mother had loved me, and she had died for no reason I could discern, and was never coming back.

I would cry often for Mamma's loss, as children are wont to do—but I could never have guessed that my own melancholy would lead to discoveries which once more dashed my world from its orbit.

The event which caused me fully to embrace my true nature took place some six months later.

By this time, I had come to know many facets of Lowan Bridge School. I knew that Taylor was secretly terrified not of being a governess but of being married to someone tyrannical, as her mother daily hid fresh bruises under flounces and lace; I knew that the curse of Fiona Fiddick's life was that she was the funniest creature on earth, which meant that she weighed a stone less than she ought to have; I knew that under Fox's dour attitude hid a girl who somehow always had an apple in her pillowcase, and never kept it for herself.

I knew that there were stables, unlocked ones, and horses available for caressing. I knew that the roof above our dormitory was accessible if one crept carefully, and that Clarke's eyes as she mapped the swath of glittering black not obscured by the reek of London to the south of us were mossy pools in the moonlight, and that though she seldom laughed, she laughed at a stolen glimpse of the night sky most blithely of all, and her laugh was like the treble of a silver flute.

Sunday was both beloved and dreaded, for while we had no classes and were allowed to play on the lawn or read in quiet nooks, we were compelled to attend chapel. As we marched towards the elegant stone building on the day my life altered forever, a parade of dull blue soldiers plodding under stony November skies, the casual observer might have supposed we were going to be executed.

Sunday, after all, was the day Mr. Munt performed a *weekly* Reckoning, in order to catch out any sins we might have foolishly neglected to mention.

"Steele, will you help me with the Catullus assignment?" Fox's ungainly form landed beside me in the third pew. "I can't make heads or tails of it, and even if Miss Werwick doesn't have a cane—"

"Of course," I agreed. Censure from Madame Archambault was humiliating and painful, but Miss Werwick of all the teachers relished referring us to Mr. Munt, as if we were chess pieces (or, better still, ninepins).

Clarke sat upon my other side. "Anything immediate, mi'ladies?"

Clarke was wont to trill when she was well fed, as if beginning to compose a folk tune, and I adored her for it. I was about to answer in the negative when Miss Lilyvale advanced to take her seat before the pipe organ and commence our two hours of agony.

"With a true spirit of praise, girls, sing with me!" Miss Lilyvale called out.

A veil of authorial privacy will be drawn here; it would behove neither the reader nor the author to dwell upon musical atrocities which reside wholly in the past and cannot now be remedied.

After the initial three hymns had been sung, Mr. Munt ascended to the pulpit. Vesalius Munt was never more happy than when every student's attention speared in his direction, fixed to him like nails as he stood before the crucifix.

"Happy Sabbath to you, my girls," he announced, beaming, and the *my* stuck in our thorny throats, for it was the truest sentiment he would admit to all morning. "I encourage you to rest peacefully upon this holiest of days, and repose knowing that Christ died to save you from your own ignorance and infamy. Let us proceed with our weekly Reckoning, that we might cleanse our souls."

A hand raised. Mr. Munt devised a demeaning punishment for the accused—and often for the accuser. There were no rules in this jungle, no trails we might tread so as to escape the tiger's tooth. We were paying as much mind as we ever did, Fox and I and Clarke, ears pricked for danger, when I startled at the sound of my name.

"Steele *means* well," my bedmate was drawling exhaustedly from two pews distant. "And she's as clever and helpful as everyone says, and oh, it's *dreadful*, but she . . . she doesn't mean to, and I *hate* to say it."

I turned to gape at her. Taylor's face was bloodless, a mere illustration: black hair thickly inked, eye and lip hinted at in delicate pen strokes. Her beauty had been marred of late by her uselessness at memorisation, and she had forsaken sleep in favour of struggling alone over data which meant nothing to her; now she embraced the only option guaranteed to merit a hot meal. I did not marvel that it was me—I was a proximal target, even a sensible one, already having earned a reputation for lying my way out of scrapes.

"What is it that Steele did not intend to do, Taylor?" Mr. Munt rested a poised arm against the pulpit.

Taylor's round eyes flew to my queer tilted almond ones. "She dreams."

"What in God's name is Taylor doing?" growled Fox.

"It's my fault," I assured her quietly. "I didn't notice she had got so frail. She has every reason to lie about me."

"She isn't lying," I thought Fox muttered.

"Steele has simply *terrible* nightmares about her mother," Taylor declared. "She doesn't mean to scream, but she won't *stop*."

My heart stuttered.

Yes, I often awoke covered in sweat and raw-throated as a carrion crow and, yes, I dreamt of my mother; but I did not *scream* for her. Did I? Once or twice had I bitten back cries, but these were rarities, accidents.

Rising, I clasped my hands before my white apron. "I'm sorry for giving any trouble, but my mother died recently."

"Over half a year hence," Mr. Munt corrected.

"Mourning her is only *natural*. But please forgive me for disturbing the peace."

"Natural?" Mr. Munt struck the flat of his hand against the podium as if smiting sin itself. "Let our hearts go out, girls, to this wayward lamb, who meditates on death when in the midst of God's abundance."

I bit the inside of my lip until I could taste all I had left of my mother, which was her blood.

"Steady," Clarke chimed softly.

"Let Steele," intoned Mr. Munt, "come to thank You, Lord, for your grace in orchestrating her removal from her mother's evil influence."

My hands gripping the pew had transformed into bleached bones.

"And let us never give up the hope that she may return one day to honest Christian practices!"

"Steady," Clarke squeaked, gripping my skirt.

"Mourning my mother is not dishonest!" I cried.

I may as well have set off a bomb in the chapel; every eye

swept to me in dismay. Contradicting Mr. Munt was tantamount to suicide; unfortunately, I had not yet grasped that suicide was the topic.

"Your mother," Mr. Munt enunciated, relishing every syllable, "was a debauchee who perished deliberately by means of self-administered laudanum. She was thus buried with minimal services by the only minister willing to overlook her Gallic Catholic affiliations and willful self-slaughter, and your sainted aunt spared you the indignity of witnessing such a barren sight. Tell me, why should mourning your mother be praised as any sort of virtue when her tainted spirit so obviously haunts your own immortal soul? Your mother was a disgrace to the natural order—an embodied disaster."

He had known all along, I realised.

There had been no mourners in crepe at my mother's funeral, I understood: only the overripe aroma of earth unwilling to accept yet another unpaid houseguest. Suicide was high treason, for what greater violation existed than thwarting God's will?

My sentence (a week of missing dinner) was announced and Taylor invited to rejoin the ranks of the fed; but the pit of my stomach swelled into a cavern long before hunger descended.

Mr. Munt had won; I had not been prepared for the truth. A small hand interlaced with mine.

"You don't cry out so *very* often," Clarke whispered, wide-eyed and earnest.

"I will now," I managed hoarsely before disengaging myself and opening our prayer book with palsied fingers.

I have learnt since that a great many people are ill intentioned and yet behave well. I might have followed suit—winked into the mirror of a morning and worn a white sheep's coat all the livelong day. Jane Eyre was told to pray to God to take away her heart of stone, that she might be gifted a heart of flesh; but my heart of flesh bled for my mother, my mother whom I would apparently *never see again* if I was good.

The wind howled that November night as if mourning a lost love; and the decision I reached in my hard bed with Taylor's cold toes prodding my calves, sobbing as silently as I could, went as follows:

If I must go to hell to find my mother again, so be it: I will be another embodied disaster.

But I will be a beautiful disaster.

EIGHT

"I might have been as good as you,—wiser,—almost as stainless. I envy you your peace of mind, your clean conscience, your unpolluted memory. Little girl, a memory without blot or contamination must be an exquisite treasure—an inexhaustible source of pure refreshment: is it not?"

It would have been possible for me to survive Lowan Bridge for longer than the bleak seven years I spent there had Mr. Munt not taken it into his head to kill Clarke.

Oh, we were subjected to daily indignity, each Reckoning more creatively vicious than the last; but small moments of happiness touched us deeply. In a mansion, blessings are lost amidst bric-a-brac; in a pit, they shimmer like the flash of dragonfly wings.

There was Miss Lilyvale's boundless capacity to ruin even the simplest music. There was Fiona Fiddick's faculties for both humour and sewing, which enabled her to hide the words *FEED ME* in an embroidered nosegay of coral peonies which Miss Sheffleton proudly hung upon the classroom wall. There were horses, and riding lessons, and I learnt to love galloping through the daisy-dotted meadows, pretending I need never return. There were the holidays, when Mr. Munt was out lecturing, and there was Clarke's fierce, small-lipped smile when she arrived back after Christmas with her carpetbag and delivered an impetuous peck to my cheek.

Reader, I had miraculously acquired a companion; Clarke's existence owned me, opened me, left me helpless with stifled giggles at midnight. Becky Clarke was brilliant and ridiculous, an effortless scholar who insisted on honour when honour led only to missed meals; she was three years my junior, so I could shrug her off as an irritating protégée the instant anyone raised an eyebrow; and she responded to both compliments and criticism with the same casual piping responses, as if baffled anyone had noticed she was there at all. Her simplicity was droll, her mind captivating—had anyone asked whether I thought her a genius or an idiot, I should not have had a satisfactory answer.

"Would you like to watch the sun rise?" Clarke would ask when the weather was fine, and madly I would accompany her to the roof, yawning and cracking sluggish joints, and we would sit there quite contented, always gazing at the murky haze of London not so very far away from us, and seeming—as was perfectly true—nearer to its outskirts every year. She would hum soft songs whilst gazing at the firmament, and her head would find its way to my shoulder.

Meanwhile, we all grew longer limbs and harder hearts every year.

Granville passed away during the fever which swept through our school when I was eleven years old. Taylor wept dreadfully, saying that Ettie Granville had been the only person ever to understand her; I raided the charity salvage pile and delivered her monogrammed kerchief to my bedmate, who clutched me about the shoulders for all the world to see.

Influenza claimed Fox when I was thirteen; I orchestrated the theft of a bushel of apples to store in her memory and was caught out during a vengeful Reckoning. Clarke smuggled me broth in a hot-water bottle and watched me guzzle it as we both hid behind the bed frame.

We became adept at grieving, suffering agonies for a day or two, and then returning to our altered orbits. I grew accustomed to the facts of my mother's death more slowly, the horrible truth that she had finally managed the trick she must have attempted long before, which was to die. The others treated me predictably poorly for a spell—who can escape the stigma of a lunatic for a mother—but we all hated Mr. Munt so ferociously, with every red pulse of life, that we had not time to hate one another.

All fell to pieces, however, when I had been at Lowan Bridge for seven years, and Clarke's preoccupation with honour swerved from pleasant foolishness into fatal lunacy.

There we stood before Miss Lilyvale's desk, awaiting instructions.

"Would you girls please study . . . oh, goodness, I'm that scattered . . . the piano part, Steele, and this soprano vocal part, Clarke, for the end-of-year gala? I can think of no one better able to demonstrate our talents. Won't you say yes?"

We glanced at each other; excelling at any course was a coveted position, but evidence suggested that our favourite teacher's praise was not so complimentary as her censure. Meanwhile, Clarke was an outstanding vocalist—her tones were dizzyingly high, hovering midair as if a magical harp had been strummed. Students came to a bewildered halt in hallways whenever she practised her scales with that mathematical precision which was so innate in her.

"Of course." Clarke took the small bundle of songs.

Then a strange thing occurred: head folding, Miss Lilyvale leant forward against her desk briefly. Her rosy cheeks had lost their blush during the course of the past two years, as if she had been bid to shoulder a stone up an endless mountainside; every month Miss Lilyvale became more of an automaton with something terribly pleading beneath the waxworks. She drew her fingers along the knob of her drawer, eyes briefly falling shut.

"Do you want something else of us?" Clarke asked.

She answered softly, "I can never have the things I truly want."

"Are you all right, Miss Lilyvale?" I inquired, concerned.

"Oh! Heavens yes, I was only . . . distracted. Thank you for being so obliging," our teacher said, smiling, and the strange moment was shattered.

"It's in the desk," Clarke announced as Miss Lilyvale bustled off to see that some younger girls were given appropriate parts. I was sixteen, Clarke thirteen, and thus as model pupils we were often left to our own devices—save for the inevitable Reckonings.

"What's in the desk?"

"Whatever is haunting Miss Lilyvale." Clarke studied her music. The charm of her distraction lay in the fact it was genuine; Becky Clarke could not lie if her life hung in the balance, and I shall soon cite statistical evidence to this effect. "This is rather high even for me, though I do like G major."

"Never mind music," I whispered as we quit the classroom. "Miss Lilyvale is stretched as tight as the catgut on her violin strings. You really mean to say you know what ails her?"

Clarke lifted the choral part as we walked. The birds outside the gloom-shrouded staircases were dumb that April afternoon, the carpets mute beneath our footsteps. "I went into the music room at half four yesterday because I thought I left my sketchbook, and Miss Lilyvale was reading a letter. When I appeared, she shoved it in the drawer she just touched so sadly."

"And you think her correspondent is making her *ill*?"

"No one can say," Clarke owned, tossing her flaxen curls though they were restrained under her chaste cap. "But if ever it looked as if a letter were strangling someone . . ."

The ensuing silence fairly crawled with questions.

Does Clarke wish me to intervene? I wondered, heart thrumming eagerly.

I had countless times thwarted hunger at Lowan Bridge, taking as much joy in naughtiness as in success; I had forged grades, pilfered supplies, told positively operatic lies. Queerly, Clarke had never minded these untruths, though I supposed that was thanks to her natural compassion, or else her practicality. In any event, I had learnt the principle swiftly: if I lied to Mr. Munt (or anyone else to do with the ultimate act of lying to Mr. Munt), I would be praised; if I lied to Clarke—all of these accidental falsehoods, bred of forgetfulness—I would be shunned until her ire burnt itself to cinders and she nuzzled into my shoulder like a cat seeking company.

So I had lied, and grown still better at it—for myself, and for my fellow prisoners. It only followed, since Miss Lilyvale was our unquestioned ally despite being a teacher, that I ought to ferret out what was wrong with her.

I wonder about the verb *to ferret* now I am grown. If a conjugation of a similar verb, *to snake*, existed, I believe that would have been closer to the truth—for my slithering, slinking capabilities had been honed by age sixteen to a nearly reptilian pitch.

I did not dream of inviting Clarke to raid Miss Lilyvale's office that night, which in hindsight was a monstrous error; had we made the discovery together, we might have talked through what was best to be done.

Quietly, I eased my coarse frock on and skipped the apron, that material being too pale for untrammelled moonlight. I flinched as the door creaked, but no one stirred; if the girls knew one thing, it was that my disobedience tended to benefit the majority. Shutting the door behind me and risking further noise would have tempted Fate, so I stepped into the hallway, leaving a draught of air in my wake.

It had cost me two weeks' practice with a bent nail to pick my first lock at the age of ten, aptitude for larder raids being a highly esteemed skill. As I knelt before Miss Lilyvale's music-room door, however, I felt strangely inept—my fingers were clubs, my ears abuzz with fanciful susurrations. At last, I prised open the lock and was greeted by the predictable midnight sight of an empty room within a sinister stronghold, its shuttered windows and watchful walls.

The desk was also locked. After fiddling with the nail, I substituted a hat pin, which swiftly worked its magic, and I pulled open the drawer.

As Clarke had suggested, a stack of letters rested there.

I lit the lamp with a lucifer from my dress pocket, hid the light under the desk, and sat upon the floor Indian-style. At first glance, I thought the letters must have dated back at least a year or two, for how else could some of the eggshell-coloured paper have deepened to pale yolk in tone? The envelopes were blank save for the addressee, *Miss Amy Lilyvale*, and I frowned in concentration as I slid the thin foolscap out.

Then my lips parted ways as I gazed upon the contents of what seemed the oldest correspondence.

They were *confessions.*

Dear Miss L——

I can suffocate no longer under this mask, nor daily live a falsehood when such misplaced secrecy makes hypocrites out of honest Christians. I do beg your forgiveness for what I am about to say, and indeed, begging your forgiveness ought to have been a duty I performed years previous; if I cannot confess all to you now, however, my integrity is meaningless, and my boundless love nothing finer than a canker eating away at my swollen tongue.

I long to put my mouth upon you; yes, your lips, but I confess to far more fervidly desired locales. I wish that when your eyes met mine, they travelled a slow route to my trouser front. I wish that I could taste you where you must ache for me as I do for you. My mouth upon your sweet flesh, and then my journey back up your body, and your face when I finish the first slow thrust into you, the one I compelled you to beg for; these images soak my dreams until there is nothing left of my free will, and I urge you to answer me: Are you innocent regarding my torment?

My hope is that you will not shun me after these disclosures. I am your employer, after all, and so must promise that your reputation as well as my own rests in my careful palms—safe from the censure of a prurient world, I assure you. I only hope that you can help to absolve me now I have disclosed my desires, and that we may unite forever as one flesh, or else live as forthright and forgiving siblings in Christ.

In brotherly love,
Vesalius

After blinking for what seemed hours, I edged under the desk beside the sour-smelling metal lamp with what I have subsequently learnt was a pile of ripe erotica.

Reading the second letter took me ten minutes, as half my body physically shrank from looking; reading the remaining thirteen took half an hour; I was, in this as in all other vices, a fast learner. I hoped that subsequent missives would deplore his initial one, but they were all of a kind, save that vocabulary like *breast* and *cunny* and *arse* and *rut* liberally seasoned later disclosures.

When I had finished, I scrambled out and leant over the desk, feeling a profoundly strange admixture of nausea and high-pitched excitement like the sensation of dismounting after a hard gallop.

Had this been what Edwin had meant?

You're every bit as bad as I am. You liked it.

I did *not* like this feeling, this unsettled tingling wrongness; I felt it with Clarke sometimes at the edge of the rooftop when I thought, *How easy it would be to simply step off,* and my heartbeat soared, and I flinched away from the edge, unspeaking and ashamed of myself and giddy with quicksilver nerves which fired from scalp to spine and lower.

I did not strictly *dislike* the sensation either, however.

I stole the letters and stole back to our dormitory. Crawling into bed next to Taylor following questionable excursions by now carried no risk, and she snored through my manoeuvres; Clarke, however, was aquiver with attention in the next bed, her eyes dancing over me in the grey not-light as I pulled back the coverlet.

"I was right, wasn't I?" she asked.

At a loss for words, I passed Clarke the letters and curled up with my back to her golden curls.

This was not my first mistake, but would prove to be the most careless—no matter how confused I was by the strange pulse of blood in my groin. Sharing my findings with Clarke seemed the only option; the thought of digesting those letters alone, without her to partake in the disgusting yet exotic meal, revolted me—I girlishly wanted someone else to be as agitated as I was.

And yet, it was more than that. Clarke made me mindlessly, achingly happy. I wanted us to share in everything; I wanted us to sail to faraway China, for us to attend a lavish costume ball, for her to be threatened with a pistol and for me to throw myself in the path of the bullet. Often as I fell asleep I fantasised she had been forced to name me as a murderess in a Reckoning, so that I might be sentenced to starve in a frigid straw-lined aerie, and as I lay dying she would visit and we should watch the stars fading through the window and I should whisper in the shell of her ear with my last breath, *Never mind.*

I forgive you.

I didn't mind.

That never happened, but apparently the worst things I can imagine still fall short of reality.

. . .

At the next daily Reckoning, we were witness to an act akin to watching a tree sprouting from the sky, or rains bursting forth from the grounds like perverse fountains. I have never been so shocked; and were you, reader, to suggest greater surprises are in store for me, I should suggest you invest in the purchase of a strait waistcoat without delay.

"I name Mr. Munt," Clarke said soberly.

The remark was so unreal that I laughed, choked, and then planted my palm firmly over my lips.

To say that Clarke turned heads would be an understatement. The announcement slammed into my chest like a physical blow. I have been thrown from a horse, attacked by multiple men, fallen down a flight of stairs; none of these events ever struck me so hard, because none of them so explicitly announced, *this is your fault.*

Mr. Munt initially could not believe his own ears. "Whom do you mean to name, Clarke?" he inquired.

"I already did. You've subjected Miss Lilyvale to unwanted attentions, Mr. Munt. Say you're sorry."

Mr. Munt's handsome face paled. He glanced at Miss Lilyvale, who was not looking at him, because Miss Lilyvale was looking at me. I understood then what I had not before: she had *wanted* us to find the letters. Miss Lilyvale was vacillating and weak, and Clarke and I were neither, and others had noticed. Miss Lilyvale's lake-blue eyes dimmed in shame as the other teachers whispered *oh my* and *but it can't be true, can it?*

"Clarke." Mr. Munt by now seemed outwardly composed save for his throat, which was ropy with rage under his white collar. "Do you truly mean to falsely accuse your headmaster when your own situation here is so precarious?"

"I don't understand," Clarke said, lifting her chin.

"Oh, I should never have troubled you with the information had you not made a mockery of the Reckoning," Vesalius Munt hissed. "Your parents have told you they publish books, I presume? That they are among the literary set?"

Clarke said nothing.

"I believe in the value of education for every child, including even *females*, a position which has garnered me much criticism!" Mr. Munt cried with an arm raised. "And here this beggar at the gates of paradise accuses *me* of misconduct! Her parents print lurid erotic fiction, which it pains me to say in your company, ladies," he added, flushing nicely before the rapt teaching staff. "They donated beyond Clarke's fee to consign their daughter to my care; I accepted, hoping to save the child from heinous influences; and now she—the viper!—tells me that I have made Miss Lilyvale the subject of my *unwanted attentions*?"

"Oh my *God*," breathed Taylor, morbidly fascinated.

We watched as Miss Lilyvale clutched at her voiceless throat and fled the room. When I think of the anger I felt, I will always recall ice and not fire, the way snow sears into one's flesh.

Clarke's face was rigid save for the tremor in her tiny lips.

"Yes," said she, "that's exactly what I mean to tell you."

"Excellent," said Mr. Munt, enjoying himself again. "You can confine yourself to porridge at breakfast for the foreseeable future. Next confessor?"

NINE

"I am very happy, Jane; and when you hear that I am dead you must be sure and not grieve: there is nothing to grieve about. . . . By dying young I shall escape great sufferings. I had not qualities or talents to make my way very well in the world: I should have been continually at fault."

Within a fortnight, Clarke was a shade haunting hallways where no one saw or spoke to her, carrying such slight weight that the desk seats must have thought her a spring breeze. Her skin grew ashen, her lips cracked, her eyes mirrors.

"I am so ashamed of myself," Miss Lilyvale whispered.

We were in the choir room on a Sunday before the service, only she and I, for I had left a note in her drawer demanding she meet me. Outside, the merry May breezes wanted only blithe girls with ribbons for their dance to be complete, and I pitied Miss Lilyvale for the necessity of my company a little; she had already endured unwanted attentions, veiled threats, and now a scheming schoolgirl. The choir room was neat and orderly, save for a dainty rug under the practice piano which had been gnawed by mice and reminded me of my music teacher.

"What can be done?" I urged, outwardly calm and inwardly

frantic. "And what did you think *would* be done, anyhow? You must have wanted us to find them, but I can't imagine what—"

"And I can't either!" she cried, eyes wild, before her mouth pressed into a tormented dash. She hugged her own arms. "You must forgive me. No—no, you mustn't, I've no right to even ask. My father is a country parson, my mother an industrious invalid, and they are happy when they've oxtails for their soup. Their parish is just outside London, but poor and plain for all its proximity. I learnt piano, thinking I could give private lessons. Well, I'm an utter shipwreck at music, and Mr. Munt when visiting our parish lecturing hired me anyhow, I arrived just a year before you did though I was far older, and this position pays—oh, don't look at me, I can't bear it."

"You think you're lucky to have the place." I tentatively touched her forearm.

"I think he wanted me and not my music—who could want my music! He courted me for years without ever proposing before the letters started, and now I'm trapped, for what decent woman would have kept a job of all things with such correspondences plaguing her?" She shuddered. "Last month, he stopped me in a deserted corridor to, to *pray* for me, and he put his palms on my brow and here, over my heart."

I required answers, and so increased the pressure on her arm. "Have you spoken with him since Clarke's Reckoning?"

"Not a word. Did you burn the letters?" Miss Lilyvale whispered. "I thought them proof of his disgusting attentions, but that was unspeakably foolish—they are merely evidence of my complicity. Did you destroy them?"

"Yes," I lied.

It was better than saying *I reread them nightly because I do not understand their effect on me and I am studying it in the cause of science.*

"Thank you. I was . . . terrified, paralysed."

"We've tried everything," said I, implacable. "We've shared, we've stolen, we've foraged spring greens when we were meant to be playing hopscotch. Clarke *will not* survive. What can we do?"

Pressing her sleeve to her eyes, Miss Lilyvale glanced in naked fright at the clock in the corner. "God forgive me. I'm your teacher, I ought to have . . . Yes, there is one thing to be done. Mr. Munt is his own bookkeeper. If you altered his accounts, and then took food on the day of its delivery, he would not know you had done so. Tomorrow the farm will deliver the week's eggs and produce."

The information echoed like the clap of a gong, for Clarke that morning had confessed herself bedridden. Porridge, lawn weeds, and rare stolen roast potatoes would no longer suffice.

"I take it I'm meant to perform this little magic trick," I could not help but mention.

"Oh, Steele—"

"Never mind. I'll do it. Does he keep the ledger in his study?"

Miss Lilyvale nodded, righting her hunched posture. "He invited me there for tea once. I shall never forget that occasion, no matter how I try."

"When girls refuse to return their food, they're told to visit his study, and no one speaks of it afterwards," I said lowly. "Why?"

"He tells them who he thinks they really are, and what they must sacrifice to save themselves from hellfire," Miss Lilyvale answered against a raw throat. "Sometimes he shows them pictures, suggests things . . . things he accuses them of secretly longing to do. For hours. Can you imagine?"

I could, but the service was about to commence. "I must know why you placed me in this position."

Two feverish blots glared from her cheeks. "Please understand that I never meant for Clarke to—"

"Do the idiotic thing she did. I still deserve an explanation."

Miss Lilyvale was a sweet, toothless, impressionable creature, but she was also an honest one, and finally she looked me straight in the eye.

"I know your past is . . . chequered. I also know that you forgive others more readily than anyone I have ever encountered, and I cherish it—you have a great talent, you know, for accepting people. Have you ever kept a secret," Miss Lilyvale asked me, all the blood in her body seeming to drain straight through the floor, "which was not precisely your fault, but which would—if discovered—ruin you? Have you ever awoken to nothing save dread of daylight?"

"You know I have," I answered, comprehending that she spoke of my mother's bad end.

"Mr. Munt means to destroy me if he cannot have me," Miss Lilyvale murmured. "Please forgive my inexcusable actions. I only . . . I simply couldn't do it anymore."

Watching her, I thought about secrets. One can grow accustomed to carrying unseeable scars, as if the tattoo one wears is inked in flesh tone over flesh tone; but nevertheless one is still covered in *secret*, painted with secret, stained by it. I would have done anything to shed Edwin's dead eyes glazed fish-scale grey.

Solving Miss Lilyvale's problem and saving Clarke at once would have to suffice, however, lest I defy the restful nature of the Sabbath.

"I'll be in Mr. Munt's study during the service." I turned on my heel. "If you might make any excuses necessary which prevent my being looked for? That would be rather the least you could do."

Shadows are curious entities; they are lightless and yet cast a shape into the world, just as I do. As I ventured through the empty hallways, I did not think of myself as *myself* at all but as another Jane, a shadow given form. This curious phenomenon echoed the way I had come to think of my cousin's murder—Edwin was no more, due to regrettable events somehow removed from the Jane Steele who had mastered translating Cato and gliding along with a spine straight as a pikestaff. My mother was also no more, but that was another matter, I thought as I tiptoed, flinching at each creak. I had been wicked, in an impulsive fashion; I had been devious, in minor targeted ones.

This time I would invade a headmaster's private office, forge records, and escape, which would be a sure step on the road to perdition.

The unlocked door to Mr. Munt's study swung open. The shelves were crammed, boasting titles from phrenology to poetry, and the dwindling fire's aroma mingled with book must and tobacco. I had visited the coffer-ceilinged chamber twice—once, I realised to my own horror, as a trusted messenger delivering Vesalius Munt a note from Miss Lilyvale; and once, after our late lamented Fox had insisted upon eating, I was sent there to escort the sobbing girl back to our dormitory.

Fox refused to say what had happened—they all did—but I heard her whimper *I'm not as feckless as I am ugly* in my memory as I stepped over the threshold.

The record lay wantonly open next to an ink pot, pen, blotter, and gleaming letter opener. A silvery charge shot through me, and I dived for the thing; my stomach rose up my gullet as I examined the record of purchases never meant for us to consume:

20 lbs. cod, alive—at 2d. a pound
50 bunches turnips—at penny a bunch
13 pints dried figs for pudding—at 1d. a pint

Biting my lip, I reached for his pen and dipped it in the inkpot. Keeping track of foodstuffs was rightfully the cook's province, but considering the profits Mr. Munt made by selling our strength away, it was unsurprising he sought complete control. Meals were planned a month in advance, with decisive check marks next to the supplies that had already been paid for.

My hands were steady as I hovered over the order to be delivered the next day. It would have been a fatal mistake to cross anything out and rewrite it, so some thought was required; but within three minutes, I had changed *70 bunches cress* to *20 bunches cress, 90 lbs. potatoes* to *80 lbs. potatoes,* and *7 dozen eggs* to *4 dozen eggs.*

Granted, I should have to ascertain how to make off with fifty bunches of cress, ten pounds of potatoes, and three dozen eggs, and then hide these items, and then cook them, but these steep obstacles to me seemed mere irritants. The fire languished, and the smiling moon of the standing clock leered at me. My altered numbers were rather strange, but not so very unlike Mr. Munt's other characters, and I blew upon the page to dry my falsehoods, imagining *a great steaming plate of fried eggs and potato hash and cress salad for—*

"I wonder just what you think you're doing—and then again, I don't."

Dropping the pen as horror gripped me, I sent a bloodlike spatter across the page.

Mr. Munt stood in the doorway, half smiling as if he were greeting a friend in a tea shop. My dismay was quickly buried under an avalanche of frozen rage.

"She meant for me to be caught," I found myself hissing.

"The kindhearted Miss Lilyvale?" Mr. Munt shut the door and approached with even strides as I backed away. "Come now, I'm not going to hurt you. When have I ever hurt any of you? Madame Archambault is a fine French instructor, and her ways are set, but despite the Bible's injunctions to spare not the rod, I confess I find violence crude."

"What are you doing here?" I demanded, too angry to prevaricate. "What about your sermon?"

Mr. Munt placed his Bible reverently upon the desk. "The village prelate is delivering his marvellous message upon original sin. One must grasp the squalorous condition of the unredeemed soul in order to be duly grateful for Christ's intercession. As for your accusation regarding Miss Lilyvale, that is more complicated. I may have mentioned to the cook that I was grateful she was so honest—for were this ledger to be tampered with, I should never know whether our deliveries had arrived intact. Miss Lilyvale may have heard me say so, for she was nearby, though I should never imply she is capable of eavesdropping."

Hatred thrust like a stake through my heart.

"I took advantage of my colleague's visit in order to settle the books. I ought to have locked the door, in retro—"

"You planned all of this!" I cried. "This is another of your cruel games."

"Cruel?" He feigned hurt, his fine features twisting. "Steele, is your heart so hardened that you can invade my private office—"

"You left the door unlocked."

"Falsify my accounts—"

"As you indirectly suggested!" I fairly shrieked.

"Plan to steal food from the mouths of your fellow students—"

"You're killing Clarke." Outrage transformed effortlessly to begging. "Please, even you cannot justify death by starvation."

Mr. Munt walked round his desk, the smug uptilt to his lips intact; I have never seen a man enjoy himself so much. "Heavens! Where on earth would you have stored these items, and how would you have cooked them?"

"I would have found a way," I spat, but the bitterness lay in the fact that he was correct.

This had been a fool's errand, and Miss Lilyvale and I the fools.

Mr. Munt sat before his ledger. He was dressed for Sunday, wearing a grey waistcoat which made his pale eyes gleam, and a high collar; his garb ever hinted at the parsonical whilst still accentuating his Byronic appearance. Running a hand through his black curls, he emitted a sigh.

"You will have to be severely punished for this."

"Do what you like," I snarled, confidence bolstered by loathing. "I'll fight back. Only please," I added as his sad look shifted into annoyance, "don't deprive Clarke anymore. I was the one who read the letters first, not she. You know Clarke is half mad, and anyway she's learnt her lesson."

"Half mad," Mr. Munt reflected, pulling his index finger and thumb along his lower lip. "Do you know, Steele, I don't think the half-mad one is Clarke."

A poisonous silence fell, one which burnt my skin.

"Do not pretend that this is about my mother."

"It is not about your mother. It is about whether you are capable of rational behaviour, or whether the devil works his will through you."

"I'm only here to save one of your own students!"

He laughed, showing straight white teeth. "So you will fight me, you say, and in the next breath you plead the case for the daughter of smut purveyors?" Standing, Mr. Munt strode past me to the opposite wall. "Ah, here we are. *The Garden of Forbidden Delights,* author anonymous, published in serial by Whittleby and Clarke. Borrow it, and then tell me whether you think Clarke's judgement of sincere affections is sound."

A small red volume, unmarked on its cover but bearing the frontispiece *The Garden of Forbidden Delights,* was in my hands an instant later. Mr. Munt raised an eyebrow, stony resolve in his granite eyes, and I queasily slid the object into my dress pocket. I saw many more books like them—I saw an entire shelf, as a matter of fact, enough to be termed a collection.

"Do show that to Clarke when you've finished," he added with a cold smirk.

He's actually insane. His power had flooded his brain, eroding it piecemeal. I recalled the phrases I had studied in such repulsed confusion, *the thought of your mouth against my cock-stand,* and *I would lick my way down your spine and lower until—*

"Miss Lilyvale has seemed most upset since you touched her private things," Vesalius Munt chastised, returning to his desk. "She carelessly left a letter lying out, I take it?"

I drew a quick breath. "I was in the teachers' wing looking for food, and one of your letters caught my eye. I told Clarke about the contents. She never . . . It was all *my doing*, Mr. Munt."

"Perhaps so—I blame myself, you realise. It's clear as day that Anne-Laure Steele's unchecked rebellion, her cunning, her willingness to spit in the face of God Himself, all have been passed down to her only child. Pity. Do you long for death too, Steele? Do you think of the Reaper as you would a suitor, turning away from God's myriad blessings?"

Hours of conversation with Mr. Munt, I thought, was indeed too hard a bargain when set against a single hot meal.

"That is why I am contemplating committing you," Mr. Munt concluded, examining his shirt cuffs.

The words hung before me like a corpse displayed for public view.

"It would sadden me beyond words should one of your classmates fall prey to your wild moods." Mr. Munt's eyes gleamed, a powerful king protecting his realm from embodied disaster—disaster by the name of Jane Steele. "You could hurt someone, Steele; you could destroy someone, I believe."

Vesalius Munt could not possibly have known my secret, but my knees turned to water anyhow; he had seen something in me—a sparking flint where there ought to have been a soul, perhaps. Asylums by all accounts, meanwhile, were handy places to be chained to a bed covered in your own filth, subjected to ice baths and mercury doses and leeches on shorn scalps, and fed rather less than was customary at Lowan Bridge School.

"Don't expel me," I breathed. "I'm, I'm not mad—you know that I am not. I'll behave. Only feed Clarke and I shall do just as you say."

Mr. Munt crooked a finger over his full lips as he cogitated. Most would have seen a headmaster wrestling with a convoluted decision; I saw a despot to whom suffering was as amusing as a penny concert.

"I am moved to be merciful," he concluded, "but Clarke's punishment must stand if you remain at Lowan Bridge. The pair of you are potentially harmful to the others when acting together. If you agree to the asylum, Clarke can return to regular meals. If you prefer to remain and repent, her rations shall remain as they are."

When I opened my mouth, it was empty—save for my heart, which lay aquiver in my throat. He was inclined to be *merciful*, and thus was offering me a choice of my life or Rebecca Clarke's. The seconds elongated, an out-of-tune music box winding ever more slowly to its finish; Mr. Munt, smiling, picked up his pen as if to correct my altered numbers.

I was not inclined to be merciful, however, and thus gripped the letter opener and plunged the sharp point deep into my headmaster's neck.

My earlier metaphor had been wrong, I discovered. The splash of ink from the pen dropping onto the page looked nothing like a spray of blood at all.

TEN

... like any other rebel slave, I felt resolved, in my desperation, to go all lengths.

There is a passage in *Jane Eyre: An Autobiography* which puzzles me mightily; and because it only tickles at the edges of my understanding, I cannot help but read it over, sitting with a glass of dark sherry as the sun grows teasing and hides behind the elms:

> *All said I was wicked, and perhaps I might be so: what thought had I been but just conceiving of starving myself to death? That certainly was a crime: and was I fit to die?*

I present to the reader an enigma: my mother rushed the giddy business of dying along and was almost universally reviled for it. Speaking as a woman who has deserved to die since the age of nine and often thinks death a charming notion anyhow, I burn to know: When Miss Eyre demands philosophically, *and was I fit to die?* is she asking whether she is wicked enough to earn capital punishment, or holy enough to merit release from the torments of her browbeaten life?

And if she wanted to die . . . did she deserve to any longer?

. . .

Few among us are aware of how much blood the human body contains—surging in thick waves should it chance to be spilt.

I had spilled it, meanwhile, and therefore drastic measures were required.

Mr. Vesalius Munt was felled by a strangely skilful blow—as if I had studied the act, when in fact I had simply decided that he should stop being alive. He gurgled a disbelieving shriek, eyes ablaze with wrath and fear, looking perversely more alive than ever, each muscle taut with severest alarm. He even got halfway to his feet, reaching for me, rich gore soaking the fateful ledger.

Then his lips bubbled crimson, his blazing eyes hardened, and he slumped forward over the desk. His fingers, so graceful in life, twitched like the poisonous insect he was; his back ceased to shudder.

I cocked my head and gauged his condition: dead.

I paused to be medically certain; but as he continued dead, I heaved a breath and looked around me, beginning with the mirror above the fireplace.

The spray of crimson across my school uniform was not inconsiderable, and another plume of blood had feathered my hand; I carefully wiped these drops on Mr. Munt's own sleeve. Using the late Mr. Munt's coat the way one would a handkerchief was an act of sufficient disrespect that I turned away giggling, the giggles followed by a hysterical peal of laughter.

A bottle of amber spirits sat upon the side table. *In for a pound, in for a penny.* I poured. The taste was much harsher than the laudanum I had once pilfered from my mother's dressing table; the sear returned my senses and, after spluttering awkwardly, it occurred to me that I was in a not-insignificant amount of danger.

My heart pattered a rhythm like spring rain upon a roof; according to the tall clock, I had nearly an hour before the close of Sunday services.

I rifled through the secretary as well as any drawers I could open without shifting my latest victim, scattering papers and pens. When my pockets contained coins in the neighbourhood of five pounds, a dented silver watch tucked away for repair bearing the initials *VOM*, and the almost-forgot volume published by Clarke's family, I shut the door of the study behind me and raced silently down the corridor.

Reader, would you prefer me to have felt remorse in the aftermath of my second slaughter?

Though the brutality of the act sent fearsome tremors through my small frame for days and weeks afterwards, never have I regretted ending the life of my headmaster.

Dressed in a too-large brown travelling suit stolen from Miss Lilyvale's wardrobe as by then I owned nothing save school-issued clothing, having wrapped my bloodied uniform in paper and stuffed it in my trunk, I was raiding the pantry an hour later when Clarke discovered me.

A small cough sounded, and I whirled around.

I stood in the windowless room aghast with a single rushlight flickering, shoving bread and fruit into my trunk, preparing to abandon everything I knew—but caught out.

"I went to his study," Clarke whispered.

A word of advice: do not ever kill for love, or you will find yourself tethered, staked to the ground when your cleanest instincts require you to run for your life without a backwards glance. Killing for love is one of the most tangled acts you can commit, reader, in an already twisted world.

She looked so small, this beautiful friend of mine. Clarke's madcap blond curls hung loose and tangled, her miniature lips chalk white. Inexplicably, she was dressed in her holiday travelling clothes, an emerald woollen suit and a cap appropriate to her age. I blinked dumbly; Clarke was the colour of goose down, so I promptly deposited her onto a stool.

"You discovered Mr. Munt, didn't you?" Her seaweed-green eyes flooded with brine. "I dragged myself to chapel to make a point in front of everyone, but he wasn't there, so I tried to catch him alone. I had meant to beg him, it was shameful, but I found—did I find what you found?"

The silent steel cogs of my mind ticked.

"Yes." I clutched her to me, cherishing her still-warm bones. "Oh, Clarke, I meant to plead with him myself. But there were drawers open and thieves must have—it was horrible. I'm so sorry you saw it too."

Lying had never been easier. Either I informed Clarke that I had shoved a letter opener in Mr. Munt's throat, or I kept my beloved companion for another half an hour; the decision did not trouble me overmuch. She set her head against my shoulder and quaked as she cried, whilst I attempted to determine the most efficient way never to set foot upon a scaffold. Swift escape seemed the best option; but swift escape had been delayed by my partner in defiance.

Meanwhile, I reminded myself harshly, Clarke was still dying.

"Here." I tore away from her, hands landing upon some plain bread and shoving it unceremoniously into the white butter pot, tearing her off a portion. "Eat slowly. You know when we don't, it—"

"I know," she answered before devouring the hunk in mouselike bites.

I continued my travel preparations; a paper packet of cheese, a fistful of nuts. For leave I must, and I felt a knife in my own throat when I thought of final separation from Clarke. I wondered why on earth she was wearing ordinary clothing when we were all due at cold Sunday supper in uniform in an hour.

"Where are we going?"

Turning, I regarded my friend, who had slid off the stool and was reaching for a lone apple in a basket full of onions and braided garlic heads. Her freckles still glared dark as tiny bruises from the pallor of her cheeks, but her voice was stronger.

"Clarke, I haven't anyone to go *to*." Telling her the truth was always pleasurable, as if I were apologising for the glaring omissions. "My aunt loathes me, and until I'm of age . . . I simply can't go back, not to her. You have a family, you can—"

"They told me they were publishers of poetry and plays." Clarke's eyes glinted hard and gemlike. "The older I grew, the more I thought it odd that they had sent me here. When I was home, they barely entertained or received any callers. For a day it would be splendid, and every hour afterwards I would feel more like a guest, Mother making the rounds at her Bohemian salons, Father at his office and clubs, them glancing at the clock during supper. I would ache to know what *you* were doing—I thought of you whenever they slighted me, whenever they heard my step and seemed almost . . . disappointed. Every visit, I told them we were tormented here, and every time, they said that school was difficult, and how could I move in artistic circles without an education? *Artistic* circles," she repeated in disgust. "By the time I left after a visit, they could barely contain themselves for joy."

"You can't—"

"They *lied* to me, Jane." The name, after so long without hearing it, stole my breath. She blinked in her oddly deliberate manner, polishing the apple against her sleeve. "They sent me away when I was *six years old*. And now you mean to send me away yourself."

"But I—"

"Please don't leave me behind to survive this school without you, I couldn't bear it. Who knows what sort the replacement headmaster will be? We'll find a new place to live." Doubt pinched the corners of her mouth. "But perhaps you don't want—"

"Of course I do." A weightless feeling soared inside me, a flock of starlings scattering into flight. "I only—I've about five pounds and a silver watch that was my father's, but that won't get us far."

Smiling slowly, Clarke took a bite of the apple. "You'll think of something." Pivoting, she fetched her carpetbag, which I had not even seen previous. "You *always* think of something—you're terribly clever, the cleverest one. It's nearly three—let's be off before the cooks arrive to assemble the cold supper. When they find what's in the head's office," she added with a shudder, "there will be hell to pay."

It may have occurred to the reader that allowing Becky Clarke to flee the scene of a murder—with the murderess, no less—was not my most shining instance of altruism. I was sixteen years old, however, sixteen and nigh berserk to escape, delirious with the old instinct to run which had brought me to Lowan Bridge in the first place. Only this time, I would not be friendless and bereft; this time, I would have someone beside me who wanted, however inexplicably, to be there.

If sixteen-year-olds are accounted selfish generally, then reader, how much greedier was I in the face of freely offered loyalty?

"London," I breathed in Clarke's ear as I took her hand. "Where else would we go save for London?"

We fled on foot to the main road, fearing to look behind lest the hornet's nest had upturned and sent swarms flying after us. The alarm had not yet been raised, however, and the grounds proved as empty as they always were of a Sunday—or had been ever since Granville and Taylor had been caught fleeing years ago and were returned by an obliging seller of trinkets who thought the sight of two unescorted girls demanded his immediate assistance.

The fact that Granville had died soon afterwards, though Taylor had scarcely been punished at all, surely does not require explanation at this late juncture. As for Clarke and me, we scaled the pocky wall next to the black wrought iron gate and tumbled to the ground with no worse consequences than scuffed shoes—or no worse consequences *yet*, unless I acted with miraculous rapidity.

Clarke threw her apple core at Lowan Bridge School, a final gesture of defiance. Half a dozen times, perhaps, we had all visited the village a quarter mile away to inflict Miss Lilyvale's Christmas hymns upon the town square, and only gradually did I realise I was taking us there. London sent out new filaments continually, cast shimmering tendrils like the spread of shattered crystal—we had seen this from the roof every year, when London swelled and burst and swelled and burst again—but it was hardly feasible to walk there. Not with Mr. Munt stiffening over his desk.

"Who do you think it was?" Clarke asked.

Swallowing a spike, I shook my head. "The room looked ransacked. Robbers?"

My friend angled her head, curls twice gilded with late afternoon sunlight. "Maybe so."

My heart constricted painfully. "Why couldn't it have been?"

"Oh, it could. It's just that . . . possibly someone wanted to find something other than money."

"What sort of something?"

"Well, you never returned Miss Lilyvale's letters. I read them, and then you . . . kept them. As protection, I assumed. But you never returned them."

At the thought of whey-blooded Miss Lilyvale plunging a makeshift dagger into the cords of Vesalius Munt's throat, I laughed so hard that a fox or a badger or some such went crashing away through the bracken.

"All right, she isn't the bravest woman I've ever met," Clarke agreed, half smiling in a way that sent me into further fits. She slapped my arm. "Jane, *stop*."

"If she was looking for the letters, she took an unnecessary risk in slaying him, for I burnt them," I gasped. This was factual, but Clarke need not know that I had shoved them in the dormitory fireplace after stabbing our headmaster. "In any case, why should I have given them to him?"

"What I mean to say is, we hated Mr. Munt—every student, better than half the teachers, the domestics. Isn't it much more likely that someone he wronged took revenge?"

"He ought to have been at the sermon during that time," I insisted, abruptly no longer amused, "so it would have been the perfect occasion to burgle his sanctum. It was a complete accident that he was present at all. Someone else was there, someone up to no good, and Mr. Munt caught them."

My words skated so close to truth telling that I sliced my eyes to Clarke; shrugging, she nodded.

"You're probably right, but I'm right too—that person could have been any of us."

I pretended to ponder this theory—as if I were upset at the implication that such a monster could hide in the skin of a young girl or a teacher undetected, when in fact I was upset at the fact we could at any moment be dragged back by our hair. The village inn rose before us, half-timbered and sagging at the roof like the shoulders of an ancient farmer, a comfortable pile of lumber emitting a faint aroma of meat pie. Clarke sagged in concert with the building, swallowing audibly in her ravenous state, even as I stiffened.

"What is it?"

"An idea," said I, gazing with impetuous hope at the vehicle resting on the cobbles. "Come along, we're filling you with a hot meal."

As Vesalius Munt was only my second murder, in the immediate aftermath I imagined that a black reaction would set upon me with razor teeth; such was not the case, however. My mind was piercingly clear, and I recognised the shabby manure-spattered coach which had carried me to purgatory at age nine as soon as I glimpsed it, thinking, *Here—if we are very lucky—perhaps is an ally.*

The instant we entered the tavern, Clarke leaning weakly against my arm, I spied him: Nick, the driver who had conveyed me here so long ago. Swiftly, I ushered us to a table. A cheerful wench wearing an apron which perhaps had been used to muck out the stables previous to dinner service grunted at my order and, upon her departure, I leant across the table to grasp Clarke's frail hands.

"Eat your curry when it arrives, *slowly*. I need to speak with someone."

"Who could you possibly know here?" Clarke asked, but I was already striding towards the coachman.

Nick sat, nursing a pint, staring at grooves carved in the bar by time and dissolution. The same forces had done a workmanlike job with his face, for his mouth was bordered by stark crevasses, and his once-red nose had abandoned its unheeded alarums and subsided to a sulky yellow.

"Nick, I think." I nearly coughed at the ripe cloud surrounding him. His boots were worn, which gave me hope, and his fingernails were cracked. "It's a long time ago we met, but I hope you—"

"I dun't know ye," he slurred, slurping at the beer. "I live on the highway, Lunnon to Manchester, Manchester to Lunnon, picking up fares. Never a respit', never two nights i' the same bloody place. Unless yer a sprite after hauntin' my carriage, and ye *look* a sprite right enough, by Jesus, I dun't—"

"You brought me here when I was a girl. I gave you a potted rabbit luncheon I couldn't eat for nerves."

"Chestnut—he's a horse, mind—knows me better than me own pillow, us having spent considerable more time together, and I've never clapped eye on ye before. I tell ye, I *never stop moving*—"

"'The world is a hard place, and I live in it alone,'" I whispered.

Flinching, Nick narrowed red-rimmed eyes at me. "By George," he husked at length. "Is that ye in the flesh, then? The wee miss wi' the tragic eyes I dun brought here from Highgate House? Yer alive?"

"And in need of your help."

Nick spat, recalling to my mind his alacrity at this skill. "*Help*, ye say? What daft breed o' thickheaded are—"

"I gave you a basket full of food once. Now I'll pay you six shillings to carry my friend and me to London."

"Stomached enough o' Lowan Bridge, then?" he puzzled, wiping his brow with his wrist.

"You couldn't have chosen a more appropriate phrase."

"And now I'm meant to risk my hide when Vesalius Munt hasn't let a charge disappear in nigh—"

"He's dead." My eyes brimmed—for myself and Clarke, for dread of shackles and scaffolds. "There will be no consequences to you, Nick, upon my honour."

Were I to picture my honour, I imagine it might resemble a less attractive than usual tadpole; Nick owned no inkling of this, however, and his bleary eyes boggled.

"Mr. Munt dead? The shite-arsed bastard what bilks the factory lads from here to three counties hence?"

"Bilks them?"

"Bilks them!" Nick cried, livening at last. "Aye, he never delivers a meal at discount save he's less ten portions promised. Says as benefactors can't give beyond their means or they'd turn paupers themselves! I'd love to see that feller stuck through the—"

"Someone beat you to it. Oh, please, Nick! We can't go back, and you know how hard the world is."

Nick considered, thoughtfully gathering spittle. I thought then that kindness had not deserted him, and I think now that he needed my money, for he did not look well. We are all of us daily decaying, after all; the speed is our only variant.

Nick spat; Nick finished his beer.

"I'll oblige ye, after I've rounded up the other fares what have already paid." He took my coins and dropped them straightaway upon the bar as he nodded to the serving lass. "But if ye thought the world was hard before . . . cor, will Lunnon ever throw ye to the wolves. She were suckled by a wolf mother, they say," he added with a faint flash of his old dire humour.

"At least she was fed," I muttered as Nick called for the bill to be settled.

When he departed, I returned to our table and passed a gentle hand over Clarke's pallid brow, promising to return upon the instant after using the privy and imploring her to be patient as she finished her modest meal. The pressure within my cranium had grown nearly unbearable by then; half-frantic with fear, sidling behind her so that my semi-conscious friend might not see, I bore my trunk to the outhouse, barred the door, and deposited my bloodied uniform therein. It was not a perfect solution—but it was foul enough to serve, and anyhow, I reminded myself grimly, it seemed that most of my solutions to conundrums fell considerably shy of the mark.

By nightfall, Clarke and I were seated together upon the same threadbare object masquerading as a cushion on which I had ridden to Lowan Bridge seven years previous. Across from us sat a lean farmer and full-bosomed girl with a fresh cap and apron who I thought must be seeking domestic employment, as she looked such equal parts terrified and jubilant.

"London," Clarke whispered, resting her head upon my shoulder. The meal had thoroughly drained her, her body flummoxed by bounty; lacing our fingers together, she settled our hands in her lap. "We'll find a new home, a better one. Anyhow, you're home."

Wincing freely since Clarke could not see me with her head tucked under my chin, I squeezed her fingers. I ought to have felt trepidatious, reader; I ought to have felt both culpable and contrite.

I felt thrilled in knowing that upon the morrow, a worthy battle could be fought—even if I, poor leaky vessel of the devil's and never of God's, was chosen as its champion. No less, I felt achingly grateful, and I watched the blue sweeps of blood through Clarke's emaciated wrist for an hour or more. Knowing that home was hateful to us both, I imagined that her calling me by the word meant I was expedient, or sturdy; but if I could only keep her hand in mine, I knew I would give my four limbs and my heart for the privilege, becoming instead four walls and a roof.

ELEVEN

Women are supposed to be very calm generally: but women feel just as men feel; they need exercise for their faculties, and a field for their efforts as much as their brothers do; they suffer from too rigid a restraint, too absolute a stagnation, precisely as men would suffer; and it is narrow-minded in their more privileged fellow-creatures to say that they ought to confine themselves to making puddings and knitting stockings, to playing on the piano and embroidering bags.

Shortly, reader, you shall experience chronological leaps which may startle the timid. *Jane Eyre* contains the delightful passage, *A new chapter in a novel is something like a new scene in a play*, thus I likewise embrace abrupt shifts even as I abhor the imminent subject matter.

We arrived in London, Clarke and I, homeless and horridly inexperienced, as coral dawn lit the charred air draped over the centre of the British Empire.

"Oh!" Clarke snatched at me as we crossed a deep wheel gouge, further slowing the already painfully lethargic Chestnut.

I steadied my friend, but said nothing; for never had I fathomed such a sight as passed before me like a parade through the coach window.

Some cities bustle, some meander, I have read; London blazes, and it incinerates. London is the wolf's maw. From the instant I arrived there, I loved every smouldering inch of it.

A lad hunched against a shoddy dressmaker's dummy slumbered on, cradled by his faceless companion. The atmosphere was redolent—meat sat piled up to a shop door's limit of some six feet, the butcher sharpening massive knives before his quarry. Yesterday's cabbage was crushed underfoot, and tomorrow's cackling geese were arriving in great crates, ready to kill. So early, the square we passed through ought to have been populated only by spectres. Instead, sounds reverberated from all directions—treble notes from a bamboo flute; the breathy scream of a sardine costermonger; the bass rumble of a carrot vendor, his cart piled with knobby red digits, shouting as his donkey staggered in the slick.

It was not welcoming, but it was galvanising. Arguing with London was useless; she was inexorable, sure as the feral dawn.

"Where *are* we?" Clarke fretted. "This is nowhere near where my parents live."

"I haven't the faintest notion." Bending, I touched my brow to hers. "Are you ready, though?"

Clarke grinned—an easy grin which made me long to buy her hearty sausage and pastry breakfasts. The carriage halted before a dingy public house with a small paved yard. Clarke stumbled out with her carpetbag and I followed, sharp pinpricks running up and down my legs.

"Thank you," I called up. Nick sat like a turtle in his shell on his high plank seat. "I hope that one day—"

"Neither of us hope to see t'other again, ye mad child." He took a long pull from his flask.

"I'm grateful, though. With all my heart, I am."

"Then let it be fer this advice. I've food enough and drink enough to keep what they call a life, but that's all's I can say on the subject.

Treat yerself better—keep yerself a good girl, and sleep in a bed wi'out interruptions. Can ye manage that?"

"Yes." I stepped back, passing an arm around Clarke's horridly small waist. "I can, I promise."

Nick had already snapped the jangling reins and pulled away—a man who lived not much better than his horse did. Meanwhile, I knew precisely which vice he was warning me against, and in starker detail than he might have imagined; words like *virtue* and *chastity* and *fallen* were lobbed over our heads like so many shuttlecocks at Lowan Bridge, but I had read Mr. Munt's "love letters," and so understood the mechanics of the practice.

Some form of employment had to be found, and at once, for when I caught Clarke's bright green eye and thought of all which could befall her—rough hands against her freckled shoulders, chapped lips at her slim throat—a swell of disgust rose. Becky Clarke, in a way which had not been true since my mother's sad, soft-edged smile and her cool hand against my cheek, belonged to *me*.

"First, a celebratory breakfast," I decided. "The man across the street with the sign for hot ham sandwiches—doesn't he seem like an expert toaster of cheese and meat?"

"Indeed. And after eating the best ham sandwiches in all of London?"

I lifted my luggage as the smile faded from my face, willing myself not to say, *I haven't the faintest idea.*

Dark days followed, and far darker nights.

After inquiring after lodgings, all priced too dear, we passed the night in the back room of a public house, Clarke's flaxen hair mingling with the straw strewn across our shared pillow. We passed a night in the spare room of a cottage outside town when we retreated;

but we could think of no employment thereabouts and returned to the city. We passed a night hemorrhaging precious funds upon a cheap hotel, knowing we had no means of replacing the currency. We passed a night propped one against the other on an empty crate, dozing fitfully, until a peeler arrived to tidy the red-brick alleyways he imagined belonged to him.

Sssshriiiek! cried his whistle, and off Clarke and I went like arrows from a bow, both knowing that we could not live this way for long.

For five days we wandered, growing steadily, silently despairing, washing our faces with rainwater trapped in old cisterns and weathered statuary. We were not wretched, nor were we rich. We simply did not appear to be trustworthy—we were blue dirt, green clouds—nothing about us made sense. Over and over, we crossed the fat, sombre river seeking new neighbourhoods, but all were either putrid hovels with mutton bones scattered about for the snarling dogs or else brick buildings with maniacally pristine windowpanes, and both frightened us. If approaching a cheery town house with a few cracked vases in the window and a ROOMS TO LET sign, we were turned away for want of references. Should we broach a wreck reeking of sewage and solitude, we would be sent packing on suspicion of thievery (which was, I own, a fair criticism).

"It isn't like I thought," Clarke said.

We had crossed London Bridge again, and I believe now that we were in Southwark, for though the street names blurred feverishly, I recall the thick sparks and steam and soot of the train station and the tooth-jarring clatter of the engines. Having located a squat public house with dull brass fixtures, we had stopped for a pot of tea, and were now loath to leave the place, instead having rested upon an empty wine barrel in the alley behind, the remains of trampled lettuce surrounding us.

"It isn't like I thought either. There's so . . ."

"So much of it," Clarke sighed.

Her skeletal arm slid off my waist when I stood. "You rest here—you look positively done and I've a lucky feeling. I'll be back directly."

Clarke wanted to believe me and did not, which hurt horribly; she watched me quit the corridor.

"Don't leave me." For the first time, she sounded frightened. "You wouldn't, would you?"

"Never," I called back.

I meant it, but which direction was I to take? Clarke and I were educated innocents, a condition resembling stupid clerks or intelligent kitchen slaveys, which is to say useless. Cognisant we would be desperate enough to sell practically anything unless we found regular employment, and terrified of watching the small nest egg I had stolen crack and dribble away, I ploughed through piles of mismatched boots and discarded nut husks, knowing that I had never yet failed to find an opportunity when I set my mind to it and still at age sixteen foolish enough to trust myself.

My stomach was empty, my mind echoing its cavernous snarl. The twisting streets with the brown water trickling between the stones led me farther from Clarke, and it occurred to me then that, were I a good person, I should leave her. Becky Clarke would live better without the hindrances of my demons and my doubts. Surely, were I to vanish, she would return to her parents, and surely being ignored was preferable to being penniless? Kicking through clamshells as I neared the great sluggish foul river, I hesitated.

Do I love Clarke enough to say good-bye to her?

I did not, I realised.

Then I heard a strange voice calling out.

"Most 'orrible and beastly murder done! Most haudacious and black crime committed!"

A man of middle age stood with a sheaf of yellow papers, crying out the latest atrocities. He was bent over—I hesitated to call him hunchbacked, but he flirted with the appellation—a heavy, downward-leaning human whom I could imagine tracking rabbits like a bloodhound. He owned a bloodhound's jaw too, a great slab on either side of his face framing his crooked teeth with fleshy drapery. His hair was russet and his eyes a hard yellowish hazel like petrified wood.

"Murder most 'einous!" he cried. "Murder most hunnatural! Penny a page, miss."

Blinking in astonishment, I reached for the broadside. He growled and I paid him belatedly, walking a few paces away to read:

MOST FOUL AND DELIBERATE MURDER
OF A COUNTRY SCHOOLMASTER.

Mr. Vesalius Munt, a most upstanding gentleman of E—— parish, was found stuck like a pig through the gullet and left to die in a pool of his own red gore. The villain what competrated this most perspicable act, an act sufficient to strike thunderific fear into the hearts of even the most auspicillary citizens, remains at large. Many schoolgirls of Lowan Bridge have gone missing; thirty or so have vanished into the idyllious countryside, two hundred more staying under the most dutiful and meritransible guard of their teachers, the rest having returned home.

Mr. Munt was lauded as the most distinguished philanderist, and a knife was shoved so far into his throat that his molars suffered renumerous damages, according to experts. The most authoritive and ingeniable Inspector Sam Quillfeather has been assigned the task of hunting

his killer, and the townspeople are most certifitive that his quest will end in the stringing up of the traitorious fiend's neck like the most veriable chicken.

A finger snapped beside my ear.

I had not fainted, but a murky tide swam before my eyes, all grey silt and shrinking terror. The patterer's fleshy face—for he was a patterer of dark deeds, and I had been identifying every way possible to obtain money whilst preventing my legs from parting company—hovered over mine, seeming at once fascinated and annoyed that I had been so affected. He wore funereal black, but had enhanced this theme with a scarlet cravat and trousers to answer, the effect being that one grew fretful over whether he had just been stabbed in the throat and the legs.

"What ails you?" he demanded.

"I went to school there," I murmured, scarcely knowing what I was saying.

Secrets, reader, are tidal—they swell and recede, and my greater misdeeds had forced this lesser intelligence from my lips, a river spilling over its bed; at the unexpected name *Sam Quillfeather*, the constable like an embodied question mark who had peppered me with queries after Edwin's death and apparently been promoted, my spine turned to jelly. The only good news the article contained was that so many had disappeared, for our absence—should it occur to Inspector Quillfeather that a schoolgirl was capable of stabbing her headmaster—would thereby seem much more natural.

"Eh?" he exclaimed. "You were there, ye say?"

"I merely—I was confused. I'll just—"

"A man in my line o' work would pay dear in order to print someone's hinsider perpinion, 'specially if you saw the cold dead corpse, like. Did you?"

He winked, and then I understood—he expected me to lie in order to earn a commission in exchange for the tale.

"Yes," said I, attempting to appear a bad perjurer, which is a bemusing trick and not one I recommend the layman acquire.

The man chuckled, jowls quaking. "Name's Mr. Hugh Grizzlehurst. And yours?"

"Miss Jane Steele."

We shook hands, I and this purveyor of tragedy, as an idea gently hatched in my brain.

"There's another Lowan Bridge girl with me, and we've need of lodgings for the night. I'll exchange my story for our board."

Mr. Grizzlehurst nodded. "If it's an hextraordinary story, I'd not begrudge two nights. Tell Bertha—Bertha's me wife—that 'appy circumstance sent you, and I'll be along when I've hexpleted my stock. The 'ouse is twelve Elephant Lane, Rotherhithe—if you hespy the White Lead Manufactory and the Saltpetre Works, you've gone too far."

Weak with shock and relief, I shook hands. Meeting Mr. Grizzlehurst seemed one of those felicitous coincidences which occur so seldom in fiction—for in fiction, such blessings can scarce be believed, whilst in life they are shared with future generations as thrilling tales of danger averted and luck seized.

I say that it *seemed* just the gift we had been seeking; I have since grown more cautious. Nature's boons are equally plentiful and random, but I have never yet encountered a more capricious mistress—save perhaps for her daughter, madly mercurial London.

Clarke and I, pulses thin with nerves, trudged past warehouses and shipyards, past a harelipped Italian organ boy whose eyes followed us soulfully as he ground his instrument, past earnest geranium boxes tucked under begrimed windows, and finally entered Rotherhithe where it perched upon the edge of the Thames. A whaler, salt in his beard and a blue marine glint in his single eye, directed us to Elephant Lane and trudged away as we knocked at number twelve.

The door creaked open. Mrs. Grizzlehurst stood there, blinking—a dull woman with flat greyish hair and an overbite which rendered her resemblance to a rodent more profound than she might have ideally preferred. Bertha Grizzlehurst's close-set eyes were amiable, however, and her dry lips even spasmed in a theoretical smile.

"I am Miss Rebecca Clarke and this is Miss Jane Steele," Clarke introduced us.

No answer emerged.

"We're looking for Mrs. Bertha Grizzlehurst?" I explained.

The woman who was probably Mrs. Grizzlehurst continued affably saying nothing.

The wind from the Thames scraped across our necks as I glanced worriedly at Clarke; we had made our way from the bridge through market gardens and occasional meadows, rejoicing as the stench of refuse faded and the aromas of maritime saline and humble beds of mint met our nostrils. Rotherhithe was actively being bullied by the metropolis, however; upon nearing the waterfront, the sunlight failed to reach the cobbles as the rickety buildings grew thicker and taller. Huge draught horses lugging wagons of timber passed, making us feel even tinier than we did already. I badly wanted a meal and a bed, and the same for Clarke.

"Your husband asked for our testimony regarding a recent murder," Clarke attempted.

Mrs. Grizzlehurst's smile spread towards her ears; this time she stepped back, and we followed.

The place was shabby, but so impeccably kept that no one could sneer at it; the hearthstone shone like a riverbed, and the irregular panes of glass fitted into the windows had been carefully cut, sparkling in a frenetic rainbow of tonic greens and medicinal ambers and bottle blues. The chimney leaked smoke in a friendly fashion, as if it wanted to join in the conversation, and a misshapen iron pot was just coming to the boil.

"Lodgings." Mrs. Grizzlehurst jerked her head upwards; her voice proved harsh but friendly, like the buzzing of a bee.

"Excuse me?" I replied.

"Low rates, breakfast gratis. He's only been gone these two days, has Mr. Buckle, but I've cleaned it plenty thorough." Mrs. Grizzlehurst waved her knife at a narrow staircase, then dropped a coarsely chopped onion into the pot. A pair of lobsters from a basket followed, flailing against their demise as they were boiled alive.

Clarke and I ascended the staircase, confused but equally curious. There we found a half-height garret room complete with bed, pot, washbasin, and—wonder of wonders—a skylight through which the coral and violet sunset yet gleamed. My friend sucked in a happy breath.

"Might we—"

"I hope so," I agreed instantly.

"But how will—"

"I've a plan," I discovered.

Our hostess, when we returned downstairs, lifted a cleaver as she prepared to make two lobsters do for four bellies. In our absence, a skillet of roasted potatoes had appeared along with a cask of porter, two glasses already poured.

"Day after tomorrow," Mrs. Grizzlehurst concluded, as if she had been conducting a conversation between her ears.

"Beg pardon?" Clarke requested.

"He'll trade two nights for two accounts. You can start paying the day after tomorrow."

Holding up my hands, I said, "We've only modest—"

"The room can't be empty." Gooseflesh sprang to life along Mrs. Grizzlehurst's wiry arms. "You'll pay the day after tomorrow."

I took this to mean that the Grizzlehursts danced upon the lip of penury. My conscientious Clarke had just opened her mouth to explain our own lack of gainful occupation when Mr. Grizzlehurst burst through the door, booming exultations in great volleys.

"If I never see such a day for hexceptional sales, it ain't my fault." Laughing, Hugh Grizzlehurst showed teeth resembling indifferently worn pencils. "This young lady with the fey looks is a good homen, Bertha—a positivical homen, I tell you."

His wife set out potatoes and a modest pat of butter.

"Is this the other heyewitness?" Mr. Grizzlehurst captured Clarke's delicate hand, which I found myself irrationally resenting. "An 'onour, miss."

"Likewise," Clarke managed.

"Mr. Grizzlehurst," I interjected, "I should like to propose that we lodge upstairs; in exchange, rather than pay you directly, I would assist you."

A silence fell; our host's twiglike masses of eyebrows descended.

"'Ere now." Mr. Grizzlehurst thrust his face into mine, jowls swinging like pendulums. "True enough Mr. Buckle hasphyxiated down at the granary, but you've habsconded from school by your own hadfession. Now I'm to suffer the keeping o' you?"

Clarke bristled, and I pressed her toe with my boot.

"You write up murders for a living," I reminded him. "Well, I've read the *Newgate Calendar* back to front, and I've been educated by the renowned Mr. Vesalius Munt. I know you didn't believe me, but it's true. I offer stylistic improvements and new material in exchange for room and board."

"'Eavens above us, hexisely what manner of improvements are

you a-thinking of?" Mr. Grizzlehurst growled. "My customers dote on my turn o' phrase."

"Think what fields we could expand into together!" I coaxed. "Gallows ballads, last confessions!"

"They live upstairs and will work for breakfast," Mrs. Grizzlehurst said.

Hugh Grizzlehurst slammed a fist upon the table, still vigorous despite his bowed back and drooping face. "Why them? We've money enough for the room to be hempty a few nights."

"They live upstairs," Bertha Grizzlehurst insisted, though her face paled to match the lobster flesh peeking from the shells.

"I've no need o' hassistance when it comes to my broadsides! My broadsides is known 'ither and yon and every street betwixt!"

"I don't think *positivical* is a word," Clarke observed.

"Can you prove positivically that it hain't?" he shouted in high dudgeon.

"No," I hastily owned, "but wouldn't it be better to employ words which actually exist?"

"Hexistence *nothing*." He regarded me with an outraged eye. "You lot will hexplicate how Mr. Vesalius Munt came to have his neck spitted like a guinea fowl, and then—"

"The room *can't be empty*!"

The shriek—high but thin, like the feral cry of a shrew—rendered all three of us mute. Following this decree, Mrs. Grizzlehurst, three plates balanced on her left arm and a fourth in her right hand, set the meal upon the table.

When finished, she sat and stared at her husband; a silence of grotesque dimensions ensued.

"We'll sup first," Mr. Grizzlehurst said contritely, "and then—*then*, mind—we can talk about halternatives."

Clarke and I ate as Mr. Grizzlehurst slurped from a lobster shell;

Mrs. Grizzlehurst only gazed at her plate, relief softening her ratlike features. After supper had ended, I jotted down an account of Mr. Munt's murder, prudently leaving out my guilt whilst doubling the gore. I did not need to ask whether it would suit; it was a mingling of my memory and imagination, and as such was criminally engaging.

Hugh Grizzlehurst read my work, snorting in approval.

"I decide which crimes deserve hadvertisement," he admonished.

"Of course."

"You get not a cent—just lodgings, that's *hessential.*"

"Absolutely."

"And what'll *she* do, then?" he demanded, pointing at Clarke.

"Teach music lessons," Clarke said dreamily. "All we must do is find a piano, and I shall partner with the owner quick as thinking."

"Well," said Mr. Grizzlehurst. He regarded his spouse as if struck by sudden melancholy. "They live upstairs, then, it's settled."

Smiling, Mrs. Grizzlehurst cleared the plates and uttered not another word that day . . . nor the day after that, nor the day after that, which ought to have set off plentiful warning bells in my ears and did not, more's the pity for everyone involved.

Clarke set out to partner with a pianist upon the morrow. A week later, having failed in many attempts, she disappeared one morning and sent me into a hair-tearing panic—wondering whether she had met with misadventure, wondering whether she had tired of me. She materialised ten minutes after supper ended (which Mrs. Grizzlehurst always served us whether we had paid her the extra fourpence or not) with three shillings, which she pressed into my palm.

"I stood upon the street corner, practicing, before meeting with Mr. Jones, but I needn't bother over using his piano." Her smile engulfed her pretty face despite the small scale of her lips. "I always thought I had a knack for music, though Miss Lilyvale's praise wasn't precisely encouraging."

"You made this much warming up your voice?" I stared stupidly at my hand.

"Imagine what I'll earn when I'm doing it on purpose," she concluded, skipping upstairs to wash.

Thus Clarke settled into an unlikely occupation as a street singer, trilling "Cherry Ripe" and "Poor Old Mam" whilst I penned atrocities; had we not been educated at Lowan Bridge School, learning daily despite our sorrows, I shudder to picture what would have become of us. She was even happy, I think, warbling like a strangely technical songbird, whilst I took heinous tales from my employer and translated them to actual English, with sufficient spilt viscera to please everyone.

These might have been idyllic circumstances, but they were not.

Mr. Hugh Grizzlehurst's behaviour when drunk owned peculiarities which it failed to evince when he was sober; furthermore, these whimsical quirks tended to be visited upon the person of Mrs. Bertha Grizzlehurst. In fairness, Mr. Grizzlehurst only imbibed when he had been unsuccessful, and—as my help and his experience rendered us jointly successful—this was seldom. When every other month, however, the British Empire had been distressingly peaceable, Mr. Grizzlehurst would arrive home with a jug of gin which could either have been imbibed or employed to strip the paint from the chipped green rocking chair.

When Clarke and I had retreated upstairs, ducking to avoid the low slant of the ceiling beams, we would hear shouting. At times, the shouting would prove the climax, and we should find at dawn Mr. Grizzlehurst snoring upon the knotted rug. At other times, shouting would prove insufficient to Mr. Grizzlehurst's purposes, and the sharp crack of a slap or two would follow, and Clarke's entire body would flinch alongside mine as I set my teeth hard against each other.

"What can we do?" Clarke whispered the third time this happened, shifting up on one elbow to stare at me with her nightgown slipping over her shoulder.

I did not know. Bertha Grizzlehurst was silent for days on end, ugly as her husband, and relentlessly calm; and now that I knew the reason for her insistence upon our lodging there, I suspected we were already doing the task she had planned for whatever tenant occupied the garret: we were witnesses, which went a long ways towards stopping a real crime from ever occurring.

"Nothing," said I. "We are here to prevent things going too far. It isn't our business."

Clarke settled her head between my neck and collarbone, smelling of starlight and lavender as she always did, and murmured, "Then whose business is it?"

Pondering, I sifted her hair through my fingers. I was not, even at age sixteen, foolish enough to suppose that love and marriage always kept company; my mother had loved my father to distraction, but I had never seen it, and as for the union our former music teacher might have enjoyed, the topic was best left unexplored. Theoretically, however, some form of affection was meant to be involved—and though I could only love hungrily, I could not imagine ever striking Clarke if I had been a man and she a woman, no matter what she may have done.

No, it is not my business, I concluded.

But it could be, I thought next, shifting and afterwards falling into a troubled slumber.

TWELVE

"Dread remorse when you are tempted to err, Miss Eyre: remorse is the poison of life."

If early reading of the *Newgate Calendar* carved a mark upon my girlish character, I was for two years grateful for the scar.

We were housed thanks to me, kept in ribbons and pub fare thanks to Clarke, and when our presence leashed the mongrel inside Hugh Grizzlehurst, so much the better. Mrs. Grizzlehurst never failed to greet us with buttered porridge or Sunday eggs and herring, so I supposed that her scheme was working, despite occasions when the lilac circle beneath one eye looked darker than the other. Clarke and I hemmed loudly at the occasional nocturnal scuffle, stomping to fetch a glass of water, returning to bed in the widening pool of quiet.

There are households which would have considered this arrangement paradise—and in retrospect, at times, I did myself.

In the frigid January of the year 1845, Mrs. Grizzlehurst grew thicker about the middle and began to whistle when she was not speaking (which was nearly all the time). Jane Eyre insists, *Human beings never enjoy complete happiness in this world,* and I agree with her—but as Mrs. Grizzlehurst slowly swelled with child, I thought what a lucky chance it was that humans do not often suffer complete unhappiness either.

Mr. Grizzlehurst produced clownish smiles as he bent to kiss her cheek in the morning, his expressions tinged a helpless shade of ash when he went through his account books in the evening. He began to toss me worried glares, meaningless winks and clucks, a pleading slackness hanging heavy in his chops before he whispered:

Miss Steele, hadvantitious as this 'ere week has been, is there nary another penny we might'a misplaced somewhereabouts?

This verse is downright halliterative, Miss Steele, and I happlaud you. . . . Can we not keep it to a single page? Paper is that dear these days, and we don't want to look 'eathenish.

Just before everything fell apart, he handed me this gem:

MOST BRUTAL STABBING RIPS HOLES
IN NUBILOUS YOUNG VICTIM—.

Sighing, I dipped my pen; I sat at the rickety table in our garret in the coral glow of a February afternoon, preparing myself to rescue our native tongue from worse than death once more. The chipped yellow vase which I generally filled with weeds—Queen Anne's lace and wild flowering parsley—sat empty in February save for some whimsical thistles Clarke had brought me to cheer my spirits when English had been dealt cruel blows.

> **We discover a most unforewitted tragedy struck in Church-lane, St. Giles's, shocking even the most hardened of that irascilacious realm. A comely lass of seventeen years was most untimely struck down by a delinquitorious scallywag, a blade thrust twixt her ribs some scores and dozens of times, and left to bleed. Whilst chances the scurrible fiend will be brought to justice are most**

uncertificable, the humble author prays that he will be left to dangle like the most inconseterial string of garlic.

Since two years previous, "Grizzlehurst's Daily Report of Mayhem and Mischief" had trebled in sales as far afield as Southwark and Deptford, thanks to my style and to Hugh Grizzlehurst's genuine talent for scouting out the rankest misdeeds imaginable; had it occurred to me to be proud of the fact, I should have tried it out. Still—I watched Bertha Grizzlehurst gather up scattered flour from her breadboard as if it were gold dust, listened monthly for the sound of the landlord's hobnailed boots and his rat-a-tat, and understood her husband's wheedling for "Just an extra three days, guv'nor, as yer a charititious Christian." I worked as many hours at the "Daily Report" as he, longer if it sold quickly, and there were four of us in that dear, dingy house, Clarke helping with laundry and mending and mopping, so our hosts never asked us for rent even if they wanted to. At the time, however, I had little notion of what a drinking habit cost, nor did I realise that some landlords considered the worth of their tenants more relevant to pricing than the square footage of their lodgings.

Small wonder, not knowing how hard the world truly was, I sat so peaceably over my paper and nibs in those final hours; small wonder that I lost something when I never knew what I had in the first place.

I felt Clarke's graceful steps entering. Her feet sounded satisfied, her gentle shutting of the door weary; she had passed a good day in the Rotherhithe marketplace, crooning sweet ballads and the occasional comedic patter song. Her forearms met my collarbone as she rested her chin upon my head; I was ludicrously smaller than she when seated, for where the younger Clarke had grown tall and willowy, I had remained a slight, sparrowlike creature.

"How bad is it?"

I shut my eyes since she could not see me, simply grateful for her; I thought us sisters, partners, the perfect duo save that I was unworthy of her affections. Tapping my pen against the word *irascilacious*, I nuzzled my head against her neck like an overgrown cat. She chuckled into my crown.

"That is almost too inventive to edit out."

"You're an evil temptress and I shun your wiles," I returned in a passable impersonation of the late unlamented Vesalius Munt. It thrilled me to call Clarke evil when the reverse was true—as if every time she laughed, I knew my own secrets remained buried.

Of course, murder was not the only secret I kept from Clarke.

By the time I was eighteen, I had read her father's publication *The Garden of Forbidden Delights* an indecorous number of times—always in the sleepy midmorning, when Clarke was out singing and I had spent half the night replacing gibberish with words, dependent upon Mr. Grizzlehurst's voluminous lungs to sell our goods each morn. Unlike Mr. Munt's letters, the erotica printed by Clarke's family failed to sicken, only caused a joyous, clamorous sensation I could not help but mistrust, since it meant that Edwin was right about me.

I liked it.

The people in the slim red book thirsted for closeness, unfolded themselves in turgid metaphors like the petals of a spring rose. Everything they did, they did for wild love—women practically scooped out their hearts and passed them to one another, men discovered these Sapphic passions and assisted in their explorations, brothers-in-arms aided one another when the women were exhausted by pleasure. Even quarrels ended in a dizzy swell of bosoms and trouser fronts; I blame my superb memory on the fact that I had memorised entire chapters.

At age sixteen, it had been too much to take in, let alone tell Clarke about; at age eighteen, I had kept the secret for so long that I should no longer be presenting Clarke with a fresh discovery, a tomcat delivering a mouse—I should be informing her that I was perfectly capable of keeping mum. Though I could not be disgusted over their stock in trade, I could understand Clarke's hurt over being snubbed by her parents, and this delicacy led to my complete failure to bring the subject up at all. As the reader has never faced a similar predicament, I warn the tempted: secrets decay, as corpses do, growing ranker over time.

"Mr. Grizzlehurst seemed disturbed," Clarke reported. She passed a glass of port over my shoulder. "What did he print yesterday?"

"Oh." I sipped, leaning into Clarke's—now blessedly filled out—torso. "Tripe about a robber who stole a boat along with its cargo of sardines. None of the people interested in that story can read, but never fear, I'll set it all right tomorrow."

I had never been more mistaken.

That night, rather than the high percussion of slaps, the deep thud of blows met our ears.

Clarke and I both were out of our bed instantly, praying for the sound resembling a rolling pin striking a veiny beefsteak to stop; it did not stop.

"What are we to do?" Clarke whispered. She dived for her robe, mindless magnanimity surging through her. "I'll go down and—"

"You're not going anywhere!" I captured her elbow.

My throat was tight with *he could so easily harm you*—by mistake, in the braying torrential rage from which some men suffer; but Clarke tore from my grip.

We heard, "Get up, you haudacious piece of baggage!" and luckily we were already tearing down the staircase, for God knows what He might have allowed if we had not done so.

When I reached the ground floor, Clarke stood with her fingers hovering before her own mouth. Mr. Grizzlehurst had wheeled to face her, chest brokenly wheezing and fists knotted. Mrs. Bertha Grizzlehurst lay upon the floor exercising her habitual silence with her arms clutched around her belly and her temple bleeding . . . *but no, not just her temple,* I thought, *for there is so very much—*

"Bertha." Mr. Grizzlehurst looked as if his favourite toy had somehow come to life and bitten him—as if *he* were the one hurt.

Mrs. Grizzlehurst made a sound through her nose, more a whisper than a whimper, which caused a strange calm to descend as if a cannon had fired next to my ear.

My fingers circled Clarke's wrist and I pulled her back, keeping the link between us gentle. The blades in my eyes I saved for Mr. Grizzlehurst and, when I swept them to him, sweat broke out over his shaking jowls.

"Get out," I ordered. "I'll take care of everything, just don't hurt her anymore. Get out."

We bundled an unsteady Hugh Grizzlehurst out the door, Clarke and I; he blubbered a bit, stumbled, groaned as we pushed him into the street.

His wife made not a sound until the heavy bar across the door scraped into place, and we had gathered flannels and hot water and the shallow hip bath, and I had scrubbed the too-solid stain from the floor; then we all wept long and low at the waste the world produces, and the way in which a baby might have been born to a doting mother but was not.

All is colourful flashes when I remember that night—scraps of scarlet emotion, the pale violet sound of soft keening. I think of Mrs. Grizzlehurst's grey head as Clarke cradled it, rocking, and the throbbing sensation that I ought to have been doing more: as if I had been summoned there following a terrible incantation, a spiteful Greek goddess dressed in radiant sapphire and Mrs. Grizzlehurst the supplicant at my altar, offering more blood than I ever wanted to see again for the rest of my life. It was easier to think myself an observer from another realm than merely a parentless child who had just watched something unspeakable take place.

So I scrubbed the floor thrice and made everyone tea with extra brandy and milk, and I soaked rusty linens and watched the sun rise and periodically glared down from our garret window to check for Mr. Grizzlehurst's return, not feeling anything.

When I think of that morning, I remember how I felt, however; I remember that morning very clearly indeed.

People vary widely in their opinions of female usefulness; my aunt Patience, for instance, preferred them to be approximately as useful as antimacassars. I had, in the wake of two murders, no illusions about what I was capable of—and Clarke, when we retreated to our room that dawn after settling Mrs. Grizzlehurst in bed, seemed to be developing dangerous faith in our combined capabilities.

"He's no better than a murderer."

Clarke paced as the moon dissolved like a sugar cube in the spreading sunlight. At fifteen, she was strikingly lovely, with her champagne curls pinned up into a cloud and her freckles grown more populous from singing in the midday square. I watched her, a queer ethereal creature myself, fretting as she stalked from wall to wall with a rose-patterned robe tied over her nightdress. Beyond the horrible fact Bertha Grizzlehurst's dreams had been shattered, Clarke's vexation pulled at me with the drag of a hundred tiny fishhooks.

"He's . . . a little better than a murderer, Clarke," I corrected, lighting two tapers on my desk.

"He just killed his own baby!" she hissed.

Pondering how easy it was to lose control, I developed an intense interest in retying my grey dressing gown.

"She has to leave him! Jane. Jane, are you listening? She has to get away from here, she'll never be able to look him in the face again without knowing—can you imagine the torment?"

I sat upon the edge of the bed so as to concentrate on the tie, which was proving unexpectedly taxing.

"We have to help her," Clarke decided.

"How?"

"Surely she can seek out a relative—have you ever heard her speak of parents or siblings?"

Raising an eyebrow, I wordlessly reminded Clarke of the number of sentences we had heard Mrs. Grizzlehurst utter.

"We'll just have to ask—and if she has somewhere to go, we can help her. I have it now!" Clarke exclaimed, clapping her hands.

Diving at the bed we shared, Clarke pulled my trunk from beneath the frame. I recall the exact set of her shoulders, the quizzical turn of her head as she searched, the way I sat watching her, not understanding, until the instant I did understand, and horror clawed at me, and I stupidly gasped, "Wait, don't—" just as Clarke chirped, "Here!" and darted to the brightening window with her prize.

"Don't touch that," I growled in the voice of a cornered beast.

Clarke had already lifted the dinted silver watch to the light, however; at my outburst, she nearly dropped it, but she had seen the initials *VOM* etched onto the metal. Pushing a curlicue of hair away from her eyes, she slowly turned.

"You said you had a silver watch of your father's when we left." Her high voice was considered but flat, as she had sounded when working out algebraic equations, which positively wrecked me. "This . . ." She stopped, her head whipping up. "This is Vesalius Munt's watch, isn't it?"

Desperate, I cast my mind in all directions for a lie which might serve, any lie, every lie, the *right* lie.

"Yes. I . . . I was leaving school, alone I thought, and had hardly any money."

"What else do you have of his?" Clarke's tone had frosted, placid as a winter lake.

Stomach churning, I pulled out *The Garden of Forbidden Delights*. Clarke took the book, pursing her lips in puzzlement. I committed this insane blunder for two reasons which, in my distress, seemed actually sound. First, aware that Clarke possessed zero tolerance for my falsehoods when directed at her, I offered her a secret like a penance; and second, it seemed prudent to remind her that I may have had a lunatic mother and a history of stealing from dead headmasters, but was her own father not also subject to trivial quirks of ethics?

As Clarke flipped through the pages, her grip began to tremble; we had encountered the obscene on London's streets before, but never produced by her own parents. I darted to her, tossed the book away, and took her hands, kissing one and holding the other over where my heart ought to have been.

"It's all right, their business doesn't affect my opinion of you," I breathed. "Oh, please don't look like that! I took the watch thinking I would be friendless and I'm sorry I lied to you, but you're so particular. That book—you should never have seen it. Mr. Munt wanted to turn me against you, but I never loved you any less."

I fell silent as Clarke's eyes grew swollen with dread. She snatched her hands away, staggering back, knocking one of the candles over; wax spattered the floorboards, began to congeal and to harden.

"Wait, I only meant to say that you—you're family to me. Are you hurt? What's come—"

"He gave this to you that day, to spite the pair of us?"

"Yes, but it didn't work, I told—"

"When you found Mr. Munt in his study, you said he was *already dead*, Jane!" she shrieked.

Time seemed to ripple, an eddying effect which left me reeling. Clarke shook her head back and forth, back and forth, like a metronome without any *click, click*.

"It's not what you think," I whispered.

It was, however.

"I never realised," she said hollowly. "I thought how natural it was that the same thing should happen to both of us, we were always so kindred, but it never entered my mind that . . . you . . . and you scour the papers for crimes every day and they never found his killer, Jane, never found any clue."

This was not precisely true; Sam Quillfeather had released a statement that, thanks to the complete lack of witnesses, his privately held suspicions could never hold up in court, and thus should remain unspoken for the sake of peace and healing. This ambiguous, insinuating news had eradicated my appetite for four days, which I explained to Clarke as a nasty attack of *la grippe.*

"You murdered him." Clarke swayed, pulling at handfuls of her curls.

"Sit down, you'll hurt yourself," I pleaded. "Oh, Clarke—"

"How could I never have worked it out?" She collapsed on the bed with rote obedience.

"Well, it wasn't the likeliest scenario on earth, was it?" I laughed, and she looked at me as if I had turned lupine, as if all my absences during the full moon now made perfect sense.

Kneeling before her, I seized her elbows. "Listen to me. You've always listened to me, and I'm sorry I lied about the watch, and—"

"Being sorry for lying about murdering our headmaster might be more—"

"He was *killing you.*" The tears which had risen were not lies, reader. "He would never have let you eat again, and I went to the study, meaning to alter his food supply records, and he caught me, and I never meant to hurt him."

"By hurt him, do you mean *stab him in the neck with a letter opener?*"

Laughing again did not help my cause. "I'm sorry, that was—I'm so sorry. Please understand, I had to choose between being sent to an asylum or watching you starve. What could I have done?"

"Attempted escape?" she offered hoarsely. "I would have gone with you, you know. Into the woods, the faraway cities. I would have gone with you anywhere."

The past-tense construction of this sentiment spread invisibly around us, graphic as a battlefield.

Disengaging herself, Clarke pulled off her robe and her nightdress; I stayed on the floor, too numb to move as I watched her cover her creamy skin with her underthings and one of her daytime frocks, methodically shoving the others hanging in the wardrobe into her carpetbag. When this horrifying ritual had been completed, she retrieved a few songbooks and snapped the latch on the bag, which sounded to me like a pistol shot.

"Please don't do this," I begged.

Clarke paused, looking down at me almost regretfully. "Do you remember what I just said about Mrs. Grizzlehurst?"

A sob rose in my throat, for I did.

She'll never be able to look him in the face again without knowing—can you imagine the torment?

"I lied at school every day." I sounded angry; but I was not angry, never that, only trying to haul myself out of the rubble. "I lied for you constantly, lied for everyone—and even if you never lied, you stole, and if I would lie for you, and you would steal for me, why . . . why not this too?"

Clarke's eyes had grown dragonfly bright, but there was something else there, an emotion I could not pinpoint, one which looked like shattered glass.

"Because I don't know who you are," she rasped. "You were always so cunning at school, but so gentle, as if you couldn't bear to watch anyone go hungry. Even the beastly ones, like Taylor—yes, she *was*, Taylor was horrid, only you never noticed—and, oh, I so admired you. You have a terribly romantic air about you, you know. And I knew you carried secrets, you've no notion of how sad you look at times, but I thought that if I took enough care, you might trust me one day. I only wanted to know you, the heart of you, for you to *show me*. But . . ."

Trailing off, Clarke glanced at the desk where a stack of half-finished broadsides sat, my odes to every variant of death and damnation.

"I saw that room, after the murder," Clarke said softly. "And I don't know you at all."

She turned to go. At the last moment, she snatched up *The Garden of Forbidden Delights*, hastily shoving it amidst her clothing as if the binding were aflame; then she departed, closing the door behind her.

I did not go to bed; instead I dressed and, at seven in the morning, I brushed a hand over Bertha Grizzlehurst's arm. She seemed alert in a way she had not been the night before, absent-eyed and weeping like a lost soul.

"Has the bleeding stopped?"

She nudged her head against the pillow, indicating it had.

"Have you anyone to go to? Clarke has received terrible news," I lied. "Her mother is poorly—I intend to offer what solace I can, I'll be quite at home there, and that means we shan't be living in the upstairs room."

Bertha Grizzlehurst absorbed this information. Had she not been quite so mousey or quite so silent, she might have been a friend, I thought, for she took in blows and bitter news with a stoicism her husband entirely lacked.

"What happened last night—that changes everything. Now he has wounded you, who is to say how far he can go?"

She said nothing, but her face grew whiter than the leadworks dust which blew down Elephant Lane.

"This is for you." I pressed the cursed silver watch into her hand, exactly as Clarke had wanted me to do. "No, no! You've been feeding us supper for two years without payment. I ought to have made you take it before now—forgive me. If you pawn this, you should have enough money for travel expenses and some left over to settle elsewhere. After, you'll have to take life as it comes, but we all do, don't we?"

She gave me a thankful blink; I brushed her cheek and she took the watch, tucking it into the bosom of her dress.

"My brother has a farm near Canterbury." Her voice always grated unexpectedly in my ears, as if a toast rack had spoken. She sat with an effort; apart from her other unspeakable injury, her lip was fat as a bloodworm and her ribs much abused.

"I'll help you sort everything. Come."

"What will Hugh think?" She sounded as if he were a small boy who needed minding.

"I'll take care of Mr. Grizzlehurst," I vowed. "You may count upon that."

You will see Bertha again soon enough. She needs time to recover," I soothed, pouring two more generous glasses of head-splitting gin.

Hugh Grizzlehurst had returned to find me cooking supper, a jug of gin on the table. He was rheumy-eyed, his jowls hanging like nooses and the whites of his eyes nearly as crimson as the puddle I had cleaned. It fell to me to improve his spirits: thus the gin and the two beefsteaks and the mashed turnips with butter and thyme.

"Poor Bertha." He snorted back tears and mucus; I had set about returning him to blind drunkenness and was by seven in the evening approaching success. "I never . . . I 'ate to think of 'urting my girl. It was an haccident, you savvy?"

I spooned gravy over the plates, seating myself. "Bertha understands. *I* certainly do as well. I only regret that Clarke had to leave so precipitously."

We ate, Mr. Grizzlehurst sniffling into his beefsteak; when we had finished, I placed both my palms upon the table.

"This house is too empty without Clarke and Mrs. Grizzlehurst." I traced the wood with my finger, playful. "Finishing this gin at Elephant Stairs would be just the ticket—the stars are out, and the night is quite clear."

You used to watch the stars through the skylight with Clarke wrapped around you, lazy as a pair of kittens, just as you did back at school on the rooftop, and now you won't feel the weight of her arm over your waist ever again.

Hugh Grizzlehurst hoisted the half-empty gin bottle; he had far outpaced me, and his mouth wore a slack, wet quality. "Gimme 'alf a tick to fetch me coat."

It was a three-minute walk to the waterfront, which was littered with crumbling stairways to the Thames—Princes Stairs, Church Stairs, Rotherhithe Stairs; so late, the streets had cleared and the air lost the graininess of a long day's labour in an ashen metropolis. A single dustman passed us, tipping his flat cap, and a vague, chill sweetness overlay the perennial aromas of fish and refuse.

Hugh Grizzlehurst and I sat at Elephant Stairs with the treacly brown water lapping at our feet, and Mr. Grizzlehurst lapping up the gin. He would make it all up to Bertha, he claimed; he would buy her trinkets, take her on holiday to Brighton, compose poems in her honour. His arms swept like scythes, winding down in a jerky, mechanical fashion until he collapsed against the stone step.

"What that woman is, she is *hexceptional.* The habsolute

devotion—and after losing two wee ones. Well, never again, Miss Steele, I can hassure you."

"Two?"

Dread crawled up my neck as I recalled her silence following a very important question.

Now he has wounded you, who is to say how far he can go?

Hugh Grizzlehurst returned to the theme, muttering in spasmodic fashion that he would forgive her for running from him.

"And if she tries to stay haway again, well." Mr. Grizzlehurst shook his head regretfully. "Then I'll 'ave to learn the bitch twice over that marriage is a sacramentation. She'll not hescape me, not my Bertha—never you fear for that."

We fell silent. The waves churned and I thought of going to bed that night alone, thought of the many times when I had jolted awake shaking and felt Clarke's soft lips murmuring against my shoulder, remembered the way she would reach up to trace loving patterns on my collarbone until I fell asleep again, and that she never chided me come morning. Then and there I vowed that Clarke should escape me; I should never seek her out, never threaten her fragile freedom, for all that my chest felt as empty as the wide spaces between the stars she so adored.

When my employer lost consciousness, I was not surprised; and when it was discovered by fishermen that Mr. Grizzlehurst had been deep in his cups and fallen into the Thames, drowning, I was not surprised either, for I had pushed him.

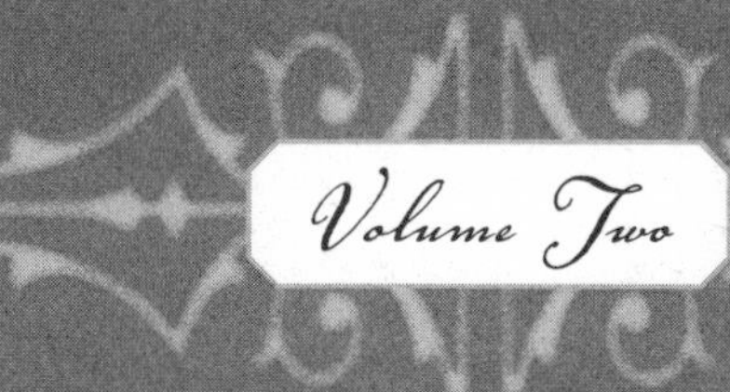

Volume Two

THIRTEEN

"Know, that in the course of your future life you will often find yourself elected the involuntary confidant of your acquaintances' secrets: people will instinctively find out, as I have done, that it is not your forte to talk of yourself, but to listen while others talk of themselves; they will feel, too, that you listen with no malevolent scorn of their indiscretion, but with a kind of innate sympathy. . . ."

A partial veil must be drawn over the subsequent period, reader—not because I wish to conjure a false portrait, but because redundancies are the enemy of narrative, and I rehearsed the same self-annihilating scene long after Clarke's departure.

After killing Hugh Grizzlehurst, for instance, I carried the remainder of the gin home and drank my fill. Upon the morrow, my skull felt as if a horse had kicked it, and my stomach practically leapt into my chamber pot, but *there's more gin where that came from*, I thought, and Clarke was gone, would be gone always, and I only faced what I deserved.

Days followed, then weeks; I had a yellow velvet purse which I had stuffed with spare coin, and the supply rapidly dwindled after I paid our landlord for a further month's rent (with tears in my eyes for poor, unlucky Mr. Grizzlehurst).

Did I mourn him? After a fashion, and this baffled me; where

Edwin's demise had devastated me, and Mr. Munt's was a pinprick, I found myself morose over murdering Hugh Grizzlehurst, as if I had smashed a spider which ought to have been shooed out the door. I felt an echo over him of the anguish I once suffered for letting my misbehaving kitten out of doors, and to this day, I sometimes daydream that he approaches me insisting, *Cannivoristic habsolutely is a word, by Jesus, Miss Steele, a genuine word.*

Meanwhile, I concluded: love is a terrible reason for committing murder. I adored Clarke because she was good, and that very goodness had stolen her from me.

Your badness stole her from you.

Sleepless in the hollow hours, I meditated on her love of the night sky, her wonder at vast, unknowable things; I obsessed over her facility at music, her mathematical precision tied to ethereal tones. I thought to write broadsides, but there was no one to hawk them; I thought to follow my former employer into the Thames.

Instead, I walked the streets, passing the sky-piercing spire of St. Mary the Virgin at a beggarly pace, hoping that I could garner solace outside a church if not inside; this did not work, nor did it assuage the hunger I studiously avoided thinking about. Instead of eating, I supped on gin and melancholy, and watched my shillings disappear.

The day before rent was next due, I struck out for more dismal pastures.

Quoting the fictional Mr. Rochester seems simplest: *In short, I began the process of ruining myself in the received style; like any other spoony.* I slept on mice-gnawed mattresses in public houses, wrote more broadsides, hawked my wares until I sounded like a saw against a board, and then understood what Mr. Grizzlehurst meant when he said, *I've a hunnatural talent for 'awking—not the most dulcedious tones, mind, but I never wear out.*

I did not thank my alma mater for propelling me into the world with expert skills in deportment, Cicero, and decorative needlework, for I could find no crying need for any of these disciplines along the docksides. In the depths of my melancholy, I fear it did not even occur to me to be equally grateful to Lowan Bridge for its tutelage in thieving, swallowing unpalatable food, and hiding from authority figures, though these proved more useful talents. When I could not sleep in public houses, I slept on the floors of the desperate and the greedy; when I could not hawk, I stole. Discovering that some men pay scant attention to waifs hovering near their pocketbooks, I relieved them of their banknotes. Often these men were cherry cheeked, laughing bright whiskey clouds, and to these men I apologise; others had eyes the colour of scaffolds, muddy and vicious, and to them I simply say thank you.

Through it all I loved Clarke, and wanted her back. When I was caught by a costermonger and he gave chase, clutching at my sleeve and tearing it, I wanted her back; when I took to sleeping rough, half-stupefied with gin and risking the law as I settled under gorse bushes, I wanted her back; when I began to be invisible, strangers' glances sliding off my tangled hair and my veiny eyes, I wanted her back. When I was accosted by leering men, fighting each off with a fury that I think astonished them, I wanted her back.

I ought to have died, reader, but I did not.

'Ere, what in Christ's name d'you think you're doing?" Tilly laughed, slapping my forearm as I stole her pipe from her; I inhaled, dark fumes and buzzing light filling my lungs.

"Helping the day along, just as you are," said I, passing it back.

We were at home before my crackling fire, sipping honey-coloured dreams. It was tobacco mixed with scant enough opium to be perfectly respectable, as neither Tilly nor I had any intention of overindulging—or not on that occasion, anyhow.

Reader, we find ourselves six years later, in December of 1851, when I was twenty-four years of age, and you doubtless wonder whether I ignored Nick the coachman's admonishment and was an unfortunate, as we call those not always entirely unfortunate women who pleasure men for frocks and food.

I was not; I was friendly, however, with those who lodged in my building near Covent Garden. Tilly Cate was my favourite, because Tilly was fond of me, the daft sot. Tilly was big bosomed, with yards of wiry dark blond hair, her complexion porous but rosy; and she was motherly, which characteristic made perfect sense when one learnt she had a daughter named Kitty Cate (an appellation which the child, I am thankful to report, did not deserve in the slightest degree).

My bedchamber contained two maroon damask chairs with a bedraggled green ottoman between, a bed beneath a window overlooking Henrietta Street, and a greying basin with funereal lilies edging the bowl. Secondhand books lay piled along the peeling green-papered walls, and my desk with its pen and ink was tucked in the corner.

The desolate period following Clarke's departure ended when a cartman whose pocket I picked, rather than whistling for a bobby and thereby bestowing upon me a stint in Newgate (which I was not fascinated enough by to fancy living there), instead gave me two cracked ribs under a dank archway in Whitechapel. As I recovered from this blessing in disguise, I realised destitution was growing tiresome and—selfishness restored—schemed over how best to earn my bread and cheese. Single pages were all I could afford to print, so I tried my hand at "last confessions," which were the fanciful one-page admissions of the recently executed.

It will surprise no one to learn that I was *marvellous* at them.

Last confessions were quite a different thing from broadsides and from gallows ballads; with our broadsides' contents you are familiar, but as for gallows ballads, here is an excerpt from "Mary May," that you may determine why I did not go in for that line of work:

Before he long the poison took
In agony he cried;
Upon him I in scorn did look,—
At length my brother died.

Since I laughed myself silly over them, I thought it imprudent to write them myself. But oh!—the confessions! The soaring imagination I lent them, the lecherous details, the pathos I could render as if it had been splayed upon a rack before me. I chose my subjects with alacrity and experience; I did not want Samuel Green, who drunkenly bludgeoned a guardsman, but I did want Hezekiah Pepper, a new father who strangled a maiden on the outskirts of St. Giles. The stories were all that mattered—how dark the deed, how deep the despair. Writing them required two to three hours of ink rippling over pages to the tune of my black heartbeats and the street soprano below, who—despite her great rolls of belly fat—reminded me achingly of Clarke.

"Me little one's off raising 'ell, I shouldn't wonder." Tilly ventured to my window to see if she could glimpse Kitty playing amidst the lost violet blooms and the chestnut shells; it was freezing, but Kitty was a reckless, towheaded thing with thick mittens, and no weather could touch her.

I shifted in my chair, wrapped in a brown dressing gown with lace at the collar, sifting through newspapers as the draught of poisoned smoke trickled into my brain.

"You know I'll buy next time," I mentioned, regarding her pipe. "If you're short of chink—"

"Not I, I'm rich as butter." She winked, adjusting a tatty purple shawl over the friendly spillage of her bosoms. "Nay, it's . . . we're nigh out o' hard up, and I've Judge Frost arrivin'."

My friend Tilly's speech was thick with local slang, which made me wish I were more fluent, since I rather adored the dialect of society's underbelly (though I certainly understood *hard up* meant *tobacco*). Meanwhile, most of Tilly's clientele were no more dangerous than horseflies—pimpled youths with sweaty hands, hawkers who had sold their stock of Barcelona nuts in the market below, sad widowers with silver hair; but Judge Frost was what Tilly liked to call a right scaly customer.

I gasped sharply, and Tilly pivoted. "Lord, Jane, you done give me a turn. What's up, then?"

Folding my lips together, I reread:

> **WANTED, at Highgate House,——shire. One young lady to see to a nine-year-old ward. Estate recently taken possession of by Mr. Charles Thornfield, heir of the Barbary family, late of the Sikh Wars, whose household requires the services of a qualified governess. Compensation——— pounds per annum with room and board, apply care of Mr. S. Singh, with references.**

"Ye look like someone just slapped ye in the quim with a fish."

I restored myself to my full senses with a hard shiver. "It's nothing. But . . . I used to live there, you see those words—Highgate House. They want a governess."

The previous August, I read with passionate interest the obituary of Mrs. Patience Barbary, who died abroad; Highgate House had passed into the care of that most universally respected profession, the law. My aunt's death hurt shallowly, like a mishap made peeling potatoes—she had never searched for me, never even advertised, an omission which made me equal parts grateful and furious.

Meanwhile, the thought of Highgate House provoked a queer unease. My mother insisted that it was mine, but died before explaining how or why. I was not unhappy in London; I adored the metropolis, the way I could disappear in it, but approaching a group of gouty men wearing pince-nez had not seemed wise. I was not destitute, but neither was I remotely respectable any longer; I wore jolly frocks with the fronts cut low and slung brightly coloured shawls about my elbows, teased my favourite costermongers with vocabulary that would have quite soured my aunt's digestion. Neither did I have paperwork, nor any means whatsoever of proving I was the Jane Steele who had disappeared so long ago, and thus the idea of knocking up a powder-wigged gentleman to say *How de do, may I have this estate, please?* frankly frightened me. In any case, ought I claim to be Jane Steele when Inspector Sam Quillfeather could be waiting with his ear to the ground, a hunter wise enough to allow his prey to trap herself and save him the bother?

Now, however—the thought of a stranger inhabiting the place smouldered in my stomach. Was the cottage occupied? Was my bedroom? Was Agatha yet living, and would she even know me if she was?

"Lived at a place named Highgate House!" Tilly teased. "Well, I never. Ye was a genuine lady, like, with silks and velvets and a stick up yer arse."

"No velvets. No silks." I folded the paper.

"But the stick?"

"Of course, they equip us with bum sticks from the cradle."

"I'll bet ye had a great bed wi' acres and acres o' white sheets," she surmised dreamily.

"All you ever think about is linens. It's actually impressive."

She shrugged. "Never 'ad naught but a straw tick, so, aye, it occupies me mind."

"Admittedly if I spent as much time in bed as you do . . ." Her face clouded. "Tilly, I'm only joking—you know I'm no better than I should be."

"How *is* Jeremiah, come to that?"

She passed the pipe and I took another slow puff. "I've thrown him over. He snores, and he wasn't much cop at . . . well, anything. He may as well have been winding up his watch."

"Bloody hell, if ye net a guppy, toss 'im back in the river." Tilly giggled.

At my lowest tide of spirits and highest of gin swilling, I had discovered that I enjoyed the practice of lovemaking as much as the theory. My swells were acquaintances from Rotherhithe, mainly—the curly-haired boy from the saltpetre works, the tap man at the Mayflower Pub. By giving the lads some fun, I could at least make a human being happy for a quicksilver moment; and once I had got the knack of pessaries and slow touches and the faint scrape of teeth over hipbones, I enormously enjoyed myself, just as I had imagined I would when gasping alone in my bed with *The Garden of Forbidden Delights*.

"I'll find someone else soon enough," said I.

"Yer doin' it wrong, ye realise," Tilly repeated, shaking her head. "They're meant to pay for the privilege."

Clattering on the stairs interrupted us, and in tumbled Kitty Cate. She had turned twelve in June and moved with that coltish energy of girls who are about to shoot up like fireworks; her great wiry corkscrews of hair were flecked with snow, and she held a golden ribbon.

"Look at what Mr. Frost done give me, mum," she exclaimed, waving it. "'E said as it would bring out me eyes."

Tilly's mouth wrenched to one side. "Judge Frost done give that to you? In the street, like?"

"Aye." Kitty stroked it, studying the colour. "Won't it look smart, though? I've that green frock, when the weather turns, and—"

"Good afternoon, all," a nasal voice sounded.

Judge Frost stood in the open doorway, belatedly rapping at the wood. Tilly often visited me, "taking the air," and thus I was familiar with her regular customers; I liked Judge Frost so much less than the others that the figure landed in the negative. He was thin and wispy, with dandelion fluff sprouting from his cheeks and neck and ears. Indirectly, he was useful, as he had caused scores of people to be hanged at Newgate and Tyburn; directly, he was petulant and insinuating.

"Well, and do you like your Christmas gift?" He chuckled, rubbing his hands. "Frills and baubles, purses and petticoats, I've a niece myself and she thinks of nothing else. I've chosen well, my pet?"

"'Tis lovely," Kitty said, beaming, and then I noted that Tilly had gone pale.

"That's to the good, then! Now, you'll excuse your mother and me whilst we have a little chat?"

Judge Frost had a voice like chalk squealing, and he was directing all his quivery attention at Kitty, who twisted the ribbon in her fingers as she pelted off downstairs again.

Tilly forced herself to smile. "Shall we pass the time in my room?" she husked, linking arms with the judge and shutting my door behind them.

I was left with an anxious feeling like tiny waves across the sea before a squall. I frowned as I crossed my feet on the ottoman, and my eyes fell back to the advertisement: *Highgate House.* The place seemed like a dream at times, at others a nightmare, but it was *mine,* I thought again with alarming intensity.

Remember when you ran to your aunt Patience with roses and your ears were boxed for ruining the gardener's chances at the flower show.

Remember when you visited the horses with carrots, preferring their company because they wouldn't warn you against hellfire.

Remember when Mamma let you take her hair down before bedtime and the firelight painted it red and gold and copper.

I did not want to remember very much of my life—but when I thought of Highgate House, its shape shifted in my memory that day, its stark lines tangling with ivy and sentiment and something disturbingly like fanatical ownership.

The decision that I would apply for the governess position by creating false references, instructing that replies be addressed to pedigreed London post offices to be left until called for, was made as I walked home through Covent Garden three days later. The market was packed to bursting so close to the holiday, donkey barrows edged nose to tail, the mournful-eyed creatures strapped to their carts with everything from knotted handkerchiefs to braided string. The air bit like an errant pup, and I skirted impossible configurations of cabbages and salted fish, smelling the barnyard ripeness of fresh-killed chickens and the sweet sap of the festive pine boughs.

My plan was nearly formed when gaslights began blinking to life under the Pavilion, and by the time I reached Henrietta Street, it was complete; the fact that the solicitors had named Charles Thornfield next of kin (doubtless due to petty machinations set in place long ago by Aunt Patience) would not be a problem if Charles Thornfield was dead. I did not precisely *want* to kill him, mind—thus far I had reserved murder for those I had actually met—but I *could* kill him, and that was a comfort. Meanwhile, my mother left me woefully unprepared; there would be papers to recover, lineage to trace, but the occupation of governess (for which I was eminently qualified) would enable me to spy from within. I had convinced myself that if anyone remained who might recognise me, it would be my own Agatha—and surely I could explain to my old caretaker why I had left, and stayed away, and returned home once more.

After striking the snow and walnut shells off my boots, I ascended the stairs. When I saw no paisley kerchief tied to the knob (our signal she was working), I banged my way into Tilly's rooms and found her alone with a mug of hot whiskey and honey, sitting at the table next to her place of business, its pillows lovingly fluffed.

"Tilly, I know it's sudden but—I'm leaving," I announced breathlessly. "I'm going to try for the job at Highgate House."

Tilly Cate burst into tears.

"Oh, God." I rushed to pull another chair over, spreading my fingers over her back. "Tilly, I. What—"

"He's going to take her."

"I don't . . ."

Tilly slumped into my side, her heavy chest heaving. "Judge Frost. That filthy cove's been after eyein' my Kitty fer six months and more, askin' if she takes after 'er mum, askin' if she likes 'im. I says to 'im, *Kitty's only a girl*, but he bullied and fussed and finally *no,* I says, and he says smug as a cat, *I'll have ye arrested fer whorin', and then she'll need a friend anyhow, won't she?* Oh, Jane, I 'ave to tell her . . . I 'ave to . . ."

Collapsing, Tilly wept as if her heart had shattered.

"Tilly," I said into her coarse hair. "Shh. No one is going to hurt Kitty. We'll think of something, you and I."

"If she'd turned bad as I did—later, on 'er own, like—I couldn't ha' judged, but this is unnatural cruel, and there's naught to think on. He'll take me and then take her."

I have never longed for children. At times, I suspect this curiosity is due to the fact I have learnt to find Death beautiful—and if I had children, then perhaps I should not think so anymore. The idea of Judge Frost with his pale flesh glowing like a maggot in the light through Tilly's window as he enjoyed a virgin Kitty, however, was not to be endured.

"All right, Tilly." I released a small sigh. "We'll not think of something. You stop fretting; *I'll* think of something."

FOURTEEN

On a dark, misty, raw morning in January, I had left a hostile roof with a desperate and embittered heart—a sense of outlawry and almost of reprobation . . . The same hostile roof now again rose before me: my prospects were doubtful yet; and I had yet an aching heart. I still felt as a wanderer on the face of the earth: but I experienced firmer trust in myself and my own powers, and less withering dread of oppression.

When the carriage pulled up the drive before Highgate House and I beheld it again a week later, it was with a wardrobe suited for a governess (staid blacks and greys with high necks and infuriating buttons) and a keepsake in the form of a newspaper (the *Pall Mall*) containing an obituary:

> **DECEASED, Judge Arthur Polonius Frost, aged 66 years. Judge Frost was a pillar of the legal community, an advocate for harsher sentencing of those he termed "irredeemables" or that segment of society which makes peaceable living so dangerous for the honest and upright. He died of heart failure following a violent nervous attack in his home in Westminster.**

The reader may not be shocked to learn that following Tilly's account, I blackmailed Judge Frost via a street Arab's verbal message, demanding he meet me after giving his servants a half day. When I arrived, he announced his intention to see me hanged. I should have been fidgety over this save for the fact the blackmail was a ruse; I feigned a fainting spell in order to drop arsenic, charmingly known as "inheritance powder," into his half-drunk glass of brandy when he went for help disposing of me.

Did I regret this latest casualty of my nature, reader?

No; I did not regret it at all.

My nerves shrieked like a steam whistle as I alighted from the carriage, however. Highgate House seemed unreal, as if someone had told me a fairy story and I dreamt of the castle that night. The countless windows like eyes, the sinister forest—I could have visited a witch's lair and been more easy. The air numbed my fingers, and my breath came in ghostly gusts.

A man walked out the front door; he was tall and the colour of strong tea, and a tingling in my spine informed me that here was a presence which would somehow influence my life—for better or for worse, I could not say.

"I am Sardar Singh," said he.

Mr. Sardar Singh was strongly but efficiently built—he seemed a whip tensed to crack, all poise and precision. His nose was regal and hooked, his black beard long, and his head was wrapped tightly with a pale blue strip of muslin so that it resembled a beehive; otherwise, he was dressed in quiet English black.

"I am the butler here. You are Miss Jane Stone?"

I nodded, having thought it prudent to conceal the other name. Briefly, I wondered whether I ought to shake hands; but he turned to take my luggage from the coachman, so I simply followed him into the house.

And what an astonishing sight met my eyes! Lips parted, my

head slowly revolved. I left behind a staid British manse, all mauve ruffles and china dogs; here were hanging cloths of crimson and gold and indigo, a beautifully carved wooden figure wearing a bronze-painted shawl, an ivory writing box on the hall table, so many potted plants I might have been in a jungle.

Mr. Singh made for the parlour, and I raptly pursued; where once was an open sitting room now a screen stood half blocking the settee, detailed with women carrying water, their hips as curvaceous as their mesmerising eyes. A peculiar smell permeated the place—part clove and part sweet herb, and I soon divined that it emanated from the glowing brass chandelier which hung in the shape of a great starburst above us.

"Welcome to Highgate House, Miss Stone," said Mr. Singh. "Might I bring you anything to refresh your spirits?"

I sat, removing my gloves. "A little wine would be welcome, thank you—the road was long and cold."

"So often the way with roads," said he, crossing to unstop a crystal decanter.

Mr. Singh's voice owned a light lilt, but his diction was crisp and clear. As he poured the claret, I saw that he wore a single steel bracelet, a sort of cuff. Additionally, there was a silver comb wedged into his hair just below the pale blue turban, glinting dangerously.

"Sardar? What on earth are— Oh, but I see she's arrived," a crisp new voice interrupted.

Here I was introduced to Mr. Charles Thornfield. It would be inaccurate to say that my heart skipped—nothing whatsoever happened to that poor excuse for an organ. My breath quickened, however, and my hands fretted, and all other outward manifestations manifested.

Charles Thornfield was neither tall nor short, with a face that seemed almost ferocious in its ruggedness; there was an elegance about the tanned cheekbones, however, and a refinement to the chiselled jaw and straight nose, which suggested diplomacy. He bowed infinitesimally, the effect as much ironic as polite. Like his foreign butler, he wore a metal ring about his right arm, and his hair had not been shorn in quite some time—far more remarkable, it was white as snow, though he looked no older than five and thirty, and he wore it tied behind with a short black ribbon. His attire was sedately rich: a navy frock coat with a grey cravat and trousers, grey gloves, and he was shod in a pair of well-worn riding boots, which endeared him to me immediately. His brows were sable and sharply arched at their outer edges, his eyes an oceanic blue, and they glimmered as they took me in.

"This is Miss Jane Stone, I hope," said he. "Charles Thornfield, at your service, supposing ever I can be. I've so looked forward to greeting young Sahjara's governess, I can hardly express my enthusiasm."

My rival's voice was a baritone with all the complexity and smoke of a good whiskey; yet it was not sombre—the sardonic edge I had seen in his bow likewise seasoned his greeting, and I fought an inappropriate smile.

If I were to kill this very intriguing man, I wonder how difficult he would make the task?

"Is my charge's name Sahjara, then? I am pleased to meet you, and shall be still more pleased to meet your daughter."

"You shan't, actually." Mr. Thornfield corrected. "Sahjara is her name and you may even be pleased to meet her, nothing is impossible, but the sprite is my ward. Frankly, there were irregularities about your application which drew me to you."

My heart gave several futile thumps as I took the glass of wine from Mr. Singh.

"I'm afraid I don't—"

"You see, I could not recognise any of the references you gave, though all returned my correspondence with the highest praises. My hope was that you worked in other . . . eccentric households. Capital, here she is! Sahjara, this is your new governess, Miss Jane Stone."

A honey-skinned, poised little girl entered the room, led by a woman of an age and complexion close to Mr. Singh's; this matron wore a drab dress after the manner of housekeepers, and thus might have been unremarkable—save for a white scar which blazed across her brow like a line dashed through text. At the sight of her, my crackling nerves settled a little. This seemed an entirely new household to the previous—and if they had retained any of my aunt's staff, they were highly unlikely to be people who had ever paid me the slightest attention.

My charge, meanwhile, was attired in ivory muslin perfectly suited to her own golden complexion, wherein I divined the reason for Mr. Thornfield's choosing me: she must have been half-born of foreign parentage. Sahjara's eyes were black and darting, and her thick black hair had been braided into a queue—upon closer inspection, I thought her closer to eight than ten. I felt immediate relief that I should not have to manage anyone who fit more neatly into society than I did.

"I am Miss Stone," I introduced myself, rising.

"Sahjara Kaur," said she, curtseying.

"Miss Stone, may I present the Young Marvel," said Mr. Thornfield dryly, pouring himself a whiskey. To my surprise, he did not remove his close-fitting gloves, an egregious breach of etiquette.

"What sort of horse do you ride?" Sahjara asked next.

"Actually," I replied, stopping there.

"Behold the first spectacular feat of the Young Marvel!" Charles Thornfield leant against the sideboard. "She can take any topic—or no topic whatsoever, working from merest air—and shift the conversation to horses."

"Because you see," the child continued doggedly, "I've nearly outgrown my pony, and Charles says that if I'm *very* cautious, I might try a small mare."

"Brava!" Mr. Thornfield set his drink down to clap neatly gloved hands. "A pitch-perfect performance, and unasked for, as all the best are." Though he was clearly the most sardonic creature alive, perversely his gaze twinkled with affection.

I sat, taking her hands; I had thought long over whom I should model myself after, and tried to say as warmly as Miss Lilyvale would have, "I've never owned a horse, though I love them and used to visit the stables at Lowan Bridge School whenever I could."

And the ones just off your own east wing, come to that.

Sahjara's jaw plummeted in horror. "No! But how horrid. Don't you ride, then? You can have one of our horses, save Charles's stallion."

Mr. Thornfield chuckled. "In astonishing succession, Miss Stone, with such dexterity the mind reels, you have just witnessed the second remarkable facility of the Young Marvel."

"Which is?"

"Giving away my property to whomever she pleases, whenever she pleases."

Sahjara tossed her head; I noted with fascination another ornamental silver comb, this one flowery and delicate, and as she set a hand to her hip in a most un-English gesture I found delightful, a silver bracelet flashed in the firelight.

"Tedious *bhisti*,"* she accused her guardian, but there was no heat, merely warmth.

"Tiresome changeling," Mr. Thornfield returned, winking at her.

This harmless exchange so perversely reminded me of being spitefully called *vermin* and *scavenger* in the same room that a small

---

* Water-carrier, a lowly menial occupation on the battlefield.

knot rose in my throat; I hastened to change the subject. "What is your third great skill, Sahjara?"

"Oh, I haven't really any others," the girl demurred, though her gaze found Mr. Thornfield's through her winglike eyelashes.

"Blatant fibs are considered unfashionable in British *chicos*,* so don't tell 'em." The master of the house dropped a mock-gallant kiss inches above her hand, as if she were royalty. "She can ride as if she were born in the saddle—always could do, from before she could walk, and I promise you, Miss Stone, it is damned infuriating."

As Sahjara blushed dusky rose, Mr. Singh returned. "All is in readiness, Mr. Thornfield, with your baggage packed and Falstaff saddled."

"Thank you, Sardar. Please explain to the new governess the limits placed upon her movements within the house."

"Of course, sir."

Whether my hackles rose faster than my curiosity, I could not say.

What limits should be imposed upon my movements, when I am to this very manor born?

"Miss Stone, I hope you shall be happy here, though happiness is hardly typical of governesses, I take it, and we no more fashionable a household than the nearest costermonger's—consider any hope of glimpsing society maidens at lavish balls hosted here crushed." Draining his spirits, Mr. Thornfield offered me his hand, yet sheathed in expensive kid.

Astonished, I rose and took it, he observing my discomfiture. "You'll pardon the necessity of my going gloved, I hope? Or are you the severe breed of Englishwoman, the sort who abhor vice and irregularity equally and shall devote your night to prayers on behalf of my immortal soul?"

---

* Children.

Englishwoman? I thought, for what else should I have been?

I replied truthfully, "The journey was a trying one, sir, and I am fatigued—I've no intention of praying for you at all."

Mr. Thornfield took half a step closer, eyes narrowing. Though he was not tall, I was diminutive, and he peered down his straight nose with one side of his mouth twitching—whether into a frown or a smile I could not tell. His manner was so rudely scrutinising, I at last extricated my hand.

"You're oddly honest, for a schoolgirl turned domestic dependent," he asserted.

As is so often the case at the worst possible times, I laughed. Quickly subduing myself, I amended, "Merely weary, sir—I've no wish to offend."

"Possibly not," he mused, stepping back again. "You'll do, Miss Stone—supposing you can keep up with the wild beast in your charge. *Idderao,** Sahjara." His ward threw her arms around him. "I'll return in a few days' time."

"Sooner," she protested, half-muffled by his coat.

"Will you listen to her?" He sighed. "Is there anything else I can do for you, small tyrant? Should you like a war elephant? The moon, perhaps?"

"Sooner," she insisted, pouting.

"If I can, darling." He pulled away, straightening his waistcoat and glancing at the standing clock, one of the few familiar objects in this bewildering sea of opulence. When next he spoke, his soft tone had regained its bite. "Sardar, bring Falstaff round to the gate."

"Of course, sir."

Sweeping up a tall hat from the piano bench, he tipped it to the pair of us.

---

* Come here.

"Do not burn down the house," he commanded sternly as he swung up an accusing index finger, lending me yet another shock.

Sahjara took my elbow. "I was reading late, and some curtains caught fire," she whispered. "I was dreadfully sorry."

"You were merely disappointed at the interruption; had I cut off your hands, you should have been sorry," Charles Thornfield growled—but it was a lion's purr, not its roar. "Until next week, then! Good riddance to the pair of you. I can tell I'll have twice the deviltry to reckon with now."

Too true, I thought as he disappeared; but when Sahjara turned her teeth up to flash me a grin, I confess I could not sense a scrap of wickedness—in her, at least—at all.

Sahjara wished to sit up late talking of riding (and of foaling, breeding, racing, and the horse species in the abstract). What ought to have been an annoyance felt a balm; I liked hearing her earnest chatter; I liked the bizarre dishes served alongside our tea—buttered sandwiches, yes, but also a curry-scented bread which drove memories of Aunt Patience's arrogant tiered refreshments straight from my mind.

At nine o'clock, when we were both nodding, I recalled that I was a severe governess, the hired instructor of a rich man's charge, and rang the bell. Sahjara went meekly enough with the scarred woman when I promised to take a full tour of the stables upon the morrow, and I found myself in the company of Mr. Singh, blinking exhaustedly at the indigo tapestries which had replaced the choleric portraits along the staircase.

"Your room has been made ready and your trunk brought up, but do not hesitate to ring," Mr. Singh said as we ascended. I did not have to feign unfamiliarity with my surroundings—the bones of Highgate House remained, but its skin had been shed.

"I expect the coach shall have worn me clean through."

"So often the way with coaches," he intoned.

"Is Sahjara a relation of Mr. Thornfield?"

I imagined slight hesitation before Mr. Singh replied smoothly, "No. Miss Kaur is the daughter of an old friend. As I said, if you need anything, ring for Mrs. Garima Kaur—our housekeeper, whom you saw before—and she will attend you. Though she speaks little English, she will understand you if you make a request."

Pausing, I asked, "Sahjara is . . . her daughter?"

Mr. Singh turned on the landing, his candle illuminating the edge of his tall turban and the hollow crescent of a smile. "Ah, no indeed. Sikh men take the name Singh, as I do, and Sikh women the name Kaur. It is our custom."

"Are all the domestics Sikhs, then?" I asked innocently, my heart tensing for his answer.

"Indeed we are, Miss Stone. I hope that will not prove a problem."

"Oh, of course not," I assured him as I thrilled with satisfaction. "I hope to learn a great deal more."

We continued up the staircase from which the oil portrait of my uncle Richard Barbary had used to stare cunningly. At last, Mr. Singh swung a door open. They had readied Aunt Patience's room for me. It was not Aunt Patience's room any longer, however; the silver lamps gleamed, the corners were full of ferns, the heavy velvet hangings on the bed replaced with magical violet and lilac ones in such dye shades as I had never before seen, and where once a few niggardly coals had gasped for breath, the hearth laughed and crackled.

Wrenching my stupefied gaze from the silent white tiger skin roaring at me from the floor, I turned to thank Mr. Singh.

"Oh, and . . ." I added. He stopped, raising his chin. "Mr. Thornfield spoke of limits regarding where I'm allowed to go within the house?"

Mr. Singh's beard bobbed. "The cellars are under construction, and it is hazardous to explore them. The rest of Highgate House, including the attics should you require storage, is at your disposal—it is only the underground which is kept locked whilst alterations are in progress."

Obviously, the house was much changed; and yet, the back of my brain still prickled at this. When Jane Eyre first tours her new home and hears the tragic laugh she supposes Grace Poole's, the author writes, *but that neither scene nor season favoured fear, I should have been superstitiously afraid.* I was not afraid; but the fierce possessiveness I felt for Highgate House made me long to relearn it from plaster cracks to stone foundation. Being barred from a portion felt galling.

"I shall conduct all remaining introductions in the morning—say, after Sahjara has shown you the stables?" Mr. Singh prompted when I said nothing.

"Yes, of course. Here I stand peppering you with questions which can wait for the morrow—though of course those questions will likely only lead to fresh ones."

"So often the way," said he, and this time I knew it for a subtle jest, "with questions."

A key reposed in the lock and, dizzied at the prospect of experiencing genuine privacy for the first time in my life, I turned it.

Revolving as I crossed the room, drinking in pillows edged with seed pearls and the filigreed birds hanging upon the walls, I suppressed a shudder.

The last time I was here, I requested to be placed in the hands of Mr. Munt.

So much had changed; I now knew myself a thousand times better, as if I were a textbook I had studied, but being at Highgate House conjured everything from the graceful dips above my mother's clavicle to Edwin's damp palms.

One memory at a time would be a welcome diversion: so many together are agonising.

With arms of lead, I tossed some water on my face from the pitcher and braided my erratic waves of hair, donning my nightdress. On an impulse, I went to the window and drew back the sheer amethyst curtains—there was the diagonal line of our cottage's gable in the moonlight, seen through silhouetted trees. Biting my knuckle, I studied it until I knew that I must turn away or else pretend to have caught a head cold come morning.

As my eyes shifted, they snagged upon the drive, a ribbon of heather within the slate, and I thought of Charles Thornfield.

Indeed, once my mind latched upon him, I stood for several more minutes, wondering what business my mortal enemy had that would take him away from his clearly beloved ward; I at last collapsed, worn to a bone shard, upon my deceased aunt Patience's feather bed.

FIFTEEN

It is a very strange sensation to inexperienced youth to feel itself quite alone in the world: cut adrift from every connection; uncertain whether the port to which it is bound can be reached, and prevented by many impediments from returning to that it has quitted.

I have no doubt but that you will find your way," Mr. Singh assured me, pouring a cup of clove-scented tea at the kitchen table. "We cannot be what you expected to find."

The December morning had been frigid, a pristine lace veil draped bridelike over the grounds. Sahjara had met me before the stables, wearing her riding habit, raven's-feather eyes gleaming. Her enthusiasm for equestrianism was no hardship—I felt pure satisfaction when I tugged back the familiar wooden gate, splinter prone and rust smelling, and entered the stable. After Sahjara gathered that horses were neither averse to me nor I to them, she blithely wondered did I always look so happy when I stood beside a stallion's muzzle, smiling at its single visible eye?

The answer was *yes*, of course, but then Sahjara departed to work with her riding coach, and I rendezvoused with Mr. Singh in the kitchen only to behold the entire domestic staff.

Agatha, I thought, suppressing a fresh gush of panic despite assurances the household was entirely foreign. *She would say nothing, surely—she would never betray my confidence, once she learnt I meant to claim what's mine.*

Agatha, however, was nowhere to be seen.

"I hope meeting us all at once was not too terribly overwhelming." In the satiny winter light of midday, I realised that Mr. Singh was younger than I had supposed; he could not have exceeded Mr. Thornfield's five and thirty. The beard framing his mouth lent the impression he was always mildly smiling or lightly frowning, both somehow solicitous expressions.

"Oh, no." Sipping my tea too soon, I scalded my tongue. "It was lovely."

It was not; I was wholly ignorant of how governesses are expected to behave. We had been groomed for the profession at Lowan Bridge: so was my first step to steal food, tell lies, or thrust a letter opener into someone's gullet?

"They were gratified by your open nature, fearing a traditionalist. You already seem quite at ease with Sahjara. I don't suppose I need tell you she is beloved by us all."

I smiled, shaking my head. I had now formally been introduced to Mrs. Garima Kaur, the housekeeper with the terrible white mark on her brow, who indeed spoke scant English but listened with such care it hardly mattered; Mrs. Jas Kaur, the cook; and eight additional Singhs and Kaurs, the remaining house servants and grooms, all of whom fascinated and overwhelmed in equal measure.

During some confusion I gathered had to do with the cellar workmen, Mrs. Garima Kaur leant into my face as if consulting a mirror and murmured, "Quiet. Afraid?"

"Why would—no," I stammered. "Only anxious."

Garima Kaur was a gaunt woman with severely stark bone structure, her cheeks hollow beneath dark eyes so deeply set one could not help but see the skull beneath. Without the silvery streak across her brow, and with a stone more flesh on her skeleton, she might have been beautiful—as it was, she was only striking. She stared straight into my mind, or so it felt.

She cocked her head, the scar glinting at the same instant as an unreadable smile. "Mr. Sardar Singh—good. Nothing bad. You, how in English?"

I had no notion.

"Safe. Mr. Singh. Do not worry, do not worry," she repeated, using a phrase she must have just learnt.

It might have been dreadfully alarming, save that it was not; butlers have the run of every estate, and to be assured by the housekeeper that ours would not infringe upon my virtue was rather companionable.

"I won't worry," I assured her, touching her sleeve, and I noted she wore no wedding ring. It was common practice for housekeepers to go by *Mrs.* without husbands, however, as a token of respect. "You are unmarried, then, Mrs. Kaur?"

Her lips pursed. "Yes, Miss Stone. You?"

"I can't think of anyone who would marry me," I joked, and Mr. Singh returned to finish the introductions.

Now we sat alone in the kitchen, Mr. Sardar Singh and I. All the hanging copper pans and cast-iron pots remained the replica of my memory's; they were augmented, however, by queer skillets and glazed vessels, and where once only salt and pepper had reposed, a sunset blaze of glass-jarred spices sat next to a heaping bowl of onion, garlic, and gingerroot, all emitting a perfume so overwhelming that I had already sneezed twice. For good measure, I did so again.

"Bless you," my companion said smoothly. "I already informed you last night we must keep away from the cellars, Miss Stone."

Yes, and now I am determined to visit them.

"And now you know everyone here by name."

Would that were true.

"Should you have any further questions, I am your man," he concluded, mouth tipping upwards as he spread his hands.

"Mr. Thornfield is a most . . . peculiar individual," I attempted, feigning interest in my teacup.

"So often the way with individuals."

Chuckling, I added, "He treats Sahjara like a princess."

"Well, she is a princess, so that is quite natural."

My eyes shot up to find that Mr. Singh's were equally mirthful. "You cannot—no, it is impossible."

"Not merely possible but true." Mirroring me, the butler watched the vortex created by his spoon. "We Sikhs call ourselves the pure ones. You were bemused by our names last night—men belonging to the religion are baptised, you would say, with the surname Singh, which means *lion*. Women are baptised with the surname Kaur, or princess."

"Every Sikh female is a princess?"

He took a sip of tea. "You must think us altogether mad."

"No!" I exclaimed so fast that droplets splashed into my saucer. Embarrassed, I set the cup down. "I mean to say, I think I could grow fond of Sahjara, and I intend to do well by her."

"That is gratifying to hear. Mr. Thornfield is not incorrect in calling her the Young Marvel, though he sounds ever in jest—her name means *daybreak*, and she truly does throw the curtains open, doesn't she? You seem too restless for tea, Miss Stone—no, no, I taxed you with social necessities. Might you enjoy a short tour?"

Eagerly, I agreed, and we pushed back our chairs that I might enjoy a tour of my own estate.

"The music room remains relatively intact, but some minor alterations have been made," said Mr. Singh, sliding back a glass-paned door a few minutes later.

The walls were covered with scores of minuscule framed artworks which had been rendered in such fine detail that I imagined I peered through an enchanted telescope. In one set, the same cottage was depicted in high summer, brilliant autumn, blue winter, and lush spring; in another, a saint with a beard and turban stared as if the viewer's soul were being weighed upon his scale; in others, lovers clasped each other with such enthusiasm any governess ought to have been shocked.

I barely remembered to flare my nose in dismay.

"This is Mr. Thornfield's collection of Punjabi miniatures." Mr. Singh either had not noted my pretended disapproval or did not care, for he smiled as he reached my side. "His eye for worth is exceptional, having been raised in Lahore. See this portrait of Maharajah Ranjit Singh, the way the furnishings are patterned so lovingly, but his face most carefully rendered of all?"

"Mr. Thornfield is from Lahore?" I asked, latching on to undeniably the most intriguing word in this statement. "How is that possible, the East India Company only having arrived there some five years ago? Or so I read in the newspapers—I supposed Mr. Thornfield English."

Again I sensed a tick of the clock before Mr. Singh spoke. "He was born there, to a British entrepreneur, but he studied medicine at the British and Foreign Medical School and then Charing Cross Hospital before he returned to the Punjab. Ah, you would not have known he belongs to the Royal College of Physicians and Surgeons of London, of course. Yes, Mr. Thornfield is a man of medicine. This particular painting is moving for us—Amritsar, the Sikh holy city where our sacred book resides."

It was a gilded palace at the end of a pure white pier surrounded by sapphire waters—an impossible place, a dream breathed from a dawn pillow.

"To have left this behind—you must miss it very much," I mentioned, wisely refraining from commentary regarding homes from which I myself had fled.

"God has his seat everywhere," Mr. Singh returned without inflection, as if quoting a text.

"I thought from the advertisement that Mr. Thornfield had been in the wars?"

An invisible shutter closed over Mr. Sardar Singh's face. "Who has not been in a war? Yes, Mr. Thornfield trained as a doctor but obtained an army commission after military training at Addiscombe."

Mr. Singh strode off and I pursued, anxious lest I had given offence on my second day. We turned left down a corridor, right down another, until I knew we stood before the billiards room, and he rested his fingers upon the door handles.

"Forgive me, I never meant to—"

Air burst into my face as the butler revealed the room; but I could not enter, such was my astonishment at the narrow fraction I beheld.

"After you, Miss Stone," Mr. Singh demurred.

A steel palace, the inside of a diamond—how shall I best describe a billiard room transformed into a war display? Swords—straight, curved, broad, tapered—lined every wall, polished to a sheen echoing the pain of the blade itself. Their handles were inset with ivory carvings, their hilts embellished with golden flourishes, their points angled into queer triangles or hollowed into deadly sickle shapes. Shorter daggers hung above the liquor cabinet, and the hearth was festooned with weapons I could scarce comprehend—tri-pronged silver objects with needlelike points, axes so beautiful I could not fathom using them, bizarre metal circlets which gleamed at us like eyes. I had never viewed such a fascinating collection of murderous devices.

"Oh," I breathed, delighted.

"Do they interest you?" Mr. Singh sounded pleased. "These are the weapons of the Khalsa, and I'm afraid we are all quite adept with them."

"Mr. Thornfield has a cuff like yours," I noted, too alight with inquisitiveness to care whether I was being rude.

"You are observant. Yes—he is a Sikh, just as I am."

"However is that possible?"

"There is no Hindu; there is no Mussulman," he answered, and I again had the impression he quoted scripture. "If there is no Hindu and no Mussulman, and all can form a single brotherhood, then there is no Christian either. I beg your pardon, as that is not a popular opinion in this country."

I could reach only one conclusion: Mr. Charles Thornfield was improbably born in the Punjab, took medical courses, gained a military commission, and at some point embraced an entirely foreign culture. The master of the house (temporarily, anyhow) was the pitied and often despised sort who had allowed his Britishness to fade in the searing desert sun, politeness and gaslight and snobbery leached into the dunes. During my newspaper scoutings, I had often glimpsed accounts of such hapless folk, as we were forever at war with *somebody*: London was pockmarked with men who professed a respect for the Buddha, women who had converted to—horror of horrors—vegetarianism.

"I shock you, Miss Stone."

I laughed. "You don't, on my life you don't. Which of these are you best with?"

Mr. Singh emitted a happy puff through his nostrils, pointing at one of the shining metal circlets. "That is a *chakkar*—a steel throwing ring honed into a blade. Members of the Khalsa used to hurl these at their foes before enemies rode within striking distance. Now experts are almost unheard-of."

"Save yourself."

"I am considered passable," he demurred, but his eyes sparkled.

My attention snagged upon something still more extraordinary, and I approached where it hung above a rack of billiard cues. The object had a rosewood sword grip; where the blade was meant to emerge, however, a metal band was coiled in upon itself and tied with thick black leather, so that it resembled a hilt attached to a lengthy ribbon of steel wound into a tidy ring.

"What on *earth* . . . ?" I stretched to the tips of my toes to look more closely.

"What excellent taste you have in exotic weaponry, Miss Stone." Instantly I relapsed onto my heels, wondering whether it was too late to affect disapproval. "No, no, I cannot fault your appreciation for what may be the most extraordinary collection of Sikh artefacts in England. This is an *aara*, and only highly advanced warriors are trained in them. Essentially, you regard a combination of a whip and a sword—when unrolled, the metal strip divides flesh as if it were butter. I need hardly add that foolhardy fascination with this weapon leads only to missing fingers or worse."

I allowed my pupils to lose their focus in the *aara*'s shining whorls—half recalling all the times in London when a strange man had approached, the jaundiced light of malice in his eyes, and imagining that I could have snapped the blackguard's head off from twelve feet distant.

"Will you show me, sometime, when your schedule permits?"

"I regret I must decline." Mr. Singh held the door open for me, signalling a need to return to his tasks. "I was once considered formidable with the *aara*, I admit, but fell out of practice. For that pleasurable spectacle, you will have to await the return and good humour of Mr. Thornfield."

I've finished, I *promise.* Now I must see that Dalbir's hoof has been tended properly."

Five days later, Sahjara and I sat in a converted schoolroom which would have elevated most eyebrows—draperies of orange and amber embroidered with flowering trees lined the walls, conjuring an impossible forest when outside all was grey and snow-softened. There were also chalkboards, paper and ink, drawing utensils, plentiful books, and a pianoforte which look neglected and obligatory.

"If you've finished translating the entire passage, I'll correct it—then of course you may check in on Dalbir."

Sahjara's pony, Dalbir, was named "brave soldier," a moniker I should have thought droll for a pony had he not been more along the lines of a petit dragon, dappled-grey and wonderfully irritable with everyone save Sahjara and myself; the unfortunate beast had suffered a badly chipped hoof that morning.

My pupil ambled over with her French essay, handed me the papers, and then unselfconsciously sat upon the luxurious carpet with her head against my knee.

I patted her awkwardly at first, then drew my fingers over glossy braids smelling of the almond oil she used to smooth out the tangles. Sahjara was demonstrative with everyone, adorably so, and it did not mean anything, I told myself; she probably expected a tyrant, but I recalled tyranny and preferred rebellion. Anyhow, I had neatly solved the problem of attention to her lessons by making each and every subject horse themed. She painted horses in watercolours, explored their anatomy, learnt geography specific to legendary cavalry marches, and translated French passages about horses, as she was doing now.

"We *will* be great friends, won't we?" she mused as I shifted to correct her work.

"I hope so. Did you expect a shrivelled old crone with a cane and a pocket Bible?"

Sahjara shrugged against my calf. "Not precisely. I feared someone who would think me unnatural, though."

This gave me pause, even as I marked an improper conjugation of *avoir*: she was almost exactly the age I had been when I left Highgate House, and Sahjara in five short days had already revealed her character; she was headstrong, impulsive, recklessly affectionate, and had gifted me with thirteen possessions of Mr. Thornfield's to date. What did a murderess four times over care if Sahjara was browner skinned than I, forward in her speech, and was familiar with the housemaids? If surnames were to be taken as given, they could be her aunties for all I knew.

"Would you have seemed unnatural at home—or do you remember?"

"That's a hard question," Sahjara said slowly. "The Punjab comes out all jumbled when I try to remember. I see pictures without any story to them."

"Do any of the pictures stand out?"

"The flap of the tent was ripped by a sword, and I was afraid of who would come through the gap, but it was Charles, and he carried me away and fed me. I was very hungry, I recall. And soon after, I was sent to England for safety's sake. I was five."

Well, there is a remarkable fragment indeed.

I pressed, "Did England improve matters?"

"Oh, yes!" she exclaimed. "Yes, before England, men had always been asking me questions. How was I faring, but also *Where is it?* and I hadn't the faintest, you see, and so kept quiet. Keeping quiet made them very cross."

"I can imagine."

Where is it? is a very specific question. Had Sahjara been caught in the middle of the First Anglo-Sikh War and interrogated at so young an age as five? A startling surge of protectiveness coursed through me. I liked Sahjara and wanted her to erase the other little girl, the one who had wandered these halls suffocating on her aunt's hatred.

"Look, I've scored eighty percent!"

"You have indeed. What were the men looking for?"

"A trunk," said she, taking her translation and glaring at the errors. "It had my dolls in it. Though they couldn't have wanted my dolls, so perhaps they thought something else was inside—there was a terrible row when it went missing, I know. I just wanted my dolls back, as I was only a *chico*."

"Perfectly natural."

"I was very upset over losing them."

A trunk.

I swear upon my copy of *Jane Eyre* that my interest in Sahjara's tale was based in both fascination and goodwill; I wanted to know more about her, and I badly wanted to know more about Mr. Charles Thornfield, who had callously flouted my poor pupil's request and stayed away longer than a few days.

"What else do you remember?"

Her eyes grew unfocused, as if peering through fogged glass. "Our house in Lahore, its balcony. It smelled like livestock and incense in the streets, which were very busy with all the Afghani horse traders, and the merchants bargaining over oranges and goats, and the fortune-tellers at tables divining from maps of the stars. I remember huge walls with heavy guns, white mosques like turnips." She charmingly screwed her face into a pucker. "It's still an awful muddle. I don't even know what the wars were *for*."

Mindful of my role, I cudgelled my brains and drew embarrassing blanks. The Sikhs' Khalsa army was by all accounts a ferocious one—sharp as a pistol crack, and just as keen to hack our East India Company to bits after the first war ended as they had been at the starting gate. Predictably, they had emerged thirsty for blood two years later, and countless British and Punjabi soldiers had blown one another's pates off before the Sikh Empire went the way of the Roman one. I knew this meant outrageous riches for Her Majesty; when I opened my mouth to unmuddle the situation for my pupil, however, I found I knew nothing whatsoever else.

"Did Mr. Thornfield never recover your trunk?"

"No, though he tried." Sahjara stretched upon the rug like a lean little cat. "It must be lost forever now."

Voice quite composed, I said, "Sahjara, I know we're strangers, and you needn't speak of your parents, nor the past—but you may if you wish, all right?"

She stood, outlined now against the dimming December sunset, for we had not turned up the lamps. "Oh, were you curious over my parents? Charles says my father was a Company man and my mother a Sikh princess. It's horrid but I can't recall them. There was the sword through the tent flap, and the trunk went missing, and I had horses to tend to, I think—but I don't recall much from the Punjab other than Charles."

Sahjara fetched her warmest cloak from where she had thrown it two hours previous, her governess too slovenly a creature to have noticed.

"Give Dalbir my best," I instructed.

"If Charles returns, send someone to fetch me?"

"Of course."

"Charles likes you," she added as she skipped towards the door. "I've never seen him like anyone so fast. He actually shook your hand."

Following this obscure observation, she disappeared, and I was left once more to ponder the enigmas of my new household. Then, lacking other occupation and knowing I had an hour till supper, a subtle electric pulse thrumming in my boot soles, I likewise donned my warmest things and quit the main house in the opposite direction, marching silently for my cottage and whatever—whomever—I might find there.

SIXTEEN

It is one of my faults, that though my tongue is sometimes prompt enough at an answer, there are times when it sadly fails me in framing an excuse; and always the lapse occurs at some crisis, when a facile word or plausible pretext is specially wanted to get me out of painful embarrassment.

If you expected to find yourself in a Gothic snowscape, reader, ears tickling with spectral whispers as the plucky protagonist breaks into a cottage haunted by the shades of her past, regrettably you are mistaken.

The door was already unlocked. Opening the panel of the small lantern I had brought, I discovered that my erstwhile home was carpeted in grit and vermin droppings, and furthermore that spiders are the most industrious creatures alive.

Slowly, my ears adjusted; no ticking of clocks greeted me, no exclamations of alarm. The place had been emptied, and not merely of its few antiques—even the bedding and the better chairs were dispatched. A pang struck me at the thought of faithful, nonsensical Agatha turned out to pasture—or worse, deceased—but I could do her no better service than to press on, so press on I did.

The kitchen was mouldering, the parlour decrepit, my mother's bedroom sacked and empty, which hurt my chest terribly, and still I could not bring myself to quit the place. Creeping up to the garret was a whim; I knew I must be back soon to sit with Sahjara over another brilliantly orange curry, swallowing questions down my gullet.

I will have a peek at the attic space, then be done.

And what did I behold but my mother's old wooden trunk, resting in a corner. I dived for its dust-soft handle and heaved open its lid; an explosion of dry grime and a short stack of letters met my gaze, and my fingers discovered the papers were indeed corporeal. I think I had been half expecting leprechaun gold in that cottage, or at least small, strange men proposing dangerous quests. Instead I held foolscap with ink scrawled over it, ink which might very well tell me what I had inherited and what I might venture to do about it.

To escape with the sole prize I had come seeking, save Agatha herself, seemed altogether too good to be true: but I did, and twenty minutes hence had stowed my treasure under my mattress without a single person knowing I had left the main house at all.

"What became of the original staff?" I asked, sniffing at a plate of heartily spiced potato and cabbage with mustard seeds. "Surely this place was populated by English servants, before."

"I regret to say that they were made to feel rather unwelcome." Mr. Sardar Singh spooned out portions of chicken curry and saffron-scented rice to Sahjara and me; twice before he had dined in our company, and I found myself avidly hoping he would do so again. "We brought with us an unknown master, foreign tastes . . . their defection was natural."

"But never forced?" I questioned, envisioning my elderly Agatha scrubbing floors in some rot-ridden dispensary.

"Of course not—heavens, I hope none of them ever felt so. Some had family they wished to return to, others dreams of travel. They were all of them dismissed with a thousand pounds, after all."

"A thousand . . ." I echoed. It was the sort of money a titled landholder or a City purveyor of stocks might have brought in yearly, and it was a princely figure to a domestic worker.

"Miss Stone, I hope that I haven't overstepped the bounds of English propriety. The figure is irre—"

"Of course it isn't irrelevant—Mr. Thornfield could have got away uncensored distributing bonuses at a hundredth the price."

"The master of the house saw no need to be parsimonious," he returned, but I saw he was pleased.

"Not often the way," I quipped, "with masters. Please do sit down."

Mr. Singh laughed, seating himself several places distant and helping himself to the steaming dishes. "At any rate, there were alterations to be effected, and long-time occupants are always dismayed at usurpers renovating their domain."

Mr. Singh was correct; the cellars, at least, were being subjected to significant changes, and it dismayed me. Workmen arrived before I rose in the morning, greeting me with the distant invisible *clink, clink* of chisels and spades as I walked to the morning room to breakfast with Sahjara; at five in the afternoon when I released her, they filed by me out the servants' entrance, anointed with mineral-smelling mud. Twice had I begun marching down the dank stairs I already knew so well, but a member of the staff always materialised with a cordial *Might I assist you?* and all attempts at reconnaissance rendered thereby impossible.

The work rankled. Our cellars had been inhospitable, the remnants of ancient foundations—neither crypts nor vaults, simply stones and pillars. I did not know what Mr. Thornfield could possibly want with caves not even fit to store wine properly (a failing of which Aunt Patience was surpassingly proud).

"When did the cellar renovations commence?"

"Three months ago," Sahjara replied. "Six months after we moved in and began redecorating—the place was dreadful, all stuffy chintzes."

I smiled, for I agreed with her. "Is the cellar to house a wine collection? Mr. Thornfield seems to own a connoisseur's soul."

"He does indeed," Mr. Singh agreed.

This was less than forthcoming.

"Is it for storage, then? This household—the exotic spices, the incense—it must be difficult to maintain here in England?"

"Not so difficult as you might imagine. Mrs. Garima Kaur, who is a highly competent individual, travels monthly to London to meet with merchants who import Punjabi essentials. She sees to it that Mrs. Jas Kaur is kept in basmati and dhal and so forth, and the rest we can easily buy from neighbouring farms."

"Then perhaps a Sikh chapel for your rituals?" I ventured next.

"Oh, I'm sure he has plans for the place, Miss Stone." Mr. Singh smiled effortlessly, passing me a dish of what appeared to be yogurt. "I myself shall be contented when these local stonemasons—good men but rather untutored—stop tracking filth through Mrs. Jas Kaur's kitchen. I knew her in the Punjab as a saintly woman, and here in England, she is ready to dissolve into fits."

As am I, I thought, *over lack of headway.*

A few hours later, I washed my face and hung my sober black dress and sat in Aunt Patience's room with the letters from the cottage in my hands, nearly in silent tears already at the prospect of voices from beyond the grave. Wrapping my dressing gown tighter, I edged my chair towards the fireplace. This first missive was written in an older, more palsied version of Agatha's hand:

Dear Missus Jane, supposing ever you return,

Your aunt weren't about to do the job herself, but know that I searched and searched for you. Should you find this, well and good, I've done what I'm meant to. Should you not, I hope no harm to anyone who may come across it.

That school was as awful as awful can be, I'd wager, and I don't fault your quitting the place—send word, and we'll all be just as happy as fish in a lake. I'm to go to——Court,——shire to be with my sister, who's always been my elder and thus an old woman now in need of some comfort.

This new fellow what owns the estate, Mr. Charles Thornfield, seems both a decent sort and terrible peculiar. He has his winning ways, and his peevish ones, but there's no faulting a soldier for quirks—they catch them abroad, and there's an end to the matter.

Mr. Cyrus Sneeves can explain something of the papers. Write to him should you have any questions, but supposing you want to leave well enough alone, I shouldn't fault you either.

Best of luck always,
Agatha

I examined the rest of the stack. Here were more correspondences between Anne-Laure Steele and Cyrus Sneeves and, like the ones I had read so long ago, they dealt mainly with ensuring our claim to Highgate House; my mother's penmanship appeared next, her faintly accented voice in my ear as I read:

Rue M——,
2nd Arrondissement,

TUESDAY

Dear Mr. Sneeves,

I wish to thank you for having granted me such a thorough understanding of our situation. The difficulty as I see it lies in the honouring of our arrangement in perpetuity. Patience Barbary is dead set against us—and when I imagine myself in her shoes, I cannot bring myself to censure her. On ne peut rien y faire, *however, and it only remains to discover a trusted party willing to visit consequences upon Mrs. Barbary should she ever attempt to disinherit my Jane.*

Suggestions to this purpose will be met with gratitude; in the meanwhile, please move forward as discussed.

Je vous prie d'agréer,
Mrs. Anne-Laure Steele

The hairs at my nape bristled. My mother had regarded Patience Barbary with as much affection as she held for dung stuck to the sole of a heeled French boot; yet I read a curious reluctance in her wording, regret over the fact Aunt Patience would be angry, which I had never glimpsed in life.

The reply told me little, meanwhile:

Rue du R——,
1st Arrondissement,

WEDNESDAY

Chère Mme. S——

Trust that our regard for Mr. S——'s memory will allow nothing less than perfect diligence regarding this most delicate of subjects. A local agent must be appointed to make real the fact that thwarting our designs will only lead to unpleasantness, and I should be ashamed to suggest anyone of less standing in the firm than my partner, Mr. Aloysius Swansea. I shall make haste to apprise him of all details, but should you ever require direct contact, he may be found at:

SNEEVES, SWANSEA, AND TURNER
No. 29C Lisle Street, Westminster

Humbly,
Cyrus Sneeves, Esq.

I think it took me eleven seconds to locate a pen and paper and begin a letter to Mr. Aloysius Swansea:

Highgate House,

December 20, 1851

Dear Mr. Swansea,

My name is Jane Steele, and I recently came across documents suggesting that you conducted business with my father, Mr. Jonathan Steele, and my mother, Mrs. Anne-Laure Steele. I would be grateful for any information you could give me upon this topic, and should the written form prove too cumbersome, I can travel to London. Letters will reach me here, but I beg that you address them to Miss Jane Stone, as the unfortunate circumstances of my mother's unhappy end have necessitated caution in revealing my true origins.

Gratefully,
Miss Jane Steele

The remaining correspondence confirmed what I already knew. I must needs await further instruction—supposing instruction would come. Stuffing the papers beneath my mattress again, I lay down, waiting for sleep to arrive.

No such guest called, however; ants seemed to crawl beneath my sheets, and the dawn greeted a weary soul. Head thinly humming, I stumbled out of bed and splashed enough frigid water over my face to appear human at breakfast.

After all, Mr. Thornfield may have returned.

He had not, though, and I smiled sunnily at Sahjara across the table, a sealed letter resting in the pocket of my dress ready to be posted at my earliest convenience.

Every brittle, branching fork of each bare tree seemed frost-spangled sculptures worthy of auction at Christie's private parlour that afternoon. Sahjara had insisted I take to riding again—in particular a bay mare far too perceptive for her own good, for she kept questioning me, and I was not accustomed to surrendering the reins to anyone.

The three-year-old bay's name was Nalin, or "lotus," and on the sixth day following Charles Thornfield's departure, she flew over rills and creek beds as if we had crafted a fragile truce. I sincerely hoped so, for I was remembering the beauty of Nature and questioning why I had abandoned it for the narrow streets of a soiled city. Having a horse beneath me again made me feel as if the wide world and myself were more akin than separate, and that as much as I remained a poisonous creature, I was related to the contrary being under my legs. Admittedly I had no proper riding habit, which vexed me only marginally less than it vexed Sahjara; still, my plain grey governess's disguise, when topped with a cape-backed cloak and a cloth cap, suited well enough for the countryside.

I had given Sahjara a Sunday holiday, so I never thought of returning to Highgate House until my letter had been posted and the sun sagged and the skies—of a woollen complexion all day—began dusting me with powdery motes of ice. These were not the fat snowflakes one so loves to see in wintertime but the ground glass which stings one's skin, and thus I cut across a familiar clearing to take the road home rather than risking the half-obscured thickets.

The daylight was nigh expired, but the moon had risen, and the lane to Highgate House was scarce ever used save by the occupants—so I never considered how foolhardy it was to steer Nalin into a leap over a stunted hedgerow until it was too late.

We landed, a shadow materialised, and Nalin reared as she emitted a shrill neigh.

My own sharp cry echoed hers as I fought to regain control; but when she bucked the second time, I flew through the air and landed with a heavy thud upon the frozen dirt.

Bloody hell, I thought, and then yelled it aloud, and then enunciated several more expressions learnt in London.

Crunch, crunch, crunch.

The shadow approached me; its steps blended with the mocking trill of the last birds left awake in the thickets.

Had I possessed a superstitious spirit, I should have been terrified to look, lest the traveller prove a goblin or a ghoul. One of the advantages to being a cold-blooded killer, however, was that I thought nothing in the woods much more dangerous than I was, so I heaved myself onto one elbow, panting with shock and exertion.

"Stay back!" As if lightning had illuminated my peril, I realised the footfalls were a man's, and I incapable of flight. "I've no money, and a knife in my skirts!"

Happily, this was nothing save God's truth; a pause ensued, but the menacing steps resumed with greater speed.

Wrenching myself fully up on one arm, I had the blade aimed at the stranger two seconds later; there are commodities some men want on deserted pathways which have nothing to do with currency.

"By all means, come closer, you whoreson bastard," I shouted. "I'll cut you to ribbons and laugh at your funeral!"

"Miss Stone, we haven't been long acquainted, but I had hoped I inspired in you a fonder spirit of camaraderie than *that*," came a deep, pleasantly grainy voice.

My heart lurched. I forced myself to breathe, replacing my knife in the pocket obscured by the pleat near my waist.

As Mr. Charles Thornfield approached, still snow-obscured save his broad shoulders and the white gleam of his hair beneath his hat brim, I debated whether instantly switching personas would be canny or dense. I had cursed, threatened, and brandished a weapon when I could simply have screamed.

You never scream when you're meant to, you dunce.

"I think I'm hurt." Indeed, my ankle seemed to have burst into flames. "Forgive me, please, I couldn't see you properly. Is Nalin all right? Are *you* all right, sir?"

The muffled clop of hooves sounded, and I glimpsed Mr. Thornfield quickly tethering Nalin's reins to a thick hedgerow branch. Once the mare was secured, his silhouette turned to face me with the moon rising behind him.

"If you never speak to me again, it'll prove difficult to sack me." I rolled to my hands and knees and a bolt of brimstone shot up my leg. *"Oh."*

He strode swiftly towards me. "The devil take your impatience!"

Attempting to stand, I insisted, "I only—"

"Wait a moment or you'll make all worse than it need be. Here, please sit down—*sit.* That's right. Heavens, but you're a feral soul at heart, aren't you? No, stretch your legs out straight."

Sitting upon the ground with icy granules accumulating in the folds of my skirts as I sprawled awkwardly, I allowed Mr. Thornfield to clasp me round the torso. The wind cut at my ears, and the stones bit through my petticoats. It had not been the reunion I had anticipated; in fact, I had amused myself by anticipating every possible reunion, from schoolroom tranquillity to defending the house from marauding seekers of mysterious boxes, save this humiliating one.

With him at my back, I managed to get my hands round my knees and wrench both limbs to the front, shaking with effort and pain.

"All right, hush now. We'll be fit to conquer the subcontinent in no time."

"Why hush? I didn't say peep."

This earned me a startled chuckle. "'Pon my life, there's some truth there. No plans on blubbing, or swooning, or stabbing, come to that?"

"Not at present."

"Capital woman," said he. "Now, I saw how you landed, and damned if it weren't a smasher—feel along your legs to the ankle, very carefully, unless you cannot and wish me to do so."

His scruples, for which I ought to have been grateful, seemed merely irritating. "A highly considerate question coming from a sawbones—I heard you were a medical man, sir."

Mr. Thornfield huffed, still bracing my spine. "And I heard you were a governess, but not many of that set can say *bugger* with quite so much purity of conviction."

A fresh wave of embarrassment washed over me. "I am not yet myself, Mr. Thornfield, but I think my legs remain intact."

"Blast, what a shame! I was so looking forward to having 'em off here in the road. Would've been like old times, I can hear the drum and the fife even now. Make certain all is well, please."

My brains were addled, my pride dented, and my ankle probably sprained, but nothing permanent had befallen me; that is, supposing I did not lose my position upon the morrow.

"All my bones are inside. I do beg your pardon, sir—had it been someone other than you there in the roadway, I don't know what I should have done."

"Called some other whoreson bastard a whoreson bastard, I expect."

Fully five seconds must have passed with my neck craned round to look into his eyes before I burst into helpless laughter. I waited for dismay to manifest, but Mr. Thornfield only smiled crookedly, and I wondered what could produce that lopsided mirth again.

"I'd every right to expect the worst of you," I complained as he lifted me easily upright. "Whatever were you doing out here in the middle of an empty dirt path?"

"I requested the local inn to house Falstaff for the night to take a weight off my conscience, for the old fellow was fatigued enough as was, and I trust them, and my mind needed clearing on the route homeward anyhow. My mind, Miss Stone, is now clear as holy water. Shall we see about getting you home?"

I used Mr. Thornfield's support to take a few steps, nearly gasping at the pangs shooting through my ankle. The joint was already swelling—and I left to the mercy of the man I had just threatened with a pocketknife.

"I think I can ride back," I suggested.

"Yes, come to that, what are you doing jumping hedgerows with one of my most expensive mares?"

"Attempting to prove myself to Sahjara—we study nothing save horses in every subject."

For a few lengthy moments, the only sound was the snow crushing under our soles as I limped towards my disappointed steed; Nalin, one of the most intelligent and yet Puritanical horses I have ever met, tapped her right hoof as if to say, *You are a disgrace.*

"Supposing you desire Sahjara's respect, shall I assume you don't want your corpse to be discovered with a snapped neck?" Charles Thornfield asked, regaining his testiness.

By the time we had reached Nalin, my entire body was confused—an ankle ballooning, breath taut and hoarse, rough but kind fingers imprinted upon my torso, roiling anger in my belly at being caught out in such a pathetic state, a strange echoing sweetness in my ears at, *Shall we see about getting you home?*

"I'll lead Nalin," Mr. Thornfield proposed, linking his fingers together and leaning to make a step for me. "Quick, now, before you indulge the urge to faint at last."

This barbed remark proved all that was necessary to effect a complete cure.

Setting the boot of my uninjured foot in Mr. Thornfield's hands, I hoisted myself onto Nalin. My other ankle pulsed bubbling tar, but it would keep; as jauntily as I could, I dipped my head in imitation of his first snide bow and calculated the distance from the hedgerow to Highgate House.

A quarter of a mile, I thought: close enough for me to make it without danger of falling; close enough for the master to make it on foot.

"I fear this injury should be seen to speedily, Mr. Thornfield," I called down. "I'll send one of the grooms back to fetch you."

With this insane parting jibe, already anticipating my return to London and imminent penury, I set off on my master's horse for my own ancestral house.

SEVENTEEN

I both wished and feared to see Mr. Rochester on the day which followed this sleepless night: I wanted to hear his voice again, yet feared to meet his eye.

I retired straight to my aunt's former room wretchedly humiliated and at once sipped at the laudanum bottle I had packed as a precaution against melancholy or sudden disaster. I awoke to an ankle blazing like a lighthouse beacon, a small breakfast tray of broth and cold green rice, and a folded communiqué written in Sahjara's friendly scrawl:

Dear Miss Stone,

Thank you for seeing to Nalin, as I was ever so worried when I heard there was an accident and the more so for your sake but I was yet glad you returned her to the stables unharmed though you were harmed yourself. Charles has returned! Happy day! He says not to disturb you, but only send you this note and ask that you ring for Mrs. Kaur when you awaken so she might treat your ankle properly and he won't let me see you as he says you must rest but know I am thinking of you every second.

Very sincerely affectionately
and kindly,
Sahjara Kaur

This brought a smile to my face; but, hark—here was another missive below the first, penned on much more masculine paper and in a matching hand:

Dear Miss Stone,

As you refused my offices so far as to flee the scene entirely and barricade yourself against enemy encroachment, I will not crudely offer them again but rather suggest that Mrs. Garima Kaur has a working practical knowledge of the whereabouts of the human ankle and a steady hand, since I've no wish to further alarm you. A repast has been provided, lest your strategy be to remain in your fortifications, but I assure you that should you emerge under the white flag of truce, the natives—though savage and frankly even heathen—will greet you with unparalleled interest.

Your servant,
Charles Thornfield

Groaning aloud did me no tangible good, reader: and yet, groan aloud I did. I rolled over with a twofold whimper—half because it hurt my ankle, half because stupidity (particularly my own) hurts my heart.

Knock, knock, knock.

"Just a moment," I called.

A glance at the ivory light through the window told me it was already ten if not later; duly considerate of my responsibilities, I stepped out of bed and promptly collapsed.

The door flew open to reveal Mrs. Garima Kaur's feet. If feet could be amused, I have no doubt but that her toes would have laughed, such was the indignity of my position.

"All right?" she asked, eyes narrowing.

"No," I admitted.

She entered, tension marring the straight sweep of her scar. After she had got me safely seated on the rumpled bedclothes, she searched my face; this was not simple concern, but rather a critical study—or perhaps I only thought so because her own physiognomy was so very apparent, her face resembling nothing so much as a handsomely clothed skull. Though she spoke English poorly, Mrs. Kaur's eyes positively radiated intellect, and I wondered what heights of nuance she could achieve in her native tongue.

"Hurt with Mr. Thornfield?" she prodded.

"No, he found me in a ditch." I pushed my posture straight with my fists. "I was hurt *near* Mr. Thornfield. He was unhurt, thank God."

"You . . . not want his help? Do not like him?"

Answering this question truthfully would have been impossible. "I don't like anyone at the moment. Save you, I think, depending on what you have there."

"Poultice." She lifted one hand. "Bandages," she added, raising the other.

"Bless you," I sighed, relief provoking bald sentiment.

"Do not worry," she answered quietly, casting her eyes down.

Some ten minutes later, Mrs. Kaur had gifted me with medical attention, and spiced tea I enjoyed very much, and a crutch I did not in the least appreciate.

"Ready?" she asked when I had fully dressed with her assistance and regained a bit of my colour.

"As I will ever prove," I agreed.

I walked step-thunk, step-thunk, step-thunk down the narrow carpeted strip upon the staircase. I was terrified to meet Mr. Thornfield; when I had not been pathetic the night previous, I had been glib, and when I had not been glib, I had been obstreperous, a truly heady concoction of undesirable traits.

Upon my arrival in the dining room, however, I discovered the household preoccupied; where I imagined my disaster of the night previous would be the sole topic, instead I found master and ward glaring daggers at an unknown person—one who beamed at my arrival and half stood, making an awkward bow.

"Augustus Sack!" he exclaimed, offering a pudgy hand. "Mr. Augustus P. Sack, and this can be no one save Miss Jane Stone. Might I be pardoned for expressing my *absolute* delight that you've rallied valiantly enough to join us for a late breakfast?"

Propping my crutch against the chair's arm, I clasped his clammy fingers. "Pleased to meet you, Mr. Sack." I sat, wincing.

"The captive emerges," Mr. Thornfield drawled. "What can she have been through, this poor prisoner, trapped behind enemy lines after such a daring escape?"

The tone may have been gently needling; but he was up in an instant to fetch me a tasselled footstool, which he deftly slid under the table, where I might take advantage of it.

"Oh, Miss Stone!" Sahjara commiserated. She was clad in sage green with her dark hair hanging loose. "When I imagine what could have happened to you—it's *too* dreadful."

"My dear Young Marvel," Mr. Thornfield put in, seating himself, "what *could* have happened was my trampled corpse, followed by a closed-coffin ceremony."

"Charles, don't!" Tossing her head, Sahjara added under her breath, "He thinks because he served in campaigns in the Punjab, he has the right to be dramatic."

"He does indeed, and correctly so!" Mr. Sack spoke in the style of a compliment; it was received in the manner of an insult, however, for Mr. Thornfield's eyes furiously darted to the pine trees just visible at the top of the windows, and there they remained.

"Well, I feel as terrible about what could have happened to Mr.

Thornfield as he does—anyhow, I'm fine, Sahjara." I lifted my napkin as Mrs. Jas Kaur appeared, placing fried breakfast cakes smelling of rose water upon my plate.

"Miss Stone is undoubtedly fine," Mr. Thornfield agreed, "or we should be informed otherwise in highly colourful language."

I promptly redirected attentions. "You arrived this morning, Mr. Sack?"

"You are as observant as you are beautiful, Miss Stone, I state so with absolute conviction."

Hardly a compliment.

Mr. Augustus Sack was a portly fellow—tan as Mr. Thornfield, but budding pink at the crests of his cheeks, the tips of his ears, and the end of his nose. He wore a dark green jacket with a brown velvet waistcoat, accented by an emerald tie, and if he wished to appear more thoroughly English, I honestly have no notion how he would have gone about working the miracle. His face was a plump oval, beaming relentlessly, and this disturbed me, for Mr. Thornfield looked enraged and Sahjara ill.

"Have you some business with Mr. Thornfield, or may I congratulate you upon a trip devoted to pleasure?"

He chuckled, an oily sound. "I fear it is a private matter. Old friends, you understand, and what with Mr. Thornfield having so recently taken possession of this magnificent estate—I absolutely had to see him, and dear Sahjara as well."

Mr. Thornfield's fingers tensed as if a poisonous insect had appeared, one in need of smashing.

"I thought it had been some nine months since," I observed.

"Correct, as you doubtless always are, Miss Stone. I encountered Thornfield here at my former assistant Mr. John Clements's funeral four days ago; I was *most* distressed that he had not sought me out sooner, as I've been back in London since August."

Mr. Thornfield threw down his napkin. "That's the worst thing about funerals—not only is someone you once liked dead, but there's an indecorous number of people you don't like swarming about."

Augustus Sack only smiled; if a grubworm had smiled, it would have looked similar.

"I should have offered you condolences, had I been aware," I ventured to Mr. Thornfield.

"Are you offering 'em now, or merely filling uncomfortable silences?"

It would have been easy to take offence at this, but the master of the house took no pleasure in the dig himself. His long white hair was neatly tied, his collar and jacket perfect, his slab jaw smooth—but he ought to have been regaling our houseguest over tales of my clumsiness, and instead he appeared almost frightened.

Augustus Sack began to nod as if a profound point had been made. "Miss Stone, Thornfield here values discretion to the point that he errs on the side of secrecy. Mr. John Clements was my assistant, as I mentioned already—he was most instrumental in helping Thornfield regain his health following the Battle of Sobraon. Four of us, in fact, were close as brothers during the first war, serving at the behest of the Director: Thornfield, myself, Clements, and a David Lavell, who was Sahjara's father."

When I turned to her in surprise, Sahjara's face was angled downward. "I don't remember him at all. It's *shameful*."

"That's the least shameful facet of your character, you magnificent nitwit." Mr. Thornfield rapped his knuckles twice against the table. "Sack, I must suggest that, having conveyed your best greetings, you now—"

"It pains me to think how few of us remain from the small set of British in Lahore before the regime fell." Mr. Sack affected an air of wisdom, but it looked merely as if he were about to sneeze. "Matters were so confused—who was friend, and who foe? Who amongst the Khalsa did not scheme, and who amongst the Company did not plot?"

The master of the house pushed back his chair. "We aren't discussing this here," he said, but it was his teeth speaking, pressed tight with rage.

"Of course, your . . . unusual closeness to Sikh affairs rendered your own judgement so much more *nuanced* than that of the other members of the British regime. I know the Director always thought so."

"Stop talking in riddles, it's nauseating. I don't have what you're after, so what more do you want from me, damn you?" Mr. Thornfield's fist clenched as it struck the table, but a distressed sound from Sahjara caused him to soften a second later.

"Want?" Mr. Sack swivelled his pink countenance, smirking. "Only to reminisce—poor John Clements's death, oh, you'll find it excessively sentimental, but I couldn't bear to think your own call to immortality might come, Thornfield, with so much left unsaid between us."

"Mr. Sack, your carriage has been brought round front."

Mr. Sardar Singh stood at the end of the dining table with his hands clasped behind him, wearing a sympathetic frown as if he were the bearer of unfortunate news. Sahjara shifted, eyes darting anxiously, whilst Mr. Thornfield's expressive face set in a look of quiet determination.

"Ah, there you are," Mr. Augustus Sack purred. "What's this talk of carriages? No indeed, I've a great deal to discuss with you both."

"Your coachman is under unequivocal instructions to take you wherever you should care to go."

"Of all the—*whose* unequivocal instructions, you scoundrel?" Mr. Sack snarled. "Confound it, you're the entire reason I—"

"Mine, sir."

The already stifling tension twined about our necks. Mr. Sack spluttered, then emitted a laugh which sounded like the yapping of a wild fox.

"Thornfield, any man who once juggled so many export concerns is doubtless most effective at household management, but is this really your idea of a proper butler? His joke is in decidedly poor taste."

"Do you know, Sardar hardly ever jokes," Mr. Thornfield replied, shaking his head sadly. "A deficit in foreign breeding, I've always assumed."

"I am remiss in the arena of humour more than any other." Sardar Singh placed one hand regretfully over his heart.

"That man could run an empire, but when it comes to puns? Satirical drolleries? He's positively dismal."

"After many fruitless attempts at improvement, I have abandoned hope."

"What the hell are you two playing at?" Mr. Sack snarled.

A natural unspoken understanding crackled among Mr. Thornfield and Mr. Singh and Sahjara, fast and ferocious as a thunderstorm, and I felt a surge of irrational jealousy.

"A brick," said Mr. Thornfield, the glimmer of a wicked smile now lurking behind his mouth, "could be on display in the warm glow of the stage footlights and garner more chuckles than Mr. Sardar Singh."

"You will *rue the day* you ever dreamt of mocking me," Mr. Sack growled, lurching up.

"No, no, that's the crux of the thing!" Mr. Thornfield cried. "When Mr. Singh says that your carriage is ready—"

"And that you are about to travel away in it," the butler added, idly examining his fingernails.

"Then it's absolutely inevitable."

It happened so quickly that I must have blinked and missed it—

one second, Mr. Augustus Sack's rosy cherub's cheeks were purpling, and the next, all the blood drained from his visage as he beheld the knife in Mr. Singh's hand.

"You pack of bloody infidels!" Mr. Sack cried. "Do you honestly think you can threaten a Company man?"

"Oh, 'pon my word, yes." Mr. Thornfield had risen now, and another knife glinted from his slack, practiced grip.

"Don't test them," Sahjara warned, arm extended, and I saw that what I had always imagined merely a silver hair ornament was also a blade.

"Sahjara!" I threw out a protective forearm.

"Miss Stone has a knife too, Sack," Mr. Thornfield drawled. "It's part of our dress uniform, don't y'know."

"You cannot seriously intend to defy me!" Mr. Sack backed towards the door, soft hands trembling. Strangely, he seemed to address Mr. Singh.

"It's as serious as a Turkish prison," Mr. Thornfield hissed.

"I'll have it out of you one way or another," Mr. Sack spat, jabbing a finger at Sahjara. "That nasty puppet—"

"Get out," Mr. Singh commanded, and now his voice was harder than the metal in his hand. "I'll not ask again."

Mr. Augustus Sack bared his teeth and turned on his heel. For several tightly stretched seconds we waited; then the grind of carriage wheels reached our ears, and I snatched up my crutch and limped to the window, staring with Sahjara under my arm as the neat black coach exited the grounds of Highgate House.

Faintly, I asked, "Do many of your guests depart at knifepoint?"

"Oh, I should not say *very* many." Mr. Singh sat, drawing a pot of porridge near and spooning himself a portion. "But when they do, inevitably I find my appetite improved."

We were all quiet, a quiet as odd and yet as comfortable as any I had ever experienced, before I succumbed to helpless laughter. Mr. Thornfield likewise chuckled, and pressed his glove to Sahjara's temple when she went to him, sliding the silver comb back into her hair.

When his eyes met mine, however, they were grave blue pools—I confess myself likewise sobered, and my ankle began to send invisible darts into my calf.

Mrs. Garima Kaur appeared, short of breath and eyes flashing. She fired off a rapid series of questions to Mr. Singh in their own language; his replies did not seem to please her, however, for she snarled and gestured at the outer door. Mr. Thornfield interjected in the same tongue, but she would have none of him, aiming another volley at Mr. Singh. When he had reassured her once more, she hissed in frustration and quit the dining room.

"Garima is understandably unsettled—Augustus Sack labours under the delusion we have something of value. A trunk of Sahjara's went missing long ago, and the deuced cur can't cease thinking on it," Mr. Thornfield said to me quietly, causing my ears to prick. "Our friend John Clements's death dredged all this up again—the ghastly affair is long past, but Sack is equal parts cunning and stupidity, a combination peculiar to a certain breed of East India Company executive, damn 'em. I apologise, Miss Stone. Had I not been cowering before the tip of your own blade last night, I should perhaps have worried over offending your notion of a civil breakfast."

"I can't even remember why I don't like him." Sahjara's eyes were wide and wet. "It was all so long ago and far away. I don't like him, though."

"There's the Young Marvel for you—sharp as a bayonet." Mr. Thornfield framed her cheeks with clothed palms.

"Was I awful, though—ought I to like him?"

"You don't like him, darling. You like him as much as you like black pudding. Are you all right?"

"Yes, I think so. Miss Stone's accident, Mr. Sack coming to

call—it's too many troubles at once," she lamented, drying her eyes with Mr. Thornfield's kerchief.

"So often the way," Mr. Singh said under his breath, "with troubles."

"Sardar?" Mr. Thornfield said softly.

"Mr. Thornfield."

"Might I speak a word in your ear—say, after supper, in the drawing room?"

"Nothing could please me more." Mr. Singh ducked his frothy beard to us, cleared his small bowl of porridge, placed the remaining soiled china on a tray, and disappeared.

For several seconds, I stood at a complete loss as to how a human being should behave under these specific circumstances; thankfully, Mr. Thornfield spoke.

"Sahjara, I require your absence. Flee, fly, flit. I need to speak with Miss Stone about a few cautions relevant to the new mare you're to begin riding on Monday." Mr. Thornfield smiled, and it struck me that when he was not bored over his own jokes, his smiles were as warm as a fireside.

"Truly? Oh, thank you, *thank* you! That is, if you think me capable."

"What is she playing at?" Mr. Thornfield pressed his fingertips to the bridge of his nose in mock chagrin. "Young Marvel, thank you for defending me against a *badmash*.* Now be gone, that I might inform Miss Stone of your new riding regimen."

Sahjara curtsied, so happy her head might have split from her grin, and quit the room.

I went to the window, attempting to calm myself; but hardly had I arrived before I saw the master hesitantly approaching, a stiff-backed reflection in the prophetic windowpane.

"Miss Stone, are you quite well?"

---

* Villain.

His awkwardness put me at once at my ease. "Very well, sir. How are you?"

"Oh, don't mimic my pretences to English manners, for God's sake, it's hardly sporting." Flashing a grim smile, he continued, "You've questions, no doubt; and I am willing to trade the commodity, for though I did seek an *unusual* governess—"

"You hadn't anticipated the scope of my abnormality." I sought the cool of the glass and leant my head against it, as much to mask my fright as in genuine fatigue.

You've scarce had time to dash off a letter to your mother's solicitor and you're already being tossed back into the gutter.

"And therefore I propose you dine with me this evening."

"Of course, I can hardly blame—" I broke off. "You propose what?"

"Dining. You've, ah, heard of the practice? It takes place in the evening hours more generally—at least, north of the Sutlej it does."

"Mr. Thornfield," I announced, "you owe me dinner at the very least over the vast number of weapons displayed just now."

"Of course." A peculiarly endearing crease appeared at the edge of his right eye, encroaching upon his temple. "I've had a blow, Miss Stone. Sack's appearance was entirely unexpected. I should never have wished you to see—"

"I accept your invitation with great enthusiasm, sir."

Mr. Thornfield crossed his arms as I limped towards the hall.

"There have already been multiple moments which cause me to suspect your true self a giant deliberately casting a small shadow," he reflected just as my crutch passed the threshold.

Pausing, I struggled to reply.

"Oh, never fear the ramblings of a former soldier, Miss Stone." He drew a hand over his neck exhaustedly. "We're cracked to a man. Go on, I've business to attend to."

So I shuffled, step-thunk, step-thunk, out of the room and away, reflecting upon the three most immediate tasks before me:

—comfort Sahjara and learn what you can of what threatens this household

—navigate dinner with Mr. Thornfield

—learn to walk silently upon a sprained ankle and thereby perhaps learn a very great deal indeed afterwards

I lay atop my quilt for twenty minutes, taking tiny sips of laudanum, fretting that not only did I understand nothing of the workings of Highgate House but also that I possessed no precedents to guide me.

Are small girls always as formidable as Sahjara? I wondered.

Perhaps they were not; but I had been. The fact that we shared a particular home at a particular age was accidental; how then did I find it so binding, as if she were my responsibility not due to the lie which had brought me here but the truth I was discovering—that I liked these people and wished for them to like me in return?

When is a butler not really a butler?

Gingerly, I flexed my foot. My experience apart from London and Lowan Bridge School, each savage places, was limited to Mamma's midnight picnics beneath the rustling leaves. At the thought of a butler ejecting a guest, however, and all the happy times Sardar Singh had sat with Sahjara and me whilst Mr. Thornfield was gone—something irregular was afoot. And what was Mr. Singh, if he was not the butler?

What has Mr. Augustus Sack to do with a trunk missing from the Punjab?

This seemed a rather more dangerous question, but one which required answering—and to that end, I sat upon the edge of my bed and shifted my weight until I stood fully.

"Bugger," I gasped.

Hobbling as far as my mirror was excruciating; leaning against the edge of the dressing table, I examined myself. At twenty-four, I had not gone far towards matching my mother's undomesticated beauty, and thus I did not often seek my own reflection. My dark hair still undulated irregularly no matter how much care I took in pinning it up, my eyes were as large as a feline's but still the same plain brown, and my face still invited comparisons to the enchanted creatures which left England long ago.

I pinched the colour back into my cheeks, as I had no wish to alarm Sahjara further . . . not when I was so badly in need of answers and she the best purveyor of that precious, perilous commodity. The past, no one knows better than myself, is a silent stalker, and I headed for the schoolroom with the express intention of seeing her pursuer more plain.

EIGHTEEN

"I see, at intervals, the glance of a curious sort of bird through the close-set bars of the cage: a vivid, restless, resolute captive is there; were it but free, it would soar cloud-high."

"Oh, that was so dreadful—and I didn't understand what Charles meant by joking that you had a knife, but I hope you aren't vexed." Sahjara had put on a brave face, but I insisted that we were too rattled for lessons; so we sat in the bow window, pillows stuffed behind our backs, our feet tangled together like schoolmates, gazing at the grounds.

I pulled the small folding blade from my pocket and tossed it once, quickly returning the weapon to its hiding place. "It wasn't a joke—London is dangerous. As for Mr. Sack, he was most insolent to your guardian."

Sahjara rolled her head against the wall tiredly. "He is not Sikh like Mr. Singh and Mr. Thornfield and myself, only an East India Company man."

"I meant to ask whether knives were de rigueur for your people," I teased.

"Oh goodness, yes! The pure ones wear five articles of faith."

"Your comb is a religious symbol? And the metal bracelets as well?"

"Yes, these are the *kanga* and the *kara*—the comb and the wristband. We're also meant to wear a short sword called a *kirpan*, but here in England we find knives more convenient because even though the wars are over, we must remain invisible. And Charles says that if we have to hide in plain sight, then we must make allowances over what will make us look noteworthy to Britons, and fix the symbols to suit us here in England. At first Sardar was a bit uncomfortable over changing tradition, but later he agreed since the *kachera*—those are our knee breeches—would make us look absolutely ridiculous here, Charles says, and God is in the Guru after all, not in outward forms."

We must remain invisible, I thought, wondering at her words. *We have to hide in plain sight.*

"You said five?" I asked aloud.

"Oh yes, long hair—*kesh*."

"It looks more natural on you and Mr. Singh than it does on Mr. Thornfield."

Sahjara regarded me with the eyes of a kitten tracking a string. "I've never seen him without it, so I couldn't say. But I do think Charles handsome—don't you?"

"He's everything a gentleman ought to be, I'm sure." Unsettled, I cast my eyes out at the lingering snowfall, the spun-sugar dust coating the bare limbs of the trees. "Are his gloves also religious, then?"

My charge frowned. "I don't think so."

"Perhaps they could hide burns or marks?"

"Heavens, that would be awful." She shrugged. "I almost forget they're there. They must look awfully peculiar to an Englishwoman."

Englishwoman, I thought warmly; now I knew more of their history, the appellation was magnificently sensible, as they all originated in the Punjab and regarded me as the foreigner.

"Mr. Singh and Mr. Thornfield seem like fast friends."

"Yes, they grew up together!" Sahjara smiled, tapping the edge of her boot against my skirts. "Charles was born in Lahore, you know, and Sardar—well, that isn't his name, but anyhow—Sardar's family traded in indigo and jaggery. They were frightfully rich before the wars."

"Sardar isn't his name?" I repeated, mystified.

"Oh, no." Sahjara hopped out of the window, idly twirling her skirts. "All that rubbish Charles was talking about Sardar being incapable of jokes couldn't be further from the truth. Mr. Thornfield said that for us to live without much remark here in England, he would have to be the butler, and he changed his name not ten seconds later to mean 'high commander.' May I just run downstairs and see whether Dalbir's hoof is any better? Mr. Sack's visit left me so flustered that I might almost have forgot."

This soup is delicious."

I sat across from Mr. Thornfield in the dining room. After admonishing myself not to gape, I reminded myself *you've never been here before*, and then gaped as I pleased. Every placid English landscape in which the dogs had contemplated the sheep and the sheep contemplated the dogs was replaced with decorative mirrors. There were as many gilt-edged and silver-embossed mirrors as there were days upon a calendar, multiplying us ad infinitum until there were a thousand Jane Steeles and a thousand Charles Thornfields.

"Is it?" he answered.

Mr. Thornfield's voice, I noted, sounded much the richer for what it did not say. It occurred to me that I wanted to know what his favourite summer had been like, whether it happened in England or the Punjab, hot desert sandscapes versus gleaming green afternoons, and then it occurred to me this topic was egregiously far afield from my true mission.

I waited for him to speak; no overtures were forthcoming.

"I think the weather will hold now the snow has stopped—don't you?"

Mr. Thornfield chuckled. He wore a swallowtail coat and a thick rust-coloured cravat—which I thought hardly fair, since my best governess disguise was a drab thing of dove-grey satin striped with a cream pattern and topped with a high lace collar, and it is beastly to be seated across from a bluntly handsome fellow when one looks about as captivating as gravel. Had we been in London, and I my nefarious self, I would have found a secondhand dress of rose silk and filled my hair with tiny yellow tea roses.

"Though of course, your estate is charming covered in white—it looks like a fairyland."

When again Mr. Thornfield said nothing, I smiled, my heart shivering in my chest; was he wary, even angry? He returned the amiable look, however, and I reached for a second helping of the blistered bread Mr. Singh had left.

"I imagined that you would be more talkative since you seemed eager to speak with me, sir."

"Good Lord, no—that would be dreadful strategy." Mr. Thornfield poured me more claret. "I've a knack for silence. I'll remain quite closemouthed and simply await developments."

"May I ask why?"

"Well, I've two topics on my mind—but if you truly would rather pretend all governesses carry knives, then I admit England would be the livelier for it. And if you won't mention the fact that priggish Company executives aren't often driven out of breakfast rooms with the same weapon, then I choose the topic of soup over snow."

I wished that I could have been Jane Steele and laughed, and flirted; since I was Jane Stone, however, I chose my words with care. "I cannot explain the latter, but I will certainly explain why I carry a knife."

Charles Thornfield's sun-burnished face gave me the sly look of encouragement I have seen many rogues attempt, all having failed miserably by comparison.

I sat forward. "Mr. Thornfield, I am here under false pretences."

The master of the house angled his bullish chin at me and took a generous sip of wine.

Lies, honest reader, are organic—they can shift from outright falsehoods into half-truths and even truths, generally when you like the person to whom you are lying, in the way wormlike creatures become butterflies out of sudden inspiration. I was inspired on that evening by knives and tiny paintings and the fond glances Sahjara and Mr. Thornfield and Mr. Singh all cast at one another.

"To boot, I am probably not fit to be a governess."

Mr. Thornfield snorted sceptically.

"My initial letter to you was correct in every salient particular, of course—I attended a school called Lowan Bridge." My heart beat a hornet's-wing tattoo. "But I did not mention that, when I was young, I was accosted in an ungentlemanly manner by my cousin. I think his presumptuousness and later our headmaster's cruelty may have endowed me with a certain fear of men. I go armed due to these experiences. I have been called many things, Mr. Thornfield—pigheaded, wayward, brazen—and yet, no one feels the grievousness of my shortcomings more keenly than I." Unexpectedly raw-voiced, I stopped.

It was hardly a thorough confession; it was a gift, however, a small piece of my saga. If gaining his regard meant I turned over my entire history, I could never oblige the gentleman—but I could proffer a biography with neither shadows nor colours, a vague outline of the person I wanted him to know but did not dare to reveal. Should I expose all, he would surely hate me, and then where would I find myself?

If Mr. Thornfield was mortified, I never saw it; instead, he shifted with a thoughtful finger edging his temple.

"You'll want to know about the swearing as well?" I asked timidly.

Mr. Thornfield laughed—the laugh of a soldier who has brushed the sands of the Sutlej from his trousers, told jokes which should have made any woman blush. "Of course I want to know about the swearing—it was damned expertly done."

My pulse tingled in the tips of my fingers. "When I left school, I went to London because I'd no family who would take me. Have you any experience with distant relations yourself, Mr. Thornfield?" I added slyly, gesturing at our surroundings.

"This place was empty when we took possession, and we should not be here had it been otherwise, Miss Stone." He shrugged, watching his wine swirl gently. "At the risk of sounding a deuced ingrate, it was a stroke of luck not to have made their acquaintance, if y' follow."

"Of course," I hastened to assure him, fearful of pressing. "I quite understand and meant only that penury requires one to live among coarse people, which is the other reason I carry a knife, and the reason I have an atrocious vocabulary—if you worry that I might endanger your ward, Mr. Thornfield, having already endangered your person, I cannot blame you; but I can admit I am not a typical governess and hope that my present candour brings you some mollification."

I awaited judgement as if being sentenced to Newgate.

Mr. Thornfield let his spoon clatter to the dish with a ring of finality. "If you think I'm intimidated by your weaponry, you've clearly not visited the billiards room. And there are practically stars in the Young Marvel's eyes when she speaks of you, so . . . consider me mollified. You must feel odd being the only knife-brandishing governess outside of London?"

I tipped my glass to him, endlessly thankful he could not see my knees knocking.

"Yes, sir. You must feel odd being the master of a Sikh stronghold in the English countryside."

"Pish—when I feel odd, it's certainly not on that account, as I'm hardly the master of anything. You've ridden Nalin, you know of which I speak. I could threaten to have the whole pack of these lunatics, horse and human alike, sold for glue, and they'd all laugh in my face."

"And how," I ventured, my nerves calming fractionally, "did that strange circumstance come to pass?"

His severely arcing brows tensed below the pristine hair. "Frankly, I find myself a terrible topic for conversation."

"I feel the same about myself, but I'm deeply interested in your household. How did you come to be acquainted with Mr. Singh, for instance?"

The tension in his shoulders melted. "We were practically schoolfellows, before. Shall I be shocking, Miss Stone?"

"Oh, yes, please."

"Where on earth did she come by the cheek? London alone couldn't have managed the feat," Mr. Thornfield muttered. "You are aware from the advertisement I was involved in the Khalsa conflicts. You may know that I was born in Lahore?"

Silence befitted Mr. Thornfield; so I tried it out myself, blankly encouraging.

"Well, how I came to be born there prior to British annexation is brief in telling and rather broad in ripple effect generally, so I'll out with it: my parents were complete scoundrels, Miss Stone."

"Mr. Singh said your father was an entrepreneur?"

"So are pirates, according to the dictionary."

I laughed until I could hardly breathe. Mr. Thornfield rumbled with amusement himself until I had calmed.

"Nathan Thornfield—that's my father, mind you keep up—

started life as a merchant in the loosest sense of the word," Mr. Thornfield continued. "Genteel as a baronet, all polished monocles and pinches of snuff. But really, he was what romantics call an adventurer and cynics a rapscallion. Travelled like the pox—Australia, China, even America, the daft old crust. The codger ought to have been locked in a cage lined with pillows, if you take my meaning, but instead he made and lost several fortunes before settling in the Punjab with my mother, née Chastity Goodwill, and if that name don't beat the Dutch, Miss Stone, the Dutch will rule the globe."

Patience Goodwill and Chastity Goodwill. My pulse thumped against my drab grey dress as I recalled my aunt's maiden name. *Sisters—there is the connection.*

"Mum wasn't *quite* mad, by the by," he added wryly. "She must sound so, gallivanting about like that with a complete knave. But the yellow fever had got hold of her altogether, and she was a passionate collector—Chinese vases, Bengali silks. When my father decided that Lahore was absolutely the ticket, I believe he bartered their way into the Punjab with French wine and Turkish opium; the Sikhs were sceptical, and he conducted one or two discussions on the wrong side of a *tulwar.** Once he was in, they realised he'd a positive genius for getting them anything they wanted, and the Sikhs ain't Quakers, mind. A hotter hive of lechery and treachery you've not seen since the Vatican."

"It sounds dangerous."

"So does war." This time his words boxed my ears gently. "But people do it anyhow."

"Were Mr. Singh's family your neighbours, sir?"

"Indeed so. My family was in the import-export line, and Sardar's were trading indigo and suchlike."

"I think he said jaggery?" I lied, for Sahjara had told me.

---

* Sikh sword.

"Yes! Great brown cakes of sugar and great blue cakes of indigo, and they were so rich they could have used solid gold piss pots if they'd— Oh, I beg your pardon."

"You really needn't, you understand."

Mr. Thornfield coughed, amused. "I am beginning to. Well. We grew up playing at cavalry in the streets of Lahore, daring each other to run beneath the legs of the war elephants when the Khalsa paraded, quarrelling like fishwives over which had to be the villainous Afghan and which the conquering maharajah, manly pursuits of that sort. Sardar would—"

"I've been given to understand that is not his actual name?"

"Oh, a snake in the grass! You've clearly been pumping the Young Marvel for gossip."

I might have quailed, but Mr. Thornfield's tone remained a happy one, a low instrument playing in a major key, as was ever the case when he spoke of his ward.

"She gushes with the substance when the poor girl remembers anything of those days; but in this case, she is entirely correct. Mad as a crate of ferrets, Sardar, and if he was going into domestic work, by gad, he meant to do it in style. What could I do but shrug my shoulders and call the man Commander?"

"Mr. Singh possesses a magnetic presence. He seems a very decent sort."

"He's a saint is what he is, and we were very close as boys, and after I returned to the Punjab, we didn't fancy the notion of parting. Have you ever had a friend, Miss Stone, and thought that if this particular person were absent, you should forever miss a piece of yourself?"

I remembered my quiet, quizzical Clarke and nodded.

"Well, Sardar may not have always called himself Sardar, but he has always been extraordinarily good to me. He took great pains to see the stuffing wasn't thrashed out of me when I was a stripling in

Lahore—and he has made certain that Sahjara was safe, always, no matter the circumstance."

"Was it during the wars that Mr. Singh took risks for Sahjara?" I asked with care.

"Yes. We were not at war, however, when he took risks for me." Mr. Thornfield smirked, tapping the tablecloth with gloved hands. "I'm not certain whether fighting or fornicating is the skill Sikhs have mastered the better, but they work terribly hard at both, y'see, and thus as a young *wilayati*,* I had plentiful scuffles to survive."

"Do not Easterners wish to befriend the British in the interests of trade?"

Mr. Thornfield twisted his lips. "Nothing like a friend for a knife in the back."

"Is that true of Mr. Augustus Sack?"

Mr. Thornfield hesitated; but at last he bit the inside of his cheek, shrugging.

"Fair play, Miss Stone—it's only proper etiquette to explain sudden confrontations with knives, as you have so kindly done for me. Mr. Sack and our dead friend Mr. Clements and Sahjara's father, Mr. Lavell, were all Company men when the conflict with the Sikhs broke out. So was I, nominally anyhow. To say the Sikh empire was rich is to say the sun does a jolly decent job at lighting the planet. Mr. Sack figures that some ripe booty which scarpered off God knows where can be found if only he plunders the Young Marvel's head, and I won't have it. Neither will Sardar, as you saw. And that's all I have to say on the blasted subject. Oh, look, here's Mrs. Kaur with the roast."

The cover was lifted, the air flooded with cinnamon-spiced mutton, and not another word would Mr. Thornfield speak regarding adventures abroad. Instead he spoke of the new mare, and warned

---

* Foreigner.

me lest Sahjara knock her head off, and pretended that he had just told me everything I desired to know.

Through it all the gloves remained; and I watched him, riveted.

My instant fascination with Charles Thornfield puzzled no one so profoundly as myself. I had taken enough lovers to know that he was not conventionally handsome, his visage too worn with crags of care to compare with my strapping young working lads. Come to that, he was acerbic and peculiar in equal measure, and he could raise an eyebrow as if raising a middle finger.

I had already borne firsthand witness to his capacity to love, however, thanks to his ease with his ward and the heightened circumstance of Mr. Sack's visit, and as a needy, greedy thing, I was curious as to how one would go about stealing a fraction of it.

"Good night, Miss Stone, and do take care with your ankles," was his send-off when we had finished. I think courtesy—even his rough version of it—had exhausted him. "Should you ever desire a bigger knife than that hatpin you're carrying, seek out the billiard room."

Smiling, I returned his farewell and made a great racket with my crutch as I went upstairs.

For Mr. Thornfield intended to meet with Mr. Singh after supper; and I knew every inch of Highgate House, the creak of each stair and the groan of each floorboard. If I was going to solve the twin mysteries of the forbidden cellar and the missing trunk, I was going to have to add eavesdropping to my vices.

NINETEEN

"A deal of people, Miss, are for trusting all to Providence; but I say Providence will not dispense with the means, though He often blesses them when they are used discreetly."

My boundless affection for the protagonist of *Jane Eyre* has already been established; and yet, I cannot resist stating that she made the most dismal investigator in the history of literature.

Consider: she discovers Edward Fairfax Rochester practically in flames. Upon the morrow, whom does she meet but Grace Poole, the assumed culprit; and when Jane suspects the vile Grace of sounding her out over bolting her door? Jane, wise woman that she is, proceeds to deliver all her intentions regarding door-bolting to the dour nurse, in detail, upon a silver platter.

Apparently there is nothing like telling murderous fire-starters exactly what they want to know about locked doors when they ask you—it confuses them, most likely.

After dinner, I made such a purposeful din going up the stairs that Mrs. Garima Kaur's face appeared at the bottom, eyes sharply inquisitive within the enormous bowls of their sockets.

"No, no, I'm all right," I called down, panting. "Nearly there, anyhow!"

"Nothing bad?" she insisted.

"Nothing bad whatsoever. Mrs. Kaur, are you concerned over something in particular?"

"Do not worry," she said, though the quizzical look had not left her eyes.

"Good night, Mrs. Kaur."

"Good night, Miss Stone."

She stood there with face uplifted, watching me until I had turned my back.

When I made it to my room, I locked the door and cast the crutch aside; I was nearly certain my plan would work, but only so long as I could execute it. After a few hobbling circuits, wincing dreadfully, I confirmed that I could walk, provided nearly all my weight was upon my left leg.

Breathless, I sat down and stared at my mantel clock.

Though not well versed in Mr. Thornfield's habits, I did know Mr. Singh's, and we had concluded our dinner during the time the butler checked the doors and windows; I had only to wait for him to finish sealing the house like a crypt, and then rush to the drawing room without my crutch, hoping I had not missed anything.

Schooling myself, I chose a time: eleven twenty-four in the evening. Milksops mewl that sin corrupts the willpower, but I have that in spades—so I sat until the minute exact and set off.

The corridor presented little difficulty, but the fourth step upon the first flight always bellowed as if someone were tormenting a calf: I avoided it. My ankle burnt, but not unbearably so, for I held both hands to the rail and proceeded with a sideways step-hop, step-hop motion. I remembered just in time that the banister squeaked above the second landing: I put my hand against the wall and gingerly set my sprained ankle upon the final step.

Pain lanced through it, and I pressed my free hand over my mouth. I managed, however, jaw screwed tight, and resumed my ludicrous progression to the ground floor.

Once in the hall, I paused, and yes—a muted glow from the drawing room combined with the muted thrum of male voices told me to hurry, or all would be for nothing. The lights were out, a single pretty bell-shaped lamp of fractured rose glass remaining; by daylight, it was one of my favourite sources of illumination, for it made the drear midwinter light blush charmingly. Now, in the surrounding darkness, all seemed feverish and bruised.

"—thrash the dog from here back to Calcutta, and then good riddance, says I," growled Mr. Thornfield.

My entire frame snapped to alertness.

This was not Mr. Thornfield's usual baritone—it was a voice meant to carry across dunes and canyons, bereft of pretension, barely even English though he possessed no foreign accent. This was who Charles Thornfield actually *was*, or at least had been, when living under vast Eastern skies.

"For heaven's sake, Charles." Mr. Singh sighed. "You always say that first, and it has never been helpful. Not a single time."

I limped close enough to the slightly open door to hear them clearly.

"I haven't another solution," Mr. Thornfield insisted. "Sardar, I need hardly tell you the man is a menace in the extremest degree—and who knows what *burchas** he has in his employ."

"Which is why I cannot comprehend why you indulged in his request to see Sahjara."

The voice was so stern that my scalp prickled.

"I was wrong to try it," Mr. Thornfield answered instantly. "Pray don't be angry, I've already taken myself to task. But what if meeting Sack again had . . . jostled something loose in what seems to be a fixed state?" A wistful pitch of yearning had crept into Mr. Thornfield's voice and I pictured him as I knew he must look, muscled

* Ruffians.

shoulders taut and dark brows threatening his stately nose. "What if seeing him had made a difference?"

"Charles, Sahjara is not an experiment!" Mr. Singh hissed. Then he sighed once more, and I heard liquor being poured, and I craned my neck further. "That was uncalled-for and yet I delivered it, rather an unforgivable sin in a *khansamah,** wouldn't you say? Accept my apologies. Tell me your object in letting Sahjara within five miles of Sack, then."

"We will never be safe until a permanent solution is found!" Mr. Thornfield rasped. "When he arrived, shocked as I was, I imagined that if she saw his face again, his own plan might snake round and bite him in the arse. That she might—"

"Ah," Mr. Singh said sadly. "You thought Sahjara might recall everything, maybe even the trunk. Which would allow us to—"

"Grant the vermin king Sack's wishes like simpering djinn—"

"And send him on his way, and then we could live as we please."

"Not that the exquisite scoundrel wouldn't have been practically invited to rob us blind in that case, which would chafe me terribly."

"Yes, Charles, we kept horses and hounds once, but *now* . . ." Mr. Singh trailed off, exasperated.

"It's not about the money!" A pause occurred, and Mr. Thornfield's voice was calmer thereafter. "No, no, this blasted huge draughty *English* house is . . ." I bristled. "This house is wild and weird and cold, bloody cold and wonderful. Sahjara loves it, and I am finding it ever more charming that my bollocks clack against my teeth when I piss."

"Are you? My bollocks have not yet quite got accustomed to making the leap past my kidneys."

"But now Highgate House is ours, you understand that Sack will never stop," Mr. Thornfield ended in a much lower tone. "I told

* Butler.

him I inherited it, but he must not have believed me. He must have thought we still have the trunk, that I bought the estate. What else could explain it?"

"I don't know," Mr. Singh confessed. "The fact of his being here was, I agree, the greatest mystery of all."

Briefly, I heard only the crackling of the fire; when Mr. Thornfield spoke next, it was almost too deep and too soft to catch.

"Sardar, if I have arrived at the point where I think experimenting with Sahjara's brains is reasonable, then perhaps it's best if—"

"No," Mr. Singh said calmly.

"No?" Mr. Thornfield's voice grew ever more serrated. "You don't even—"

"No, you are not embarking upon a crazed quest to murder Augustus Sack, who has assured us that the entire scandal will come out via any one of a dozen solicitors if we so much as touch him. Neither are you murdering a dozen solicitors."

"So the scandal comes out? Who is affected?" Mr. Thornfield had risen, for I could hear his boots striking the carpet. "This is a Company affair. Sack dies mysteriously, my shame is aired for all to see, I throw myself upon the mercy of the Director and face some sort of court-martial and five or ten years in gaol, and—"

"And you still miss Sahjara's entire childhood, emerging broken by hard labour with a ruined constitution."

"Is that worse than perennial torment?"

"Yes."

"Why?"

"Because you wouldn't be here, and she needs you." Mr. Singh sounded three shades beyond exhausted. "I need you, for God's sake."

Mr. Thornfield sat, breathing hard.

"Mark me," Mr. Singh said carefully. "That you want to go to gaol for a crime we both committed long ago, simply to save the rest of us, is both typically thickheaded and typically noble. However, you are not thinking this through. Who was your accomplice when you committed the deed?"

"You were," Mr. Thornfield said testily.

"Now. Supposing the Company doesn't actually want to tar and feather you? The white prodigy raised in Lahore who journeyed back on their commission and was rushed through Addiscombe to do so, they were so eager?"

"Well—"

"Why, yes, Charles, I believe the Director would find a scapegoat if he didn't want to sully the papers with ill repute of the Company."

Mr. Thornfield thought this over, shifting in his seat.

"I wonder who might suit."

After a longer pause, Mr. Thornfield admitted, "You *are* rather brown."

"How brown am I, Charles? Take a good long look now."

"Darkish, though a sight short of black."

I did not know what they had done, of course; but my heart gave a rabbity leap at the thought of Sahjara without either of them. As self-sufficient a child as she was, she fed off love as if she were a walking siphon, and both Mr. Thornfield and Mr. Singh quietly, almost without gesture and never with words, delivered the substance to her in staggering quantities.

"All right, throwing myself upon my sword is out," Mr. Thornfield said pettishly. "Your advice is loathsome, Sardar, and it disendears me to you."

"So often the way with advice," Mr. Singh muttered.

"Well, I think it's deuced unfair, really." Mr. Thornfield lightened the tone. "Sack seeing me at the funeral by accident when I'd no idea he was in England at all seems like cheating."

"It is regrettable, though it does not entirely explain his swaggering into our home with such complete confidence. Thankfully we have both been upon our guard—"

"Of course we've been on our guard! But the die is cast. And a sight too soon after arriving here, if you ask me."

"Undoubtedly." I heard the sound of a vesta being struck. "I meant to take up cricket."

Mr. Thornfield snorted, then guffawed, and then the pair of them wheezed together as I leant against the wall, smiling.

"Oh, I don't know what to do." Mr. Thornfield sighed as the laughter faded.

"Fight back," Mr. Singh said. A chair creaked. "The same as we always do."

"And to think that if the good Sam Quillfeather hadn't posted me, we should never have known John Clements had died at all. It's a hard push whether to be grateful or vengeful."

My back was already against the wall, thankfully, or I should have fallen as the fear seized me—Sam Quillfeather, the policeman who questioned me after Edwin's death? Sam Quillfeather, the inspector who had drawn unspoken conclusions over Vesalius Munt's?

"It's a lucky chance," Mr. Singh agreed. "Enough to make me wish to meet him one of these days. Considering your new arrangement, doubtless I'll make his acquaintance quite soon."

My vision swam; I was in a crazily tilting corridor lit the colour of blood.

"You'll like him—he takes more care with his profession than any man I've ever seen. Makes a point of keeping his investigations utterly quiet unless he has the evidence necessary to prove a party's guilt, not like these boorish peelers who bully their way to solutions, pissing on every water pump they see. Certainly of all the lads going in for medicine at Charing Cross, I liked him best, for he'd no business being there and I felt as if neither did I. I was still sweating curry, and here's this mad *chowkdar** twenty years my senior taking desultory anatomy lessons. The mind reels, Sardar, that such wonders exist."

"I'd be less shocked at a courteous tax collector."

"Imagine if he had taken the tiger by the tail and joined the Royal College instead of merely brushing up on his tibia versus fibula."

"Incredible. A constable who also just happens to be a doctor of medicine."

"Because he thinks it will make him a better police officer."

They were both laughing helplessly again, and a good thing too, for I was struggling noisily for breath. The notion that the Sam Quillfeather I had known would take an anatomy course upon a whim was directly in character—the man was the definition of inquisitive, which is why I felt sick at the mere mention of his name.

"Is it certain, then, Charles?" Mr. Singh's voice had grown grave. "Are you positively certain John Clements was murdered, without question?"

My eyes, which had been shut in terror, flew open again.

"Certain as daybreak." It was a complex tone, layers of sadness and regret. "Poor old Johnny, with that puppyish way he had about him. Remember when he used to sniff around your secretary as if she were Cleopatra?"

"The poor woman must have put him off a thousand times—I asked her if she wanted my help over it, but she said there was no more harm in him than a mule. I've never met a more credulous person."

"True enough. Johnny had sand where his brains ought to have been, but he certainly didn't deserve to be served cyanide with his tea, or however Sack managed it."

---

* Constable.

"You seem very sure of yourself."

"Consider!" Mr. Thornfield admonished. "Clements and Sack return from the Punjab together to rub elbows with the Company nabobs and kiss their grannies and such before being reassigned. Quillfeather gets called in as a special consultant after Clements expires mysteriously in his rooms, as Quillfeather is madder than a flock of loons but can both solve a murder and keep quiet, and the Director wants to know why they lost Clements. Sardar, you recall the poor blighter—he was tanned same as us, but he weren't never *ruddy*, and his corpse was flushed something awful, not to mention the fact he was in the prime of life and a heart episode seems very unlikely. Cyanide is the military poison of choice, and who save Sack would be coward enough to stir prussic acid in his brandy rather than killing him like a man would do?"

"Yes, but where's the motive? You said Quillfeather called you in initially because of some papers he discovered Clements was working on?"

"Aye, Johnny was looking up David Lavell's record, and naturally there were our names in stark print—reports from his superiors, correspondence, journals. What cause could Johnny possibly have to investigate a scoundrel dead since the first war unless he suspected something amiss?"

"He wanted to know why we did it, perhaps." Sardar said softly. "He knew we were guilty—he wanted to know why."

"And Sack found out he was digging."

"It doesn't quite wash, Charles. Even supposing he discovered Lavell was a blackguard, what difference should that have made?"

"Puts a whole different colour on the affair, don't y' see? It's one thing to harass a pair of footpads, quite another to persecute old friends—Johnny Clements was an intellectual ant, but he was damned decent to the end. The more he knew of Lavell's character, the less easy it would have been for Sack to keep him leashed."

They fell silent. I was breathing easier by this time, yet still hardly myself; I had wanted information, but this variety led only to more questions, and the notion that Mr. Thornfield had an arrangement with Inspector Quillfeather was nothing short of horrifying.

"How was dinner?" Mr. Singh inquired.

My feet sidled closer to the door.

"Very passable. Jas Kaur always did have a way with sheep."

"Charles," Mr. Singh chided.

"Oh, you mean how was the *governess*?" He was smiling, I could hear as much. "She gave me a straightforward explanation without much prompting. Hard living and harder men made her cautious, and the same circumstances led to the saltiest tongue I've ever heard in an English head."

I should not have taken pride in this; and yet, I could not help myself.

"She's a remarkable woman," Mr. Singh replied. "I did my best to take the measure of her whilst you were away, and I confess I did not get far. Miss Stone seems a clear enough pool on the surface, but glimpsing the bottom is another matter."

"I can't put my finger on it either," Mr. Thornfield said quietly. "You ought to have seen her when she was thrown from Nalin. Popped up again like a jack-in-the-box, not even knowing how badly she was hurt. If she weren't so thoroughly British—that pale elven look about her, those lustrous eyes—I'd have thought her raised north of the Sutlej. She doesn't just carry a knife, she knows how to hold it. If I'd meant her any disrespect, I'm fairly sure she'd have made mincemeat of my bollocks."

"She interests you," Mr. Singh mused, and there was a twist to his tone which made me long to have seen his face as he spoke.

"Of course she does, she would interest anyone," Mr. Thornfield retorted. "Not to mention the fact I've had nothing to occupy me all this while, save your company and that of a child whose every third word is *horse*."

"You'll feel better when the dead start speaking to you again."

I had been listening with such rapt interest to the topic of myself that this shocking pronouncement startled me terribly; and further, I realised that the men had risen from their chairs and would find me with my ear to the door in a matter of moments.

"All locked up, then?"

"Snug as a noose," Mr. Singh answered, and I heard the rattling of an iron in the grate.

Whirling towards the staircase, I made as much soundless haste as possible. My ankle felt as if a spike had impaled it, but I forced myself to limp faster.

"I can't bear the feeling there is nothing to be done," came Mr. Thornfield's voice, and now they were at the threshold of the drawing room door.

"We shall consider further. Be at peace in the meanwhile."

"At peace with both eyes open."

"Quite so."

They're coming, I thought in a blind panic, and I had only made it halfway up the first set of stairs, and my ankle was ready to give way under me; getting up a staircase, it seemed, was another matter altogether than getting down. They would see me, they would know. I faced either being caught like a rat fleeing a refuse heap, or . . .

That is a terrible idea, I informed myself.

"Sahjara starts on the new mare tomorrow. She's named it Harbax."

"God's gift," said Mr. Singh as they neared the start of the staircase. "Excellent choice."

"Clever little creature," Mr. Thornfield agreed fondly. "Though *Charles's gift* might have been more appropriate."

"Even you, my friend, are moved by the will of God."

There was nothing for it; I made an about-face, went as limp as I could, and fell down half a flight of stairs.

"What in the name of the devil!" Mr. Thornfield cried.

An inarticulate groan emerged when I had got my breath back from the wind being knocked out of my lungs. My left side was bruised, my limbs twisted, and my brain rattled into oblivion; beyond this I could not tell where I was hurt, though hurt I knew I must be. Mr. Singh was speaking urgently now, and so was Mr. Thornfield, and there were warm, careful hands on my shoulders. Then one of them shifted and a soft, thin glove with a heartbeat inside it cupped my cheek and drew it away from the carpet.

"Miss Stone! Dear God, Sardar, what has she— Confound it, Miss Stone, look at me."

"She's breathing steadily," Mr. Singh's tense voice added.

"Miss Stone, can you hear me?"

I could; I could feel him as well, feel the pressure of his fingers beneath the glove, and thought for a lunatic instant that apart from having just thrown myself down a staircase, I felt surprisingly happy. I opened my eyes.

"Christ, there you are." Mr. Thornfield blew out the breath he had been holding. "'Pon my soul, you gave us a fright. Can you move at all? It would greatly endear you to me."

Shifting, I found that I could, but stifled a cry when I discovered that my knee had been badly wrenched, and this time on my previously uninjured left side.

"Easy, easy now, that's it," he admonished, sliding a hand under my back.

"Oh God, I feel such a fool," I gasped as Mr. Thornfield helped me to sit. "I left my book in the morning room, and I make such a horrid clamour with that crutch—I thought I could manage without."

"You feel a fool because you *are* a fool," Mr. Thornfield growled. "What in hell did you think you were about? You could have woken the whole bloody house with reveille on the trumpet for all we—"

"Mr. Thornfield," put in Mr. Singh, his butler persona back in place, "might I suggest you help Miss Stone back to her bedroom and that you cease swearing at her? Miss Stone, what were you reading?"

"*La Rabouilleuse*," I lied.

"I shall fetch it up to you with a bit of brandy." Mr. Singh smoothly disappeared.

Mr. Thornfield was still on bended knee, glowering at me as if I had fallen down the stairs on purpose and little knowing I had done exactly that. When I raised my brows, he opened his mouth, shut it again, and composed his features by scrubbing his hand over them.

"May I?" he asked.

"I don't think I can walk," I admitted. "I'm sorry, sir. This grows tedious."

"You find falling from potentially fatal heights tedious?" he returned, but now the tone was less strident, and if I painted it with my own imaginings, it might almost have been called tender.

So Mr. Thornfield effortlessly carried me up the stairs, and when my arms were about his neck, I smelled not only the cigar he had smoked with Mr. Singh but also a faint, clean sandalwood aroma which must have been the man himself, and made me think of steep hills overlooking dry plains, and the sweetness which must surely linger in the air after the monsoons have passed beyond the Sutlej.

TWENTY

I felt at times, as if he were my relation, rather than my master: yet he was imperious sometimes still; but I did not mind that; I saw it was his way. So happy, so gratified did I become with this new interest added to life, that I ceased to pine after kindred: my thin crescent-destiny seemed to enlarge; the blanks of existence were filled up; my bodily health improved; I gathered flesh and strength.

A month passed, reader, before my investigations progressed, partly because for the next fortnight I could not walk.

If you have never lain in bed in your dressing gown, your ankle and knee shrieking as you try to confine yourself to a reasonable amount of laudanum, teaching a bright, babbling girl sitting at the end of your bed by day and fretting by night why the master of the house's spirits will be improved when the dead start to speak, then I am glad for you. I was full of restless energy which could be discharged nowhere, as if I were a kettle coming to boil lacking lid or spout, and if I had exploded, I should not have been the least surprised.

For a week I suffered, uninterrupted by any save Sahjara, a maid bearing meals which included an improbable dish of plum pudding on the day I reasoned must have been Christmas, and Mrs. Garima Kaur, who delivered poultices I suspected came from Mr. Thornfield. These smelt of sage and vinegar and worked wonders for swelling. If I had been an object of wonderment to the housekeeper previously, now I was a nuisance, for she coolly assisted me with an air suggesting my falling down stairs was in poor taste. The fact that the master of the house had not visited chafed terribly, but I supposed it would hardly be proper for him to pass the hours in my bedroom, and he seemed to harbour a horror of making un-English blunders in my presence.

Meanwhile, I wanted him to make certain blunders very much indeed.

By day I taught Sahjara, who brought me unceasing small presents ranging from orange flower cakes to bouquets of jolly red berries; by night, I imagined my employer making the sort of inappropriate advances which would have made most governesses flee the estate forthwith, and in graphic detail, complete with bare thighs and calloused fingers and the diagonal notches which rest so sweetly above the hipbones when a gentleman is in training, as I had no doubt whatsoever Mr. Thornfield was.

Then one morning when I was fidgeting in my sheets, silver sunlight knifing through my curtains, I heard pounding steps hurtling down the corridor which could only have meant Sahjara. A knock preceded her entrance, but she did not wait for me to say "Come in," and the words thus overlapped with her banging open the door.

"Miss Stone!" she cried, her dark eyes alight. "There's a chair!"

I struggled to ascertain the import of this phrase.

"Charles has just brought it back in the carriage. A chair with wheels! He went to the village to get it, I think, and you're to make yourself ready and then you can come down!"

I swiftly dressed in plain governess black with my hair pinned as tidily as my hair ever allows; no sooner had my small charge carefully tied my boots than Charles Thornfield appeared within the open door. Seeing him again after nearly a week without was a disproportionately stirring event, for I should not have cared so much over beholding a man with whom I had passed less than twenty-four hours' time. He crossed his arms and leant against the frame, a sardonic quirk to his lips.

"Hullo, Young Marvel. Behold the Female Prodigy," he announced. "She can tutor the pure ones, wield knives, and fall from dangerous altitudes with equal grace."

I opened my mouth, glanced at Sahjara, and rolled my eyes instead.

"By Jove, is she trying not to swear at me in front of the child?"

He was correct, so I laughed. "Did you really find me a wheelchair, sir?"

Mr. Thornfield straightened, advancing. I have written that he was a man of medium height, not so tall as Sardar Singh, yet it seemed there was not sufficient space for him in this wide room, so great was his effect on me.

"It took rather more reconnaissance than I'd have liked, but the village physician had one in his attic, positively wreathed with cobwebs. One could scare tell it was a chair at all. Mrs. Garima Kaur has dusted it, naturally."

"I'm so glad you'll be downstairs with the rest of us!" Sahjara exclaimed, throwing her arms round my shoulders.

Blushing is not a habit of mine, but I am unused to raw sentiment being lobbed in my direction. As Mr. Thornfield took in this awkward scene, his ward clinging to me and then unselfconsciously racing away to do whatever Sahjara Kaur does when she isn't on horseback, he looked uncertain whether to be delighted or dismayed, drawing a hand over the back of his neck in what I was learning to be a habitual gesture.

"She's spontaneous," I offered. "It means nothing, I'm well aware."

"It doesn't mean anything like nothing, not to anyone who knows her." Mr. Thornfield shook off whatever uneasy thought plagued him. "I could carry the chair upstairs, but then there remain stairs when we reverse course—should we carry Mahomet to the mountain instead?"

"Whensoever you like," said I.

Again I was lifted—respectfully, more's the pity—by my employer. The journey, reader, was too brief for my liking; but once I had arrived at the ground floor and saw the charming vehicle, all wicker and softly curving wood painted a demure black, with carefully placed cushions, I positively glowed as I was set into it.

"I can't tell you how grateful I am for this." I looked up at Mr. Thornfield, who surveyed the results of his labours with satisfaction.

"Yes, well, do let me know if I should retain possession of it, supposing you decide to fly out the attic window."

"No, I mean . . . thank you. Hardly anyone has ever bothered to take care of me."

I paused to reflect, scarce registering that I had just confided an intimate fact to a near stranger. A list emerged:

—Agatha

—Clarke, when I was not taking care of Clarke

It may seem strange that I did not include my mother; but my mother was a butterfly's wing, too fluttering and fragile to take care of anyone, and though we loved each other . . . she had left me, had she not?

Mr. Thornfield's rough features smoothed into disbelief. "Whatever circumstance you're speaking of, there ought to have been fifty lined up for the job."

I sliced a look at him, unsure if he actually believed such nonsense; but he strode behind me, gripping the handles of the chair. Admittedly I might have wheeled the thing myself, but since Mr.

Thornfield pushing me meant Mr. Thornfield a foot distant, I should have been a dunce to defend my independence.

"Where to, Miss Stone? I admit I had not thought so far, only feared that you were like to suffocate if you stayed in the same room any longer."

"May we go to the morning room?"

"Think of this not as your chair but as your chariot, Miss Stone," he proclaimed sarcastically, and I could not help but wonder whether Mr. Thornfield, on occasion, hid truth in falsehoods just as I did.

The master of the house and I forged a pattern when I was not at lessons with Sahjara; in the mornings and evenings, he would carry me downstairs so I could dine with what I was coming to understand was the family—the aforementioned individuals plus Mr. Sardar Singh—and after Sahjara had been led off to bed by Mrs. Garima Kaur, and Mr. Singh had adopted an introspective look and excused himself, the pair of us stayed up later and later and progressively later. I loved these strange sessions, for Mr. Thornfield, despite his prickliness, seemed to love them too, though it was a hard push not to blurt out *What crime did you and Mr. Singh commit in the Punjab?* or *Why should the dead speak to you?*

One night five days into my convalescence, Mr. Thornfield wheeled me into the drawing room after supper, I having confessed that good Scotch and I were not strangers, and when we were both equipped with this lovely commodity, I ventured to ask him a question. We should have been the picture of English domesticity, the firelight in Mr. Thornfield's pale hair and I nestled into my cushions, if only I held a needle in my hand and not a glass of whiskey.

"Is Mr. Singh really the butler?"

Mr. Thornfield's chin shot up. "By the Lord, is she actually interrogating me now?"

"He doesn't sit with the servants at meals," I insisted. "He doesn't count the silver or manage your wine collection or berate the rest of the staff. I should venture to say that his only jobs are answering the door and locking the windows of a night, and those because he likes the control."

Mr. Thornfield frowned. "Are you an inspector, Miss Stone? I shall have to look out over pinching extra kippers at breakfast and telling Sahjara lies about not being able to afford two mares for her instead of one."

"That was a very neat way of not answering my question."

"Oh, what's the use—you've found us out." Mr. Thornfield smiled, and this was an effortless one. "You know that Sardar and I were practically brothers growing up. The rest of the household, other than Sahjara of course, were his own servants in Lahore—we brought them with us, as he'd no wish to sack 'em all and they'd no wish to see the back of him. The man inspires affections left, right, and sideways—it's a foul thing to watch."

"So Mr. Singh is not a butler?" I pressed.

"Of course he is, supposing you want to keep meddling English busybodies out of our hair. But, no, you're quite right—when Sardar vanishes, he is either studying the Guru, taking long constitutionals, or fiddling with Jas Kaur over replicating Punjabi dishes in the kitchen."

I chuckled over my glass. "So though this is your estate, an argument can be made he is the master, since the servants are *his* domestics and not yours."

"We couldn't very well have made off with my parents' household, could we, would've strained relations something frightful. You're near to correct, but one of them—Mrs. Garima Kaur—was Sardar's confidential secretary back in Lahore."

This surprised me. "I thought she knew very little English?"

"Spoken like a true colonialist—didn't matter a fig back then, there were only a pocketful of us. She probably figured it beneath her, never did warm to whites much, come to think of it. She speaks Punjabi, Hindi, Arabic, Farsi, Turkish, and Pashto something spectacular, and that's all Sardar required."

"And now she's a housekeeper."

"Well, what with Sardar a butler and all, she can't be too miffed."

Smiling, I leant my head against the cushion of my chair. "Tell me more."

"More of what, you impudent elf?"

"Anything. Everything. Your parents survived the wars, I take it, since they still needed a staff? And why did you leave them in the first place—why study medicine?"

"Miss Stone," he drawled, "if I did not know better, I would think I intrigued you."

"You do intrigue me."

I said this without a trace of guile. A British chap might have been chagrined over such an open display, but Mr. Thornfield only settled farther back into his armchair.

"Do you know, Miss Stone, that you are exceptional?"

"I have been told so, but never in complimentary light."

Mr. Thornfield's jaw twitched. "That was undeserved on your part, and therefore I will answer you. My parents are still in Lahore, and survived both wars without so much as a scratch. I should be proud of them if it were the done thing to be proud of privateers bleeding Company executives dry; I ought to be delighted, in fact, as it all comes to me in the end and now they have ten times the population of expatriates to drain to the dregs. Pardon, you might mistake me; I cherish my parents, but they are not suitable subjects for small talk."

"Neither are we."

This time he laughed freely. "Quite right, Miss Stone—if misfits cannot converse amongst themselves, then who can? Very well, my parents are brazen criminals and I elected to study medicine because I have always been fascinated by the impermanence of the human body. Does that answer your question?"

I shook my head, waiting for him to continue.

"Becoming a charlatan and a cheat never appealed to me," Mr. Thornfield admitted. "My parents are crafty rather than malicious, but damned if I share their tastes—medicine meant studying mortality, in a sense. The Sikh holy book contains plentiful passages about flesh, and since my parents were about as interested in religion as they were in sobriety, I learnt from Sardar and his family. 'We are vessels of flesh. . . . The soul taketh its abode in flesh. . . . Women, men, kings, and emperors spring from flesh.' Sikhs are very—how shall I put it delicately?—straightforward about flesh. It was a comfort to me that they thought souls separate from lungs and livers, this sack of bones and blood we daily maintain, and I thought there was romance in medicine's efforts to stave off the inevitable. This was when I was young and thick as a marble bust, you understand," he added with a dour expression.

"I adore the macabre," I confessed. "I used to supplement my governess's income by selling last confessions in tea shops and the like."

"Good Lord! Miss Stone, I find it difficult to picture you peddling gallows doggerel."

"No more should you, sir, for it was prose, and I always chose the most poignant subjects, as if by placing hard words upon a page, like so many stones, my own heart would not be so heavy."

Mr. Thornfield ran a finger over his chin. "If your writing was half as good as what you just said, Miss Stone, then I should very much like to read it."

"Oh, they're long gone," I demurred, though my eyes must have shone at the praise. "They harmed no one and interested me—what sort of occupation could be better?"

"Well, there you have it. Medicine was honest work, and I had always wanted to see the place where my parents met, so I fled the Punjab at precisely the wrong time, in order to pursue a career which I've never practised outside of a war."

"Surely you saved lives when you returned?"

He made no reply, his face so fixed that I imagined that I had turned him to stone.

"A few, perhaps," he said at length.

I knew better than to press this point. "What did you think of London?"

Relieved I had shifted topics, Mr. Thornfield answered readily. "It's filthy, and wet, and hides a brutal soul behind majestic walls. Its people are alternately snobbish or base, and if I didn't come from a culture of warriors, I'd say it was the most savage city I'd ever seen. I thought it glorious, of course, from the instant it sullied my boots."

"I loved it as well."

"Yes, and if there are bits of yourself which you should prefer to toss in the gutter . . ."

"You can shed your skin."

"And no one the wiser."

"Still. It was by far the most crowded place I've ever been lonesome," I added, staring into my glass.

"That ought not to have been the case, Miss Stone," he said quietly. "I know very little about you, but I know you would be absolute rubbish at solitude. Your relish for companionship is clear as print."

Tripping steps sounded, and Sahjara entered the room with her face alight, wearing a dressing gown over her nightdress. Rushing to Mr. Thornfield, she tugged at his sleeve. "Charles, I've had the most *wonderful* idea, and Sardar says he'll only do it if you promise to join him, and of course I will as well though I'm not so good as either of you, but I'll make up for it on horseback I'd wager, and Miss Stone will be so pleased after having been cooped up indoors for so long."

"What is she jabbering about?" Mr. Thornfield asked irritably, swallowing a measure of Scotch. "She speaks English, I know she speaks English, she learnt the tongue in the Punjab from my parents and perfected its nuances here when she was five."

"Charles, don't be dreadful, we're going to put on a demonstration!"

"A demonstration of *what*, you ill-mannered imp?"

"Of everything!" She turned to me, her smooth cheeks flushed with enthusiasm. "Riding, in my case, and perhaps archery. The *chakkar*, the *tulwar*, the *aara*—"

"Has she lost her mind?" Mr. Thornfield exclaimed. "You want to stage a mock fight Khalsa-style in the middle of the British countryside?"

"Yes!" She clapped her hands together decisively. "Yes, the way Sardar says you used to practise outside Lahore's gates, only we'll do it on the grounds, and Miss Stone will *love* it."

"Miss Stone will be entirely put off by our foreign antics and will quit the house in high dudgeon."

I burst out laughing at the transparent falsity of this excuse.

"Have I not given you steeds?" Mr. Thornfield demanded, rubbing his temple. "Have I not given you fine frocks and an English mansion? Have I not given you a governess—"

"Please, Charles." Her smile meant she expected to get her way. "Sardar said yes."

"Sardar spoils you so obscenely it's all I can do not to throw myself in the nearest river."

"Please?" I interjected, grinning. "It would be so educational."

Mr. Thornfield's glower was fast losing strength; finally he gave a martyred sigh, finished his whiskey with a snap of the wrist, and said, "I'm no match for the pair of you martinets."

"Hurrah!" Sahjara exulted, taking his gloved hand and delivering a peck to it. "Tomorrow?"

"Oh, certainly, supposing you prefer me headless. I've not practised with the *aara* in years."

She swung the hand she still held. "Next week."

"You'll be the death of me yet. Fine."

"It really is a marvellous idea," I said, smiling at her.

"It's a ridiculous idea." Pushing himself to his feet, Mr. Thornfield brushed a wisp of hair off Sahjara's brow. "Go back to bed, darling, and thence to sleep, so that you'll be unable to hatch any fresh schemes to gall me."

"Insufferable gaffer," she said affectionately.

"Impertinent brat."

Sahjara disappeared with a toss of her head. Mr. Thornfield returned our empty glasses to the sideboard, looking contemplative. I had begun to better cherish his silences, for he possessed many shades of stillness and sharing them with me meant he was at ease in my presence; this was a blue quiet, as deep as his eyes.

"I wish that whatever you are thinking, you did not have to dwell upon it," I told him.

"You've a generous nature, Jane." He stopped, turning back to me. "Apologies, I don't know how that slipped, only I've come to think of you . . . Blame it on my upbringing, if you please."

A sting pierced my chest; hearing my actual name was meaningful, as if he had taken my mask off and glimpsed my real face.

"You may call me Jane if you like."

He cocked a brow. "You don't find it overfamiliar?"

"Not from you."

Had he been anyone else, I should have dreaded making so bold a declaration; as it was, my heart thrummed major chords within my ribs as I watched him blink.

"Thank you—as you might gather from the Young Marvel's example, you may call me anything you damn well please." The empty expression he affected did not hide the fact his mouth was pinched at the corners. "Jane, I've apparently a deal of unnecessary physical training to undergo tomorrow—shall we retire?"

Breathlessly, I agreed; but he only carried me up to my room and bid me the usual polite *Good night, then, Jane,* and I pretended the strange sweetness upon my tongue when I bid him the same was due to expensive whiskey. I then assured myself that my symptoms merited a diagnosis of simple lust, and I fell asleep repeating that Charles Thornfield had stolen nothing more serious than my attention.

The air crackled and clawed the afternoon of Sahjara's demonstration; it had snowed again, and an inch of powder lay glimmering upon the grounds, awaiting the performers as the pale January sunlight bent down to kiss the top of the trees. I sat in my wheeled chair wearing my cloak as well as two blankets, hot-water bottles at my lap and feet, upon the terrace at the side of the house; surrounded by Singhs and Kaurs, who spoke excitedly to one another in Punjabi and stamped their feet against the cold, I awaited the performers.

I will not attempt to describe the dexterity with which Sahjara on Harbax navigated the jumps the grooms had built and strewn about the lawn. She was dazzling, and Mr. Thornfield's face as he watched her mirrored Sardar Singh's in a potent combination of glad mouths and strangely anguished eyes. Neither can I conjure the impassioned cries of "*Khalsa-ji!*" from the Sikh household as Mr. Singh, left arm loaded with serrated metal circles and right forefinger spinning a disc in the air, threw ten *chakkar*s in rapid succession, cutting ten distant poles into splintered halves. His servants screamed their approval, and I thought I glimpsed a tear in Mrs. Garima Kaur's eye, reflecting sunlight just as her scar did.

Should I not at least essay to capture the spectacle of Mr. Thornfield wielding the *aara* outside my childhood home as the sun sank, however, I should consider this entire memoir a failure. He joined Mr. Singh on the lawn with a set of double-tongued metal whips about five feet in length, both wearing very loose cotton trousers fastened at the calf and nothing more, bare shoulders gleaming like cliffsides, and at a nod from his friend, they began what can only be called a dance.

They did not merely flick the deadly tongues at targets, for there were no targets; they leapt from foot to foot, sweeping the flexible steel over and under and above themselves, vicious blades passing within inches of their heads and arms. The snow exploded as they struck it, plumes flying with the sharp snaps of a thousand firecrackers, and the servants and Sahjara screamed encouragement in their native tongue. Faster and faster they whirled, sometimes falling bodily back to catch themselves, sometimes balancing on a palm after throwing themselves forward headlong, and all the while the *aara*s sang and snapped.

Mr. Sardar Singh was the superior; his lightness of foot and the detached technicality with which he performed a madcap dance was unsurpassable.

I could see, however, why he wrongly claimed Charles Thornfield was his better when it came to the *aara*, because he was riveting; he silently snarled as he flayed the ice and mud, surged from foot to foot as if a demon possessed him, and following this onslaught of fury, could flick the tip of the blade to send a scant few snowflakes delicately soaring.

I can assure the reader that I did not do anything so asinine as to fall in love with Mr. Thornfield by watching him demonstrate the *aara*; I had already fallen in love with him, and on that day, a feverish sheen upon my brow despite the winter's chill, I elected to admit it, if only to myself. For the thought of confessing as much could only mean confessing far more about myself, if I truly cared for him, and I could not bear the idea that he should ally himself with evil unawares.

TWENTY-ONE

It had formerly been my endeavour to study all sides of his character: to take the bad with the good; and from the just weighing of both, to form an equitable judgment. Now I saw no bad. The sarcasm that had repelled, the harshness that had startled me once, were only like keen condiments in a choice dish: their presence was pungent, but their absence would be felt as comparatively insipid.

Perhaps the most touching passages in *Jane Eyre* are those after she discovers she loves Mr. Rochester and before she discovers he loves her in return. There is little unwieldy pretension and still less saccharine sentiment; she simply loves him, as I loved Mr. Thornfield, and is woeful because one cannot uproot love any easier than one can force it to flourish.

I wrestled with the identical problem, although my tactics during this period would have positively curled Miss Eyre's hair.

A week later I was out of the wheelchair with my ankle tightly wrapped, my knee quite healed, limping gamely, and Mr. Thornfield must have supposed himself haunted by a familiar when my mobility was restored. I took his elbow when he asked me if I cared for a walk; I drew my fingertip down the silver cuff he wore; I shone in every way I knew how, and lastly, I told him the truth.

Truth in my case must needs have been partial, but I thrilled at each new self-exposure.

"Sahjara lived with my father's sister in Cornwall when she emigrated, until Sardar and I arrived early this year," he answered my question after a curried fish supper.

"I hated my aunt." My nerves whistled in high alarm, but I soldiered on. "She called me cruel names and snubbed my mother perennially."

Mr. Thornfield scowled around his cigar. "If she had such poor taste as that, failing to hate her should have been shirking, Jane."

Further examples abound; for instance, Mr. Thornfield and I often granted Sahjara's wish that we might all go riding together, precious windswept occasions on which water sprang to my eyes at the keen wind and the joy of galloping over hillsides; and on the first of these rides, I made the acquaintance of Mr. Thornfield's horse—a great rusty-black stallion.

"I just adore him, I can't help it," Sahjara crooned, pressing the flat of her hand up the beast's nose.

"I assume he is called Falstaff because he is so funny and charming?" I asked, smiling.

Mr. Thornfield coughed dryly, his breath clouding in the cold. "He is called Falstaff because given the choice, he would eat oats and sugar until his belly exploded and he was strewn all over Christendom."

I laughed, as did Sahjara, and Mr. Thornfield shot me another of his queer appraising glances, the ones which sent liquid warmth pooling through my torso.

"There were times when the comfort of communing with horses was all I had," I admitted.

"I think the same was true of me, before. I can't remember. Oh, Charles, say you'll give Nalin to Miss Stone—she's better on her than anyone!" Sahjara entreated.

Mr. Thornfield tugged at her cloak's collar until it lay flat. "Young Marvel, ordinarily I should have to box your ears for squandering my assets and forgetting Miss Stone is not in a position to keep her own horses." He glanced at me. "But supposing that I can retain the honour of feeding and sheltering duties, Jane should consider Nalin entirely her own."

Can I be blamed for strewing my secrets like seeds when they blossomed into such kindly responses? A fortnight had been expended on the practise before I began to run dry of tasteful confessions, and then, reader, I invented them like the lying devil I am.

"I should like to read the Guru Granth Sahib," I declared. "It would explain so much about your character." Mr. Thornfield sat writing a letter in his study as I watched him, pretending to be reading Balzac.

"There is neither an adequate explanation for my character, nor a copy of the Guru in the English language." He dipped his pen without raising his head. "Apply to Sardar, he can recite damned impressive heaps of the stuff."

"I shall. I can't give any credence to the Bible because so many villains quote it."

This was not true; I simply wished for something freshly shocking to tell him. Though the Bible dictated my mother and I would be listening to each other's skin crackling for eternity, and my former headmaster had been cruelty incarnate even as he called upon God's Name, I thought many of its teachings beautiful.

Mr. Thornfield's eyes narrowed in amusement. "Never read the thing, though Sardar has lobbed plentiful passages at me—my parents are more for cheap novels when they can get 'em. Whale blubber and seal pelts and nor'easters. Damsels, you understand." He coughed charmingly. "Heaving bosoms."

"There are plentiful bloody bits, and even some sensuous parts, I suppose," I said idly, passing fingers along my hairline. "Song of Solomon is about a pair of lovers. 'Let him kiss me with the kisses of his mouth!' It's quite salacious material."

"I've heard better. Now kindly shut your head whilst I finish congratulating my father on his latest swindle."

Helpless to stop myself, I tried again the next day, discovering him reorganising books in the library and (predictably enough) offering my assistance.

"Are there any Punjabi books in the house?" I wondered, sorting through several volumes of Medieval spiritual poetry I suspected belonged to Mr. Singh and not Mr. Thornfield.

"Oh, certainly." He craned his thick neck upwards, wearing a frown as he lifted a stack of unbound folios. "But they kept turning up missing, don't y'know, great gaping holes in the collection, and when Sardar found 'em circulating at a jaunty clip in the servants' wing, we installed proper shelves where they were wanted."

"That was good of you."

"Of course it wasn't. I can march over there whenever rereading *Chandi di Var** tickles me, can't I? I have legs, and so does Sardar."

Finished, I began sorting through the Renaissance plays. "Your servants are very interesting. They must know you both well, I take it, since they worked for Mr. Singh before? Mrs. Garima Kaur, for example, seems most devoted to him, even for a confidential secretary."

Mr. Thornfield glanced up from where he was kneeling, eyes lit with the wistful shade of earnest. "You know how she came by that extra bit of facial ornament, then?"

"The scar? How should I?"

"She saved his life once."

"No!" I exclaimed, kneeling to mirror him. "Oh, do tell me how."

"Nasty business," he owned, frowning. "Sardar was twenty-

---

* A poem written by Guru Gobind Singh in the classic Punjabi heroic ballad style.

three, I believe. He was overseeing the delivery of—what was it, indigo or ivory? damned if I can recall, ivory it must have been—across town by the Bright Gate, and he was set upon by thieves. Not your friendly book-borrowing type either, the picking-their-teeth-with-*tulwar*s kind, and Garima was accompanying him to keep records. Sardar is a tiger, but it was five on one, and incapacitating suits his delicate sensibilities better than slaughter. Anyhow, Garima threw herself into the fray and did him a few good turns with the knife she carried before taking that slash over the brow. She'd be dead but for his skill, and he'd be dead but for her help."

He fell silent, sifting through titles.

"I would fight like that, if I cared enough for the person," I confessed with endless devotion in my eyes.

Mr. Thornfield quirked a smile, granting me the merest glance. "*You* would have eaten their hearts in the marketplace afterwards. Just fetch me the magnifying glass on the desk there? Damned if I can make out this inscription."

So it went; day after day he gave me smiles rather than scowls, and at times I tilted my head up at the perfect evening angle when he passed my chair to refill our glasses of Scotch, and still my lips went unkissed and my questions unanswered. Despite these obstacles, I was achingly fulfilled over the simple act of wanting—having passed so much time seeking necessities, a combatant in an arena where to lose is to die, possessing the leisure to lie awake yearning after caresses I did not merit felt like an extravagance in and of itself.

That is, until work upon the cellar was completed a fortnight after Sahjara's weapons demonstration.

The pinging of distant hammers and circular progression of workmen hauling rubble out the back exit had been a torment, and I do not mean in the sense of peace disrupted; I yearned to know what was below; and when one day I came downstairs for breakfast to discover profound silence save the ticking of the standing clock, I quickly inferred that the men had, at last, finished.

"Congratulations." I took the tea Mr. Singh offered me, containing a splash of milk and one lump of sugar, exactly as I liked it.

"Might I ask upon what account, Miss Stone?"

"The completed renovations downstairs."

Mr. Thornfield stirred his coffee, transfixed by the newspaper; Mr. Singh nodded graciously, whilst an uncaring Sahjara yawned over her bowl of spiced porridge.

"The immediate dangers of an unsafe substructure have been seen to, yes," Mr. Singh reported, "but it remains best to consider the place entirely unsafe, ladies. That is, supposing you value your lungs, for the place is yet a haven for mould and damp."

Sahjara's nose wrinkled; Mr. Thornfield made a remark about the weather.

Unsafe, my shapely white arse, I thought.

That night, I heard a tread in the corridor outside my bedroom which was neither Mr. Singh's stately glide nor Sahjara's heedless prance. It was Mr. Thornfield's vigorous stride, at four o'clock in the morning.

A frontal attack seemed best, as the cellar was now kept locked during the day—and should I catch Mr. Thornfield at whatever nocturnal activity he had been indulging in, I could claim to have been frightened of intruders sent by the odious Mr. Sack. At any rate, I did not fear my nominal master's wrath, for he now showed me every courtesy, including the caustic teasing I had come to relish. Two days I waited; then a long crate was delivered to Highgate House and quickly spirited away.

Tonight, I determined, and after pleading the excuse of a headache, I lay awake and fully dressed with my ears tinnily ringing, so hard did I listen for the faintest whisper of sound. Midnight chimed, then one o'clock; at last, a bit before two, I heard a man's steady footfalls. As I had done when eavesdropping upon his conversation with Mr. Singh, I waited a few minutes until I knew Mr. Thornfield was fully engaged and then slipped from my bedchamber with a fitfully flickering candle.

When I reached the door to the cellar stairs, again I heard the suggestion of movement below; this was all to the good, however, and—finding it unlatched—I opened it.

Where once only rubble and the columns of the house's foundations stood, here a polished wooden staircase plunged below the earth. Though I glimpsed wall sconces, they were unlit, and the breath seized in my chest at the thought of my taper going out, for the terrain was now an uncharted one.

Step by step I advanced, careful of the faint echoes of my healed injuries, eyes watering as I peered into the gloom. The noises grew louder—what was he doing, this unexpected love of mine, that he waited for the dead of night and hid below the earth's surface?

I reached the bottom and stopped, suddenly fearful; a queer, sweet reek like badly mouldering apples coated my throat. Shaking minutely, I turned the door handle.

Several horrible things happened at once.

There had been a lamp lit, for its amber ribbon had lined the threshold, but upon my opening the portal, the room was subsumed in darkness. This would not have been frightening had I not been pretending false confidence when I threw the door wide, which snuffed out my own flame . . . but not before I had glimpsed an unholy tableau. A muffled male curse pierced the black curtain at the same time I emitted a strangled squeak—nothing so dignified as a scream—and dropped my candle entirely.

All was sable midnight surrounding me, and I shared the room with Mr. Thornfield and a naked corpse.

I clutched the doorframe to orient myself. More curses followed, then slow, confident steps, until an arm wound about my waist and an urgent hand caught my shoulder.

"Jane, please—are you hurt, or only frightened? Jane . . . I turned down the lamp to prevent your seeing anything you wish not to, but you're quite safe."

When I opened my eyes—for in my insensible startlement I had witlessly shut them—I discerned that I could see after all, as the lamp still held a spark of life, though its ghostly sphere now illuminated only Charles Thornfield's face, the familiar worried line between his brows, and the edge of a great table like a butcher's where a carcass lay supine.

"I'm all right," I managed. "The light gave me a turn when it went out, and . . . the . . ."

The truth was, reader, that—though I had created four corpses—I had never lingered over my accomplishments; this specimen was well past its prime, and the candied egg smell was overwhelming enough to choke me.

"Confound it, Jane, you've no business here!" Mr. Thornfield snapped. "I gave explicit orders—"

"I heard noises. Pray don't be angry, I was thinking of thieves, I—"

"And when you supposed ruthless *badmash*es had invaded, rather than wake the menfolk—who are, I will take the liberty of reminding you, deucedly clever when it comes to sharp objects—you marched down here to challenge 'em to a duel with a bloody pocketknife?"

My mind was a storm cloud, all static and hurtling thoughts. "I was half sleepwalking. I'm sorry." I steadied myself and gripped Mr. Thornfield's forearm, looking down.

This was when I noticed: Charles Thornfield was not wearing his frock coat, and neither was he wearing gloves. My lips parted as

I studied his fingers spanning my waist; he retreated now I seemed in no danger of falling, but not before I could see that his hands were positively shocking.

There was not a mark on them. Unscarred wrists, one adorned with a silver cuff, led to subtly veined skin, splitting into slender phalanges with well-shaped knuckles. It felt obscene that I could not drag my gaze from them—as if I had happened upon him naked in a woodland pool and refused to turn my back as he fetched his small-clothes.

"What is it, Jane?"

"Your hands, sir. They're not scarred."

"I never said they were."

I wrenched my eyes up. "You must think me a hateful busybody."

"You haven't the vaguest idea what I think of you."

"Forgive me." My enterprise now seemed detestable. "I'll not broach the subject again, I don't care what you're—"

"Yes, you do!" he exclaimed, shoving a hand over his high brow. "Damn it, I— If we are apologising, then I apologise for accidentally besetting you with waking nightmares. Now, do you wish to see something of my work, or shall I escort you upstairs?"

"Oh, please, if you will have me, I should prefer to . . . to stay."

Mr. Thornfield studied me as the devout study God; then he softened the hard spread of his shoulders.

"I have told you that I've not practised medicine save in two wars?"

Nodding, I straightened my spine.

"I have told you that I've a friend called Sam Quillfeather who is a police inspector?"

Again I inclined my head; Mr. Thornfield stepped back as if testing how much of the view I could manage.

"Behold the Highgate House Mortuary." His voice rang clear as a brook, but I could not discern any pleasure in the telling. "There isn't a single decent deadhouse between here and London, and Inspector Quillfeather is a monomaniac when it comes to collecting evidence. I had him round for dinner not two weeks after arriving here and told him I should require an occupation or else succumb to despair. This morgue, with me as its coroner, was his notion, and the men have been hard at work for three months."

He asked more gently, "If I turn the lamp up, will you swoon?"

"Bugger swooning," I replied, meaning it.

Mr. Thornfield smiled and reached for the tab; the brightening lamp revealed an incongruously lovely sight. The floors had been finished with wood stained quite dark, the walls plastered where before there was only stone. The air made my arms tingle, cool as a cave, and the rough-edged pillars remained; but lining the walls were cabinets and tables, and a set of medical tools was arranged upon a counter. I spied a chemistry apparatus, a formidable hacksaw, and what I would later come to understand was termed a rib spreader.

I forced myself to view the corpse, taking a few steps closer. The stranger was of medium build, with a weak chin and ruddy side-whiskers, aged over forty years, and he lay upon a huge slab of wood with grooves carved along the edges.

"I ought to have had a look at this fellow some two days hence, but was delayed by the family's protests. Chap dropped dead in his barley field, and Quillfeather understands that the bucolic countryside ain't precisely free of murder," Mr. Thornfield observed, watching me carefully. "He and I studied together, so he knew that I always had an uncanny knack for autopsies. It was as if they told me the stories of their final moments—I never once got it wrong."

You'll feel better when the dead start speaking to you again, I recalled Mr. Singh telling him, and could not suppress a shiver.

"Aye, it takes one like that at first." Mr. Thornfield's gloves rested next to a delicate chisel, and he pocketed them as if the sight were too private for sceptical eyes.

"You said that you only used your training when you were at war. Why not start a practice rather than aiding an enthusiastic policeman?"

"Because I touch only the dead, never the living."

Having experienced a fair number of shocks in my time, I gave no outward indication when he said this.

The silence, however, grew around us like a cancer.

"No, not always, not before, I'm not . . . it's a sacrifice," he told me. "For my sins."

"For a period of time, sir?"

"For the rest of my days."

I do not know how it feels when the trap drops and the noose crushes the windpipe—but though I stood perfectly still, staring at the pained crease thickening above his nose, I imagined the sensation was similar.

"I'll take you on a brief tour, as the facility is modern as possible."

Mr. Thornfield wanted me to attend, and I wanted to settle his spirits; so I listened dumbly to short lectures. Absently he said, *this is a microscope*; absently he said, *this is a bone saw.* The morgue was constructed with an attentive eye for detail—there were grooves in all the tables, drainage, plentiful basins, no white tile even a hairsbreadth out of place. When he was quite through, Mr. Thornfield turned, and the face which ought to have been emblazoned with pride looked near as pale as the body he was about to dissect.

"You are mute, Jane. When we walk out of this place, will we two still be friends?" he asked.

Words formed on my tongue and dissolved like dreams; but I already knew what I wanted to say. Striding towards him, I gripped the bend in his forearms where only shirtsleeves separated us, and his hands lifted to mimic mine as if they were not his own.

"You are either asking me that because you mistakenly think having a morgue under the house would upset me, which it doesn't, or because you know I seek an explanation for your present distress in your past trials. Mr. Thornfield, I . . . I should prefer to risk all than to inflict further torments on myself. May I ask you three questions?"

"You may ask them, but whether I will answer is another matter."

Shaking my head, I pressed warm skin beneath cool cloth. "Have you ever loved?"

"Yes." The reply was immediate, just as I thought it would be.

"Are you now claimed by anyone who made her pledge in exchange for yours?"

"God, no."

"Do you find me objectionable, sir?"

My feelings were at such a high pitch that he could have said anything and pleased me better than what he did: he released the grip he had on my forearms, pulling himself respectfully away.

"Jane, if anyone ever finds you objectionable, direct me to his house that I might test my crop upon his sorry hide. Please believe that I do not, and forgive me for having befriended you; I ought to have calculated the effect that our conversations might have upon an English—"

"I do not speak this way because I am a confused Englishwoman!" I cried. "You know that I have fallen into past errors and have admitted as much yourself. Despite this, or perhaps because of it—damned if I know whether 'tis one or the other—I understand you, and that understanding led to admiration. We are scoundrels, are we not? Please don't turn your face, I am not through! I should not like you to suppose you were endeared to me because I thought you as deficient as I am, or because your past is chequered: that would be a gross misrepresentation of my sentiments. I care for you wholly, entirely, not piecemeal, therefore I charge you to be honest with me regarding your feelings if not your history. Only tell me whether . . . tell me whether you value me too."

This last was delivered upon the thinnest breath of air, and then truth telling could bring me no further: I had unravelled myself, and had only to await his reply.

"Jane." Reaching, Mr. Thornfield trailed his fingers over my shoulder.

"Don't stand there deciding whilst I watch you." Tears were forming, and I forced them back.

"Such a fragile soul she turns out to be after all," he said softly. "Grievous injury frightens her not, yet my standing here without a yes on my lips quite shatters her. How you look, Jane—don't allow me to hurt you so. I don't deserve the privilege, I might venture to say no one on earth does. For God's sake, be the wild creature I found in the lane, free of ties that will only pull you to pieces."

"I won't be torn apart at all, supposing you stay near, sir." Forcing the words from my swollen throat, I added, "I only want to be closer still. You are unattached, you said as much—where is the harm to anyone in claiming me? Whatever you have done, it cannot be so terrible that you must deny yourself human contact forevermore."

"There you would be surprised."

"No, I honestly wouldn't be!" I cried.

He lightly took me by the shoulders, gazing down with such a look of mingled fondness and misery as I have never witnessed.

"If you knew the immensity of my blunders, if you knew how *culpable* I was, you'd be sore tempted to spit in my eye. But that's neither here nor there—I know, and the knowledge will never cease to haunt me," he hissed. "I took small comfort in the fact you were happier here than whatever bloody hellhole you used to occupy in London, the fact I could keep you fed and safe among people who relish your company, but do you really want a partial man, a grotesque carnival figure? The gloves are only an outward symbol of an inner deformity. Please, darling, I hate to see what harm I've already caused you. It's agonising—say only that we can be friends again."

I could say no such thing; my mind felt full of smoke, my ears muffled with the word *darling*, my veins laced with laudanum though I had taken none. Meanwhile, his eyes could or would not stop roving—from my own, to my lips, to my throat, and back again.

I decided that I would look desperate if I said anything more, and thus my next words were not calculated; they were like slipping off a ravine's treacherous edge.

And as long as you still mark me, I don't care.

"You study me, Mr. Thornfield." I placed a shaking hand over his breast. "Do you find me beautiful?"

Slowly, Charles Thornfield pulled his gloves from his pocket and slid them back on; then, looking as flayed as anyone I have ever seen, he strode for the stairs and disappeared within the house.

Not such a very long period passed between his exit and my lifting myself from the cold floor where I had curled into the hard shape of a shell, my sobs buried in my skirts; soon enough my pride had reared its haughty head, and I dragged myself back to my room to pour the salty confessions into my pillow.

That Mr. Thornfield could not desire me would have been devastating, but a clean cut—that he *would* not desire me was a ragged gash indeed. I imagined that no night would ever prove worse, and thus it came as an unpleasant surprise when the following proved very much more hideous indeed.

TWENTY-TWO

There was nothing to cool or banish love in these circumstances; though much to create despair.

The next morning, I resolved to break through Charles Thornfield's walls as if I were a battering ram; but gently, over the course of years, and in the meanwhile I might see his white head bent over a harness buckle he was adjusting for Sahjara, and hear him casually cursing. This plan greatly improved my spirits, and I set to filling Sahjara's pate with horse-related facts, feeling quite myself again by the time we parted.

I ought to have noted something malevolent in the air, for the skies were heavy as lead. Still favouring my ankle, I went into the hall to sort through the mail and discovered an envelope postmarked from London, addressed to Miss Jane Stone.

The slender ivory packet crackled in my grip, but I made no move to open it; the missive could only be from my solicitors, and if they reported I had no claim on Highgate House, then nothing would change. Alternately, if I did own the property, I already lived here, and the thought of Highgate House without Mr. Thornfield was now as appealing as London sans Clarke.

"Have you a letter, Miss Stone?"

Mr. Singh approached, and his features beneath the wiry sweep of his beard were grave.

"Apparently so. No one ever writes to me, so I'm at a bit of a loss."

"We missed you this morning at breakfast."

"I was a trifle unwell."

"Then I am glad to see you looking hale now. Miss Stone . . ." He hesitated, adjusting the cuff upon his wrist. "Did anything distressing happen last night?"

"I found the mortuary," I owned. "I've no aversion."

Provided I have ample warning every time Sam Quillfeather pays a call.

"Oh, marvellous—we feared distressing you, and if you don't mind failing to mention it to Sahjara, we are unsure how she'll take it. When she is older . . ."

"Of course."

"And nothing else occurred? Mr. Thornfield is not himself today."

"Is he all right?" I felt stricken—if he were morose, I was culpable. The next instant I felt glad—if he were affected, hope was not lost.

"Yes," Mr. Singh replied, but the word was too lengthy for one syllable.

"He told me about the, um. The penance. The gloves."

"Ah." A frown formed beneath his nobly hooked nose. "Did he elaborate upon why he abstains?"

I shook my head.

"The Guru contains passages about abnegation—fasting, meditation, the renunciation of wealth, but in my opinion, Miss Stone . . ." He lowered his voice. "Such a profound sacrifice is not required by God. The pair of us made a mistake long ago which led us into terrible circumstances, but Charles—I beg your pardon, Mr. Thornfield—"

"It's all right. I know you're not the butler."

"Do you?" he exclaimed.

"I imagine you're a sight better as a commander," I teased.

"Well." He made a small bow, after which his eyes crinkled in distress once more. "Charles, then, feels so culpable that he denies himself touch as a form of self-mortification. I have not yet directly attempted to prevent him, thinking he needed time more than any other balm—but his heart is wide, and bleeds from many hidden wounds."

"So often the way, with hearts."

Brushing a hand over his beard, Mr. Singh passed me, inscrutable, heading towards the front door. I remembered Mrs. Garima Kaur's early assertion to me that he was good, and was grateful, for I knew no one else in whom I could confide.

"I am for the village to settle our bill with the mortuary workmen. Miss Stone, know that I do not take discussion of Charles's heart lightly, and forgive me if I've overburdened you."

"You haven't. He has mine, you know."

Mr. Sardar Singh lingered even as his hand pulled the ornate brass handle of the door. I could not read his face well in any light, so obscured was it by his beard, but now he was quite masked by the cold glow beyond.

"Yes, I thought he might," he admitted. "I will charge him to guard it, Miss Stone. On my honour."

"The Sikh people seem to me very honourable indeed."

Though wintry gusts pelted us, Mr. Singh paused again, and a look steely as his *chakkar* sharpened his features. Since my initial conversation with Garima Kaur over his character, he had never frightened me; now, however, a chill shot down my spine which had nothing to do with the freezing draught.

"There you are mistaken. Which is worse, Miss Stone, if you will pardon my crudeness—a rapist or a pimp?"

"I . . . I can hardly answer that." Crescendos of arctic air whirled into the house. "I should abhor either one."

"Consider the East India Company the rapists, Miss Stone, and the Sikh ruling class the pimps supplying them." He pulled his collar up. "Forgive me . . . you've no desire for a history lesson. Keep yourself well. Charles and I will not return until tomorrow—he met Inspector Quillfeather at his home some miles distant to raise a glass to the mortuary's completion, and we both plan to pass the night there. Thank you for being so free with yourself, as you have given me much to consider."

The door closed, and I watched as the snowflakes turned into teardrops upon the floorboards. Something about this exchange nagged at me—something which I did not understand but felt like awakening in a lightless room with the fanciful certainty that one is not alone.

Soon, I walked upstairs with the unopened letter; it seemed a breathing creature in my hands, and in a way I have always thought that words are alive a little, for they can whisper sweet nothings and roar dragon flame with equal efficiency. After all that had taken place the previous night, I could not even imagine what I wanted it to say, and when I had closed the door to my room, I placed it on the table and stalked about it in circles as if contemplating a chained beast. If I learnt I was not the true mistress of Highgate House, would I prove so spineless as to simply accept Mr. Thornfield's scruples and live as his lovesick shadow for the rest of my days? If learnt that I was the rightful heir, would I prove so horribly low as to use my power for leverage against his wishes? Both outcomes made me ill; one or the other must inevitably be contained in the envelope, scratching to escape with malicious claws.

At length, I simply hid the volatile missive in my bedchamber; I did not want it now, could not even look at it calmly, but I could not read my future in my teacup either. The remainder of the day was uneventful, closed by a hesitant spill of Scotch I poured for myself in the spreading silence and an hour spent in my bed over a book of Irish poems.

I ought to have been grateful for the tranquillity; tragedy would not strike upon that night, as it happened, until one o'clock in the morning.

There was no sound at first, merely a sense; I snapped awake, *feeling* him downstairs, my eyes stuffed with sleepy cotton.

Dread crawled over my skin an instant later when an unknown object audibly shattered.

When I remember these swift seconds, I was up almost before the china had finished splintering, knowing that Mr. Singh could never be so clumsy and that if Mr. Thornfield had staggered and fell, then he must be drunk, and it was my responsibility to see he was not hurt, for I must have been the one who hurt him; and even if what I was telling myself was nonsense I still yearned to be near him in every capacity, so I threw my dressing gown on and slipped my small knife into its pocket and flew for the ground floor.

If it sounds foolish to race towards a clumsy housebreaker, I had ample reason; Mr. Thornfield was all I had thought of for weeks of fever dreams and halfhearted plotting, and even if we were both poorly stitched together creatures made of scar tissue and regrets, I wanted only to find a way to live in his world more fully. So I tumbled into the front hall and came face-to-face with the remains of a vase and a man unlike any I had ever previously met.

I could not tell what race he was, for his eyes were dark and his skin burnished, side-whiskers bright red in the light of his portable lamp; his trousers boasted a loud check pattern and his secondhand coat was wine-coloured velvet. He swayed, emitting acrid whiskey clouds as he panted like the lousiest Company cur north of Calcutta, as Mr. Thornfield would have put it.

Unfortunately, Mr. Thornfield was not present.

"What are ye?" the ruffian snarled, sounding pleased.

The accent was nigh-impossible to parse, but I thought it might have been the result of a Scottish lilt applied to already-musical Indian intonations.

"The governess."

I considered screaming for once in my life; but Mr. Singh and Mr. Thornfield, who slept on the same floor I did, were from home, and the servants inhabited another wing. Apart from Sahjara three doors down from my bedroom, whom I prayed would *not* come downstairs, I was alone.

"D'ye always keep such midnight hours?" he purred, revealing yellowed teeth.

"Get away from here! I'll call the master of the house."

He slanted a canny look at me. "And why haven't ye already? I suspect he ain't here to come when ye do shout."

Morbidity is not the same as stupidity, so I wheeled and made for the kitchen, intending to shriek my face off for whichever Singh or Kaur could hear me; but I found my throat caught in a vise, hashish-laden breath creeping across my cheekbones.

"I meant t' question the half-bred lass, but ye might be a sight better," the rotting relic of foreign wars spoke in my ear. "Tell me now where the trunk is and ye can sleep sound and safe."

"They don't have it!" I choked. "Let me *go*!"

How long we wrestled in that entryway I cannot recall, though I know I landed a number of ineffective blows. I was once more a being of edges and angles, fighting viciously to preserve not only the little girl upstairs I hoped was not roused by our clamour but the woman downstairs, making it.

"That's the most whoreson lie I've heard since leaving Delhi," his fat lips spoke against my ear.

Howling now, though to no one in particular, I fought to free my hands; he had caught both under one burly sweat-smelling arm.

If I could get to my knife.

I can get to my knife.

I will *get to my knife.*

Laughing in cruel wheezes like the rasp of a hacksaw, he shoved me facedown over the arm of the sofa in the drawing room after he had dragged me there, filling my nose with sweat and leather and lust, and I knew what happened next, had already faced the prospect. His bones bruised my wrists where they were pinioned, his other hand clumsily jostling at my skirts as he raised them.

"D'ye squeal like cows hereabouts, or just eat 'em?" he asked, rancid teeth brushing my neck.

I heard the approach of measured footsteps on the drive, and the front door opening.

Reader: I screamed, and if I could have screamed loud enough, I would have pierced him clean through.

"Damn ye straight t' hell," he growled.

A scorching pain blazed through my head as my assailant seized me by the follicles and led me into the shadows of the large chamber; the noises from the hall ceased.

"I'll see the whole lot o' ye vipers in hell," my captor hissed.

He pressed pocket-warm metal against my gullet, and I had no choice save to follow as he dragged me by the scalp. When Mr. Thornfield and Mr. Singh burst into the room, I yet supposed the weapon a dull knife, but after the brute brandished the thing, I saw that it was a pistol in his hand.

Upon glimpsing my assailant, both men's faces distorted as if a sword had met their bellies.

"How is it possible you're yet alive?" Mr. Thornfield cried, unsheathing the blade he carried.

"Oh, aye, always so shocked when the rent comes due," crooned the man holding me hostage. "Give me the small one who knows where the bounty is buried—or else the trunk, better still—and we'll argue nae further."

"We don't *have it*," Mr. Singh protested urgently. "And Miss Stone knows nothing of your monstrous intrigues. Let her loose or—"

"Or what?"

"They aren't lying to you," I croaked, still feeling the phantom clench of a fist round my throat.

"It's nae in the Punjab." He rubbed against my cheek, boar's bristles abrading me. "It's nae in jolly old London town. And ye claim it's nae here, but mayhaps a bullet will jog someone's faculties."

"No!" Mr. Thornfield cried.

"Oh, d'ye prefer this aimed at you, then?"

The scorching grip against my hair blazed into a bonfire even as the *badmash* removed his gun from my neck and swung it in the direction of Charles Thornfield.

Mr. Singh, whose movements were generally so calculated you could have set your watch by them, lifted a futile palm in horrified protest; the master of the house looked endearingly relieved, as if having a pistol aimed at his forehead was preferable to its being aimed at mine. My immediate circumstances branded themselves upon my memory—the setting half-moon, the distant scuffles as the servants were roused, the fact Mr. Thornfield was gazing into my eyes rather than the barrel of the weapon now levelled at him. The sheer horror of the scene nearly finished me.

It did not, however—because the blackguard now had one arm devoted to a gun cocked at Mr. Thornfield and the other to tearing my scalp from its moorings; so I whipped out my knife and stabbed blindly backwards with all the fervour men devote to war.

I do not know whether the casual reader of novels is acquainted with an anatomical curiosity known as the femoral artery; without too much medical meandering, although you might suppose that cutting a man's throat would be the fastest way to slaughter him, a good jab to the thigh will do.

Fainting in front of Mr. Thornfield and Mr. Singh was never my object, but faint indeed I did for the second time in my life. Not due to fright—pain swept me under its carpet. It must have been a brief respite, however, for when I came to, I was tucked deep in the settee with a blanket covering me, and Mr. Thornfield was shouting for towels, hovering over the pitifully whimpering brute. Mrs. Garima Kaur was there, looking haggard, twisting her fingers in violent worriment before running to obey the master of the house.

Walls tilted and furniture swam, and perhaps ten minutes later Mr. Thornfield was not shouting for anything anymore, merely gazing with dark satisfaction at what seemed a corpse and a crimson pond upon our floorboards.

The fact of my fifth murder at first slid off my consciousness like water from a goose feather; but I knew instinctually I could not remain in the same room with the dead man lazing in the pool of blood. Wrenching myself upright, I attempted a graceful exit.

"Wait a moment, Jane!" Mr. Thornfield cried.

"I can't stay here."

"You're reeling from hurt and shock, you'll injure—"

"Don't touch me!"

We stared at each other, I in astonishment I had rebuffed him and he in chagrin he had startled me so. His thin grey gloves were covered with the other man's gore, his shirt and waistcoat too, for he had been practicing his profession automatically, I believe, tending to the injured in spite of everything, and I was ready to splinter into a thousand mirror shards reflecting every memory of my own ugliness. Mr. Singh arrived bearing a mop and a bucket of soapy water and stopped, taking measure of the situation.

"Charles." He passed his friend the cleaning supplies. "Miss Stone, will you let me walk beside you to the morning room?"

I started to speak, but clutched at his elbow rather than continue.

Mr. Singh ducked his cloth-bound head against my throbbing scalp in a glancing touch; Mr. Thornfield spread his arms as if in supplication, but since I could not speak, neither to protest the tainted innocence of accident nor beg forgiveness for guilt, I walked away. Mr. Singh accompanied me and, when we were in the morning room, I crossed to the divan and collapsed.

I could not see the shadow which tangled with mine as Sardar Singh hovered over me; I smelt him, though, warm nutmeg and the clean wintry sweat which accompanies a trek on horseback in January, and I fought not to weep at the strange comfort of it.

"Miss Stone, I am no doctor, but Charles will be here shortly, and in the meanwhile you've nothing whatsoever to fear. Are you injured in any sense we're not aware of?"

"No."

"Thank God for that, then," he said as his footfalls grew fainter. "And thank God we were early in returning—we should have been here around midday tomorrow had we not been loath to leave the property unprotected."

He knelt on the carpet before me with a glass of brandy when he returned; I swallowed it, and the searing of my bruised throat brought me back to myself. When I could focus, I saw that Mr. Singh regarded me as he might a casualty of a war he had started, and I did not think I could bear that expression.

"All this will pass," said I, unsteadily.

"I am glad you think so."

I wanted to elaborate—in this impossible future, I would not have just murdered yet another man, Sahjara would break mighty stallions, Mr. Thornfield would love me, and everyone would lose the look we had of folk waiting for the axe to fall.

"I think about many things that aren't true, even say them sometimes," I confessed instead, and his mouth tugged fathoms deep.

"Miss Stone, there is nothing I can do to relieve your pain over what just occurred. But I had a sister once, and in a way—in a very *English* way," he amended, "you remind me of her. I don't think that anyone who reminds me of my sister ought to feel so melancholy about herself, though I understand you must be in a state of extreme distress."

You really cannot imagine what sort of state I am in.

"Did I kill him?"

"Yes," said he.

I bit my lip, that sharp hurt dulling the ache in my chest. "Was your sister beautiful?"

Mr. Singh smiled. I have visited many churchyards, both as inspiration for gallows ballads and for perverse pleasure, and it was the smile I had found on the carved angels' faces—peaceful but eroding.

"Indeed she was. Her name was Karman, and do you know, that sealed her fate, I think."

"What does it mean?"

"'Doer of deeds.' Charles will never tell you this, but I was always a pacifist at heart. Oh, I am a skilled warrior, as is our honour and the will of God. But 'Let compassion be your mosque,' the Guru states, and if you were to discuss compassion with a Khalsa *naik** today . . ." He shrugged.

I tucked my arm under my pulsating head. "But your sister was a fighter?"

"The great Maharajah Ranjit Singh would have been hard-pressed to win a battle with my sister," Mr. Singh reflected. "Karman, from the time she was small, was wildly passionate. She loved the Khalsa in the new ways, with sharp swords and fat jewels and daring feats, whilst I loved it in the old ways, with meditation and acceptance.

---

* Corporal.

'Whom should I despise, since the one Lord made us all?' If you were to have asked Karman, she would have spat, 'The British and the Bengali strumpets who service them.' Then she would have laughed and shouted, '*Khalsa-ji!*' and you may have thought it merriment, but there was war in her eyes from the age of five, and later, men adored her for it. I did not blame them. I loved her before they did, after all."

"You were a good brother to her."

"Oh, yes," he scoffed. "I taught her to fight with the *tulwar*, the *chakkar*, just as I did Charles, when I ought to have taught her meditation."

"Did it grieve you, that you were so different?"

"A little—but people cannot help being who they are."

"They can help the things they do because of who they are, however."

"Are you merely shaken, or are you often distressed by who you are?" Mr. Singh inquired gently.

"Either." I laughed. "Both, perhaps. I don't know."

"'If I say I am perishable, it will not avail me; but if I truly know I am perishable, it will.' Miss Stone, pardon me for asking, but . . . do you ever think about death?"

Only of the many deaths I've caused, and my mother's, and my own, and every day.

When I held my tongue, Mr. Singh pressed my wrist. "You do, I see. Then you are far closer to God than you think you are. I must go help Charles."

"Mr. Singh," I called after him with tears in my eyes, "will you tell me what your name was? Before?"

Hesitating, he replied, "Aazaad was my name. It means 'free of care.'"

"And why did you change it?"

This time, he did not pause.

"Because it did not suit me anymore, Miss Stone," he replied, shutting the door softly as he went.

Rolling onto my stomach, I buried my head in my arms and wept. I have seen, employed as a literary phrase, that characters *wept as though the world were ending*; the world ending, I thought, would be better than continuing to deceive compassionate people, lying from dawn to dusk because to stop lying would mean ceasing to be entangled with them.

When I awoke, I felt perfectly at ease though my pate shrieked with pain, and someone was tenderly cleaning the wound with a damp cloth.

I think Mr. Thornfield sensed my wakefulness due to my stilling rather than stirring. A knee was wedged behind the curve of my lower back, and the quilt covered me from neck to toe. I quickly realised it was impossible for him to work with such delicacy of touch whilst still wearing blood-crusted gloves.

The sea could have parted in the centre and it would not have felt as open as I did then, the whorls of his fingertips parting my already scattered tresses.

"Jane, please speak a word if only to berate me. You've done a damn sight more than I tonight, but grant me this single further favour."

I could think of nothing to say, however.

"Darling? Jane, for heaven's sake, only live and let fly at me with all the abuse you like and you'll make me a happy man."

My lungs produced a frightful sound, and he crossed one arm over my torso diagonally, as if protecting me from falling.

"Will you pardon me for murdering someone in your drawing room?" I breathed.

"Oh, Jane." His voice was wracked, vibrating through me, but I shook for more reasons than I liked to think about.

He handled my hair with bare hands, though he never brushed my skin, and I registered sharp hurts, and glass draughts smelling of herbs and strong spirits against my lips and my head. He dried the tear in my scalp, and washed the blood from my locks in a porcelain bowl, and as dawn approached he lifted a tendril of my hair up to his lips even as I fell asleep in his arms, kissing it as though his heart were breaking.

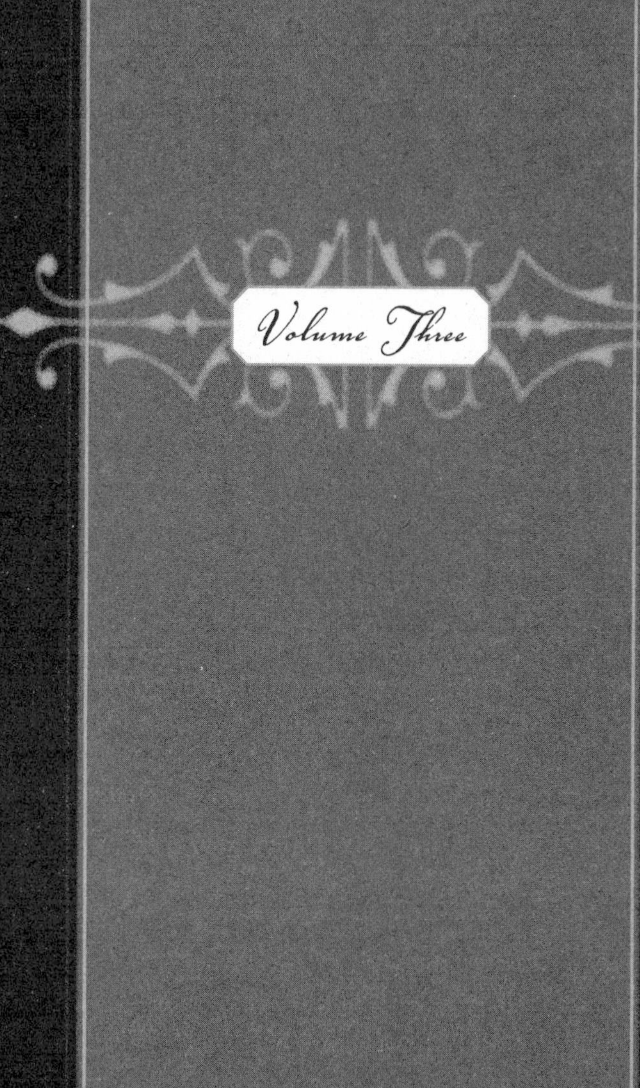

Volume Three

TWENTY-THREE

Mr. Rochester did, on a future occasion, explain it.

I did not awaken for many hours, though neither did I sleep; my consciousness thinned into a filmy half-awareness, and when I did feel the slow burn of sunlight drifting across my face, I heard a chair creak.

"Jane?"

"Is there water?"

"Of course."

Mr. Thornfield seemed never to have quit the room. Thirst quenched after the glass had been held to my lips, I discovered I was not as hurt as I had supposed. Yes, I had killed a man in front of two respected friends; yes, I had then acted like an abominable weakling; but, no, my cranium had not cracked, only torn, and I found myself staring glassy-eyed at a haggard Mr. Thornfield.

It would do him discredit to pretend he was unmoved, but I hesitate to set down how distressed he was in fact, his countenance as pale as if he were the one who had been strangled.

"I thought when I saw you with that pepperbox* against your

---

* Pistol.

throat . . ." He made an abortive movement. "Jane, I hardly know how to speak to you."

"As the governess would suit." I sighed, shifting my knees.

"No, it bloody well would *not.* As the woman I acted a cad towards in the morgue downstairs, or the woman who saved my skin last night?"

"Please don't, sir. You never acted a cad, and I never saved you."

"You saved me sure as God saved Isaac."

My mind could not seem to light upon important subjects, only trivial ones. "How do you know that story?"

"Sardar could write a book entitled *A Thousand and One Useless Meditations.* He knows all when it comes to retribution and forgiveness."

"Not all, or he'd have taught us both to stop hating ourselves. Who was it I killed?"

"Jane, I am hesitant to—"

"Don't I deserve to know? Sahjara and I both were at risk, and had you not arrived when you did . . ."

His flinch told me he knew I was right, but he took his time: pouring a pair of neat Scotches, passing me one.

"I am all attention, sir."

Mr. Thornfield's chest gave a small heave, and then he abruptly drew his hand over his mouth and sat down close beside me on the divan.

"Where should I begin?"

"Try the beginning."

"What was the beginning? The wars were years in coming," he said softly. "Believe me or don't, or ask Sardar, but it didn't even occur to the British to conquer the Punjab until the Sikh ruling class started dangling it in their faces as if they were *cunchunees.** It was

---

* Dancing girls.

too well fortified, y'see. The Khalsa army was the best in the world, and they *wanted* to march—on Delhi, on London. Geography was never their top marks, bless 'em, but so long as they stayed in the Punjab, they were unbeatable."

"Yet they were still beaten." I sipped the amber liquid. "Mr. Singh called the Company rapists, and the Sikh royalty their pimps."

Mr. Thornfield nodded as his knuckles met his lips. "I can still see the Khalsa parading on the *doab** when I was thirteen: a hundred thousand strong marching in such perfect order a Geneva watch would have dashed itself to pieces forthwith. Sapphire turbans, red feathers thrusting from round steel helms, emerald jackets and scarlet jackets and indigo jackets, every jab of the light infantry's bayonets into the sandbags precise enough to kill a gnat. If you've never seen dozens of war elephants draped in crimson, there ain't a way to describe what happens to your stomach. As for the horses—if you watched their white chargers at parade exercise, you could almost grasp why 'He made intuition his horse, and chastity his saddle' is in the Guru."

"How could the monarchy have wanted to throw away its own empire?"

"They didn't want to throw away their empire, that would have been *ridiculous*," he drawled. "They wanted to keep it—keep the palaces and the stuffed coffers and the all-night debauches with man, woman, and donkey—and throw away their army. You build a fighting force that strong, what do you suppose they're keen to do after breakfast and a spot of coffee?"

"Fight," I realised.

He nodded, staring at his sleeve. "When the royals figured out they'd created an uncontrollable army, they got the trots, and arranged for John Bull to slaughter 'em."

---

* Dry land between the five rivers of the Punjab. The word *Punjab* itself translates literally to "five rivers."

"You cannot mean that is truly what happened?" I exclaimed, horrified.

"I can, I was there. Anyhow. There were too many ghastly betrayals to recount, and when the Director of the Company understood that the area was about as stable as a rocking horse, years before the fighting started, he began to send . . . emissaries."

"Spies," I supplied.

"Oh, Jane," he said warmly, and for a spear-flash moment, he was here with me and not long ago and far away. "Spies, yes. The Company soldiers always rather despised the politicals because the latter gorged over greasy state dinners and the former got shot full of holes, but some of these were good eggs."

"John Clements," I suggested, remembering the half story I had been told regarding the funeral.

"Aye, save he'd the brains of a fly whisk. In any event, Lahore grew a bit thicker with white men, though never so's you'd notice unless you were British yourself." The smile he attempted fell yards short of the mark. "I noticed, though, and my mother and father—didn't *they* fleece the sheep. 'Oh, have you seen the Pearl Mosque yet?' and then, 'If a pipe's in your line, guv'ner, won't you share one with me?' and before long they were rooking the lot. One of these Company interlopers was, as you know, a consummate worm by the name of Augustus Sack. Sack's assistant was John Clements, and the third player in this happy pantomime . . ."

"David Lavell," I supplied. "Sahjara's father."

"Yes." Mr. Thornfield coughed. "Yes, he was that as well. So. David Lavell . . . he was five years older than I when he arrived in Lahore, ostensibly to conduct border discussions, but really to take the measure of every toady he could tattle back to Delhi regarding. My family was brown as a nut by then, and Augustus Sack cut too ridiculous a figure for the Sikh to credit him—and if the superior is absurd, why should they mind John Clements trailing after him like a spaniel? But David Lavell was one of your strapping soldier types. For face furniture, the man was a palace. Adonis's brow, blinding teeth, you see the portrait I'm painting."

As I did not trust myself not to say, *he could never be so handsome as you,* I kept my peace.

"He was also charming." Mr. Thornfield spoke the word as if it cut his lips. "Lavell could talk an elephant in *musth** out of charging and, in a cunning way, there were brains in his head. Witness him flatter the jewels off a *kunwar*† one moment! Gape as he drops a hint and ruins an officer's chances for advancement the next! Two-faced? Whoreson bugger had a hundred of 'em, and you hardly minded when your pockets were empty and your mother cashiered."

"You didn't get on."

"Is she truly teasing me?" He sighed fondly. "No, Jane, we didn't get on, but when he discovered that the Thornfield family was quite close to Sardar's, and that loot flowed down our street like rain down a gutter, he began popping round uninvited."

"That is how you and Mr. Singh and the other two British politicals all became acquainted?"

"Yes, and would the Director had sent the devil himself to Lahore first." Mr. Thornfield's face darkened, as if I could see the spiritual bruise beneath the sun-bronzed features. He shifted, seeming to steel himself, drawing a knee up to rest on the sofa beside me. "Did Sardar ever mention to you he had a sister?"

Oh, I thought, my heart breaking for them.

"Karman Kaur," I replied, proud that I kept my voice steady.

Charles Thornfield's lips wavered, but he did not shrink. "I knew

---

* A highly aggressive, violent madness which can occur seasonally in male elephants.

† The son of a maharajah.

her from the cradle, as she was my closest friend's sibling and was always besting me at sword fighting. Sardar's physiognomy has been hidden under that magnificent bush ever since he was old enough to grow one, that's their custom—but you can guess at it, can't you, and she looked very like him."

"Brown skin, grey eyes, slender nose with a fine crook to it, full lower lip. Yes, I can see her."

"I'm glad, Jane," he said, equally low. "It was laughable how arresting she was. Karman was all fire and fight, and if she had been Maharani instead of Jindan Kaur,* tens of thousands of the Khalsa would be alive today, because she would have crushed any army who dared to say boo to her."

"Mr. Singh implied that she was considerably more combative than he."

"Wasn't she just!" A smile died before it reached Mr. Thornfield's lips. "But she had a soft side; deucedly handy with children, not to mention horses—you see where Sahjara caught the itch, at least that's part of it—and a laugh that carried clear to Kandahar. Sardar always preferred studying the Guru to the *chakkar*; he just happens to be damnably talented. Karman, though—the three of us once forded all five rivers of the Punjab on horseback as a dare to ourselves, seeing as Ranjit Singh had managed it. Sardar was half a man by the end, I nearly drowned twice, but Karman? I think the daft girl wanted to do it again."

"You loved her very much."

"Not enough for her to notice," came his answer. "But yes."

A silence followed, one tempered by the whispering of the fire and the knowledge that outside, the sun was rising and the wind singing arias to the elms. Mr. Thornfield's sadness must have been

---

* The regent of the last Maharajah, her son Duleep Singh.

excruciating; but mine was strangely sweet for, though it pained me, the mere fact of the melancholy meant that he had taken me into his confidence, and so I wrapped myself in it all the tighter.

When I returned from my reverie, Mr. Thornfield was passing me another large glass of spirits. "To your health, Jane."

"And yours, Mr. Thornfield."

"Where to continue? Ah, David Lavell. The cur took a shine to Karman, because he had eyes in his head, and Karman took an equal shine to Lavell, thanks to that perverse rule of Nature which causes pearls to cast themselves before swine. As a female yourself, can you account for this oddity of science, Jane?"

"In some cases, it's because the pearls know themselves grains of sand at heart, though I cannot imagine that should have been the case for Karman."

Pained laughter escaped Mr. Thornfield's chest. "No, her opinion of herself was middling favourable. Perhaps they shared that in common, and God knows that when it came to flattering the Sikhs, to the point of convincing 'em defeating the Company would only be a matter of three or four cavalry and half an hour's botheration, Lavell was a master. From the moment they took up together, I was an object to be pitied, which is a state I do not care for."

I remembered the cracked cloud cover of a London sky a few months after Clarke left me—brain pulsing fit to leak out my ears, covered in dew, observed by a silent beggar whose legs had been lost at the knees and had likewise slept rough in the park. "I understand."

"It was piss on the wound that it was my own fault." Mr. Thornfield took a hearty swallow. "The three of us had been inseparable—studying, shooting, riding out to the Jupindar rocks to drink French brandy filched from my parents and laugh until we were sick. I had assumed her mine already. I was a dunce, carousing with flighty *houris** who meant nothing to me and then smoking *bhang*† with Sardar and Karman—they were family, and I expected it all to remain the same. After three months of pining, I announced to my parents that I meant to take up medicine and packed my bags for London."

"Afterwards you needed a legitimate way back into the Punjab, though, and so signed up for military training at Addiscombe. What happened in the interim?"

"Sardar's letters had been played plenty close, but I could tell something was rotten," he answered. "He mentioned that Karman and Lavell had actually married; he also said she gave birth to a baby named Sahjara, but I was too melancholy for more detail. After Charing Cross and the Aldersgate Street Dispensary were through and I'd earned a place at the Royal College, I spent a single year at Addiscombe because I knew the Punjab was about to blow like a powder keg, and I'm not puffing myself up but complimenting Sardar's early tutelage when I say that was record time. The Company sent me straight back to Lahore, and when I arrived . . ."

I watched as his face turned to stone.

"Lavell was living it up royally. Relations there aren't the same as in England, the elite have plentiful concubines—even the women take lovers. But Karman's husband was hilt deep in every back-alley cat he could find, and when he wasn't drunk, it was hashish or opium. My parents were appalled and shut him out, but it isn't as if buying double the shite poppy can't sustain the habit. Meanwhile, he was practically setting fire to Karman's money, and the last straw came when Sardar spied one of these sloe-eyed tarts waltzing through the marketplace wearing a necklace that belonged to his sister. Karman

* Beautiful women.

† Indian hemp.

had the typical Sikh taste in baubles, by which I mean she had a disgusting pile of 'em. It was an emerald choker that got away."

"Did Augustus Sack do nothing about this?"

"Sack wasn't his superior, and anyway he was winning a fortune off Lavell at poker—Karman's fortune. Lavell couldn't sink low enough for Sack's taste."

"I imagine you wanted to thrash the hide off him."

"Oh, I threatened to, Company be damned, but we went to Karman first." Mr. Thornfield's mouth wrenched regretfully. "She wouldn't hear a word against the blackguard. She was drunk when Sardar and I arrived, which wasn't exactly surprising, and she was glad to see us as ever, but she waved it all off, saying when the Khalsa marched to Delhi we would all have twenty fortunes to spend, that he was the father of her child and a man who liked to take his pleasure where he found it, and that she was no better, and that we were a set of old hens."

"What did you do?"

Mr. Thornfield placed his brow in his hand. "We stole her jewellery collection."

This, then, was the terrible crime; perhaps it was the Scotch, I pray so, but I laughed. An instant later, Mr. Thornfield was chuckling in the helpless way people have when it is either that or put a pistol in your mouth.

"I know," he groaned. "Jane, Jane, Jane. We thought we were protecting her, and the war broke out the next day. This was December of eighteen forty-five, and the Khalsa army began their march to Ferozepore. Lavell was still stationed in Lahore at the time, and raised all holy Hades when he discovered his candy dish missing."

"What did Karman have to say about it?"

"That's not a tale worth the telling." His jaw clenched briefly. "Sardar hid the jewellery in a Khalsa military-issue satchel in a secret compartment in his own rooms. Then everything fell apart. The war scattered us, for all it was only three months long. Sardar, bless him, was never part of the Khalsa army and remained in Lahore doing business. Lavell went to Amritsar, the capital, and the Director ordered Sack and Clements to consult with the generals at Ferozepore. After the Company won Ferozeshah, thanks to the Sikh royals castrating their own military, I was called to Ludhiana to provide my services as a medico and Punjabi translator. Are you following me clearly?"

"Yes," I answered, thinking only, *What terrible fate befell Karman Kaur that you will not speak of?*

"I was involved in the Battle of Sobraon, which was decisive." His voice was brittle as glass, and suddenly I remembered Sack's words, his implication that Mr. Thornfield had been severely hurt in the conflict. "Sack and Clements arrived just as the fighting ended, in an advisory capacity, though I can't speak as to their movements because I had been injured—sweet Jane, don't look like that, it was only a scratch from a *tulwar* across my back and upper shoulder, just here, but the blasted cut was infected and I spent a hellish fortnight hardly aware of myself. Clements was at my side whenever he could be. I never forgot that. It was a kindness."

"Then I am grateful to him," I whispered.

Mr. Thornfield's eyes creased in acknowledgement. "After I recovered, as treaty preparations were finalised, I returned to Lahore. Both Lavell and Karman had been killed in the interim. Lavell played one dirty trick too many and ended up with a sliced throat in Amritsar, and when I have occasion to meditate upon that, Jane, my heart is filled with gladness and song."

"In future, so shall mine be, Mr. Thornfield."

Mr. Thornfield sat forward again. "Lahore was filling with dangerous types in the vacuum naturally caused when a region destabilises. I'm afraid Sardar and I then made a decision still more stupid than stealing his sister's unholy stock of jewels; fearful of the thieves swarming the city, we decided to hide 'em in plain sight, and employed Sahjara's doll trunk. Sardar's mum and my shameless buccaneering parents passed a delightful afternoon stuffing dolls with diamonds we'd pried out of their prongs and decorating their little bodies with precious stones. Sahjara was only five, but she had the finest French doll collection outside Paris, and when they were through, you might not have noticed it was anything but a trunk full of the most opulent *chico*'s toys on Earth."

Raptly, I questioned, "Who did notice?"

"Augustus Sack," Mr. Thornfield snarled. "We had told Sahjara that her trunk was forbidden for the time being, which was a fantastic error—she scarce ever touched those dolls in the first place, but we had reminded her of 'em, you see. When Sack returned to Lahore, the maggot, he went to Sardar's house to pay respects and there she was, playing with a doll covered in rubies. Instead of waiting for Sardar, he asked Sahjara if she would show him the doll's sisters, which she was happy to do. Sack recalled Lavell's hysterics over Karman's missing treasure, he added two and two together, and he decided they spelt blackmail."

"How did he go about it?"

"Ah, there's the clever part, that thrice-damned son of a bitch. He told Clements that Sardar and I must have stolen Karman's jewels before the war broke out, recalled Lavell's lamentations to Clements's mind, and asked Clements, as honourable Company men, what should be done about it considering we were all such close mates? Then Sack suggested that, since Karman and Lavell were both dead, why should they not confront us privately, without bringing the Director into it, seizing the trunk and holding it in trust for Sahjara until she came of age? You can imagine how that would have played out."

"How *did* it play out?"

"Exactly as they wanted it to, save for the fact the trunk had disappeared!" he exclaimed, slapping his palm against his thigh. "We had been keeping it quite in the open, not knowing Sack had designs on it. It was gone. It remains gone. Some lucky *burcha* came in through the window and is whoring his way through Kashmir to this very day."

"What happened afterwards?"

"Sack thought that between Sardar, myself, and Sahjara, *someone* was playing the crooked cross, and *someone* knew where the trunk was." His voice was full of stones. "He bullied us, threatened us, talked of *chowkdar*s, of driving me out of the Company and Sardar out of Lahore."

"You rebuffed them."

"We thought that best."

"Was it?"

Mr. Thornfield studied his stiff scarlet gloves where they yet lay upon the table, and not once did he look up until he had finished. "Sack ordered Sahjara abducted a week later by a half-caste *badmash* named Jack Ghosh he sometimes used for his dirty work. You not six hours ago killed Jack Ghosh, an act which I assure you deserves a medal and a pension. Sardar and I practically lost our minds when we had word that Ghosh would feed her when we had delivered the trunk to a secret locale. We, I remind you, did not have the trunk."

My lips parted in horror. I thought of Sahjara—her complete candour, her keen black eyes—and could not help but shudder. She had never come downstairs, so I lived in hope that the events of the previous night had not touched her.

"How long did it take you to find her?"

"Four days," he rasped. He pressed his hand over his mouth, then continued. "Clements knew nothing of the scheme, thinking Ghosh had acted alone after hearing of the trunk from Sack, so he was of no use in finding her, though he aided all our efforts—as for Sack, he made certain to be away from Lahore at the time, or I should have knocked her whereabouts straight from his skull. Sahjara was locked in a desert stable when we found her, by which I mean a tent with horses in it, all alone, her captor fled. Ghosh had kept her quiet by having her feed and brush and water the animals, telling her when she was finished, she could eat. She was never quite the same afterwards."

Tears were streaming from my eyes. "Oh, Mr. Thornfield."

"It's not the worst event I've ever caused." He laughed unsteadily. "Enough of this. We retrieved her. Of course we realised who was behind it all, but there was no evidence—only Sack's knowing little smirk when I stormed into his offices raving over the kidnap. The Company was in full force by that time, secretaries and clerks thick as fleas, but Ghosh had fled and I couldn't accuse Sack without exposing the original theft. So I went to my superior officers, begging for Ghosh to be found—they laughed in my face. What was the disappearance of a half-caste villain to the subjugation of an empire?"

"Did they offer you no assistance?"

"The most they would do was provide a guardian to send Sahjara to my paternal aunt's house in Cornwall, for she started at every shadow in Lahore, and I was still in the employ of the Director. Sardar thought of accompanying her, but his mother was ill at the time, and fresh fighting loomed, so we put Sahjara in the frankly doting care of a wounded lieutenant returning to his family. That put Sack off long enough for the second Sikh war to break out, and there you have it. After I inherited this place, I sold my commission, and Sardar and I were bumping across the desert from Suez to Cairo in the back of a wagon to take the steam route here from Alexandria."

I pulled at my hair, wanting the dull ache. "Do you think Sack tired of waiting and sent Ghosh on this occasion as well?"

"Very likely. I'm only glad he's stone dead in the morgue downstairs."

"Did Sahjara ever wake?"

"Yes, but we bundled her off with Garima Kaur, so she's quite snug, thank heaven. If anything should have happened to her here . . . Jane, I am forever in your debt. I've never managed to do as much for her."

"You gave up your home for her, sir. You gave up everything."

"Ridiculous. Christ, if I never see the Punjab again, it'll be too soon. I have her, and Sardar, and this house, and that's a deuced sight more than I merit."

I thought of Clarke long ago, our fleeing to London and her telling me I was *home*, and was so deep in lightless conjectures I nearly missed Mr. Thornfield saying, "And now a true friend in you, Jane."

Suddenly nauseated, I shivered. A wall which has been well constructed with strong stones and good masonry can defend against many a dire circumstance; but put a single crack in that mossy edifice, and a former fortress is as good as a pile of rocks.

They knew me for a killer; Clarke's words regarding Hugh and Bertha Grizzlehurst rang in my ear as if her lips were pressed to the lobe.

She'll never be able to look him in the face again without knowing—can you imagine the torment?

"Jane, wherever you've gone to, please come back to me, or anyway what's left of me at the moment," a rough voice pleaded.

Standing unsteadily, I shook my head. I must have looked a fright, traces of blood on my gown, mermaid hair snaking its brown waves all about my waxen face. I set the glass down and made for the door.

"Let me—"

"I'm fine on my own."

"You most certainly are not."

"Alone, I want to be alone."

"You really do, and for the first time I've ever observed. Is this to be the end of the peculiar smile I see form whensoever you spy me? I can imagine it all too easily—no warm tilt of your head, no spark of light in your eye. Do you think me a blackguard following that terrible account, Jane?" he questioned raggedly, the edge of his sleeve painted ivory by the brightening dawn rays bleeding through the curtains.

"I think you an eyewitness," I gasped before I could stop myself, but he did not know what I meant, he could never ever know what I meant, so I ran from the room and up the stairs and locked the door and did not emerge again that day.

TWENTY-FOUR

He who is taken out to pass through a fair scene to the scaffold, thinks not of the flowers that smile on his road, but of the block and axe-edge; of the disseverment of bone and vein; of the grave gaping at the end: and I thought of drear flight and homeless wandering—and oh! with agony I thought of what I left!

After a sleep which felt more like drowning than rest, tempests tossing me, I awoke to discover it was dark. Silently, I crept to the door, gazing out into the corridor; no one was there, but a tray of bread and cheese and fruit had been left, and a bottle of wine, and I quickly collected these, shutting myself in once more.

Tying my messy hair into a painful braid, I stoked the fire which had burnt down to coals. The sustenance was accompanied by a note:

Dear Jane,

I should have set myself as guardian over your gate forever, save that I cannot know whether I inspire feelings of safety and security in you or dampen them, and immediate arrangements must be made. You shall not be disturbed, I vow, and should you wish to disturb any of us, a bell rung will be answered upon the instant. I cannot help but live in hope I might be called for personally, but already owe you far too great a debt to make any further presumptions.

Sahjara is from home, staying with Mrs. Garima Kaur in the cottage with the grooms rotating watches over them. Whilst investigating last night's siege, we thought it best; should you wish to repair there, arrangements would be made with all haste, and the place has been thoroughly cleaned and heated.

It grows less and less bearable to consider denying you any wishes, come to that, save only those beyond my power—if you can imagine a way I might ease the burden a good woman like yourself should never have had to bear, I beg you to command me.

Your servant,
Charles Thornfield

Laughing at the depth of this miscalculation, I forced myself to eat food which turned to cinders on my tongue, washing all down with half the bottle of wine and a larger dose of laudanum than I had taken since my London days, for my head felt as if a glowing poker had struck it.

It was not, I ought to clarify, troubling to me that Jack Ghosh was no longer numbered among the living; he had hurt a little girl I had grown to love, and in any case, he had not precisely inspired esteem during our brief acquaintance. No, he could rot for all I cared, and he would, too—but he had smashed my dam and now the seawater was up to my neck.

I could live a complete lie, I comprehended as I sorted through the knotted threads of dread in my chest; I could not live a partial one.

Already, falling in love with Charles Thornfield had meant dropping truths in his path like so many bread crumbs, and though he may have approved my stabbing Jack Ghosh, however could I justify four previous killings? The number was outrageous. I could neither lie, nor could I confess; and I could neither pull down his walls without candour nor risk baring my hollowed heart.

When Jane Eyre understands that she must depart from Mr. Rochester or else become his mistress and not his wife, her eyes remain entirely dry, and her former fiancé surmises that her heart must have been weeping blood before he begs her to stay. I admire this passage for a number of reasons—not merely because it is beautiful, but because I can be moved by it even when recalling my own experience of leaving Highgate House, and my reasons for doing so, and want to shake the other Jane's damn fool head off for leaving a gentleman who loved her so, and was remorseful for his error. For I understood that night—not with a dry eye, either—that as much as I had come to adore Sahjara and esteem Mr. Singh, I could not love Mr. Thornfield every livelong day without having him.

I could have lived off my fingers in his white hair, or my brow against his collarbone, or the whole expanse of our bared skin nestled together in sleep, or my lips against his rugged temple. I had done far worse things for love than entwine fingers or kiss the nape of a neck, had I not? The prospect of total famine, however, dying of thirst and nothing betwixt me and the glass of water resting on the table—I cannot imagine that anyone could have done it.

Very well, I determined around midnight, my eyes crimson and my head pounding. *You will live as you used to, and life is a tenuous thing after all, so one day inevitably the hurt will stop.*

There was still the matter of Highgate House, however, so I located the fateful letter from London and opened it with shaking fingers.

SNEEVES, SWANSEA, AND TURNER

No. 29C Lisle Street,
Westminster

Dear Miss Steele,

Though you addressed your letter to Mr. Swansea, that gentleman passed away six years hence, necessitating my own return from abroad; thus, know that it is Mr. Cyrus Sneeves who addresses you. If you are able to call upon me at the above address, I believe I can make your position clear to you; in fact, I consider it my duty to do so, as I may have an unexpected opportunity to right a wrong which I had begun to consider permanent.

I regret the loss of my partner but rejoice in the fact your appeal found me. Forgive my reticence but the matter is of such delicacy that to confide it to ink and paper would be unforgivable. There even exist solicitors who abhor scandal, if you can credit me, and I number myself among them.

Humbly,
Cyrus Sneeves, Esq.

My blood seemed to thin as a weightless excitement filled me.

No longer did I delude myself that I could usurp Highgate House from people I had grown to love; but if the property were clearly mine, perhaps I should not have to pen gallows ballads, or perhaps I could pen them from the relative luxury of a small Chelsea flat. I should not ask Mr. Thornfield for any staff or horses: merely enough of an allowance that I might live well, and my other expenses should be supplied by my writing. Mr. Thornfield had, after all, given a thousand pounds each to the white servants who had left his employ;

surely I, a woman for whom he harboured a slight attachment, could request assistance when Highgate House was legally mine?

And think that twice yearly—no, once a month, you might insist upon once a month—a cheque would be delivered to Mr. Sneeves and perhaps a letter with it! If you had his letters, you could have as much of him as here at Highgate House.

I dried my eyes. This would not be an ideal life, living with a tiny gouge where my heart had once been; but it would be a possible one, one which would make waiting to die more tolerable.

Since he could not touch me, what was it to him if I was here or in London? I had been accounted a good enough writer to earn my stout and oysters by it; if the endearments I showered him with, all the languidly falling petals of my shaken tree, were written rather than spoken, so much the better—he could read them over whensoever he liked, shove them in a drawer if he preferred, and my love would have some permanence, the way whispers made in the dead of night do not.

I retained his first letter by accident, the one regarding my ankle—I had set it upon the mantelpiece and simply forgot to bin it. Standing, I went to fetch the artefact; for a few seconds, I studied the curve of his *e*'s, and then I carefully refolded this as well as the latest note and placed them in the grey reticule I had bought at a slop shop off Covent Garden, thinking it would suit a governess.

Then I went to the mirror to survey the carnage; my features were so petite that eighty percent of them were blotchy, and my eyes so large that the whites appeared bloody pools. Washing my face in cold water helped a bit, and—when I beheld myself again—I realised that there was a third reason to go to London other than escaping Mr. Thornfield and finding Mr. Sneeves.

If I could settle this dark affair for the residents of Highgate House, would that not be a fine thing?

Resolved, I took a quiet moment to regard Aunt Patience's old room with all its lovely new trappings, the draperies in impossible shades of lavender and plum, the melancholy patina of winter moonlight . . . and then I set to packing.

Getting my things in order was not difficult, and I spent the rest of the night in a downy laudanum haze, only stopping the small doses when I collapsed into bed a mere few hours after quitting it. A brightly scouring sun woke me early, for I had forgot to draw the curtains; this was for the best, however, and I did my hair up carefully but looser than usual. Lifting my trunk, I carried it downstairs and left it in the hall.

The coward in me wanted to avoid Mr. Thornfield entirely and simply ask one of the Singhs in the stables to drop me in town. When I thought of the crags of his cynical brows, however, I knew I must explain myself or go mad to the tune of hearing, *Do you think me a blackguard following that terrible account, Jane?* So I went to the parlour and dining room and, finding them deserted, approached his study and knocked.

"Enter."

I peered in; Mr. Thornfield was writing a hurried correspondence, but he levered to his feet, rounding the desk. Either his gloves had been cleaned or he owned multiple pairs, for his linens were spotless and his cravat a rich flourish of burgundy; his cheeks below their sharp angles were sunken, however, and his eyes clearly questioned whether he was about to receive a greeting or a curse.

"The heroine emerges." The accompanying smile was a faintly glinting sickle. He approached me. "Oh, Jane, have you been crying all this while?"

"Some."

"God help us, you have every right, only I cannot bear to see it. You are unaware, I think, of the effect your misery has upon me."

"Perhaps so," I owned as another drop escaped.

He brushed it away with an almost reverential touch, then gestured at a chair and abruptly returned behind the desk. "Had you been a precious lamb and I a doting shepherd who found it rent by wolves, I couldn't feel any more harrowed over this—but you are not a lamb, thank Christ for that, you are a lioness and have no need of my bloody incompetent safeguarding. I shall make this all up to you in any way I can, however."

"I wondered . . ." Lowering myself into the chair, I hesitated. "I would appreciate an advance upon my wages."

"Of course." He was already pulling the cheque-book from the drawer. "How much?"

"Whatever you think fair, Mr. Thornfield."

An efficient scratching sounded. "Will a hundred pounds do?"

"You don't owe me a hundred pounds!" I exclaimed.

"Must I listen to her talk utter tripe so early in the morning?" he muttered, gripping the blotter. "Here—payment for initial services rendered, including delivering historical, scientific, deportmental, and elocutionary lessons translated into equine form, not to mention reparations for medical disasters. If you want more, you have only to say."

Swallowing, I placed the cheque in my reticule with the two letters. I did this, reader, because the most idiotic thing that Jane Eyre ever did other than to leave in the first place was to depart without her pearl necklace and half Mr. Rochester's fortune, which he would gladly have given her. If she had been eaten by a bear upon fleeing penniless into the wilderness, I should have shaken that bear's paw.

"How cheerless you look still," he reflected, stormy eyes feathering at their corners. "Come, ask me for something else so that I can say yes, saving only a trunk containing half a million in bauble-draped dolls, for damned if I've got it."

"So much?"

"Yes, blast the cursed thing."

I cleared my throat. "Mr. Thornfield, I came to tell you my things are packed."

He scarcely seemed surprised, and soon I fathomed why. "Do you prefer to take a bite of breakfast with me first, or shall I carry 'em over to the cottage so you can dine with Sahjara? I'll be glad of your company provided you can stomach mine, but you must wish to see her."

I twisted my fingers together in my lap. "Mr. Thornfield, I am quitting Highgate House. I cannot stay here."

Mere seconds had passed since he had called me a lamb he should have dreaded to see injured; even were I to etch the words I am now penning straight into the flesh of my arm, the slices would not cut me so thoroughly as his expression did. Far from protesting, Charles Thornfield froze in surprise, then seemed to crumple, as if taking a blow which was not unexpected.

"No, it isn't that," I pleaded. "It's not your story, nor the distress I was caused—I want to hear all of your woes, and I'd wield a knife for your sake a thousand times over, but you honestly cannot want me to have charge of your ward."

"Why the devil not?" he demanded hoarsely.

"Because . . . because you know me to be a murderer."

"For Christ's sake, Jane, that makes a neatly matched pair of us. We'll set up snug as salt and pepper cellars and Sardar can give sermons to us in the garden of a Sunday."

Mr. Thornfield's shoulders bristled after this statement was hurled at me; but it was all bravado, for he searched my eyes as if all his many missed turnings were mapped in them.

"I . . . But of course, you were in two wars," I stammered. "That isn't the same thing at all."

Charles Thornfield drew a stuttering breath—but instead of speaking, he brushed a hand over his lips, shutting his eyes in despair.

"This is why I cannot stay," I cried. Rushing to the desk, I took both his gloved hands, which shook like the fine tremor in the bow after the arrow has flown. "You could tell me all and never diminish yourself in my estimation, but these half confidences are like Solomon's suggestion of cutting a child in half. I understand what it is to feel so myself, for you *know* I have secrets, and it would never be enough, sharing fractions when I'm the greediest soul in shoe leather. I should blurt it all out, every sordid sin, and want the same of you, be petty and selfish and the most hateful person you've ever known when you deny me."

"That is the most whopping pack of calumnies I have ever heard," he husked, shifting my hands in his and studying them where they sat cradled. "Take 'em back this instant. You could never be hateful. And Sahjara will . . ." He shook his head, still not raising his eyes. "I hardly know what to say to her. Or to Sardar, either."

"Tell them I ruined everything, that I always ruin everything."

"Stop this," he growled. "It was my own wretched fault. You are a young woman—intelligent, beautiful, vibrant. Why should you wish to live with a pair of ruined men in a house full of ghosts?"

"But I never minded that! Only you ought to be free to see ghosts without my demanding to know where the bodies are buried. I've always wanted too much, sir—your not wanting me back doesn't make you culpable."

"I never said I didn't want you."

"You could say it now," I requested, heart hammering.

"No." He glanced up at last. Whatever gnawed him, it had burrowed through to the bone. "I could *not* say that, Jane."

"Heaven help me, this is madness." I leant forward, half-seated on his desk and inches from his weathered features. "The whole truth, is that what you want—*my* truth in exchange for your own? It could quite literally cost me my life, I . . . You know what happened when Ghosh attacked me, and—"

"That was self-defence, you raving—"

"But I'd not care, I wouldn't, not so long as you loved me. I should be the happiest woman on earth if you did. Anyone would be."

"The last one wasn't."

I suspect something else would have happened there in that cosy study, our lips parted and eyes ablaze with both craving and restraint, had we not heard steadily approaching footfalls.

"Jane!" he protested when I pulled away, but I turned my back as he rose, composing myself, and so it was in the mirror above the hearth that I first saw the door swing open following a confident knock and Inspector Sam Quillfeather enter the room.

I did not scream; it was a near thing, however.

"Oh, gracious me, what was I thinking barging in so?"

Teeth set tight as a ship's hull and eyes glued to the mirror, I took in Mr. Quillfeather. He had aged, but not diminished, and the perennial forward sweep of his spine and the exaggerated arches of his nose and chin and brow would already have imparted an impression of relentless momentum without the additional trajectory of his steel-grey shock of hair as he swept off his shabby beaver hat.

"Quillfeather." My employer quickly forced his features into neutrality, but this only left him resembling a tattered shoreline after a squall.

"I'll come back after surveying the cellar?" Mr. Quillfeather proposed, voice retaining the old questioning lilt. "I'm before my time, I see—yes, three full minutes! Won't you forgive me? I'll just—"

"No, no, it's all right." Mr. Thornfield coughed. "Inspector Sam Quillfeather, may I introduce Miss Jane Stone, Sahjara's governess?"

There was nothing for it: I forced my fists to unclench and turned to face the gallows.

He might not recognise you, not after so many years and so much sorrow, I told myself.

Gallantly, he made a neat bow over my hand; and then his eyes met mine, variegated hazel and canny as ever, and a spark flared to life, and I was caught. For Highgate House had been mine before my disappearance and here I was again, and he could not help but know me.

"Mrs. Stone, I take it?" he clarified. "It is very good to see you again in these parts. A country widow and so young?"

"No indeed, she comes to us from London."

Mr. Quillfeather studied me, and then Mr. Thornfield added his curious gaze to the already potent atmosphere, and I was just considering the benefits of throwing myself into the fireplace when the inspector waved his hand in the air.

"Of course, of course, I must have momentarily mistook her? The older I get, the more everything and everyone manages to remind me of, well, of something or someone else entirely? Pleased to meet you, Miss Stone."

"Likewise," I managed.

The floor was opening like a pit beneath me, gravity turned upside down.

"Was Miss Stone affected by these dreadful events?" Mr. Quillfeather asked, politely addressing Mr. Thornfield.

The trail of bodies, oh God, he knows, he must know, first Edwin for certain and then Vesalius Munt in all likelihood, and now there just happens to be another carcass needs burying and here I—

Mr. Thornfield hesitated not a whit. "Miss Stone arrived downstairs first following the crash which alerted us, and suffered injury at Jack Ghosh's hands—but thankfully, he was already bleeding out. I'll show you the window and the glass, naturally, but it's all quite straightforward. Hoisted upon his own petard at last, if you'll pardon my satisfied tone, Quillfeather."

"Nothing to pardon, my good man! You suspect Sack's behind this?"

"I should be a simpleton not to."

"Yes, yes, we'll work it out between us, won't we? How was the young lady injured?"

"Torn scalp. It bled considerably, and she nary made a sound. If you ask me, the blackguard could have died for that alone and I should have said good riddance," Mr. Thornfield droned in his haughtiest tone even as his eyes dared me to contradict him.

"Might I see, Miss Stone?" Sam Quillfeather asked gently.

What could I do? I bent my head, and Mr. Thornfield cupped my nape in a tender touch I did not think planned, and Mr. Quillfeather tutted, "Shameful, Thornfield, simply shameful," and I raised my face after a gentle press to my neck preceded both men stepping back.

"What luck it was only a minor insult?" Again Mr. Quillfeather turned to Mr. Thornfield for confirmation, and the latter nodded curtly. Then the inspector glanced back at me.

"A painful hurt, and a lucky escape," he repeated. "Frankly, it . . . reminds me of something, Miss Stone?"

A torn sleeve and a cousin dead at the bottom of a ravine. My mouth turned instantly dry.

"Jane, why don't you lie down for a little?" Mr. Thornfield suggested, the gash between his brows thickening. "These have been trying times, and for no one more than yourself. Go to the parlour and try the settee—I'll be along after I post Quillfeather here, all right?"

"Just the thing—can you make it unescorted, Miss Stone?" the inspector asked, bending forward solicitously.

"Yes," said I. "Please don't concern yourselves."

"We'll talk further soon," Charles Thornfield said, voice as tight as it was fond. "Sleep if you can, but we shouldn't be more than an hour."

"Take your time. Excuse me, gentlemen."

When I walked into the corridor, I paused for only a second; one glance at the packed trunk persuaded me to leave it behind. It contained nothing I wanted, not without Mr. Thornfield, and I carried the cheque and my collection of letters in my reticule. Walking at first, then sprinting, I raced for the stables and ordered Nalin saddled and after stealing the horse he had given me, I rode hell for leather towards the village.

TWENTY-FIVE

Some say there is enjoyment in looking back to painful experience past; but at this day I can scarcely bear to review the times to which I allude: the moral degradation, blent with the physical suffering, form too distressing a recollection ever to be willingly dwelt on.

I left the spirited mare in the care of the inn, leaving explicit instructions that it should be returned to Highgate House and whatever man they sent would be compensated; this transaction complete, I booked a seat on the next coach with coin collected writing gallows ballads, which stock had not been depleted. Then I bought a penny roll and sat upon a bench outside the inn and began numbly to eat, knowing the miles ahead to be slow and dreary as the Thames.

I had an hour's worth, more or less, of a head start, and the gallop had taken a mere ten minutes. The coach, meanwhile, should leave in half an hour, and *perhaps Mr. Thornfield has not yet been told by Mr. Quillfeather I pushed a child over a cliff and speared a headmaster through the neck, perhaps—*

"Miss Stone?"

Thankfully I had forced the last of the roll down, else I should have suffocated; there stood Mr. Sardar Singh, warmly bundled, a sheaf of papers tucked under his arm, his the only head in the sluggish trickle of pedestrians which had been wrapped in an elaborate configuration of sky blue (which doubtless accounted for the hostile stares). He was accompanied by Mrs. Garima Kaur, who was recording something in a small pocketbook; her gaunt face looked still more stark than usual, her eyes lost in the curves of her skull.

"Oh!" I exclaimed, shrinking. "What are you doing here, Mr. Singh?"

"Picking up blank death certificates for Charles from the village physician—we're not quite outfitted fully, and are to meet with Mr. Sam Quillfeather today."

"Yes, he's there at the house."

I knew I did not sound right; I hated that I did not sound right. Mr. Singh turned to Mrs. Kaur, conferring in Punjabi. She looked at me so oddly, a mingling of inquisitiveness and something I could not identify, that I averted my eyes; thus I only saw in my periphery that, after a muted request, Mrs. Kaur began walking briskly back in the direction of Highgate House.

"We are quite alone, Miss Stone, unless you wish it otherwise," I heard Mr. Singh state.

My vision blurred until I was seeing from the bottom of a lake; then the bench squeaked and a hand was at my elbow.

"What in heaven's name is— Has something else happened, Miss Stone?"

"Nothing to speak of."

"Miss Stone, please know I would hold any confidence from you under eternal lock and key."

"It isn't that I don't trust you."

"Then please assure me that you're all right," he insisted more strongly.

Several seconds passed.

"I'm not all right," I choked at last. "I cannot remain in Mr. Thornfield's company."

Ascertaining what the stuffy, sausage-smelling citizens of that hamlet thought of a Sikh dressed as an Englishman wrapping his arms around a governess as she sobbed soundlessly into his coat would be quite impossible, for I could see nothing whatsoever. However many stares we garnered, the activity served a dual purpose; my heart was breaking, so the simple comfort was appreciated; and if I keened over cruel fate and lost love, I should not have to explain I was also running away to London to escape execution.

"Yes, there . . . that's better," he said as I calmed. "Miss Stone, may I ask what brought matters to this state?"

His grey eyes were bright with compassion when I pulled away. After he had passed me his handkerchief and sat there patiently as the quaking in my shoulders lessened, I found I did indeed wish to speak with him, and still had fifteen minutes before my coach departed.

"Forgive me for making such a scene."

"Not at all."

"It's just . . . the night I killed that scoundrel, Mr. Thornfield told me about your sister and Sahjara's abduction and the trunk, and it's horrible you were dragged into such a nightmare, and I know you both to be honourable, but he says he's a murderer and he won't say how or when, and he won't say he doesn't want me, he won't say anything at all of consequence, nor touch me, nor trust me, and I *cannot bear it* any longer."

"Ah," he said. "Then your sorrow is partly my doing, and I have been gravely at fault."

"Regarding?"

"Charles's refusal to touch living people."

My mouth must have gaped overlong for, passing his fingertips over his beard, he continued after a brief reflection.

"Charles emulates me, always has done. Even when I have tried to prevent him. But the specific point I am making, Miss Stone,"

Mr. Singh said, measuring his words, "is that I am both devout and monastic, and I think Charles may well have confused the two. I have never been married. I have no interest in marriage or its accompanying joys."

I stared, yes, but he did not seem ruffled. "You have never loved, then?"

"That is not remotely what I meant," he corrected mildly.

"Oh. You are . . ."

I trailed off, helpless; after he had registered shock, he shook his head.

"No," he answered firmly. "Ah, I see why you—I beg your pardon. Yes, of course I love Charles, but no."

I thought a little longer. "You are like a priest? Devoted to God and to study?"

"There we have it," he approved before the shadow returned to his face. "But you must understand, it is very easy for someone who is not tempted by flesh to be celibate, and I have always been so—content to watch the moon rise, to try a new spice, to practise the *chakkar* but never use it to harm. When I was small, I dreamt of sitting under a tree, waiting for God to possess me with divine knowledge which would incinerate my very soul. If God told me to give up strong coffee, I would feel that loss keenly, and God would thus honour my sacrifice. But I do not actually long for the thing I abstain from—which is not abstinence at all. So I am simply wondering whether, in my own infinite ignorance, I contributed to this great error Charles has made."

"Nothing you've said implies you were gravely at fault in any way."

"Then I have not helped so much as I ought to have done."

"Why should you help me?"

"Why should I not? Help Charles is what I meant, however." He sighed. "His life, his body—I have told you already such sacrifices occur in the Guru, but this is a needlessly raised shield after the battle has already left one bloody."

"You've plenty to fear yet, it seems," I reminded him, feeling Jack Ghosh's fingers crushing my soft throat.

"That is a new battle," he corrected, frowning. "I never dreamt of the old battle haunting us here save in ways you have already mentioned—our own. It's most peculiar, if you ask me. This trunk business must have an end put to it, for Sahjara's sake if not ours."

And I shall help in any way I can, I vowed to myself.

Mr. Singh's face took on the quality of a death mask. "Did Charles tell you whom he murdered, if neither how nor when?"

I shook my head.

"Do not believe him, then, when he claims to be a murderer," he said hoarsely. "Unless he has been killing other people than the one I am thinking of, he is not to be trusted on the subject."

"I don't know how many subjects he is to be trusted upon—he said he should never miss exile from the Punjab, for instance."

"He and I are agreed." His voice scraped now, a blade being sharpened upon a stone. "I loved Lahore, but to watch an empire sabotage itself so? We were all meant to be lions, but some of us proved unshorn dogs. Why do you suppose we are warriors, Miss Stone? It is because our Gurus have been sat upon red-hot iron plates and covered with scorching sand, sewn into raw hides which shrank and broke their bones, had pegs thrust in their heads and their brains removed when yet alive. My people have been slaughtered like animals, our cities sacked, children's bellies slit, our sacred pool filled with our hacked-apart bodies, and for what? So we might throw away the richest land in all of Asia?" His hands spasmed into fists. "I was not exaggerating when I said my sister should have been maharani—instead, the Company butchered us like cattle. There is too much blood in the sands of the Punjab, Miss Stone."

I did not know what to say. We watched the inching progression of a sweet-faced crone on the arm of her grandson, listened as the church's bell sang salutations to the heavens, marked the stares slitting towards us in charcoal shadows of doubt and disgust.

"Mr. Thornfield implied that as long as you and Sahjara are here, he has all the home he requires."

A smile barely brushed the corners of his lips. "He does us honour, then."

Nodding bleakly, I checked the inn's entrance. The carriage had clattered into the manure-strewn yard and I rose, indicating it to Mr. Singh with my eyes; he stood, looking appalled.

"But—*now*? Where is your trunk, where your farewell to the household, why—"

"I can't." I forced back the tears which newly threatened. "Please tell Sahjara I love her, and ask her forgiveness. If—when I see her again, I'll be glad of it. Mr. Thornfield gave me a hundred pounds. I'll be fine. I still have my knife to protect me from *badmashes*."

I did not achieve a second smile, but the set of his lips did grow a shade less alarmed.

Clasping my hand, he said, "In that case, farewell, Miss Jane Stone, and send us word of your whereabouts at once. Should you ever wish to trade the name Jane Stone for Jane Kaur, however, you should make a wise and courageous Sikh princess, and must return to us immediately. I beg you to consider it—the return, at least, if not the new moniker."

Walking towards the coach was like pulling my own skin off, but Mr. Singh helped by stepping back courteously.

"Keep them safe," I called when I reached the tall step. "Parting from you, from Sahjara, from Mr. Thornfield—well, the poets are liars. It isn't sweet sorrow at all, it's like dying a little."

Mr. Singh turned towards the half-timbered hostelry and Mr. Thornfield's waiting carriage. "So often the way," he agreed sombrely, "with partings."

. . .

My journey to London was a clanking, frigid stretch of dull farms and weathered church spires during which none of the other passengers so much as snored in my direction. When I at last arrived in the city, still shaking from the road's vibrations as well as nerves, I knew myself too sensible simply to crawl to a low lodging-house in Drury Lane and forget the sour bedclothes with the help of a pint of rum; so I walked for a few miles, stopping before the door of a seedy theatre for a ham sandwich with mustard and a tin cup of coffee.

Restored, I recalled a guesthouse called the Weathercock in Orchard Street, Westminster, where I had lived for a few weeks high on the hog with the best-paid and best-educated literary patterers. As I was already near Marylebone, travelling there by foot would be easy as blinking, so I thanked the sandwich man and set off.

All was as I remembered it, a pretty white-painted building with gas lamps aglow at either side of the broad front steps, and men of letters guffawing over politics in the lobby. When I rang the bell, the clerk expressed dismay at my lack of luggage; however, as I had the commodities of both tears and money at the ready, pleading railway thieves, I had soon obtained his sympathies, and he vowed to send the boots round for toiletries, laudanum (my pate ached something terrible, as did my heart), and a packet of tooth powder.

The Weathercock had a lending library for the consideration of 1d. per week, to be paid upon Sundays, but I further endeared myself to the establishment by paying for this privilege immediately, made a selection based upon the volume having slipped down against its cohorts in a defeated diagonal posture, and took a glass of hot brandy and lemon to my room.

After a desolate time spent nursing that toddy—though no tears, for the rest of them had taken up residence in Mr. Singh's coat—I had produced a plan of action. This was three-pronged, and intended the following goals be achieved:

—Remove all threat from the lives endangered by Augustus P. Sack
—Ascertain whether you are the heiress of Highgate House
—Escape the clutches of Mr. Sam Quillfeather and avoid the noose

Penning this last, I shivered. Inspector Quillfeather may well have forgot everything, may well have indulged his friend Charles Thornfield, may well even have wanted to see the corpse before leaping to conclusions; but I had witnessed his absolute recognition of me, had heard him suggest I must have been a widow in a polite effort to explain why he was addressing a Stone and not a Steele. Sam Quillfeather was decorous and might even be kind; Sam Quillfeather was not stupid, however, and he had just examined the body of yet another chap slaughtered by my hands.

By my calculation, knowing where I stood upon these matters now that I had vanished would take me no more than a fortnight; resolving them, no more than a few months. I had enough money to live for some two years with only the hundred pounds Mr. Thornfield bestowed, provided I practised economy, and meanwhile the boots had delivered a fresh evening edition to my room with my other requests, and the paper was chock-full of executions. With hard work added to the formula, it would be enough; I might linger here, and so bury myself in projects that no one should see I was transparent by daylight, a ghost with a soul of smoke and secrets.

Once resolved, I picked up the edition I had selected upon a whim, and began the novel.

There was no possibility of taking a walk that day. . . .

. . .

It will seem peculiar to the reader, doubtless, but I awoke to my exile feeling much refreshed the next morning.

After all, I had a set of purposes; the frenzy of fright I had been driven into by the reappearance of Sam Quillfeather was quite dampened here in the world's greatest cesspool; and the daily agony of seeing Charles Thornfield as if through a glass case in a museum display had ended. Additionally, London crackles and buzzes; it spits and it decays and it shines. I had missed it without knowing, so engrossed had I been by my new companions, but now I felt afresh the energy a metropolis can infuse into its strivers.

The first thing to be done was to purchase new—by which I mean secondhand, but far more opulent—togs, which would further two out of my three schemes.

I obtained a glass of porter and a good penny plate of bread and fried haddock at a pub first, and then took a crowded omnibus towards Aldgate. Far from Highgate House, my abandoned frocks were recalled as spinsterish and depressing rather than merely dull, for I had never dressed so in the city; I had sometimes been destitute and never wealthy, but it must have been my French half insisting upon the richest plaid capes despite their threadbare edges, the daintiest buttoned boots.

Aldgate was a veritable sea of plate glass, a thousand welcoming eyes reflecting happy glints from the gas jets. Even in the wet grey mire of winter, the countless shops were a cheery sight—but I had no intention of making purchases on the main thoroughfare. Instead I veered towards St. Paul's by way of Fenchurch Street, and after traversing salt-strewn cobbles for a few blocks, I found the haven I had sought: a nondescript window gleaming citron and edged with holly branches, with no sign posted save for PRIVATE ALTERATIONS UNDERTAKEN. I rang the bell.

So close to Aldgate, secondhand shops kept as demure as middle-class whores, but this was the best of them, and soon I was prattling away with two familiar saleswomen who cooed and clucked over my present drab attire, waltzing about to find something of the sort I had used to like. When I explained money slipped easier through my fingers of late, and that I must dress more like a lady than my previous blithe showiness, our budding friendship was sealed—I suspect they imagined I had a dalliance with the master of the house where I tutored, a hypothesis only vexing because I had failed to do exactly that. I departed the shop with my arms full, promising to return for three more frocks they were altering to my shape.

Next stop after another omnibus ride was the Soho Bazaar, where the rosy-cheeked craftswomen rent stalls inside the row houses at the northwest of Soho Square. By the time I quit this fairyland—equipped with new gloves and a stole and several hats—I was fagged enough to take a hansom back to the Weathercock, drawing a sly but amused stare from my new friend the clerk when he saw me dressed colourfully as a child's top and laden with plunder.

My room, after I had piled my twine-adorned parcels and be-ribboned hatboxes upon the bed, seemed much the barer for the additions. Mr. Thornfield may not have known my real nature, but he had spoken compass-true when he observed I sought companionship as bees do nectar.

Restlessly, I pulled off my gloves and hung my new powder-blue hooded cloak, and surveyed the afternoon dress I wore in the long glass.

It was the finest dress I had ever owned: dull silk, of a colour as much green as it was brown that made my eyes gleam like mahogany, painted asymmetrically with vines of delicate vermillion roses; along the bosom, the cinched waist, and the fully draped sleeves were barred pairs of emerald stripes. A single cascade of tiny buttons dripped from neck to waist, and it occurred to me, seeing the mischievous tilt to my lips, that I had never looked better.

I am far too vain to even attempt the prevarication this brought me no foolish pleasure; but my eyes soon prickled because there was no one of importance to see me, and I turned hastily away to store my new belongings.

That task accomplished, I sat down to write a pair of letters. The first need not be recounted as it was merely the request for an appointment with Mr. Cyrus Sneeves, eagerly informing him I was now in London; the second had required more imaginative plotting.

Room 26,
the Weathercock,
Orchard Street,
Westminster

Dear Mr. Augustus Sack,

I hope you will remember meeting the governess, one Miss Jane Stone, upon your dramatically terminated visit to Highgate House not two months previous. My note concerns matters confidential in nature, for I gather through your own curtailed speech and hints dropped by the always sinister Messrs. Charles Thornfield and Sardar Singh that acquaintances were renewed at Mr. John Clements's funeral which rekindled old grievances.

I hereby confess that I was so frightened by their display of weaponry that I embarked upon my own private investigation. As a governess, I was in no financial position to quit any master even if he should be a scoundrel—pray exercise your empathy, Mr. Sack, when I tell you I was determined to learn all I could in the interests of my own safety.

Pausing, I poured myself a glass of the claret I had rung for, reading my lies back over. It should not do to lay it on too thick;

however, Sack had seemed more of a vicious bully than a master criminal. I dipped my pen once more.

The results of this amateur exploit have been most fruitful—indeed, I may well have learnt the whereabouts of a long-lost object.

Letters to me can be sent to the above address under the name Miss Jane Smith, as bloody deeds were enacted which precipitated my flight from Highgate House. Speak to no one of Miss Stone, if you would be so kind; a Mr. Jack Ghosh, or so I have been told he was identified, broke in during the small hours and died of some misadventure. Singh and Thornfield give out to the police inspector that he cut his thigh upon a piece of window glass when entering, but I cannot believe this account, and when I made the discovery which enabled my departure, the devil himself could not have spirited me away quick enough.

It is this matter of finances of which I wish to speak with you. Do not entertain the idea of coming to my lodgings, for I am not in immediate possession of the item in question; send me a summons for an appointment, however, and we may be able to assist each other.

Expectantly,
Miss Jane S——

I addressed the envelope to Mr. Sack in care of the undersecretary at the Company's headquarters, which was the intentionally imposing East India House in Leandenhall Street. Having passed it before, I realised it suited what I knew of the Company itself: opulent, powerful, and cold as marble.

An equally frigid smile touched my lips at the thought I might soon enter its stone maw, a predator in the guise of a slender young woman.

TWENTY-SIX

The fact is, I was a trifle beside myself; or rather out of myself, as the French would say. . . .

Days of preparation followed, reader, ones which left me in a strange daze of commingled purpose and despair. By now, I thought I might actually expire without Mr. Thornfield, sudden heartaches piercing with the lances of a hundred Khalsa cavalry; at others, I felt haler to know I served him still. I read my borrowed novel twice through, then bought a copy at a quaint bookstall—I have not yet got *out* of the habit of reading *Jane Eyre*, come to that—and idled, and schemed, and awaited answers to my letters.

I had only to wait one day to hear from Mr. Sneeves; he was from home, the message having been forwarded, and so I must wait two more days to meet with him. Hastily agreeing to this via his clerk, I gnawed my thumb and hoped for a missive from Mr. Augustus Sack.

I got one, too, on the very morning I was to meet with my solicitor, and it read as follows:

East India House, Leadenhall Street

My dear Miss Smith,

Of course I recall the pleasure of your company, a boon which rendered bearable an otherwise profoundly distressing journey. I confess that, though I may have an inkling of the matter to which you refer, the less said in written form the better, for this is very much a Company affair, and therefore I propose you visit me in my office. My hours are from eight to seven, but a request from you could find me there at any time.

Very sincerely &etc.,
Mr. Augustus P. Sack

My lips twisted into what resembled a smile, but may have invested the casual observer with more fear than mirth.

Then I donned another of my new frocks in order to properly present myself to Mr. Sneeves. This costume was all of the same patternless fabric, a shimmering fawn colour, but the detailing was exquisite—ten deep pleats, a plain band of the same fabric at the waist, and then it blossomed into fold after fold, like a modern woman's dream of a Renaissance belle.

My eccentric looks did not quite do the workmanship justice; but next I added a calculated finishing touch, a demure but real set of necklace and earrings, the stones of which the jeweller assured me had travelled straight from the Punjab. I had sixty pounds of Mr. Thornfield's advance remaining, and I assured myself that the rest of the money could not possibly have been better spent.

The first sense engaged upon entering Mr. Sneeves's offices was that of smell; the reek of snuff greeted me long before the man himself did, though he was scrupulously prompt. Mr. Sneeves introduced himself in a reedy voice, hastened me into his consulting room, and shut the door.

As soon as we were alone, he lifted a teak snuffbox. "You don't mind, I hope?"

"Not at all."

I must waste no time over describing the chamber—the usual maelstrom of ledgers, untidy bookshelves, and the like—for Mr. Sneeves had my passionate attention. He was a little man with a great round balding dome covered in freckles, as if his shoulders had sprouted a mushroom. Though of fine quality, his black coat was in no way ostentatious, and I realised that—apart from the almost dizzying aroma of snuff—Mr. Sneeves preferred his clients to forget they had ever required his services at all.

"You are most accommodating. Thank you." Mr. Sneeves set the snuffbox down and commenced staring at me with pale eyes beneath thistly brows.

An interminable period passed, during which my sweat began to seep forth like morning dew.

"Pardon, Miss Steele, but you stir up old memories," Mr. Sneeves concluded at last, sitting back in his chair. "You resemble your mother, you know, save in colouring—that is entirely upon the paternal side. What should you prefer to drink?"

I sat there, dumb; resembling my adored mother was enough news, leaving me hotly aglow, without the fact that I apparently took after my unremembered father as well. Meanwhile, Mr. Sneeves was already headed for the sideboard with a shuffling gait. I reminded myself of the role Jane Steele was to play today—a moderately interested but well-off woman, that she might get all answers not generally imparted to a beggar at the door.

"Thank you, but I—"

"You must have a taste of something fortifying, Miss Steele, for I fear I may shock you. There are a few solicitors, you will find, who are actually aware their clients possess sensibilities. Sherry?"

"Please," I said rather faintly, "though . . ."

"Brandy, then," he curtly suggested. "Considering your background, it must have been administered as a restorative at one time or another, and once having had brandy, one ought not go backwards."

The man, for all his resemblance to your more affable variety of fungus, was riveting. I drew my soft blue cloak, which I had neglected to shed, closer about my frame as Mr. Cyrus Sneeves planted a brandy snifter before me; he deposited half as much before himself and resumed his place behind the desk.

I soon came to understand from his complete silence that I was expected to make an overture.

"Mr. Sneeves, thank you for seeing me—you must have wondered at my letter's contents."

"Heavens, no." Mr. Sneeves took another great pinch of snuff, making my own eyes water. "No, Miss Steele, I only wondered who told you about me."

Faltering, I removed my gloves. "My mother left a few letters—"

"May I see them?"

Turning over my mother's letters felt a strangely intimate act, for all that my solicitor would learn nothing he did not already know; I had so little of Mamma left that all my relics were magical, more talismans than mementoes. At last, finished, Mr. Sneeves scrubbed a hand over his mottled pate.

"Miss Steele," he questioned, "do you know more of your legal standing beyond what I have just read?"

When I shook my head, he rapped his desk, as if signalling the start of a race. "I was first recommended to your father in Paris, where Englishmen often preferred to do business with a firm operating upon both sides of the water. His concerns had to do with his status as a landholder. Highgate House was in good repair, but your father desired to settle minor liens and generally ascertain whether keeping the manor was feasible; I am happy to state that he was doing very well indeed in Paris, no less than were his partners in London, and so my advice was, if the property gave him pleasure, to keep it. It was not only matters of his estate upon which he consulted me, however."

Mr. Sneeves waited as my heart pounded a brisk martial beat.

"And these other matters?"

"Were matters to do with your mother." His voice softened, and he smoothed errant grey wisps behind his ears. "Mrs. Anne-Laure Steele was such a woman as you do not meet twice in life, Miss Steele—beautiful, charming, and artistic. Sadly, not long after your first birthday, your father fell prey to an inflammation of the lungs, and your parents wished to know your precise legal standing in Britain should the worst happen. I was tasked with setting measures in place to ensure both you and Mrs. Steele were protected. You remember your aunt, Mrs. Patience Barbary?"

"Naturally."

Mr. Sneeves, dappled head bobbing, made quick work of gathering papers. "She was very strongly against your and your mother's residing at Highgate House—and your father proved to be ill with consumption at an advanced and virulent stage, so your parents were forced to act quickly. Here is the marriage license between Anne-Laure Fortier and Jonathan David Steele; here also is a special contract they devised to be signed by your aunt as a dowager, stating that Highgate House should be your sanctuary for life."

I examined the documents. Rather than clearing the mists, however, the atmosphere thickened—*sanctuary for life* did not mean *inheritance.* For the first time, I examined my mother's statements against the backdrop of what I knew to be true as an adult woman. Unmarried females scarce ever inherited, particularly when wills were disputed; my mother had assured me of my place time and again, but had never explained the whys or wherefores.

Meanwhile, supposing it was mine, why should Mamma and I have lived in the cottage, why not the main house, why should not Aunt Patience and Edwin have lived in—

"Miss Steele, do you know the man in this picture?"

I found myself holding a sketch from a French newspaper describing a series of audacious trades enacted at the Palais de la Bourse.

"Of course—this is my uncle," I answered readily. "Richard Barbary."

"That is your father," Mr. Cyrus Sneeves said, "who for a time—when courting your mother in the guise of a rich gentleman of leisure—went by the name Jonathan Steele."

"No, no." The words emerged before I even had thought them. "That's impossible."

Mr. Sneeves made no answer; I stared at the artist's rendering, all breath ripped from my lungs.

Richard Barbary's portraits had occupied many places of honour at Highgate House before the arrival of Mr. Thornfield, and here he was in starkly inked miniature: a calculating businessman with an air of mischief about him. Effortlessly, I recalled how those portraits had beckoned to me, with their brown eyes like mine, their mocking half smiles, their air of roguish mystery.

I felt as if my bones were curling up inside my body.

"It can't be," I whispered, knowing it true.

Mr. Sneeves took a fortifying pinch of snuff.

"Mr. Richard Barbary was one of our best clients, Miss Steele, and when he informed us of the . . . situation, we strove in every way to accommodate him. Initially, he had only sought an affair with your mother, who was quite destitute save for the odd sou made from her street portraits and work as a cabaret dancer in Montmartre, which I believe is how the pair met. But when Anne-Laure Fortier and Richard Barbary had lived together for over six months and she informed him of her pregnancy, he impetuously determined that her pleas for wedlock be indulged, and he married her under the false name he had given, fearing to reveal all and lose her regard. This was no light task, but your father was a rich man, and so managed the necessary documentation—he avoided mentioning the fact, of course, that he had already left a wife and child behind in England."

Fighting dizziness, I marked him, the words falling as lightly upon my ears as the patter of rain upon a window.

My half brother. Edwin, who tried to rape me, was not my cousin, he was my half—

"Here you are, Miss Steele," a smooth voice intoned.

I drained the brandy Mr. Sneeves had thrust beneath my nose and watched as he poured another, setting it within easy reach. Memories untangled themselves before my eyes, twisting and contorting—Aunt Patience's calling my friendship with her son *family feeling,* my mother's open disgust for Edwin, my aunt's visible loathing of me. Sickened, I tasted the spirits again.

"Tell me," I rasped. "Everything. Please."

Mr. Sneeves sniffed, not unkindly. "I fully intend to. Miss Steele, when your father first fell ill, another event threatened the tranquillity of his, ah, French family life: your mother found a portrait of Patience and Edwin Barbary amongst his belongings. These led to a frenzied quarrel, but your father soon fell into agreement with his illegitimate second spouse: he had no intention of abandoning you, not even in death, for a match begun in the sort of lies wealthy men tell had developed into profound mutual devotion. Mrs. Barbary, I ought to mention, was dealt a bad hand—she was an arrangement made by your paternal grandfather in the interests of money and pedigree, and though your father never loved her, I believe she loved your father, or so Anne-Laure Steele led me to conjecture."

Recalling all the times my aunt begged my mother not to speak of Jonathan Steele, recalling in my mother's own letter to the firm her reluctant, *when I imagine myself in her shoes, I cannot bring myself to censure her*, I felt as if my world had been blasted to shrapnel, and I left clutching the shards with bleeding fingers.

"Why did my father create such a wretched quagmire?"

"As much as in looks you resemble your mother, Miss Steele, you have your father's direct manner about you, and I find I must battle nostalgia in your presence."

"I cannot begin to imagine whether or not that is a compliment," I rasped. "Please continue."

"Very well, then. Mr. Barbary was the heir to an estate which might once have proven impossible to maintain; he was told to marry Patience Goodwill, whose holdings after her elder sister, Chastity, eloped were considerable. After he proved himself an expert trader here at Capel Court and her wealth proved superfluous, the marriage, already fragile, fizzled despite the birth of a son named Edwin."

"Is that the reason he fled to France?"

"I believe so, though the story given out emphasised the professional benefits of his temporarily relocating. In any case, Mr. Barbary travelled to Paris when offered a liaison with one of la Bourse's officially licensed *agents de change*, and he presented himself to your mother as a gentleman of leisure named Jonathan Steele. You were conceived, your parents were married, your father fell ill, your mother found out his true marital status, and he and your mother threatened Patience Barbary with exposure of all his sins should she refuse to cooperate—your father blackmailed his wife with his own ill-usage of her, knowing the second marriage illegal."

It fit everything I knew, and it hurt accordingly—from my scalp to my soles, I was altered.

I am not who I thought I was.

Neither had Edwin been—he was my dear, repellent, spoilt brother rather than my dear, repellent, spoilt cousin. What other grotesque errors had I made in my life that I should find myself sitting in an office being told my own father's name?

Meanwhile, my mother—oh, my *mother.* It had been a love match; I had not needed Mr. Sneeves to tell me so. She had been mad with grief over him, and now I understood that Aunt Patience had been similarly afflicted; two women, both in love with a different name, forced to live with revolting insults right before their eyes. It would have been sensible to have hated my aunt Patience all the more now I knew she had kept me in ignorance, to have loathed my father as a philanderer and my mother as a blackmailer; rotten as my own core had proven, all I could do was pity the lot of them.

As for my half brother, I reflected with the cold scrape of an icicle down my spine, *the less contemplation of Edwin the better.* Everything I knew about my blood and bones had been stripped from me, leaving me bare.

"Is my name even Jane Steele?"

"If you like—we've no documentation save that name, so if it suits you better than Jane Fortier . . ."

"It does." I sighed, draining the second brandy. "Mr. Sneeves, supposing as the illegitimate daughter of Richard Barbary I can do nothing whatsoever regarding Highgate House, what is the wrong you meant to put right?"

Mr. Sneeves wheezed in disbelief. "I should have though that was obvious."

"It isn't," said I, with some asperity.

"Miss Steele, I am sorry for what you have learnt today," Mr. Sneeves replied, clasping his fingers together. "But the wrong I meant to right was that you should *know* who you *are*, as I had strong suspicions that no one ever bothered to tell you. You are not without inheritance."

"Oh." It was all I could summon.

"You have an allowance of three hundred a year." Cyrus Sneeves wrote a note to himself, as if that clinched matters. "You do not possess any part of Highgate House, but your independence is assured, as guaranteed by Mr. Richard Barbary. I have your current address here from your last correspondence, I take it? Very good. I shall lose no time in setting up an account for you to draw upon and transferring your yearly allotments there, which after all this time amounts to a tidy nest egg. Lacking your whereabouts but hoping you lived still, I held the funds in trust. Now. Is there anything else I can do for you?"

Dazed, I glanced again at the newspaper sketch of my father. As a child, I had felt about his portraits as I would an imaginary friend; trying to summon greater depth of feeling now, however, I found the task impossible. He was a collection of pen strokes who resembled me vaguely. I ought to have felt grateful to know him at last; instead, I felt grateful for his money.

"Yes," I said quietly. "Burn any evidence of their wrongdoing save documents attending to my stipend, including the letters I brought you from my mother. All of it—and then tell me your fee."

By the time I left my solicitor's office, I was no longer dwelling upon my mother's attempts to escape the cage she had locked herself within, nor my father's inability to ponder future catastrophes of his own making.

No, reader: by then I was mourning the death of my world entire. I did not even know my own name.

Oh, I knew who I *was*—a scarlet-toothed tigress, one forever burdened by the iron weight of her own black stripes. I was apparently also the illegitimate daughter of a two-faced stockbroker (as if there were any other kind).

Until something has been taken from you, it is difficult to gauge what sort of holes will be left by its absence. Guessing that Clarke's departure would make a yawning cavity would have been obvious, the loss of Charles Thornfield an equally predictable pit; but I hope, reader, that you have never lost something you took entirely for granted, like your name.

Returning to the Weathercock in Orchard Street was a blur of draughty omnibuses and crooked roads, a dreadful numbness settling over me. All I wanted was to call for a hot bath and read Mr. Thornfield's letters. Trudging into the lodging house, I waved a vacant hand to the clerk who had come, however contrarily, to like me.

"No visitors of any kind, please!"

"Wait, Miss Smith!" he called, but after the strangely painful thought *that isn't my name either*, I paid him no mind.

My alias rang out twice more, and urgently too, but my eyes flooded and I fled—up the stairs, half stumbling in my beautiful new dress, desperate for sanctuary. When I reached my room, I fetched the key from my reticule and was surprised to find the door already unlocked. Hesitant, I felt for the knife in my skirts with one hand and turned the knob with the other.

"Hello, Miss Steele," Inspector Sam Quillfeather said when I discovered him occupying my own room.

TWENTY-SEVEN

Much enjoyment I do not expect in the life opening before me. . . .

Discovering the man who could see me hanged sitting on my striped chaise, smiling peaceably with his hat in his hand, might have been unbearable had I been in a merry humour; I am sure I could never have withstood the shock had I not just learnt I was the bastard child of a philanderer and an extortionist, which had invested me with a certain flexibility.

"Mr. Quillfeather," I whispered.

"You are surprised to see me?" He rose and bowed, gangly limbs folding inward. "But . . . no, I see that you are dismayed? Forgive me, but I was eager to have a discussion with you, a very *frank* discussion, and you quit Highgate House quite precipitously. It was clear that I was the cause, Miss Steele, and I found myself unable to rest until I had located you?"

"How . . ." Swaying, I hid my weakness by leaning on the door as I shut it.

"Only by the most careful searching, Miss Steele! I knew after speaking with Mr. Sardar Singh—interesting man, that, and I'm glad to have made his acquaintance—you had taken the coach to London, and there the trail went quite cold. But doggedness, you will find, works miracles, and I canvassed every respectable guesthouse I could locate where single women of independent temperament might lodge, asking if a woman of your description had recently taken rooms. When I learnt a young lady named Jane Smith had lived here for precisely the right amount of time, could I ignore the possibility it was you?"

Broken in every way imaginable, I turned away from where I had stood with my head bowed before the door.

"Miss Steele!" Mr Quillfeather exclaimed. He crossed quickly to me, hand extended. "Have I already upset you so?"

The ground seemed to heave. For the briefest of moments, I considered a knife to his heart and a mad flight through alleys and over stiles until I had reached another sort of freedom, a true outlaw's comfortless existence—but it was not Sam Quillfeather's fault he was a police inspector, and it was entirely my fault I was a killer.

So I stayed my hand and reached for his instead.

"I know your mind, Miss Steele," he said quietly. "I will share mine with you, and we will reach an understanding after many years of poisonous secrets—does that suit you?"

Such an overwhelming dread possessed me that I thought my faculties must shatter. I opened my mouth, and just as I was about to make an idiot of myself, Mr. Quillfeather urged, "Oh, please, Miss Steele—won't you sit down before you do yourself an injury?"

I obediently sat upon the chaise he had vacated, neck tingling with terror.

"Now, Miss Steele," said he, seating himself upon the chair opposite and leaning forward in his sweeping fashion. "I have some hard words, and want you to understand—I don't wish to say them? But I simply must, and I frankly regret not having said them to you when you were a little girl. I know, you see, why you lied to my friend Thornfield about your name, why you ran without even taking your luggage. You must know . . . I told him nothing? He believes you to be Jane Stone still. But I know the entire contents of your biography, and of your secret fears."

"This is about Edwin, then." My voice was parchment thin.

"Could it be about anything else?" he asked softly.

Yes, I thought, and swallowed what felt like a bullet.

"The fact is that I know . . . everything, Miss Steele, absolutely everything, about the events leading up to your cousin's unfortunate demise."

My eyes fell shut; so I was to lose my name, my claim to Highgate House, and my freedom, all in a single afternoon. In a way, I thought, it was kinder—in a way, it was better than I deserved.

"You were so young then, so . . . vulnerable? I never saw such a sensitive little girl in all my days. Now I have found you, however, and you have grown into such a lovely young woman, could my cowardice *still*, to this *very day* prevent my speaking out?"

A strong wind seemed to blow, a strangely silent one, and I was a leaf floating upon it.

"Oh, Miss Steele, please don't take on so!" To my shock, I opened my eyes to find Sam Quillfeather's beaked nose inches away, his dry, calloused hands grasping mine. "Listen here, my girl—take a few deep breaths, if you can? *Very* good. I must say the words now, and you can hear them bravely, can you not?"

A faint nod was all I could manage at this point.

"I know that your cousin, Edwin, attacked you, and the nature of that attack."

I waited; I continued to wait. When he said nothing further, I heaved a breath as if I had been drowning. Inspector Quillfeather nodded, squeezing my limp fingers. He continued to say nothing of murder, and I continued to gape at him, utterly speechless.

"There, I knew that would be difficult. Shall I go on?"

Shaking my head in disbelief, I managed to husk, "Yes," after which contradictory signals Sam Quillfeather smiled paternally.

"I cannot help but feel that I have done you an . . . injustice? There was evidence, *so much* evidence, but how can one conscience putting a mere child through such trials? Had I to do it over, I think that I should have acted differently? I can only claim misplaced propriety, though I hope you lived the better for my choice, I truly do."

"Evidence," I echoed.

"Oh, evidence in *spades*!" he cried. "The torn button upon your cousin's clothing might have been explained as you suggested, by the idea that you were playing. However! Though I do not claim to be the world's finest policeman, I can assure you that I *aspire* to be, and the tear in your dress sleeve combined with the bruising beneath? Shaped, even what little I could see of it, like a handprint?" Inspector Quillfeather's already clifflike brows surged into bolder protrusions. "Miss Steele, you never got *that* injury playing a game, that was as plain as the nose on my face!"

"Very plain indeed, then," I accidentally said aloud.

"Ha!" exclaimed the policeman. "Oh, may I state how gratified am I that even after such unspeakable liberties being visited upon your person, you retain your sense of humour?"

Pressing my hands a final time, he released them and sat back, though between the hair and the brows and the nose and the chin, this did nothing to diminish the impression that he was a train hurtling towards me. "If you could know the nights I've kept vigil over this affair, would you wish to? No, don't answer that; I think not. But your very attitude that day, Miss Steele—your ramrod posture, your *obvious* terror, your inexplicable distress which, like a puzzle piece which is the right colour but the wrong shape, did not match grief over the death of your cousin . . . The truth was obvious. I asked myself so often, *What can I do?* Such cases of unspeakable violence, particularly against the young, are impossible to prosecute."

"I see." I pressed my still-shaking hands into my skirts.

"Yours would have been, I assure you. And with the perpetrator of the assault, who was likewise the second principle witness, *dead* by tragic accident? Imagine! A nine-year-old girl dragged through the assizes, pointed at, questioned, shamed, her reputation forever soiled, her heart broken, her mind subjected to not merely a single gross indignity but multiple others? *No,* I said—not when the guilty party could not be punished by a mortal court."

"I didn't scream," I blurted out.

"I beg your pardon, Miss Steele?"

"I didn't scream." Suddenly the tears were an ugly waterfall, hot and gushing, and *someone has to know after all this time*, I had to tell *someone.* "He . . . Edwin made a mistake, you see, because I was so shocked that I stayed quiet, which misled him, so it was entirely my fault, you understand, that he . . . that he . . . because I didn't scream."

If a man can look simultaneously exquisitely gentle and boiling with rage, that man is Sam Quillfeather. He pursed his lips and curved towards me.

"You listen to me, Miss Steele, and you listen *ardently*," he grated. "That a lady's succumbing to shock at exposure to such villainy could ever be considered a black mark against her—put the thought from your mind this very *instant*, do you hear?"

Opening my mouth, I was prevented by a sharply upraised hand.

"Mark me now!" Inspector Quillfeather ordered. "It is a gentleman's greatest privilege to protect the fair sex, and when he abandons that privilege, when he casts it aside in favour of *lechery*, why then he is no longer a gentleman, and therefore the lady in question owes him *nothing*, because he is a coward and a blackguard, and for a lady to doubt her own behaviour in the presence of a coward and a blackguard is *lunacy*, I tell you, from stone silence to violent caterwauling, because she owes him *no interaction whatsoever* from the instant he discards his honour, and I won't have it. Promise me something?"

"Um," I said. He was handing me his pocket handkerchief, I

realised, and I took it, though the flow of tears had dried under the blast of his vehemence. "If I can."

"Promise me," he urged, eyes shining, "that you will put this aborted scream from your mind forever?"

"I . . . well . . ."

"You owe your attacker *no debt*, Miss Steele. It is, as I have proven, a logical impossibility? Promise to *try*?

"Yes," I whispered. For the second time in as many hours, I felt as if I had been blown apart and put back together again. "I promise to try."

"I can ask no more of you than that." He stood to his full scarecrow's height, setting his hands against his scrawny hips as if satisfied that a hard task had been seen to. "Well, I think we can both agree I have taxed you enough, yes, Miss Steele? Please forgive me for any harm I may have caused you inadvertently. Now I must return to work, for there are several urgent matters which require my attention, and I have neglected them in favour of finding you. You have eased my mind, Miss Steele."

"Here is your handkerchief," I said, offering it.

"Handkerchiefs should remain where they are needed, don't you agree?"

Weakly, I laughed at this, and Inspector Quillfeather beamed at me as he retrieved his hat and gloves from the table.

"I hope you will trust my complete sincerity in vowing never to reveal your secret to Thornfield?" he pressed. "I ought to say, however, that should you elect to reveal your true name to my friend, I believe he would treat you honourably."

I haven't any true name, I thought in despair, *and he treats me too honourably by half.*

"Forgive me—my words pain you. Here is my card, should you wish to contact me for any reason, great or small? You are looking well, very well indeed, Miss Steele, and I see by your attire that you have no need of governess work. But in any case, don't stay away from Highgate House on my account?" he added kindly.

"I won't." Mr. Thornfield's likeness appeared in my mind's eye, deep-blue eyes and pure-white hair, and I banished the image. "I promise."

He turned to go. We had not finished yet, however—nothing could be this simple. Though the thought of deliberately broaching the subject sent leeches slithering through my belly, I could not allow him to exit without truly mapping the miracle of my safety.

"Mr. Quillfeather, did you know that I was at Lowan Bridge School when . . ." I forced myself to look at him. "When Mr. Vesalius Munt was murdered?"

He lifted his overhanging brows, and the neat set of horizontal lines appeared along his forehead. "Miss Steele, I regret to say that I did, for you were included in the roster of some thirty missing girls? I always wished you well, you know, and I did seek you for a time."

My heart slammed against my rib cage as if attempting escape. "Did you ever suspect anyone in particular?"

"Ah, that would be telling, wouldn't it?" he mused. "But between us, yes, there was a clear suspect."

"You cannot mean it!"

"I must assure you I do."

"For my own peace of mind, then, I beg you to inform me who the culprit was."

"It won't upset you to hear the truth?"

"Not after that . . . other truth," I replied in a hushed tone, and he smiled at me.

"Quite so. Do you recall Miss Amy Lilyvale?"

"Very clearly."

"Yes, she gave me testimony that every single girl without exception had been present at chapel that fateful day, which quite clinched the matter."

"Did it?" I questioned, feeling sick again.

"Oh, I should think decisively?" He began ticking people off on cadaverous fingers. "Miss Rebecca Clarke was not present—ill-usage, I gather, was the cause; you were not present, doubtless comforting your friend; and Miss Davies was laid up with a bad case of the croup. Therefore, Miss Lilyvale was not actually at chapel to check, and wished not to falsely throw any students under suspicion. Other teachers claimed she was there, but the inaccuracy of her attendance report convinced me they were lying in order to shield her." Scowling, Mr. Quillfeather passed his hand forward over his head, a familiar gesture that made him resemble a ruffled bird of prey. "Your headmaster, Miss Steele, was no saint. He kept a diary? Oh, yes, I found it! In it he recorded, in the foulest language, the most disgusting perversions he could conjure, planning to visit all upon Miss Lilyvale. He wrote that he had been sharing such filth with her for years, the villain . . . One is not gladdened by any death, but some touch the heart rather less than others, do they not?"

"Undoubtedly."

"Miss Lilyvale it was, that is certain, but I make a habit of never pursuing an unwinnable case, you see? I cannot find the good in it? And the evidence was *so* circumstantial! Nothing could be done."

"Surely the diary counted for something?"

"Oh, the *diary*." He made a subtle bow of acknowledgement. "Yes, that would have gone a very long way indeed, but sadly it was lost."

"However did that happen?" I marvelled.

"I fear that *I* lost it, Miss Steele," he declared, eyes twinkling. "In a lit fireplace. Clumsy of me, I know—can you imagine? And they call me a steady policeman!"

So saying, he donned his hat, tipped it, and walked straight out the door.

. . .

I had planned to pay a call upon Augustus Sack that evening regardless of the outcome of my meeting with my solicitor; however, the reader will likely empathise when I confess I was too prostrate with nerves following my identity exploding in multiple fashions to infiltrate the East India Company. A message dispatched via the boots conveyed my intention to call upon the morrow. Moving as if in a dream, I unfastened my fine jewellery, brushed and hung my clothing, donned my soft new nightdress, and crawled into bed with a wineglass full of whiskey and *Jane Eyre* within arm's reach.

I was a rich woman now, even without Mr. Thornfield's assistance. Time drifted sluggishly, distorted by the whiskey and the warmth. Everything about me had changed, and yet I could see the slender bend of my wrist at the end of a white forearm, looking the same as it always had, could see the tiny mole between my left thumb and index finger, assuring me that I was still myself.

I was not myself, however. I was a Jane with an imaginary surname, one who apparently was not to blame for failing to scream. It was too mad to comprehend in an instant, or even an hour, so I burrowed farther into the bedclothes to puzzle over it all. My life's sole mission had once been a simple one: to carve out a tiny sliver of human affection, having none of the commodity for myself. For all that I so thoroughly disapproved of my own character, however, Mr. Sneeves and Mr. Quillfeather had proven that day I was capable of grievous errors upon the subject of Jane Steele.

I rolled clumsily onto my belly, reaching, and flipped to a passage from my new copy of my favourite book:

To this crib I always took my doll; human beings must love something, and, in the dearth of worthier objects of affection, I con-

> *trived to find a pleasure in loving and cherishing a faded graven image, shabby as a miniature scarecrow. It puzzles me now to remember with what absurd sincerity I doted on this little toy; half-fancying it alive and capable of sensation. I could not sleep unless it was folded in my night-gown; and when it lay there safe and warm, I was comparatively happy, believing it to be happy likewise.*

Upon first reading, I had found it bizarre that the adult Jane Eyre regarded this exercise as either puzzling or absurd; upon subsequent readings, I marvel still more at her derision. Lacking interest in dolls, I had once—not unlike my poor, sweet Sahjara—gathered crumbs of pleasure by spoiling horses. This seemed to me neither worship of a false idol nor a quirk of an infantile mind; it did no one any harm if I treated a horse well, and made my days less miserable.

Did I deserve misery for the things I had done?

Yes, of course I did. Even apart from being the tainted bastard offspring of a suicidal mother and a lying father, I was a murderess five times over.

As I seemed incapable of turning myself in, however, would any harm come to the world if for the moment I thought of this newly reborn Jane—Jane without legitimate parentage, Jane without legitimate surname—as a creature worth treating gently?

There was no one else volunteering for the task, after all.

Brisk footfalls outside my bedroom door woke me at eleven the next morning; the anonymous movement dragged me from a weirdly sweet slumber. The sun was high, however, and breakfast long concluded, and the whiskey's solace had left me with an empty belly, so I clambered from bed and washed. Then I donned another of my fashionable frocks, a floral silk with a dramatic shawl collar, all save the white lace sleeves emerging from fabric printed in grey and silver and a blue which reminded me of Mr. Thornfield's eyes.

Today is for you, I thought, *wherever you are and however you fare,* and was seized with such a longing that my breath caught.

My set of modest Punjabi diamonds completed the picture, and I deftly swallowed the remainder of last night's whiskey, fortifying myself as I quit the Weathercock.

Noontide bells rang as my soles struck the cobbles. I had been too disoriented to give Mr. Sack a specific time the day before, so I did not feel rushed. Luncheon was the first order of business, and I knew of a beautiful tearoom Clarke and I had used to frequent mere blocks away from East India House; I was seized with a longing to see it again, its gliding servers and polished brass rails, so I hailed a hansom and directed the driver to the City.

Cox's Tearoom was just as I recalled it when we pulled up before its door, and by the time I had paid the driver, both the wind and my stomach bit sharply. A liveried gentleman led me to a table, where I was soon equipped with Darjeeling and a tower of sandwiches. After a few sips and bites, however, I thought I should be more comfortable with a newspaper; I visited the rack and selected a late-morning edition, glancing at the headlines as I returned to my table. Nearly colliding with a waiter, I looked up, murmuring an apology.

I stopped dead, staring in astonishment.

Rebecca Clarke sat at a table by the window, shafts of illumination waltzing through the golden corkscrews of her pinned-up hair.

TWENTY-EIGHT

But I ought to forgive you, for you knew not what you did: while rending my heart-strings, you thought you were only up-rooting my bad propensities.

My heart, so egregiously taxed of late, rung in my breast like a great gong—I thought it must have been audible, so painfully glad was I to see my schoolmate, my companion, nay, my *sister*, again after so long a time.

Once the initial shock had worn off, I ceased marvelling and allowed happiness to spread like a virus through my chest. We had shared the same tastes once, Clarke and I, moved in twin orbits like binary stars. It was not very surprising, therefore, that in this labyrinth of a town I should stumble upon my lost great friend, particularly considering I had sought the place out because it reminded me of her.

Clarke was twenty-one years old, and where once she had been thin and ethereal, now she was beautiful—as freckled as ever, with the tiny mouth of an inquisitive porcelain doll. So many times had I pictured her starving that the sight of her hale was a gift, the unlooked-for sort which pierce deeper than the expected. Her clothing was fine but eccentric: a long bronze skirt, a close-fitted ivory waistcoat, a dark copper jacket with tails and lapels to it, a golden cravat. This elegant but oddly mannish ensemble was completed by a miniature top hat, and she peered through a pair of half-moon pince-nez at the afternoon edition of the *Times.*

My feet had carried me farther than I realised during this reconnaissance, and I found myself before her, my eager shadow brushing the hem of her skirt.

"Just put it on my account, if you—*oh!*" Clarke exclaimed, her cup clattering into its saucer as she glanced up.

Say something, I thought.

Nothing emerged.

I've missed you terribly and deeply regret the fact you learnt I am a homicidal maniac.

I hesitated.

Not that.

"It's good to . . ." I swallowed, for Clarke had turned as pale as the milk brought for her coffee. "That is—we needn't speak, only I saw you, and . . ." I battled the urge to prove myself the pinnacle of urbanity by throwing myself in her lap and sobbing. "You look well, and I'm glad."

At this juncture, I considered that a sound from Clarke—any sound—would be taken as a boon. Instead, she stared at me with wide green eyes, her hands vibrating hummingbird-fast.

"I'm upsetting you." The admission stung. "I can't tell you what it meant to see you again. I'll just—"

"No." Clarke trapped my wrist with the strength of a steel manacle. "Sit down." She blinked, hard. "I mean, won't you sit down?"

Slowly, she released me.

I sat down.

Clarke folded the newspaper with care; then she took a long breath and sat back, nodding at the silver coffeepot. "Would you like a cup?"

"Please."

A waiter came with an additional service and poured, a civilised piece of pageantry which enabled us both to pretend we were friends meeting for coffee to discuss our summering plans, rather than friends meeting for coffee to discuss whatever we were going to discuss. My teapot and sandwiches appeared, and I gestured for her to help herself; Clarke shook her head, eyes wide under pale lashes, and I looked away.

"You look well too," said she.

"Hmm?" I had been studying my coffee with more interest than that beverage had ever previously inspired.

Clarke smiled—the indulgent one which meant I had journeyed too far into the wilderness of my head. "You look very smart. I'm happy over that, your clearly having plentiful coin. So often I wondered whether—"

"Me too, every single day," I blurted.

When she blushed, she looked more herself again, for her previous pallor had been alarming. Clarke had never blushed often, however, and never lacking a sound purpose, so I wondered at the expression.

"Well." She pretended to polish her pince-nez as I pretended to add sugar to my coffee. "I probably did not wonder quite as much as you did, for I used to hear news of you."

"You have the better of me, then," I marvelled. "How?"

Clarke's head found the much-loved angle it adopted when thinking harder than usual; as if remembering something, she spoke. "'I always knew my grip upon the thread of time was tenuous, and the harder I clutched, the sooner it would break. Therefore, do not weep for me, my tender sweet love—we must all resign ourselves to the final snapping of that bond between soul and breath, and though it is a present unworthy of your grace and beauty, you must know that I gift my soul to you.'"

Jaw dropping, I laughed. Clarke gave me a faint smile.

"I wrote that!" I exclaimed. "John Jacob Holdworth, hanged at Newgate in eighteen forty-seven."

"Precisely so. When your gallows confessions started selling at newsagents' and tea shops, occasionally I would purchase them, though I never caught a glimpse of you delivering the papers or picking up your earnings."

"But of course my name wasn't on them, only the names of those executed—however did you know it was me?"

"That wasn't very difficult," she said quietly. Brightening, she attempted to adopt a brisk air. "And now what are you doing with yourself? Good Lord, that frock and those jewels—I didn't suppose last confessions brought in ready enough chink for those togs."

I glanced down at my new dress, and my pulse sped, for she was right.

"I had better not say," I confessed softly. "It's complicated."

The set of her shoulders grew brittle after she shrugged. "You always did keep secrets, and everything is complicated these days."

Extraordinary contradiction, I thought, *that she could always condone even the most operatic of my falsehoods, so long as none were directed at her.*

"I'd tell you if it didn't mean betraying another party."

My friend took rapt interest in the traffic outside the window. "It's all one to me."

"Where did you learn slang?" I teased, wanting the light to return to her eyes. "You always spoke so properly, even in Rotherhithe."

"We were speaking with each other mainly, so it was easy to keep pure back then." Surely I imagined the dryness in her tone, having spent too long in Mr. Thornfield's company.

"Oh, *won't* you say what you've been doing?" I begged. "The matter which brought me to London doesn't involve just myself, you see. Pax, please. I'm desperate to know—you never bought that rigging with street-chaunting coin either, and my vocabulary is every bit as disgraceful, and you really must take pity on me. We were so lucky, when we arrived here, to find shelter so quickly, and afterwards when I pictured you . . ." Faltering, I cleared my throat. "If anything had happened to you, it should have been my fault."

Clarke's gaze grew a shade less hard.

"No." She sighed. "I was the one who left, after all."

"But what came next?"

"I continued singing, but finding lodgings was harder than I imagined, since for all those years you'd taken care of me—I was sharp enough at school, but a complete ninny when loosed to the streets. At times, I slept in doss-houses with the dollymops, and it was . . . Don't frown like that, Jane. Most of them were kind, for all that they were filthy and coarse. I could have gone straight back to my parents. I did, for a fortnight," she admitted, wincing. "When they seemed only half relieved to see me, I asked them for a few pounds and struck out again. They claimed what I was doing was 'admirably Bohemian.'"

She sounded so bitter at this last that I hastened to inquire, "How did your fortunes change?"

A wistful look glazed Clarke's eyes. "I was singing near to Elephant and Castle when a woman—Mrs. Priscilla Pellanora is her name—stopped to speak with me. She asked if I had ever sung in a company before, harmonies and the like, and of course I had at Lowan Bridge, and she offered me a place in the chorus of her production."

"But that's absolutely wonderful!" Laughing, I imagined Clarke in a wooden-walled theatre, her freckles blurred by the faint glow of the footlights, the smell of peanuts and ale thick in the air. "You excelled, of course, which is why now you are so fashionable."

Clarke lifted one shoulder, though she seemed pleased; she had always been peculiarly uninterested in her own talents, the same way she viewed everyone else's attributes and shortcomings as stamped in the stars, inevitable. "Mrs. Pellanora is an excellent tutor."

"Oh! May I come see you? Do please say yes. Are you at the Olympic, or maybe the Delphi?"

Biting her lip, Clarke shook her head.

"The Lyceum, then! I know you must think . . ." I stopped, eyes prickling. "That is, I don't know what you must think of me, but I should so love to hear you sing again."

"I'm not at the Lyceum," she husked strangely.

"Do you sing for penny concerts, then? I'll come to the Surrey side to see you, only tell me which it is. The Victoria? The Bower Saloon?"

"Jane, I sing at Mrs. Pellanora's private club," she snapped.

My ears buzzed in the ensuing silence, drowning out the soft clinking of tableware and the susurration of strangers' voices. A man with a Yorkshire accent was demanding to know where his pudding had got to as the words *private club* echoed in my skull.

"Oh, for God's sake," Clarke groaned, then abruptly lowered her voice. "Surely this cannot be *quite* so surprising as some of your own past revelations. Wipe that expression off your face, if you please—no one touches me, the stage is gorgeously appointed, I've room and board with a set of bang-up girls, I'm petted and toasted all over town, and the costumes are nothing like what you're picturing. They're not far off from what I'm wearing now, come to that, only more . . . theatrical, and with trousers, and apt to get kohl stains."

"I'm sorry," I protested. "I wasn't thinking anything, only that you were always so scrupulous, you see, but now I comprehend it's all quite aboveboard."

"No, it isn't either," she hissed.

"I don't understand."

"It's outrageously bawdy, the content of the programme."

"Oh," was all I could muster.

"That must please you, that I work in a dirty cabaret."

"No! I mean I'm happy—so long as you are."

"You don't *look* happy, Jane."

"I'm delighted for you, only . . . surprised, I suppose. You were always so honourable."

"Well, honour wasn't doing anything for me." The waiter had

dropped a salver on the table and she signed her bill with a flourish. "Mrs. Pellanora's establishment does."

"I don't think any the less of you," I said fiercely, panicked at the thought of losing her again so soon—here one heartbeat, gone the next. "I could *never* think less of you."

Wincing, Clarke shook her head. She was so striking in her boyish clothing, the curve of her throat and the flash of her eye beneath the glass half-moons, that save for the skirts and the curls she really did seem a young rake cooing over watch fobs and walking sticks in Regent Street.

"I've an appointment to rehearse with our pianist in half an hour." She tugged on a pair of gloves. "You should know I don't regret seeing you, Jane, and that I don't any longer harbour a . . . Hang it, nothing I say will do any good to anyone. When I think of you, it's altogether fondly."

"Clarke, please don't—"

"Will you say my name at least?" Flushing again, she adjusted her pince-nez. "I don't know why you do that, I never did. Rebecca is my name, Becky what my parents called me, Becca what the four other company girls call me. Take your pick. Why should you want to remind us of Lowan Bridge?"

Because the only shaft of sunshine in all that endless midnight was meeting you.

"Rebecca." The name tasted strange, like salt where sugar was expected. "Let me contact you, please. Have you an address?"

"That would be unwise."

Desperate, I snatched up her bill and stole the pencil from the salver, scribbling my room number at the Weathercock and the street address. I thrust it at her.

After breathing tensely through her nose for a few seconds, she took it. Clarke placed the paper in a pocket beneath her jacket lapel and pressed her lips together.

"I always loved you as a sister." My hand was so near to hers that taking it was a thoughtless act, the only right one.

My old friend cocked her head at our joined fingers, cogitating; she was a self-made woman, a singer of questionable provenance, and otherwise she had not changed a whit since she was six years old, and I was speaking the truth: I had always loved her.

"I never loved you so," she said.

Clarke freed her hand from my tightening grasp as two tears fell soundlessly from beneath the pince-nez. Had she trussed me up like a slaughtered buck, I might have thought it my just deserts for the web of lies in which I had entangled her—this, though, seemed to exceed the boundaries even of cruelty. When my breath hitched, she rose to depart.

"Do you recall the book you had—the one my father published? *The Garden of Forbidden Delights*?"

My mouth must have worked; but sepulchres cannot produce sound, and I was a monument to wishes ungranted and tenderness left to rot unused.

The whisper of fingertips touched my cheek, and then Clarke was kissing me.

It was only a brief press, but it was neither dry, nor chaste, nor seeking. It was the kiss of a person who has thought about variants of the same kiss for a very long time, as if it were a hundred kisses, all of them passionate and all of them hopeless. I was startled and—in the moment—grateful enough even to reciprocate, did so before even thinking why I should not, and I tasted years in that kiss. I tasted years of dying hope, and the sweet bellyache of longing, and coffee, and Clarke herself, before she pulled away, running her thumb over my open lips.

"That was how I loved you," she told me.

Women often embrace, sisters often kiss, and no one regarded us as she bowed her head, closing her eyes for a fleeting instant, and then turned and walked out of the tea shop.

I floated to the window, following her as she strode into the street. She did not look back, gauging the traffic at the corner with a practised tilt of her head; therefore I was the one turned to salt, and not Rebecca Clarke, when I watched her hand leave the front of her bodice and drop my address to the cobbles, the paper fluttering prettily before it landed in the filth and the straw.

For minutes which stretched before me like miles, I stood at that window, still seeing the ghostly afterimage of her slim back and gleaming hair the instant before I lost her for the second time. Carriages and buses clattered over the bill, no longer visible in the road, but that was for the best—I had never wished Clarke harm in all my days, and if seeing me grieved her, I renewed my vow never to seek her out.

An unexpected peace flooded the air around me.

Some tragedies bind us, as lies do; they are ropes braided of hurt and bitterness, and you cannot ever fully understand how pinioned you are until the ties are loosened.

Other tragedies free us, as Clarke's confession freed me.

You cannot know what it means, reader, to have thought yourself despised for your unworthiness for a period of years—to have supposed your very nature poison, and your friend right to have thus abandoned you—and to learn thereafter that you were loved not too little but too well.

East India House was a fortress; the building loomed over me like a conqueror, the lower two floors absurdly high-ceilinged, and the entrance guarded by six positively enormous Ionic columns. A frail wind whined in my ears, tugging the tailcoats of the men dancing about with their arms full of papers in a chaotically choreographed tribute to wealth. Never had I set eyes on a place which so pungently reeked of power and money, and I hesitated, fearing the consequences should I provoke the lion in its den.

Better you than the residents of Highgate House, I thought. *You have been Jane Stone, Jane Smith, and today you will be Jane Steele—the only woman suited to this task.*

I adopted an aloof air and entered the front hall.

If the shareholders were already assured of the Company's ruthless dominance by the exterior of East India House, the interior hammered the point home; everywhere I looked was marble and crystal and carvings and paintings of faraway lands. Finding Augustus P. Sack's office would have been daunting, but a clerk with waxed grey moustaches escorted me, somehow exuding hauteur and deference simultaneously. A knock produced an instant reply of "Come in!" and the stranger presented me to Sack, making a prompt exit.

"Well, well, Miss Stone," Augustus Sack purred, quitting his desk to drop a kiss above my outstretched hand. "I was very intrigued indeed by your letter."

"Yes, I suppose you must have been."

"Do sit down. Tea or a little wine, perhaps?"

"The latter, if you will join me."

"Miss Stone, a beautiful woman need hardly ask that question—and may I state in addition that your present costume quite takes my breath away?"

It had not escaped my attention that Mr. Sack's shrewd eyes had examined my attire, landing with a spark of lust upon the Punjabi diamonds.

"Governesses are expected to be such drab creatures. It is a life of terrible drudgery even when one is not living in fear of one's employer, Mr. Sack."

"Frightened you, did they, the scoundrels?" Mr. Sack commiserated. "Happily, you are safely under the care of John Company now, Miss Stone."

Mr. Sack poured claret from a decanter on a carved mahogany sideboard; he was just as I remembered him, doughy and pink faced, with gleaming cheeks and fat fingers. Now I saw that his rich attire—a maroon coat on this occasion, with a yellow silk necktie—matched his office, for everywhere I looked were signs of needless expense. From ivory cigar box to silver-chased gasogene, Company executives seemed to display wealth like peacocks spreading their plumage.

He ushered me into a chair, equipped us with wine, and perched on the front of his desk. "First, Miss Stone, let me offer my solemn oath that you may tell me anything in complete confidence—I gather that you departed Highgate House in great anxiety, which I confess does not surprise me, considering the dark history of Thornfield and his shadow, Singh. If we are to be friends, we must trust each other."

So I am already promised immunity for stealing the trunk, I thought, delighted.

"I am yours to command, Mr. Sack, so harrowed was I by my recent experiences."

The sympathetic frown he manufactured was revolting, so sharply did his eyes cut from my necklace to my face and back again. "We speak of desperate men, Miss Stone. Please—tell me everything."

I did not tell him everything, and several of the things I told him were bold-faced lies.

Tremulously, I informed Mr. Sack that after the knives had driven him away at breakfast, I had feared for my life. However, I had determined to wait at least until I was given my first quarterly wages, having no other means of returning to London. In the meanwhile, I had launched a secret investigation of the house's occupants and learnt what Mr. Sack had been doing visiting Highgate House thanks to covert eavesdropping (not untrue); thus had I heard the story of the trunk and its contents.

"The tale sounded to me quite preposterous, but I continued in my quest to discover all I could," I informed him shyly. "There seemed no other choice if I wished to escape their clutches."

"None at all, none in the *world*, Miss Stone—you did quite right," the Company diplomat soothed. "Please go on."

Leaving out the pieces of the story which reflected badly on Sack was simplicity itself. I knew my employer had robbed David Lavell and his wife, Karman Kaur, but said nothing of Sahjara's kidnap; I knew John Clements and Jack Ghosh were both dead, but implied Mr. Thornfield or Mr. Singh were to blame. The Company man's ruddy cheeks creased in sympathy whilst his stare bored into me with all the gentility of a bullet.

"This Jack Ghosh person's death was the final straw," I lamented. "Oh, Mr. Sack, it was so horrid—their claims it was an *accident*, the blood on the floor. I redoubled my search for the trunk, and . . ." I allowed myself to blush.

"And enterprising woman that you are, you found it, and you took it in order to escape the clutches of these fiends," he said softly.

Pretending a coquettish version of guilt, I said nothing.

"The trunk was hid amongst Mr. Sardar Singh's things, I imagine?"

Dumbfounded, I blinked at him.

"Why do you say so, Mr. Sack?"

"Because it's that posturing heathen who taunted me with word of it upon my arrival back in England. This was before the loss of John Clements, of course—wretched business, that, and I don't know that this Inspector Quillfeather will ever get to the bottom of it, more's the pity. I thought Thornfield to blame at first, and told the Director so, but now I have reached another conclusion."

These assertions sounded nonsensical—that either man would ever stoop to poisoning anyone (as I had once done) was ludicrous, I thought, and the notion that Sardar Singh had made any communication to Augustus P. Sack whatsoever beggared belief.

"I don't understand . . . Mr. Singh seemed so contemptuous of you," I faltered. "You claim he was a correspondent?"

"He did hate me, the swaggering savage, and wished me to live knowing his crimes would go unpunished. See for yourself."

Going behind his desk, Mr. Sack produced a folded letter. This he passed to me, and upon opening it, it was all I could do not to recoil in horror. Many a time had I watched Mr. Singh as he wrote, and many a time posted letters for him; these were his exact characters, from angular downstrokes to oddly spiked capitals. It read:

Dear Mr. Sack,

As little as I desire ever to see your face again, I can no longer live without informing you that I picture it often upon your making the discovery that you have been thoroughly bested. All subterfuge is futile at this point: we do indeed have the trunk, and should you ever attempt to recover it again, know that I will not hesitate to destroy you utterly.

Your Company has raped my entire culture in systematic fashion; what is in my possession will remain there, and any attempt by you to steal it will result in your bloody death. Highgate House is a fortress, and I its guardian. Lacking any other avenues by which to make you suffer for your arrogance, I send this letter; think upon its contents often, Mr. Sack, for the treasure you seek will never fall into your hands the way our great Empire did.

Charles knows nothing of this and would not believe your lying tongue should you attempt to tell him—it is partly for his sake that I write you, indeed, for you have brought a good man to the brink of mental ruin. Live in discomfort, Mr. Sack, knowing that once, at least, one of the pure ones snatched a bone away from an English cur.

Your enemy, and your better,
Mr. Sardar Singh

My head spun; for it sounded like him, not the usual mellow-tongued Mr. Singh but the warrior whose voice abraded my ears that day in the hall, when he stood in the snow-swept entrance hall and called the Company rapists and the Sikh royals their pimps.

Meanwhile, my entire plan was ruined; I had intended to draw any imminent fire away from Highgate House by proving that the trunk existed and offering it to him myself. The glad news which was to have distracted Sack, bought me time whilst I thought of the perfect way to kill him, was not news after all.

It was not news because apparently Mr. Singh had been lying to us.

"You see how they blame me for their woes." Mr. Sack sighed. "I only wished to see justice done regarding the trunk's recovery, you understand—David Lavell was a Company stalwart, and he would have wanted this fortune to be held in trust by the Company for Sahjara when she comes of age. Had Mr. Singh merely hated me as any guilty party hates the law, he may not have been angry enough to risk such a foolish correspondence; but all is tangled in his mind with Charles Thornfield's subsequent madness, you see, and the pair are quite devoted to each other. It is easier for Singh to blame me for everything than to consider that the fault lies squarely upon their shoulders."

"Madness?" I echoed, stricken. I quickly corrected myself. "Do you mean to say I was living under the authority of a . . . a lunatic?"

"Oh, but then you don't know what happened to Charles Thornfield at the Battle of Sobraon," Mr. Sack crooned. "Clements did, and so do I, you see. We were there."

TWENTY-NINE

The answer was evasive—I should have liked something clearer; but Mrs. Fairfax either could not, or would not, give me more explicit information of the origin and nature of Mr. Rochester's trials. She averred that they were a mystery to herself, and that what she knew was chiefly from conjecture. It was evident, indeed, that she wished me to drop the subject; which I did accordingly.

Reader, I did not drop the subject; and I confess that, greatly as the letter from Mr. Singh had disturbed me, all thought of him was crowded out at the prospect of Charles Thornfield's bloody biography being revealed at last.

I hardly needed to feign my agitation. "Won't you please explain? It would soothe my conscience so to know that I am right in coming to you."

"Let there be no doubt whatsoever about *that*, Miss Stone!" Mr. Sack exclaimed. "David Lavell was a friend, and his treatment at the hands of these reprobates—shocking, simply shocking."

I recalled Mr. Thornfield's account of the same circumstances and gritted my teeth into what I hoped was an encouraging smile.

Sack wasn't his superior, and anyway he was winning a fortune off Lavell at poker—Karman's fortune. Lavell couldn't sink low enough for Sack's taste.

"Oh, do make all clear, I beg—he unnerved me, but I never thought him mad."

Mr. Sack puffed air into his rosy cheeks; he made a show of considering, checking his watch against the richly gilded clock, whilst I channelled my real anxiety into breathless anticipation. Thankfully, I knew I had him, for he was the breed of braggart who enjoys imparting salacious information to delicate-seeming females.

"There really is no putting off a lovely young lady when she makes a fair request of me," he concluded with a sudden air of gallantry.

"Only you can ease my mind, Mr. Sack."

"In that flattering assessment you are correct, Miss Stone," he simpered, and I could see the half-humble, half-preening attitude he took with foreign dignitaries and their wives. "Though I must confess part of my knowledge comes secondhand—my former colleague John Clements helped to nurse Charles Thornfield and was thus the audience to his most ghastly ravings. I am of such a tenderhearted nature myself that I can hardly bear to see anyone suffer, and yet . . . sometimes, I think God visits punishments upon the living as well as the dead, and Charles Thornfield was greatly culpable regarding his own disastrous circumstances."

At least fractionally, this was true, for Mr. Thornfield had told me himself—an infected slash across the back of his shoulder, a long convalescence spent in Clements's company.

"Any man who would rob his closest friend's sister has much to answer for," I agreed.

"Aye, there's the crux of it!" Mr. Sack's ability to swagger whilst stationary cannot be exaggerated. "Between you and me, Miss Stone, Charles Thornfield was desperately in love with Sardar Singh's sister, Karman Kaur. I shock you, I see—forgive me. Jealousy of her husband, David Lavell, caused him to take the crudest measures, and ones which led, as crude measures so often do, to tragedy."

I folded my hands primly. "I gathered that Mr. Thornfield and Mr. Singh preferred to rob their own loved ones than allow them to live as they pleased."

"Precisely so, Miss Stone." Mr. Sack ran a fat finger over the lip of his wineglass, reflecting. "Lavell was a dear friend as well as a colleague—a handsome devil with an adventurer's appetites, and his wife adored him. Oh, we sowed a few wild oats in the Punjab, but you must understand, reputations abroad *shatter* if a gentleman cannot keep pace with the local elite! The Director knows this to be true. What are a few card games, a few harmless flirtations, when failure to carouse with the natives leads to their instant censure?"

Nodding, I twisted my lips into a gracious frown.

"Thornfield couldn't stomach it despite being born and bred there," Mr. Sack huffed. "Pitiful really, how he doted on Karman Kaur when she would have none of him. She was a goddess, Miss Stone, a warrior queen, and all hell broke loose when those miscreants stole what was hers to share with her husband as she pleased. What, allow him to default on his gambling losses? What self-respecting woman would dream of such a thing?"

"Strange that a woman so loyal to the Khalsa should marry an Englishman."

"Not at all! She had grown up with the Thornfields, and Lavell had nothing but praise for the Sikhs—a political of the highest order, he was, and the first man to say that the East India Company didn't stand a chance against the Khalsa on their own ground. These bastards made their own artillery, you understand, based on English designs, and when you've your own foundries, you're your own master. All the better if your army is a hundred thousand strong! As I recall, the line Lavell took was that once the Khalsa had trounced John Company, the world's greatest armies would join forces and rule the territories from Calcutta to St. Petersburg. He was very popular in Lahore, and not just with Karman Kaur."

I swallowed bitter disgust, for this confirmed all my friends had told me—Company spies flattering the Sikhs whilst infiltrating their empire, Sikhs defying the Company whilst their leaders betrayed them.

Small wonder that Sardar Singh longed for vengeance.

"Anyhow, Karman wouldn't have cared a fig about Lavell's politics. It was, how shall I put this, a *love* match, Miss Stone," Mr. Sack added in a greasy tenor. "Screaming fights, tender reconciliations—they burnt the candle at both ends."

"What did she say when the theft was discovered?"

"Now mind, we never learnt *who* pilfered her treasure until I discovered Sahjara's trunk," Mr. Sack boasted with a hand over his breast. "But we all knew what happened after it went missing—Karman Kaur ordered a Khalsa cavalry uniform altered to fit her, sharpened her *tulwar*, saddled her best horse, and joined the army to seek a new fortune for herself and Lavell."

I forced myself to relax clenched fists.

"She did not consult anyone over this step, I take it."

"Not her!" He chuckled. "Magnificent, she was, Miss Stone, a stunner of the first water. So she had lost a tidy sum—why whinge when the Khalsa were poised to annihilate John Company in the name of the Guru? Lavell was called to Amritsar to negotiate, and Karman was off like a shot to Ferozepore after sending word to her brother to look after his niece. By the time Sardar Singh and Charles Thornfield discovered her plan, she had already joined a Sikh encampment, to the delight of all the men she met there. She distinguished herself in action at Ferozepore as well as at Aliwal and Sobraon."

"The Khalsa did not win the Battle of Sobraon."

"No, they were slaughtered," Mr. Sack returned cheerily.

He moved to refill our wine; by the time he had passed the glass back to me, my spine tingled with horror. It did not matter that Karman Kaur may well have joined the ranks of the Khalsa anyhow; it did not matter that Mr. Singh did not think Mr. Thornfield a murderer. Mr. Thornfield saw every step leading to her decision like paces towards a gallows, saw the fateful instant when the loss of her treasure propelled her into a harrowing war, and he thought himself wholly responsible. It did not matter that I knew any woman would be lucky to be loved by him—would, as I had put it, be the happiest woman in the world.

The last one wasn't, he had told me, for he had set her death in motion.

"The Battle of Sobraon was butchery at its most primitive," the political continued almost gleefully. "It had been pouring rain for days, and the Sutlej River was as bloated as a pagan prince. The Khalsa had been pummelling our Bombay brigades with heavy artillery for hours when the order came to return the bombardment. When that failed, the Bengali troops as well as the King's Light Dragoons launched counterattacks which the Khalsa repelled like true barbarians—hacking down the wounded, finishing the dying as if they were cattle in an abattoir. After confronting them from the west and the south and the east, the Sikh line began to collapse, which is when the true carnage began."

"It sounds sufficiently apocalyptic already, Mr. Sack."

Mr. Sack adopted an introspective look. "All those rains, Miss Stone—the surging of the Sutlej's waters, the vulnerability of their position. One pontoon bridge linked the Khalsa back to the Punjab. Think about it—a single thread of boats leading to the only possible escape after the fords had flooded. The Company may have had . . . friends, let us say, on the Sikh side, friends who understood the value of this bridge. Or they may not, and God Himself may have weakened the moorings linking the line of ships—who can say for certain?"

My stomach turned over.

"Can *you*, Mr. Sack?"

"I, a mere diplomat? You compliment me extremely, Miss Stone."

"Go on," I urged.

"The bridge of boats collapsed and took the Khalsa with it," he mused. "It was never a retreat, for they fought madly every second . . . but it was a reckoning. They had murdered our wounded, and the generals thought it best that an example be made."

"What sort of example?"

Augustus Sack lifted his wineglass, swirling the liquid within as a gentle smile touched his lips. "I did not arrive until the Khalsa had been conquered, but this was the colour of the Sutlej when I saw it after the rout. We fired every weapon we had into that river. Ten thousand Khalsa men and one woman died that day, either drowned or shot whilst in the act of drowning."

"That's horrifying," I breathed because I could not help myself.

"All the more so for Thornfield." Mr. Sack sipped his vintage, clearly unperturbed by its shade. "The woman I refer to is Karman Kaur. Thornfield was in the thick of it and, in his later delirium, it became clear to my man Clements that upon spying Karman in the watery massacre, Thornfield tried to save her. The fool got sliced in the back for his trouble. He nearly drowned in blood and gore before he made it to Karman on a riverbank covered in corpses, but she was so full of holes that only meat remained of her. Head half blown off, body riddled with grapeshot. Pity. She was remarkable. He spent over twenty hours on that beach with her remains amidst the carnage, unable to move from blood loss. Oh. Have I delivered too graphic an account for your taste, Miss Stone? My apologies."

In truth, I did feel faint—with rage, with grief. "Blood has always upset me, and imagining . . ."

"Here, a bit more claret will restore you."

Crimson liquid splashed before me. "Mr. Thornfield was delirious afterwards, you say?"

"He had suffered a large wound which went untreated for a full day after taking a literal bloodbath, so that is hardly surprising." My eyes shot up to the political as I realised Augustus Sack was actually enjoying my distress. "Thornfield was on the brink of death for a fortnight. I was busy planning terms of the treaty with the Director, but Clements was with him for much of it. The illness was an ugly one, Miss Stone. Fever visions, night terrors—often you could hear his screams, before Clements had managed to calm him."

If Mr. Thornfield had been the one to relate the story, I should not have been able to bear it; seeing his face, his attempts at a wry brow, his guilt like a gouge through his breast, his natural stoicism—all should have conspired to tear me in two. Learning the details from an utter villain, however, one I knew had ordered a child kidnapped and starved, that was a simple matter of endurance. Mr. Sack could smirk knowingly all afternoon, relate any repulsive tragedy which had befallen Mr. Thornfield, and I could sit there, blithely picturing my knife in his guts.

"Tragic, no doubt, and yet I cannot fully sympathise when the man so unnerves me," I owned, downing half the claret. "Thank you. Mr. Sack, I feel much restored."

I had puzzled him, for he beamed in approval whilst his eyes narrowed to cruel slits. "Forgive me—I should never dream of upsetting a lady of your myriad charms intentionally. Where was I?"

"Mr. Thornfield was ill, but . . . I have heard nothing to indicate he was mad?"

"Ah, yes!" The portly diplomat settled himself back in his chair. "I first knew Charles Thornfield as a strapping young medico with a head of hair so black it was nearly as blue as his eyes. After the battle, he was finally brought back to our camp by a Bengali company, and the wretch was so covered in dried gore that an orderly shaved his head. When he could walk again, and speak a little, after three weeks' time, the new growth was white as goose down. The entire camp was unsettled by it—they thought him possessed by a devil.

And perhaps it was something to do with the circumstances in which he found his lady love, but he developed the most extraordinary aversion to touch thereafter. Clements clapped Thornfield by the bare arm one afternoon whilst he was shaving and nearly got a razor in his eye. He began wearing gloves soon thereafter, even when the Director demanded his services in the second Sikh conflict. I don't suppose you've ever seen a man performing surgeries whilst wearing gloves, Miss Stone? Madder than a full March moon, and he has never fully recovered."

"Clearly not," I said, half smiling. "Not if he couldn't manage to puzzle out that his closest friend kept the trunk under his nose all that while."

"You most eloquently return us to the topic at hand, Miss Stone." Mr. Sack tapped all ten fingers of his hands together. "I confess to having been testing you—I know it was early days for you at Highgate House when I was present, but nevertheless I could not help but wonder whether a connection formed between you and Charles Thornfield. How foolish would I have been to take into my confidence a confederate of his, sent to sound me out? But now I see that you, like him, are merely a thief."

His words, warm at the outset, deepened to a sickly-sweet growl.

I glanced at the time and then at the window, where scattered snowflakes drifted to their sooty demise. No one, I realised, knew I was here save Sack and the grey-moustached clerk who had shown me in; suddenly I wanted someone else present, anyone else.

Draining my wine, I shrugged. "I am not accustomed to being called names, Mr. Sack, but you can see my dress and the necklace for yourself, so I can hardly contradict you. Anyhow, I have already made my full confession. What do you want from me?"

"I should think that obvious, Miss Stone." Mr. Sack's lips thinned, a predator's expression in a piggish countenance. "I want the trunk. What do you want?"

"A satisfactory recompense for having delivered it to you. And to know all that you do about the circumstances of Clements's and Jack Ghosh's deaths, for I must understand whether forces continue to threaten my welfare. Did you send Ghosh to Highgate House after you were driven off yourself? Mr. Thornfield suspected as much, I overheard."

Augustus Sack snorted in contempt. "Jack Ghosh had his uses, but I should never have sent him *alone*, Miss Stone, not into that household—I should have been a fool for trying. An armed guard of Company officers to search the place whilst the occupants were locked in the cellar, on the other hand? I was organising just such a campaign."

Then I was only just in time.

"Ghosh acted on his own recognisance?"

Mr. Sack tilted his head back and forth, considering. "He has been in this office on many occasions and could easily have found Mr. Singh's correspondence, so that is the most likely explanation. He was a brute and a snoop and the world is well rid of him."

The words were delivered so carelessly that they seemed altogether true. The waters I had dived into were far murkier than I had imagined.

"What about John Clements? You said you no longer suspected Mr. Thornfield of murdering him—why?"

"Poison simply doesn't seem our dear Charles's style, does it?" The diplomat sighed. "Clements had been looking into the circumstances surrounding David Lavell's unfortunate murder in Amritsar, but my late colleague hadn't the intellect God bestows on sheep. He was low over the project, over his lack of progress. Then he saw an old love of his briefly, and he sank further into melancholy. Honestly, Miss Stone? I believe he took the soldier's way out. Now you will tell me where the trunk is."

The moment of truth could not have come at a worse time.

"I cannot tell you where I have hid the trunk yet, Mr. Sack," I demurred firmly, "not for lack of trust, but because I wish to know what you plan to give me as a finder's fee."

Mr. Sack, far from looking miffed at my insolence, grinned. Rising, he approached me where I sat, rubbing his hands together like a benevolent uncle out of a Dickens novel. An equally avuncular glimmer came into his eyes as his hand rose, seeming about to whisper a caress of fingertips over my hair.

Mr. Sack ripped the necklace from my spine.

I shrieked briefly, but soon mastered myself. Had I been less frugal and bought a sturdier chain, I might have had my neck snapped—as it was, the metal gave before my bones did, and I was left a shaking huddle on the floor, battling not to whimper as I observed the first red drop of blood trickle from my shoulder onto the creamy carpet.

Mr. Sack squatted, dropping his hand to lift my head. The fiery pain produced when my posture shifted was shocking, and I gasped.

"Miss Stone, I do not think that we quite understood each other when I said this was a *Company* matter," he hissed. "Here is what I propose: I assume the trunk is somewhere nearby. If by midnight tomorrow you supply it, and I find it contains what I am looking for, I will give you a gift. If you do *not* supply it, I warn you that I know every fence and pawnbroker in London, not to mention every ship's captain who might be tempted to sail away carrying a mysterious female passenger. The Company owns this city, Miss Stone, and you have stolen from us—so now I own *you*. Your rooms will be watched, you will be followed, and when you have given me what I seek, my gift to you will be that I shan't rip those earrings from your lobes."

Augustus P. Sack leant forward, close enough to bite me, close enough to kiss, laughing as I scrambled away. He tossed the bloodied necklace in the air, caught it, and put it in his trouser pocket. We stood facing each other, my breath heaving as more jewel-bright liquid seeped into the bodice of my dress.

"Put your cloak on and lift your hood so that no one need glimpse any blood, least of all your own sweet self," Mr. Sack suggested, ringing a bell to see I was escorted out. "Thank you for your visit. And, I assure you, I look forward to our meeting again with the very *greatest* pleasure."

My hooded cloak served his purposes just as neatly as Mr. Sack had imagined, and I arrived at the Weathercock without a single glance of concern darting my way. This is not to suggest that eyes did not follow my progress; shadow-obscured figures trailed after me as I exited East India House, for I saw their doubles in the windowpanes, and when I had reached my lodgings, I peered through the curtains and saw men with hats pulled low, studying newspapers as they idled against the brickwork.

These small impediments served solely to bait me.

I called for linens and hot water. Viciously harsh with the key, I locked my door and pounded a single fist against it, unspeakably vexed both at myself and the *badmash* who had dared to treat me so.

My requested supplies arrived well before an hour had passed, and I barricaded myself in again and stripped all away, sinking into the bath. Gingerly, I cupped my hand and splashed at the line Mr. Sack had torn through my skin, which had already stiffened into a fiercely throbbing counterpart to the tear in my scalp. I then lay back to wash all clean.

Soaking, drifting, I sifted Mr. Sack's fresh details in my mind. Some were valuable wholly in the sense that I loved Charles Thornfield, others in the sense that I wanted him safe. Sack's words could have been false, I told myself, but they had not sounded like any sort of prevarication I had ever encountered—what, therefore, would it mean if they were truths?

Nothing to the good, I thought at first. My feelings upon theorising that Sardar Singh was a liar were, in ascending order: shame, hurt, and dismay. I hesitate to tell you that lies, reader, are a very easily learnt knack, so I did not for an instant marvel over whether he could have retained possession of the precious trunk, crossing oceans with it no less, without confiding in anyone.

Yet I could not reconcile what I knew of Mr. Singh with the fresh sketch which had been inked—and neither could I reconcile his epistolary posturing with his obvious chagrin at Mr. Sack's visiting Highgate House, his love for Sahjara Kaur, and his fury that Mr. Thornfield might have exposed her to evil influences.

At the thought of what Mr. Thornfield must have seen on the battlefield, his childhood love blown apart and swept ashore like so much river flotsam, I was tempted to weep.

No weeping, I thought furiously. *Thinking is more useful than weeping.*

I allowed my mind to drift farther afield; after all, this whole mess had begun in the Punjab.

Who is to say the key to it could not be found in the Punjab?

Lest one mistakenly consider me a close reasoner, I am only a close observer of human nature, my own being defective. On this occasion, however, I had lit upon a valid idea. Streaming bathwater everywhere, I leapt out of the tub, hastily drying myself before throwing a dressing gown over my shoulders. The steam had become soporific, and I needed to wrest nagging hints from the hind of my brain to the front.

After an hour's chaotic sprawl in my bedsheets, I thought I had got somewhere. It was hardly evening, and yet the sunlight had utterly decayed, winter's dreary gleam just visible through my curtains.

Eagerly, I hastened to write a letter to one Inspector Sam Quillfeather.

Solving the murder of Jack Ghosh was irrelevant, for I had killed him; solving the murder of John Clements was impossible at the moment. A grisly trail of blood across the continents, however, had been left behind by those associated with Karman Kaur's vast fortune, and I thought that, all other avenues being barred, I might glean some leavings from an earlier—much earlier—misdeed.

I had to solve the murder of David Lavell—in Amritsar, all those years hence.

It is of the utmost importance that I see the papers regarding Mr. Lavell that Mr. Clements was studying. . . .

This I wrote to Inspector Quillfeather, followed by:

If I am correct in my conclusions, I must confess to you that I have committed a terrible crime, and must be brought at once to justice.

THIRTY

I leaned my arms on a table, and my head dropped on them. And now I thought: till now, I had only heard, seen, moved—followed up and down where I was led or dragged—watched event rush on event, disclosure open beyond disclosure: but now, I thought.

It's a lucky thing I left my card, isn't it, Miss Steele?"

The sun had long since set, the eleventh hour dolefully chimed, and Mr. Quillfeather's bright hazel eyes were creased with fatigue as he passed me paper after paper from a battered black case. Some were written in Punjabi, which I placed in a separate pile. Others were reports from Lavell's superiors, however; some were letters writ in my native tongue; and a few were journals written by Lavell himself, which I snatched up eagerly.

"You were very frank with me, Mr. Quillfeather, and you seem a true friend to Mr. Thornfield, so I must learn to be at ease in your company. Thank you for bringing these so quickly—you've no reason to trust me, after all."

"I have reason to trust myself, Miss Steele, and you have always struck me as a most scrupulous young woman?"

Smiling at this outrageous compliment, I touched the black buttons at the neck of the high-collared coral dress I had donned to hide my fresh battle scar. I had always thought Inspector Quillfeather remarkably affable for a policeman, and it was shocking to realise that speaking with him felt like conversing with an old friend.

"I will thank you for saying so by taking you entirely into my confidence—for I need you, Mr. Quillfeather, both you and your police wagon."

"Yes, you mentioned having committed a crime?" Inspector Quillfeather's prominent brows wriggled in disbelief. "Surely you do not expect me to believe—"

"Let me tell you the story from the beginning. You first called Charles Thornfield to examine the body of John Clements because you knew Clements had been studying Lavell, and that all these men were acquainted in the Punjab?" He nodded. "Would it shock you to learn that Mr. Thornfield has taken me into his confidence regarding that subject?"

"Certainly *not.*" He sniffed. "Forgive my candour, Miss Steele, but may I remark that Thornfield seemed quite, er, *aware* of your presence, very aware indeed?"

My heart leapt skyward at this, but I forced myself to focus. "And you still have no suspects regarding the Clements poisoning?"

"None, though I am convinced that a man in the midst of an investigative effort is very unlikely to commit suicide."

"Then may I ask whether you know the story of the lost trunk?"

"That has rather an air of romance, doesn't it? I fear I do not."

I thought of Mr. Quillfeather losing Vesalius Munt's lust diary in a fireplace, steeled myself, and heaved a great breath.

"If I were to tell you of a mistake that Mr. Thornfield and Mr. Singh made long ago in the Punjab, would you hold it against them? If what they did to protect someone they loved was not . . . entirely legal?"

The tufted brows now swooped like carrion birds towards his

nose. "Charles Thornfield is the very *best* of men, and any friend of his, especially for so long a period, must be exceedingly well chosen. Please continue?"

Telling the tale of the trunk took us to the midnight hour. Mr. Quillfeather, positively twitching with interest, paced as I sat painting a crimson picture of a bloody history for him. When I had nearly concluded, after confessing all my prevarications at East India House in an effort to protect my unlikely friends, I began unbuttoning my frock, and he froze in astonishment.

"This is what Augustus Sack did when he saw even a taste of what he thinks is coming to him," I said, revealing the ugly stripe.

"The brute!" he exclaimed.

"We haven't time for outrage," I protested, quickly righting my attire. "Without your help, I am lost, Inspector, and I have an intuition that the trail, though cold now, leads back to Amritsar and David Lavell's demise. You see why I must help you to solve it, and before midnight tomorrow? I've only a day, and the pieces don't fit. Please say you'll assist me."

Mr. Quillfeather flung a long arm out, palm up. "Miss Steele, can a man make a greater blunder than to ignore the intuition of a woman? When our mutual friend has been wronged unspeakably, yourself injured, and a child shamefully abused? I am your man to the marrow!"

"We have only until tomorrow," I breathed, "and if you make an enemy of Mr. Sack, you could—"

"Sleep is for the weak, and what is an East India Company bureaucrat to a seasoned peeler?" He landed in the chair opposite, somehow still conveying the impression he was in motion. "We begin work at *once*, and I shall tell you all about these documents, and we shall see what we can accomplish."

I opened a bottle of claret, Mr. Quillfeather finished emptying the case, and the clock ticked inexorably onward.

So commenced a strange stretch of hours during which I consulted with the man I had once feared as I do the gallows. Inspector Quillfeather saved me time reading by detailing what the officers' reports contained, outlining the contents of the Punjabi documents, and summing up the early diaries. David Lavell, it seemed, was every bit as thoroughgoing a scoundrel as his crony Augustus Sack. His superiors commended his ruthless ability to worm his way into any society he wished whilst revealing, even in their compliments, their distaste at his complete lack of principles. The Company men relied on his insinuating ways as well as his connections to Karman Kaur's family: between them and the Thornfields, the few scattered politicals north of the Sutlej when the fighting broke out were still kept in French wine and aged Scottish whiskey. Lavell's throat had been cut in his own rooms, which led the Company to imagine that one of his many dalliances had grown jealous of Karman, or that a Sikh acquaintance had been fleeced one too many times at the tables.

"The domestic setting means it is extremely unlikely that Lavell should have been killed by a stranger?" Mr. Quillfeather thrust his jutting chin as if to inquire whether I agreed.

I did, and we continued. Lavell had bled out quickly, and there were no witnesses; he was found cold in his bed a week before the Battle of Sobraon.

"Sahjara Kaur inherited, of course," I mused.

"Quite right, but inheritance could not have been the motive, even if the heir had not been a little girl. Despite her mother's assets, her father had amassed considerable gambling debts?"

"Was no one ever suspected?"

Mr. Quillfeather drummed spindly fingers on the tabletop. "I don't believe so? The housekeeper was questioned, and said Lavell had returned, after picking up another delivery of imports and contraband to buy the goodwill of the Amritsar elite."

The clock's hands spun too swiftly, dizzying me. A second bottle of claret became necessary at three in the morning, and at six we called down for toast and kippers. Try as we might, we could find no clue—and if Lavell had died at the hands of an anonymous *badmash*, then I was wrong, and the murder in Amritsar meant nothing, and barring a miracle I would fall into Mr. Sack's clutches upon the morrow.

"We're going about this wrong," I sighed at nine o'clock, squinting balefully at the sunlight shearing through window. "We must consider who *wanted* Lavell dead."

"I fear there are too many options to narrow our choices?"

"Any number of people hated him, but if unrelated to the trunk, they don't help us, so we can discount them anyhow," I answered, shuffling papers. "Mr. Clements could have had nothing to do with it, for he died trying to solve the crime just as we are. Mr. Sack needed him alive if he wanted to keep bleeding Lavell of Karman Kaur's money. Mr. Thornfield had cause, but he was already at war. Mr. Singh . . ."

My eyes flew open again as I gasped aloud.

"Miss Steele?"

No, it cannot be. My stomach fluttered weakly with horror.

Yes, it can.

"Lavell picked up a shipment of goods to use for bribes that day, you said. Did any of the officers' letters mention what he employed to curry favour or with whom he did business?"

"He did business with his wife's family, naturally," Mr. Quillfeather said as the colour left his gaunt face. "But by all accounts, Mr. Singh was in Lahore throughout the First Sikh War?"

I thought about Sardar Singh—his history, his noble bearing, his monkish preference for a solitary life of few friends, simple comforts, and quiet study; I thought of his almost casual celibacy. I thought of his distinctive handwriting, the paper Mr. Sack had thrust before my eyes reading, *Your Company has raped my entire cul-*

ture in systematic fashion; what is in my possession will remain there, and any attempt by you to retrieve it will result in your bloody death, and swallowed black bile.

"I think I have it," I whispered.

"What is it, then, Miss Steele?" Mr. Quillfeather pressed.

I told him, hoarsely but efficiently, precisely what it was. The policeman's hollow chest leant towards me until I thought he should fall from his chair, and his hand ruffled his hair in appalled disbelief.

"All this time?" he marvelled when I was through.

"All this time." I pressed my hand over my breast, for it ached beyond bearing. "Oh, Mr. Quillfeather, there is only one thing to be done."

"What is that, Miss Steele?"

I held out my wrists. "I'm a hardened criminal—write a note to the nearest station house and have a police van sent round at once. You've a pair of darbies, about you, I assume?"

Plentiful hay littered the back of the wagon, which clanked as it traversed the ancient streets. There were also blankets and, though they smelled of mildew, I managed awkwardly to wrap one about myself with my hands shackled together, for my lovely blue cloak could not protect me from the freezing draughts gushing through the iron-barred windows. Once bundled, I fell to the straw and rested my head, for by now it was ten o'clock and, for all that I was strung tight as a violin, my eyes kept fluttering closed.

So weary was I, and so overwhelmed, that no blackness resided behind my lids; rather, a kaleidoscope of colours whirled. My scalp ached and my neck throbbed, but these tangible discomforts were as nothing. I knew what must be done and loathed to do it; I knew what must be said, and the words pierced, cold as icicles in my throat.

Oh, Mr. Thornfield, how little do you deserve all that has been done to you.

Nature will have her way, however, and I did sleep for an hour despite being fettered and fretful. The scratch of rough wool and the whispers of the hay were crude lullabies, but comforts nonetheless, for they distracted me from the fear of failure and the near equal fear of success.

"Miss Steele?"

My name brought me back to myself, but it was the scrape of the key in the locked door of the wagon which startled me into full consciousness; shivering, I sat up just as a man's fingers gripped the bars and opened the box I had been penned inside. The blanket slipped from my shoulders as I blew a wisp of hair from my eyes, aware that however unruly it habitually looked, now my coiffure must be positively outrageous.

"Were you warm enough?" Inspector Quillfeather inquired.

"No." I managed to get to my feet with my hands on the nearer bench; my legs prickled, and my limbs felt weak and coltish. "Where are we?"

"Well outside of London—not far from Waltham Abbey?"

I must have tottered on my way to the door, for Mr. Quillfeather gripped my waist with hands that looked absurdly long wrapped round it and swung me to the ground. We were in a stable yard outside a hostelry, and I blinked against the glare as my captor released me from the rust-scented handcuffs.

"I take it the plan worked."

"Never did I doubt it would, but may I admit to some initial anxiety, Miss Steele?" Mr. Quillfeather dropped the darbies into his satchel and swung shut the door. "Happily, my fears were unfounded. You were *most* convincingly distraught as we left the Weathercock, and I observed two men who seemed, as you suggested, to be keeping a watch on the boarding house? They conferred quickly and departed in haste after you were shut in the conveyance."

They will go straight to Sack with news of my arrest, I thought with dark satisfaction. *He will search all the London gaols, and when he comes to the division which liaisons with Inspector Quillfeather when they need him in London, the sergeant will confirm my arrest.*

I would not, however, be allowed any visitors; I pictured the apoplexed face of the Company diplomat when told by a placid bobby that he could under no circumstances see Miss Jane Stone before she had been thoroughly questioned, and could not help but smile.

"We've bought ourselves a bit of time," I said, "but how long?"

Mr. Quillfeather called for the constable to drive off; gesturing to a much faster one-horse trap, my ally helped me into it.

"Enough, Miss Steele?" he answered gravely. "It does not matter precisely how much time, provided it is enough."

Nodding, I watched the hedgerows blur as we quit the hostelry at twice the speed we had employed upon arrival. We covered our laps with layers of wool nearly as thick as my finger; silently, as if we had long been close companions, we shared bread and cheese from Mr. Quillfeather's satchel. Keeping a fast pace, stopping once to change horses, we could be at Highgate House by dawn.

It only remained to determine whether I was more frightened of the accursed treasure I would encounter there, or of its keeper.

As it happened, our trials were to commence before we so much as set foot upon the property.

Mr. Quillfeather had at first met my suggestion of driving with resistance; but when I pointed out that a man yawning every ten seconds surely could not mind the roads closely, he thanked me, wondered aloud if there were a finer woman in all of England, tipped his hat brim over his eyes, and commenced snoring. Our horse was sturdy country stock which needed little minding, so I allowed my thoughts to drift; a fox barked mournfully in the distance, and I heard the soft hooting of owls, but these nocturnal companions were as nothing compared to the friend in my mind's eye.

You are about to see Charles Thornfield again.

How would he look, after these weeks apart? *Identical to the way he looked before,* I thought, but then questioned the assumption. Jane Eyre, when leaving her fiancé to find her own way, writes:

> *As yet my flight, I was sure, was undiscovered. I could go back and be his comforter—his pride; his redeemer from misery; perhaps from ruin. Oh, that fear of his self-abandonment—far worse than my abandonment—how it goaded me! It was a barbed arrow-head in my breast: it tore me when I tried to extract it; it sickened me when Remembrance thrust it further in.*

Charles Thornfield and I had only skimmed the rippling surface of an attachment which went, on my part, deep as the Atlantic; despite his refusals, I could not pretend my departure had affected him not at all. Mr. Singh had begged me to return, and even Mr. Quillfeather had sensed an "awareness" of me on the part of my former master. To this I could add the evidence of my own experience. Mr. Thornfield, upon learning I planned to leave Highgate House, had neither wept nor blustered; he had shrunk, this impossibly large presence curled in on himself as if acknowledging I was right to seek elsewhere for happiness and affection, for loyalty and love.

He had been wrong—but did he know as much? Would the absence of my face at the dinner table cause him to push his plate away? Would he have wasted, would he have—wonder of wonders—*missed* me?

It will likely make little sense to the reader that seeing my sad, sweet Clarke again had invested me with new hope of winning Mr. Thornfield; but she had transformed me into a creature who, rather than being loved solely by a madwoman, was loved by a madwoman and a precious friend. I grieved for her, I regretted her sorrows, and yet they inexplicably heartened me. Never had I doubted her devotion prior to her flight, but as to the nature of it—if Clarke could long for the touch of my hand, could not Mr. Thornfield learn to?

Brooding made the time pass more quickly than I should have thought possible, and the birds were chirruping in the yew trees outside of the familiar village when Sam Quillfeather awoke with a punctuating snort. The horizon flamed red-gold, and our second horse, which had given admirable service, snuffled tiredly.

"Nearly there, I believe?"

"Very nearly, Mr. Quillfeather."

"We shall soon get to the bottom of this affair, eh?"

Twenty minutes later, we pulled into the village, and there was the sleepy half-timbered inn, there the post office, there the white steepled church, and there the road leading to Highgate House.

In the next instant, my gaze lit upon something foreign, however, something that emphatically *did not* belong.

"Get down, below the seat," Mr. Quillfeather hissed. "Quickly!"

I threw myself to the floor. A band of half a dozen splendidly uniformed men approached the inn on horseback, presumably seeking eggs and sausages; I had never seen East India Company soldiers in the flesh previous, and yet I should have known one anywhere. These wore white breeches and white waistcoats with gold buttons, black neck stocks with scarlet sashes to match their brilliant blood-red cutaway coats.

"Mr. Sack planned to storm Highgate House for the trunk if he did not have his way," I whispered loudly. "Do you think—"

"I do not know what to think, but we are taking no chances!" Mr. Quillfeather thrust his hawk-nosed face down at me. "Once they are indoors, you shall drive as fast as you can to Highgate House. If you can locate the trunk before giving the alarum, then your story will be strengthened by hard evidence. I fear they may not believe you otherwise, or that the guilty party may fly? I shall learn what these men are planning. Be of good courage!"

Forcing myself to breathe, I nodded. The inspector brought the trap into the yard and swung from it with his stork's legs akimbo, waving away offers from the stable boys to wipe down and water the horse, telling them his niece had need of the vehicle. When Mr. Quillfeather had disappeared into the inn, the lads stared in wonderment as my head popped up like a jack-in-the-box; but I did not linger for conversation, snatching up the reins and setting off at as brisk a clip as the fagged horse could produce.

Mr. Sack's words echoed, their urbanity laced with the tinny sneer of the school yard bully.

The Company owns this city, Miss Stone, and you have stolen from us—so now I own you.

If the Company owned London, its vast power feeding itself like a deadly serpent forever swallowing its own tail, how far did its reach extend? India, of course; China, certainly; the Punjab, without question—but a sleepy hamlet a day's hard ride from the metropolis?

Did Sack mean to wage a literal battle against the warriors of Highgate House? And if so, was he brilliant or simply obsessed?

My joints ached with fatigue when I pulled up to the gate, tethering the horse to the scrollworked iron. I wanted to treat the poor animal better, but I could not risk my approach being heard, and so caressed its ear and assured it of further attentions directly.

Skirting the main house along the edge of the forest was a simple matter, the dew wetting my boots as I strode round the back. The sun was well up, and my nerves sang so dissonantly with hope and apprehension that I wished only for it to be two hours from now, ten hours from now, when all was settled one way or the other.

I should never have wished such a foolish thing, so in part I blame myself for what took place that morning.

The kitchen door would be unlocked, I knew, for Mrs. Jas Kaur was always up with the dawn, grinding whole spices into blends and rubbing yogurt into cubes of freshly killed sheep. She was there when I appeared like a vision from the mists, pulling the feathers from a chicken, and she gasped out something in Punjabi before smiling at me.

"I'm sorry to have startled you—I'm afraid I wanted my return to have an element of surprise."

Jas Kaur, who spoke no English whatsoever, chuckled and shrugged and waved a down-covered hand at the door, bidding me go about my business.

I did so, stepping into the wider hall of the servants' wing.

The air here was cooler than the kitchen, thin and still; I had walked for perhaps twenty yards before I remembered the night prior to my quitting Highgate House, the terrible attack by Jack Ghosh and what came afterwards, and I knew I was heading in the wrong direction.

The treasure would be close to its possessor, and its possessor had recently moved.

Turning, I ran back the way I came and out the door, provoking another mild exclamation from Jas Kaur.

Sahjara will be having her morning ride, I thought, *and everyone else wide awake and working, and only one guard set to impede you.* I sprinted across the grounds, lungs burning in the cold, cloak flapping about my bright rose skirts. *I will find the treasure, and give it to Mr. Thornfield, and all will be well, though it will hurt terribly.*

When I reached my destination, to my surprise no bearded and turbaned Singh whatsoever awaited me. Having planned simply to wave my way through—as I was known to all the servants despite my terrible facility with their names—I hesitated momentarily. When I realised that Sahjara was the true commodity to be watched over, however, and decided her guard must surely be out riding with her, I gripped the door of the cottage and found it locked.

This, though not precisely surprising, was vexing—until, that is, I remembered my late mother's enormous facility for losing keys, and recalled that Agatha had kept a spare underneath a loose flagstone a few yards from the entrance. It took a few minutes to recognise the right one, but barely a minute had passed before I stood there triumphant, with dirtied fingernails and an eroding key.

It fit, and the door creaked open.

I began the search with the bedrooms, but soon thought better of this and ran for the attic; up, up, up I went to the place where I had read Mamma's letter so long ago. When I reached it, I took in the steep-roofed chamber, all its draped furnishings like censorious guards.

A large wooden crate which had not been there before rested under the round window.

The lid came off easily and revealed paperwork—written in Punjabi, but the neatly lined columns indicated records. I scattered them to the floor, heedless of the mess I was making. I had not tossed many aside before I found a thin piece of wood, and I clawed the false bottom from the crate.

Reader, no dolls rested within.

There were jewels, however—set jewels and loose ones, sapphires wrapped in velvet and topaz tumbling loose, an emerald bracelet which spanned wrist to elbow and a ruby tiara which would have caused the Queen of Sheba to swoon. There were ropes of pearls, golden chains, and the effect was nearly laughable in its opulence: so I did what I always do at inappropriate times, and I laughed.

"I shouldn't celebrate prematurely, Miss Stone."

I turned, electric with fright; there stood Garima Kaur, her once-handsome face set, holding a curved and long-bladed knife in her hand.

THIRTY-ONE

I requested him to shut the door and sit down: I had some questions to ask him. But when he complied, I scarcely knew how to begin; such horror had I of the possible answers.

Her words were free-flowing, practically accentless save for the same familiar lilt Mr. Singh owned, which made my very marrow quiver.

"I had supposed you didn't speak much English?"

This amused the housekeeper, but the twitch of her lips was not even hinted at in her eyes. Where Mr. Quillfeather appeared affably cadaverous, all appendages and hooked nose, Garima Kaur looked as if her flesh had shrunk too tight to fit her, the sleeves of her drab housekeeper's black loose around her pale brown wrists. Save the unsightly scar, one might wonder if she were a shade casting an illusion which only appeared to be human skin.

"Having deceived far better minds than yours, I cannot fault you for thinking so. Do not worry, do not worry," she parroted, and then laughed, her lips stretched over her teeth. "I speak six other languages and worked with Sardar from the time we were both fifteen; he and Charles spoke Punjabi half the time, English the other—I could only have avoided learning your ugly tongue had I stuffed my ears with cotton."

There were things about her I had slowly gleaned, reader, and things I had only just come to understand; I had not, however, expected her capacity for deception to exist on so global a scale, and could not help but admire her.

"And you never let on that you were fluent?"

"Why should I want to deal with every loutish *ferengi** Sardar traded with?" she spat. "They only wanted to rob us, as you do now—Charles was raised better, but the exception proves the rule, as you say. Take the knife from your skirts and leave it in the trunk, covering all up again."

Of course she knows about the knife, for we had been speaking English as she drifted the corridors all that while, and I never thought twice about it. Peering at her cruelly curved blade, I dropped my paltry weapon in the tangle of treasure at my feet; against a Sikh fighter, it may as well have been a berry spoon.

Lacking even that token means of defending myself, however—every hair on my crown stood on end. I returned the false bottom and the papers to the crate, fitted the lid, and then turned to face my captor.

"Please." I raised my hands in supplication, "I mean you—"

"Surely you are not about to tell me that you *mean me no harm*," Garima Kaur interjected, and again the shift of her mouth did not affect her cavernous eyes. "Do you really mean to suggest that you intend to leave that fortune in this garret and walk away from Highgate House?"

Deliberately, I exhaled. "There are half a dozen East India Company soldiers in the village sent by Mr. Sack, ready to raid the premises—it's time this was ended."

Conversely, her eyes burst now to life, as if I had turned up a gas lamp.

---

* A derogatory term in India for a Western foreigner.

"Are there?" she said softly.

"Yes, so you see—"

"Then you are correct, Miss Stone. It is time this was ended."

Garima Kaur's voice was a scalpel, and a small wound in the rational world opened; I had assigned many characteristics to her since that morning—brilliant, vengeful, and ruthless all figured prominently.

Not once had I suspected her mad.

"You cannot mean to fight them," I pleaded. "The people you care about will be hurt, maybe even killed, and the wars are over, you cannot bring the battlefield to England and expect—"

"How came you to be here?" she interrupted, swinging the long knife in a lazy, expert circle around her index and middle fingers before palming it again.

"I think you killed David Lavell."

She laughed. "Remarkable. What else do you think?"

"I think that John Clements was in love with you, and when his colleague Mr. Sack received a taunting letter from Sardar Singh, I think . . . I think he suspected you were the one behind it. All those years he trusted you, fed you information without realising that's what you wanted him for. And I think when he concluded you had stolen the trunk, and had finished Lavell, I think he confronted you, and you poisoned him in his rooms in London."

Her mouth worked again, but now pain warped the derision, and she paused before speaking. It was an expression I knew well and, though kissed by madness thanks to my mother, I did not think I lived in its embrace as Garima Kaur did, that obsessive desire to right *the single great wrong* which has swept your life off its course. We could have been sisters otherwise, for our propensities; we could have been friends.

Her silent shock confirmed my suspicions, albeit superfluously—I had only to recall the single thread connecting the dead men to know I was right.

Mr. Sack was the one who had first stimulated my interest, when he had said of John Clements, *He was low over the project, over his lack of progress. Then he saw an old love of his briefly, and he sank further into melancholy. Honestly, Miss Stone? I believe he took the soldier's way out.*

Half a clue is as useless as none at all; but then I recalled a scrap of conversation which illuminated a dark landscape.

Poor old Johnny, with that puppyish way he had about him, Mr. Thornfield had said to Mr. Singh the night I had eavesdropped on them. *Remember when he used to sniff around your secretary as if she were Cleopatra?*

Garima Kaur, of course, was that secretary—a woman loved by a British political she used and despised, a woman capable of copying her employer's penmanship and imitating his voice even in a language she loathed, writing, *Your Company has raped my entire culture in systematic fashion.* Mr. Singh had remained in Lahore throughout the First Sikh War guarding Sahjara, I was certain, for it fit all I knew of him, but his secretary—the loyal princess with the accomplished knife hand—had made at least one delivery to David Lavell in Amritsar, and she had left him with a gash through his neck.

"I think you may have tipped Jack Ghosh as well," I mused, "but I'm not entirely certain of that. Did you?"

"Yes." She had recovered her poise, though the sunken pits of her pupils were glassy. "I contacted him through Clements—he was staying in the village. I waited until Sardar and Charles were guaranteed to be absent, and then I sent him word they were away from home."

"Why?" I demanded.

"To be rid of him. I could have finished him for us. And to be rid of *you.*"

"I don't . . ." I faltered. "God in heaven. Why should—"

"I removed the jewels from Sardar and Charles's keeping, yes, having heartily approved their taking them." Her voice was as smooth as a river stone and twice as cold. "They were keeping it *unguarded,* in a *child's trunk.* I was on my way to meet Sardar when I glimpsed Sack leaving the house in a sort of ecstasy. Sahjara confirmed she had shown him her dolls—I was forced to act quickly. I buried the trunk in the depths of the warehouse the Thornfields shared with Sardar, wedged between cracked jades and silks from poor dye lots, where no one would ever look. When Ghosh took Sahjara . . ." She directed a series of guttural curses in an unidentifiable tongue at the sloped ceiling. "They ran off like puppies, did not tell me what was troubling them, or I could have given them the trunk. Her mind was forever altered, and I love that little girl as if she were mine. How could I *not* vow to kill Jack Ghosh? I waited for years, until the perfect opportunity arose. I meant to do it with my own blade—after he had finished you, of course, but that did not go as planned."

"Yes, but as for myself—"

"I said, *I love that little girl as if she were mine*!" she screamed.

The air turned to ash between us—thick and hot in our throats, as if a volcano had erupted.

"Oh," I breathed, comprehending.

She laughed miserably, the scar across her brow raised in disbelief. "In an English way, you are quite clever, Miss Stone; but in an English way, you are also very stupid. When Sahjara was sent away, my heart broke—she was all I had left of my friend Karman, and *oh*, Karman was like a shaft of God's light striking earth. Lavell wasn't fit to clean her boots with his spit, and the instant I heard of her demise, I slaughtered him in Amritsar and was back in Lahore before anyone there so much as knew he was dead. He would have alternately ignored and bullied Sahjara, that precious girl."

"Her father would have mistreated her. But not Sardar Singh," I murmured, understanding still more.

"Not Sardar—Sardar is a good man. When she was sent to England, he used to tell me to have patience, tell me that we would all be together again soon. For a while, Miss Stone, I thanked God for my new home here at Highgate House. I was teaching Sahjara Turkish, Pashto, how to sharpen a sword and how to balance accounts. Then Charles hatched a truly foul idea with Sardar—and in English, no less, though they did not know I minded them."

"He wanted an English governess. I'm so sorry."

"No, you aren't," she growled, gesturing with the knife's tip. "You adore the pair of them, and they love you back, they . . . they can *see* you."

A sob escaped her, and she panted, clutching the knife's handle so hard I thought her fingers must break.

"It was bad enough not to work with Sardar any longer—passing the time with him on long journeys, going over inventory, dining with his sister," she seethed. "As his confidential secretary, I negotiated for him, flattered for him, foresaw every difficulty and prevented it happening at all. Here I was sent to the *servants' wing*, none of my efforts with Sahjara were given more than passing praise, Sardar lost all interest in my company, there was no meaningful work to distract me, and then they determined to advertise for a white governess. I wrote to Mr. Sack the next day."

"How could you do such a thing if you truly loved Sahjara?"

"To remind them of *who we really are.*" Her death mask's face tilted up, challenging. "I was wasting away, misery robbing me of flesh by the pound, and they didn't even *notice.* They needed something to fight for, Miss Stone. We all did—it's in our blood. My friend Karman was eighteen years old when she had her first Khalsa cavalry uniform tailored—we were born to fight, destined by God, and she would have despaired at seeing them so emasculated."

This account of Karman's uniform rang like bells; but before I could comprehend why the detail was important, I was being given my marching orders.

"Now, come here, slowly—and walk down the stairs, slowly. If you fail to do exactly as I say, this knife will be in your kidney."

The *slowly* portion was easily managed, for I dreaded accompanying her. My limbs moved stiltedly, as if they belonged to Sahjara's long-lost dolls, but my senses were keenly attuned to the familiar creak of the staircase, the velvety wood of the aged bannister. The only thing to do was to keep her talking—but I could not for my life imagine what to say to a woman who wished I had never been born.

"Why didn't you tell them about Karman's fortune after Sahjara was rescued?" I asked.

"At the start of *another* war?" she sneered from behind me.

"After that war, then?"

"In the midst of transporting an entire household across the continent?"

I stopped, hands visibly limp at my sides, and turned.

"You knew it was wrong," said I. "You don't want to find out what Sardar will think."

"He stole those jewels in the first place, you fool," she spat, but her lip trembled. "Go on, out the back door and head for the forest."

"What are you going to do with me?"

"I haven't decided yet. I am curious, though, how after all you have seen and discovered, that you could dream you mean me no harm."

I stepped outside. The fresh air was like a slap across the cheek; it warned that, unless I was very fortunate, I was about to die. I would not, I had already determined, fall to my knees and allow the guillotine to fall. If this was to be the end, I would fight with tooth and claw at the edge of the woods; but before those methods were employed, I elected to try persuasion.

"We could invent a story," I said, and it was not a lie: it was a *possibility*. "Do you wonder how I came to go armed?"

"No." The tip of her knife caressed the edge of my cloak. "I was listening outside the dining room. Faster now, towards that copse."

The woods loomed before me, the thicket from which Edwin

and I had burst, all the starkly bare-limbed beeches and the forbidding pines near to the edge of the ravine, and I did not want to die where Edwin had, could not stop my skin from crawling when I felt his unmoving stare pinned to my face.

"Then you know I have faced hardship," I insisted. "I will tell you more, something I have never deliberately told anyone: I am your equal in infamy. I have murdered—more than once. I can lie for you, only tell me what your reasons were."

"You suppose a false confession will save you?"

This, of all strokes, was surely deliberately arranged by God to needle me.

"It isn't fal—"

"Never mind. I will tell you anyhow what my motives were," Garima Kaur added, and I could sense the gathering snow as the avalanche gained speed, hurtling towards the ravine. "I killed David Lavell because had he never existed, we should all be at peace. I maintained ties with John Clements because thereby I kept my finger on the pulse of the activities of Augustus Sack and Jack Ghosh. I killed John Clements because, imbecile though he was, he knew enough about my movements to grow suspicious after I forged the letter. And I forged the letter because—"

"Garima! And can that possibly be Miss Stone?"

I could have collapsed at the sound of that voice—indeed, I staggered, and Garima Kaur gasped.

We turned as one animal to see Sardar Singh. He seemed puzzled but delighted at the sight of me and said something in Punjabi to Garima Kaur, who had clearly masked the knife in the fold of her skirts upon the instant she heard him call from behind us.

She answered readily enough; but I, much closer to her, could see that her hands shook, and knew that what had previously been a perilous situation was now absolutely a deadly one.

"Miss Stone!" Mr. Singh exclaimed. "What a happy moment I

seem to have chosen for a long winter's walk. I have passed many a frank hour in Charles's company since you departed, but had hardly hoped you would return after you sent no forwarding address. Welcome home—or so I hope you think of it."

Garima Kaur aimed a painted puppet's smile at him even as her eyes flooded with tears.

Not long after my mother's death I had a nightmare I actually remembered, the screaming sort which led Taylor to single me out in the Reckoning: a creature came to the doorstep of our cottage, and I knew without seeing, as one does in dreams, that it was a rabbit, and I picked up the small animal thinking to pet its fur. Only after I had lifted it did I realise that it had already been skinned by a hunter, and begun to be butchered as well; deep knife marks were scored along the spine, and only half its head remained, as if the brains had been reserved to tan the pelt. Though it moved as if alive, nuzzling my chest, I knew it must be in unfathomable pain, and I awoke shrieking about needing to kill something because in the dream I had no proper weapon.

I had not thought of that nightmare in years; but Garima Kaur's expression brought it immediately to mind.

"Mr. Singh," said I, stepping two paces away from her.

"Whatever is the matter?" he asked, frowning. "Have I interrupted you?" These questions were followed by what I assumed was the Punjabi equivalent.

Garima Kaur waited to see what I would say, her attention flicking rapidly between us.

For the first time in my life, I decided that truth was preferable.

"She speaks English," I announced. "Very well indeed, and she has the treasure—look in the garret of the cottage, under the false bottom in the crate of records."

Several expressions fought for supremacy on Mr. Singh's face, the winner proving disbelief. "Miss Stone, I cannot imagine—"

"You don't have to; you can find it yourself. She wanted to protect your sister's fortune, but now there are Company soldiers in the village, Mr. Quillfeather is keeping them at bay, and she killed David Lavell in Amritsar all those years ago. I know you won't mourn him, but she's the reason Sack was here—she sent him a letter in your name."

Garima Kaur's fleshless face reacted not at all to my betraying her secrets, but she swayed slightly. I had told only a fraction of what I knew, and only what I thought Mr. Singh and Mr. Thornfield might forgive. Slanting my gaze, I willed her to understand me.

I will never tell them you killed John Clements, nor that you sent Jack Ghosh—not if you and I can both survive this.

Sardar Singh stood there motionless, taking in my words with eyes wide; I saw the exact moment when he believed me, for he flinched. Then I remembered that—unlike Mr. Thornfield, who seemed to expect trouble to find him magnetically—Mr. Singh had always known that the key to the conundrum lay in how Mr. Sack came to be at Highgate House in the first place.

The fact of his being here was, I agree, the greatest mystery of all.

"Garima, is what Miss Stone says accurate?"

"Yes." The tears spilled down her bony cheeks. "But it was all for you, for *us*. Why should I have told you I speak English? You would talk of your problems to Charles, and I solved them without your ever asking me to—I was your djinn, your secret granter of wishes. You used to need me. How can you think you don't need me any longer?"

"We all of us need one another," he said softly, but she was a rudderless ship close to capsizing.

"Sahjara and I were fine, we were all *fine*, until *she* came!" Garima Kaur may as well have been brandishing the knife, for her words slashed through the air between us. "So you didn't seek me out any longer, banished me to the servants' quarters, and never thought to visit—none of it mattered whilst I still had our sweet girl to tutor. But you took even that pittance and gave it to *her*, and never noticed I was fading away right in front of you."

Mr. Singh raised his hands, seeming as contrite as he was appalled. "We shall set all this right. Do you hear me, Garima? Please—I am to blame, you are correct, but as to Augustus Sack's coming here—how could you even consider bringing such a plague upon us when he had thought Karman's treasure lost in the Punjab?"

"Because the only time you ever loved me was when I was fighting beside you!" she cried.

A ghastly silence fell. I took in her terrible scar, her posture like prey caught in an iron trap. I did not blame Mr. Singh for being celibate, nor for being stupid, because I am apparently remarkably dim-witted myself where Clarke is concerned. Imagining the eternal desert Garima Kaur had walked through all her life, however—next to the man she loved but never near him—repelled me on her behalf. I had chosen to leave Charles Thornfield, and she had locked herself in a prison with a view of paradise through the window.

Mr. Singh, meanwhile, seemed to have forgot his own mastery of our language—any language—regarding Garima Kaur as if he had never truly set eyes on her previous.

"There were five of them, and they came on us, thirsting for blood and spoils, and you'd no heart to take their wretched lives, but I was there, and so we lived," she said brokenly. "We *survived*, Sardar, and for two terrible, magnificent minutes, I wasn't invisible. And after it was over, after they'd marked me and my chances at marriage to anyone else had vanished, I disappeared again the same way my hopes did. So courteous you were, so distant—I may as well have been your shaving mirror."

Had she whipped the blade from her skirts and slit his belly, I do not think Mr. Singh's expression would have differed.

Then I did something entirely brainless, and thus set a number of dreadful events in motion. What I ought to have done was to bolt whilst her attention was fixed on the object of her affections; I ought to have sprinted to the main house shrieking for Charles Thornfield, and many ghastly consequences would have been avoided.

Unfortunately, I scarcely ever scream when I am meant to.

"I think we must—"

The instant I opened my lips to offer an unsolicited opinion, Garima Kaur bellowed in rage and swung her knife at my throat.

There was not enough time.

Had there been enough time, I could have evaded her; had there been enough time, Mr. Singh could have drawn a weapon. Had there been enough time, Garima Kaur would not have been almost unhampered in her decision to send me to hell.

I say *almost* unhampered.

Sardar Singh emitted a wordless sound of protest and leapt, using what I only then realised was a final recourse when lacking other shields, and blocked her blade with his metal cuff. The knife slid with a horrid scraping noise down the sheath and then soundlessly sliced off his right hand.

Garima Kaur emitted a despairing groan, dropped her weapon, and ran.

Mr. Singh roared in pain and fell to his knees; I whipped off my cloak, bundled it, and I buried the gushing stump within. The hand with its severed tendons and its white gleam of bone lay to my left, pointing in the direction whence its butcher had fled.

"I'm sorry, I'm so sorry, I— You saved my life."

Mr. Singh's lips were pressed so hard within his mouth that nothing save beard remained; he had not lost enough blood yet to faint, but the shock did battle with his consciousness nevertheless.

"Please, you'll be all right. You have to be. *Please*."

I think my uselessness roused him, for he ordered, "Help me to stand."

Between the two of us, we managed, though I nearly toppled under his weight; the instant he was upright, he was striding for the main house with his good arm about my shoulders, I pressing the ball of my cloak against his stump.

"Can you make it?"

"I don't know, but I needn't," he gasped. "Not if you fetch Charles to wherever I collapse."

The journey, I am sure, took less than three minutes; if ever three minutes were drenched with horror enough for three lifetimes, it was those. We burst through the front door like marauders, interrupting Charles Thornfield as he came from his study into the hall, dropping several pieces of mail on the table.

"What in the name of the devil—" he began, and then paled. "Is this our Jane returned? Oh my God—Sardar, what has—"

"We'll talk about it later, Charles," Mr. Singh said, breath heaving. "If you could stop me bleeding to death in the meanwhile . . ."

Mr. Thornfield's cry of dismay was the only signal I had that Mr. Singh was about to topple like a felled tree; I was dragged a bit by his bulk, but Mr. Thornfield caught him round the waist and together we made it into the parlour. Mr. Singh landed on the settee and lay back, all his limbs quivering.

"Jane, whatever are you doing here?" the love of my life demanded. "Who dared to lay a finger on—"

Mr. Thornfield tore off the makeshift bandage of my cloak and saw what had been done.

"No." He closed his eyes and shook his head as if the sight could be erased. "For Christ's sake, no. Sardar—"

"No!" I cried, lurching towards the window.

Mr. Singh managed to raise his torso, and the three of us watched as Mrs. Garima Kaur, saddled on Nalin, galloped past the bay window with Sahjara seated between her knees and exited the estate through the gate where my forgotten horse was still tethered with its trap.

THIRTY-TWO

"I could dare it for the sake of any friend who deserved my adherence; as you, I am sure do."

What in hell is the meaning of all this?" Mr. Thornfield shouted as he tore off his coat and rolled his sleeves up, dropping to his knees. "Where is Garima off to with Sahjara?"

"Go," Mr. Singh gasped, eyes on me. "Please bring her back. It is unfair to ask it, I know, but—"

I was already running; the last sight which met my eyes before I flew out the parlour door was that of Mr. Thornfield viciously cursing at the spectacle of an arm without a hand attached before tearing off his gloves.

There was no time to think about what that meant as my feet and lungs propelled me towards the stables, my ears burning in the cold. Homelike smells of leather and manure assaulted me as I charged into the refuge of my childhood, my exhalations hanging in the atmosphere like malevolent ghosts.

The Sikh grooms stared at me in astonishment. There might have been some trouble over procuring a mount; but as it happened,

Sahjara's new mare was still saddled, having just returned, so I swung myself up onto Harbax, tearing out of the stable as if Satan were at my heels. For the first five minutes of my pursuit, I despaired of catching up to them before we reached the village, for Nalin was the fastest steed in Mr. Thornfield's stables, and young Harbax the most unpractised.

Gift of God. Sahjara named you that, and Mr. Singh supposed it important, though Mr. Thornfield joked about the meaning. Please, please prove to be a gift of God.

I caught sight of them—a silhouette, really, just an outline in the gathering crystalline fog. Recalling with a thrill of hope that Nalin was the least tractable of her species I had ever encountered, I urged the more docile Harbax onward, feeling the mare surge as she sensed my distress.

Garima Kaur heard her pursuer and craned her head to glance behind, her emaciated form looking dangerously fragile atop such a powerful beast. Nothing of Sahjara could be seen save her rhythmically swinging feet; but reader, I loved her then, for she was the victim of blighted hopes and blind circumstance, as so many are, as I am, and Garima Kaur did not have a knife any longer, and I would return Sahjara to the people who quietly, carefully cherished her if it cost me my own right hand—or worse.

Abruptly enough that I feared snapped necks would result, Garima Kaur reined Nalin, and the mare emitted a wild, wary sound; she turned the horse with difficulty, and then it was that I saw Sahjara's lovely face—uncomprehending and panicked.

"Miss Stone!" she gasped. "Where is Charles? Mrs. Kaur says we are to escape to London, that there are Company soldiers making for Highgate House."

"Mrs. Kaur," I cried through the mist, "there is no one more sympathetic to your situation than I. I beg you, however—"

"You will ruin more lives, but you will not ruin mine entirely," Garima Kaur snarled. Nalin's nostrils flared, her hooves agitatedly stamping the ground.

"I seek to ruin no one, I swear to you upon any holy book you like." Harbax, conversely, was an island once halted, perfectly quiet. "Only let me take Sahjara home."

"Sahjara is *mine*!" she cried with the cracking voice of a breaking woman.

At times disaster visits us when we least expect it; and at others, we see the fraying rope and know that the hour of peril is nigh. I did not know what form disaster would take, but I knew then that Garima Kaur would not be returning to Highgate House, knew it with every fibre of my being.

I should have loved to stop the inevitable, but there was nothing whatsoever I could do.

Nalin reared—triumphant, angry, frightened. One never quite knows what a horse is thinking, but I like to imagine that horses are able to sense what people are thinking.

My frantic cry as Garima Kaur was tossed like a flour sack from the fractious horse was not so loud as the hammering of my heart when I saw Sahjara begin to slide after her kidnapper. Dismounting to catch her was impossible, and riding to meet her would cause Nalin to career off until she found the horizon.

Helpless, I flung out an arm.

Falling, Sahjara did the same.

Except she did not mirror me, not quite; she hooked her arms round Nalin's neck, swung a leg over, and tumbled almost gracefully, a pendulum swinging within a clock. When she dangled from the mare's neck, dropping to the ground a few seconds later, I could have wept for relief; she had Nalin by the reins immediately, thanks only to instinct. Then she viewed the tragically contorted body of Garima Kaur and began to cry.

How long I held her there in the road after dismounting Harbax, I cannot say; how long Garima Kaur took to die I can, however, for she was stone still by the time I had reached Sahjara. Not wanting to leave any erstwhile friend of Sardar's crushed and discarded, I instructed Sahjara to mind both horses and not look at me as I hid the sickeningly light shell of a body under a holly tree.

When I emerged again, I was a wreck and Sahjara similarly blasted. We embraced for a long while, each supporting the other, until I realised that I was freezing to death.

"We must get back to the house," I grated. "Ride Harbax, and I'll take Nalin?"

"Miss Stone," she sobbed. "We can't leave Mrs. Kaur so. What if—"

"There are no more *what ifs* for her, darling," I said, hoping Mr. Thornfield's favourite endearment might calm her. "She is sleeping peacefully, and no one can hurt her ever again. Ride back with me—the gentlemen are worried sick over you."

"Because of the Company men?" she asked, touching the knife in her hair.

"Yes," I lied. "We're going home now, as fast as ever we can."

"Miss Stone?" She raised her tearstained face. "You won't tell Charles that I learnt to hang from the neck of a horse—"

"Oh, Sahjara," I gasped, pulling her back to me. "I'll never tell. You're alive, and you've a secret—well and good. Live as long as you can, and have as few secrets as possible. Mr. Thornfield wouldn't last a day without you—remember that, for all our sakes."

When we arrived back at Highgate House, my first task after guiding Sahjara to her bedroom was to take Sam Quillfeather's neglected horse and trap to the stables. The grooms were absent, probably speculating as to what the deuce had happened to Sardar

Singh; so I rubbed the beast down and afterwards stood, silently weeping, with my brow against its ribs.

I simply did not wish to face learning that anything disastrous had befallen Charles Thornfield—for he would equally be lost without Sardar Singh, and I had begun to suspect that I might be similarly affected by his absence.

After cursing myself for a weakling, I hurried to the main house, tapping upon doors and tumbling through them as if I had a right to be there. They had made me feel as if I had a right to be there, after all—they had made me feel as if I had a home.

At last I found Charles Thornfield in the kitchen, speaking urgently to Jas Kaur as he washed his bare hands; they were already clean, but his crusted shirtsleeves told a gruesome story, and his white hair was liberally speckled with blood.

"How is he?" I questioned. "Did he tell you . . . did he—"

"Jane!" Mr. Thornfield dived for a cloth, drying his fingers; seeing them naked again was peculiar, as if I ought to turn away and grant him privacy. "Say that you found Sahjara, I beg of you. If she—"

"I'm here," came a small voice, and I saw that the commotion had brought Sahjara out of hiding; she stood in the hall just outside the kitchen, eyes puffy and strained.

I am not proud of many of my actions; most were committed for selfish reasons, and bringing Sahjara back ought to be numbered among these, for I could not bear the thought of losing her. However, the look on Mr. Thornfield's face as he crossed the flagstones in a frantic leap and swept her up into his arms, cradling the shivering child's face against his shoulder without any barrier between them, I thought might be cause for celebration.

"Mr. Singh?" I asked again. "I must know how he fares, and what he told you. Please—"

"He told me, in brief, everything. And he will live, thank God. I was just arranging with Jas here to steep claret with oil, rosemary, and oregano to prevent infection. Supposing that fails us, I'll resort to pine pitch, but Sardar is an accommodating bastard, so I don't suppose he'll put me to the trouble if he can help it. I've knocked the poor fellow cold with laudanum, so now it is merely a matter of vigilance. All right, darling, hush," he spoke against the crown of Sahjara's head. "I was sick with worry over you, but I was busy saving your uncle's life."

"My uncle?" she repeated, dazed.

"Yes, I know you don't remember," he returned tenderly. "Your uncle Sardar he has always been, and ever will be. I didn't quite know how to introduce the topic. Forgive me?"

"Of course," she murmured. "What happened to him?"

"He was hurt." Mr. Thornfield shifted as if to set her down, but she clung to him. "All right, all right, Young Marvel—he'll be fine. Everything is fine now."

"It isn't fine," she choked, clutching his collar. "Garima was thrown from Nalin. Miss Stone dragged her out of the road, but she's . . ."

Charles Thornfield had endured such atrocity in his life that he simply glanced at me and then closed his eyes, nodding after he had seen the answer there. Yes, his jaw tightened painfully, but he gave no other sign. I do not think he meant to be stoic; he had already suffered so deeply, however, and gained so much back in a single hour—Sardar's life, Sahjara's safety, Karman's fortune—that news of Garima's death caused him to bend rather than break.

I shall never forget, however, that after he turned to Jas Kaur and told her the news in Punjabi, she sat at her worktable and split in two—sobbing, palms upwards in helpless anguish before her, her breaths like a death rattle.

It was a lesson, and a welcome one, that one member of the household had not been indifferent to Garima Kaur's existence; it was a lesson that everyone—even myself, I dared to hope—would be mourned by one fellow traveller.

Mr. Thornfield pressed her shoulder warmly and carried Sahjara from the kitchen. As I likewise exited, granting Jas Kaur some privacy in the rawness of her grief, I called, "Mr. Thornfield, there is much which I can explain to you, if you will allow it."

"Allow it?" Despite all which had occurred, a spark of gallows humour entered his eye. "Jane, I think it is safe to say I shall insist."

He was about to take Sahjara upstairs when a forceful knock sounded; instead, he set her down with a quiet, "Stay with Jas, darling," whisking her behind the kitchen door and shutting it firmly.

It is a testament to how well used to this household I had grown that I did not even blink when he pulled a short sword with a carved ivory handle from its place upon the wall. When I snatched up a dagger from farther down the corridor, however, he hissed, "What the devil can you be thinking? That could very well be half a dozen Company soldiers."

"Your point, Mr. Thornfield?"

"For God's sake, Jane, I—"

"Mr. Singh is incapacitated, and if you think I am going to allow you to face *badmashes* alone, you're cracked in the head. Sir."

Mr. Thornfield pronounced several exasperated curses, barked, "Keep *well* back, do you understand me?" and then strode for the entrance, where our visitor was creating still more of a racket than previous.

When he threw wide the door, however, I dropped the blade upon his pile of correspondence there on the table, weak with relief; Sam Quillfeather stood at the top of the steps, his aquiline nose thrusting urgently indoors. Mr. Thornfield gripped his hand even as he turned to cast a concerned eyebrow at me.

"Inspector, I hardly dare inquire as to what happened between you and the Company men—though last I saw you, this pixie vanished seconds later, and that sits poorly enough in my gut. We have much to discuss."

"Yes, upon this very *instant* lest disaster befall you!" Mr. Quillfeather returned. "And Miss Stone will correct me if I am mistaken, but I think she and I have reached an amicable understanding? Good heavens, Thornfield, whose blood is that?"

Mr. Thornfield gripped his neck, rubbing exhaustedly. "Sardar's, I am sorry to say. He will live, thank heaven, though 'tis a grievous injury. There are tales to be told."

Mr. Quillfeather's fingers clenched around his tall hat. Stepping within, he scuffed his boots upon the rug.

"Then shall we pour a spot of brandy, sit before a fire, and tell them?" he suggested. "Perhaps if we are wise enough, there may be a happy outcome after all?"

"I don't think after all this anyone will accuse me of possessing a speck of wisdom, but I can certainly contribute the brandy and fire." Mr. Thornfield sighed, taking the inspector's place before the door. "Only let me quick march to have men sent for Garima's remains and I'll join you in the parlour."

"Remains?" Mr. Quillfeather asked softly when Mr. Thornfield had vanished. "Oh, Miss Steele, what must you have seen today?"

"Enough," I admitted, drying my eyes. "But far less than some."

We talked much that afternoon, and though I explained that I had schemed to outwit Mr. Sack—much to Mr. Thornfield's belated but vocal dismay—I said nothing yet of my greater history with Inspector Quillfeather, nor did that gentleman press me into broaching the subject. The most difficult moment, therefore, occurred when we had reached an understanding and regarded each other in the pale amber glow of the dying fire, knowing we could postpone the inevitable no longer.

"I shall glance at Mrs. Kaur's remains and fill out the death report, as the task would pain you, Thornfield," Inspector Quillfeather kindly offered. "There is, if all I have heard is true, no need for an autopsy?"

"I should not be offended," I assured them.

"No need." Mr. Thornfield tapped his fist against his brow, the curve of his wide shoulders slack with grief. "I just stitched up what Garima did to Sardar—she could have been in no state to manage Nalin. I only thank Christ you were there, Jane."

Mr. Quillfeather rose. "I shall also get a message to Mr. Sack, and arrange for the village physician to be here by morning. Time this was ended, don't you think?"

"High time," Mr. Thornfield grated, donning his hat and coat as we three exited the parlour.

Mr. Quillfeather headed for the underground mortuary, Mr. Thornfield and I out of doors. The stars were a cold spill of glass shards in the darkening sapphire canopy, sharp and treacherously beautiful; I wondered whether they looked the same in the Punjab, and if Garima Kaur thereby had at least the same sky to wish upon, or if they were hung at another angle in England, and the housekeeper thus entirely alone. Mr. Thornfield, seeming to see me for the first time, shook his head in annoyance.

"You'll catch your death without an overcoat, you mad thing." He passed his own round my shoulders and coughed, abashed. "Your cloak is quite irretrievably ruined, by the by."

"I should think so."

"You'd not have wanted it again in any case, I imagine."

"No, Mr. Thornfield."

"Your new frock suits you much better than governess weeds, though you did 'em better justice than most."

"Thank you, sir."

"Is that what you wanted the advance in wages for—to convince Sack you were a thief?"

"No . . . well, yes, but I've also had an inheritance. I shall tell you about it when we are through."

"Confronting Sack in such an audacious fashion—I hardly know what to make of these extraordinary efforts upon your part." He gazed upwards as if only the firmament were equally unfathomable. "You could have found a far better recipient for your loyalty, you realise, than a ruffian with a curse upon his house."

"I don't agree," I said, and all my heart was in those words.

"Jane, blast it to pieces, I don't know whether I can do this."

"At least you need not do it alone," I breathed, wanting only to reach out and fold my arms around him.

Charles Thornfield shifted upon the grass, shoved his hands in his trouser pockets, and strode towards the cottage.

I hastened after. We traversed the grounds in lockstep, lit a lantern within the cottage's sitting room, carried it with us as we trotted up the stairs; the door to the garret remained open and Mr. Thornfield made at once for the crate, flinging the lid aside and digging through papers until he arrived at the false bottom and tore it open.

The treasure gleamed with the too-saturated colour of poisonous vipers and venomous toads—a rainbow's spectrum of danger, those jewel tones which Nature employs to warn *keep away*.

"Yes, these are Karman's," Mr. Thornfield said, and it scored my heart to hear his voice breaking. "Oh, Jane, so much suffering, and for this pile of trinkets? You cannot know how I loathe myself, little friend, and the only riddle left to solve is why Sardar doesn't detest me as well."

Then I recalled one of Garima Kaur's last confessions, and why the seemingly trivial detail mattered.

"Garima Kaur said that Karman had her first Khalsa cavalry uniform altered to fit her when she was eighteen."

"What?" Mr. Thornfield's rugged face tilted in confusion.

"She wanted to fight long before her jewels went missing." My entire frame was taut with nerves and desperate hope. "Garima told me so. So now you know it had nothing to do with you—she would have risked all for glory anyhow, can't you see? No object is served by flaying yourself over the circumstances of her departure. War was in her blood and bones, and *doer of deeds* is what Mr. Singh said her name meant, and perhaps you left the Punjab to escape your heartbreak and made mistakes afterwards, but maybe the rest of it—the death, the *loss*—that was only what happens to us after we are born, and not a punishment at all."

"How do you know she died in battle?"

"Mr. Sack told me."

"Damn his eyes." Mr. Thornfield drew a shaking breath. "Jane . . ."

"I learnt in London that there was no subject upon which I was more mistaken than that of myself, sir." Brushing my fingertip over the blood still soaking his sleeve, I met his tearful gaze with my own. "Of you, however, I have made a close study, and I vow that I think no man more deserving of a measure of happiness, and that if I could fetch it for you, I should travel the globe."

"What if my remaining here whilst you travelled the globe would rather hamper my contentment than enhance it?" he answered after weighty pause.

"Then . . . I should stay here," I whispered. "With you."

Mr. Thornfield dashed his fingers over his eyes. "You've had an inheritance, you say."

"Sir?"

"An endowment, a legacy, a *bequest*, you contrary sprite."

"Yes, and a generous one."

"So you've no need of gainful employment any longer? You are an independent woman of means who requires no assistance to make her way in the world. Pressed duck served on fine china, Belgian lace edging your lowliest handkerchief, servants used as ottomans—all this, and without the necessity of drudgery. No longer need you talk horses for six hours daily to earn your bread and cheese."

I saw what troubled him then, and thought to tease him; instead, I laughed, and drew a step closer.

"I like horses," said I, lungs tight with feeling. "I always have done."

"Do you like dreadfully draughty English country houses?"

"I did not always, but I have grown to."

"What about curry?"

"Everyone likes curry, sir."

"Could you like a former Company medic who keeps a morgue in the cellar?" He smiled with such tender sadness that it nearly felled me.

"I don't like him—I love him. You aren't wearing gloves."

"So it would seem. Jane," he said, and then neither of us was speaking, for his mouth was sweetly, reverently pressed to mine, his hands at my nape and on my cheek, and when my lips parted and I tasted all the affection he had kept so long buried, I knew that no words could possibly have served as well as his kiss did.

"You don't know what it did to me." Breaking away fractionally, he clenched a fold of my skirt in his right hand. "At least before, I could hear your step upstairs, or know you were riding, or catch your laugh when passing my study. One is not always directly regarding the full moon, Jane—but should it disappear, the oceans would rot. I was rotting already when you found me, and then your tide pulled, and you were gone so long. A mere matter of weeks, but still . . . how long till you leave me again?"

Kissing him once more seemed the right answer, but I could manage it only briefly. Realising as one that others' needs should be seen to quicker than ours, we hastened out of the cottage where I grew up, and back to the main house, the sky a faint lavender like a bruise almost forgotten.

. . .

The following day, preparations had been made for Charles Thornfield and myself to travel to London with all possible haste; Mr. Quillfeather had made our position clear to us, the village doctor fetched to tend to Sardar Singh in the meanwhile. I breakfasted with Sahjara and Mr. Thornfield, all of us sombre despite our victories. When I laid down my fork, I looked up to discover blue eyes studying me as if I were some sort of miracle, and an irrepressible smile spread over my features.

After the kiss, we had parted, and I believe Mr. Thornfield sat up with Mr. Singh for most of the night. Still—there was a crackling in the air between us now, something electric and wanting.

"May I see Mr. Singh alone?" I asked him. "I feel I cannot leave without thanking him for my continued existence."

"Of course. By extension I owe him my own, for I should have borne the loss of you with very bad grace."

Sahjara looked up curiously, lips curving. "Are you staying, then, Miss Stone?"

"If Mr. Thornfield will keep me after we conduct an important conversation, then yes."

"Naturally I'll keep you, we're all of us deuced keen to keep you—we've considered the benefits of shackles," he huffed. "A conversation on what subject?"

"My name, sir. But first I must see Mr. Singh, and then we must be off, and after all is settled with Mr. Sack, then I must tell you a story."

Charles Thornfield scowled, and shrugged, and said it was all very good if I wanted to play games with him, that I was incapable of changing his mind, and then he swept off to see our carriage was packed. I kissed Sahjara atop her dark head, and then I hurried upstairs to the bedroom where Sardar Singh lay recovering.

Knocking first, I entered; the injured man was propped upon pillows in his darkened bedchamber, his arm bound in a sling with copious bandaging at the end of it. I could smell herbs and wine from the poultice, incense from a small metal holder in the corner of the room. The walls here—my father's old bedchamber, I realised, thought to be my dead uncle's—had been converted almost entirely into shelves containing score upon score of books, many cracking like so many ancient stone tablets.

"You needn't look like that, Miss Stone." Mr. Singh's voice was rusty but sure. "Charles stitched me up again, and I cannot imagine anyone taking greater care."

"Without gloves, no less."

"A triumph borne of misfortune, yes. He managed on the battlefield with far cruder measures, going so quickly from fallen to fallen."

I perched upon the edge of the bed. Mr. Singh's brow was strained, though not yet feverish, and his head was bare; his long hair glistened faintly, but seemed almost dry, and he smiled at my speechlessness.

"There was blood in it," he rasped. "Highly dishonourable—it felt almost worse than my arm. One of the servants will be along shortly to tie it up again, for this . . ." He waved at his injured limb.

"Oh, I cannot tell you how sorry I am. Please forgive me," I begged.

"For the loss of my hand?" He shook his head. "There is nothing to forgive—you were the one truly endangered, after all. At last I am able to offer a true sacrifice: a disfigurement upon the altar of justice. Or so I tell myself. Monkishness is second nature to me, but as to my hand—I was quite attached to it."

"So often the way with hands," I agreed, and then we were laughing like overwrought children, wrung to the highest pitch of nerves, and there were tears in my eyes when I added, "I am also sorry for the loss of your friend."

"Yes, Charles told me." He sighed, a devastated look clouding his strong features. "This is on my head, not yours."

"You ought not blame yourself any more than Charles ought to blame himself for your sister's demise."

"I shall have to teach myself that wisdom slowly, Miss Stone, as did he."

I wanted to ask if he had suspected Garima Kaur loved him, but thought the question cruel.

"What does the name Garima mean?" I asked instead.

"There isn't quite an equivalent in English." Shifting, he settled farther back into the nest of pillows. "A crossroads between dignity and pride, perhaps."

"Do people's names always seal their fates, or only in the Sikh culture?"

He smiled again, though it did not erase the lines of suffering etched upon his brow. "I sound superstitious, don't I? I do think that when God gifts a parent with insight, a child's name will reflect their soul. Take Jane Stone, for instance—it suits, does it not?"

"It's the plainest of given names and an adopted surname," I confessed.

"Ah. Is it really? Nevertheless, I believe you mistaken. We are so locked within ourselves, we often lack perspective on these subjects—I take it to mean a rock, an island in the midst of perilous seas, and Jane is from the Hebrew, you know."

I had not known. "What does it mean?"

Mr. Singh's eyes, though laced with red spider's silk, twinkled thoughtfully. "Gift from a gracious God. I have found it, you will pardon me, not unfitting."

Rather than stem my tears, this spurred more. "You are far too kind to me."

"It is a great privilege, to have the opportunity of being kind to anyone. What is your real surname, if you'll pardon my asking?"

"I don't precisely have one—but it used to be Steele. I mean to tell Charles the whole story after Sack is dealt with; I shall give you a full account then, I promise you. Rest well."

"Steele," he mused as I quit his bedside. "Better and better—strength, resistance, a fighting spirit."

"I'll need all I have just to enter East India House again," I said from his threshold. "Mr. Sack is a brute and I shan't relish seeing him again, even with Mr. Thornfield there."

"So that is the meaning of all this bustling." Sardar Singh's eyes narrowed into knife blades. "You are off to London. What do you mean to do there?"

"To give up the treasure," said I, gently shutting the door.

THIRTY-THREE

"No—no—Jane; you must not go. No—I have touched you, heard you, felt the comfort of your presence—the sweetness of your consolation: I cannot give up these joys."

"Are you mad?" Augustus P. Sack circled his own desk like a jackal.

He was discomfited; I, Charles Thornfield, Sam Quillfeather, and Cyrus Sneeves had descended on him without warning. Freely do I admit that we brought the treasure he sought, and freely did we give it—expecting at any moment the arrival of another guest.

Mr. Sack, for a man who had been seeking a single prize for so many years, did not seem sufficiently glad to have it in view. Soon, I understood this was due to the fact he had loved tormenting Messrs. Thornfield and Singh with that the same glad viciousness which had caused him to tear my necklace from my throat; in addition, he suspected something amiss with the generous overture.

He was perfectly correct.

"Our demands are entirely reasonable, sir," my solicitor droned. To Mr. Sneeves's immense credit, confronting the East India Company sounded as if it were the duller sort of business to conduct on any given Thursday. "You are welcome to this box so long as you never reveal from whence it originated. Mention of the Punjab is acceptable, but this gentleman is to be released from all liability regarding the ownership of these gemstones. To that effect, you shall simply sign this paperwork exonerating Charles Thornfield of any wrongdoing, and I shall have it copied and delivered to any litigators in your employ."

"Surely you will comply, Mr. Sack?" Mr. Quillfeather pressed. "You now have my full report regarding the unsolved murder of John Clements, and the killer is beyond the punishment of mortals. All this, and a fortune in recovered property—what could be a happier circumstance?"

Charles Thornfield, meanwhile, continued to say nothing. When we had learnt the true intentions of the Company soldiers from Inspector Quillfeather, he had expressed profound relief; the sight of Augustus Sack, however, predictably wreaked havoc with his digestion. He sat expressionless before the political, one finger framing his temple, boring holes into the enemy with his pupils.

"You've forgot your gloves, Thornfield," the Company man hissed.

"Lucky for you, or I would be challenging you to a duel with 'em," Mr. Thornfield drawled. "Are you ready to steal a little girl's property, Auggie, or shall we keep gassing? The box sits before you. You've won. It's the last pound of my flesh and Sardar's you'll be taking."

"And exactly how does *she* come into this, then?" Mr. Sack's full lips curled in a sneer. "Miss Jane Stone, governess, who claimed to have robbed you of the trunk and then was hauled off in a police wagon. What am I to make of it?"

"A profit, I had presumed," said I. Footsteps sounded in the hallway outside. Glancing from Mr. Quillfeather to Mr. Thornfield, I could not suppress a tiny pursed smile.

There was no knock. There was no warning. There was simply a tattoo of approaching footsteps and then the door banged open, revealing a half dozen Company soldiers and the man they all referred to as the Director.

"Oh, thank heaven," Mr. Thornfield sighed, crossing his legs. "I was on the verge of physical violence."

"Sir," spluttered Mr. Sack. "I . . . You are most welcome. To what do I owe the honour—er, pleasure—of this visit?"

The soldiers from the previous day, resplendent in their white and red coats, formed a neat file behind their leader. The Director was a tall man, impeccably dressed in sober black with silver trimmings; he carried a cane but seemed not to require its use, and his face called to mind a dignified greyhound, lean and efficient. He tapped twice with his cane upon the carpet.

"Inspector Quillfeather, I offer you my congratulations." The Director's voice was high but firm. "Charles Thornfield, it has been too long, too long indeed, sir. It is a pleasure to see you in better health."

Mr. Sack sank back into his desk chair like a deflated balloon.

"By the Lord, you're in fine fettle, sir." Mr. Thornfield offered his hand to the head of the Company. "Thank you for meeting us."

"You have made it well worth my while." The Director smiled coldly. "I was informed by Mr. Quillfeather here that you were being . . . how shall I put this . . . meddled with by certain of my staff. I at once launched my own internal investigation, and I have it on good authority that you are a wronged man. Naturally, the happy recovery of the item in question also sparked my keen interest, and I lost no time in sending a small body of troops to your residence after I had discovered the truth. Thankfully, I am told they were not required to defend you and Mr. Singh. Your services to the Crown and your family's favours in the importation line have not been forgot and indeed continue to be valued overseas."

"I'm damned grateful for your memory, sir," Mr. Thornfield replied.

"Do you hold fast to your decision to turn these spoils of war over to the Company?" The Director tapped the crate with his cane, eyes gleaming with avarice.

"If I never see 'em again, I'll die happier than I ever expected to."

"We were just discussing the remaining formalities and awaiting Mr. Sack's signature," Mr. Cyrus Sneeves intoned, taking a large pinch of snuff to fortify himself.

Augustus P. Sack's rosy features had paled during this exchange beyond a shade I had thought possible; he now gaped, fish-mouthed, as the Director stared at him with all the tender affection of a mongoose eyeing a snake. The soldiers at the back of the room stood at parade rest, eyes forward.

"Of course, of course." Suddenly Mr. Sack was scrabbling at the documents on his desk, as if being asked to address them for the first time. "I shall be only too happy to sign."

"See that you are." The Director nodded to the soldiers; two sprang neatly into action, lifting the crate. "Take this directly to my private chambers—I shall be informing the prime minister I require a word with him this afternoon. Inspector Quillfeather, we are grateful for your efforts on behalf of Mr. Clements; Mr. Thornfield, thank you for your cooperation."

"I was only too happy," Mr. Thornfield parroted at Mr. Sack.

"There is one other small matter," said I.

It was, of course, highly unlikely that the Director had ever been detained by a woman within the very walls of East India House, but a man who is a veteran of foreign wars ought to prepare himself for the unexpected, I reasoned. Dumbfounded, the Director tapped his cane against the rug again, frowning darkly, as Mr. Sack's complexion shifted from white to green.

"Mr. Sack was under the mistaken impression that he confiscated a piece of Karman Kaur's treasure from me, when it was in fact my property. I should like the misunderstanding rectified, and the necklace returned immediately."

Mr. Quillfeather hid a smile, and Mr. Thornfield chuckled.

My solicitor's speckled head bobbed dutifully as he suggested Mr. Sack send the item round to his offices.

"Do as she says, Mr. Sack," the Director commanded. "And afterwards, you can clear out your belongings and quit this establishment permanently. You need not expect a reference of any kind from us—I will not tolerate conspiracies fomenting under my very nose. Unless, that is, I am invited to take part in them—trumped-up politicos with delusions of importance have toppled entire empires. I think everyone here knows to which I refer specifically. Deliver Miss Stone what you owe her, and pray to God Charles Thornfield doesn't whip you through the streets like a stray pup. He would certainly, I daresay, have ample cause."

We found ourselves, Charles Thornfield and I, walking slowly down a wide avenue in Westminster after finishing a celebratory repast with Sam Quillfeather. The high-hung moon was as pearly as the oysters we had consumed, and the cold wind whistled along the cobbles. It was the sort of silver-lit midnight which always reminded me of my mother, and made me wish there had been more picnics before she left the cottage and our garden forever.

Not having been sure of the outcome of our adventure, we had made no plans; now we strolled under winter plane trees, their inky fingers grasping at the stars, watching the lights flickering from within the pubs and the parlours. Mr. Thornfield was quiet with the uneasy calm of learning a long ordeal was behind him, as if not quite believing his fortunes had altered; I was equally still, but with apprehension.

My desire to never be parted from him was as ardent as my desire for breath; but I knew, should I fail to broach the subject of my past,

I could become a puppet Jane, all wooden limbs and painted smiles. Reader, I do not foolishly suppose any one person can ever achieve perfect eloquence regarding their memories and affections and fears; if I did not take courage, however, I should always be viewing the man I loved through four eyes instead of two, ever cognisant of the monster hid deep in the back of my head.

"You are troubled, Jane."

I looked down in some surprise; his hand had caught mine within the folds of the cloak I had borrowed from Sahjara, as I had never made spectacular achievements in the realm of height and did not care it failed to quite reach my ankles. The fact that we were both gloved against the chill did little to diminish the pulse which surged through me.

"If this—if I—am unwelcome," he attempted, "please tell me so quickly. I recall your feelings as stated with exact clarity, I promise you, but I am overwhelmed. When a chap announces, 'I fancy that star in the sky,' and the star is actually amenable—'tisn't likely to be true, you see."

"I resemble no star, sir."

"Well, you've clearly never heard of mirrors, then. I'll teach you to use 'em, they're easy as anything."

I gripped his hand harder and stopped us, staring up at him, *because this all might be lost at any moment*, and the idea broke my heart. His roughhewn face was tilted down in concern, his pale hair agleam in the light of the lamp, and he was everything to me, so if I was not to hear his gruff voice in the morning, in all the mornings, I wanted to paint a mental portrait of him on a London street corner with his hand in mine.

"Jane, you look as though you're saying farewell, and it's deuced disconcerting," he said.

"Far from that." I brought the back of his hand to my cheek, and we resumed walking. "Only I said I had to tell you a story, first. Before you kept me."

"It is only the amount of needless secrecy I've subjected you to which prevents my laughing in your lovely face. If shackles won't do it, I've half a mind to try iron bars. Just here," he added, pausing uncertainly before a neat, narrow row house. "I bought this when I first inherited so we should always have a place to keep our heads out of the rain in the city. Garima used to use it . . . well, before. Should you like to come in, and speak with me? If not, I'll find a cab and take you to your lodging house."

My answer was a rather breathless yes, I should very much like to come in, because anxiety and hope were wrapping thick vines about my throat. I found myself in a pleasant sitting room with yellow and green Sikh tapestries upon the walls and a profusion of richly tasselled cushions on the furniture which the neighbours would have found highly disreputable. After carelessly tossing his greatcoat over a chair, Mr. Thornfield poured spirits into crystal glasses for us as he always did—though now we both removed our gloves—and I placed Sahjara's cloak on a tree in the hall.

When I chose the armchair nearest the fire, he endearingly pulled up a footstool directly before me and sat, our heads now near upon a level. Before I knew what I was about, I stroked my fingers over his temple and he smiled with the roguishness of a tomcat. He placed our glasses upon the carpet.

"You invest me with hope you shan't be punishing me for my asinine refusals with your absence." He caught my fingers and wove them with his own. "All other punishments you care to mete out will be met with better bravery. Now. Let's have your secrets. This house was heated and aired this morning, but I ordered all the servants away."

At times, the swiftest cut is the cleanest, so I announced, "The name I gave you is a false one. As a girl, I lived at Highgate House.

I am the illegitimate daughter of your aunt Patience Barbary's husband, Richard Barbary, and a French dancer who went mad and took her own life."

Mr. Thornfield's dark brows are dashing enough to perform great sardonic feats, but I had never before seen them execute such acrobatics. Then his eyes brightened nearly to sapphire and his lips parted. "You don't mean to tell me that you're really Jane *Steele*?" he exclaimed.

"I . . . I do, actually. How—"

He slapped his knee, barking a laugh. "Mum used to mention you from time to time, the French changeling whose mother wormed her into an English estate. Awfully thick situation for Aunt Patience to swallow, but Chastity and Patience Goodwill never got on, you understand—Mum thought it rather a ripe coup d'état. Why didn't you say something?"

Flushing beet red, I replied, "Your inheritance was unexpected. I wanted to live there again, thought that it may have been . . . mine."

"And so it is!" he crowed. "Every brick, every weapon, every bloody blade of grass is as much yours as I am, darling, supposing you'll give me a pallet in the stables and a crust from time to time. Are you *quite* mad?"

"I don't want you to live on a pallet." My tears spilled, and he painted his fingertips over my jaw. "I want you to live in my bones, but how can you not be angry I lied?"

"I'm a scoundrel, Jane. Born of scoundrels, bred of 'em to boot. Not to mention a whoreson bastard, as you yourself once called me, and I remember the occasion with great fondness save for the part where you toppled off a horse."

"Oh, but there's more, there's—"

"Breathe, darling." Running his palms down my arms, he cupped my small hands in his large ones as we had once done in his office. "Please, I'm drowning just looking at you. Have a spot of pity and breathe for me. So you're a scoundrel too, I take it—I'd suggest we make matching uniforms, but that quite sabotages knavery, you see, and should thwart our purposes. What else?"

"I'm a murderess, sir."

"Does she suppose me deaf and blind?" he cried incredulously. "Does she suppose I simply forgot that she—"

"Five times over."

Charles Thornfield began to say something. Then, brushing his thumb under my damp eyes once more, he began to say something else. Finally, after puffing a vexed sigh, he muttered something else entirely, by which time I was prepared to die on the spot. I think my heart must have only commenced beating once more when the wry creases around his brows smoothed into softer seams, as he looked when he spoke with Sahjara or picked up a delicate antique volume from his library—as he looked when he wanted to take especial care. He passed me his kerchief, counting on his left hand.

"The first?" he questioned, and his rough voice had gentled.

"When I was a girl, my half brother tried to rape me and I pushed him," I whispered. "He died. I used to— I no longer think that was entirely my fault; but it was the most important, for it was the first, and made me who I am."

Mr. Thornfield's eyes frosted over entirely. "Oh, my darling Jane. Next?"

"My headmaster gave me the choice of watching my friend starve or being sent to a madhouse. I stabbed him with a letter opener."

He whistled, continuing to count. "Much more impressive. The third?"

"My landlord beat his wife until she lost their unborn child, so I pushed him into the Thames."

"It's not many corpses as can foul the Thames, bless 'em. You accomplished a miracle. Go on?"

"A judge wanted to buy my friend's little girl and turn her into his dollymop. I gave him inheritance powder and he died dreadfully."

"Not so dreadfully as he should have done. And I know Jack Ghosh personally, my darling, so does that make up the full roster?"

"Yes."

Reader, I wanted with every cell in my bloodstream to fly from the room and weep for days, but I was prevented; the grim line above his clear-cut nose appeared, and he pursed his lips sternly.

I waited, frozen in terror.

"I don't think much of your list, y'see," he declared, and though his eyes were warm they were wet as well. "A more sorry lot of rubbish than you've dispatched I've not heard tell of. Why, in battle, Karman killed dozens of strapping British and Bengal gents who'd not have pissed on these dregs if they were on fire. We simply must raise your killing standards, my darling, because I'm frankly ashamed at the quality of chaps you've—"

We were both laughing through tears by the time I had flung myself the short distance into his lap and was kissing him, so warm and so real underneath me. His shoulders under my questing hands were at first as tense with worry as mine, I think, for I had alarmed him; but soon, they calmed, and he cradled me more softly, and dropped his lips against my neck with a breath like a prayer.

"That was egregiously unfair of you," he murmured against my skin. "I thought you were about to confess to fatal consumption, or a fellow whose company you prefer, or the fact you've been called back to faerie, something bloody *important.*"

"Do you know that you're entirely insane?" I had pulled the black ribbon from his head and buried my hands in his hair.

"Yes, actually, but this form of madness is far preferable to that of a fortnight since, don't y'agree?"

"God, yes." I calmed myself. "And I never thought that mad, only tragic."

He set his hands softly at my waist, frowning in thought.

I passed quiet fingers over his hairline and waited, wondering whether his torment had been constant or more like owning a heart which had stopped like a broken watch; I wondered whether he knew himself.

"I hated the hands which couldn't help her," he concluded hoarsely. "And all those dead, Jane . . . Even after coming here, when I would walk into a pub or a square, I couldn't look at humans without seeing them as corpses." He shook his white head. "Then I saw you. You are so *alive*, Jane Steele, you make my breath catch, as if a glowing creature from the depths of the forest had lit upon the end of my finger. You had already endeared yourself to me by greeting Sahjara so courteously, as if somehow it were a happy circumstance for you to accidentally enter our madhouse. When I saw you fall from Nalin that night, I knew you were dead, my darling, I knew it with such certainty, because how could anyone I had liked so well from the first survive such an accident? Then you sprang up wielding invective and knives and I adored you. I thought it lunacy that you should take such a frank interest in my history."

"Only insomuch as your history makes you who you are today. I dreaded your knowing mine, sir."

His eyes, so wistful seconds previous, narrowed in amusement. "Had you not better call me Charles?"

Laughing, I pressed my forehead to his. "I love you, Charles Thornfield."

He placed his hand over my heart, and I could not help but wince at the sting; where once he had been about to speak, he stilled in chagrin, and I realised any further intimacy would reveal the injury inflicted by Mr. Sack. This was distressing. I wanted no words on the subject of the Company to distract us; I wanted fewer articles of clothing between, and ideally a bed, though the nearby sofa would do, or the rug barring that.

"It's nothing, only a scratch."

"A scratch from what manner of animal?" he demanded.

Clearly I was to be thwarted in any attempt to keep the injury secret; I unbuttoned my dress at the neck a few inches, and then several inches more than was necessary, and watched as my love's heated gaze darkened to black. The gash was indeed an ugly one, a crusted purple line.

"Very well, precisely whom am I meant to murder this evening?" he snarled.

"I thought I was the expert on that activity."

"Jane, I demand satisfaction!"

"Might we employ other avenues in our search for satisfaction?" I said in his ear.

"There have been too many outrages upon your person in our brief acquaintance, and it will *not* be tolerated a moment longer, not while I have breath, do you hear me?"

I placed my hands along his stony jaw, set upon having my own way.

"Charles," said I. "While you have breath in your body is, I hope, a long period of opportunity. Now, if you will forgive me for being coarse, I should like your breath on my body. I am a wicked woman, and I should like for us to go upstairs and wash this blasted scrape, and see that my head is mending well—because that will please you upon a professional level, and because you enjoy being tender with me—and then I should like for you to express that tenderness in positively filthy fashions."

The scowl did not vanish, but now his sculpted mouth and eyes both softened at their corners. "Is that truly how you wish to pass the night?"

"Oh, I do, sir."

"Had I not better ask you to marry me?"

"I don't know. Do you want to?"

Finally, he chuckled and drew me closer, pulling slack lips over the hollow of my throat. "Yes."

I shivered. "I don't see any ministers here, do you?"

"Drat, we seem to have run dry of prelates. Happens at the worst possible times. Jane, we are doing this all out of order."

"Are we?" My nose crinkled in confusion.

"Indeed so." His voice lowered, its warm burr scraping over me softly. "I love you, Jane Steele. I love you. I've loved you since you fell from my horse. I love you, and I'm a damn fool. That should have been said by this time. Now, I've a confession to make." He rose easily to his feet, and I rose with him, for he had slipped his arms round my back and under my legs. "You, my darling, must vow to me on your honour never to fall down another staircase. But you've no idea how cruel it was to have you in my arms like this every night, thinking you should only ever be my friend Jane, so I shall indulge your desire to shift our plans from murder to other sins."

We did exactly so.

At first there was great tenderness, and kissing until our lips were supple and rosy whilst he was still learning for himself that I was all right; and if later there was passion, and muffled cries, and Charles's *No, I want to hear you, please let me hear you,* and expanses of skin being tasted until we were both panting with exertion and simple love, then it is not the polite place of autobiography to address the subject.

When we had more than once exhausted ourselves, however, and Charles in sleep rolled to his belly and I spent long minutes tracing the scar marring the muscles of his back, I thought that this would be the memory I would treasure best, and I was right. As soon as I could leave off stroking his skin, I touched the mark at my own neck and blessed it; for we are doers of deeds, he and I, and as such lose parts of our flesh along the way, and can only pray to meet friends and lovers who can help to stitch us back again, and that we can make them whole in turn.

I did not marry Charles Thornfield until some few years after I began sharing his bed.

I am today Jane Thornfield, née Steele—but I am also, though few outside the household saving Mr. Quillfeather know it, Jane Kaur. Sardar Singh performed the ceremony in June, in the garden at midnight as my mother would have wanted, as Charles and Sahjara looked on proudly. Mr. Singh filled a ceremonial iron bowl with clear water and then poured into it a quantity of sugar; this he stirred with one of the swords from the billiards room, a double-edged one, as he called out in his lion's voice, "*Sri Wahe Guruji Ka Khalsa, Sri Wahe Guruji Ki Fateh.*"

The passage is a pretty one, even in English: "The Khalsa belong to God, and God's truth will always prevail."

Charles says that he does not care what sort of Jane I am so long as I am his Jane; Sardar says that he does not care what sort of Jane I am so long as I am my own Jane; Sahjara says that she does not care what sort of Jane I am so long as she is my Sahjara. Thus I am daily three Janes, and so the luckiest of all.

When corpses arrive at Highgate House, they speak to Charles, and he reports to Sam Quillfeather—sometimes they died naturally, but sometimes not, and these occasions are much preferable, for we share adventures, and I cannot imagine a happier circumstance than leading a life spiced with murder and intrigue alongside the man I love.

I hope that the epitaph of the human race when the world ends will be: *Here perished a species which lived to tell stories.*

We tell stories to strangers to ingratiate ourselves, stories to lovers to better adhere us skin to skin, stories in our heads to banish the demons. When we tell the truth, often we are callous; when we tell lies, often we are kind. Through it all, we tell stories, and we own an uncanny knack for the task. In *Jane Eyre*, the wise author writes, "Reserved people often really need the frank discussion of their sentiments and griefs more than the expansive." I have lived this—should we neglect the task of expressing our passions, our species should perish upon the vine, desiccated and desolate.

Mr. Rochester after being married to Miss Eyre announces that their honeymoon "will shine our life long; its beams will only fade over your grave or mine." As I am not a prognosticator, and have been witness to myriad calamities, I can make no such claim regarding my own marriage. Confident I remain, however, and I find myself hopeful as well—if the world is wide enough for me to find someone, who knows what miracles lurk behind each and every closed door? Charles Thornfield and I are far from perfect; but we are perfect for each other, and perhaps in the end, our chains bind us more closely than anyone who has never been a prisoner can imagine.

Historical Afterword

While *Jane Eyre* needs no introduction, I should mention that Charlotte Brontë's preface to the infamous second edition thrilled me from the instant I first set eyes on the quote, "Conventionality is not morality. Self-righteousness is not religion." While the author continues to lob great Molotov cocktails of scriptural invective at her critics for perhaps a trifle longer than necessary (if Brontë lived today, it wouldn't be impossible to picture her replying to troll tweets and one-star Amazon reviews), the spirit of the thing is marvelous, and to anyone who has read the novel without the preface, know that it was a major inspiration for this satirical riff off the classical Jane.

The position of women in the nineteenth century was notoriously fraught with economic peril and rife with class divisions, and nowhere is this more evident in *Jane Eyre* than when the haughty Blanche Ingram rails against governesses as if they are repulsive insects children have every right to squash ruthlessly. Marriage to a rich man was a respectable way to make a fortune—but to be educated and servile at once, raising the children of others simply due to reduced circumstances, was considered a ghastly fate. Richard Nemesvari, who edited the careful scholarly edition of *Jane Eyre* I myself used, suggests regarding Blanche's tirade announcing "half of them [governesses] detestable and the rest ridiculous" that:

> *On one level this is purely a rude attempt to put Jane in her place, but it is also an attempt by Blanche to establish her own place . . . It is absolutely essential for Blanche to despise all governesses, because only in this way can she ensure (in her own mind and others') that there is no connection or potential relationship between them.*

Naturally, this made the notion of writing a serial killer governess who was also in all likelihood a wronged heiress cracking good fun, and while Jane Steele is a far more egalitarian soul than Blanche Ingram, she also has no strong objection to pretty frocks, good whiskey, large estates, expensive horses, or marriage to a brooding Byronic hero.

It would be ludicrous to pretend that I could have grasped Sikhism after only six months' research, but a few books in particular were of immense help. First, *The Sikh Religion* by Max Arthur MacAuliffe (1842–1913) was written by an Englishman whose love of the Punjabi religion was roundly ridiculed by his associates within the Indian Civil Service, who really didn't think converting was quite the done thing, by gad. Responsible for producing the first UK translation of the Sikh holy book, the *Guru Granth Sahib,* MacAuliffe continued to pen English-language volumes about Sikh history with the help of Pratap Singh Giani, a brilliant linguist and calligraphist who among other prestigious accomplishments worked as a scripture-reader in Amritsar, the holy city. Second, *The First and Second Sikh Wars* was commissioned by the British Army in 1911, and military historian Reginald George Burton executed his mission with tremendous care and detail—for which I'm grateful, as it's nigh impossible to picture a battle when you've never been in one.

Thirdly, *The Sikhs*, written by political activist, magazine publisher, and scholarly author Patwant Singh, proved crucial. While

Charles Thornfield and Sardar Singh are romanticized versions of nineteenth-century warriors, the bloody battles and corrupt politics were real, and long continued to plague the region. Patwant Singh attempted to intercede for peace during a tragic modern-day confrontation (the 1984 crisis at the Golden Temple, in which three hundred fifty extreme Sikh separatists and seventy Indian soldiers died), and he worked tirelessly to present a faithful and well-rounded picture of a much-misrepresented culture. An entire chapter of *The Sikhs* is titled "Grievous Betrayals, 1839–1849," and describes how gross mismanagement—or more likely, outright treachery—by powerful Sikhs led to the slaughter of the Khalsa, and the eradication of what had once been an opulent empire. Based in personal sacrifice and responsibility, monotheism, pacifism, meditation, but also military prowess, the people who were once massacred for rejecting the inhumanities of the caste system grew into a legendary army, and Patwant Singh did us an incredible service by placing these disparities in vivid context. His books have my highest recommendation, as they are full of what he refers to as the "invasions and inquisitions, triumphs and tragedies, piety and sense of divine purpose, devotion and depravities, loyalties and betrayals, courage and convictions" of his religion.

Finally, it would be disingenuous of me to suggest that this book isn't rather ridiculous, and be it known that its ridiculousness is based in both truth and in fiction. While Mr. Squeers, who "had but one eye, and the popular prejudice runs in favor of two" was not real, the terrible school called Cowan Bridge that Charlotte Brontë claimed took the lives of two of her sisters was. While George MacDonald Fraser's fine novel *Flashman and the Mountain of Light* is almost too deliciously ridiculous to exist, the defeated Sikhs were in fact required to hand over the Kooh-i-Noor diamond to Queen Victoria, which was cut from 186 carats to 105.6 carats and is now part of the

Crown Jewels. And while it may appear ridiculous that an accidental avenger should find a home with refugees from Punjabi battlefields, as Nicholas Nickleby mentioned to his friend Smike, "When I speak of home, I speak of the place where—in default of a better—those I love are gathered together; and if that place were a gypsy's tent, or a barn, I should call it by the same good name notwithstanding."

Acknowledgments

For reasons that are obvious to everyone kind enough to read this book, I dedicated it to Jane Eyre and Nicholas Nickleby, who have given me many hours of literary joy since childhood (and who unfortunately led quite parallel lives of undeserved squalor and questionable headmasters). Jane has often tugged at my heartstrings, however, while Nicholas once caused me to guffaw aloud on the New York subway system, which drew incredulous stares. I'd be remiss if I failed to mention Jonathan Small and the gaunt, devoted Mrs. Danvers to boot; thus, thank you endlessly to Charlotte Brontë and Charles Dickens, as well as to Sir Arthur Conan Doyle and Daphne du Maurier, whose smudgy literary fingerprints are likewise all over this volume.

Thank you to every stunningly fabulous talent at William Morris Endeavor, first and foremost the magnificent Erin Malone, who fixes my mojo when it frequently nosedives. From the moment I first emailed her about Jane Steele years ago, she has been waving magic pom-poms every step of the way. Tracy Fisher and Cathryn Summerhayes, you are splendid midsummer goddesses, as all my foreign publishers (to whom I am also deeply grateful) are well aware. To everyone at WME who has been of such tireless assistance, I am forever grateful.

I had the honor of working with Kerri Kolen on my debut novel, and it feels sublime to have such a fantastic and kindly powerhouse in my corner again. Though she is but little, she is fierce—and brilliant, and I adore her. Thank you as well to Ivan Held, Katie McKee, Alexis Welby, Ashley McClay, and every other person who makes my employment by Putnam and Penguin Random House feel like such a privilege. Grateful thanks to Claire Baldwin and Sherise Hobbs at Headline, whose notes and encouragement were equally appreciated.

My family, as ever, have heaped support on me to the point I'm beginning to resemble an overbuilt skyscraper—but I need it all, and I thank you. My friends deserve a collective vacation to Aruba for talking me down whenever I flounder; to every school chum and coworker and actor and Sherlockian and just plain fellow nerd, thank you from the bottom of my heart. My husband, Gabriel, quietly makes me fish tacos with homemade corn tortillas when the writing is going poorly and I'm being a complete jackass, which is probably the definition of devotion, so I thank him most of all.

Finally, as ever: Reader, I thank you. Your collective existence will forever baffle and delight me.